Radiation Therapy

A Guide to Patient Care

Radiation Therapy

A Guide to Patient Care

Marilyn L. Haas, PhD, RN, CNS, ANP-C
Nurse Practitioner
Mountain Radiation Oncology
Asheville, North Carolina

William P. Hogle, RN, MSN, OCN®
Clinical Manager
University of Pittsburgh Medical Center
UPMC Passavant Cancer Center
Pittsburgh, Pennsylvania;
Adjunct Faculty
La Roche College
Department of Nursing
Pittsburgh, Pennsylvania

Giselle J. Moore-Higgs, ARNP, PhD(c), AOCN®
Coordinator, Breast Cancer
University of Florida Shands Cancer Center
Gainesville, Florida

Tracy K. Gosselin-Acomb, RN, MSN, AOCN®
Director, Oncology Services
Duke University Hospital;
Clinical Associate
Duke University School of Nursing
Durham, North Carolina

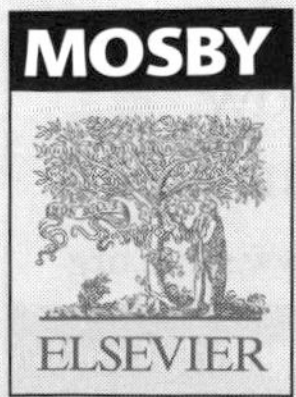

Contributors

Terri S. Armstrong, DSN, APRN, BC
Clinical Assistant Professor Target Populations
School of Nursing
University of Texas Health Science Center
Houston, Texas;
Advanced Practice Nurse
MD Anderson Cancer Center
Houston, Texas
6. Central Nervous System Tumors

Anita Axiak, RN, BSN, OCN®
Case Manager—Radiation Oncology
William Beaumont Hospital
Troy, Michigan
25. Accelerated Partial Breast Irradiation

Micke A. Brown, BSN, RN
Director of Advocacy
American Pain Foundation
Baltimore, Maryland
31. Pain

Susan D. Bruce, RN, MSN, OCN®
Associate Director of Education and Program Development
Duke Oncology Network
Durham, North Carolina
24. Stereotactic Irradiation

Heather Lynn Brumbaugh, RN, MSN, ANP, AOCN®
Nurse Practitioner
Duke University Medical Center
Durham, North Carolina;
Clinical Associate
Duke University School of Nursing
Durham, North Carolina
16. Hodgkin's Disease and Non-Hodgkin's Lymphoma

Kathryn Burrows, BA, MA
Research Analyst, Palliative Radiation Oncology Program
Department of Radiation Oncology
Princess Margaret Hospital
Toronto, Ontario, CANADA
14. Spinal Cord and Bone Metastases

Jormain O. Cady, MS, ARNP, AOCN®
Nurse Practitioner, Radiation Oncology
Virginia Mason Medical Center
Seattle, Washington
4. Diagnosis and Staging

Elise Carper, RN, MA, APRN-BC, AOCN®
Director of Nursing, Radiation Oncology
Continuum Cancer Centers of New York
New York, New York
7. Head and Neck Cancers

Carrie F. Daly, RN, MSN, AOCN®, APN
Oncology Nurse Manager/Advanced Practice Nurse
Rush University Medical Center
Chicago, Illinois
22. Radioprotectants

Georgia M. Decker, MS, RN, CS-ANP, CN, AOCN®
Nurse Practitioner
Integrative Care
Albany, New York
41. Influence of Complementary and Alternative Medicine

Judith A. DePalma, PhD, RN
Associate Professor
Department of Nursing
Slippery Rock University
Slippery Rock, Pennsylvania;
Professor
Nursing Doctoral Program
Rocky Mountain University of the Health Professions
Provo, Utah
38. Evidence-Based Clinical Guidelines

Pamela Devine, RN, MSN
Clinical Nurse Specialist, Radiation Oncology
Philadelphia Veterans Administration Medical Center
Philadelphia, Pennsylvania
11. Urinary Cancers

Joni Dunn, MN, RN, CNS, AOCN®
Level IV Clinical Nurse
Department of Radiation Oncology
University of Colorado Hospital
Denver, Colorado
26. Total Body Irradiation and Total Lymphoid Irradiation

Constance Engelking, RN, MS, OCN®
President
The CHE Consulting Group, Inc.
A Resource for Healthcare Delivery Education and Research under The CHE Group, Inc.
Mt. Kisco, New York
34. Radiation-Induced Nausea, Vomiting, and Diarrhea

Christine Flynn, RN, BSN
Brachytherapy Nurse Clinician
William Beaumont Hospital
Royal Oak, Michigan
25. Accelerated Partial Breast Irradiation

Mary Longnecker Garrett, BSN, RN
Clinical Research Nurse
Abramson Cancer Center
University of Pennsylvania Health System
Philadelphia, Pennsylvania
40. Geriatric Considerations in Radiation Oncology Nursing

Mark R. Gilbert, MD
Professor of Neurology
Deputy Chairman
Department of Neuro-Oncology
Houston, Texas
6. Central Nervous System Tumors

Tracy K. Gosselin-Acomb, RN, MSN, AOCN®
Director, Oncology Services
Duke University Hospital;
Clinical Associate
Duke University School of Nursing
Durham, North Carolina
27. Hyperthermia
29. Total Skin Electron Beam Therapy

Marilyn L. Haas, PhD, RN, CNS, ANP-C
Nurse Practitioner
Mountain Radiation Oncology
Asheville, North Carolina
8. Lung Cancer
28. GliaSite Radiation Therapy System

Christie M. Hancock, APRN, BC, OCN®
Advanced Practice Nurse
Highlands Oncology Group
Fayetteville, Arkansas
6. Central Nervous System Tumors

Laura J. Hilderley, RN, MS
Clinical Nurse Specialist, Radiation Oncology *(retired)*
Greenwich, Rhode Island
1. Evolution of Radiation Oncology

William P. Hogle, RN, MSN, OCN®
Clinical Manager
University of Pittsburgh Medical Center
UPMC Passavant Cancer Center
Pittsburgh, Pennsylvania;
Adjunct Faculty
La Roche College
Department of Nursing
Pittsburgh, Pennsylvania
13. Male Genitourinary Cancers
15. Skin Cancers
28. GliaSite Radiation Therapy System

Jean C. Holland, RN, MSN, AOCN®
Clinical Nurse
Fox Chase Cancer Center
Philadelphia, Pennsylvania
10. Gastrointestinal Cancers

Norissa Walter Honea, RN, MSN, AOCN®, CCRP
Senior Clinical Research Nurse
Arizona Oncology Services Foundation
Phoenix, Arizona
36. Nursing Research and Clinical Trials

Annette Lea Jones, RN, OCN®
Oregon Health Science University Student
Portland, Oregon
22. Radioprotectants

Sarah H. Kagan, PhD, RN, APRN, BC, AOCN®
Professor of Gerontological Nursing
University of Pennsylvania School of Nursing
Philadelphia, Pennsylvania;
Gerontology Clinical Nurse Specialist, Secondary Faculty
Department of Otorhinolaryngology: Head and Neck Surgery
Hospital of the University of Pennsylvania
Philadelphia, Pennsylvania
40. Geriatric Considerations in Radiation Oncology Nursing

Karen Snow Kaiser, PhD, RN-BC, AOCN®
Clinical Practice Coordinator
University of Maryland Medical Center
Baltimore, Maryland;
Adjunct Assistant Professor
University of Maryland School of Nursing
Baltimore, Maryland
31. Pain

Colleen K. Lambertz, RN, MSN, FNP, MBA
Family Nurse Practitioner, Radiation Oncology
Mountain States Oncology Group/Mountain States Tumor Institute
Boise, Idaho
37. Advanced Practice Nurses in Radiation Oncology

Catherine M. Comeau Lew, RN, BSN
Staff Nurse
Department of Radiation Oncology
Brigham and Women's Hospital
Boston, Massachusetts
26. Total Body Irradiation and Total Lymphoid Irradiation

Kim L. Light, RTT, CMD
Chief Dosimetrist
Department of Radiation Oncology
Duke University Hospital
Durham, North Carolina
5. Simulation and Treatment Planning

Sandra L. Luthringer, RD, LDN
Clinical Dietician
The Regional Cancer Center
Erie, Pennsylvania
33. Nutrition Through the Continuum of Cancer Care

Maurene McQuestion, RN, BA, BScN, CON(C), MSc
Advanced Practice Nurse
Radiation Medicine Program
Princess Margaret Hospital, University Health Network
Toronto, Ontario, CANADA
3. Radiation Protection and Safety

Katen Moore, MSN, APRN, BC, AOCN®
Nurse Practitioner, Radiation Oncology
Department of Veteran's Affairs
New Jersey Healthcare System
East Orange, New Jersey
20. Combined Chemoradiation Safety

Giselle J. Moore-Higgs, ARNP, PhD(c), AOCN®
Coordinator, Breast Cancer
University of Florida Shands Cancer Center
Gainesville, Florida
2. Basic Principles of Radiation Therapy
9. Breast Cancer
12. Gynecologic Cancers

Martha Polovich, MN, RN, AOCN®
Oncology Clinical Nurse Specialist
Southern Regional Medical Center
Riverdale, Georgia
20. Combined Chemoradiation Safety

Annette Martin Quinn, RN, MSN
Program Manager
Department of Radiation Oncology
University of Pittsburgh Cancer Center
Pittsburgh, Pennsylvania
24. Stereotactic Irradiation

Kellie L. Ritari, RN, BSN, OCN®
RN Specialist
University of Florida
Gainesville, Florida
17. Soft Tissue Sarcomas

Mary Ann Robbins, RN, BSN, OCN®
Nurse Manager
Department of Radiation Oncology
Duke University Hospital
Durham, North Carolina
18. Nonmalignant Tumors

Carmel Sauerland, MSN, AOCNS®
Clinical Nurse Specialist Oncology
Westchester Medical Center
Valhalla, New York
34. Radiation-Induced Nausea, Vomiting, and Diarrhea

Judith A. Shell, PhD, RN, AOCN®, LMET
Medical Family Therapist, Marriage and Family Therapist
Osceola Cancer Center
Kissimmee, Florida
35. Sexuality and Sexual Dysfunction

Sheila G. Sparks, RN, MSN, OCN®
Oncology Nurse Practice Consultant
Gardendale, Alabama
30. Radiodermatitis

Susan Vogt Temple, RN, MSN, AOCN®
Senior Clinical Educator
GlaxoSmithKline Oncology
Philadelphia, Pennsylvania
23. Radiopharmaceuticals

Dianna Wellen Traylor, RN, MSN
Clinical Content Specialist
IMPAC Medical Systems, Inc.
Mountain View, California
39. Clinical Outcomes and Documentation

Wendy H. Vogel, MSN, FNP, AOCN®
Nurse Practitioner
Blue Ridge Medical Specialist
Bristol, Tennessee
19. Chemoradiotherapy

Rita J. Wickham, PhD, RN, AOCN®, CHPN
Associate Professor
College of Nursing
Rush University
Chicago, Illinois
34. Radiation-Induced Nausea, Vomiting, and Diarrhea

Eileen Maloney Wilensky, RN, MSN, CRNP-C, CNRN, CCRN
Director, Neurosurgery Clinical Research Division and In-house CRNP/PA Program
University of Pennsylvania Health System
Philadelphia, Pennsylvania
28. GliaSite Radiation Therapy System

Diane Williams, RN, BScN, MN
Advanced Practice Nurse
Palliative Radiation Program
Princess Margaret Hospital, University Health Network
Toronto, Ontario, CANADA
14. Spinal Cord and Bone Metastases

Mary Ellyn Witt, RN, MS, AOCN®
Clinical Research Nurse
University of Chicago Hospital
Chicago, Illinois
32. Mucositis

Diana H. Wortham, MSN, RN, OCN®, CNS
Oncology Clinical Nurse Specialist
Mission Hospitals
Asheville, North Carolina
21. Interventional Radiology Procedures

Reviewers

Elaine DeMeyer, RN, MSN, AOCN®
President and CEO
Creative Cancer Concepts, Inc.
Rockwall, Texas

Julie M. Earle, RN, BSN, OCN®
Nursing Supervisor, Radiation Oncology
Mayo Clinic
Rochester, Minnesota

Marjorie J. Gould, RN, BSN
Director, Cardiac Imaging
University of Pittsburgh Medical Center
UPMC Passavant
Pittsburgh, Pennsylvania

Pamela H. Haylock, BSN, MSN
Oncology Consultant
Doctoral Student
School of Nursing
University of Texas Medical Branch
Galveston, Texas

Lauren D. Kelly, RN, MPH, OCN®
Nurse Intake Manager
Francis H. Burr Proton Therapy Center
Massachusetts General Hospital
Boston, Massachusetts

Paulette Komarny, RN, BSN, OCN®
Radiation Oncology Nurse *(retired)*
Radiation Oncology Department
Virginia Hospital Center—Arlington
Arlington, Virginia

Jennifer Jean Seimens, RN, BSCN, BEd
Concene Health Services
Thunder Bay, Ontario, CANADA

Anne Marie Shaftic, MSN, NP-C, AOCNP®, OCN®
Nurse Practitioner, Oncology
Regional Cancer Center
Holy Name Hospital
Teaneck, New Jersey

Patti Simmons, RN, MB, CHPN
Assistant Professor of Nursing
North Georgia College and State University
Dahlonega, Georgia

Tamara M. Ware, RN, BC, OCN®, MSN
Visiting Assistant Professor
Shepherd University
Shepherdtown, Wyoming

Preface

> "Enthusiasm is one of the most powerful engines of success. When you do a thing, do it with all your might. Put your whole soul into it. Stamp it with your own personality. Be active, be energetic and faithful, and you will accomplish your object. Nothing great was ever achieved without enthusiasm."
>
> Ralph Waldo Emerson

This textbook was developed by editors and writers who share an enthusiasm for radiation oncology and the profession of nursing.

The nurse's role in the evolving field of radiation therapy has grown from care coordinator to active caregiver, educator, advocate, researcher, and navigator. As a result of this ever-expanding role and advanced technology, there was a serious need to develop an updated reference text on which to base the practice of radiation oncology nursing. It was the editors' intent to put forth an updated text based on sound scientific principles and evidence-based practice to provide safe and appropriate care to oncology patients who receive radiation therapy and their caregivers.

This textbook, *Radiation Therapy: A Guide to Patient Care,* expands on the first two editions of *Nursing Care in Radiation Oncology* by Karen Hassey Dow, Jennifer Dunn Bucholtz, Ryan Iwamoto, Vickie Fieler, and Laura Hilderley. Nurse experts from various clinical and administrative settings were asked to combine their clinical knowledge and expertise to provide an in-depth discussion on the principles of radiobiology, adjuvant and special treatment modalities, while including nursing care of major cancer sites highlighting evidence-based symptom management and follow-up care as well as additional dimensions of clinical practice.

Section I begins with the overview of the science. The reader will gain an appreciation of the evolution of radiation oncology and how the field has advanced to include three-dimensional conformal therapy, intensity modulated therapy, and frameless stereotactic radiotherapy. After understanding the basic principles of radiation therapy, the reader will then recognize the recommended protection and safety guidelines, which must be followed when caring for this patient population. Section II contains two new chapters that highlight the foundation of diagnosis and staging of oncology patients. In addition, the simulation and treatment planning phases are detailed and expanded upon to create a better understanding of these critical components of radiation therapy. Section III provides an in-depth discussion about major cancer sites, reviewing the anatomy and pathophysiology, clinical manifestations, diagnostic studies for work-up, pathology and pattern(s) of metastases, treatment modalities, nursing interventions and education, and additional resources. Section IV illustrates the newer adjuvant therapies that are offered to radiation oncology patients. Section V also presents the special treatment modalities that are available beyond external beam irradiation to destroy cancer cells/tumors. Section VI expands on the special supportive nursing care with six major issues for patients receiving irradiation. The final section, VII, covers special dimensions of clinical practice, including research, clinical trials, evidence-based clinical guidelines and outcomes. Special issues for advance practitioners working in radiation oncology are presented, along with special topics related to geriatric care and complementary medicine as they relate to radiation oncology.

Readers are encouraged to also pursue other oncology literature as the field is rapidly moving forward in its use of advanced technology, adjuvant pharmaceuticals, and improved application of scientific evidence-based management of patients receiving radiation therapy. It is our hope that this text, *Radiation Therapy: A Guide to Patient Care,* will meet your needs in caring for this patient population for whom we all share a special affection.

It is enthusiasm that drives our passion. Together we bring you the experts who are willing to share their time, talents, and expertise in the field of radiation oncology nursing.

Marilyn L. Haas, PhD, RN, CNS, ANP-C
William P. Hogle, RN, MSN, OCN®
Giselle J. Moore-Higgs, ARNP, PhD(c), AOCN®
Tracy K. Gosselin-Acomb, RN, MSN, AOCN®

Acknowledgments

The task of assembling the leading textbook for radiation oncology nurses requires enthusiasm and collective commitment from numerous individuals. A special thanks to my contributing editors, William Hogle, Gigi Moore-Higgs, and Tracy Gosselin-Acomb, for their expertise, time, and talents given to this project. Without their thoughtful insights, we could not have offered a comprehensive resource for radiation oncology nurses and other members of the multidisciplinary team. Their devotion to content accuracy, and special needs of the patients/families were extremely helpful to this project. Also, there were forty-five authors, beyond the editors, that all deserve special recognition for their dedication to this project. For without their investment of time, clinical expertise, and writing skills, published knowledge beyond the original textbook, *Nursing Care in Radiation Oncology*, would not exist. Special gratitude to our Elsevier publishing staff: Sandra Clark Brown, Senior Editor, Nursing Editorial; Sophia Oh Gray, Senior Developmental Editor, Nursing Editorial; and Catherine Harold, consultant, who all shared the same goals in helping others learn about radiation oncology.

Marilyn L. Haas, PhD, RN, CNS, ANP-C

Foreword

Thirty years ago, in 1977, Linda Knight Morse and I were lone nurses working in separate radiation therapy departments in Boston. We weren't necessarily lonely as we each had a caseload of about 40-50 patients receiving radiation therapy daily. Each of our departments was located far from in-patient or out-patient care units. In those days, we called them out-patients; today we call them ambulatory patients. Nevertheless, most of my out-patients walked a lonely road past hospital green walls to the radiation therapy department that was located in the basement, next to the laundry. Some patients' families were terrified of accompanying their loved ones to radiation. They saw the steam emanating from the doors and thought it was radiation, not the laundry. Needless to say, I did a lot of basic patient education, supported families, and allayed their fears about radiation.

In our department, we had one 6MV linear accelerator (linac), three radiation therapy technologists, three radiation oncologists, two or three radiation oncology fellows, one receptionist, two secretaries, one unit manager, and one nurse. When the linac needed tune up or repairs wait times increased astronomically and most patients sat stoically waiting for several hours. It was probably during these most stressful times in waiting that I began to learn so much about my patients and families—their lives, hope, fears, needs, and their suffering.

Radiation therapy was very much considered the stepchild treatment in those days. Most of my fellow oncology nurses worked in the inpatient unit or the hematology oncology unit giving chemotherapy. They would look at me quizzically and ask, "Why would you ever want to work in radiation?" Patient needs were so high and the nurses so few. I couldn't imagine working anywhere else. But patient and family needs were truly hidden far in the recesses of a department isolated from other patient units.

In 1978, I had the great fortune to hear Laura Hilderley deliver a presentation about nursing care in radiation therapy at an American Cancer Society meeting. I sat in rapt attention hanging on to her every word about nursing, about radiation, and about improving patient care. I immediately asked if I could spend time with her in her radiation therapy department, learning about how she managed acute side effects such as radiation skin reactions, nausea, vomiting, hair loss, anxiety, communication problems, and patient travel issues. Ever gracious and welcoming, Laura agreed. So Linda Morse and I traveled about an hour from Boston to Warwick, Rhode Island and spent a day in radiation oncology with Laura. I like to think of that meeting as the first informal SIG gathering of radiation oncology nurses.

That was then, and this is now. Radiation oncology is a tremendous specialty within oncology. The Radiation Therapy SIG enjoys one of the largest memberships in the Oncology Nursing Society. Textbooks, monographs, papers, abstracts, and conferences have been dedicated to radiation oncology in the ensuing 30 years. Most modern radiation oncology departments actually have windows and even soothing gardens that patients and families can enjoy while waiting for treatment. Countless patient education materials are available in written, audio, and internet-based formats, not only English, but other language versions as well. These are the works of dedicated radiation oncology nurses who are passionate in their endeavors to continue to improve the quality of life of patients and families.

I am so very pleased and honored to write the foreword to this very important textbook, *Radiation Therapy: A Guide to Patient Care.* Within the following pages, the reader will find a tremendous wealth of information about the evolution of radiation, its role in cancer treatment, types of cancers treated, exciting developments in adjuvant therapies (both old and new), supportive care issues, and the ever changing role of nursing in radiation oncology. May we all continue to find wisdom in these pages, learn from one another, and share our experiences with others.

Karen Hassey Dow, PhD, RN, FAAN
Professor & Beat & Jill Kahli Endowed Chair in Oncology Nursing
University of Central Florida, Orlando, Florida

Contents

Unit I

Overview

Chapter 1

Evolution of Radiation Oncology

Laura J. Hilderley

HISTORY OF RADIATION ONCOLOGY

Although radiation therapy began in the late nineteenth century with discoveries made by such eminent scientists as Roentgen, Becquerel, and the Curies, the groundwork for their discoveries had been laid long before. In 460 B.C. Democritus proposed the idea that tiny particles called *atoms* were the building blocks of all materials. Medieval alchemists were intrigued by fluorescence, a chemical property of certain elements that played a significant role in Roentgen's discovery of x rays. Similarly, early work by Sir Isaac Newton (1642-1727) and Benjamin Franklin (1706-1790) on the nature and production of electricity provided vital information that lead to the development of generators, motors, and transformers to produce the current for Roentgen's experiments almost a century later. One additional development, the vacuum tube and subsequent cathode ray, attributed to Sir William Crookes (1832-1919), was to play a major part in the discovery of x rays by Roentgen.

Wilhelm Konrad Roentgen (1845-1923), a German physicist at the University of Wurzburg, was particularly interested in working with cathode ray tubes. Late in the afternoon of November 8, 1895, Roentgen was at work in his laboratory experimenting with a fluorescent barium compound, when he made his renowned discovery. An electrical charge was passed through a cathode ray tube that had been shielded with black cardboard; it produced a fluorescent glow extending a few feet from the tube. Because cathode rays were known to have limited distance, Roentgen concluded that a new type of ray was being produced and continued to investigate its penetrating power. This powerful ray was given the designation *X*, the scientific symbol for the unknown. Roentgen was subsequently honored with the first Nobel Prize for physics and by the naming of this new science as *roentgenology*.

Paralleling the events in Germany that led to Roentgen's discovery of the x ray were the activities of Antoine Henri Becquerel (1852-1908) in France. Becquerel was particularly interested in the chemical properties of the elements; he is credited with the discovery in 1896 that uranium is naturally radioactive. Becquerel's publication on this phenomenon caught the attention of Marie Curie (1867-1934), who was looking for a subject to research in her pursuit of a doctoral degree. With her husband and fellow scientist, Pierre Curie (1859-1906), Marie determined to explain the origin of this newly recognized energy produced by uranium. Although the answer to that question eluded the scientific community for many years, the investigation conducted by the Curies led very quickly to the discovery of polonium and radium in 1898. For the next 35 years Madame Curie concentrated her efforts on the investigation of radium and radioactivity, until her death from aplastic anemia in 1934.

RADIATION ONCOLOGY IN THE TWENTIETH CENTURY

During the early 1900s the therapeutic use of x rays became widely popular. In Chicago, Emil Grubbe developed dermatitis on his hands while working with x-ray tubes. He then decided to apply this tissue-damaging effect to a patient with an ulcerating breast cancer and claimed, years later, that the treatment improved the lesion noticeably.

Although the discovery of radium and its ionizing radiation paralleled the discovery of x rays, application of radium in medical practice evolved more slowly, largely because of the great difficulty in extracting even small amounts of radium from pitchblende. However, by 1900 sufficient amounts of radium were being prepared, and its widespread therapeutic application was underway. Interstitial radium needles were implanted, and the first reports of tumor sterilization were issued.

In the first decade of the twentieth century, radiation was employed in the treatment of benign as well as malignant disease. Thyrotoxicosis, rheumatism, herpes, and gout were treated with the same vigor as that applied to the treatment of cancer. Radium's apparent curative powers soon had the public and the scientific world hailing it as a restorative, rejuvenating panacea. Over the next decade, growing concern was expressed about the adverse effects of radiation and the documented cases of radiation-induced cancer. Cures were also documented, but results could not be duplicated because there was no way of measuring a given dose of radiation. Technical development continued, and more penetrating x-ray machines were produced.

Between 1920 and 1940 the development of deep-therapy x-ray machines with a range of 180,000 to 250,000 volts allowed treatment of more deeply seated tumors with maximum tumor destruction. Such doses, however, frequently caused destruction of normal tissue as well, sometimes resulting in tissue necrosis and death. Lung damage following the treatment of breast cancer was recognized, and attempts were made to devise methods of avoiding lung tissue by rearranging the direction of treatment beams. Treatment reproducibility and dosage measurement were still problems. The use of skin erythema as a biologic indicator of dose was a common but unsatisfactory method, particularly to the radiologists.

During this period, radium was available in many forms such as creams, powders, and suppositories; the mail-order business in radium products was booming. Radon toothpaste was advertised as a plaque preventive by a German manufacturer.[1] It was not until the mid-1930s that the American Radium Society declared that mail-order distribution of radium treatments was unethical. Despite such seemingly unscientific applications of this new technology, radiation therapy was beginning to be recognized as an established science. An international dose unit for x ray was defined and called the *roentgen* or R *unit.* With this definition, the search for a method of measuring dose in air and in tissues was launched. Radiobiology also emerged as a science concerned with the effects of radiation on all tissues (Figure 1-1).

The development of the atomic bomb during World War II was among the most significant events of the 1940s because of its effect on all of society as well as on the science of radiation. Following the war, medicine and engineering combined to produce high-powered treatment machines, including the betatron and linear accelerator. Radioactive isotopes resulting from neutron bombardment of stable elements, such as cobalt and cesium, helped to refine nuclear medicine for both diagnostic and therapeutic purposes. The cobalt teletherapy machine became standard equipment in most radiation treatment facilities, generating high-energy gamma radiation from the radioactive cobalt-60 source.

Use of megavoltage equipment became a practical reality between 1950 and 1970. Computers were employed to calculate isodose distributions and later for analysis of data when controlled clinical trials were introduced in the late 1950s. In 1953 the Seventh International Congress of Radiology met in Copenhagen and adopted the *rad* as the unit of absorbed dose of any ionizing radiation. Combined therapy and efforts to increase the radiosensitivity of tumors led to remarkable improvement of results in the treatment of some tumors.

By 1970 radiation therapy was an accepted, highly scientific, and still growing discipline within the practice of oncology. Advances and improvements in machine design, refinement of techniques, and ever-increasing application of computer science brought about remarkable progress in cancer treatment, while sparing normal tissue and minimizing side effects. The trend toward the use of the term *radiation oncology* to describe the practice of radiation therapy reflected the greater emphasis on all aspects of the study of malignant tumors and not just the delivery of ionizing radiation. Terminology also underwent changes when the term *Gray* replaced *rad* (1 Gray = 100 rad) in 1985. Other changes in terminology adapted in 1985 by the International Commission on Radiation Units and Measurements included *Becquerel* in place of *Curie,* and *Sievert* instead of *Rem.*

During the 1980s and early 1990s oncology care was enhanced by attention to the team approach to cancer management. Quality radiation treatment became increasingly available outside of hospitals and medical centers, as private, freestanding practices were established. Nurses were recognized as valuable members of the team and were employed in many more radiation oncology centers. Advanced practice nurses were acknowledged as collaborative partners in radiation patient care.

Period	Events
Late 1800's	• Roentgen's discovery and naming of x rays (1895) • Becquerel's discovery of radioactivity in uranium (1896) • Marie and Pierre Curie identify radioactive polonium and radium (1898)
1900-1920	• X rays and radium used to treat many benign as well as malignant diseases • Radium hailed as panacea
1920-1940	• Development of orthovoltage x-ray equipment • Reliance on "erythema" dose to determine treatment parameters • International x-ray dose unit defined as "*Roentgen*" • Introduction of protracted course of therapy
1940-1950	• Therapeutic radiation administered by diagnostic radiologists • Post World War II development of the Betatron and Cobalt teletherapy machines
1950-1970	• First dedicated Radiation Oncology training program (1952) • "*rad*", as unit of absorbed dose, replaces "*roentgen*" (1953) • First linear accelerator employed routinely for RT in Western hemisphere (1955) • Megavoltage equipment, and low dose-rate brachytherapy in common useage • Introduction of clinical trials • Combined RT and chemotherapy introduced • Computers used for isodose calculations and statistical analysis
1970-1990	• "*Gray*" replaces "*rad*" as International measure of dose (1985) • Technologic and radiobiologic focus on Clinical Trials: 3-D treatment planning, hyperthermia intraoperative RT radiolabeled antibody therapy high dose-rate brachytherapy stereotactic radioneurosurgery Gamma Knife
1990-2000	• 3-D treatment planning in common use • Hyperfraction-ation • IMRT • Multileaf collimator • Radiation therapy as primary treatment for specific cancers
2000-2006	• 4-D conformal therapy • Stereotactic *body* radiation • Newer equipment and techniques including: MammoSite, GliaSite, INTRABEAM, Cyberknife

Figure 1-1 Historical Perspective of Radiation Oncology.

Intraoperative radiation, hyperthermia, and the use of radiolabeled antibodies underwent careful scrutiny in clinical trials.[2-8] Brachytherapy techniques, particularly high dose rate brachytherapy, were optimized, allowing treatment on an outpatient basis.[9-11] Further refinement of stereotactic radioneurosurgery using either the gamma knife or specially adapted linear accelerators provided an option for treatment of some intracranial lesions that were previously not accessible by standard radiation techniques.[12,13] Conformal radiation therapy, which allows increased intensity of radiation by reducing the volume of normal tissues within the overall treatment volume, was given continued and renewed attention, especially with the development of three-dimensional treatment-planning computer programs and equipment.

As the twentieth century drew to a close, oncology science and technology was experiencing an exponential rate of growth, particularly in radiation oncology. Treatment planning became even more sophisticated using computed tomography (CT) scanners linked electronically to linear accelerators. By the mid-1990s intensity-modulated radiation therapy (IMRT) became available with the introduction of the multileaf collimator, reducing dose inhomogeneity in the target site.[14] This is accomplished by modulating the number of fields as well as the intensity of dose anywhere within a field. IMRT is considered by many to be the most significant development in the science of radiation oncology in more than 30 years.

Treatment planning software continued to evolve, yielding highly sophisticated plans for IMRT. In contrast to standard two-dimensional and three-dimensional (2-D, 3-D) treatment plans, IMRT planning can take up to 2 weeks to complete.

As 3-D planning and treatment matured, recognition of an acknowledged but largely unaccounted for fourth dimension grew. During treatment, patient movement and normal digestive and respiratory activity can alter the dosimetry and potentially the effectiveness of treatment.[14] In an effort to account for this movement, the development of four-dimensional (4-D) conformal radiation therapy was launched. Combined positron emission tomography (PET) and CT are being explored in the refinement of 4-D treatment planning.

Stereotactic radiosurgery (SRS) for treatment of brain tumors was a product of the late twentieth century. As the new millennium arrived, so too did refinement of stereotactic body radiation or SBRT.[15] This new application of SRS has evolved through application of meticulous physics and technology, treatment planning, and treatment delivery. The CyberKnife (Accuray, Sunnyvale, Calif.) is an example of a stereotactic radiosurgery system capable of delivering SBRT and cranial SRS.[16,17] The CyberKnife is a self-contained unit consisting of a 6 MV linear accelerator, nonisocentric treatment-planning capability, image guidance technology (capable of tracking patient movement and the position of the target lesion during treatment), and a robotic arm with multiple targeting nodes.

The development of new treatment devices and refinement of treatment planning have fostered continued interest in intraoperative radiation therapy for breast and other cancers. One such device is the Intrabeam (Photoelectron Corporation, North Billerica, Mass.). This equipment operates from a 50-kV electronic generator and uses an intraoperative cone selected to fit the tumor bed after excision of the lesion.[14] The intraoperative treatment can be given as a boost dose or as the primary treatment.

RADIATION ONCOLOGY: TOMORROW'S FUTURE

Radiation treatment for breast cancer has seen a number of changes in the early twenty-first century. Shortened treatment time achieved through innovative brachytherapy application has become an option for many patients. The MammoSite Radiation System (RTS) (Cytyc Corp., Marlborough, Mass.) delivers high dose rate (HDR) brachytherapy by means of a balloon-tip catheter implanted into the operative site after lumpectomy.[14,18] This method of HDR brachytherapy is usually delivered twice daily for 5 days, in contrast with standard external beam treatment given 5 days per week for approximately 6 weeks. A similar system, the GliaSite Radiation Therapy System (Cytyc Corp., Marlborough, Mass.) was introduced in 2001 for treatment of brain tumors.

The first decade of the twenty-first century is one of continued interest and research in all of the oncology disciplines. Radiobiologic principles are being explored and exploited as research reveals greater understanding of the mechanisms governing cell survival and cell death. Radiation is known to trigger defensive cytoprotective action and inhibition of apoptosis. Manipulation of the timing and dose of radiation is being explored in efforts to counter the cytoprotective response.[15] Research continues on the use of radiosensitizers and radioprotectors in pursuit of maximum tumor destruction with minimum damage to healthy tissue, the goal for all radiation treatment.

REFERENCES

1. Grigg ERN: *The trail of the invisible light, from x-strahlen to radiobiology*, Springfield, Ill, 1965, Charles C. Thomas.
2. Cox JD: Clinical applications of new modalities. In Cox JD, editor: *Moss' radiation oncology: rationale, technique, results*, ed 7, St Louis, 1994, Mosby.
3. Stelzer KJ, Koh WJ, Greer BE et al: The use of intraoperative radiation therapy in radical salvage for recurrent cervical cancer: outcome and toxicity, *Am J Obstet Gynecol* 172(6):1881-1888, 1995.
4. Gunderson LL, Nagorney DM, Martenson JA et al: External beam plus intraoperative irradiation for gastrointestinal cancers (Review), *World J Surg* 19(2):191-197, 1995.
5. Johnstone PA, Sindelar WF, Kinsella TJ: Experimental and clinical studies of intraoperative radiation therapy (Review), *Curr Probl Cancer* 18(5):249-290, 1994.
6. Macklis R: Radioimmunoconjugates and other target-selective therapeutic radiopharmaceuticals. In Mauch PM, Loerner JS, editors: *Radiation oncology: technology and biology*, Philadelphia, 1994, Saunders.
7. Oleson JR: Hyperthermia. In Mauch PM, Loerner JS, editors: *Radiation oncology: technology and biology*, Philadelphia, 1994, Saunders.
8. Waldmann TA: Monoclonal antibodies in diagnosis and therapy, *Science* 252(5013):1657-1662, 1991.
9. Arterbery VE: High dose rate brachytherapy for carcinoma of the cervix (Review), *Curr Opin Oncol* 5(6):1005-1009, 1993.
10. Hilaris B: Evolution and general principles of high dose rate brachytherapy. In Nag S, editor: *High dose rate brachytherapy: a textbook*, Armonk, NY, 1994, Futura Publishing.
11. Orton CG: High and low dose rate remote afterloading: A critical comparison. In Sauer R, editor: *International radiation therapy techniques-brachytherapy*, Berlin, 1991, Springer-Verlag.
12. Flickinger JC, Lunsford LD, Kondziolka D: Radiosurgery. In Mauch PM, Loerner JS, editors: *Radiation oncology: technology and biology*, Philadelphia, 1994, Saunders.
13. Thapar K, Laws ER: Tumors of the central nervous system. In Murphy GP, Lawrence W, Lenhard RE, editors: *Clinical oncology*, ed. 2, Atlanta, Ga, 1995, American Cancer Society.
14. Bucci MK, Bevan A, Roach M, III: Advances in radiation therapy: conventional to 3D, to IMRT, to 4D, and beyond, *CA Cancer J Clin* 55(2):117-134, 2005.
15. Song DY, Kavanagh BD, Benedict SH et al: Stereotactic body radiation therapy: rationale, technique, applications, and optimization, *Oncology* 18(11):1419-1436, 2004.
16. Quinn AM: CyberKnife®: A robotic radiosurgery system, *Clin J Oncol Nurs* 6(3):149-156, 2002.
17. CyberKnife® (website): www.accuray.com/ck/how9.htm. Accessed March 24, 2005.
18. Hogle WP, Quinn AE, Heron DE: Advances in brachytherapy: New approaches to target breast cancer, *Clin J Oncol Nurs* 7(3):324-328, 2003.

Chapter 2

Basic Principles of Radiation Therapy

Giselle J. Moore-Higgs

Radiation oncology is the term used to describe the clinical as well as scientific discipline dedicated to the treatment of a person with cancer using ionizing radiation. As a clinical discipline, radiation oncology focuses on treatment of the individual while providing care and support for the individual patient and family. As a science, radiation oncology encompasses the education of personnel, research, and other academic pursuits designed to increase knowledge and further refine the application of ionizing radiation in malignant disease. *Radiation therapy* refers to the treatment modality used in radiation oncology. The success of radiation therapy depends on the delivery of an adequate dose to the entire tumor volume without causing severe damage to the surrounding tissues.[1] The goals are to achieve the highest probability of local and regional tumor control with the lowest achievable incidence of side effects and to prolong the life of the patient with the best possible quality of life. Achieving this therapeutic ratio requires application of the many clinical and scientific principles of radiation oncology, including physics, radiobiology, pathology, radiology, surgery, medicine, and nursing. It is also most successful with a multidisciplinary team approach.

INDICATIONS FOR RADIATION THERAPY

Irradiation is an effective modality in the treatment of many patients with cancer and can be used as the primary treatment for certain cancers (e.g., early laryngeal lesions and prostate cancer), as an adjuvant therapy to ensure local control of a cancer (i.e., after lumpectomy for breast cancer), and to provide palliative relief to patients with incurable cancer (e.g., pain from bone metastasis). In the adjuvant setting, radiation often precedes or follows definitive surgery to ensure local control. Radiation also may achieve long-term control when cure is not possible. Treatment for palliation of symptoms (pain, bleeding, obstruction, neurological compromise) constitutes approximately 50% of all treatments given in radiation facilities. Radiation also may be used in some benign conditions that may not respond well to other types of treatment. Examples of benign conditions include Grave's exophthalmos, orbital pseudotumor, keloids, heterotopic bone formation, and gynecomastia.

When planning the course of therapy, the radiation oncologist must consider the individual patient's needs, desires, and life expectancy as well as the principles of physics and radiobiology.[2] Generally, the treatment course is shorter when the intent is palliative, giving only enough radiation to accomplish palliation of symptoms without causing undue side effects. When life expectancy is short, the quality of that life must be maximized, and this would be incompatible with a lengthy course of radiation.

When cure or long-term control of cancer is the goal, total radiation dosage is increased and the length of the treatment course is longer. Differential doses are used because the primary tumor may require a higher dose than lymphatic drainage sites that require prophylactic treatment. Planning is more complex than that required for most palliative treatments, and one is usually more willing to risk inducing acute side effects. Of course, with the anticipation of increasing the patient's life span, the risk of late (chronic) side effects also must be weighed.[3]

LIMITATIONS OF RADIATION THERAPY

A variety of factors can lead to the failure of radiation therapy to eradicate a tumor. Perez and Purdy[1] classified the factors into three areas: clinical, physical and technical, and biological. The clinical factors include (a) inadequate appraisal of the full extent of the tumor in the surrounding tissue or lymphatics; (b) clinically unrecognized distant metastases at the time of initial treatment; (c) inaccurate definition of gross tumor volume (GTV), clinical target volume (CTV) and planning tumor volume (PTV); and (d) inaccurate definition or difficulty determining critical normal structures. The physical and technical factors include (a) inadequate treatment planning with inhomogeneous dose distributions; (b) dose exceeding tolerance of critical normal structures; (c) unreliable patient immobilization techniques resulting in faulty reproducibility in daily treatments; (d) lack of adequate verification-dosimetry techniques; and (e) inadequate dose prescription. Some of the key biological factors include (a) large initial cell burden; (b) limited tolerance of normal tissues to irradiation; and (c) variation in radiosensitivity throughout cell proliferative cycles. Other factors include the general condition of the patient, presence of comorbid disease, overall nutritional status, metabolism, and immune response to the treatment.

ASSESSMENT AND EVALUATION

The decision to treat with radiation therapy should be preceded by a thorough patient work-up. History and physical examination, laboratory and diagnostic radiological studies, and pathological confirmation of tumor type are considered essential. On rare occasions, radiation therapy may be given without biopsy-proven disease when the tumor is either inaccessible or when the possibility of serious injury occurring in attempting to obtain a biopsy specimen is a risk.

SELECTING TREATMENT MODALITIES AND INTENT

A multidisciplinary tumor conference may be employed to help in the decision to treat and in determining the best plan of therapy, particularly in the present era of multimodal therapy. The choice of treatment appropriate to an individual patient's needs is a product of three components: (1) the tumor type, (2) the stage of the disease, and (3) the therapeutic objective (i.e., neoadjuvant, adjuvant, prophylaxis, control, or palliation). When radiation therapy is to be preceded by several cycles of chemotherapy (e.g., in treatment of small-cell carcinoma of the lung) or is to be given after resection of an operable lesion (e.g., breast cancer), it maybe beneficial to have the radiation oncologist and other team members meet and examine the patient before the chemotherapy or surgery starts. From the patient's perspective, meeting the various specialists and visiting the radiation facility before any treatments are given allows an opportunity to ask questions and explore the risks versus the benefits of the proposed treatment. This is particularly true if the patient has some reservations or bias regarding radiation or has two treatment approaches to choose, one of which includes radiation.

PRINCIPLES OF RADIATION PHYSICS

Understanding ionizing radiation requires a basic understanding of atomic and molecular structure. All matter is composed of atoms, and atoms combine to form molecules. An atom consists of a central core or nucleus containing positively charged protons and neutrons that have no charge. Orbiting about the nucleus are negatively charged electrons equal in number to the number of protons. The atom maintains a stable state through the balance between the number of protons (+) and electrons (−).

Electromagnetic energy is characterized by vibrations of electric and magnetic intensity in space called *electromagnetic waves.* The distance from the peak of one wave to the peak of the next wave is called the *wavelength. Frequency* refers to the number of wave vibrations in 1 second. Electromagnetic waves are a form of energy, and as the length of a wave increases, the intensity of its energy decreases. This is explained by the fact that the farther an electromagnetic wave (beam) travels from its source, the wider the area over which its energy is spread. The electromagnetic spectrum is made up of energies of decreasing wavelength. The spectrum includes radio waves, infrared light, visible light, ultraviolet light, and ionizing radiations. Ionizing radiation, then, is electromagnetic energy with very short wavelength and very high-energy intensity.

Therapeutic radiation is either electromagnetic or particulate in nature and is capable of the ionization of matter. Electromagnetic radiations are characterized by high energy and absence of mass. They can be thought of as bundles of available energy. X rays and gamma rays are two forms of electromagnetic radiation that are roughly equivalent and differ only in their means of production. X rays are generated electrically by machines

Table 2-1 Teletherapy Equipment and Its Use

Equipment	Emission	Beam characteristics and biological effects	Clinical application, advantages, disadvantages
KILOVOLTAGE			
40–150 kV	X rays	Superficial, limited range, poor skin tolerance	Skin cancers or other very superficial lesions, if electrons are not available
ORTHOVOLTAGE			
150–1000 kV	X rays	Deep penetration, high skin dose, high bone absorption	Limited because of poor skin tolerance and potential for bone necrosis
^{137}Cesium radioisotope teletherapy (600 kV)	Gamma rays	Large source size with wide penumbra	Long half-life Low energy and output Used in head and neck treatment
MEGAVOLTAGE/SUPERVOLTAGE			
^{60}Cobalt 1.25–2 MeV	Gamma rays	Deeply penetrating Skin-sparing as a result of maximum dose buildup beneath the skin	Deep-seated tumors Ease of mechanical operation
		Produces penumbra area at edge of beam that receives less dose	Slower dose rate (longer treatment time) as source decays
LINEAR ACCELERATORS			
4–20 MeV	Photons	Deeply penetrating Skin-sparing Increased versatility and precision of dose distribution	Deep-seated tumors Large field capability Complex electronics with tendency for "down time"
6–30 MeV	Electrons (optional)	Electrons give maximum dose on skin and a few centimeters beneath, falling off rapidly thereafter	Skin lesions, chest wall recurrence, superficial nodes
BEATRON			
10–30 MeV	Electrons	High-velocity electrons with deep penetration	High dose rate with shorter treatment time Limited field size
18–40 MeV	Photons	High-energy photons	Bulky equipment Low dose rate photons

(e.g., linac, betatron, orthovoltage, kilovoltage) and are also referred to as *photons,* particularly as generated by megavoltage machines (Table 2-1). Gamma radiation is produced through spontaneous emission by radioactive materials undergoing nuclear transition. Radioactive cobalt and cesium are the primary sources of gamma emissions used for teletherapy.

Electromagnetic radiation interacts with matter at the molecular level, causing a disruption of the atom's stability through three potential processes known as the photoelectric effect, the Compton effect, and pair production. The *photoelectric effect* occurs when an incoming photon undergoes collision with a tightly bound orbiting electron. The photon transfers its energy to the electron and ceases to exist. The electron departs with most of the energy from the photon and begins to ionize surrounding molecules. The *Compton effect* is the most important photon-tissue interaction for the treatment of cancer. A photon collides with a free electron (i.e., one not tightly bound to the atom). Unlike the photoelectric effect, both the photon and electron are scattered. The photon can then continue to undergo additional interactions with a lower energy. The

Table 2-2 High Linear Energy Transfer and Heavy Charged Particle Beams

Energy source	Beam characteristics and radiobiological effects	Used in clinical trials
FAST NEURONS		
16–50 MeV deuterons	Fixed field size and beam position Wide penumbra Absorbed dose decreased exponentially with depth Low OER RBE higher with small dose increments	Advanced cancers of the head, neck, and pelvis, gliomas, and melanoma Esophageal cancer and osteosarcomas
PROTONS AND HELIUM IONS		
600 MeV	Precise dose distribution with ability to deliver very high tumor dose with sparing of adjacent normal tissues RBE and OER similar to that obtained with gamma and photon sources	Pituitary tumors, chondrosarcoma, chordoma, abdominal and pelvic tumors Soft tissue sarcomas Head and neck tumors
NEGATIVE PI-MESONS		
40–70 MeV	Absorbed dose increases slowly with depth, then rises sharply Lowered OER Enhanced RBE	Tumors of the head and neck, brain, prostate, pancreas Skin metastases

OER, oxygen enhancement ratio; *RBE,* relative biological effectiveness.

electron begins to ionize with the energy given to it by the photon. *Pair production*, the third potential action of ionizing radiation with atoms, involves interaction of the photon with the nucleus of the atom (as opposed to its orbiting electrons), producing two electron particles, one with a positive charge and one with a negative charge. Electromagnetic energy (the photon) has then been converted to particulate (electron) energy. Because the electron pair have opposite and equal electrical charges, they do not affect the net electrical charge of the atom, and therefore ionization does not take place at this point. As the electron pair continues to seek a stable state, the two electron particles may subsequently produce ionization through interaction with other atoms.

Particulate radiations that are used in therapy include electrons, neutrons, protons, helium ions, heavy ions (carbon, neon, argon), and negative ions (Table 2-2). As noted earlier, electrons are the most commonly used form of particulate radiation. The interaction of electrons with atoms is one of direct collision. The electron (characterized by its properties of mass and low energy) loses energy constantly through many collisions with matter, thus expending its energy after penetrating only a short distance within the target substance.

BIOLOGICAL EFFECTS OF IONIZING RADIATION

Radiobiology is that aspect of radiation oncology that examines and integrates the principles of mammalian biology with the physical and chemical effects of ionizing radiation. The effects of radiation on mammalian tissues should be viewed as a succession of processes extending from microseconds to months and years after exposure.[4] Principles of radiobiology are an essential part of radiation therapy planning and constitute a major part of the specialty training for radiation oncologists.

Whereas the goal of radiation treatment is to destroy or inactivate cancer cells, a parallel goal is to preserve and maintain the integrity of the normal tissues being treated. Any local tissue change caused by ionizing radiation can have systemic effects with alterations occurring in various physiological processes. For example, mediastinal radiation is likely to cause esophagitis—a local tissue reaction. The resulting dysphagia, however, can affect the patient's intake and compromise nutrition and ultimately result in permanent fibrosis of the tissues and decreased function. Similarly, high-dose radiation for a squamous cell carcinoma in the head and neck region can produce an intense skin reaction; in addition to the local discomfort of this reaction, moist desquamation alters the protective mechanism of the integumentary system. Late effects may include skin fibrosis and protracted healing after injury.

Understanding and integrating radiobiological principles into nursing care helps to assure the desired patient outcome. As clinicians assume greater responsibility for managing treatment and disease-related symptoms and side effects, the science of radiation oncology becomes integral to the entire process.

Cell Survival/Cell Kill

Ionizing radiation kills cells by producing secondary charged particles and free radicals in the nucleus, which in turn produce a variety of types of damage in DNA. Ionization may cause breakage in one or both chains of the DNA molecule, faulty cross-linking of the chains after breakage, damage or loss of a nitrogenous base (thymine, adenine, guanine, cytosine), or actual breakage of the hydrogen bond between the two chains of the DNA molecule. In addition to the direct effect on chromosomal structures, a complex chain of chemical reactions takes place in the medium (mostly water) surrounding the cells. The ionization of water results in significant toxic changes that ultimately affect the cell's function and survival. Loss of the cell's reproductive capacity is considered to be the most biologically significant end point of radiation damage.

Cellular Response to Radiation Injury

The relative radiosensitivity of a given tumor is closely related to its proliferative activity. Radiosensitivity is an expression of the response of a tumor to radiation in terms of degree and speed of response.[5] Some tumors may therefore be classified as very radiosensitive, but this does not necessarily correlate with radiocurability, which is the local or regional eradication of tumor. For example, although non-Hodgkin's lymphoma is very radiosensitive, it is not necessarily radiocurable. Adenocarcinoma of the prostate requires high-dose radiation and may not regress for months after a course of treatment, yet it is considered radiocurable.

Following radiation, a given population of cells in any tumor will sustain lethal injury, and some cells will maintain indefinite reproductive capacity. For the fatally damaged cell, several possibilities are present. Immediate lysis or interphase death without an attempt at mitosis may occur. The number of cells undergoing immediate lysis increases with the dose of radiation. Other cells, which have not undergone postradiation lysis but have sustained lethal damage, will exhibit the lethal effects after one or two attempts at mitosis.

The radiosensitivity of normal tissue encompassed by the radiation beam is vitally important. All tissues within the body have a known degree of radiosensitivity, and it is this characteristic of the healthy tissues surrounding the tumor site that largely determines the maximum dose of radiation that can be given safely as well as the expected side effects (Table 2-3).

Table 2-3 A Compilation of Tissue and Organ Sensitivities

	Injury	$TD_{5/5}$, Gy*	$TD_{50/5}$, Gy*	Field size
CLASS I ORGANS				
Bone marrow	Aplasia, pancytopenia	2.5	4.5	Whole segment
Liver	Acute and chronic hepatitis	30	40	Whole
		50	55	1/3
Intestine	Obstruction, perforation, fistula	40	55	Whole
		50	65	1/3 or 1/2
Stomach	Perforation, ulcer, hemorrhage	50	65	Whole
		60	70	1/3
Brain	Infarction, necrosis	45	60	Whole
		60	75	1/3
Spinal cord	Infarction, necrosis	47	—	20 cm
		50	70	5 or 10 cm

Table 2-3 A Compilation of Tissue and Organ Sensitivities—cont'd

	Injury	$TD_{5/5}$, Gy*	$TD_{50/5}$, Gy*	Field size
Heart	Pericarditis and pancarditis	40	50	Whole
		60	70	1/3
Lung	Acute and chronic pneumonitis	17.5	24.5	Whole
		45	65	1/3
Kidney	Acute and chronic nephrosclerosis	23	28	Whole
		50	45	1/3 or 1/2
CLASS II ORGANS				
Oral cavity and pharynx	Ulceration, mucositis	60	75	50 cm²
Skin	Acute and chronic dermatitis, telangiectasia	55	65	100 cm²
Esophagus	Esophagitis, ulceration	55	50	Whole
		60	70	1/3
Rectum	Ulcer, stenosis, fistula	60	80	No vol effect
Salivary glands	Xerostomia	32	46	1/3 or 1/2
Bladder	Contracture	65	80	2/3
		80	85	1/3
Ureters	Stricture	70	100	5–10 cm length
Testes	Sterilization	1	2	Whole
Ovaries	Sterilization	2–3	6–12	Whole (age dependent)
Growing cartilage, child bone	Growth arrest, dwarfing	10	30	Whole
Mature cartilage, adult bone	Necrosis, fracture, sclerosis	60	100	Whole
Eye—retina	Blindness	45	65	Whole
Eye—cornea		50	6	Whole
Eye—lens	Cataract	10	18	Whole
Thyroid	Hypothyroidism	45	150	Whole
Adrenal	Hypoadrenalism	60		Whole
Pituitary	Hypopituitarism	45	200	Whole
Peripheral nerves	Neuritis	60	100	
Ear—middle	Serous otitis	30	40	No volume effect
Ear—vestibular	Ménière's syndrome	60	70	
CLASS III ORGANS				
Muscle—child	Atrophy	20	40	Whole
Muscle—adult	Fibrosis	60	80	Whole
Lymph nodes and lymphatics	Atrophy, sclerosis	50	70	Whole node
Large arteries and veins	Sclerosis	80	100	10 cm²
Articular cartilage	None	500	5000	Whole
Uterus	Necrosis, perforation	100	200	Whole
Vagina	Ulcer, fistula	90	100	Whole
Breast—child	No development	10	15	Whole
Breast—adult	Atrophy, necrosis	50	100	Whole

From: Hall EJ, Amato JG: *Radiobiology for the radiologist,* ed 6, Philadelphia, 2006, Lippincott Williams & Wilkins, pp 334-335. Based on a combination of Rubin P, Casarett GW: *Clinical radiation pathology,* vol 1, Philadelphia, 1968, Saunders; and Emami B, Lyman J, Broun A, et al: Tolerance of normal tissue to therapeutic irradiation, *Int J Radiat Oncol Biol Phys* 21:109-122, 1991, with permission. Table compiled by Dr. Richard Miller.

*The minimal tolerance dose ($TD_{5/5}$) refers to the dose of radiation that could cause no more than a 5% severe complication rate within 5 years after treatment. The maximal tolerance dose ($TD_{50/5}$) refers to the dose of radiation that could cause no more than a 50% severe complication rate within 5 years after treatment.

The Oxygen Effect

Although the exact mechanism of the oxygen effect is not fully understood, it is generally agreed that oxygen acts at the level of the free radicals. As radiation passes through biological material, ion pairs are formed that very quickly progress to the production of free radicals. These free radicals are highly reactive molecules that then break chemical bonds, trigger chemical changes, and ultimately stimulate the chain of events leading to biological damage. Oxygen (if available) reacts with free radicals, binding them into organic compounds that essentially make them unavailable for reparative function.

Oxygen Enhancement Ratio

The oxygen enhancement ratio (OER) describes the magnitude of the dose required to produce a given level of biological damage under oxygenated versus hypoxic conditions. For most cells the OER is around 3.0.[6] Low linear energy transfer (LET) radiations, which are sparsely ionizing (x rays and gamma rays), require 3 times the dose under hypoxic conditions as under oxygenated conditions (OER of 2.5 to 3). Neutron therapy (intermediate ionizing density) has a very low OER of 1.6, thus making this a more effective treatment under anoxic conditions than x ray or gamma radiation.

Sublethal injury may be repaired after an initial cycle delay, allowing mitosis and regrowth to occur. Sublethal damage repair also may be faulty, with chromosomal aberrations resulting. If the surviving cell is capable of undergoing mitosis, the chromosomal damage is likely to result in genetic mutation.

As the science of radiobiology developed, certain phenomena were observed that led to the increased ability to achieve eradication of the tumor while sparing healthy tissue. The biological factors that influence the response of normal tissue and tumors to fractionated radiation therapy are summarized by the "four R's of radiation therapy"[7]:

- *Repair*—as evidenced by cellular recovery during the few hours after exposure (i.e., the ability of cells to recover from sublethal radiation injury).
- *Reassortment*—cell-cycle progression effects, otherwise known as *redistribution*. Cells that survive a first dose of radiation will tend to be in a resistant phase of the cell cycle and within hours they may progress into a more sensitive phase.
- *Repopulation*—during an extended course of radiation therapy, cells that survive irradiation may proliferate and thus increase the number of cells that must be killed.
- *Reoxygenation*—the process in which radioresistant hypoxic tumor cells become radiosensitive aerated cells between doses of a fractionated course of radiation therapy.

Measuring Radiation Absorption

The dose of radiation absorbed correlates directly with the energy of the beam. An accurate measurement of absorbed dose is critical. The basic unit of radiation absorbed dose is the amount of energy (joules) absorbed per unit mass (kg). This unit, know as the gray (Gy) has replaced the unit of rad used in the past (100 rads = 1 Gy). One rad is equal to one centigray (cGy) (1 rad = 1cGy). This has resulted in mixed usage of the two terms in the radiation therapy literature.

Fractionation

A single dose of ionizing radiation produces a greater effect on tissue than that same dose divided into several fractions (fx) or treatments. This can be viewed as both a positive and a negative effect when considering the concept of therapeutic ratio in planning a course of radiation therapy. If the goal of treatment is to eradicate tumors while sparing normal tissues, then fractionation becomes crucial to achieving this goal.

Fractionation of total dose is planned to take advantage of the four Rs of radiobiology.[4] *Repair* of sublethal injury generally occurs within 24 hours and possibly in as few as 4 hours. Normal cells therefore can repair between daily doses of radiation. Tumor cells may do so initially but become less capable of repair as treatment is protracted. *Repopulation* or regeneration of healthy cells continues after repair of sublethal injury allows mitosis to take place. Tumor cells are more likely to die during mitosis as the result of lethal radiation damage.

Successive daily doses of radiation given at regular intervals help to disrupt the tumor cell cycle, causing division delay. *Reassortment* of tumor cells in their cycle theoretically enhances the effectiveness of each succeeding radiation dose because more cells are likely to be in mitosis at the same time. Healthy cells are less likely to be subject to redistribution.

Table 2-4 Comparison of Conventional Fractionation With Hyperfractionation and Accelerated Fractionation

	Conventional	Hyperfractionation	Accelerated fractionation
Overall treatment time	5–8 weeks	5–8 weeks	2.5–7 weeks
Fractions per day	1	2–3	1–3
Total number of fractions	25–38	60–80	25–38
Dose per fraction	1.2 Gy–2 Gy	1 Gy–1.2 Gy	1.2 Gy–2 Gy
Total dose	45 Gy–65 Gy	60 Gy–81 Gy	25 Gy–76 Gy

The single most important advantage of fractionation is the opportunity it provides for *reoxygenation* of the tumor cells. The presence of oxygen in the cell at the time of irradiation greatly increases the lethal effect of ionization; according to Coleman et al.[8] adding oxygen even 1/100 of a second after exposure produces no sensitization to radiation because the lifetime of a free radical is measured in microseconds.

In addition to allowing time for reoxygenation, fractionation has an advantage when treating large tumors with necrotic (anoxic) central components. As daily radiation gradually destroys the outer (oxygenated) layers of the tumor mass, the central core is thus exposed to capillary oxygenation and becomes more radiosensitive to the latter portion of the protracted course of treatment. This assumes, of course, that good microcirculation exists in the target site. Preexisting factors such as compromised circulation (due to radical surgical procedures or radiation fibrosis) and anemia can effectively reduce radiosensitivity.

Over the past two decades, studies have introduced new insights into biological factors affecting radiation response in both normal and tumor tissues.[9] As a result, various fractionation schedules have been introduced that deviate from the standard single daily fraction.

Alternative Fractionation

Daily single fractions given 5 times a week is the standard fractionation schedule for radiation therapy with a dose range from 1.8 to 2.0 gray (Gy). Alternative fractionation schemes continue to receive attention as the search continues to achieve greater cell kill and tumor control. Prolonging treatment in order to administer higher doses of radiation and spare acute reactions may, however, lead to excessive late injury. In addition, there is some evidence that prolonged treatment time allows for proliferation of surviving tumor cells.[5,10] Two strategies have been developed involving multiple fractions per day: hyperfractionation and accelerated fractionation (Table 2-4). In both approaches, 4 to 6 hours between doses must be allowed for repair of sublethal damage from the first dose before the second is given.[5,11,12]

Hyperfractionation refers to the use of several smaller than standard doses given more than once daily in the standard overall treatment time.[11] Daily dose and total dose are usually greater than that used in conventional treatment. The goal is to reduce (or at least not increase) late effects and gain better tumor control. Two and sometimes three fractions per day are administered with the appropriate time interval between each dose. Total daily dose approximates that given for the same tumor treated with a standard single fraction per day.

Accelerated fractionation refers to a shortened overall treatment time in which standard total doses are given in a shorter time period by increasing the number of standard fractions per day.[11] The rationale for accelerated fractionation is based on the fact that reducing overall treatment time reduces the opportunity and probability of tumor cell regeneration during the treatment course and therefore increases the likelihood of tumor control. As long as the overall time is not markedly reduced, acute reactions are usually tolerable. However, if overall time is significantly shortened, then total dose must also be reduced to prevent severe acute reactions. A number of approaches have been suggested for accelerated fractionation including the following:

- Short course of treatment with a correspondingly reduced total dose of radiation (e.g., whole brain radiation therapy with 3000cGy in 10 fractions).

- Short course of treatment by delivering multiple fractions per day (e.g., accelerated partial breast radiation therapy with MammoSite).
- Administering the boost as the second daily fraction during 2 or more weeks of the standard single daily dose (e.g., during whole breast radiation therapy, giving boost to tumor bed).
- A steady increase in the dose each week throughout the course of treatment.

Although alternative fractionation schemes have shown promise and potential for further study, there remains a concern for unexpected late sequelae in normal tissue, usually seen after protracted recovery from acute reactions.

Treatment Planning and Simulation

Treatment with ionizing radiation is based on a body of knowledge accumulated over many years of research. Perez and Purdy[1] have identified eight important steps involved in effective planning and administration:

1. Thorough knowledge of the natural history and pathological characteristics of the tumor.
2. Adequate evaluation of the patient and staging procedures to determine the full extent of the tumor.
3. Definition of the treatment strategy to select the best method or combinations of therapies to be applied, which may depend on the stage, type of tumor, and routes of spread.
4. Treatment planning volumetric imaging study with accurate definition of the target volume, critical normal structures, and radiation beam portals.
5. Treatment isodose (volumetric) computations and plan evaluation to determine the optimum distribution of irradiation within the volume of interest.
6. Accurate and reproducible repositioning and immobilization techniques for daily treatment delivery.
7. Applicable in vivo dosimetry, portal localization and verification procedures to ensure quality control throughout the therapeutic process.
8. Periodic evaluation of the patient during and after therapy to assess the effects of the treatment on the tumor and the tolerance of the patient.

The radiation oncologist is responsible for treatment planning, and in most facilities other professionals are involved as well. They may include radiation physicists, radiobiologists, computer scientists, radiation therapists, dosimetrists, and possibly others who may have a role in the planning process. A more detailed description of the treatment planning process can be found in Chapter 5.

PRINCIPLES OF EXTERNAL BEAM RADIATION THERAPY

The most common method of delivering radiation therapy is by external beam. *Teletherapy,* or external beam radiation therapy, refers to radiation treatment delivered by a radioactive source or electromagnetic energy from a machine placed at some distance from the target site. Teletherapy (from the Greek *tele,* meaning "from a distance") is distinguished from brachytherapy, or the use of implanted or injected radioactive sources. Teletherapy equipment can be categorized according to energy produced and depth of penetration within the target area. Table 2-1 lists the various types of equipment, emissions, beam characteristics, and clinical applications.

Before 1951, most radiation treatment units were x-ray machines capable of producing photon beams having only limited penetrability. Kilovoltage machines, with a range of 40 to 150 kV (low voltage), were some of the earliest available sources of ionizing radiation and are in use today for treating very superficial skin cancers. A kilovoltage unit that operates with only a 2 cm or less source-to-skin distance (SSD) is called a *contact unit.* Those operating at a 15 to 20 SSD are called *superficial units.*

Orthovoltage (deep therapy) equipment in the range of 150 to 1000 kV was introduced in 1920s and 1930s. Although capable of reaching deep-seated tumors, orthovoltage x rays produced severe late effects because of high bone absorption, leading to osteonecrosis. Skin tolerance was also very poor with these machines, which operated at an SSD of approximately 50 cm.

Megavoltage (supervoltage) machines evolved during the period immediately after World War II. Nuclear reactors allowed production of sufficient quantities of radionuclides for medical usage. The cobalt teletherapy unit was first introduced 1951 in Canada and became the mainstay of radiation therapy treatment facilities until the 1960s.

Cobalt machines are mechanically simple and have the ability to penetrate deep within the target site. A typical cobalt source emits gamma radiation with an energy range of 1.17 to 1.38 MeV (million electron volts) and operates at an SSD of 80 cm to 100 cm. Cobalt is a radioactive element that emits energy through a process of constant decay or disintegration (half-life of 5.26 years). Therefore efficiency of output decreases over time and the radioactive source must be replaced every 4 to 5 years. These machines are becoming obsolete in light of newer technology.

The linear accelerator is the predominant teletherapy equipment in use in most treatment centers throughout the world. The linac (linear accelerator) or clinac machine generates electrons using high-frequency electromagnetic waves to accelerate the electrons to high energy before striking a tungsten target and producing photons (Figure 2-1). Photon radiation is then directed at the target volume in a defined, shaped beam as it emerges at a very high speed from the linac. Photon energy is equivalent to gamma radiation (produced by a cobalt source) in its energy range and penetrating power.

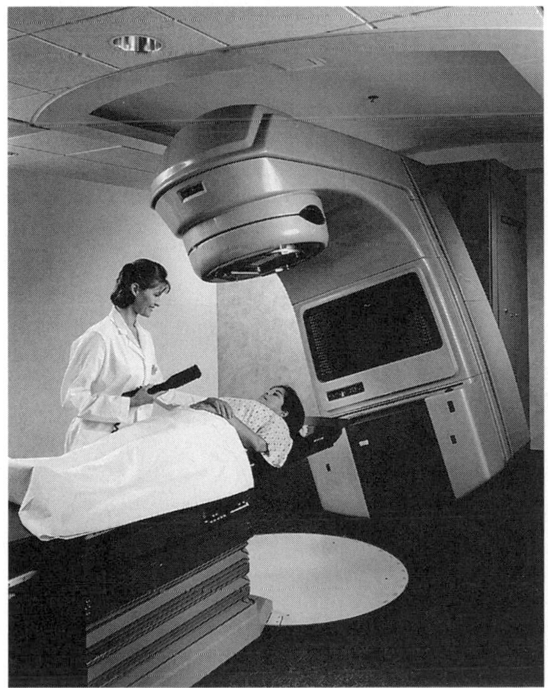

Figure 2-1 Linear Accelerator.
Photo courtesy of Medical Systems, Palo Alto, Calif. All rights reserved.

Many linear accelerators are equipped with an electron mode that allows use of the electron energy itself for treatment of surface lesions or those within a few centimeters of the surface. The electron beam is characterized by rapid dose buildup followed by rapid dose falloff beyond the target volume. Electrons are equivalent to beta radiation in depth of penetration and have useful energies ranging from 4 to 20 MeV. Because of the rapid dose buildup at the surface of the target, electron therapy characteristically produces more intense skin reactions than does photon therapy.

Radiation is currently delivered with substantially more precision than in the past because of advances in imaging and treatment planning.[13] The most advanced photon beam delivery method is intensity-modulated radiation therapy (IMRT), which can deliver higher doses of radiation to a tumor while reducing the dose delivered to selected normal tissues. This is accomplished by applying numerous radiation fields of varying intensities from different directions.[13] However, one of the concerns about IMRT is that the use of numerous fields increases the volume of normal tissue that is irradiated and that over time, this exposure of more tissue to low-dose radiation will increase the risk of a second malignancy or other unwanted late tissue effects. This concern has lead to the tremendous interest in the use of other types of radiation that may produce superior dose distributions resulting in even less damage to normal structures.

High Linear Energy Transfer and Heavy Charged Particle Beams

Linear energy transfer (LET) refers to the quality of different types of ionizing photons and particles. LET describes the rate and amount of energy, transfer of a given radiation as it passes through a target substance. High-LET beams expend most of their energy (and thus have their greatest impact) on tissues within a few centimeters of the skin surface. Low-LET sources may be of equal energy to high-LET sources but deposit or transfer that energy much more slowly as the beam passes through tissue, thus continuing to have significant effect on tissues deep within the body.

Equal doses of ionizing radiation from different energy sources do not produce equal biological effects.[5] The ratio of dose required of any given source to produce an effect equal to that of a standard dose of 250 kilovoltage x ray is known as the relative biological effectiveness (RBE). RBE increases with LET up to a certain point. However, with very high LET, a decrease or loss of RBE occurs as each succeeding lethal hit on a given cell becomes redundant.[5]

Clinical trials using protons, helium ions, fast neutrons, heavy ions (carbon, neon, argon), and negative *pi*-meso*ns* (pions) have been underway at a number of sites around the world since the 1950s. Characteristics of high-LET and heavy charged particle beans are described in Table 2-2. The two major advantages of these sources of ionizing radiations are (1) deposition of large doses of radiation in small volumes of tissue, with sparing of surrounding normal tissue (proton beams, heavy ions, and negative pi-mesons) and (2) biological advantages, including more effective killing of hypoxic cells and decreased fluctuation in radiosensitivity throughout the cell cycle (fast neutrons, heavy ions, and pi-mesons).

Introduced in the 1930s, fast neutrons, neon- and carbon-ions, were high-LET radiation that was used in radiation. Although tumor response in the early studies was encouraging, late sequelae in long-term survivors were severe enough to discourage further usage for a number of years. When in vitro cell culture techniques became available in the 1950s, neutron studies were resumed and important information regarding RBE of high-LET radiation was made clear. The radiobiological data indicate that high-LET radiations have a potential benefit for the treatment of some cancer types or sites, namely those tumors that are inherently photon-resistant because of high repair capability or marked hypoxia.[14]

Fast neutrons were the first high-LET radiations to be used, and this therapy continues to hold promise, particularly with the introduction of hospital-based neutron therapy systems with improved dose-distribution. Indications for treatment include tumors with the following characteristics: (1) hypoxic and slowly reoxygenating tumors and (2) slow growing, well differentiated, repair-proficient tumors.[14] Clinical trials were developed to evaluate the response rates in salivary gland tumors, adenoid cystic carcinoma, prostate adenocarcinoma, soft tissue sarcomas (slow-growing), and selective non–small cell lung carcinoma.[14]

Boron neutron capture therapy (BNCT) is being used to increase delivery of thermal neutrons to deep-seated tumors.[15] An isotope of boron, ^{10}B, known to have an affinity for slow or thermal neutrons is infused into the patient before irradiation. Neutron capture in the ^{10}B atoms results in a high local radiation dose to the tumor cells whilst sparing the healthy tissue. Currently, the European Organization of Research and Treatment of Cancer (EORTC) is conducting trials using this therapy at the high flux reactor (HFR) at Petten in the Netherlands.

Proton beam radiation therapy is a form of charged particle therapy that allows for excellent dose distributions with the added benefit of no exit dose (Figure 2-2). Protons have a very rapid energy loss in the last few millimeters of penetration.[13] The result is a sharply localized peak of dose, known as the *Bragg peak* (Figure 2-3). The physical and biological advantages of high-LET and heavy charged particle beams are offset somewhat by the complexity and costs of the equipment and facilities. However, a significant amount of interest in this treatment approach resulted in the development of hospital-based cyclotrons with higher energy beams capable of reaching deep-seated tumors, field sizes comparable to linear accelerators, and rotational gantries. Currently, 23 facilities are open worldwide and several more are expected to open in the next several years.

Protons have been studied in ocular (uveal) melanoma, sarcomas of the skull base and spine, benign meningioma, parasnasal sinus, nasal, and nasopharyngeal tumors, prostate carcinoma, hepatocellular carcinoma, early stage lung cancer, and pediatric malignancies.[13]

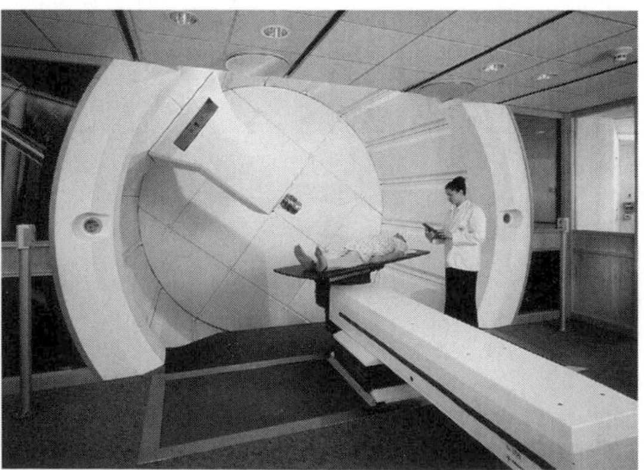

Figure 2-2 Proteus 235 Proton Therapy System. *Courtesy of Ion Beam Applications, Belgium.*

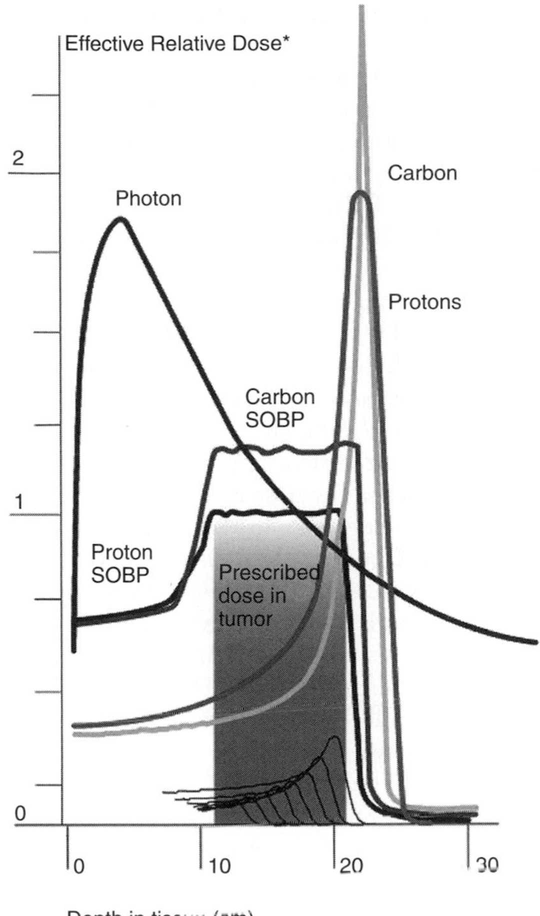

Figure 2-3 Bragg Peak.
Courtesy of Ion Beam Applications, Belgium.

PRINCIPLES OF BRACHYTHERAPY

Brachytherapy (*brachy*, from the Greek for short distance) is the temporary or permanent placement of a radioactive source very close to or in contact with the target tissue (Table 2-5). Also called *internal radiation therapy* or *implant therapy*, brachytherapy offers the advantage of delivering a high dose of radiation to a specific tumor volume, with a rapid falloff in dose to adjacent normal tissues. Implantation techniques include interstitial, intracavitary, transluminal, or mold techniques and may be permanent or temporary implants. They maybe preloaded, manually afterloaded, or remotely afterloaded, and the dose rate may be low, medium, or high. Intracavitary insertion consists of positioning a temporary applicator with the radioactive source into a body cavity in close proximity to the target tissue. Interstitial brachytherapy consists of surgically implanting small radioactive sources directly into the target tissue that remain permanently. Transluminal brachytherapy consists of inserting a temporary single source into a body lumen to treat its surface and the adjacent tissue. Mold techniques are surface dose applications used to treat superficial lesions on the skin or mucosa.

Brachytherapy has been in use since the early 1900s following the discovery of radium by Marie and Pierre Curie. Treatment with brachytherapy began with the use of surface applicators of radium to treat skin lesions. Since then, many developments, both beneficial and destructive, have occurred in the therapeutic use of radioactive sources. In the early days of brachytherapy, physicians had limited knowledge of the destructive effects from improper handling of radioactive sources. In the

Table 2-5 Brachytherapy Radionuclides

Radionuclides	Abbreviations	Placement	Brachytherapy type
Cesium	^{137}Cs	Tubes and needles	Intracavitary Interstitial
Iridium	^{192}IR	Seeds, nylon ribbon, metal wires	Interstitial
Cobalt	^{60}Co	Encapsulated spheres	Intracavitary
Iodine	^{125}I	Seeds	Interstitial
Palladium	^{103}Pd	Seeds	Interstitial
Gold	^{198}Au	Seeds	Interstitial
Strontium	^{90}Sr-^{90}Y	Plaque	Superficial ocular low exposure
Samarium	^{145}Sm	Seeds	Interstitial
Phosphorus	^{32}P	Chromic phosphate colloid	Instillation
Strontium	^{89}Sr	$SrCl_2$ IV solution	
Iodine	^{131}I	Capsule	Thyroid Cancer

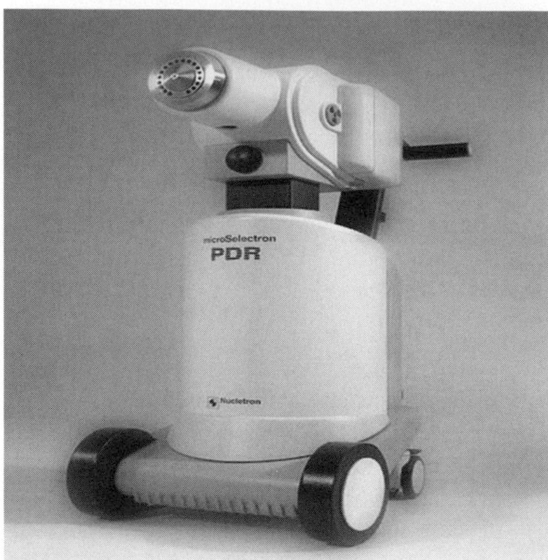

Figure 2-4 Nucletron MicroSelection PDR Afterload Brachytherapy Machine.
Courtesy of Nucletron, Columbia, Md.

1950s, afterloading methods were developed in which source holders are placed during the operative procedure but the radioactive sources are not added until later when the patient returns to his or her hospital room. This technique protected nurses and other healthcare workers from undue radioactive exposure. In the 1960s and 1970s, the development of the linear accelerator led to a decline in the popularity of brachytherapy. However, with the influence of computers and availability of pneumatic remote afterloading systems (Figure 2-4), improved safety and protection techniques, a better understanding of the radiobiology of brachytherapy, and a renewed interest in the use of brachytherapy, either alone or in combination with other modalities, has emerged.

Today, knowledge about the long-term effects of radiation exposure has led to highly regulated guidelines on the safe use and handling of radioactive isotopes. In a comprehensive study conducted by Nag et al.[16], they found that 819 facilities in the United States were practicing brachytherapy using intracavitary, interstitial, intraluminal, and plaque techniques. The most common sites treated were cervix, endometrium, head and neck, and lung. High dose rate (HDR) remote afterloading brachytherapy or low dose rate (LDR) remote afterloading brachytherapy was used in approximately 25% of the facilities that responded to the survey.

Pulsed brachytherapy (PB) is a relatively new approach to treatment. It involves the delivery of a large number of radiation pulses over a time period similar to that used in continuous low-dose brachytherapy. Pulse durations are typically on the order of 10 to 20 minutes, with interpulse intervals of up to a few hours.

Radiobiology of Brachytherapy

The basic radiobiological principles of repair, repopulation, reassortment, and reoxygenation (the four Rs) have a different tissue response when radiation is administered on a continuous basis either in high or low dose rate brachytherapy, as opposed to being fractionated on a daily basis (e.g., external beam radiation). Repair is an intracellular process that is thought to be equally efficient in both normal and cancer cells. Normally, repair is complete within a few hours after external beam radiation. Theoretically, with brachytherapy techniques, malignant cells would have a decreased ability to repair damage. Thus when external beam radiation is combined with brachytherapy, tumor cells in the irradiated volume that may survive after external beam radiation are less likely to undergo repair.

Repopulation involves the replacement of dead or dying cells through cell multiplication. Both normal and malignant cells are able to recover from radiation injury; however, repopulation rates vary with different tissues. Theoretically, continuous dose rate radiation, when targeted to a specific tumor volume, would decrease the ability of malignant cells to repopulate. The rapid falloff in radiation dose to normal surrounding tissues would have less interference with the ability of normal tissues to repopulate after radiation damage.

Reassortment of cells throughout the cell cycle occurs after a dose of fractionated radiation. Irradiated cells may be blocked in the late G2 phase of the cell cycle and are more susceptible to radiation damage. With brachytherapy, a greater percentage of cancer cells accumulate in the G2 phase. Although cellular proliferation can occur during brachytherapy, these new cells are still blocked in the G2 phase and continue to be susceptible to radiation damage. Redistribution of a significant proportion of the cell population into G2 phase can result in an increased sensitization effect.

Reoxygenation is the process in which hypoxic tumor cells become sensitized as a result of the redistribution of oxygen after radiation exposure. Reoxygenation occurs as a result of decreased tumor burden and changes in the blood flow patterns of tumors. Less oxygen is needed to sensitize cells to damage with continuous radiation. Hence, brachytherapy techniques may be more effective with anoxic tumors than is conventional fractionated external beam radiation.

Properties of Radioactive Isotopes

After the initial discovery of x rays by Roentgen, radioactive isotopes were found to emit three distinct types of radiation: alpha (α) particles, beta (β) particles, and gamma (γ) rays. Since the discovery of these radioactive elements, several other particles have been identified including neutrons, positrons, neutrinos, pi-mesons, mu-mesons, and k-mesons. Of the 103 known radioactive elements, the first 92 occur naturally; the remaining have been produced artificially.

The decay constant of a radioactive nucleus is defined as the fraction of the total number of atoms that decay per unit time. Radioactivity is defined as the total number of disintegrations per unit time interval. The curie (Ci) is a unit of activity that is equal to 3.7×10^{10} disintegrations per second. The Becquerel (Bq) is a special name for the SI unit for activity and is equal to one disintegration per second. The half-life of a radioactive isotope is the time required for the number of atoms in a particular sample to decrease by one-half.

Gamma decay occurs when a nucleus undergoes a transition from a higher to a lower energy level. During this process, high-energy photons called *x rays* are emitted. Related to gamma decay is a process called *internal conversion*. Rather than emitting gamma rays, excess energy from the excited nucleus is transferred to an electron in one of the inner atomic shells, which causes the ejection of the electron from the atom and the resulting emission of characteristic x rays.

In beta decay, a neutron within the nucleus is converted into a proton, which results in an electron and an antineutrino being emitted. With beta decay, the emitted particles vary in their kinetic energy. Half-lives for beta decay are longer than gamma decay half-lives.

Alpha decay occurs when the ratio of neutrons to protons is low and in nuclides with atomic numbers greater than 82. Alpha particles have high LET, which means that they lose their energy quickly when they collide with electrons in their path. With a high LET, alpha particles are unable to penetrate more than 0.04 mm into tissue.

Mechanism of Radiation Injury in Cells

Alpha and beta particles and gamma rays exert damage in tissue by transferring energy to living matter. They ionize molecules in cells to cause physical and chemical changes that ultimately alter the biological processes responsible for cellular reproduction. Irradiated cells are either destroyed or are left unable to reproduce. The extent of radiation injury is partly a function of the ionizing capabilities of the isotope. Alpha and beta particles are directly ionizing radiations. They are electrically charged and produce ionization at small intervals along their paths through collision with other particles. Gamma rays are indirectly ionizing and have no electrical charge. Gamma rays transfer energy to directly ionizing particles, ionize and liberate electrons in the atom with low energy loss, and proceed to ionize other particles in their path. The net result is that directly ionizing gamma rays transfers energy to directly ionizing particles deeper within tissue. Because gamma emitters posses the greatest capacity to produce damage deep in tissue, they also present the greatest hazard to healthcare providers.

Brachytherapy in Specific Cancers

Brachytherapy can be used alone or in combination with external beam radiation, surgery, chemotherapy, or hyperthermia. It is used to improve control of local disease, treat areas at high risk for tumor recurrence, enhance comfort with recurrent disease, preserve vital organ function, and spare normal surrounding tissues from damage. Implantation techniques have been used in a wide variety of cancers (Box 2-1). Information about the different brachytherapy techniques for each malignancy can be found in each disease-site chapter.

Brachytherapy in Benign Conditions

Brachytherapy techniques also have been used to treat benign conditions such as pterygium, a nonmalignant ocular condition. A pterygium is a degeneration of collagen that produces a fleshy mass in the bulbar conjunctiva that grows across the

Box 2-1 Disease Sites Treated With Brachytherapy

Bile duct
Bladder
Brain
Breast
Bronchus
Cervix
Endometrium
Esophagus
Nasopharynx
Ocular structures
Pancreas
Prostate
Rectum
Skin
Tongue
Vagina

cornea and replaces the epithelium and Bowman's membrane.[17] Although the primary treatment for this condition is surgical excision, high recurrence rates are associated with surgery. Brachytherapy can be used to decrease the recurrence rate. Treatment consists of a weekly surface application of strontium-90 for 3 to 4 weeks.[17]

Systemic Radioisotopes

Several systemic radioisotopes are currently being used in the clinical management of cancer (Table 2-6). Strontium-89 (Metastron) and samarium-153 (Quadramet) are currently approved for the palliation of pain related to metastatic disease in bone.[18] Rhenium-186 and Rhenium-188 are investigational agents available for similar bone metastasis. Radioisotopes are generally given intravenously on an outpatient basis. All four of these isotopes emit beta particles (electrons) with sufficiently long half-lives to provide cytotoxic irradiation of malignant cells localized in skeletal tissue. Data from numerous studies in patients with metastatic prostate and breast cancer provides strong evidence that these radioisotopes are effective in relieving pain in a substantial number of patients. Unfortunately, because pain is a subjective assessment and is not readily quantifiable with reproducibility between patients and studies, the data has been somewhat controversial. The variability in the assessment of pain response, the different measures used, and the timing of such measures has led to some of this confusion. In addition, other issues such as which isotope to use and on what schedule remain unanswered.

Unsealed Radioactive Sources

Unsealed radioactive sources are used for the selective delivery of radiation to tumors or target organs in both benign and malignant disease (Table 2-7). In cancer treatment, it combines the advantage of target selectivity with that of being systemic and may be used as part of a therapeutic strategy with curative intent or for disease control and palliation.[19] The basis for successful therapy is sufficient uptake and prolonged retention of the radiopharmaceutical in the target tissues.[19]

The mechanism of action of radionuclide therapy, with its low irradiation dose rate, is not well understood. Radiation is delivered selectively by the appropriate radiopharmaceutical, taking advantage of shorter range β particles or ultrashort-path-length α particles or Auger electron emitting radionuclides.[20] Calculation of the dose delivered to a target remains a challenge mainly because the distribution of the radiopharmaceutical in the target is nonuniform.[21] However, advances in antibody engineering, the identification of tumor antigen targets, and the synthesis of regulatory peptide analogues and bifunctional chelating agents are providing new opportunities for the use of these agents in oncology including radioimmunotherapy.[19] For more information on radioimmunotherapy, see Chapter 24.

Table 2-6 Radioisotopes Used for Palliation of Bone Pain

Radioisotope	Brand name	Dose	Indications
^{89}Sr-Chloride	Metastron	1.48–2.22 MBq/kg	Prostate, breast, lung
^{153}Sm-EDTMP	Quadramet	37 MBq/kg	Prostate, breast, lung, osteosarcoma
^{186}Re-HEDP			Breast and prostate
^{188}Re-HEDP			Prostate, breast, lung

MBq, Megabecquerel.

Table 2-7 Therapeutic Indications for Nonsealed Radionuclide Sources

Isotope	Therapeutic indication
^{131}Iodine	Hyperthyroidism (diffuse toxic goiter, multinodular goiter, solitary toxic thyroid nodule)
^{32}P-orthophosphate	Thyroid carcinoma (papillary, follicular)
	Polycythemia vera
	Thrombocytosis
	Malignant ascites
	Malignant pleural effusions
^{131}*I*-m–iodebenzylguanidine (MIBG)	Brain cysts
	Pheochromocytoma
	Paraganglioma
	Neuroblastoma
	Carcinoid medullary thyroid carcinoma

INTRAOPERATIVE RADIATION THERAPY

Intraoperative radiation therapy (IORT) delivers a concentrated beam of radiation to a tumor(s) while it is exposed during surgery. This technique allows the administration of high doses of radiation without exposing nearby healthy organs to radiation. A single dose of intraoperative radiation may have as much effect on the tumor as the multiple daily radiation treatments. When combined with surgery, chemotherapy and/or external beam radiation therapy in clinical trials, IORT has been shown to be affective in controlling some locally aggressive tumors.

IORT has a number of logistical and cost considerations that have limited its availability. This is a procedure that requires being in the operating room. In the past, conventional radiation equipment was heavy and required heavy concrete shielding, not available in the majority of operating rooms. This restricted IORT to a few facilities who either were able to move the patients during their surgical procedure to a room

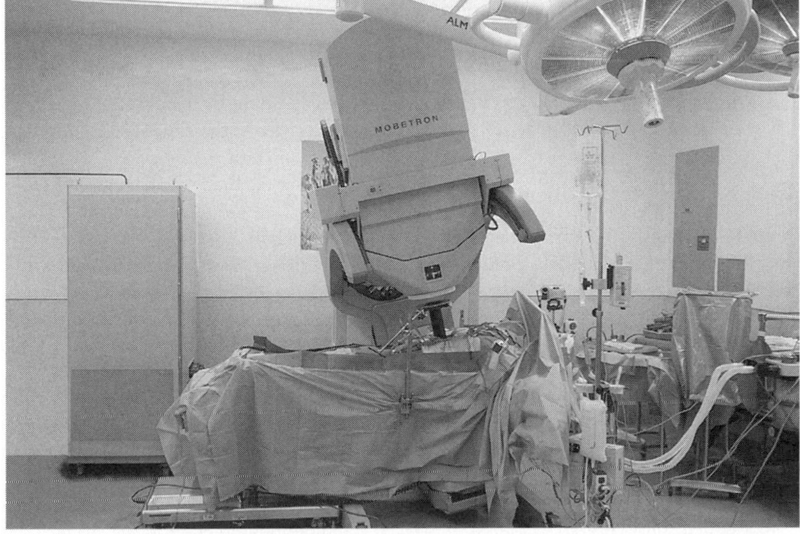

Figure 2-5 Mobetron IORT (Intraoperative Radiation Therapy) Machine.
Courtesy of IntraOp Medical Corporation, Sunnyvale, Calif.

with a radiation therapy machine or who had a dedicated radiation machine in the operating room.

However, new linear accelerator equipment with electrons were developed over the past decade that are light-weight and mobile (Figure 2-5). As a result, a number of centers are currently conducting phase II and phase III trials using this technique under the auspices of the IORT Protocol Group within the International Society of Intraoperative Radiation Therapy (ISIORT).

Two major indications for the use of IORT are (1) use with surgery to irradiate a tumor bed or areas of unresectable gross tumors and (2) as a "boost" in combination with large-field external beam radiation therapy and surgical resection. IORT has been studied in most cancer disease sites, but the primary sites have been breast, bladder, stomach, pancreas, colon, rectum, brain, extremities and retroperitoneum.

SUMMARY

In today's sophisticated cancer treatment environment, radiation oncology plays a major role in cure, control, and palliation of cancer symptoms. A substantial number of patients diagnosed with cancer receive radiation treatment at some time during the course of the disease. The person with cancer who is referred for radiation therapy can best be supported by a radiation oncology clinician who understands the history, physical and chemical principles, and biological effects of radiation therapy and is prepared to provide the education and information needed by the patient.

REFERENCES

1. Perez CA, Purdy JA: Fundamentals of treatment planning in radiation oncology. In Levitt SH, Kahn FM, Potish RA, et al, editors: *Levitt & Tapley's technological basis of radiation therapy: clinical applications*, ed 3, Philadelphia, 1999, Lippincott Williams & Wilkins, pp 30-51.
2. Lenhard RE, Lawrence W, McKenna RJ: General approach to the patient. In Murphy GP, Lawrence W, Lenhard RE, editors: *Clinical oncology*, ed 2, Atlanta, 1995, American Cancer Society, pp 64-74.
3. Ritter MA: Cell proliferation. In Mauch PM, Loeffier JS, editors: *Radiation oncology: technology and biology*, Philadelphia, 1994, Saunders, pp 525-544.
4. Steel GG: Introduction: the significance of radiobiology for radiotherapy. In Steel GG, editor: *Basic clinical radiobiology*, ed 3, London, 2002, Arnold, pp 1-7.
5. Hall EJ, Cox JD: Physical and biologic basis of radiation therapy. In Cox JD, editor: *Moss' radiation oncology: rationale, technique, results*, ed 7, St Louis, 1994, Mosby, pp 3-66.
6. Horsman MR, Overgaard J: Overcoming tumor radioresistance resulting from hypoxia. In Steel GG, editor: *Basic clinical radiobiology*, ed 3, London, 2002, Arnold, pp 169-181.
7. Steel GG: Cell survival as a determinant of tumour response. In Steel GG, editor: *Basic clinical radiobiology*, ed 3, London, 2002, Arnold, pp 52-63.
8. Coleman CN, Beard CJ, Hlatky L et al: Biochemical modifiers; hypoxic cell sensitizers. In Mauch PM, Loeffier JS, editors: *Radiation oncology: technology and biology*, Philadelphia, 1994, Saunders, pp 55-89.
9. Peters LJ, Brock WA, Travis, EL: Radiation biology at clinically relevant fractions. In DeVita VT, Hellman S, Rosenberg SA, editors: *Important advances in oncology*, Philadelphia, 1990, Lippincott, pp 65-83.
10. Fowler JF, Tepper JE: Fractionation in radiation therapy, *Semin Radiat Oncol* 2:1-2, 1992.
11. Fowler JF: Brief summary of radiobiological principles in fractionated radiotherapy, *Semin Radiat Oncol* 2:16-21, 1992.
12. Peters LJ, Ang KK: Altered fractionation schemes. In Mauch PM, Loeffier JS, editors: *Radiation oncology: technology and biology*, Philadelphia, 1994, Saunders, pp 545-565.
13. Levin WP, Kooy H, Loeffler JS et al: Proton beam therapy, *Br J Cancer* 93(8):849-854, 2005.
14. Wambersle A, Hendry J, Gueulette J et al: Radiobiological rationale and patient selection for high-LET radiation in cancer therapy, *Radiother Oncol* 73(suppl 2):S1-14, 2004.
15. Wazer DE, Zamenhos RG, Harlfug OK et al: Boron neutron capture therapy. In Mauch PM, Loeffier JS, editors: *Radiation oncology: technology and biology*, Philadelphia, 1994, Saunders, pp 167-191.
16. Nag S, Owen JB, Farnan N et al: Survey of brachytherapy practice in the United States: a report of the clinical research committee of the American Endocurietherapy Society, *1nt J Radiat Oncol Biol Phys* 31(1):103-107, 1995.
17. Markoe A, Brady L, Carlsson U et al: Eye. In Perez C, Brady L: *Principles and practice of radiation oncology*, ed 2, Philadelphia, 1992, Lippincott, pp 595-609.
18. Finlay IG, Mason MD, Shelley M: Radioisotopes for the palliation of metastatic bone cancer: a systemic review, *Lancet Oncol* 6(6):392-400, 2005.
19. Chatal JF, Hoefnagel CA: Radionuclide therapy, *Lancet* 354(9182):931-965, 1999.
20. Wheldon TE, O'Donoghue JA, Barrett A et al: The curability of tumours of differing size by targeted radiotherapy using ^{131}I or ^{90}Y, *Radiother Oncol* 21(2):91-99, 1991.
21. Humm JL, Cobb LM: Nonuniformity of tumour dose in radioimmunotherapy, *J Nucl Med* 31(1):75-83, 1990.

Chapter 3

Radiation Protection and Safety

Maurene McQuestion

The use of ionizing radiation in the diagnosis and treatment of cancer requires that healthcare professionals in clinical radiation settings have the knowledge and understanding of radiation protection principals and practices in order to ensure a safe working environment for themselves, their patients, and families. Federal and state government agencies regulate the nuclear industry and enforce radiation safety guidelines related to the development, production, transportation, and use of radioactive materials and equipment to generate radiation. This includes the setting of strict limits related to exposure, ongoing monitoring, establishing guidelines related to radiation safety training, and the documentation and reporting of any environmental or individual radiation exposure.

HISTORY AND STANDARDS OF RADIATION PROTECTION AND SAFETY

Risks associated with the delivery of ionizing radiation have been known since the late 1800s, after the discovery of x rays by Roentgen in 1894 and the discovery of radioactivity by Becquerel in 1896.[1,2] Radiation protection standards have developed in response to the increased knowledge of the biological effects of radiation and improved understanding of acceptable risk. Early limits were set based on preventing skin-related changes from radiation exposure whereas later limits were based on the risk of cancer from high dose exposure. The earliest reported dose limit, set in 1902, was 10 rad per day or 50 rem per week.[3-5] As a result radiation workers during that time received significant annual doses of radiation. By 1924 professional societies were beginning discussions about 'tolerance doses' and suggested that exposure to 70 rem per month was tolerable. Dose limits were informal and not consistently applied. At that dose it was felt that individuals did not exhibit signs of harmful effects related to the radiation. A decade later in 1934, the U.S. Advisory Committee on X-ray and Radium Protection (which evolved into the National Council on Radiation Protection and Measurements, NCRP) was setting dose limits at 0.1 roentgens per day (approximately 1 mSv per day), again based on the lack of observable harm rather than on a sound understanding of the biological effects of ionizing radiation.[5] By the 1940s, after observations of the effects of radium on radium-dial painters and plutonium on industry workers, as well as early laboratory studies of the effects of radium, limits were being based on the internal uptake related to toxicities associated with the long half-life of these elements. Following World War II, Canada, the United States, and Great Britain were collaborating and sharing research knowledge.

The first formal annual dose limits for the public as well as for radiation industry workers were set in the early 1950s, with a dose rate of 150 mSv per year. By 1957, lower limits were agreed on based on concepts of measurement including absorbed dose (expressed in rad or Gray), dose-equivalents (expressed in rem or sieverts) and relative biological effectiveness.[4,5] Dose equivalent uses a common scale, taking into account the type of radiation and the absorbed dose in order to make comparisons between doses from different sources of energy (alpha, beta, or gamma). The absorbed dose and the dose equivalent are the same for beta, gamma, and x-ray radiation. For alpha radiation, there is a twentyfold increase between the absorbed dose and the equivalent dose.[6] Today maximal permissible occupational dose limits have been set by the U.S. Nuclear Regulatory Commission, at 50 mSv (5 rem) per year for the whole body, with a lifetime cumulative dose limit of 10 mSv multiplied by age. The limit for pregnant workers is 0.5 mSv per month.[7] Recommendations on maximum annual and cumulative limits for exposure to ionizing radiation are listed in Table 3-1. The principle of

Table 3-1 Recommendations on Limits for Exposure to Ionizing Radiation

A. Occupational exposures*	
1. Effective dose limits	
(a) Annual	50 mSv
(b) Cumulative	10 mSv × age
2. Equivalent dose annual limits for tissues and organs	
(a) Lens of the eye	150 mSv
(b) Skin, hands, and feet	500 mSv
B. Guidance for emergency occupational exposure*	
C. Public exposures (annual)	
1. Effective dose limit, continuous or frequent exposure*	1 mSv
2. Effective dose limit, infrequent exposure*	5 mSv
3. Equivalent dose limits for tissues and organs*	
(a) Lens of the eye	15 mSv
(b) Skin, hands, and feet	50 mSv
4. Remedial action for natural sources:	
(a) Effective dose (excluding radon)	>5 mSv
(b) Exposure to radon decay products	$>7 \times 10^{-3} J_H \, m^{-3}$
D. Education and training exposures (annual)*	
1. Effective dose limit	1 mSv
2. Equivalent dose limit for tissues and organs	
(a) Lens of eye	15 mSv
(b) Skin, hands, and feet	50 mSv
E. Embryo-fetus exposures* (monthly)	
1. Equivalent dose limit	0.5 mSv
F. Negligible individual dose (annual)	0.01 mSv

From National Council on Radiation Protection and Measurements: Report #116, *Limitation of exposure to ionizing radiation*, 1993, Bethesda, Md.
*Sum of external and internal exposures but excluding doses from natural resources.
mSv, Millisievert; J_{H}, heat transfer factor.

ALARA (as low as reasonably achievable), initially recommended in 1977 by the International Commission on Radiation Protection (ICRP) was based on the assumption that any exposure to ionizing radiation can increase the risk of developing cancer, continues to be recommended by national and international organizations involved in radiation safety, so that exposure remains lower than the established limits.[7-9]

Currently in the United States federal and state agencies involved in the regulation of radiation protection and safety include the U.S. Nuclear Regulatory Commission (NRC) (regulates brachytherapy and systemic therapy), the Public Health Service, the Environmental Protection Agency, the Center for Devices and Radiological Health of the Food & Drug Administration (regulates external beam therapy in collaboration with states), the Department of Labor, Occupational Health and Safety Administration (OSHA) and the National Council on Radiation Protection and Measurement (NCRP). The NRC is responsible for the regulation of radioactive materials, setting dose limits for workers, monitoring and labeling radioactive materials.[1,3,10-12] Individual states regulate materials and sources not regulated by federal regulation, as well as equipment related to the production of radiation, including linear accelerators and x-ray equipment.[12] The NCRP provides guidance and recommendations on radiation protection and measurement and is responsible for determining the maximum permissible dose (MPD) equivalents or the safe limits of annual and lifetime exposure.[3] Guidelines developed by the NCRP represent current scientific knowledge and are used by medical agencies, industry, government, the general public, and other state, federal, and international organizations within the nuclear radiation industry.

In Canada the Canadian Nuclear Safety Commission (CNSC) (1999), replacing the Atomic Energy Control Board (AECB) that was established in 1946, serves as the federal regulator of the nuclear industry to protect nuclear industry workers, the public, and the environment.[13] The CNSC regulates the operation of uranium mines and refineries, nuclear power plants, nuclear research facilities, and the use of radioactive sources including the production of radioisotopes. The CNSC establishes all regulatory requirements and standards governing (1) all uses of nuclear energy and materials, (2) licensing of medical facilities that use radioisotopes in the diagnosis and treatment of cancer, (3) establishment of guidelines and strict limits on public and nuclear worker exposure, and (4) the monitoring and documentation of compliance, including leak testing of sealed sources and gamma radiation survey meter calibration.[13,14] Limits covered by "radiation safety" and regulated by the CNSC relate to equipment with energies higher than 6 megavolts (MV) and radioactive isotopes. The limits nuclear energy workers can be exposed to are set at 100 mSv over a 5-year period, averaging a limit of 20 mSv per year. This limit includes up to 50 mSv as a dose limit accounting for incidents or accidents, as long as the 5-year limit remains under 100 mSv.[15] The yearly exposure limit for a member of the public is 1 mSv. "Radiation protection" is regulated by the provinces through provincial acts of legislation for diagnostic and treatment equipment that runs at less than or equal to 6 MV of energy (e.g., x rays and fluoroscopy). Annual occupational exposure limits are the same as in the United States.

North American radiation protection agencies collaborate with international organizations, including the ICRP and the International Commission on Radiation Units and Measurement (ICRU). The ICRP and the ICRU develop recommendations on radiation protection, quantities, and measurement. Although the ICRP does not have authority in individual countries, it is respected as an advisory organization offering recommendations promoting security, health, and safety in all aspects of protection against ionizing radiation, including medical radiation. The International Atomic Energy Agency (IAEA) develops standards based on recommendations from the ICRP and the ICRU and publishes safety guides, including guides on the principles of radiation protection and safety and the protection of workers and the public.[16] International standards, guides, and codes are published on the IAEA website at www.iaea.org.

CONCEPTS RELATED TO EXPOSURE AND RISK

The greatest risk of occupational exposure for healthcare professionals in settings using ionizing radiation occurs during diagnostic procedures such as fluoroscopy, special procedures, and portable radiography as a result of the length of exposure times and potential scatter.[1,11] Although a risk of exposure remains when using ionizing radiation with an external beam to treat cancer, brachytherapy (sealed source radioisotope), and drug/systemic therapy (unsealed sources), the risk and potential exposure can be minimized and even prevented through strict adherence to radiation protection procedures and practices. Time, distance, and shielding are the three principles of radiation protection related to reducing the risk of exposure to any form of ionizing radiation.[17,18] Further, the type and amount of protection afforded depends on the type of energy being used (electromagnetic or particulate radiation and the dose activity, half-life, and type of emission of the radionuclide) and on the treatment modality.

Principles of Protection (time, distance, and shielding)

Guidelines for radiation safety and protection are based on principles of *time*, *distance*, and *shielding*. A direct relationship exists between time and radiation exposure, meaning that the greater the time of exposure, the more radiation is absorbed. Precautions include limiting time in the environment of the radioactive source or reducing the amount of time the source is exposed.[1,18,19] The concept of distance relates to the *inverse square law*, whereby the radiation intensity is reduced by the square of the distance from the source.[1,3] If an individual stands double the distance from the source, for example, he/she moves from 1 meter to 2 meters away from the patient receiving the radioactive source, the exposure is reduced to one-quarter of that at 1 meter. Shielding provides a barrier between the individual and the radioactive source, thereby preventing primary exposure through direct contact or secondary exposure through scatter radiation. Shielding to stop exposure to the radiation source may range from paper to varying thickness of lead

Table 3-2 Characteristics of Radionuclides

Element	Half-life	Energy	Half-value layer* (lead [Pb])
Radium-226 (^{226}Ra)	1620 years	1.0 MeV (gamma)	60.2 days
Cesium-137 (^{137}Cs)	30.0 years	0.66 MeV (gamma)	0.65 cm
Cobalt-60 (^{60}Co)	5.2 years	1.25 MeV (gamma)	1.2 cm
Iridium-192 (^{192}Ir)	64.2 days	0.13–1.06 MeV (gamma)	0.6 cm
Iodine-131 (^{131}I)	8.0 days	0.36 MeV (gamma)	0.3 cm
Gold-198 (^{198}Au)	2.7 days	0.41 MeV (gamma)	0.33 cm
Iodine-125 (^{125}I)	60.2 days	0.02 MeV (gamma)	0.02 cm
Strontium-89 (^{89}Sr)	50.5 days	1.46 MeV (beta)	1 mm of lead blocks (100% of ^{89}Sr)

From Ma C-MC: The practice of radiation oncology. In Watkins Bruner D, Haas ML, Gosselin-Acomb TK, editors: *Manual for radiation oncology nursing practice and education*, Pittsburgh, 2004, Oncology Nursing Society.
*One half-value layer blocks 50% of the radiation.
MeV, Megaelectron volts.

or concrete. The thickness of shielding that is required to block the intensity of the beam by 50% is referred to as the half-value layer (HVL).[20] Table 3-2 identifies the HVL of shielding for specific radionuclides. Barriers to exposure also may include the use of latex gloves as protection from radioisotopes that are excreted through body fluids.

Type of Energy and Emission From the Source

Electromagnetic radiation is generated as x rays, neutrons, or photons from a machine (e.g., linear accelerator or as gamma rays from the decay of a radioactive source, e.g., cobalt-60), respectively. Radionuclides/radioisotopes used in diagnostic and therapeutic cancer treatments emit alpha or beta particles and/or gamma rays as they decay and have energies specific to the individual radionuclide. A list of radionuclides, their half-life, and energy levels is provided in Table 3-3.

Alpha particles have poor penetrability (less than 0.04 mm) and cannot penetrate the outer layer of the skin.[17] Therefore they are not routinely used in cancer therapy. A sheet of paper or a distance of 5 cm is sufficient to shield an individual from any radiation exposure to alpha particles. Although they travel quickly (but for a distance of only 5 cm), alpha particles are an internal hazard if they are inhaled (e.g., radon gas).[21]

Beta radiation is emitted from radioactive material such as radioisotopes (e.g., phosphous-32 or yttrium-90). Beta particles have limited penetrability depending on their energy. Slow-moving beta particles cannot penetrate the skin, whereas fast-moving beta particles may cause radiation exposure and irritation to the eyes, skin, and extremities. Penetration also can occur up to $^1/_2$ inch inside the body and therefore pose an internal hazard.[6,21] Radioisotopes such as yttrium-90, which are injected into the body, require only

Table 3-3 Radionuclides and Their Properties

Radioisotope	Symbols	Half-life	Type
Cesium-137	^{137}Cs	30 years	Beta, gamma
Gold-198	^{198}Au	2.7 days	Beta, gamma
Iodine-125	^{125}I	60 days	Beta, gamma
Iodine-131	^{131}I	8 days	Beta, gamma
Iridium-192	^{192}Ir	74.4 days	Beta, gamma
Phosphorus-32	^{32}P	14.3 days	Beta
Radium-226	^{226}Ra	1620 years	Alpha, gamma
Strontium-90	^{90}Sr	28.1 years	Beta

Reprinted with permission of the National Council on Radiation Protection and Measurements: Report #40, *Protection against radiation from brachytherapy sources*, 1972, Bethesda, Md.

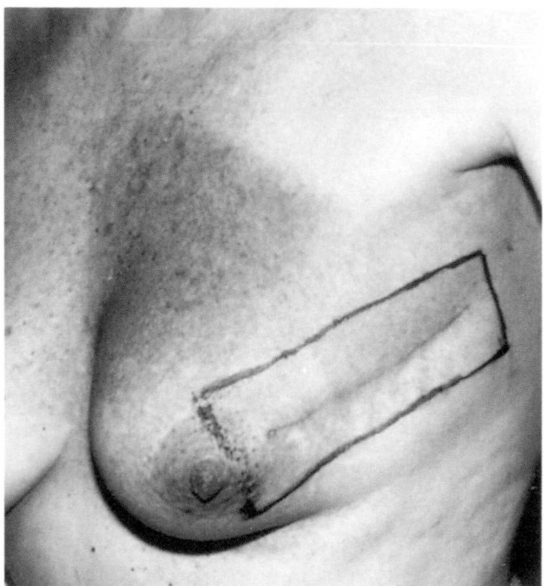

Color Plate 1 Erythema Secondary to Breast Irradiation.
From Dow KH, Bucholtz JD, Iwamoto R et al: Nursing Care in Radiation Oncology, ed. 2, Philadelphia, 1992, Saunders.

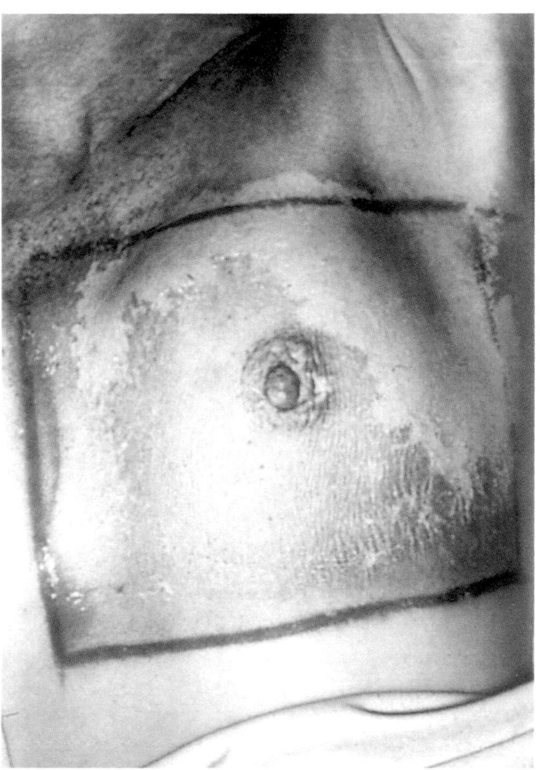

Color Plate 2 Increased Pigmentation and Dry Desquamation Secondary to Breast Irradiation.
From Dow KH, Bucholtz JD, Iwamoto R et al: Nursing Care in Radiation Oncology, ed. 2, Philadelphia, 1992, Saunders.

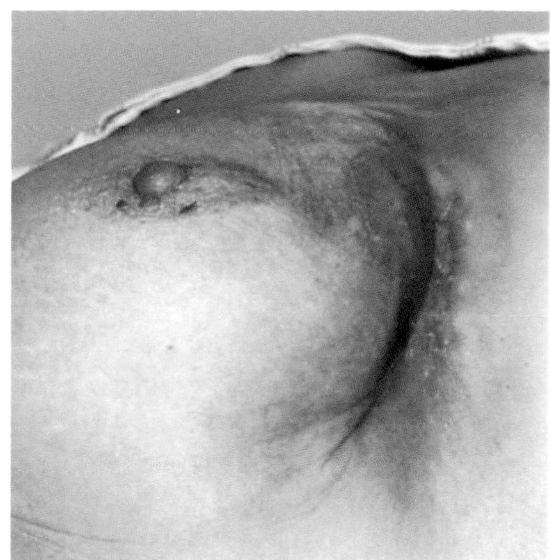

Color Plate 3 Moist Desquamation Secondary to Breast Irradiation. Note increased skin reaction in skin fold in inframammary region.
From Dow KH, Bucholtz JD, Iwamoto R et al: Nursing Care in Radiation Oncology, ed. 2, Philadelphia, 1992, Saunders.

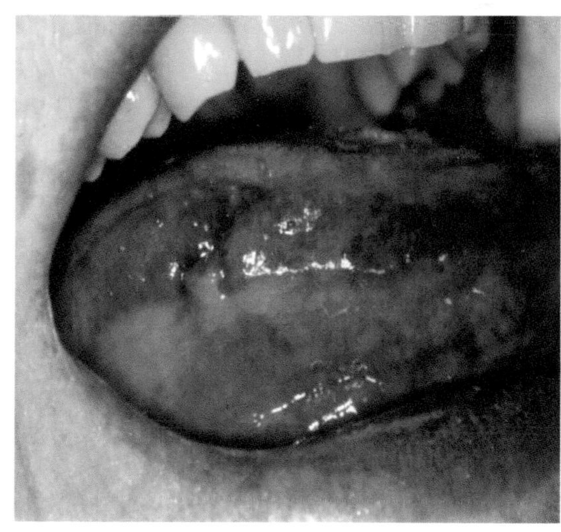

Color Plate 4 Mucositis.
Courtesy of Dr. Jonathan Ship.

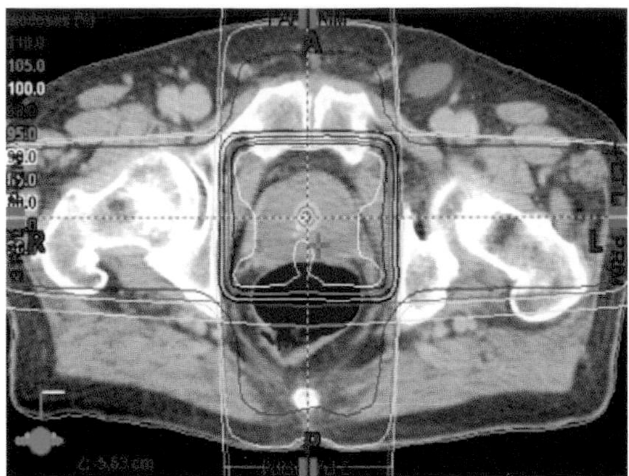

Color Plate 5 Prostate Treatment Plans.
Courtesy of Duke University Health System.

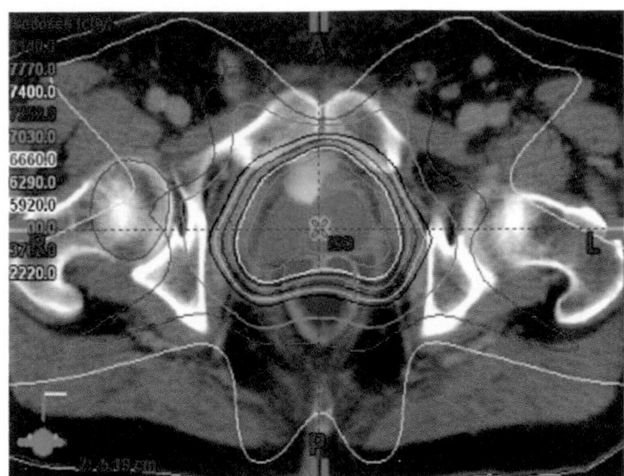

Color Plate 6 Prostate Treatment Plans.
Courtesy of Duke University Health System.

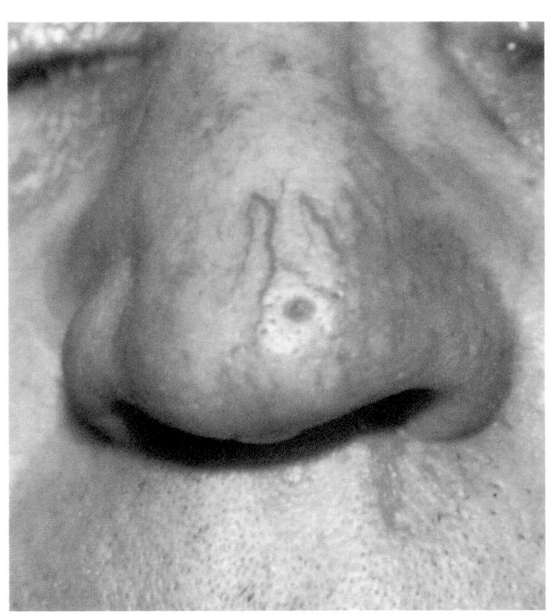

Color Plate 7 Late Skin Changes of Telangiectasia Approximately 2 Years After Interstitial Implant for Squamous Cell Carcinoma of the Nasal Vestibule.
From Dow KH, Bucholtz JD, Iwamoto R et al: Nursing Care in Radiation Oncology, ed. 2, Philadelphia, 1992, Saunders.

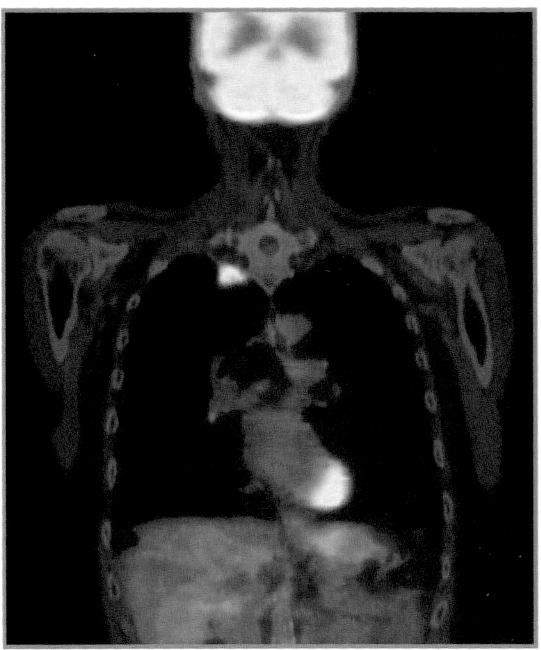

Color Plate 8 Lung Cancer.
Courtesy of Todd Blodgett, MD, University of Pittsburgh Medical Center.

an acrylic shielding over the syringe to protect the healthcare worker. The body itself provides adequate protection and prevents exposure to other people once the beta radionuclide has been injected.[22]

Gamma radiation and x rays are very penetrating waves of energy and are the most hazardous to healthcare workers, therefore requiring protective measures. The higher the source energy, such as with cobalt-60 or a linear accelerator producing 18 MV of energy, the greater the requirements are for lead and concrete shielding. Low-energy gamma emitters, such as palladium-103 used in prostate brachytherapy, do not require the same precautions and provide little risk of exposure even at close contact. The patient's body acts as the barrier and prevents exposure to others.[23,24]

Treatment Modality

External Beam/Teletherapy

External beam radiation or teletherapy is the most common method used to deliver radiation therapy, using a radioactive source emitting gamma rays (e.g., cobalt-60) or electromagnetic energy producing photons, electrons, and neutrons from a machine (e.g., linear accelerator). All activities related to external beam radiation treatment delivery, access to treatment areas, machine maintenance and repair, and changes to teletherapy equipment or sources are regulated through conditions of licensing, organizational policies and procedures, and safe work practices. Patients are not radioactive after the treatment and are not a risk to the staff or their families. Because staff is not allowed inside the treatment room while the beam is on and the radiation therapy is being delivered, risk of exposure to staff is very low. Because of the type of radiation emission (e.g., gamma rays, photons, electrons) and the penetrability of the energy, the concept of shielding is the most important principle of protection from exposure with external beam radiation therapy. The rooms housing the treatment machines require special design and usage specifications to ensure a safe working environment and prevent exposure to staff working in the area.[25] Shielding for teletherapy units may involve the use of lead and concrete or lead equivalents, such as steel or cast iron in cement. The thickness of the shielding for the walls, ceiling, and door is calculated based on the energy emitted, the direction of the incident beams, and any potential scatter within the room, in order to prevent any exposure to radiation outside the room.[25] Acceptance testing is completed before commissioning of a unit for therapeutic use. Exposure to the radiation beam or scatter occurs only during the time the beam is turned on and the treatment is being delivered. Alarms and safety mechanisms are in place to prevent the radiation beam from turning on if the room is not secure.

Sealed Source/Brachytherapy

Brachytherapy, using sealed sources of radioactive isotopes is largely used in the treatment of gynecological cancers and cancer of the prostate. It is also used in the treatment of sarcoma, cancers of the head and neck, bile duct, and penis, and endobronchial and esophageal cancers and intraocular neoplasms. Treatment delivery and the associated safety precautions depend on the radioisotope required to treat the cancer. The radioactive isotopes are contained within a protective shell to limit exposure. Sealed sources and equipment are locked up and accessible only to authorized users. Once the equipment and source have been transported in a shielded container or the isotopes have been loaded into the machine that is then moved to the location at which it will be used, restrictions are set not to exceed a safe dose rate per hour (e.g., 2.5 uSv per hour).[1,2,26]

Low-dose implant brachytherapy, used in the treatment of prostate cancer (iodine-125 or palladium-103) and intraocular cancers (iodine-125), uses radioactive seeds to deliver the radioisotope directly to the tumor. Safety precautions during and after implant procedures are related to the radioactive decay process and time that is unique to each radioisotope. The half-life of various radioisotopes is listed in Table 3-2. Low-dose implant procedures are done in a controlled operating room or procedure room environment. All radioactive sealed sources are handled with forceps or housed in special tubes, thereby preventing exposure to the radiation therapy staff preparing the treatment or the radiation oncologist administering the treatment. In the case of prostate cancer, the seeds are contained in titanium shells and emit low-level radiation, thereby providing minimal exposure to staff. By the time 3 months have elapsed, radioactivity cannot be detected in patients who have been implanted with palladium-103.[27] Studies by

Smathers et al.[24] and Michalski et al.[28] have shown that posttreatment exposure and lifetime exposure to family and household members that comes from a patient who has received prostate brachytherapy is very low and below the recommended exposure levels. In the case of intraocular tumors, the only radiation protection procedure required after the suturing of an eye plaque onto the eyeball is that of having the patient wear a lead-lined eye patch when in contact with any other individual. This is required during the 7-day period that the eye plaque remains in place.

Remote control after-loading units are used to deliver radiation treatment for interstitial and intracavitary brachytherapy. Low dose rate (LDR) treatments given continuously over several hours and days require an inpatient admission. High dose rate (HDR) treatments given intermittently may be given on an outpatient basis over a few minutes or hours a day with a minimum of 6 hours between treatments.[6] Time between treatments allows for the repair of sublethal injury to normal cells, the redistribution of cycling tumor cells, and the reoxygenation of tumor cells, thereby increasing the beneficial effects of the radiation.[29] Both low-dose and high-dose treatment methods require a shielded private room where the radiation can be delivered without risk of exposure to staff. The radioisotope is housed within a lead-lined unit and delivered through catheters and applicators to the site of the tumor. Exposure is possible when the radioactive source is outside of the after-loading unit. Safety precautions used to reduce the risk of exposure include the use of a private room, which is shielded with lead and concrete, keeping the door closed, warning signs posted on the doors, and interlocks, alarms, and lights indicating the status of the radioactive source. When the radioactive source has been returned to the after-loading unit, it is safe for staff and visitors to enter the room.[18] Interruptions for frequent care provision or visiting is avoided because the treatment must be stopped with each interruption, thereby extending the overall length of time the patient is in hospital receiving the treatment.

Although not as common today, some treatments may be given by manually loading the radioisotopes into applicators without the use of a remote after-loading machine. Low-dose exposure occurs every time the nurse needs to be in direct contact with the patient. In that situation, care activities need to be organized in order to ensure that direct care time is restricted to 30 minutes per shift, which reduces the risk of exposure to nurses caring for the patient.[19] Assessment of the patient's self-care abilities and education related to self-care measures before the start of treatment is important.[19,20] Providing care at the head of the bed, farther away from the sealed source, and assisting with indirect tasks or speaking to the patient from the doorway also limit the time care providers are in close contact with the patient and source. Observation, indirect care activities, and support also can be provided externally, away from the patient's room, through the use of the visual monitoring systems and the telephone and intercom systems, thereby reducing exposure to the source. Although it is unlikely that pregnant nurses caring for patients receiving radioisotopes would receive even the maximum allowable exposure of 0.5 mSv per month, many centers reassign pregnant nurses to other care activities or patients to avoid any contact with patients receiving radioisotopes.[30] Safety to the public includes restrictions being placed on the amount of time visitors can be with the patient. They also must remain 6 feet or more from the patient and treatment source at all times.[18] Pregnant visitors are prohibited from visiting altogether.

In situations of accidental dislodgement of a radioactive source or where the sealed source does not retract into the after-loading unit, potentially allowing for exposure to the source, special precautions for safe handling are outlined in safety guidelines and facility policies and procedures. These guidelines must be followed to ensure safety and protection to staff and the patient. Long-handled forceps only are used to touch any exposed radioactive source while it is being transferred to a lead-lined container.[18] Because of low levels of environmental radiation within the patient's room, a survey meter assessment is completed before patient discharge to ensure that any environmental radiation is within acceptable and safe limits.

Unsealed Source

Unsealed sources of radioactive materials may be in the form of liquids or suspensions that may be ingested or injected. Examples include iodine-131 for the treatment of thyroid cancer, yttrium-90, used in the treatment of non-Hodgkin's lymphoma and strontium-89 used for painful bone metastasis.

From a safety perspective, the use iodine-131 presents the greatest risk of radiation exposure to nurses and other care providers. Patients must be cared for in a single-shielded room. Authorized personnel, often a physician or radiation safety officer, deliver the unsealed source to the patient in a lead-shielded container.[2] Once the care provider leaves the room, the patient opens the container and takes the oral dose of radioactive iodine-131. During the following days, time spent in direct care activities is limited and distance is maintained between the nurse and patient for any indirect care activities that are required within the treatment room.[19] Time, distance, and shielding precautions taken with unsealed sources are the same basic radiation precautions used with sealed sources of radioactivity.

Because of low levels of environmental radiation within the patient's room and the contamination of body fluids as a result of systemic absorption and excretion of radioactive iodine-131, all personal protective equipment, gloves, linens, and any waste from the patient's room are considered contaminated. All reusable materials, including linens, must be removed and stored for about 90 days (10 half-lives) to allow for radioactive decay to a level of background radiation before reuse. Other disposable items such as food trays and personal items are stored initially, allowing for decay, and then are disposed of.[2,31,32] Disposal of radioactive liquid waste, such as contaminated urine from the excretion of iodine-131, must be handled in a manner that ensures that the amount of waste is within safe disposal dose recommendations and limits set by regulatory agencies. Direct disposal via the toilet into the public sewage system may be safe in facilities that treat only a few such patients a year and that have a large water output, thereby assuring the ability to dilute the radioactivity to an acceptable concentration. Most facilities treating patients receiving iodine-131 now use storage holding tanks to manage the liquid radioactive waste, until the end of a decay period when the waste can then be released into the public sewage system.[23] Contamination through incontinence or diarrhea poses a radiation hazard. Skin that has been in contact with the contaminated body fluids must be scrubbed with a decontamination cleansing solution. Any contamination to the floor may require the tiling or floor surface to be torn out and replaced, with the contaminated material being stored until it is safe to destroy or discard it.[31]

By 72 hours, the rate of radiation exposure has usually reduced to a safe level appropriate for the patient to be discharged (30 mCi or less; less than 1.8 R/hour at 1 meter).[31] A survey meter assessment of the individual's belongings must be conducted before patient discharge to measure the amount of radioactivity to ensure that it is safe to discharge the patient. After discharge, the patient must follow precautionary instructions related to physical contact and disposal of waste at home for about 2 weeks. These precautions are necessary to minimize exposure to family and household members and ensure that exposure limits are within the regulatory guidelines for public exposure.

Outpatient radioactive iodine-131 therapy is being offered in situations where no significant hazard to members of the public is anticipated. Dose limitations for family members who knowingly and willingly will be exposed to radiation while caring for the patient, are allowed exposure to a dose limit not to exceed 5 mSv per year, and in this case are not subject to the usual 1mSv annual dose limit to members of the public.[13,14,33] Exposure to the general public, pregnant family members, and children remains limited to 1 mSv per year. Grigsby et al.[34] measured radiation exposure levels to family members and pets, as well as environmental levels in kitchens and bedrooms, and found that exposure to household members caring for the patient receiving outpatient iodine-131 treatment was between 0.01 and 1.09 mSv, well below the special circumstance regulatory limits.[34]

Unsealed sources also may be used in radioimmunotherapy in which the radioisotope is conjugated to a monoclonal antibody. The radioisotope is delivered to the tumor cells through the attachment of the monoclonal antibody to an antigen on the surface of the cell. Iodine-131 (beta- and gamma-emitting radionuclide) and yttrium-90 (beta-emitting radionuclide) are examples of unsealed radioisotopes used this way. Safe handling and exposure precautions after radioimmunotherapy using iodine-131 are the same as precautions taken when the radioisotope is used in the treatment of thyroid cancer because it emits gamma radiation and is absorbed systemically and excreted through body fluids.[22,35] Yttrium, a beta-emitting radionuclide, requires only a plastic or acrylic shielding over the syringe to protect the individual

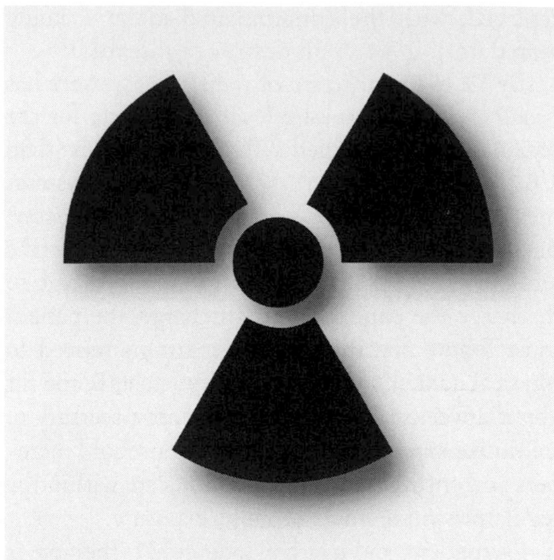

Figure 3-1 Trefoil (International Radiation Warning Symbol).
From the Canadian Nuclear Safety Commission, 2005 (website): http://laws.justice.gc.ca/en/n-28.3/sor-2000-203/154458.html.

administering the radiolabeled monoclonal antibody.[36,37] Safety precautions for the protection of family members and the public from exposure are the universal precautions adhered to with possible body fluid exposure. This includes double flushing of the toilet after use and the use of condoms for sexual activity for the first week. If exposure of family members to body fluids is possible, they should all wear gloves when interacting with the patient.[22,36,37]

Safety Labeling and Signage

All areas where radioactive isotopes are stored, used, or manipulated require labeling with radiation warning signs and notices indicating "Radioactive Material." All equipment used with unsealed radioactive isotopes also must be similarly marked. Areas where radiation is produced by a machine such as a linear accelerator or cobalt unit or rooms in which patients are being treated with radioactive radioisotopes must be labeled indicating "Radiation Hazard." This hazard sign indicates that an area could potentially become contaminated with radioactive material or that special procedures or authorization is required for entry to the area. Use of warning labels in areas where it is not necessary is not only not required but is prohibited by law. The trefoil is the international radiation warning symbol (Figure 3-1). Signs are generally yellow and maroon in color and must provide an emergency contact number. Permits issued for the use of materials must be current and visibly posted. Posters indicating the care and use of personal monitoring devices also must be available and clearly posted.[15,18]

KNOWLEDGE AND FEAR

One of the greatest barriers to ensuring a level of comfort and safety with working with patients receiving ionizing radiation treatment can be the misperception of risk of exposure rather than the knowledge and understanding of radiation protection and safety. Inadequate knowledge or fear may lead to hasty patient care with minimal interaction. It is important for nurses to understand the effects of radiation, the risk of exposure and the practices required to ensure safety for themselves and their patients. Nurses also may partake in risky behaviors, including cancer-causing behaviors, but associate those behaviors as having a lower risk of causing cancer. Some individuals may incorrectly perceive a greater risk of developing cancer from occupational exposure despite safety guidelines, procedures, and practices but minimize their risk of cancer from other causes. Risk behaviors may include smoking, alcohol consumption, unprotected sex, use of recreational and prescription drugs, use of pesticides, obesity, hypertension, lack of exercise, and sunbathing or the use of tanning studios.[38,39] A British report from the early 1990s indicated that the risk of death from other causes was greater than the risk of death from exposure to 0.3 mSv of radiation, which is significantly less than the annual occupational dose limit in North America.[38] Risk of death from smoking 10 cigarettes a day was 1 in 200, from road accidents 1 in 10,0000, accidents at home 1 in 10,000, work-related accidents 1 in 50,000. Risk of death from exposure to 0.3 mSv of radiation was 1 in 70,000.[38] Further, many nurses were exposed to chemotherapy agents before the introduction of safe handling practices and continue to live with an uncertain risk of developing cancer.[9] Having knowledge about natural background radiation, annual dose limits for both the public and occupational settings, the type of energy used in the occupational setting, the dose activity, and half-life and type of emission of radioisotopes helps nurses apply the concepts of radiation protection: time, distance, and shielding. Reinforcement of safety practices through ongoing education and the sharing of results of film badge monitoring reports may be a helpful strategy within organizations.[27]

EMERGENCY RESPONSE AND CARDIOPULMONARY RESUSCITATION

The emergency response and initiation of cardiopulmonary resuscitation (CPR) for patients receiving external beam radiation or sealed source brachytherapy using an after-loading machine poses no exposure risk to staff and would be the same as for any other patient in the treating facility. In all situations of patients receiving radiation treatment, CPR is immediately initiated. In the situation where a manual loading system has been used, the source needs to be removed as soon as possible and sealed in a lead container. The area would require meter surveillance to ensure that no other risk of exposure is present.

Although risk of exposure is low, the initiation of CPR on patients receiving unsealed sources such as radioactive iodine-131 can create a situation of increased anxiety for the responding code team. Limiting the number of unnecessary team members responding to the code limits any potential exposure to staff. Adherence to body substance precautions to prevent contamination through body fluids during the resuscitation procedure is important. Exposure for 30 minutes at a distance of 1 foot to a patient with 100 millicuries of radioactive iodine-131 would cause 100 mrem of exposure or a rate of exposure of 200 mrem/hour, significantly below safe exposure limits.[6,40] Staff and equipment need to be cleared by the radiation safety officer before they leave the room. Fortunately, most patients receiving radioactive iodine for thyroid cancer are otherwise healthy, and it would be a very rare occurrence for such a patient to have a cardiac arrest during the radiation treatment.

Monitoring Devices

Personal monitoring devices measure and record any radioactive exposure received by an individual. All staff who may be exposed to external gamma radiation at a rate of more than 200 microsieverts (μSv) (or 0.2 mSv) per quarter, are required to wear a personal monitoring device. A variety of devices are available including film badges (nuclear emulsion monitor), wrist or ring badges (thermoluminescent dosimeter detector, or TLD), and pocket ion chamber dosimeters.[19] The radiation safety officer is responsible for monitoring and reporting exposure results. Film badges absorb any exposure on a photographic emulsion housed in a plastic holder. The film provides a measure of cumulative whole-body exposure. Ring badges, or TLDs, are small and therefore useful for monitoring exposure to the hand. Electrons in the thermoluminescent powder are raised to an excited level when exposed to radiation. Staff handling radioactive seeds during preparation or implant often wear ring badges during the procedures in addition to a film badge worn routinely. The ring badge does not document cumulative exposure but will capture any exposure during the procedure. Pocket ion chamber dosimeters look like a pen and attach to the clothing. The chamber requires charging before use. Any radiation exposure reduces the charge in proportion to the level of exposure. Multiple recordings by the nurse are required including documenting a reading before entering a patient's room and upon leaving the room. Readings are not retained in the chamber, nor are cumulative exposure levels monitored.[19,41]

Individuals using personal monitoring devices are advised to wear the monitor on the body somewhere between the level of the neck and the waist. Ring devices need to be worn facing toward the source of radiation. Additionally monitors should not be exposed to high temperatures, water, direct sunlight, or fluorescent light to prevent erroneous readings. They need to be stored at the facility in an area away from any radioactive material. Lost or damaged badges need to be reported and replaced immediately.[41]

Environmental monitoring devices include the Geiger-Mueller counter. Electrical pulses are produced in the presence of ionizing particles and the monitor is reliable, sensitive, and easy to use. It does not measure exposure or dose rate and therefore cannot be used for personal monitoring. A survey meter assessment is completed before patient discharge to ensure that any environmental radiation is within acceptable and safe limits.[19] Federal regulations and institutional policies also address survey meter calibration and leak testing for sealed radiation sources to ensure environmental safety.[12,42,43]

ROLE OF THE RADIATION SAFETY OFFICER

Radiation safety officer (RSO) roles have been established in the United States for many years and are developing and expanding in other countries.[44] The role may vary depending on whether the organization is a small treatment center or a large multisite organization with a variety of cancer treatment modalities and research facilities.

Individuals in the RSO role may have a variety of responsibilities within their organization related to the use of radioactive materials, as well as responsibilities for x ray and devices that emit nonionizing radiation. The RSO often has an educational background in physics or radiation technology and needs to be aware of all of the regulatory bodies, regulations, and specific licenses that pertain to their practice environment. Responsibilities within a radiation safety program may include staff training and building a culture of radiation safety, monitoring and documentation of exposure, managing a quality assurance program, purchasing and receipt of delivery of sealed sources, maintaining lists of all sources within the organization, monitoring leak testing and equipment maintenance, and the purchase of equipment.[44]

REFERENCES

1. Passmore GG: A review of radiation protection principles and practices for workers and patients in the radiological health-care environment, *Semin Radiol Technol* 4:18-30, 45-50, 1996. Corrected—published erratum appears in *Semin Radiol Technol* 4:145, 1996.
2. Thompson MA: Maintaining a proper perspective of risk associated with radiation exposure, *J Nucl Med Technol* 29(3):137-142, 2001.
3. Dowd SB: The basics of radiation protection for hospital workers: considerations and procedures, *Hosp Top* 69(4): 31-35, 1991.
4. Meinhold CB: Lauriston S. Taylor Lecture: the evolution of radiation protection—from erythema to genetic risks to risks of cancer to...? *Health Phys* 87(3):240-248, 2004.
5. Meinhold CB, Taxchner JC, Inkret WC: Radiation and risk—a hard look at the data: a brief history of radiation, *Los Alamos Science* 23:116; 1995. Accessed May 9, 2005 at www.fas.org/sgp/othergov/doe/lanl/00326631.pdf
6. Dunn Bucholtz J: Radiation protection. In Watkins Bruner D, Haas ML, Gosselin-Acomb TK, editors: *Manual for radiation oncology nursing practice and education*, Pittsburgh, 2004, Oncology Nursing Society.
7. National Council on Radiation Protection and Measurements: NCRP Report # 107, *Implementation of the principle of as low as reasonably achievable (ALARA) for medical and dental personnel*, Washington, DC, 1990, U.S. Government Printing Office.
8. Health Physics Society: Answer to question #435 submitted to "Ask the experts," posted October 18, 2000 (website): www.hps.org/publicinformation/ate/q435.html. Accessed May 9, 2005.
9. Prasad KN, Cole WC, Haase GM: Radiation protection in humans: extending the concept of as low as reasonably achievable (ALARA) from dose to biological damage, *Br J Radiol* 77(914):97-99, 2004.
10. Agency for Toxic Substances and Disease Registry: Ionizing radiation: an overview for the occupational health nurse, *AAOHN J* 45(4):170-183, 1997.
11. Holmes S: Making sense of radiotherapy: delivery and safety, *Nurs Times* 92(27):42-43, 1996.
12. U.S. Nuclear Regulatory Commission (website): www.nrc.gov/what-we-do/radiation/reg-matls.html. Accessed May 9, 2005.
13. Canadian Nuclear Safety Commission: Nuclear safety in Canada, *Canadian Nuclear Safety Commission* INFO-0749, 2004.
14. Canadian Nuclear Safety Commission: Putting nuclear safety first, *Canadian Nuclear Safety Commission* INFO-0721, 2002.
15. Canadian Nuclear Safety Commission: Radiation protection regulations, *Canada Gazette Part II* 134:1126-1169, 2000, http://www.nuclearsafety.gc.ca/pubs_catalogue/uploads/SOR203.pdf.
16. National Council on Radiation Protection: The application of ALARA for occupational exposures, NCRP statement No. 8, *Health Phys* 78(5 suppl):S76-S77, 2000.
17. Dunne-Daly CF: Principles of radiotherapy and radiobiology, *Semin Oncol Nurs* 15(4):250-259, 1999.
18. Gosselin TK, Waring JS: Nursing management of patients receiving brachytherapy for gynecologic malignancies, *Clin J Oncol Nurs* 5(2):59-63, 2001.
19. Dunne-Daly C: Principles of brachytherapy. In Hassey Dow K, et al, editors: *Nursing care in radiation oncology* Philadelphia, 1997, Saunders.
20. Cember H: *Introduction to health physics,* ed 3, New York, 1996, McGraw-Hill.
21. Bucholtz J: Radiation therapy. In Gross J, Johnson BL, editors: *Handbook of oncology nursing,* Sudbury, Mass, 1998, Jones and Bartlett, pp 35-55.
22. Tuinstra N: Outpatient administration of radiolabeled monoclonal antibodies, *Clin J Oncol Nurs* 7(1):106-108, 2003.
23. Leung PM, Nikolic M: Disposal of therapeutic ^{131}I waste system using a multiple holding tank system, *Health Phys* 75(3):315-321, 1998.
24. Smathers S, Wallner K, Korssjoen T et al: Radiation safety parameters following prostate brachytherapy, *Int J Radiat Oncol Biol Phys* 45(2):397-399, 1999.
25. Health Physics Society: Answer to question #1094 submitted to "Ask the experts," posted August 2001: (website): www.hps.org/publicinformation/ate/q1094.html. Accessed May 9, 2005.
26. Canadian Nuclear Safety Commission: Principles of the management of radionuclide therapies, *Canadian Nuclear Safety Commission* INFO–0714, 2000.

27. Abel LJ, Blatt HJ, Stipetich RL et al: Nursing management of patients receiving brachytherapy for early stage prostate cancer, *Clin J Oncol Nurs* 3(1):7-15, 1999.
28. Michalski J, Mutic S, Eichling J et al: Radiation exposure to family and household members after prostate brachytherapy, *Int J Radiat Oncol Biol Phys* 56(3):764-768, 2003.
29. Hilderley LJ: Principles of teletherapy. In Hassey Dow K et al, editors: *Nursing care radiation oncology,* Philadelphia, 1997, Saunders.
30. Jankowski CB: Radiation protection for nurses: regulations and guidelines, *J Nurs Adm* 22(2):30-34, 1992.
31. Freeman SJ, Girolamo RF: Radioisotopes and their use in the diagnosis and management of thyroid disease, *Clin Geriatr Med* 11(2):189-218, 1995.
32. Parthasarathy KL, Crawford ES: Treatment of thyroid carcinoma: emphasis on high-dose ^{131}I outpatient therapy, *J Nucl Med Technol* 30(4):165-171, 2002.
33. National Council on Radiation Protection and Measurements: NCRP Report 116, *Limitation of exposure to ionizing radiation*, Washington, DC, 1993, U.S. Government Printing Office.
34. Grigsby PW, Siegel BA, Baker S et al: Radiation exposure from outpatient radioactive iodine (^{131}I) therapy for thyroid carcinoma, *JAMA* 283(17):2272-2274, 2000.
35. Blumel SM, O'Brien TM, Jones T: Radioimmunotherapy for non-Hodgkin lymphoma (NHL): nursing and patient perspectives, *Spotlight on Symposia from the ONS 29th Annual Congress in Anaheim, Calif, 2004* (website): www.ons.org/publications/journals/pdfs/spotlight49.pdf. Accessed May 9, 2005.
36. Hendrix C: Radiation safety guidelines for radioimmunotherapy with yttrium 90 ibritumomab tiuxetan, *Clin J Oncol Nurs* 8(1):31-34, 2004.
37. Hendrix C: Radiation safety with yttrium 90 ibritumomab tiuxetan (zevalin) radioimmunotherapy, *Semin Oncol Nurs* 20(1 suppl 1):14-19, 2004.
38. Gilmore M, Fairclough C: Putting radiation into perspective, *J Cancer Care* 1:183-188, 1992.
39. Sanoshy J: Despite hazards, oncology nurses remain dedicated to their profession, *ONS News* 15(2):1, 4-5, 2000.
40. Health Physics Society: Answer to question #1753 submitted to "Ask the experts," posted March 2002 (website): www.hps.org/publicinformation/ate/q1753.html. Accessed May 9, 2005.
41. Princess Margaret Hospital, University Health Network: TLD issue, distribution and return, *University health network policy & procedure manual: corporate radiation safety manual,* May 2003.
42. Atomic Energy Control Board: Regulatory document R-116: requirements for leak testing selected sealed radiation sources, *Atomic Energy Control Board*, 1995.
43. Atomic Energy Control Board: Regulatory document R-117: requirements for gamma radiation survey meter calibration, *Atomic Energy Control Board*, 1995.
44. Gordon K: The emerging role of the radiation safety officer, *Can J Med Radiat Technol* 30(3):106-133, 1999.

Unit II

Treatment Work-Up and Planning

Chapter 4

Diagnosis and Staging

Jormain O. Cady

PURPOSE/SIGNIFICANCE

It has been estimated that over 1 million new cancer cases will be diagnosed in the United States this year, making cancer a significant health problem facing the population.[1] The diagnosis and staging process may be full of uncertainty and apprehension for patients, therefore a thorough understanding of principles guiding practice is crucial to providing appropriate oncology nursing care for newly diagnosed patients and those with recurrent disease. Multiple tests and procedures may be exhausting and require considerable intervention, including providing explanations about the rationale for the work-up indicated, instructions for preparation, or the interpretation of information when results are known (Table 4-1). Distress, anxiety, and perhaps even the presence of the symptoms that prompted evaluation may pose challenges for the patient and render learning new information difficult until it is adequately addressed. In some instances, however, the diagnosis and staging process may be relatively straightforward. In either case, it is important to recognize the importance and impact of accurate staging, what the implications of staging mean to the patient, and that while the initial diagnostic stage may represent a snapshot in time because the actual disease state can be dynamic, the outcome of the initial staging process is particularly significant because the results will define that person's "stage" (and therefore prognosis) throughout his/her experience with cancer.

OVERVIEW

Even for a relatively straightforward diagnosis, the staging process will often involve multiple members of the healthcare team, including the primary care provider, a medical oncologist, radiation oncologist, surgeon, radiologist, pathologist, and potentially consultation with other specialists as appropriate. Communication between these specialists may be approached differently at different institutions, varying from informal inter-colleague discussions to formal conference meeting to present patients. Presentation of the patient and all available information at tumor board conferences may be required at larger or teaching institutions, members of which will make formal recommendations for either further work-up required or treatment options. Other members of the patient care team, such as nurses, nutritionists, social workers, speech pathology, research coordinators and/or case managers, also may attend tumor board conferences to gain additional information about the patient and needs that should be addressed. Smaller, or rural, facilities may not necessarily have such specialists immediately available to them and therefore may have networks in place to present selected patients at the tumor board conferences of larger facilities. Improvements in teleconferencing technology, and digital or internet access to imaging and other medical records, is greatly improving rural access to specialty consultation and care. The assessment and recommendations put forth by the tumor board members should be documented, and generally are included in the medical record.

Goals of diagnosis and staging include determining tumor histology (tissue type), site of tumor origin (primary site), and the extent of disease involvement, all of which provide information about the most appropriate modality for treatment and potential for disease recurrence.[2] Patients presenting for radiation oncology consultation may be at varying points in the staging process at the time of their evaluations, and goals of the initial visit may be different. For some patients, diagnosis and staging may be complete and the role for radiation therapy very clear at the time of consultation. Other patients may be seen before completion of full staging to obtain information ahead of time that can help facilitate the decision-making process, for example, a woman with breast cancer who is seen before lumpectomy or mastectomy. Depending on

Table 4-1 Selected Diagnostic Procedure Preparation

Test	Special preparation required
Angiogram/interventional CT	Discontinue anticoagulants (e.g., coumadin, aspirin) 7 days before procedure NPO 4–6 hours before procedure Sedation may be used
Barium enema/CT colonography	Encourage increased fluids day before procedure Light meal/clear liquid diet day before procedure Bowel prep as directed evening before/morning of procedure NPO 6 hours before exam May require laxatives after the procedure to evacuate barium Because of residual contrast, perform after other required GI imaging
Capsule endoscopy	NPO 12 hours before study, and 2 hours after ± Light bowel prep Avoid strenuous activity during the test Avoid strong electromagnetic field source (e.g., MRI) until the device is expelled
CT scan (head, neck, abdomen, pelvis)	Check recent serum creatinine level (if IV contrast) Hold glucophage 72 hours before IV contrast administration No solid foods 4 hours before exam (liquids, medications OK) Premedication administration if indicated Encourage increased fluid intake after study if IV contrast given
Mammogram	Avoid use of deodorant, powder, or body lotion before exam
MRI	Screen for incompatible implants (pacemaker, cochlear implant, aneurysm clips, or other metal objects) Instruct patient to leave jewelry at home NPO 8 hours before exam (if abdominal MRI) Claustrophobic patients may require some form of sedation
Endorectal coil MRI	Bowel prep (enema) required before procedure; use of IV glucagon during the procedure to decrease bowel motility.
PET (for cancer evaluation)	Recommend high protein/low carbohydrate diet for 2 days before exam NPO (except water/medications) 4–12 hours before exam No water within 1 hour of exam Avoid strenuous exercise 24 hours before exam Diabetics may require special instructions for glucose control at the time of the study (serum glucose must be less than 200 mg/dL at the time of the study) Short half-life of radioactive material (approx 2 hours), safe to return to community after procedure
Ultrasound	Abdominal: NPO 8 hours before exam Pelvic: increase fluids/do not void 1 hour before exam (full bladder required)
Upper GI studies	NPO 8 hours before exam

risk for more extensive disease (nodal involvement or distant metastasis), further staging studies may be ordered by the radiation oncologist to ensure that the planned treatment is appropriate (local disease) or to ensure adequacy of planned treatment field (inclusion of regional lymph nodes).

Careful consideration of the appropriate test to obtain is essential to ensuring accurate information and to avoid unnecessary procedures and cost for the patient. In test selection, effort is made to select the test that is most likely to yield the information being sought, in the least invasive and most cost-efficient manner. Availability of diagnostic equipment, third-party payor approval and goals of therapy also may influence test selection.[2] In avoiding unnecessary procedures, the test should pass the following challenge: "how will these results change the plan of care?" In some instances, further testing may provide new information, or confirm suspicions, but will not change the intervention that is planned and therefore is of limited usefulness. For example, extensive disease work-up in a patient presenting for palliative treatment would be unwarranted because evaluation and treatment in that setting are often directed by symptoms. An exception would be when the result of a test would provide meaningful information about the patient's condition or prognosis that, although does not change the course of treatment, provides the patient with information about what to expect. A patient who has received whole brain radiation therapy for central nervous system (CNS) metastasis may want to obtain a follow-up brain MRI to evaluate response to treatment. Although no further radiation would be indicated based on the results, the results might benefit patients in their understanding of the disease state and prognosis and therefore may be of merit. Tests that will only confirm known information are generally redundant and should be performed only if they are likely to enhance another aspect of the understanding of the patient's disease. As technology continues to move forward, offering an increasing array of sophisticated modalities with which to evaluate disease state, careful selection of the appropriate test for the circumstance is important to providing accurate, streamlined and cost-efficient care.

Attention to the principles of *sensitivity* and *specificity* as they relate to diagnostic tests and procedures is prudent when considering the appropriate selection of studies, and their interpretation. *Sensitivity* refers to the likelihood a positive result correlates with the presence of actual disease, whereas *specificity* refers to the likelihood a negative result correlates with the actual absence of disease. A test that is not "sensitive" for the suspected condition, carries a high risk of being falsely negative and thus risks not identifying those in whom the condition is present. Whereas a test that is not particularly "specific" for the condition being sought, if positive may not significantly narrow the differential diagnosis, thus being of limited usefulness. Familiarity with the sensitivity and specificity of studies used for specific conditions is helpful for accurate interpretation of the results. In some cases, several complimentary tests may be required to accurately stage the many aspects of potential disease involvement. Pelvic computed tomography (CT) may be the test of choice to evaluate evidence of lymph node involvement in prostate cancer; however, it is not sensitive for identifying extracapsular extension. Endorectal coil magnetic resonance imaging (MRI) would be a more sensitive test in that situation (Figure 4-1).

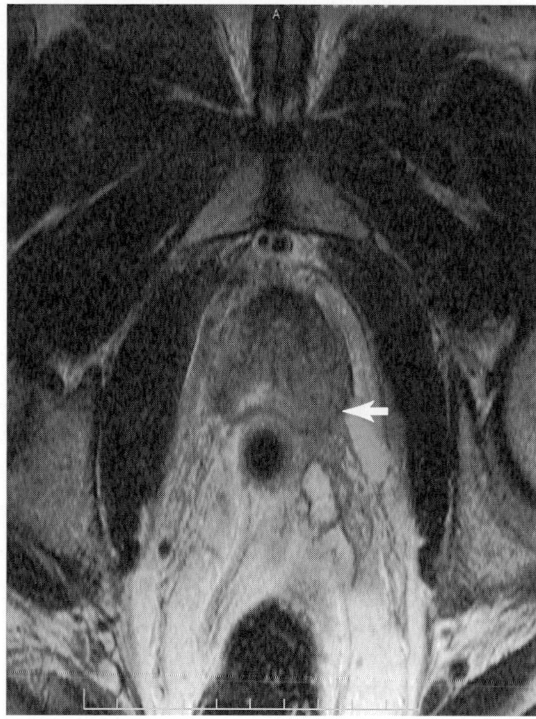

Figure 4-1 Endorectal Coil MRI. There is a subtle breach in the integrity of the prostatic capsule at the left base–mid gland, suggesting evidence of extracapsular extension.
Courtesy of Virginia Mason Medical Center, Seattle, Wash.

CANCER SCREENING

Many patients presenting for consideration of radiation therapy acquired a cancer diagnosis following presentation with specific symptoms that herald the presence of disease, prompting evaluation. However, many other patients are identified in an asymptomatic state as the consequence of having a positive cancer screening exam. Although screening is not the focus of this chapter, given the number of patients affected by the practice of cancer screening, mention of some general screening principles merits attention.

The practice of cancer screening is based on the principle that diagnosing disease in an earlier state makes controlling or eradicating the disease more likely. Although this may seem to be a relatively straightforward goal, in fact, selection of appropriate and useful screening tests may be quite difficult. It must be remembered that screening tests differ from diagnostic tests in that one is testing *healthy, asymptomatic* people, and therefore the costs and risks associated with many diagnostic exams in this setting are less acceptable. The goal of a screening exam is not to diagnose a disease, but rather to separate those people in whom disease is likely to be present from those people in whom it is not present. Because a screening test is not diagnostic, most of those who test positive will go on to have more definitive evaluation, perhaps including invasive procedures, in an effort to determine the presence or absence of malignancy and to achieve accurate diagnosis. Therefore, as with diagnostic tests, an ideal screening test must be *sensitive* (meaning a positive test correlates with a high likelihood of disease presence) to avoid unnecessary diagnostic tests in a healthy population, and also be *specific* (meaning a negative test correlates with a high likelihood the disease is absent) to avoid overconfidence in a population that they are disease free. Both untoward outcomes of screening (false positive or false negative results) may have serious outcomes for a patient, which are magnified when applied to an entire population. The *accuracy* of a screening test represents the percentage of all true test results (either positive or negative) and may vary according to the population of subjects being tested. An example of this would be reduced accuracy of mammography in younger women (less than 40 years old) in comparison with older women (those over 65 years old). To some degree, this is due to increased density of breast tissue in younger women, which makes radiographic interpretation more difficult, but also in part due to the increased prevalence of breast cancer in women over 50. The more prevalent a disease is in a population, the more likely a screening test will be correctly positive. The combination of a particular screening test's sensitivity and specificity, along with the actual prevalence of the disease in the population being tested is referred to as the test's *positive predictive value*. This reflects the test's actual ability to detect disease in the population, whereas the term *negative predictive value* reflects the ability of the test to accurately predict disease absence.

In order for a screening test to be useful, it must be relatively inexpensive, accessible to the population, convenient enough that people will participate in large numbers, and the disease must be somewhat prevalent within the community so that those identified with the disease justify the number of nonaffected people exposed to the screening test. In addition, evidence must exist to indicate that diagnosis in an asymptomatic state results in identification of disease at an earlier stage and that such identification can result in a survival benefit. Although intuitively this would seem to be evident, such is not always the case. For example, a linear progression or transformation from in situ disease to invasive disease does not occur in all cases. Many forms of low-grade cancer inherently do not behave in aggressive ways. Earlier diagnosis of these tumors may increase the amount of time someone lives with knowledge of the diagnosis but does not necessarily impact overall survival. When evaluating success of a screening test, it is important to differentiate between survival from time of diagnosis and overall survival. Increased survival from the time of diagnosis may be due only to the fact that disease present in an asymptomatic state has been identified earlier than it otherwise would have, regardless of whether this had an impact on overall survival. This is known as *lead time bias*.

In comparison with the prevalence of cancer, the number of screening exams available are relatively small, and even of some of those are controversial. Currently, widely recognized screening exists only for breast, colorectal, prostate, and cervical cancers (Table 4-2). Although it is generally not appropriate to focus on screening activities for patients undergoing active treatment for malignancy, it is important to remember that secondary malignancies can occur in patients with prior cancer histories. For previously treated patients, long-term surveillance for disease recurrence is important, along with attention to appropriate screening for other malignancies as indicated.

PRINCIPLES OF STAGING

The primary purpose of staging is to stratify risk (prognosis) based on disease extent and characteristics. Accurate staging of malignancy is critical to providing the patient with specific information about prognosis and is the basis for selecting an appropriate treatment plan. Consistency in staging criteria also allows for analysis of treatment efficacy across groups and contributes to greater understanding of prognostic indicators. Historically, many staging systems have been devised, often site

Table 4-2 American Cancer Society Cancer Detection Guidelines

Cancer site	Guidelines
Breast	Women over age of 40: Yearly mammogram
Colon	For men and women over age of 50: Yearly fecal occult blood test (FOBT) *or* fecal immunochemical test (FIT) *or* flexible sigmoidoscopy every 5 years *OR* Yearly FOBT/FIT + flex sig every 5 years (preferred over above) *OR* Double-contrast barium enema every 5 years *OR* Colonoscopy every 10 years
Prostate	For African-American men or those with a family history of prostate cancer at an early age: Yearly prostate specific antigen (PSA)/digital rectal exam (DRE) For all other men over 50: Yearly PSA/DRE
Cervix	For women from age of sexual intercourse or older than 21: Yearly PAP smear (liquid-based PAP may be done every 2 years) May be done every 2–3 years if more than 30 years old and has had three consecutive normal PAP tests

Data from *American Cancer Society prevention and detection review of screening guidelines.* Based on information from the American Cancer Society, 2005 (website): www.cancer.org/docroot/PED/ped_2.asp?sitearea=PED&level=1. Accessed February 24, 2006.

specific, which although accurate, have contributed to lack of regional standardization and can make comparison across populations or studies difficult. Although the International Union Against Cancer TNM Committee (UICC [Union Internationale Contre Cancre]) and American Joint Committee on Cancer (AJCC) defined their own independent objectives for cancer staging almost 50 years ago,[3] efforts progressed in the 1980s to create a world recognized standardization system based on end-results data to classify cancer using the TNM *(Tumor Node Metastasis)* system. The AJCC/UICC TNM classification system is currently the national and international standard,[4] and largely replaces earlier unique staging systems where possible (such the Dukes' classification for colon cancer). Some classification systems not amenable to the TNM system were adopted instead of the TNM system, for example, the FIGO (International Federation of Gynecologists and Obstetricians) for gynecological malignancies and the Ann Arbor classification for Hodgkin's and non-Hodgkin's lymphomas.[5] In the last 50 years since the TNM system was first introduced, many modifications of specific staging criteria have been implemented based on changes in understanding of disease behavior and improved accuracy of diagnostic techniques. The most recent modification of the TNM classification system was implemented in 2003, providing a uniform set of definitions and rules across disease sites to ensure standardized application in all settings.[6]

The TNM staging system classifies extent of disease before the introduction of definitive therapy based on the extent of local tumor growth (T), nodal involvement (N) and presence or absence of distant metastatic disease (M). While being a predictor of overall prognosis, TNM staging does not address the unique biological behavior (indolence or aggressiveness) of a specific tumor, and therefore other pertinent tumor characteristics also may be identified along with the TNM stage (e.g., tumor marker or receptor status, Gleason score, and others). Recognizing that TNM stage reflects only disease that is known or detectable, the accuracy depends on the sensitivity of available tests and the thoroughness of the work-up. Following a comprehensive clinical evaluation (exam, laboratory studies, endoscopic/radiographic evaluation, etc.), surgical exploration or excision, with or without nodal sampling, may change the understanding of the disease classification based on the gross surgical findings and/or pathological review of the tissue. A distinction between "clinical TNM stage" (cTNM) and "pathological TNM stage" (pTNM) is generally made because of this potential for "upstaging" after surgery. Both staging modalities are

Table 4-3 Definitions of TNM

PRIMARY TUMOR (T)	
TX	Not evaluable
T0	No evidence of primary tumor
Tis	Carcinoma in situ
T1, T2, T3, T4	Increasing size or local extent of primary tumor
REGIONAL LYMPH NODES (N)	
NX	Regional lymph nodes cannot be assessed
N0	No regional lymph node metastasis
N1, N2, N3	Increased involvement of regional lymph node
DISTANT METASTASIS (M)	
MX	Distant metastasis cannot be assessed
M0	No distant metastasis
M1	Distant metastasis
Subdivisions of TNM	
Subdivisions of some main categories are available for those who need greater specificity (e.g., T1a, 1b, or N2a, 2b as with breast and prostate)	

significant because the clinical stage will guide the primary treatment approach and the pathologic stage will determine need for adjuvant therapy and provide the greatest insight into estimated prognosis.[4]

Each category in the TNM staging system is graded according to the anatomic extent of evaluable disease (Table 4-3). Generally, extent of local disease is categorized on a 0 to 4 scale, according to criteria specific to the primary anatomic site (T0–T4), with TX indicating the tumor is not evaluable and Tis indicating in situ disease. Nodal involvement is documented as N0, N1, N2, or N3, based on the characteristics (regional involvement, discrete or bulky, mobile or fixed) of involved nodes. Metastatic disease is only categorized according to its presence (M1) or absence (M0), unless it cannot be assessed, in which case this is communicated as MX. Disease stage is a product of all three of these components in combination according to the diagnosis, rather than solely based on any one of these parameters (with the exception of M, as any metastasis implies Stage IV disease).

Staging criteria are not static. Evolving understanding of tumor biology and the ability to accurately diagnose extent of disease and biologic behavior will continue to impact these standards. Currently, the dominant focus of staging is anatomic extent of disease, with standards for classification based on anatomic site of origin. Other characteristics that may influence disease behavior and outcomes (e.g., age at onset, tumor grade and gene expression, or identification of other tumor markers) are not currently incorporated into the classification system. Identification of supplemental characteristics may substratify tumors of comparable stage into different risk categories (Figure 4-2).[6] In fact, for certain tumors histopathologic grade is more important in determining stage and prognosis than anatomic extent, such as soft tissue sarcomas and gliomas.[5] As more information becomes available, there may be significant changes in the concepts of staging that emerge. Staging criteria are periodically revised according to a specific structured process instituted by the UICC, as understanding of disease outcomes and increasing ability to detect currently undetectable disease evolve. However, frequent changes to the classification system may confuse the ability to compare response rates over time, because what would previously have been diagnosed as T2 disease, with improved diagnostic ability may now be staged as T3 disease. Therefore care should be taken when comparing longitudinal studies to ensure that comparable staging criteria have been applied.

PRINCIPLES OF DIAGNOSTIC EVALUATION

Thorough History and Physical Exam

Although malignancy for some is identified by screening, other patients are alerted to the presence

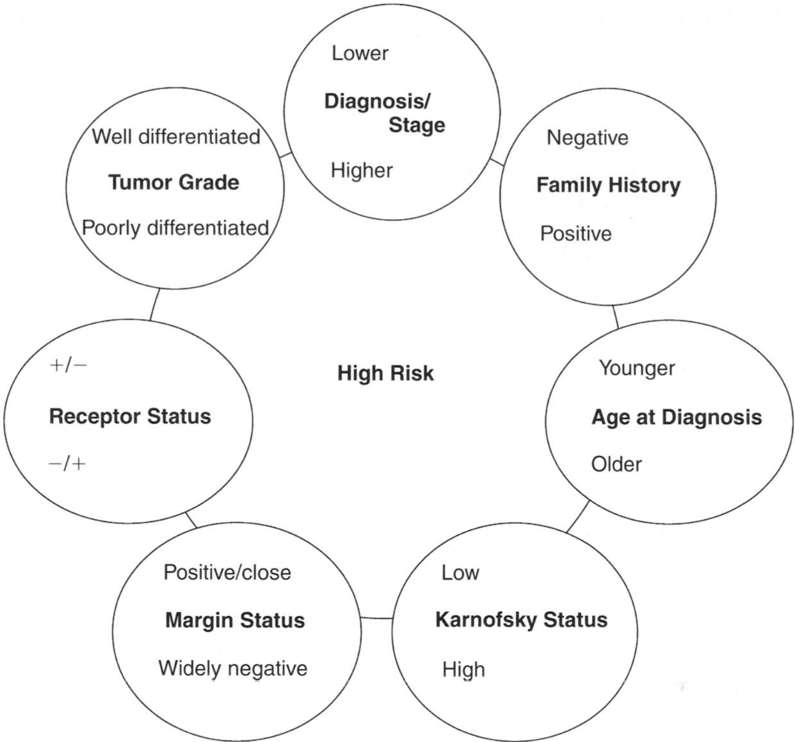

Figure 4-2 Schema of Selected Prognostic Factors (Generalized). Patients with comparable diagnosis and stage may be considered to be more or less at risk based on supplemental diagnostic information. This may affect decisions regarding need for more aggressive therapy.

of cancer as the result of a presenting symptom or cluster of symptoms, for example, cough/hemoptysis, changes in bowel habits, early satiety/weight loss, jaundice, or the presence of a palpable mass. A thorough history and physical exam (H&P) will be performed by the provider to fully describe the presenting symptom and its course (history of present illness). Other information about the patient's medical condition in general should be gathered (past medical history), as well as information about allergies and current medications. Family and social history are also important and may provide information about potential risk factors for malignancies. Initial physical examination should consist of a complete head-to-toe evaluation, encompassing the major body systems (general appearance and mental status, head and neck, lymph nodes, respiratory, cardiac, gastrointestinal, genitourinary, nervous system, and extremities). This is important not only in evaluating the extent of clinically evident disease burden but also in monitoring for undetected metastatic disease and evaluating the impact of disease burden on organ function (i.e., presence of neurologic deficit, cyanosis, jaundice, edema or ascites).

The nurse may be involved in obtaining detailed information about the patient's current complaints, past medical history, and the prior work-up that has been obtained. For patients being seen in consultation for radiation therapy, particular attention must be given to prior history of malignancy or other conditions for which the patient may have potentially received radiation treatment. This could have an impact on the current treatment plan. Manifestations of a malignant process, such as constitutional symptoms (early satiety, weight loss, fatigue, constipation), the presence of persistent or progressive pain, physical findings (e.g., a palpable mass or adenopathy), or other symptoms related to the location of disease (such as hoarseness, cough, odynophagia, obstructive urinary symptoms, thin stools or abnormal bleeding) should be assessed and documented. It is helpful to have a baseline from which to evaluate clinical response to treatment once it has been initiated, particularly when radiation is given as primary therapy or in the neoadjuvant setting.

Based on the pattern of presenting symptoms, along with information from a detailed H&P, and attention to principles of epidemiology, the differential diagnosis can be formulated. Tests will then be ordered to rule out or confirm potential diagnosis on the differential list. This will often include venous blood evaluation, radiography, and perhaps most importantly, biopsy or other histopathologic evaluation of tissue. Further diagnostic techniques may be appropriate based on risk for more extensive disease, typical patterns of disease spread for the suspected malignancy and goals of therapy. Only when diagnosis is confirmed, and thorough staging evaluation has been completed, can appropriate treatment options, radiation or otherwise, be determined.

Pathologic Evaluation

The goal of pathologic review is to specify disease presence in sampled tissue, describe the nature of disease (classification and grade) and the extent of tumor involvement (stage). Histologic evaluation of tissue is absolutely essential in establishing the diagnosis of a malignancy and relates directly to the generation of a treatment plan. Radiographic appearance, although in some instances strongly suggestive, is not diagnostic for malignancy alone, therefore tissue sampling is mandatory except on the rare occasion when it is technically not feasible. Confirmation of tissue histology is one aspect of the evaluation, but other information that can be obtained from pathologic review includes degree of differentiation, nuclear activity, evidence of invasiveness (muscular, extracapsular, lymphatic, neurovascular invasion), adequacy of surgical excision (margin status) and special staining techniques that may provide insight into responsiveness to treatment or disease behavior (receptor status, tumor markers).

Increasing availability of immunohistochemistry, cytologic and molecular genetic techniques, is increasing the complexity of appropriate test selection. Overuse of highly sensitive tests increases the likelihood of too many false positive results, whereas utilization of too many highly specific tests leads to an increase in false negative outcomes. Increasing complexity of testing techniques requires a higher level of laboratory sophistication, which may contribute to instances of misdiagnosis due to laboratory error. Algorithms and protocols that are tumor/organ specific are therefore being generated by pathologists to avoid overuse and inappropriate use of such tests, in an effort to contain costs and limit the potential for misdiagnosis due to the improper selection of evaluation technique.[7]

Classification of tumor type is often based on the microscopic appearance of tumor sections after special staining techniques.[8] Tumor classification is hierarchical, distinguishing between progressive differences in behavior, differentiation, and phenotypic expression.[7] The nomenclature of tumor classification has been standardized to ensure consistency, with periodic updates. Most tissue samples are adequately evaluated using standard microscopic techniques, however, in some instances (such as insufficiently differentiated tumors or inadequate biopsy sample) use of more advanced methodology including electron microscopy, polymerase chain reaction analysis, expression array assays, or immunohistochemical studies may be required to accurately identify certain features that are diagnostic for a specific malignancy. Application of a variety of available tissue analysis techniques may provide information about gene mutations, altered patterns of gene expression, and molecular marker expression, useful in diagnosis, prediction of disease behavior and/or likelihood of response to particular treatments (e.g., HER-2 Neu).

The *primary tumor* is the site of tumor origin and is determined by evaluating the tissue type the specimen most closely resembles. In most instances, the presenting lesion is consistent with the histologic determination of the site of origin (pulmonary nodule on biopsy found to be consistent with non–small cell lung cancer). On some occasions, however, the presenting nodule is found on biopsy to more closely resemble distant tissue and therefore represents *metastatic disease* (such as a liver nodule that on biopsy proves to resemble adenocarcinoma of the colon). Patients also may present with solid organ or lymph node disease that is so poorly differentiated that determination of primary site may be quite difficult. Thorough evaluation (potentially including CT scanning, PET scans, endoscopy, random biopsy sampling of suspected origin tissues) may be undertaken in an effort to find the primary lesion, because origin of disease is important in choosing an appropriate treatment plan. In rare instances, the primary tumor is not identifiable *(tumor of unknown origin)*, which often portends a poor prognosis. Patients with known current or prior malignancy also may present with evidence of a new tumor, either representing metastatic disease or a *second primary tumor*, which is the independent development of an unrelated malignancy. Distinguishing between the two (generally by tissue confirmation) is extremely important because treatment and prognostic implications may be markedly different (the significance of a second stage 1 tumor is entirely different than new pulmonary metastasis).

Along with determining the tissue type, complete staging also requires determination of the tumor's histologic grade. *Histology* refers to determination of the normal tissue or cell type the tumor most closely resembles. Therefore *histologic grade* describes the extent to which the tumor cells resemble that normal tissue type (differentiation).[4] Tumor cells that retain characteristics of their normal progenitor cells are referred to as *well differentiated* and therefore are given a low histologic grade (grade 1). As the tumor cells progressively lose characteristics of the normal tissue of origin, they become more poorly differentiated and are given a higher histologic grade (Table 4-4). Although for some tumors histologic class defines the tumor grade, such as small cell lung cancer (poorly differentiated) or carcinoid tumor of the lung (well-differentiated).[7] Grading criteria are tumor specific, attempting to stratify according to the prognostic significance of different patterns. The *Gleason score* in prostate cancer is the sum of both the dominant and less dominant architectural growth differentiation patterns, with a higher score indicating greater risk of treatment failure (Figure 4-3). The biologic behavior of the tumor, and risk of disease spread, is often linked to higher (i.e., greater differentiated/anaplastic) histopathologic grade, although the significance of tumor grade may vary according to tumor type.

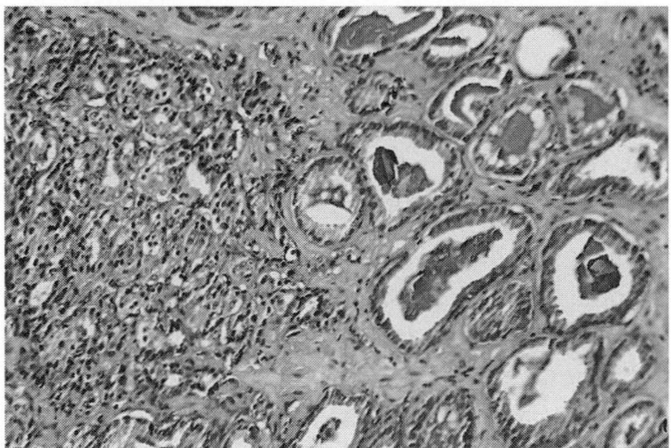

Figure 4-3 Prostate Cancer Cells.
Courtesy of the National Cancer Institute.

Table 4-4 Histologic Grading

Grading	Description
GX	Grade cannot be assessed
G1	Well differentiated
G2	Moderately differentiated
G3	Poorly differentiated
G4	Undifferentiated

Used with the permission of the American Joint Committee on Cancer (AJCC), Chicago, Illinois. The original source for this material is the *AJCC Cancer Staging Manual, Sixth Edition* (2002) published by Springer-Verlag New York, www.springeronline.com.[4]

Pathologic review of tumor stage attempts to quantify tumor extent, the size of the primary tumor (T), tumor depth or invasion, and evaluation of local extension. In many instances, pathologic contribution to identification of tumor involvement provides important staging information that impacts prognosis assessment and treatment decisions. Although work continues to identify molecular markers that have clear prognostic meaning, for many cancers, pathologic staging is paramount to assigning risk. In head and neck cancers, cervical lymph node involvement is the most important prognostic indicator for risk of tumor recurrence and survival.[9]

Molecular Biomarker Evaluation

Increasingly during pathologic review of tumor tissue, additional antigen, protein, or DNA markers are evaluated by immunohistochemistry, polymerase chain reaction or other means, to assist in diagnosis and provide additional characterization of the disease. Advances in understanding of the molecular initiation and progression of many malignancies is contributing to improved diagnostic specificity and outcomes.[10] Microarray technology has the potential to ultimately identify molecularly defined subclasses of tumor.[11] Presence of specific tumor antigens such as HER-2 Neu, p53, and rab 25, among others, may distinguish a benign from malignant process, confirm tissue histology, or provide insight into potential tumor behavior and risk of relapse. Other potential uses for molecular profiling include identification of cancer precursor lesions at risk, assessment of residual microscopic disease in the tumor bed or microscopic nodal involvement, and surveillance of disseminated tumor cells.[11] In some instances, the identified DNA abnormalities, or tumor specific receptors, not only serve in tumor identification but also may provide the substrate for novel therapies. Specific markers including estrogen and/or progesterone receptor status, HER-2 Neu, EGF receptor status, when present in tumor tissue, now influence eligibility for particular chemotherapeutic treatment modalities designed to exploit their role in tumorigenesis. It is anticipated that similar targeted therapies for a host of malignancies will emerge over time.

Molecules that may serve as targets for such markers include DNA markers (loss of heterozygosity, alleic imbalance, microsatellite instability, gene methylation, mitochondrial mutations, single nucleotide polymorphisms, and specific gene mutations), protein markers (serum proteins, plasma proteins and antibodies) and evaluation of tissue mRNA levels using reverse transcriptase-polymerase chain reaction.[11]

Immunohistochemistry, commonly performed for marker identification and tumor classification, uses antibodies to identify specific antigens, commonly tissue specific markers.[7] Tumor proliferation (indicator of aggressive behavior) also can be evaluated by immunohistochemistry techniques by identifying specific nuclear antigens expressed during cell division.

Biopsy

Biopsy is the removal of a tissue sample for pathologic evaluation. Depending on the clinical circumstance, the location of the tissue of concern, and the sample requirements that are necessary for accurate analysis, many different approaches to biopsy may be undertaken. Percutaneous biopsy is commonly performed, although endoscopic biopsy may be employed for lung or other intraluminal lesions. Additionally, various radiographic methodologies also may be used during biopsy procedures to improve safety and accuracy in tissue localization (such as CT, MRI, or ultrasound guided biopsy, stereotactic biopsy, fluoroscopic assisted biopsy) (Figure 4-4).

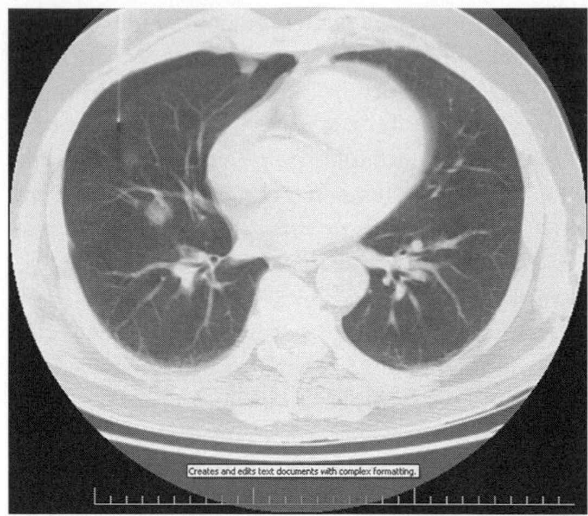

Figure 4-4 CT Guided Needle Biopsy.
CT guided needle biopsy of right middle lobe pulmonary nodule (with resultant pneumothorax).
Courtesy of Virginia Mason Medical Center, Seattle, Wash.

Various types and sizes of biopsy needles are available and are selected according to the specific needs of the type of tissue to be sampled. Fine needle aspiration (FNA) may be accomplished with a small-gauge aspiration needle (usually 22G), that provides cells and cell clusters from the mass for cytologic examination (review of fluid for malignant cells shed from the tumor surface, scrapings, or washings). Large-core biopsy cutting needles will deliver an actual piece of tissue (core) that can be analyzed by cytologic and histopathologic exam, with the advantage of preserving the histologic architecture of the tissue specimen.[12] Excisional biopsy involves the surgical removal of the entire lesion lymph node, nodule, or mass. This may be done for therapeutic reasons (such as removal of a melanoma lesion) or because the tissue obtained from prior biopsy was not sufficient for diagnosis. For very large lesions, if excisional biopsy is not feasible, an incisional biopsy (partial excision) may be obtained.

Nodal Evaluation

During the staging of most solid tumors, a decision must be made about the best way to approach pathologic evaluation of regional lymph nodes. Clinical evaluation may reveal the presence of physically palpable or radiographically detectable nodes, in which case consideration for either neoadjuvant therapy or nodal dissection (for both therapeutic and staging purposes) may be made.

In some instances, there is no clinical evidence of nodal involvement, however, the assumption that there is no regional nodal involvement cannot necessarily be made. In this situation, two questions must be answered: is there a likelihood of nodal metastasis and if so, what method of assessment in this patient with no clinically detectable disease will be thorough enough to answer this question but with the least morbidity for the patient. These questions are often answered by the pathologic information derived from the biopsy. Evidence of certain "low risk" characteristics, such as low mitotic activity, early stage, low grade, well to moderately differentiated tumors without evidence of invasive activity such as in situ disease, or invasive disease but without evidence of extracapsular, neurovascular, or fatty tissue invasion, often will not require further evaluation. However, evidence of high mitotic activity, high grade, later stage, poorly to undifferentiated disease, or evidence of invasion to surrounding structures on pathologic review, will generally require further investigation of lymph node status. Historically, this would require surgical lymph node dissection (LND), which involves sampling of lymph nodes in the immediate drainage area from the primary tumor. To adequately stage, a minimum number of lymph nodes must be dissected, which is dictated in the staging criteria by the primary site of origin.[13] LND is not without morbidity, including longer postoperative recovery, scarring, increased cost, and long-term risk of lymphedema, therefore careful identification of those patients who will clearly benefit from the procedure is critical.

Evolution of sentinel node biopsy (SNB) is increasingly being performed to minimize risk of morbidity in selected lower-risk patients. Although this technique is primarily used in staging for breast cancer and melanoma, it is proving to be applicable to the evaluation of head and neck cancers and other solid tumors as well.[14] SNB involves the injection of dye at the time of surgical excision of the primary tumor in order to identify the first node that receives lymphatic drainage from that site. The identified node (or in some instances more than one) is sampled. If this node is positive then the patient will return for LND to fully evaluate nodal involvement. If this node is negative, then LND will not be required because risk of node involvement is minimal. Identification of the sentinel node also may be used to direct limited lymph node sampling, where only the nodes most likely to be involved are sampled according to the location of the sentinel node.[15] Advantages of SNB use include avoiding unnecessary surgery and thereby decreasing morbidity in lower-risk patients; however, a disadvantage is that patients with a positive sentinel node will need to return for a second surgery, rather than having the LND done at the time of primary tumor excision as it would otherwise be done.

How best to manage the sentinel node with only microscopic foci (0.2 mm–2 mm, N1mi) of metastatic disease involvement remains a dilemma.[16] Generally full LND is not required in this setting, but the presence of microscopic disease involvement in combination with other pathologic characteristics may influence consideration of adjuvant therapy.

Other Invasive Diagnostic Techniques

Direct visualization of luminal surfaces and internal organs by endoscopic techniques can provide meaningful information about disease status, including diagnosis and assessment of staging/operability, that in many instances cannot be obtained by other less invasive means (although technology to advance CT or MRI-based three-dimensional "virtual endoscopy" techniques is growing). In head and neck cancer, *panendoscopy* has demonstrated more sensitivity for identifying mucosal lesions than other imaging modalities.[17] Access to internal spaces also has the added benefit of allowing other diagnostic assistance (such as obtaining brushings, washings, and/or biopsy for pathologic review, or directed endoscopic sonography), and therapeutic intervention (tumor laser ablation, removal of polyps, stricture dilation, stent placement, and management of hemorrhage).[18]

Endoscopic procedures may vary in degree of invasiveness or risk depending on location and may have differing requirements for sedation (ranging from conscious sedation to general anesthesia). Generally, they are considered to have an excellent safety profile, and the unique information gathered from this modality justifies the modest risk.

Evaluation of many different anatomic regions may be achieved endoscopically, using either rigid or flexible fiber-optic (or other visual modality) scopes, and use of assorted instruments designed to pass through the scope, such as probes, brushes, forceps, or biopsy needles, permits the performance of several diagnostic and therapeutic procedures. Intraluminal disease of the upper gastrointestinal (GI) tract (esophagus, stomach, and upper duodenum) is evaluable by *upper endoscopy*, whereas the distal colon and rectum are accessible by sigmoidoscopy, and the entire large intestine, cecum, and rectum are examined by *colonoscopy*.

Approved by the Food and Drug Administration (FDA) in 2001, *capsule endoscopy* is proving to be a useful modality for identification of tumors located in the distal small intestine, not accessible by gastroscopy or colonoscopy.[19] Although small intestine tumors are relatively uncommon, in certain circumstances when source of GI bleeding cannot be located, capsule endoscopy provides a means of evaluating this difficult-to-reach region and appears to be sensitive in the identification of small bowel tumors.[20,21] A disposable camera enclosed in a small biocompatible plastic capsule is ingested and travels by peristalsis through the GI tract to the anus. Images are produced at a rate of two per second and wirelessly transmitted to a recorder worn by the patient. Fasting is required before the procedure, although bowel preparation generally is not necessary. History of intestinal obstruction or stricture, or in some cases those with significant motility problems, are contraindications to the procedure.[20]

Inspection of the peritoneum may be achieved by laparoscopy *(peritoneoscopy)*, which involves the introduction of air into the peritoneal cavity (pneumoperitoneum) and the insertion of a thin scope through a puncture in the abdominal wall.[18] Examination of the anterior peritoneum, much of the liver surface, gallbladder, the greater omentum, serosal surfaces of the stomach, small bowel and colon, and the pelvic organs can be performed using standard laparoscopic techniques and is frequently employed for the preoperative staging of pancreatic, esophageal, gastric, gallbladder, and rectal tumors.[18]

Incorporation of a high-frequency ultrasound transducer into the tip of an endoscope *(endoscopic ultrasonography, EUS)* produces high-resolution images of local structures to provide more detailed information about tumor depth, evaluation of submucosal or extrinsic lesions, and for nodal evaluation, particularly for staging of GI malignancies.[22] EUS also has been used for staging of subaortic and subcarinal lymph nodes in lung cancer (transesophageal ultrasound), although use of EUS with bronchoscopy has been more difficult because ultrasound waves are not transmitted in the air-containing space (bronchi).[18,23]

Endoscopic retrograde cholangiopancreatography (ERCP) is generally performed to evaluate pancreatic masses and the biliary tree, with the option of endobiliary stent placement in the event of biliary obstruction. Pancreatic and biliary duct anatomy are visualized by the use of a scope and the injection of a contrast agent into the selected duct using fluoroscopic guidance. ERCP is helpful in evaluating extent of disease and involvement of critical structures (such as encasement of the hepatic artery) for surgical planning.

Bronchoscopy (flexible or rigid) is indispensable in the evaluation and staging of lung masses and also is useful for investigation of other upper aerodigestive malignancies. In addition to obtaining biopsy, brushings, and/or washings for cytologic evaluation, bronchoscopy also permits evaluation of airway compromise (degree of occlusion from either intrinsic or extrinsic compression from tumor) and intraluminal stent placement to maintain airway patency. Diagnostic sampling of mediastinal or submucosal structures not directly available for biopsy may be accomplished using transbronchial aspiration techniques.

Mediastinoscopy allows visualization and biopsy of lymph nodes in the superior mediastinum using a mediastinoscope passed through a small suprasternal incision. This technique is useful in lung cancer staging because it identifies patients with locally advanced disease who may not benefit from surgical resection, thus avoiding potentially unnecessary procedures. *Thoracoscopy* allows investigation of the pleural space, mediastinum, and diaphragm and is useful for the evaluation of pleural effusions and peripherally located indeterminate pulmonary nodules.

Endoscopic evaluation of the bladder *(cystoscopy)*, vagina, and cervix *(colposcopy)*, and endometrium *(hysteroscopy)* are also common diagnostic procedures in the setting of genitourinary malignancy evaluation.

Much of the time adequate disease assessment can be accomplished endoscopically by many of the above techniques and others, therefore minimizing discomfort and risk to the patient. In some instances, however, endoscopic evaluation is not appropriate, or further surgical exploration (such as lymph node dissection, thoracotomy, and exploratory laparotomy) is necessary.

Laboratory Evaluation

Inevitably during the diagnosis and staging process, patients will have laboratory studies obtained, often of blood or serum, but also potentially of urine, sputum, stool, or other body fluids (such as cerebrospinal fluid [CSF], ascites fluid, or pleural effusion) depending on the suspected diagnosis. Information obtained from this evaluation may provide support for a suspected diagnosis, may give general information about the patients overall condition, may offer insight into the impact the presence of a tumor is having on particular organ systems, may be obtained as a baseline study for comparison to evaluate treatment response, or may be obtained for any combination of these reasons.

Increasingly tumor markers are being used in the evaluation of tumor status and response to treatment,[24] and clinically useful practices for the use of tumor markers continues to evolve. Tumor markers are substances found in blood or other body fluids that are produced either by a specific tumor (tumor derived) or produced by the host in response to tumor presence (tumor associated), which may indicate presence of disease. Qualitative or quantitative measures of tumor markers may be obtained by chemical, immunologic, or molecular biologic techniques and may include any number of molecules including enzymes, hormones, antigens, proteins, genes, or receptors, among others.[25] Elevated levels of certain tumor markers may correlate with tumor burden, although not all patients will have elevated tumor markers at diagnosis, and nonmalignant causes of abnormal tumor marker levels are common (Table 4-5). Many tumor markers, such as carcinoembryonic antigen (CEA), are nonspecific and therefore overuse of them can lead to increased cost, patient anxiety, and limited useful information on which to base patient assessment.[26] Evaluation of specific tumor markers at diagnosis may be done to confirm diagnosis and serve as a baseline from which to monitor disease response to treatment or may be obtained to facilitate identification of tumor origin in the case of ambiguous or unknown primary. Tumor markers also may be obtained periodically after treatment as part of the surveillance for disease recurrence.

Table 4-5 Review of Selected Tumor Markers

Marker	Malignancy related to	Associated nonmalignant conditions
α-fetoprotein (AFP)	Liver, hepatocellular, testicular	Pregnancy, hepatitis
CA 15-3	Primarily breast cancer	Benign breast tumors
CA 19-9	Pancreatic/biliary, colon, transitional cell tumors	Gallstones, pancreatitis, liver cirrhosis, cholecystitis
CA 27-29	Primarily breast cancer	Endometriosis, benign breast disease, ovarian cyst, liver and renal disease.
CA 125	Mucinous epithelial tumors Ovary, cervix, endometrium, GI tract, breast	Endometriosis, pelvic inflammatory disease
Carcinoembryonic antigen (CEA)	Primarily colon, breast, pancreas, lung, prostate, melanoma, lymphoma, others	May be elevated in smokers, inflammatory bowel disease, pancreatitis, liver disease
Lactate dehydrogenase (LDH)	Nonspecific, metastatic disease	Myocardial infarction/heart failure, anemia, hypothyroidism, lung disease, liver disease, infection
Prostatic acid phosphate (PAP)	Prostate, transitional cell carcinoma, carcinoid tumors	Hepatitis, osteoporosis, benign prostate hypertrophy
Prostate specific antigen (PSA)	Prostate	Following rectal exam, benign prostate disease, prostatitis

Radiographic Evaluation

Plain Film Radiology

Although x rays do not often offer enough diagnostic detail to fully evaluate malignancy involvement or extent, because of their safety, ease of use, and availability, this modality is often useful in the initial evaluation of a presenting symptom or complaint. Lung cancers are commonly identified by abnormalities found on chest x ray incidentally or sometimes obtained for evaluation of cough, shortness of breath, or other reasons, for instance. However, further diagnostic imaging will then be required to more thoroughly evaluate disease extent.

X rays are obtained by generating a beam, which is attenuated by variations in tissue density as it passes through the body. As the x rays of varying intensity emerge, they penetrate a screen coated with fluorescent particles, which then emits light rays exposing photographic film and producing a recognizable image reflecting the anatomy.[27] Different structures have different radiographic densities that can be distinguished on the films generated, with air-filled spaces and low-density structures appearing darker and more dense tissues (such as bony structures) appearing lighter or white. Many soft tissues attenuate x rays to a similar degree and therefore make evaluation of various tissues difficult to distinguish by this modality. In many instances, however, bone radiographs remain quite useful.

Ultrasonography

Ultrasound is often useful in further characterizing nodules or lesions that have been identified on exam (such as a palpable mass) or on other imaging (such as mammogram) and is also used to evaluate vascular flow. Common applications in oncology include evaluation of superficial masses (thyroid, breast, testes, chest wall, etc.), liver and biliary structures, kidneys and organs of the pelvis and also are used in guiding interventional radiology procedures (such as ultrasound-guided biopsy).[28]

Ultrasound generates images detected from the echoes of sound energy reflected from tissues. High-frequency sound energy is transmitted through patient tissues, and a composite image is generated by detection of the time it takes for the echo to return to the transducer. Different structures or organs may have varying degrees of echogenicity, with fluid-filled structures generally being less echogenic than solid structures (which generate a more speckled appearance) and fatty tissues (which are generally highly echogenic). Lesions that generate less echo intensity than surrounding tissue are described as being *hypoechoic*, whereas lesions that generate greater echo intensity than surrounding tissue are referred to as *hyperechoic*.[27] Although relatively inexpensive and well tolerated by patients, ultrasound is limited by somewhat poor soft tissue resolution and inability to penetrate bone and air-filled spaces.

Computed Tomography

Computed tomography (CT) scanning is ubiquitous in evaluating the presence and extent of malignancy and is used extensively both as part of the initial staging work-up and to monitor response to treatment and ongoing surveillance after treatment for many types of cancers, including head and neck malignancies, lung cancer, cancer of the gastrointestinal and genitourinary tracts, and in the evaluation of adrenal masses.[13] It has been a mainstay of imaging in oncology because of its noninvasive approach, relative accuracy, widespread availability, and reasonable cost.[13]

Images are obtained by computer reconstruction of cross-sectional anatomic images generated from interpretation of attenuated x-ray transmission through sequential sections (or slices) of patient tissues.[27] Use of contrast agents (intravenous, oral, or rectal) may be given to enhance tissue density differences. Although generally safe, adverse reactions to intravenous contrast can occur including nausea, vomiting, hives, bronchospasm, and rarely, anaphylaxis. Caution also must be used in patients with renal insufficiency, and generally a recent serum creatinine level must be obtained before intravenous contrast administration.

In conventional CT, the images are obtained one slice at a time, allowing the patient to take a breath and advancing the table in between slices. With helical (or spiral) CT, the table is moved at a constant speed through the CT gantry with continuous scanning of the x-ray tube rotating around the patient in one breath hold.[27] Advantages are improved image acquisition times, and less artifact, particularly when imaging the lung and liver, due to variations in breath holding.

Helical CT

Helical (spiral) CT and other CT innovations such as multidectector CT are increasing the sensitivity and specificity of this modality. The development of spiral CT imaging has been particularly helpful in evaluating lesions within the thorax (due to the single breath hold technique) and also lesions of the liver, pancreas, and biliary tree, and their vasculature. Depending on the technique, spiral CT is proving to be highly accurate in identification of liver lesions greater than 1 cm (which are more likely to represent a malignant process) and can generally differentiate between characteristics more likely to represent benign (cyst, hemangioma) or malignant disease.[13] Increased ability to accurately evaluate tumor burden and large vessel involvement provides important information in determining the appropriate treatment course, as significant disease involvement of major vessels often precludes the option of surgical resection (Whipple procedure) in this population.

Multidetector CT

Continued refinements of imaging techniques incorporating spiral CT technology and advancements in computer software capability are leading to the development of novel imaging capabilities likely to have a significant impact on staging accuracy and treatment planning. For example, multidetector CT scanning, which allows control of variable slice thickness (capable of 1-mm slices), is more time efficient, may improve image detail and can be used with three-dimensional imaging techniques. Continued refinement of three-dimensional images reconstructed using specialized equipment and techniques may reduce the need for some invasive procedures, such as endoscopy and cholangiography. To acquire these images, special contrast agents are used (either oral or IV) or effervescent powders are employed to enhance air/fluid-filled intraluminal spaces, allowing for visualization of luminal surfaces and anatomic structures (virtual endoscopy).[29] An advantage of virtual endoscopy, apart from being noninvasive, is the ability to visualize beyond a stricture or obstructing mass that would otherwise be inaccessible endoscopically.[28]

Magnetic Resonance Imaging/Spectroscopic Imaging

Use of magnetic resonance imaging (MRI) has become indispensable in the evaluation of certain tumors, and advances in technology continue to improve the images obtained from this modality and broaden the spectrum of applicability. MR differs from CT in that it uses magnetic fields, rather than ionizing radiation, to produce images, and rather than interpreting only one tissue characteristic (x-ray attenuation), it analyzes multiple tissue characteristics including proton density, proton magnetization time (T1), time to loss of tissue magnetization (T2), and blood flow, providing superior imaging, particularly soft tissue contrast resolution.[27] Therefore, MRI is particularly suited for evaluation of soft tissue (although CT will provide better bone images) and CNS structures, and use in evaluation of tumors of the head and neck, breast, and prostate (endorectal surface coil MRI) is increasing (Figures 4-5 and 4-6).

Strong magnetic fields are used to induce synchronized spinning of hydrogen protons, and with application of radio frequency pulses, a computer analyzes and generates a map of proton signal intensity by spatial location.[30] Variations of the radio frequency pulses can be generated to optimize the images based on certain tissue characteristics. Therefore, *T1-weighted images* emphasize differences in the T1 relaxation times of tissues (relaxation of the net magnetized vector back to the longitudinal plane) and generally provide the best anatomic detail, *T2-weighted images* emphasize the differences in the T2 relaxations times of tissues (relaxation of the net magnetized vector back to the transverse plane) and are more sensitive for pathologic lesions, and *proton-density–weighted images* emphasize varying tissue proton density and are most useful in brain imaging.[27] Gadopentetate dimeglumine (gadolinium-labeled diethylenetriamine pentaacetic acid [DTPA]) also may be given intravenously with MR scanning to enhance differences in signal intensity, in much the same way as contrast is used in CT scanning. Because malignant tumors often have increased blood supply, the gadolinium is taken up by these tissues more readily than by surrounding nonmalignant tissues or many benign abnormalities, thereby identifying contrast enhancing lesions as areas of concern.[31]

In magnetic resonance spectroscopic imaging (MRSI), differing frequencies of signal intensity from hydrogen protons in different molecules (chemical shift) generates a map based on signal intensity (rather than frequency) and spatial location, offering an evaluation not just of anatomic

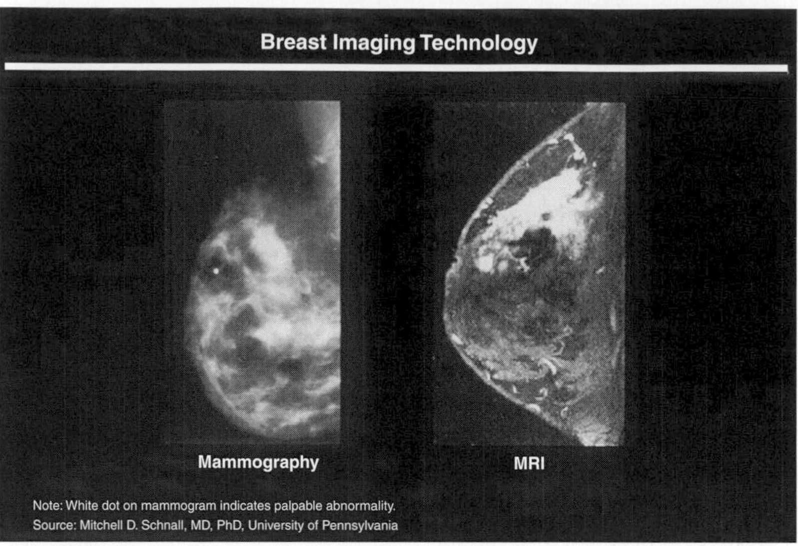

Figure 4-5 Breast Mammography Compared With MRI.
Courtesy of the National Cancer Institute.

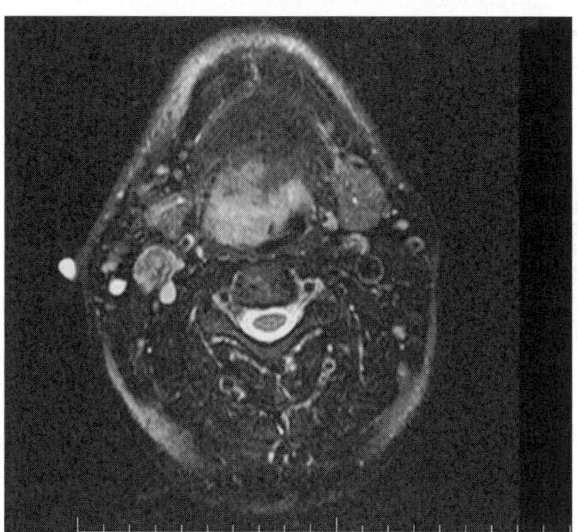

Figure 4-6 Head/Neck MRI. Large exophytic mass in right base of tongue, with skin marker placed where mass is palpable.
Courtesy of Virginia Mason Medical Center, Seattle, Wash.

information but metabolic activity.[30] Higher magnetic field scanners are required to achieve improved spectral resolution, enabling separation of metabolite signals. Differences in metabolite ratios, such as choline, creatinine, *N*-acetylaspartate, and citrate, of normal tissues and tumors can be identified.[32] Choline is an indicator of increased cell membrane phospholipids turnover, associated with increased cellularity and tumor cell growth, whereas decreased tumor choline levels have been associated with response to radiation therapy.[28] Therefore, MRSI is proving to be helpful in distinguishing active tumor from normal tissue, edema, or necrosis and may be important in defining the spatial extent and characteristics of tumors.[33]

Positron Emission Testing

Although many imaging techniques quantify anatomic presence of abnormalities, positron emission testing (PET) is unique in that it attempts to assess biologic activity. This unique metabolism-based imaging technique exploits the increased uptake and accumulation of a tracer, commonly fluorine 18-labeled fluorodeoxyglucose (FDG), by metabolically active tissue, such as tumor cells. L-thymidine, antibodies (Immuno-PET), receptor ligands, C-11 methionine, 2-O-[18F]fluoroethyl-L-tyrosine (FET-PET), and other tracers have been used in PET evaluation, but do not yet have a clear role in clinical practice.[34] The radiolabeled tracer emits positrons that are detectable by gamma camera tomography,[2] and the resultant whole body images detect regions of accelerated metabolic activity. FDG uptake is quantified and reported as the standard uptake value (SUV), which is a factor of the metabolic activity of the lesion, the weight of the patient, and the dose of FDG administered (higher SUV indicating greater metabolic activity).

Increased metabolic activity may be evident in PET studies as a result of malignancy, but also may be positive for other benign conditions characterized by highly metabolic states (such as inflammation or infection). Nonetheless, PET may be quite useful in differentiating between benign etiology of a mass lesion, such as fibrosis or radiation necrosis, and malignant tissue. PET scanning also may be useful during staging in the setting of unknown primary site and is known to be sensitive for detection of nodal involvement or distant metastasis in many circumstances. Use of PET during staging of lung and colon has proven to be particularly useful and cost-effective in identifying more extensive disease (up-staging) than other modalities identified, which has a significant impact on changing the treatment plan and avoiding unnecessary surgery.[35,36] Disease responsiveness to treatment can be evaluated using PET technology, because metabolic changes of the tumor may be evident even before structural changes are identified by other means.[37] Restaging evaluation after treatment and evaluation of recurrent disease are other potential uses for PET.[34,37] It is important to remember, however, that with both PET and MRI, uptake may be increased or enhancement for several weeks after invasive procedures (such as biopsy); therefore this should be taken into consideration during test scheduling and when interpreting results.

Although useful in evaluating disease in a number of situations, PET is limited by its relatively poor resolution in comparison with other modalities (poor sensitivity in lesions smaller than 1.2 cm).[34] Additionally, FDG uptake may differ among tumor types, with some tumors exhibiting relatively low uptake of the tracer, potentially leading to false-negative results.

PET/CT Fusion Studies

As previously discussed, CT scanning is an excellent imaging modality, but does not differentiate metabolically active from metabolically inactive tissues, whereas PET identifies areas of heightened metabolic activity but provides relatively poor anatomic precision. Technology allowing the computerized "fusion" of the two imaging modalities is proving to be quite useful clinically and appears to be more accurate in lesion localization than does use of PET independently along with CT or MRI.[38] PET images revealing increased metabolic activity are overlaid onto CT images, correlating the exact localization of functional abnormality with anatomic definition. This capability is particularly useful for surgical and radiation planning (Figure 4-7). The feasibility of using fused PET/CT images in intensity modulated radiation therapy (IMRT) planning has been investigated, and may hold promise in tailoring dose to physiologic activity and attention to areas containing proliferating tumor burden.[39]

Radionuclide Bone Scan (Skeletal Scintigraphy)

Whole body bone scan (WBBS) is a useful imaging modality when concern for skeletal metastasis exists and is generally preferred over PET for bone evaluation. Sensitivity for identifying metastatic bone involvement in non–small cell lung cancer has been reported at 87%.[40] Furthermore, bone scintigraphy is sensitive even in the presence of early bone metastasis (before development of bony pain) and often is capable of identifying lesions sooner than other radiographic methods.[41] Clinical factors that may increase suspicion of bone metastasis may include bone pain/tenderness, elevated alkaline phosphatase, and/or elevated serum calcium levels, particularly in patients with malignancies demonstrating a pattern of bone involvement (such as breast, lung, prostate, melanoma, and others).[42]

Bone scan may be performed during part of the initial staging evaluation in certain high-risk patients to ensure no evidence of metastatic disease is present before surgical resection (such as in prostate or lung cancer) or after initial treatment for evaluation of new bony complaints; it is also an appropriate test to help determine the presence of direct osseous invasion from the primary tumor. Evidence suggests that in non–small cell lung cancer, staging bone scintigraphy done routinely at diagnosis accurately identified 14% to 22% of patients with advanced disease that would otherwise not have been recognized if bone scan had been performed only in the presence of suspicious symptoms, therefore improving appropriate selection of patients eligible for definitive treatment.[40]

Skeletal scintigraphy uses injected ^{99}Tc-labeled phosphonates taken up by areas of high osteoblastic

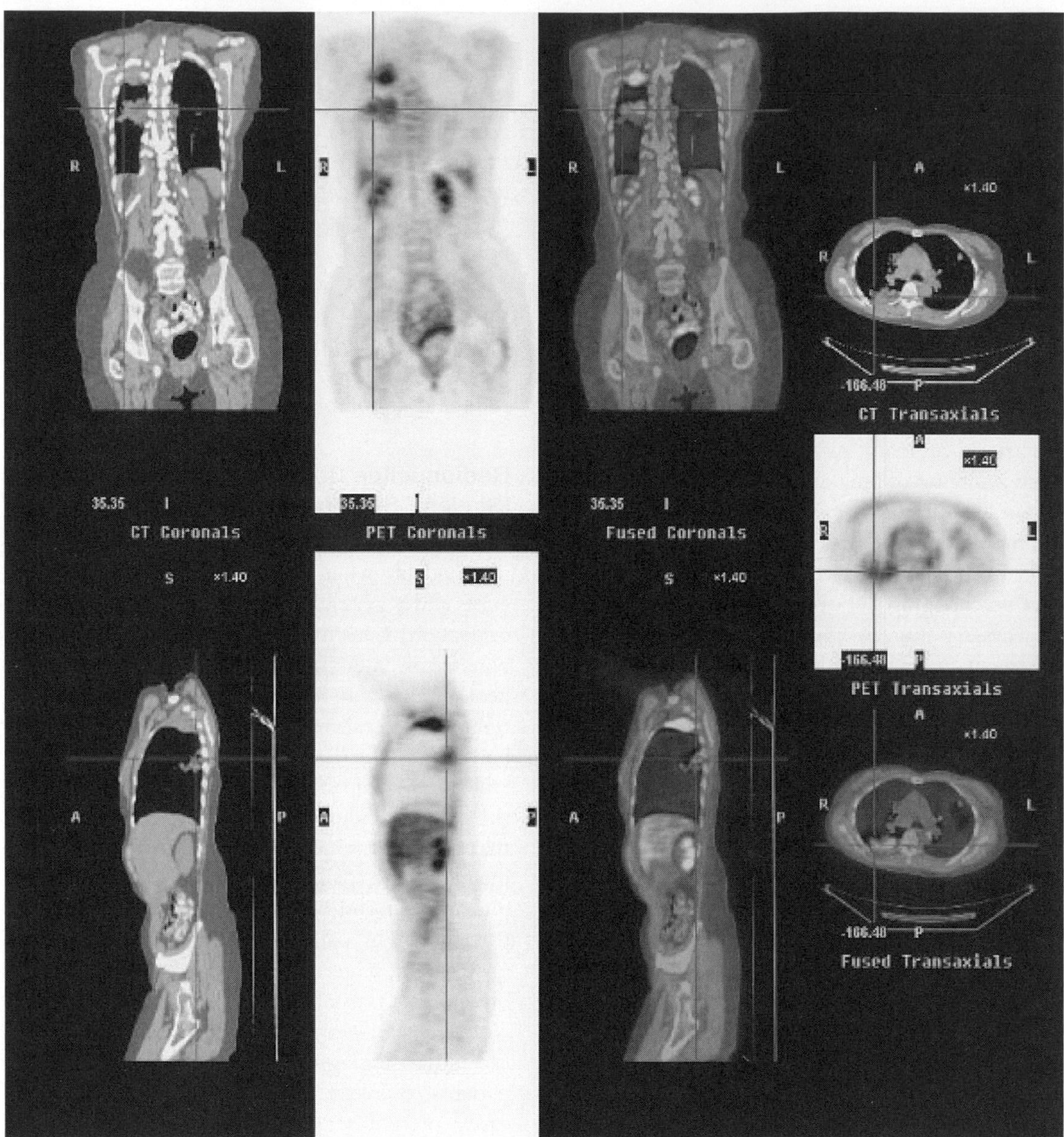

Figure 4-7 PET/CT Fusion. CT demonstrates a right upper lung mass, with PET confirming abnormal increased uptake in the corresponding region. An inferior right hilar metastatic lesion also is evident on both the CT and PET.
Courtesy of Virginia Mason Medical Center, Seattle, Wash.

(bone formation) activity, which can then be visualized. Tracer uptake is also influenced by local blood flow.[43] Although most bone lesions are osteoblastic in nature, bone scan is also effective in evaluating predominantly lytic lesions, which will induce attempt at bone repair resulting in tracer accumulation.[43] Bone scan has been proven to be more sensitive than standard radiographic imaging in detecting both sclerotic and lytic metastatic lesions.[34] Plain film radiography is generally preferred in the setting of multiple myeloma (characterized by lytic lesions), because bone scan is less sensitive in detecting small myelomatous lesions in most locations except the ribs.[44]

False-positive results may occur in the presence of osteoarthritis, trauma, surgery, and other benign bone disorders, and so results must be interpreted in a manner consistent with other known clinical history, radiographic tests, and physical exam findings.[42]

SUMMARY

Accurate and thorough diagnosis of malignancy is a team effort, often requiring the expertise of a variety of specialists and other members of the healthcare team. Oncology nurses are particularly suited to assist patients through this process, guiding and reassuring patients through what may seem to be a complicated maze of tests and procedures. Understanding the principles and rationale for diagnostic strategies, and how to prepare patients for such tests and what to tell them to expect during the procedure can be invaluable. Additionally, oncology nurses are often an important resource for patients regarding understanding the significance of test results and making sense of their diagnosis.

An understanding of the principles of staging and risk assessment are important not only for fully understanding the patient's diagnosis but also for their treatment. Staging results will guide the options available to the patient, and the oncology nurse may be important in helping the patient understand the rationale for the selected therapy. Knowledge of imaging and staging principles is particularly pertinent to radiation oncology nurses, because it is necessary in order to anticipate the prescribed treatment field to be encompassed and accurately advise the patient about what toxicities may be expected.

As technology advances and diagnostic modalities become more sophisticated, nuances in staging may become more complex. Although the current staging classification is based predominantly on the anatomic involvement of disease, the future will likely see more integration of "biologic staging" criteria as more implications of these as prognostic indicators are understood. More specific tumor identification techniques (proteomics and molecular and genetic profiling) will continue to evolve, along with the expansion of imaging modalities, including variations of functional, anatomic and three-dimensional imaging techniques. Clearly, the emerging role of biologic evaluation of malignancy (both pathologically and radiographically) promises to revolutionize understanding of tumor classification and treatment in the years to come.

REFERENCES

1. Jemal A, Murray T, Ward E: Cancer statistics, 2005, *CA: Cancer J Clin* 56(1):10-30, 2005.
2. Griffin-Brown J: Diagnostic evaluation, classification, and staging. In Yarbro, Frogge, Goodman, Groenwald, editors: *Cancer nursing principles and practice,* ed 5, Boston, 2000, Jones and Bartlett, pp 214-239.
3. Gospodarowicz MK, Miller D, Groome PA et al: The process for continuous improvement of the TNM classification, *Cancer* 100(1):1-5, 2004.
4. Greene FL, Page DL, Fleming ID et al, editors. *AJCC cancer staging manual,* ed 6, New York, 2002, Springer-Verlag, pp 3-8.
5. Rubin P, Chen Y, Brasacchio RA: Staging and classification of the cancer and the host: a unified approach versus neotaxonomy. In Perez CA, Brady LW, editors: *Principles and practice of radiation oncology,* ed 3, Philadelphia, 1997, Lippincott-Raven, pp 213-229.
6. Compton CC: Pathologic staging of colorectal cancer: an advanced users' guide, *Pathology Case Reviews* 9(4): 150-162, 2004.
7. Borowitz M, Westra W, Cooley LD et al: Pathology and laboratory medicine. In Abeloff MD, Armitage JO, Niederhuber JE, et al, editors: *Clinical oncology,* ed 3, Philadelphia, 2004, Churchill Livingstone, pp 299-319.
8. Wilbur F: Diagnosis of lung cancer: pathology of invasive and preinvasive neoplasia, *Chest* 117(4), Suppl 1:80S-89S, 2000.
9. Schmalbach CE, Chepeha DB, Giordano TJ et al: Molecular profiling and the identification of genes associated with metastatic oral cavity/pharynx squamous cell carcinoma, *Arch Otolaryngol Head Neck Surg* 130(3): 295-303, 2004.
10. Brown J, Xu H, Nishitani J et al: Potential biomarkers for head and neck squamous cell carcinoma, *Laryngoscope* 113(3):393-400, 2003.
11. Partridge M, Gaballah K, Huang X: Molecular markers for diagnosis and prognosis, *Cancer Metastasis Rev* 24(1):71-85, 2005.
12. Geschwind JH: Interventional radiology. In DeVita VT, Hellman S, Rosenberg SA, editors: *Cancer: principles & practice of oncology,* ed 6, Philadelphia, 2001, Lippincott Williams & Wilkins, pp 690-707.
13. Fishman EK, Urban BA: Cancer diagnosis: imaging. In DeVita VT, Hellman S, Rosenberg SA, editors: *Cancer: principles & practice of oncology,* ed 6, Philadelphia, 2001, Lippincott Williams & Wilkins, pp 659-719.
14. Guler SA: Sentinel node biopsy in head and neck cancer, *Am J Oncol Rev* 4(1):23-24, 2005.
15. Ross GL: Sentinel node biopsy in the management and staging of the N0 neck in head and neck squamous cell carcinoma, *Am J Oncol Rev* 4(1):16-22, 2005.

16. Reynolds T: Updates to staging system reflect advances in imaging, understanding, *J Natl Cancer Inst* 94(22):1664-1666, 2002.
17. DiMartino E, Nowak B, Hassan HA et al: Diagnosis and staging of head and neck cancer: a comparison of modern imaging modalities (positron emission tomography, computed tomography, color-coded duplex sonography) with panendoscopic and histopathologic findings, *Arch Otolaryngol Head Neck Surg* 126(12):1457-1462, 2000.
18. Kurtz R, Ginsberg RJ: Cancer diagnosis: endoscopy. In DeVita VT, Hellman S, Rosenberg SA, editors: *Cancer: principles & practice of oncology,* ed 6, Philadelphia, 2001, Lippincott Williams & Wilkins, pp 721-737.
19. Li CZ: Viewing the small intestine via capsule endoscopy, *Nursing* 34(4):70-71, 2004.
20. Scible SL, Anwer MB: Detecting a small bowel tumor via wireless capsule endoscopy: a clinical case study, *Gastroenterol Nurs* 27(3):118-120, 2004.
21. Eliakim R: Wireless capsule video endoscopy: three years of experience, *World J Gastroenterol* 10(9):1238-1239, 2004.
22. Bhutani MS, Jones Jr DV, Zwischenberger JB: Endoscopic ultrasound-guided fine-needle aspiration staging of lung cancer: is it time to go beyond cytology? *Chest* 127(2):418-421, 2005.
23. Fritscher-Ravens A, Petrasch S, Reinacher-Schick A: Diagnostic value of endoscopic ultrasonography-guided fine-needle aspiration cytology of mediastinal masses in patients with intrapulmonary lesions and nondiagnostic bronchoscopy, *Respiration* 66(2):150-155, 1999.
24. McGinley P, Kilpatrick E: Tumour markers: their use and misuse by clinicians, *Ann Clin Biochem* 40(6):643, 2003.
25. Sokoll J, Chan DW: Clinical chemistry: tumor markers. In Abeloff MD, Armitage JO, Niederhuber JE, et al, editors: *Clinical oncology,* ed 3, Philadelphia, 2004, Churchill Livingstone, pp 329-337.
26. Moss EL, Hollingworth J, Reynolds TM: The role of CA125 in clinical practice, *J Clin Pathol* 58(3):308-312, 2005.
27. Brant WE: Diagnostic imaging methods. In Brant WE, Helms CA, editors: *Fundamentals of diagnostic radiology,* ed 2, Philadelphia, 1999, Lippincott Williams & Wilkins, pp 3-21.
28. Hricak H, Akin O, Bradburg MS et al: Advanced imaging modalities. In DeVita VT, Hellman S, Rosenberg SA, editors: *Cancer: principles & practice of oncology,* ed 7, Philadelphia, 2005, Lippincott Williams & Wilkins, pp 589-617.
29. Maniatis P, Triantopoulou C, Sofianou E et al: Virtual CT cholangiography in patients with choledocholithiasis, *Abdom Imaging* 28(4):536-544, 2003.
30. Coakley F, Oavvum A, Kurhanewicz J et al: Magnetic resonance imaging and spectroscopic imaging of prostate cancer, *J Urol* 170(6Pt 2):S69-S76, 2003.
31. Davidson D: Novel breast-imaging modalities, *Clin J Oncol Nurs* 9(2):255-256, 2005.
32. Greene K, Coakley F, Kurhanewicz J et al: Endorectal MRI: when to consider in PCa detection, *Urology Times* 33(1):24-25, 2005.
33. Chiang IC, Kuo YT, Lu CY et al: Distinction between high-grade gliomas and solitary metastases using peritumoral 3-T magnetic resonance spectroscopy diffusion, and perfusion imagings, *Neuroradiology* 46(8):619-627, 2004.
34. Baum RP, Hellwig D, Mezzetti M: Position of nuclear medicine modalities in the diagnostic workup of cancer patients: lung cancer, *Q J Nucl Med Mol Imaging* 48(2):119-133, 2004.
35. Delbeke D: Oncological applications of FDG PET imaging, *J Nucl Med* 40(10):1706-1715, 1999.
36. Hubner KF: Can ^{11}C-methionine play a role in lung cancer staging? *J Nucl Med* 41(2):291-292, 2000.
37. Flamen P: Positron emission tomography in gastric and esophageal cancer. *Curr Opin Oncol* 16(4):359-363, 2004.
38. Pelosi E, Messa C, Sironi S et al: Value of integrated PET/CT for lesion localization in cancer patients: a comparative study, *Eur J Nucl Med Mol Imaging* 31(7):932-939, 2004.
39. Scarfone C, Lavely WC, Cmelak AJ et al: Prospective feasibility trial of radiotherapy target definition for head and neck cancer using 3-dimensional PET and CT imaging, *J Nucl Med* 45(4):543-553, 2004.
40. Schirrmeister H, Arslandemir C, Glatting G: Omission of bone scanning according to staging guidelines leads to futile therapy in non–small cell lung cancer, *Eur J Nucl Med Mol Imaging* 31(7):964-968, 2004.
41. Maffioli L, Florimonte L, Pagani L et al: Current role of bone scan with phosphonates in the follow-up of breast cancer, *Eur J Nucl Med Mol Imaging* 31(Suppl 1):S143-S148, 2004.
42. Erturan S, Yaman M, Aydin G et al: The role of whole-body bone scanning and clinical factors in detecting bone metastases in patients with non–small cell lung cancer, *Chest* 127(2):449-455, 2005.
43. O'Sullivan JM, Cook GJR: A review of the efficacy of bone scanning in prostate and breast cancer, *Q J Nucl Med* 46(2):152-160, 2002.
44. Sohn SK, Ahn BC, Lee SW et al: Bone marrow immuno-scintigraphy using technetium-99m anti-granulocyte anti-body in multiple myeloma, *Eur J Nucl Med Mol Imaging* 29(5):591-596, 2002.

Chapter 5

Simulation and Treatment Planning

Kim L. Light

The goal of radiation therapy is to irradiate a predefined target volume while minimizing exposure to adjacent normal tissues. However, this goal can often be difficult to achieve. Ideally, the radiation beams should fully encompass the target and avoid all the normal tissue structures. In reality, the target volume usually lies adjacent to normal tissue structures. Most treatment fields are designed to treat the target volume with a margin that accounts for treatment uncertainties such as target delineation, organ motion, and daily set-up errors. The margins placed on the target volume should be as small as possible, without compromising the target coverage, while considering normal tissues.

The radiation oncologist collaborates with surgeons and medical oncologists to determine the overall treatment course for each patient. With the aid of diagnostic x rays, computed tomography (CT), magnetic resonance imaging (MRI), positron emission tomography (PET) scans and other diagnostic procedures, the radiation oncologist defines the treatment volume and prescribes the dose of radiation to be delivered. The dosimetrist or physicist works closely with the radiation oncologist to generate a treatment plan that uses the best beam arrangement to treat the target volume and spare adjacent normal tissue. The radiation oncologist, along with the radiation oncology clinician, monitors the patient for normal-tissue reactions throughout the course of radiation treatment and also in posttreatment follow-up visits.

The treatment prescription includes the anatomic site, treatment technique, radiation beam type and energy, total radiation dose, daily radiation dose, and number of fractions. The treatment technique can vary from a single radiation field, used to treat fairly superficial areas such as the supraclavicular area, to multiple fields needed to treat deeper targets. Angled or oblique beams also may be used to avoid the spinal cord or to decrease the dose to another normal-tissue structure while treating the target to higher doses.

Radiation beams are typically either photons or electrons. Photon energies vary from 4 to 20 MV (megavolt). The energy chosen depends on the target location, patient thickness, and number of beams being used. Higher energies are usually used for thicker parts of the body whereas lower energies are used when treating thinner body parts or targets closer to the skin surface. Lower energy photons are used when treating head-and-neck cancers where nodal tissue also may be involved. Electron beam energies range from 5 to 22 MeV (mega electron volts) and decrease rapidly after reaching the maximum dose (Figure 5-1). Electron treatment is typically used to treat superficial targets, such as skin cancer or lymph nodes. Selection of the electron energy is usually chosen so that the deepest part of the target receives the prescription dose and normal tissue deeper to this point is spared. Different thicknesses of bolus material, which is a tissue-equivalent material, are sometimes placed on the skin surface to increase the skin dose. Superflab is a commonly used bolus material that is available in different thicknesses. Wet gauze also may be used. Bolus material is typically used when treating with higher-energy photon beams or lower-energy electron beams. The bolus material is pliable and conforms to the curvature of the patient's skin surface.[1,2]

IMMOBILIZATION

The treatment planning process is usually initiated with a conventional simulation, CT simulation, or treatment planning CT. The radiation oncologist decides which procedure is needed, depending on the tumor type, tumor location, treatment technique, and extent of the disease. The clinician provides an in-depth description of the simulation and planning process to the patient, reinforcing

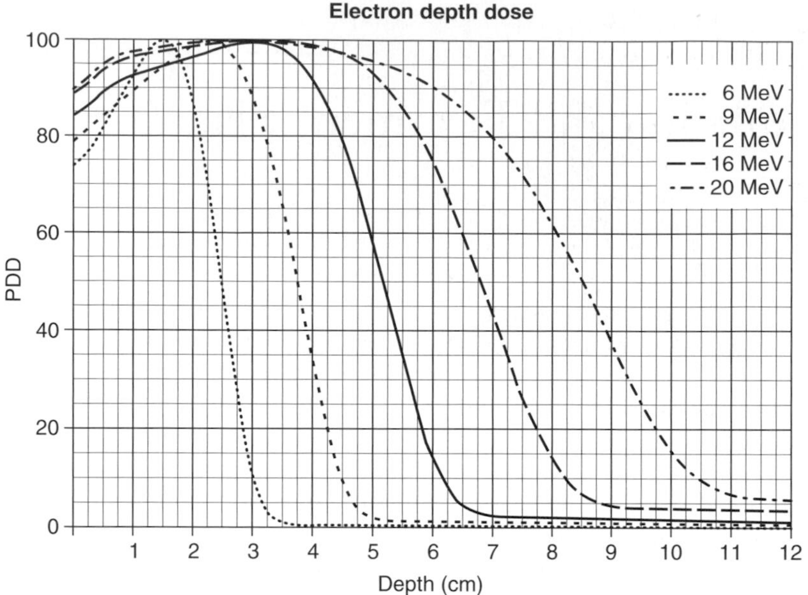

Figure 5-1 Electron Depth Dose.

and supplementing the information given by the radiation oncologist.

Regardless of which procedure is selected, it is important that the patient be adequately positioned and immobilized to ensure accurate daily setup. This is especially important with pediatric patients who may have trouble holding still during the planning stages and treatment delivery.[3] Various studies have been done to evaluate different patient positions and immobilization techniques. If the patient is not positioned properly, radiation-field placement errors may reduce the prescribed dose to the target volume. The dose-response curve for many types of tumors is steep, and a small error in dose can decrease tumor control.[4-7] Immobilization devices reduce such errors by maintaining the patient in the proper position for each treatment. A simple but important issue to consider in treatment positioning is the patient's comfort and ability to maintain the position on a daily basis. An uncomfortable position is always difficult for the patient to maintain during daily treatments, and also can be difficult to replicate for each treatment session.[8]

Immobilization devices may be simple or complex. Many commercially available "simple" immobilization devices can assist with the daily setup of the patient position. Although these devices are not customized to the individual patient, they may be adequate to immobilize a patient being treated palliatively with relatively simple treatment fields.

When the target volume is located adjacent to radiosensitive structures and the treatment plan is more complex, a more rigid immobilization device is recommended. For example, when the head-and-neck region is irradiated, multiple matching fields are sometimes used. The frequency of treatment field misalignment in head-and-neck irradiation has been well documented.[8-10] Unless the head and neck area is adequately immobilized, critical nontarget tissues (eyes, optic nerves, optic chiasm, and spinal cord) could be inadvertently irradiated, causing complications. Therefore, a customized immobilization cushion is usually made to support and maintain the patient's head and neck in a reproducible position. This customized cushion is molded around the patient's head, neck, and shoulders while the patient is lying in the desired position for treatment. In addition, a mask may be draped across the patient's face and attached to a base plate that is fixed to the treatment table. This provides a "sandwich immobilization" in both the anterior and posterior directions and allows treatment and setup marks to be made directly on the mask, instead of the patient's skin (Figure 5-2). A bite block also may be used with the head immobilization device to keep the patient's mouth open during treatment. The bite block is useful to

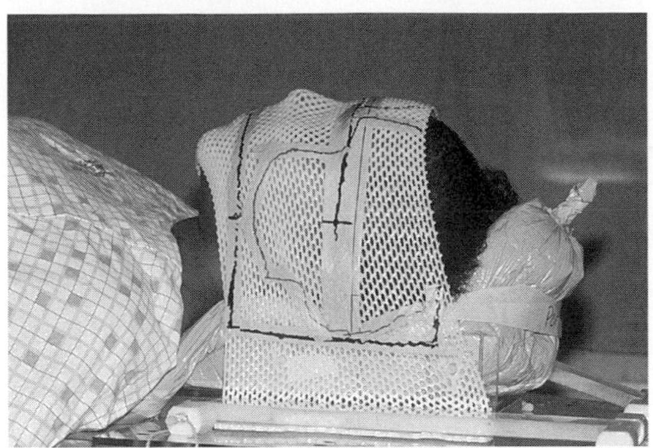

Figure 5-2 Head Mask With Treatment Marks.

increase the separation between the maxilla/hard palate and the mandible/tongue such that radiation exposure to one site can be reduced by targeting the other. For example, when treating the maxillary sinus, the bite block displaces the tongue and mandible inferiorly away from the beam. Similarly, if the floor of the mouth area is targeted, the soft palate can be spared by moving it superiorly.

For body immobilization, Alpha Cradle (Smithers Medical Products, Inc., Akron, Ohio) molds are a popular and reproducible means of immobilizing the patient. A polystyrene bag is filled with chemicals that react and expand into foam. When the patient lies down on the bag, the foam molds around the body or body part. The nursing or technical staff should explain this process ahead of time and inform patients that the chemical mixture may feel warm when they lie on top of the bag. The Alpha Cradle molds around the patient's body or extremity to create a customized immobilization device. The cradle is individually fitted for each patient and can be used only for that one patient's course of treatment. Vacuum bags also may be used to immobilize patients. Vacuum bags, consisting of a bag filled with Styrofoam or plastic beads that mold themselves around the patient, may be refitted and reused to immobilize several different patients.

These body immobilization devices can be used to immobilize patients being treated for prostate, lung, and breast cancer, as well as many other treatment areas. They are useful in positioning patients in awkward or "unnatural" positions when necessary for treatment. Extremity irradiation, used to treat a sarcoma in the leg, is an example of the need to position a patient with the extremity turned outward or in an unusual direction. Occasionally, the unaffected limb may be in the way of the radiation beam if the extremity is left in a neutral position. By rotating the extremity and adequately immobilizing it, muscle compartments may be spared. An immobilization device will help maintain the extremity in a particular position to facilitate the desired beam direction.[8,11]

Immobilization devices have been shown to slightly increase the skin reaction to irradiation when treating through them. The immobilization device can act as "bolus" and increase the skin dose. This is related to the beam energy, total dose, type of immobilization device, and treatment technique used. The degree of skin reaction usually increases when using a low-photon energy, such as 4 MV, and when treating through a thick section of the immobilization device.[8]

Customized immobilization allows alignment marks to be placed on the device instead of just on the skin, which can be mobile. Skin moves over underlying tissues, so marks on the skin may not be totally reliable. Skin marks also tend to smear and fade, even when the therapist reinforces the marks daily. The use of alignment marks on the immobilization device eliminates some of the problems with reliance on skin marks and also ensures that the device is positioned on the table the same way for each treatment. This improves patient setup and treatment accuracy.[1,2,8] Patients are not always receptive to skin markings, especially on the face, but basic alignment marks are crucial for accurate treatment setup. The nursing staff should discuss the importance of the skin marks with patients and instruct them about proper skin care in the treatment area during their course of radiation treatment. Once the treatment fields have been confirmed on the treatment machine, small permanent marks (tattoos) are made to indicate the center and edges of the treatment field. These tattoos are used for daily setup and are helpful for duplicating treatment fields if the patient returns for treatment in the future.

2-D CONVENTIONAL SIMULATION

A simulator is a machine with geometry similar to a radiation therapy treatment machine, but it uses low-energy x rays and fluoroscopy like that of a diagnostic x-ray machine. The simulator also can mimic the motions of the treatment machine that will deliver the patient's daily treatment.

During conventional simulation, the ideal patient position, treatment fields, and the optimal beam directions are selected. If needed, an immobilization device is constructed during simulation. The patient removes all clothing and jewelry in the affected area and usually wears a hospital gown, which is moved away from the treatment area before the immobilization device is constructed. It is very important that there is no clothing between the patient's body and the immobilization device when making the device because the same clothing is not worn each day. Even the small difference caused by wearing different clothing can affect treatment setup accuracy on a day-to-day basis.

BB markers or solder wire may be placed on the patient's skin before filming to mark target volume areas, normal tissue structures such as the eyes, or surgical scars. These markers are visible on the film to help with the field setup. The isocenter, or center of the treatment field (CAX), is usually placed in the center of the target volume or body structure. Two or more fields may be used to treat the target volume. Sometimes, multiple fields are matched to each other to treat larger areas, such as when the lateral necks and anterior supraclavicular area are treated. Once the treatment fields are verified, the field dimensions are marked on the device and on the patient's skin with a temporary marker.

The radiation oncologist approves the treatment fields and draws shielding blocks on the film to block normal tissues from the radiation beam. A graticle (measuring tool) inside the simulator is displayed on the films to assist the radiation oncologist in drawing the blocks after manually drawing the target on the films. The shielding blocks may be constructed from Cerrobend (a metal alloy) and then attached to a Plexiglas tray that is inserted into the treatment machine each day during treatment. A multileaf collimator (MLC) mounted inside the head of the treatment machine also may be used for field shaping. MLCs are mounted on either side of the treatment machine jaws and consist of thin leaves of tungsten. The leaves are operated by motors and can be moved to match the field shape of the desired treatment field drawn by the radiation oncologist. An advantage of an MLC over Cerrobend blocks is that the field shape can be quickly and easily adjusted, if necessary (Figure 5-3).

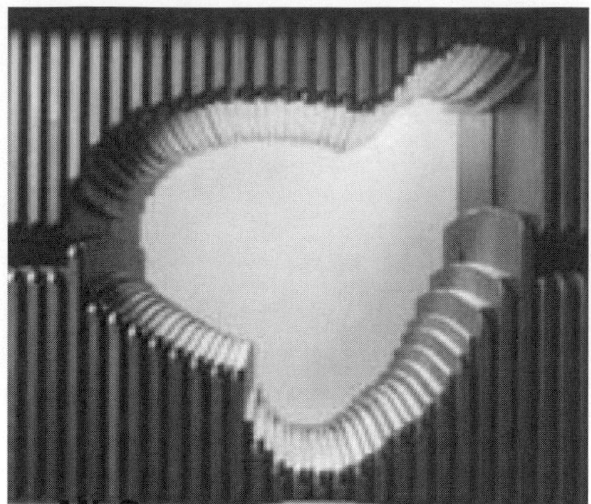

Figure 5-3 Multileaf Collimator.

Initial (primary) fields are simulated to treat the target volume and nodal tissue or areas of potential microscopic disease. The size of the treatment field is usually reduced several times to focus more dose to the gross tumor volume (GTV). If the same treatment angles will be used for the field reduction (boost), blocking is usually drawn on the same film with a different color marker to clearly distinguish sets of fields receiving different radiation doses.

CT-SIMULATION

The CT-simulation combines CT imaging and simulation into one session. The immobilization device is made in the CT-simulator room, and volumetric CT images are acquired. The CT data are reconstructed, and radiographic images are digitally generated and displayed on the computer screen. Target volumes and normal tissues can be contoured on these images and displayed in a "beam's eye view" of the treatment field for more accurate field shaping around the target area. The CT-simulation process is considered more accurate because it minimizes uncertainties in registration of CT images with conventional simulation films that are taken during two different sessions.[12]

2-D TREATMENT PLANNING

Once the simulation and/or CT procedure is completed, a treatment plan may be needed. A common field arrangement in radiation therapy is "parallel opposed fields." This technique delivers a fairly homogeneous dose from the entry point to the exit point of both beams. Multiple treatment fields also may be used to "spread" the dose out more and spare normal tissues. An example of this is a four-field pelvis treatment where the bladder and rectum can be spared more effectively in the lateral fields than in the AP–PA fields (anterior-posterior). A contour of the patient's body through the center of the fields is usually obtained from CT. The dosimetrist inputs into the planning computer the field shapes from all four fields, which the radiation oncologist has drawn on the computer or on the simulation films, and then calculates a dose distribution. Equally weighted, higher-energy photon beams (15 MV) are normally used to give a homogeneous dose through the treatment area and also to limit the dose to the normal tissue in the entrance and exit areas of the beams. When higher-energy beams are not available, unequal beam weights (unequal doses) may be used for the treatment fields to reduce dose in the entrance/exit regions and to make the dose distribution fairly uniform.

Wedges, or beam modifiers, also may be inserted within the path of the beam to improve the dose uniformity. Wedges, commercially available in various angles from 15 to 60 degrees, attenuate the beam progressively across the field. The thicker parts of the wedge attenuate the beam more than the thinner parts. The appropriate wedge is chosen to deliver the most uniform dose distribution. Each treatment day, the therapist places the wedge in the appropriate position to modify the beam.

3-D CONFORMAL TREATMENT PLANNING

Some specific tumors or treatment sites require more conformal planning than conventional simulation can provide. Difficulty in identifying the relationship between structures sometimes limits the radiation oncologist's ability to choose optimal beam angles when using a conventional fluoroscopic simulation. Three-dimensional (3-D) conformal planning attempts to limit the prescription dose to the 3-D shape of the target volume while delivering lower doses to the nontarget normal tissues.[13-17] With 3-D planning, smaller margins around target volumes are often used, thus rigid immobilization is recommended.

The immobilization device is constructed during the CT procedure. The treatment planning CT is done with CT slices ranging from 2 to 5 mm thick. Intravenous contrast is sometimes injected to better visualize the tumor and normal structures. In some radiation oncology clinics, it is the clinician's role to start the IV line and then push the contrast. Education and competency regarding IV starts, IV contrast risks, and knowledge about adverse reaction management are all important responsibilities of the clinician. Setup or alignment marks are drawn on the patient's skin and on the immobilization device. The patient may then leave the radiation oncology clinic.

The planning proceeds on a computer system, based on the three-dimensional images. During the planning process, the radiation oncologist and the dosimetrist or physicist work together to define volumes. It is important that all volumes to be considered are "drawn" on the computer during this stage of the planning process. If a structure is not contoured, it may be forgotten later during planning. The planning CT is displayed on the computer monitor, and the target and normal tissue volumes are outlined on the computer screen, using a computer mouse. The radiation oncologist may request fusion with other diagnostic studies such as magnetic resonance imaging (MRI), positron emission tomography (PET), or single photon emission computed tomography (SPECT). Fusion with a diagnostic scan is sometimes required to better define the target volume. MRI scans provide excellent soft-tissue contrast and are used for outlining target and normal tissue structures. PET and SPECT scans give detailed functional information that may be used during the planning process. The fused image is then displayed on the computer screen, aligned with the planning CT, and the radiation oncologist "draws" the target volume directly onto the MRI, PET, or SPECT scan.[12,18,19]

It is very important that the terms used during the planning process be consistent and clearly understood by everyone. The International Commission on Radiation Units and Measurements recommends standard target volume terms and definitions to be used during the planning process[20]:

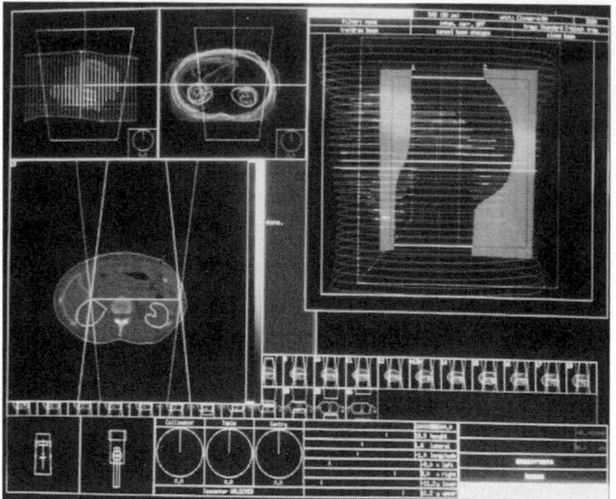

Figure 5-4 3-D Virtual Simulation.

- Gross tumor volume (GTV) = gross palpable or demonstrable tumor
- Clinical target volume (CTV) = GTV + subclinical disease, such as lymph nodes, etc.
- Planning target volume (PTV) = CTV + margins for geometric uncertainties, such as organ motion

The 3-D treatment planning system includes a "virtual simulator" that simulates all of the motions of the treatment machine. The gantry, collimator, and couch can all be rotated independently during the virtual simulation to achieve axial and nonaxial beams (Figure 5-4). Nonaxial beams often provide increased separation between a target and normal tissue, such as in lung cancer in the left lower lobe where the heart may otherwise receive an increased dose using a more conventional AP–PA technique (anterior-posterior = AP, posterior-anterior = PA). While rotating the beam in different directions on the computer, the treatment area is displayed through the beam's eye view (BEV). The BEV displays all of the anatomic structures and target volumes drawn on the individual CT images. The patient can be simultaneously "turned" in space around all three axes, making it easier to choose a beam direction that maximally avoids irradiating normal tissue. Once the beam direction is chosen, the radiation oncologist defines the field shape either by defining a specific margin around the target volume or by drawing the field shape with the computer mouse. A combination of beam energies, wedges, and beam weighting is selected in order to devise the most optimal plan possible.

The planning system performs a 3-D–volume calculation of the plan, and the dose distribution is superimposed onto the CT images. The radiation oncologist can view the dose distribution on the computer screen or on a printed treatment plan. A dose-volume histogram (DVH) of target volumes and normal tissues is calculated for review. The DVH plots the percentage of volume of the vertical *(y)* axis that receives a dose equal to or greater than the dose indicated on the horizontal (*x*) axis (Figure 5-5). Several different potential plans may be devised to determine the best treatment approach. The radiation oncologist can view the dose

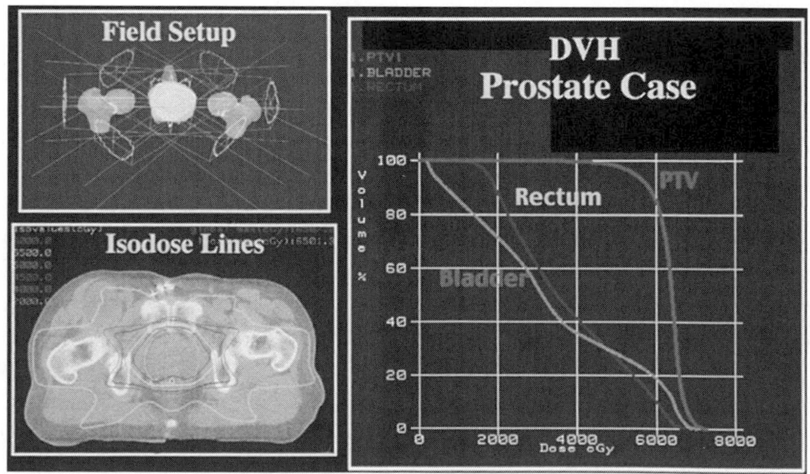

Figure 5-5 Dose Volume Histograms for Prostate.

contribution that each structure contoured will receive on the DVH graph.

Digitally reconstructed radiographs (DRR's) are generated from the CT data set that shows the field shape and structures contoured on the planning system. These are used just like conventional simulation films to document the planned treatment fields, so it is not always necessary for the patient to have a conventional simulation.[21] However, in some instances such as radiation therapy for lung cancer where respiratory movements may not be thoroughly appreciated from the 3-D CT data set, a physical simulation is also done to visualize the field and target under fluoroscopy.

If a physical simulation is not performed, the isocenter position must be checked for accuracy before the first day of treatment. Port films of the setup fields and treatment fields are taken either with the treatment machine or by electronic online portal imaging in order to verify that the patient is aligned accurately according to the plan.

INTENSITY-MODULATED TREATMENT PLANNING

In conventional 2-D or 3-D external beam radiation therapy, the radiation beams are aimed at the target and consequently may also treat normal tissue structures. As discussed, 3-D treatment planning is more complex than 2-D treatment planning, but the processes of beam selection and plan optimization for both methods are similar. With intensity-modulated radiation therapy (IMRT), the radiation is distributed among thousands of tiny beams of nonuniform intensities that enter the body from many angles to converge upon the target area and to spare normal tissue structures. Different levels of dose are delivered to different parts of the tumor. IMRT often allows greater radiation dose delivery than is possible with conventional or 3-D treatment planning because flexibility in how to distribute the dose is increased.[12,22,23] For instance, IMRT permits a higher dose to be delivered to prostate cancer targets while maintaining acceptable toxicity levels to the bladder, urethra, and rectum.[24-26] Many studies have shown that IMRT is especially useful in treating tumors in the nasopharynx and head-and-neck area.[27-35] IMRT also has been shown to improve target coverage in situations where concave tumors are surrounded by normal tissue because the treatment dose can be limited by the radiation dose tolerance of the closely surrounding normal tissue.[12,30,36-38] More recently, IMRT has been used also for breast cancer radiation treatment planning, as well as other treatment sites.[8,24,32,33,36]

The IMRT planning process also begins with the immobilization process, and a CT scan is done with 2- to 3-mm scan thicknesses. The immobilization technique used must rigidly immobilize the patient because even a small misalignment of the beams may miss the target volume and significantly increase the dose to normal tissues.[8,28,39-43] When treating head-and-neck cancer with IMRT, accurate immobilization is a necessity. Studies have shown that conventional techniques averaged a setup error of 2 to 3 mm.[8-10] This degree of setup error is not acceptable with head-and-neck IMRT because normal tissues, such as parotid glands and optic structures, may receive much higher doses than prescribed because of the steep dose gradient with the IMRT plan. The problems associated with organ motion that can cause the setup to be incorrect are even more pronounced with IMRT than conventional or 3-D treatment planning. During organ motion such as respiration, the target volume may move in and out of the high and low dose regions created with the IMRT plan. Current research is underway to investigate methods of controlling organ motion during IMRT planning and treatment.[41-44]

Next, the radiation oncologist, along with the dosimetrist or physicist, outlines target volumes and normal tissue structures on the computer. The radiation oncologist prescribes the minimum dose to the target volume(s) and also prescribes the maximum allowable dose to normal tissue structures. It is very important that all normal tissue structures are outlined so that the radiation oncologist can set *dose constraints* (dose limits). If normal tissues are not contoured and included as part of the plan optimization, these structures could receive too much dose. The process of defining doses before planning is called *inverse planning* and is different from 2-D or 3-D planning where the dose is prescribed after planning. In inverse planning, the planning computer adjusts beam shapes and intensities to conform to the target and normal-tissue prescription set by the radiation oncologist. Physical compensators or a multileaf collimator (MLC) modulate the beam intensities and can be moved while the radiation beam is on.

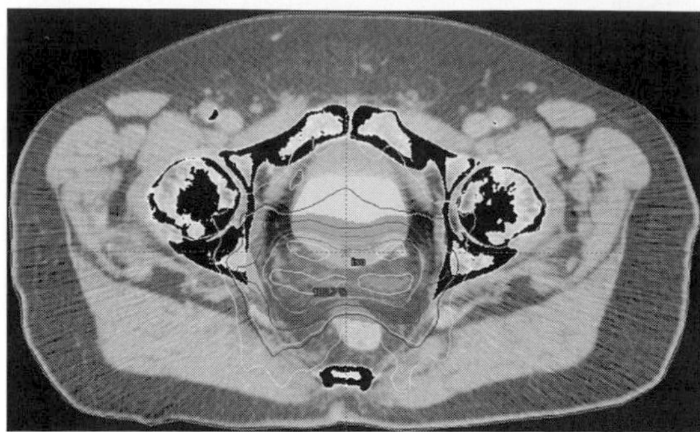

Figure 5-6 IMRT Dose Distribution.

As with 3-D planning, the IMRT dose distribution is superimposed onto the CT image at every slice level and is evaluated (Figure 5-6) along with 3-D volumetric or color-wash rendering of the dose overlaid onto the PTV and critical organs. DVHs of the various structures contoured during the plan evaluation process are also analyzed. The radiation oncologist chooses a plan and approves the field shapes and beam intensities. The medical physicist then performs quality assurance checks on the linear accelerator to verify that the treatment plan and prescription can be accurately delivered.

As discussed, IMRT is a major advance in radiation therapy that allows higher doses to be given while sparing normal tissues. However, as with any new technology, extreme care must be taken when introducing it into a radiation oncology clinic. Each step of the IMRT process must have quality assurance procedures established to ensure accurate and safe treatment delivery. The cost for using IMRT for planning and treatment is expensive. The equipment expense is high, as well as the increased amount of time needed for the radiation oncologist, dosimetrist, and physicist to do the planning. The planning process may take 10 to 12 hours to complete. For these reasons, patients and tumor treatment sites must be carefully selected for use of IMRT.

TREATMENT PLANNING/TREATMENT DELIVERY QUALITY ASSURANCE

For all planning techniques, quality assurance (QA) of the planning process and the daily treatment delivery is vital. This requires teamwork by all members of the radiation oncology clinic. Quality assurance standards written by the American Association of Physicists in Medicine (AAPM) were published in 1994 that suggest various quality assurance procedures for all aspects of the treatment planning and treatment delivery process.[45] Although all AAPM procedures may not be followed exactly in all clinics, written directives for treatment planning, treatment delivery, and quality assurance policies are still necessary.

The patient's treatment chart is used as a communication tool between staff regarding the details and flow of treatment and should be easily accessible to all members of the clinic. The actual treatment chart may be a physical chart or it may be a computer record. Treatment planning parameters, in terms of dose and the area to be treated in the radiation field, must be clearly documented in the patient's chart. The treatment parameters may be entered into a record-and-verify computer system that contains all of the information about the prescription plan. The radiation therapist uses this record-and-verify information during treatment delivery to ensure that all of the planned parameters will be used to treat the patient. Only when all of the parameters defined during setup have been met will the computer allow the treatment to proceed.

An important step in the quality assurance process during treatment delivery is that of making certain the isocenter is positioned exactly as planned. Throughout the course of radiation treatment, port films or electronic imaging are used to verify that the treatment isocenter and treatment fields are aligned correctly. Sometimes specialized QA techniques may be used to verify field placement. For example, for prostate treatment, the radiation therapist may perform a daily ultrasound to localize the prostate for each treatment delivery. Ultrasound information is used to reposition the treatment isocenter in order to follow prostate movement caused by changes in the bladder or rectum. This procedure is easy to perform and takes only an additional 5 minutes. Another localization system uses implantable gold markers placed in different locations within the prostate (ACCULOC, Northwest Medical Physics Equipment, Lynwood, Wash). Electronic portal imaging is used to precisely locate the target in reference to the gold markers. CT images are taken to ensure that the prostate target is within the treatment field for each treatment. This localization system can be used for other treatment sites as well.[46-48]

Daily QA of the treatment chart is performed by the radiation therapist, and weekly chart-check QA is performed by the physicist or dosimetrist. Weekly conferences, attended by radiation oncologists, dosimetrists, physicists, technical staff, and the nursing staff, should be held to review the treatment charts and films. Such conferences provide peer review of patient treatments and can identify inconsistencies between intended and actual treatment delivery. Treatment plans are reviewed in these conferences, as is the rationale for a particular treatment approach. Special-procedures conferences also may be held for detailed review of plans for complex cases, such as those involving 3-D and IMRT treatment.

The total quality management program of a clinic should include an ongoing evaluation of its quality assurance procedures to evaluate their effectiveness. An effective QA program helps provide the safest and most accurate patient treatments possible.

SUMMARY

The clinician is an integral member of the radiation oncology clinic who collaborates with radiation oncologists, medical physicists, dosimetrists, radiation therapists, and other key members of the healthcare team. As stated, the clinician's primary role is to educate patients and their families. The clinician sees patients throughout treatment and follow-up and orchestrates appropriate medical intervention to address issues related to the type of treatment that patients receive. The clinician should immediately communicate patient problems or difficulties to the radiation oncologist during the treatment course and follow-up visits. This is especially important with the newer treatment technologies. The increasing complexity of treatment techniques may cause unanticipated problems for patients that need to be addressed as soon as possible. For these reasons, it is important for the clinician to fully understand the simulation, treatment planning process, and treatment delivery procedures, and to become involved in ongoing clinical QA initiatives.

REFERENCES

1. Bentel CG: *Radiation therapy planning*, ed 2, New York, 1996, McGraw-Hill Publishing.
2. Khan FM: *The physics of radiation therapy*, ed 2, Baltimore Md, 1994, Williams & Wilkins.
3. Halperin EC, Constine LS, Tarbell NJ et al: *Pediatric radiation oncology*, ed 4, Philadelphia, 2005, Lippincott Williams & Wilkins.
4. Song PY, Washington M, Vaida F et al: A comparison of four patient immobilization devices in the treatment of prostate cancer patients with three dimensional conformal radiotherapy, *Int J Radiat Oncol Biol Phys* 34(1):213-219, 1996.
5. McLaughlin P, Wygoda A, Schijdak W et al: The effect of patient position and treatment technique in conformal treatment of prostate cancer, *Int J Radiat Oncol Biol Phys* 45(2):407-413, 1999.
6. Zelefsky MJ, Happersetts L, Leibel SA et al: The effect of treatment positioning on normal tissue dose in patients with prostate cancer treated with three-dimensional conformal radiotherapy, *Int J Radiat Oncol Biol Phys* 37(1):13-19, 1997.
7. Kneebone A, Gebski V, Hogendoorn N et al: A randomized trial evaluation evaluating rigid immobilization for pelvic irradiation, *Int J Radiat Oncol Biol Phys* 56(4):1105-1111, 2003.
8. Bentel GC: *Patient positioning and immobilization in radiation oncology*, New York, 1999, McGraw-Hill Publishing.
9. Hong TS, Tome WA, Chappell RJ et al: The impact of daily setup variations on head-and-neck intensity-modulated radiation therapy, *Int J Radiat Oncol Biol Phys* 61(3): 779-788, 2005.
10. Olch AJ, Lavey RS: Reproducibility and treatment planning advantages of a carbon fiber relocatable head fixation system, *Radiother Oncol* 65(3):165-168, 2002.
11. Light KL: Immobilization and treatment of patients receiving radiation therapy for extremity soft tissue sarcoma, *Med Dosim* 17(3):135-139, 1992.
12. Ling CC, Leibel S, Fuks Z et al: *A practical guide to intensity-modulated radiation therapy*, Madison, Wis, 2003, Medical Physics.
13. Hardenbergh PH, Bentel GC, Steffey B et al: Blocking the breast to spare the heart: 3D treatment planning in breast conservation therapy. Proceedings of the 40th Annual ASTRO Meeting, *Int J Radiat Oncol Biol Phys* 42 (suppl 1):247, 1998.
14. Morris DE, Bourland JD, Roseman JG et al: Three-dimensional conformal radiation treatment planning and delivery for low- and intermediate-grade gliomas, *Semin Radiat Oncol* 11(2):124-137, 2001.
15. Hatano K, Nanta Y, Araki H et al: 3D-CRT and intensity modulated radiation therapy (IMRT), *Gan oT Kagaku Ryoho* 30(13):2050-2055, 2003.
16. Marks LB, Sibley G: The rationale and use of three-dimensional radiation treatment planning for lung cancer, *Chest* 116(Suppl 6):5395-5455, 1999.
17. Brizel DM, Light KL, Zhou SM et al: Conformal radiation therapy treatment planning reduces the dose to the optic structures for patients with tumors of the paranasal sinuses, *Radiother Oncol* 51(3):215-218, 1999.

18. Jabour BA, Choi Y, Hoh CK et al: Extracranial head and neck: PET imaging with 2-[F-18]fluoro-2-deoxy-D-glucose and MR imaging correlation, *Radiology* 186(1): 27-35, 1993.
19. Scarfone C, Lawley WC, Cmelak AJ et al: Prospective feasibility trial of radiotherapy target definition for head and neck cancer using 3-dimensional PET and CT imaging, *J Nucl Med* 45(4):543-552, 2004.
20. International Commission on Radiation Units and Measurements: *ICRU Report No. 62: Prescribing, recording, and reporting photon beam therapy (Supplement to ICRU Report No. 50)*, Bethesda, Md, 1999, International Commission on Radiation Units and Measurements.
21. Sherouse GW, Novins K, Chaney EL: Computation of digitally reconstructed radiographs for use in radiotherapy treatment design, *Int J Radiat Oncol Biol Phys* 18(3): 651-658, 1990.
22. Galvin JM, Ezzell G, Eisbrauch A et al: Implementing IMRT in clinical practice: a joint document of the American Society for Therapeutic Radiology and Oncology and the American Association of Physicists in Medicine, *Int J Radiat Oncol Biol Phys* 58(5):1616-1634, 2004.
23. Wu Q, Manning M, Schmidt-Ullrich R et al: The potential for sparing of parotids and escalation of biologically effective dose with intensity-modulated radiation treatments of head and neck cancers: A treatment design study, *Int J Radiat Oncol Biol Phys* 46(1):195-205, 2000.
24. Zelefsky MJ, Fuks Z, Happersett L et al: Clinical experience with intensity modulated radiation therapy (IMRT) in prostate cancer, *Radiother Oncol* 55(3):241-249, 2000.
25. Burman C, Chui CS, Kutcher G et al: Planning, delivery, and quality assurance of intensity-modulated radiotherapy using dynamic multileaf collimator: a strategy for large-scale implementation for the treatment of carcinoma of the prostate, *Int J Radiat Oncol Biol Phys* 39(4):863-873, 1997.
26. Gerber RL, Smith AR, Owen J et al: Patterns of Care Survey results: treatment planning for carcinoma of the prostate, *Int J Radiat Oncol Biol Phys* 33(4)803-808, 1995.
27. Bubenzer V, Esfandi M, Jafari N et al: Dosage along the matchline between upper head-and-neck IMRT fields and conventional supraclavicular fields, *Med Dosim* 29(2): 104-108, 2004.
28. Chao KS, Low DA, Perez CA et al: Intensity-modulated radiation therapy in head and neck cancers: the Mallinckrodt experience, *Int J Cancer* 90(2):92-103, 2000.
29. Chen JC, Chao KS, Low D: Comparison of intensity modulated radiation therapy (IMRT) treatment techniques for nasopharyngeal carcinoma, *Int J Cancer* 96(2):126-131, 2001.
30. Fournier-Bidoz N, Giraud P, Spirous S et al: Penumbra sharpening with IMRT in paraspinal treatments (Abstract), *Med Phys* 28:1260, 2001.
31. Happersett L, Hunt M, Chong L et al: Intensity modulated radiation therapy for the treatment of thyroid cancer, *Int J Radiat Oncol Biol Physics* 48(3S):351, 2000.
32. Hsiung CY, Yorke ED, Chu CS et al: Intensity modulated radiation therapy versus conventional three-dimensional conformal radiotherapy for the boost or salvage treatment of nasopharyngeal carcinoma, *Int J Radiat Oncol Biol Phys* 53(3):638-647, 2002.
33. Peñagarícano JA, Ratanatharathon V, Papanikolou N et al: Intensity modulated radiation therapy reduces the dose to normal tissue in T2N0M0 squamous cell carcinoma of the glottic larynx, *Med Dosim* 29(4): 254-257, 2004.
34. De Neve, W, De Gersem W, Derycke S et al: Clinical delivery of intensity modulated conformal radiotherapy for relapsed or second-primary head and neck cancer using a multileaf collimator with dynamic control, *Radiother Oncol*, 50:301-314, 1999.
35. Hunt MA, Zelefsky MJ, Wolden S et al: Treatment planning and delivery of intensity-modulated radiation therapy for primary nasopharynx cancer, *Int J Radiat Oncol Biol Phys* 49(3):623-632, 2001.
36. Hong L, Hunt M, Chui C et al: Intensity-Modulated tangential beam irradiation of the intact breast, *Int J Radiat Oncol Biol Phys* 44(5):1155-1164, 1999.
37. Mayo C, Lo YC, Fitzgerald TJ et al: Forward-planned, multiple-segment, tangential fields with concomitant boost in the treatment of breast cancer, *Med Dosim* 29:265-270, 2004.
38. Huang E, Teh BS, Strother QG et al: Intensity-modulated radiation therapy for pediatric medulloblastoma: Early report on the reduction of toxicity, *Int J Radiat Oncol Biol Phys* 52(3):599-605, 2002.
39. Haslam JJ, Lujan AE, Mundt AJ et al: Setup errors in patients treated with intensity-modulated whole pelvic radiation therapy for gynecological malignancies, *Med Dosim* 30(1):36-42, 2005.
40. Sharp L, Lewin F, Johansson H et al: Randomized trial on two types of thermoplastic masks for patient immobilization during radiation therapy for head-and-neck cancer, *Int J Radiat Oncol Biol Phys* 61(1):250-256, 2005.
41. Kini VR, Vedam SS, Keall PJ et al: Patient training in respiratory gated radiotherapy, *Med Dosim* 28:7-11, 2003.
42. Langen KM, Jones DML: Organ motion and its management, *Int J Radiat Oncol Biol Phys* 50(1):265-278, 2001.
43. Mageras GS, Yorke E, Rosenzweig K et al: Initial clinical evaluation of a respiratory gated radiotherapy system, *Med Phys* 27:1419-1420, 2000.
44. Teh BS, Dong L, McGary JE et al: Rectal wall sparing by dosimetric effect of rectal balloon used during intensity modulated radiation therapy (IMRT) for prostate cancer, *Med Dosim* 30(1):25-30, 2005.
45. Kutcher GJ, Coia L, Gillin M et al: Comprehensive QA for radiation oncology: report of AAPM Radiation Therapy Committee Task Group 40, *Med Phys* 21(4): 581-618, 1994.
46. Lattanzi J, McNeeley S, Hanlon A et al: Ultrasound-based stereotactic guidance of precision conformal external beam radiation therapy in clinically localized prostate cancer, *Urology* 55(1):73-78, 2000.
47. Litzenberg D, Dawson LA Sandler H et al: Daily prostate targeting using implanted radiopaque markers, *Int J Radiat Oncol Biol Phys* 52(3):699-703, 2002.
48. Lattanzi J, McNeely S, Hanlon A et al: Daily CT localization for correcting portal errors in the treatment of prostate cancer, *Int J Radiat Oncol Biol Phys* 41(5): 1079-1086, 1998.

Unit III

Integrative Systems and Site-Specific Disease

Chapter 6

Central Nervous System Tumors

Terri S. Armstrong, Christie M. Hancock, and Mark R. Gilbert

EPIDEMIOLOGY OF CNS TUMORS

Tumors that occur in the central nervous system (CNS) are a heterogeneous group of neoplasms that vary widely by morphologic features, genetic alterations, growth potential, extent of invasiveness, tendency for progression and recurrence, and treatment response.[1] Tumors may originate from structures within the CNS (primary tumors) or spread from cancer elsewhere in the body (secondary or metastatic tumors). Metastatic tumors of the brain, occurring in approximately 170,000 persons per year in the United States, are by far the most common cause of brain cancer, having an incidence rate higher than all types of primary brain tumors combined. In comparison, primary brain tumors (PBTs) have an annual incidence of approximately 39,000 persons per year. PBTs are further classified as to whether they are low-grade (also termed *benign*) or malignant. Low-grade tumors, such as pilocytic astrocytomas and meningiomas, of the brain compose about 40% of all PBTs. These tumors are composed of slow-growing cells but can be life-threatening if located in vital areas. In addition, low-grade glial tumors often dedifferentiate to a more malignant type, with median survival of less than 7 years for certain histologic types. Malignant primary tumors of the brain, which represent 1.4% of all cancers diagnosed in the United States, tend to be invasive and fast growing. The most common type of PBTs are the gliomas, which arise from the supportive cells of the brain (glial cells). Primary tumors, whether benign or malignant, rarely spread outside of the central nervous system, and the degree of malignancy is determined by cellular characteristics and degree of invasiveness.

Risk Factors

Epidemiologic research has revealed few causal factors in PBTs. People working at certain occupations, including those in oil-refining, electrical and electronics, machining, rubber processing, airplane manufacturing, farming, and pharmaceutical and chemical industries, are associated with a higher incidence of PBTs than those in the general population.[1,2] Other occupations associated with higher incidence include artists, laboratory professionals, veterinarians, and embalmers.[3] Those with a history of exposure to high-dose therapeutic ionizing radiation to the head region are at risk for nerve sheath tumors, meningiomas, and gliomas.[4] A family history of cancer is reported in approximately 15% of patients with tumors of the central nervous system.[5] In addition, those with inherited risk factors, such as neurofibromatosis type II, ataxia telangiectasia,[6] Li-Fraumeni tumor syndrome,[7,8] and Turcot syndrome[8] are at increased risk of developing primary brain tumors.

Several agents have recently received attention regarding their relative risk of neurocarcinogenicity. These include exposure to polyoma viruses or alkylnitrosureas and nonionizing electromagnetic fields.[1,8] Biologic and epidemiologic evidence to date fails to support an association with electromagnetic fields and brain cancer, but results with the other two potential factors are equivocal.[9,10] No association between cellular telephone use and brain tumor occurrence has been shown to date.[11,12]

ANATOMY AND PATHOPHYSIOLOGY

The central nervous system is composed of the brain and spinal cord. Primary cellular components and associated tumors are listed in Table 6-1.[13] Both the brain and spinal cord are surrounded by three continuous sheets of connective tissue, the pia, arachnoid, and dura. The brain and spinal cord are surrounded by cerebrospinal fluid, located between the pia and arachnoid. The spinal cord conducts sensory information (both somatic and autonomic) from the peripheral nervous system to the brain and conducts motor information to

Table 6-1 Common Primary Brain Tumors and Cells of Origin

Cell of origin	Function	Type of tumor
Astrocyte	Supportive, controls neuronal environment	Astrocytomas
Ependyma	Lines ventricles	Ependymoma
Lymphocyte	Immune mediation	Lymphoma
Meninges	Protective covering of the brain	Meningiomas
Oligodendrocyte	Makes central nervous system myelin	Oligodendroglioma

Table 6-2 CNS Anatomy and Associated Dysfunction

Anatomic location	Dysfunction
FRONTAL LOBE	
Unilateral	*Left:* Right hemiplegia or hemiparesis, nonfluent dysphagia *Right:* Left hemiplegia or hemiparesis, mood disturbances
Bilateral/bifrontal	Bilateral hemiplegia or hemiparesis bulbar palsy, impaired intellect, dementia, emotional lability
TEMPORAL LOBE	
Nondominant	Minor spatial and perceptual disturbances; complex partial seizures
Dominant	Receptive aphasia, complex partial seizures, dysnomia
PARIETAL LOBE	
Nondominant	Focal sensory seizures; unilateral sensory changes
Dominant	Unilateral sensory changes, agraphia, acalculia, construction apraxia, astereognosis, ginger agnosia, expressive aphasia, loss of right-left discrimination
OCCIPITAL LOBE	Contralateral hemianopsia or quadrantanopia, visual hallucinations, seizures
CEREBELLUM	Ataxia, incoordination on same side as lesion Signs of increased intracranial pressure
BRAINSTEM	Dysphagia, vomiting, cranial nerve deficits, weakness, sensory changes.

the muscles and glands. The brain receives sensory input from the spinal cord and its own nerves (i.e., olfactory and optic) and devotes most of its volume to processing and initiating appropriate motor responses. Both the brain and the spinal cord are divided into gray matter, composed of cell bodies and dendrites forming the receptor end of synapses and white matter, consisting of axons, the cytoplasmic extension of the nerve cell body. Astrocytes, a form of glial cells that are the supportive cells of the CNS, are located throughout the grey and white matter. Additionally, white matter contains oligodendrocytes that generate the myelin sheath on axons.

Both the brain and spinal cord also can be divided by specific anatomic structures, which correlate to recognized areas of functional control. Table 6-2 describes the basic components of the brain and outlines dysfunction that may occur as a result of tumor growth in specific locations.[13]

CLINICAL MANIFESTATIONS

The presenting symptoms of a primary brain tumor are typically classified as generalized or focal.[14] Headache, often the consequence of increased intracranial pressure from mass effect, and seizures are considered to be generalized symptoms, whereas deficits such as weakness, language dysfunction, or sensory loss are focal in nature. Seizures are a more common presenting feature in the lower-grade tumors, whereas headache is more prevalent in patients with faster-growing, high-grade tumors. Focal loss of neurologic function tends to be insidious with low-grade tumors, a consequence of their slower rate of growth. However, acute events such as hemorrhage markedly alter the tempo of symptom onset regardless of tumor grade.

Careful review of the patient's history and consultation with family members often uncovers evidence that subtle changes have been present for months to years, suggesting either that the tumor is lower grade or, if found to be highly malignant, that it evolved from a low-grade tumor. Occasionally, patients will have undergone extensive psychiatric evaluation for behavioral changes, treatment for sinusitis, or may even have had a work-up for gastrointestinal problems because of intractable vomiting. In retrospect, however, the etiology for these varied symptoms becomes clear, and treatment of the tumor often results in prompt symptomatic improvement.

DIAGNOSTIC STUDIES

In patients presenting with new neurologic symptoms, brain imaging, typically magnetic resonance imaging (MRI) both with and without gadolinium-based contrast material, is used to evaluate brain parenchyma.[15] MRI has better resolution and is more sensitive for nonenhancing infiltrating tumors than traditional computerized tomography (CT). Figure 6-1 provides an example of CT and MRI, highlighting the improved resolution with MRI. Imaging sequences such as fluid-attenuated inversion recovery (FLAIR) and T2 are particularly good for evaluating the extent of infiltrating tumor both for high-grade and low-grade tumors. However, CT is better at imaging calcifications and bone structures.[16] For example, tumor calcification is a hallmark of oligodendrogliomas, a radiographic finding often missed with the widespread exclusive use of MRI. Although exceptions exist, high-grade tumors demonstrate contrast enhancement, whereas low-grade tumors tend to display no enhancement. Intermediate-grade neoplasms (e.g., anaplastic

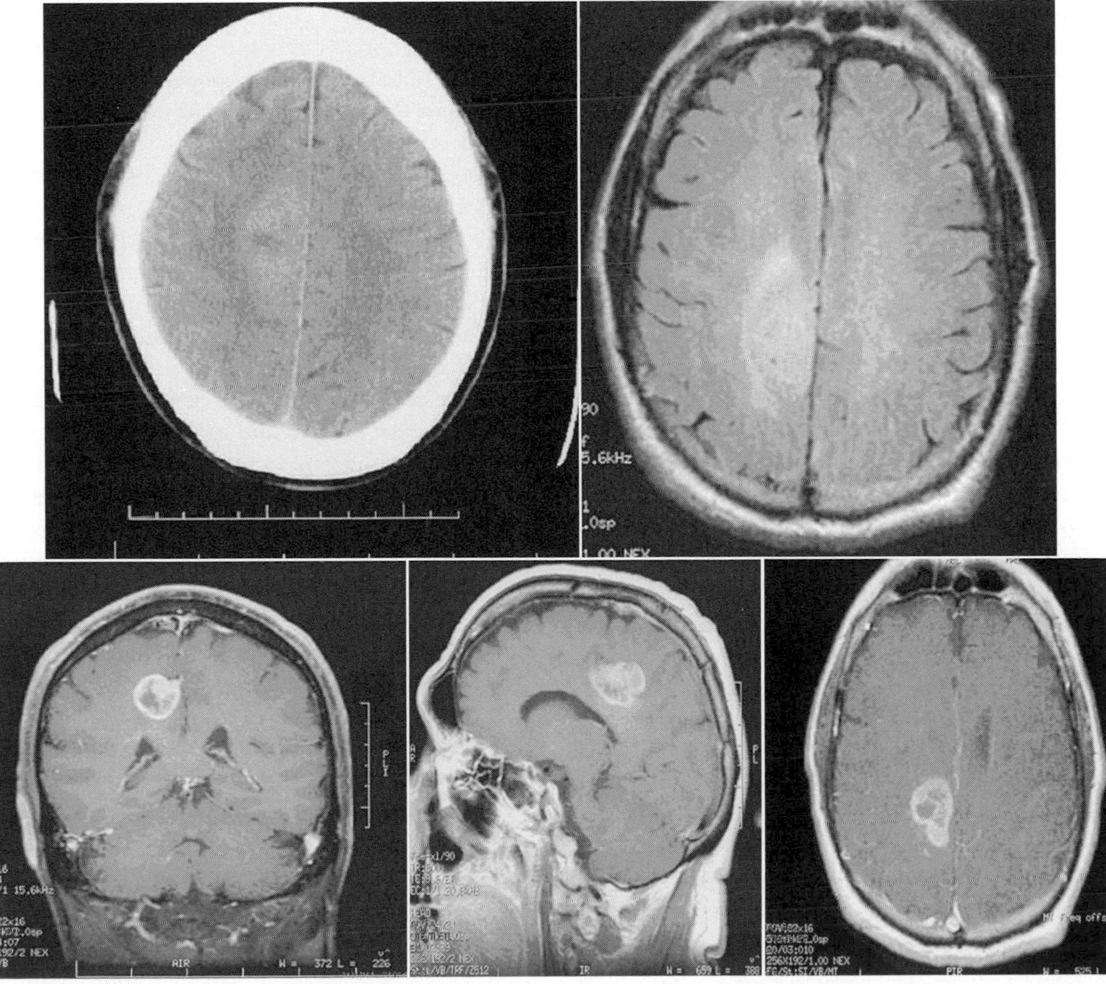

Figure 6-1 CT and MRI Images of a Glioblastoma Multiforme.

astrocytoma) tend to have patchy or no visible enhancement.[17] Often, the region of enhancement represents the most malignant component of a large tumor. The enhancing region is an area of angiogenesis and usually is the target of tissue sampling for diagnosis.

Interest in using functional imaging to assist in the diagnosis, management, and determination of response of gliomas is increasing. Functional imaging, such as magnetic imaging spectroscopy and positron emission tomography (PET) provide biochemical or physiologic data.[18,19] Currently, these technologies have not proven useful in determining tumor grade because their respective functional parameters tend to overlap. Functional imaging is more commonly used when a distinction between treatment-related necrosis and recurrent tumor is needed. Additionally, functional imaging has been useful in determining the most abnormal region of tumor to improve diagnostic accuracy when a small biopsy will be performed.[20,21] Functional imaging also has been used to define the margins of tumor for both surgical resection and radiation fields.

After discovery of a mass lesion, a tissue sample is almost always required before appropriate treatment can be initiated. Exceptions to this rule are infiltrating brainstem glioma in children and similar lesions in adults, although in the case of adults, the histologic grade and natural history of the tumor can be quite varied. Therefore, whenever possible, a tissue sample should be obtained from brainstem tumors in adults.

The decision to perform a diagnostic biopsy or tumor resection is complex. Several factors, including tumor location, the patient's overall physical status encompassing general health, number of lesions, and presence of significant mass effect (midline shift or herniation), need to be considered. Biopsy, either open or using a stereotactic technique, is well tolerated with low morbidity, and only a short hospital stay is required. However, the tumor burden is not reduced, and sampling errors in the typically small sample is a critical issue, particularly for lower-grade tumors. One study compared the diagnostic accuracy of biopsy with resection and found that nearly 50% of diagnoses changed when a subsequent (within 60 days) resection was performed after a biopsy.[22] However, tumor resection is a major operative procedure with increased risk of postoperative complications. Given the infiltrative nature of the cancer, temporary or permanent neurologic compromise remains an issue when deciding on the extent of surgical resection. Advances in neurosurgical technique, particularly intraoperative mapping and monitoring have facilitated more complete resections while decreasing postoperative morbidity. Some studies do suggest a survival benefit to extensive resection, although a prospective randomized trial has not yet been performed.[23]

PATHOLOGY AND PATTERNS OF METASTASIS

Clinical staging of cancers typically follows the TNM system in which universally accepted anatomic features, often with corresponding clinical signs are used to group patients for determination of optimal treatment and prognosis. However, the staging of primary brain tumors does not use the conventional TNM staging system. Because malignant gliomas rarely spread outside the central nervous system, the N component (nodal metastases) and the M component (distant metastases) would almost always have a value of zero. As a consequence, malignant gliomas are staged on the basis of their histologic grade. The grade of tumor is always based on the most malignant component of the tissue, even if it constitutes a small percentage of the overall tumor.

The most widely accepted grading system is that of the World Health Organization (WHO). This system was carefully reviewed at a consensus conference in 1993 and again in 2000, thereby leading to significant modifications being published as the WHO II criteria.[24] For infiltrative malignant gliomas, tumor designation begins with grade II. Grade I is reserved for noninfiltrating tumors, such as juvenile pilocytic astrocytomas, that are often cured by surgical resection. Grade II gliomas demonstrate increased cellularity, often with only mild degrees of pleomorphism and rare mitotic figures. Grade III neoplasms are marked by extensive pleomorphism and increased cellularity with mitotic figures and the absence of necrosis. Grade IV tumors are characterized by necrosis and include marked increases in cellularity and pleomorphism. The WHO II permits a diagnosis of grade IV to be made only on the basis of vascular proliferation being present without a definitive finding of necrosis, a major change from the prior classification schema (WHO I) and a change in diagnostic criteria that has not been universally accepted.[24]

Accurate assessment of tumor grade has great importance in patient management. Patient prognosis directly correlates with tumor grade, and treatment regimens have been developed using this system. The universal acceptance of the grading system permits interpretation of treatment results from a wide range of treatment groups. Most studies report survival of patients with grade IV gliomas to be in the 10- to 12-month range, grade III having a 2- to 4-year range, and grade II having a 5- to 8-year range.

TREATMENT

The treatment of malignant brain tumors requires a multidisciplinary approach with consideration of the incurable nature of the disease and the potential for treatment to cause neurologic toxicity and deleteriously impact on quality of life. Treatment regimens vary according to histologic category and tumor grade, but generally involve a diagnostic surgical procedure followed by radiation and/or chemotherapy.

Surgery

The role of surgery was discussed earlier. As stated, surgery is useful to determine the type of tumor and also can be used for cytoreduction of the mass. For certain low-grade tumors, such as pilocytic astrocytomas, gangliogliomas, and meningiomas, complete surgical resection can be curative. Safely removing as much visible tumor without causing neurologic deficit is the goal of surgery for most tumors, with a few exceptions, such as primary CNS lymphoma or with multiple metastases.

Radiation Therapy

Radiation therapy plays a primary role in the treatment of CNS tumors. Radiation therapy has been shown to extend survival time and improve the quality of life for patients with primary and with metastatic tumors. The type of radiation techniques selected for treatment and the potential dosage depends on the histology and grade of the tumor, the location of the tumor, patient status, and training of the radiation oncologist and available technologies. A combination of radiation therapy and surgery is commonly used with a curative intent for patients with low-grade tumors. Chemotherapeutic agents also may be added to the treatment regimen. Whole brain radiation therapy may be used to prevent brain metastasis or to palliate neurologic symptoms emanating from advanced disease.

Delivery Methods of Radiation Therapy for CNS Tumors

External Beam Radiation Therapy

External beam radiation therapy (EBRT) is the conventional form of treatment for most CNS tumors. It may be used after a diagnostic surgical procedure or in lieu of surgery for tumors that are either inoperable or extremely sensitive to radiation therapy. The goal of EBRT is to deliver an appropriate dose to a specifically delineated treatment field that encompasses the entire tumor volume while minimizing toxic effects to normal tissue. When only a portion of the brain is treated for a primary brain lesion, it is often referred to as partial brain irradiation. Total dose for these tumors using this technique typically ranges between 40 Gy and 60 Gy. EBRT generally involves the delivery of once daily treatments of a dosage of 1.8 Gy to 2.0 Gy, 5 times per week.[25] Lower doses of EBRT are used to treat metastatic brain tumors, with a commonly prescribed dosage of 30 Gy over 10 treatments.

The delivery of EBRT involves the use of sophisticated and complex pretreatment planning. Simulation of the brain will usually take place before treatment or on the first day of treatment. The treatment fields are designed for the patient during simulation using diagnostic studies and physical examination. A diagnostic CT scan is also used in conjunction with simulation to provide intricate detail used to facilitate accuracy and precision in developing the treatment field. The patient must be treated in the exact position each day. Individualized immobilization devices (e.g., Aquaplast face masks, head-holding casts) are used to decrease mobility and to ensure exact reproduction of the treatment position (Figure 6-2). Children may require additional immobilization devices or anesthesia for daily treatment.

The majority of brain tissue is shielded from the effects of radiation therapy through the use of blocks that are custom designed for each patient. Patients undergoing EBRT for CNS tumors will often need blocks for the eyes or other critical structures or portions of the brain not targeted for treatment. Patients receiving adjuvant radiation therapy to the brain after surgical resection will require a treatment volume that encompasses the

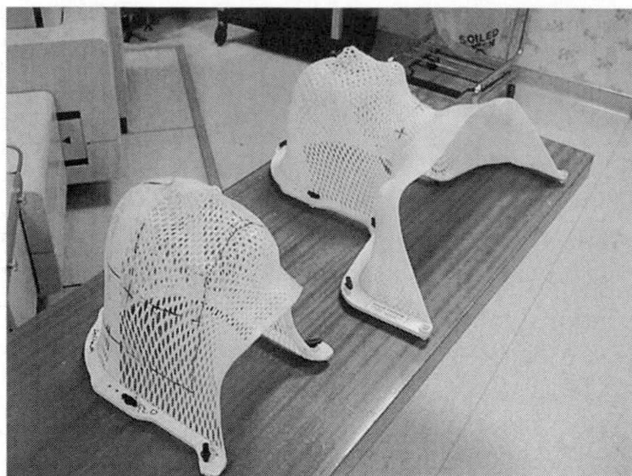

Figure 6-2 Head Immobilizers.
Courtesy of WFR/Aquaplast/Q-Fix Systems, Wyckoff, NJ.

original site of the tumor because this area is at risk for residual/recurrent disease.[26]

Additional treatment planning performed by the medical physics and dosimetry departments determines optimal dose distribution through the use of computer programs and complex data individualized for each patient and radiation delivery unit. The radiation therapy technician then ultimately delivers the treatment to the patient.[26] Whole-brain radiation therapy involves the delivery of radiation to the entirety of the brain. Conformal radiation consists of high-dose external radiation beams that are shaped or "conformed" to match the shape of a tumor. The purpose of conformal radiation is to deliver a uniform dose to the tumor while minimizing radiation exposure to adjacent brain tissue. Stereotactic radio-surgery, also known as *radiosurgery*, is the delivery of a highly focused dose of radiation to an area encompassing the tumor with minimal margin. This is generally administered in one fraction. The advantage of this treatment is that it delivers high dose to the tumor while sparing normal tissue. However, in the case of infiltrating tumors, undetectable tumor extension to surrounding brain tissue will not be targeted. For more information on stereotactic radiosurgery techniques, see Chapter 24.

Intensity-Modulated Radiation Therapy

Intensity-modulated radiation therapy (IMRT) is a state of the art cancer treatment method that delivers high doses of radiation directly to cancer cells in a targeted form. IMRT allows delivery of higher radiation doses to a specific target, sparing more of the surrounding healthy tissue. IMRT, developed in the 1990s, takes external beam radiation therapy one step further by using computer programs to design the dose distribution, control the radiation therapy treatment delivery system, and allow collimator leaves to move during treatment. The motion of the collimator leaves stop and start while the treatment is given, thereby varying the beam's intensity. This allows the radiation dose to the tumor to differ from the radiation dose to the surrounding tissue and allows for highly irregularly shaped tumors to be completely targeted by numerous beams. This theoretically reduces side effects associated with high doses of radiation.[27]

Advantages of IMRT include (1) delivery of precise radiation treatment; (2) delivery of high doses of radiation to the target with lower doses to nearby normal healthy tissues, thereby in theory resulting in fewer side effects; (3)shaping and intensity modification of radiation beams; and (4) provides a noninvasive alternative to surgery in some cases. IMRT use in the treatment of CNS tumors is still being evaluated, and its clinical value is still being defined. It is thought that the reduction of radiation therapy delivered to surrounding brain tissue can help decreased cognitive effects that can be seen months after radiation therapy is completed.[28]

Proton Therapy

Proton therapy is given much the same way as conventional external beam radiation therapy, but it uses proton particles rather than x rays to kill brain tumor cells. The major advantage of proton treatment over conventional radiation, however, is that the energy distribution of protons can be directed and deposited in tissue volumes designated by the physician in a three-dimensional pattern from each beam used. This allows for greater control and precision and, therefore, superior management of treatment. Minimum interaction with electrons occurs as the protons approach their targeted stopping point. Thus maximum energy is released within the designated cancer volume. The surrounding healthy cells receive significantly less energy than the cells in the designated volume.[29] Examples of CNS tumors treated with proton therapy include skull-based tumors, such as chordomas and chondrosarcomas, uveal melanomas, meningiomas, craniopharyngiomas, and arteriovenous malformations.[30] This treatment is available in only a few centers in the United States.

Stereotactic Radiosurgery

Stereotactic radiosurgery (SRS) is a noninvasive alternative to treatment of CNS tumors. SRS allows delivery of high-dose radiation in a single fraction to a precise area in the brain. The primary goal of radiosurgery is to eradicate tumor cells within a targeted area, yielding minimal damage to adjacent tissue. SRS is used to treat benign tumors such as acoustic neuromas and meningiomas, primary brain tumors and metastatic brain tumors, as well as arteriovenous malformations, trigeminal neuralgias, and parkinsonian tremors.

On the day of the procedure, a mechanical guiding device or frame is fixed to the patient's skull to assist with immobilization and localization of the specific area. The location of the tumor and the surrounding tissues is evaluated with CT and/or MRI. The radiosurgery team, usually consisting of a radiation oncologist, physicist, and neurosurgeon, work together to plan a procedure to precisely treat the lesion.

Variations of SRS include stereotactic radiation therapy (SRT) and CyberKnife. Detailed information regarding CyberKnife can be found in Chapter 24.

Brachytherapy

Brachytherapy, the surgical implantation of radioactive isotopes into or near a tumor, is a conformal irradiation technique that can deliver high doses of radiation to well-defined brain tumors measuring less than 5 cm to 6 cm in diameter.[31] Radioactive sources can be implanted either temporarily or permanently. Temporary treatments use sealed radioactive sources that are removed after a calculated dose is delivered to the target. Permanent treatments are sealed sources that are left in the body and give off radiation to the tumor as the source decays.[32] Various sources of radiation can be used for brachytherapy. The most commonly used temporary sources for treatment of CNS tumors are iodine-125 and iridium-192. The most common permanent source is iodine-125.

Brachytherapy is used most commonly in patients with recurrent disease who have previously received external beam radiation therapy. Brachytherapy maximizes the radiation dose to the tumor while minimizing the dose to healthy brain tissue. Treatment is limited by tumor size. In tumors larger than 6 cm in diameter, brachytherapy results in an excessive dose to the healthy surrounding brain, increasing the risk of radiation damage.[31] One type of brachytherapy used to treat certain CNS malignancies is GliaSite (Cytyc Corporation). Please refer to Chapter 28 for additional information regarding this treatment modality. The role of brachytherapy in the treatment of brain metastasis is limited. Although the size and shape of intracranial lesions make them suitable for brachytherapy, SRS is now the preferred treatment modality.[31]

Hyperthermia

Hyperthermia is a type of treatment in which body tissue is exposed to high temperatures to damage and kill cancer cells or to make cancer cells more sensitive to the effects of radiation and certain anticancer drugs. Hyperthermia enhances the effect of radiation through an additive and synergistic effect, with the most therapeutic benefit being attained when irradiation is followed by hyperthermia. Smaller tumors (less than 3 cm) demonstrate a better therapeutic outcome than larger tumors.[33] Hyperthermia is still being researched regarding its role in treatment for CNS tumors. For additional information regarding hyperthermia, refer to Chapter 27.

Other Treatment Modalities

The high failure rate of conventional treatments for CNS tumors has lead to the development of many novel treatment techniques. Some are directed at making the treatment more specific, and others are aimed at making treatment more tumoricidal.[34] Examples of these treatments include boron-neutron capture therapy, proton beam irradiation, and radioimmunotherapy. These nonconventional treatments are progressing into clinical trials and may provide promising results in the treatment of CNS tumors. Another area of research is the use of radiosensitizers to enhance external beam radiation therapy or stereotactic radiosurgery. Common chemotherapy agents such as paclitaxel, carmustine, cisplatin, and the oral agent temozolomide may prove to be beneficial when given concomitantly with radiation therapy. New radiosensitizers such as motexafin gadolinium and RSR13 are currently being studied for their efficacy.

Chemotherapy

Chemotherapy is often used as an adjunct to surgery and radiation therapy and is often the primary method of treatment at recurrence. The type and course of chemotherapy depends on tumor histology. Specific treatment approaches, incorporating information on surgical and radiation approaches in addition to standard chemotherapy for commonly occurring tumors, are discussed briefly below.

Glioblastoma

Traditionally, surgery along with radiation therapy has been the standard treatment approach for patients with glioblastoma multiforme (GBM) tumors. The use of chemotherapy in the postradiation setting, often referred to as adjuvant chemotherapy, has had a modest benefit in terms of overall survival and progression-free survival.[35] However, in a recent large randomized trial, a regimen that combined low-dose chemotherapy with the oral alkylating agent temozolomide and radiation, followed by additional months of adjuvant temozolomide, demonstrated a survival advantage over radiation alone.[36] The treatment was well tolerated with only rare complications related to the addition of the chemotherapy. Chemotherapy (carmustine [BCNU])-impregnated polymer in the form of a wafer also has been shown to improve survival in patients with newly diagnosed malignant gliomas.[37] The polymer has active drug intercalated within the chemical structure, and after implantation, the wafer slowly undergoes biodegradation, releasing active drug. This local delivery system has the advantages of minimal systemic toxicity, no limitation posed by the blood-brain barrier, and ability to deliver very high local concentrations of chemotherapy. A randomized double-blind study compared surgery with implantation of the BCNU-containing chemotherapy wafer to a group of patients undergoing surgery but with empty polymer.[37] Both groups then received radiation therapy. A statistically significant improvement in survival was reported for patients receiving the chemotherapy-containing polymer, although statistical significance was not reached for the subset of patients with GBM. Thus far, no studies have compared a systemic chemotherapy strategy with wafer treatment to determine the optimal treatment for patients with newly diagnosed glioblastoma, so definitive guidelines have not been established.

At recurrence, various conventional chemotherapy treatments are used, including the nitrosoureas, BCNU, and lomustine (CCNU) as well as chemotherapy agents such as irinotecan, carboplatin, or cisplatin and etoposide. Typically, the recurrent disease scenario is where new agents or combinations are used in a clinical trial setting. Select patients may benefit from a tumor resection, reducing tumor mass and burden before initiation of other therapies. Reoperation also permits the placement of chemotherapy-impregnated polymer wafers.[38] Patients with recurrent glioblastoma are particularly encouraged to participate in approved clinical trials in order to assess the development of more effective regimens.

Anaplastic Astrocytoma

The treatment principles for anaplastic astrocytoma are similar to those for glioblastoma. Radiation therapy is a component of nearly all regimens. However, because a concurrent chemotherapy-radiation therapy trial using temozolomide has not been performed in this group of patients, the benefit of this approach, whereas proven for glioblastoma, has not been established for anaplastic astrocytoma. Similarly, the use of the chemotherapy-impregnated wafer has not been tested in anaplastic tumors. Patients with anaplastic astrocytoma demonstrate a higher rate of objective response to systemic chemotherapy regimes than those with glioblastoma multiforme.[39] This encourages the use of adjuvant (postradiation) chemotherapy, using temozolomide or combination treatment with procarbazine, lomustine, and vincristine (PCV). However, its benefit has not been proven in randomized controlled clinical trials.

Low-grade Astrocytoma

The treatment of low-grade astrocytoma is controversial.[40] Many investigators concur with serial observation in young patients (younger than age 40) who have undergone extensive tumor resection. Older patients or patients with extensive residual tumor often undergo external beam radiation therapy. Studies confirm that time to tumor growth is prolonged in patients receiving radiation compared to untreated patients. However, most studies found that overall survival did not improve significantly.[41] Chemotherapy is not widely used for low-grade astrocytoma. Reports of small series of patients treated with chemotherapy vary widely in the regimen used and response rate.[42-45] Therefore, chemotherapy is often reserved for recurrent disease.

Oligodendrogliomas

The optimal treatment for oligodendrogliomas is rapidly evolving. The recent discovery of the prognostic and predictive treatment response related to allelic chromosomal loss on *1p* and *19q*, has dramatically impacted therapeutic decisions. Preliminary reports suggest that anaplastic oligodendrogliomas with "classic" histopathology demonstrating allelic loss of heterozygosity of the *1p* and *19q* chromosome arms have nearly a 100% response rate to chemotherapy and/or radiation therapy.[46] Nonclassic tumors without the same allelic loss have a response rate in the range of 15% to 30%. Survival mirrors the marked difference in response. As a consequence of these findings, evaluation of chromosomes in oligodendroglial tumors is universal, and most centers base treatment decisions on these findings. Of note, although a small percentage of anaplastic astrocytomas demonstrate the *1p 19q* LOH, this finding does not predict response or prognosis as it does for oligodendroglial tumors.

Similar chromosomal changes have been noted in low-grade oligodendroglial tumors, although few studies have evaluated their prognostic or treatment-predictive importance in these tumors. However, some preliminary reports suggest an association exists between chromosomal perturbations and an increase in treatment response.[42,47,48] Therefore, patients with low-grade oligodendrogliomas containing the *1p* and *19q* LOH are being treated with chemotherapy as the initial treatment. In these patients, radiation therapy is reserved for recurrence, based on the rationale that delaying the use of radiation therapy postpones the risk of radiation-induced neurotoxicity. No formal studies have compared this chemotherapy approach with the more traditional radiation therapy treatment regimen. Radiation therapy is still recommended for tumors that do not demonstrate *1p* and *19q* chromosomal changes but need treatment.

CNS Lymphoma

CNS lymphoma, an aggressive form of non-Hodgkin's lymphoma, is a rare tumor that is increasing in frequency in both immunocompetent and immunocompromised patients. If suspected, steroids are usually withheld until after biopsy, because their use may impact the ability to make a diagnosis. Additional work-up also includes evaluation for systemic lymphoma, evaluation of cerebrospinal fluid (CSF), and slit-lamp ophthalmologic exam to rule out malignant uveitis. The use of a methotrexate-based chemotherapy regimen is standard and results in improved survival over nonmethotrexate-containing regimens. Because most tumors are of a B-cell lineage, rituximab in patients with residual enhancing tumor is often added. The role of whole brain radiation therapy is controversial and is often reserved for the postchemotherapy setting or at recurrence.

Brain Metastases

Radiation therapy for brain metastasis is the most common form of treatment used. Corticosteroids are also used concomitantly with the radiation therapy to prevent edema caused by tumors. Whole brain radiation therapy (WBRT) is delivered over a 7- to 10-day period with a fraction size ranging from 1.5 Gy to 4.0 Gy daily, resulting in a tumor dose of 30 Gy to 50 Gy. Fraction size and total dosage is determined based on patient prognosis and performance status.

Chemotherapy has a limited role in the treatment of brain metastasis. Intrathecal chemotherapy can be used in patients that have no evidence of leptomeningeal metastasis. The most commonly used agents are methotrexate, cytarabine, and thiotepa. Response rates were reported as approximately 20%.[49]

Future Directions

Despite ongoing efforts by many investigators, centers, consortia, and cooperative oncology groups, new treatments are clearly needed to impact the poor prognosis that persists for patients with high-grade primary brain tumors. Innovative approaches, including immunotherapies, gene therapies, and targeted therapies that block specific signal transduction pathways, are being actively investigated in clinical trials.

ADVERSE EFFECTS AND NURSING INTERVENTIONS

Irradiation of the brain can result in the toxic effects that may be characterized as acute reactions, early delayed reactions, or late reactions. Acute reactions are those that occur during radiation therapy and are usually not severe. The most common acute reaction is hair loss, which is directly related to local dose to the scalp.[50] Regrowth usually occurs in 3 to 6 months. Permanent hair loss is uncommon with doses less than 55 Gy.[30] Other acute side effects are usually secondary to cerebral edema caused by the normal tissue and tumor reaction to radiation. Symptoms include worsening of preexisting deficits and nausea, vomiting, headache, dizziness, or problems with speech, balance, or movement. These symptoms are usually controlled with administration of corticosteroids. Multiple side effects may occur as a result of steroid use, and patients should be educated regarding these potential problems and their management. Special care should be given to patients with diabetes who require management with corticosteroids. Blood glucose levels should be monitored closely, and signs and symptoms of diabetic ketoacidosis should be reported promptly.

Skin reactions, such as erythema and dry desquamation of the scalp, resulting from brain irradiation occur commonly but are seldom severe. Intense skin reactions are most likely to occur in areas of skinfolds, particularly the ears. Symptoms are managed with skin care products commonly used in the treatment of radiation dermatitis (see Chapter 30). Most patients can safely continue their usual regimen of hair care without exacerbating skin reactions.[51]

A common acute side effect of radiation therapy is fatigue. The degree of fatigue a person experiences depends on the size of the treatment field, comorbid conditions, and their overall physical condition.[30] Interventions commonly employed in the management of fatigue, such as frequent rest periods and pacing activity, are suggested during CNS radiation therapy. Studies that have evaluated fatigue during radiation therapy indicate that fatigue is minimal at the initiation of treatment, but intensifies as treatment progresses.[52]

Early delayed reactions are defined as reactions that may occur weeks after radiation therapy. These effects are considered secondary to transient demyelination, which results from radiation injury to oligodendrocytes or through alterations in capillary permeability.[50] Radiation somnolence syndrome can occur 6 to 12 weeks after completing radiation. Clinical manifestations include somnolence, irritability, anorexia, lethargy, or an exacerbation of previous neurologic symptoms.[30] Steroid therapy may be required for neurologic problems that compromise mental/physical function. Radiation somnolence syndrome is usually self-limiting and is reversible.

Late reactions may develop months to years after the completion of radiation therapy. These effects include radiation necrosis, cognitive impairment, leukoencephalopathy, and decreased hormone production. Radiation necrosis may occur from 6 months to 2 years after the completion of treatment. CT scans may document evidence of white matter changes with edema. It is difficult to distinguish radiation-induced necrosis from recurrent brain tumor with CT scan or with an MRI of the head. A PET scan may be helpful in tissue/necrosis differentiation. Surgical intervention may be necessary in order to accurately diagnose and treat radiation necrosis. Symptoms are variable and may range from fatigue and personality changes to memory impairment and dementia.[53] Daily fractionation and total dosage are the most significant factors influencing the development of radionecrosis.

The incidence of cognitive impairment after brain radiation therapy is not well defined. Memory deficit appears to be the most common manifestation of cognitive impairment.[30] Learning disabilities are seen often in children and are most prevalent in those ages 4 to 7.[53] Multiple factors including age, radiation dose, tumor size, previous treatment, and medications may impact cognitive function. Additionally, there are multiple factors clinicians should be cognizant of when caring for pediatric patients in this setting. A pediatric consideration box on the next page provides a detailed, though not exhaustive, list of considerations for treating pediatric patients.

Diminished hormone production may occur in patients receiving radiation therapy to the hypothalamus. Growth hormones are affected but can be replaced by prescription hormone medications. Leukoencephalopathy is a late side effect characterized by disorientation, personality changes, memory loss, and dementia. Brain lesions show demyelination, multifocal coagulation necrosis, and gliosis.[50] This event is commonly described in children but also may be seen in adults treated with brain radiation therapy. Permanent neurologic damage may occur as a result of leukoencephalopathy.

At any phase during treatment, psychosocial aspects of care should be considered. Often patients are diagnosed after an acute event such as a seizure and may have permanent neurologic deficits, which impact their role performance and quality of

Pediatric Considerations

- *Does child require anesthesia for treatment?*
  Conscious sedation policy
  Staff adequately trained
  Adequate staffing available
- *Role of child life therapist*
  Family-focused care
  Parent and sibling guilt/grieving
  Sibling alienation
  Access to care
  Medical bills
- *Role of dietitian*
  Nutritional screening
  Considerations related to age, growth and development, disease process
- *Care coordination across the continuum*
  Ongoing quality-of-life assessment
  Transition from pediatric to young adult to adult practitioners
- *Age-specific milestones*
  Growth and development
  Attainment of independence
  Social skills
  Peer acceptance
  Self image
- *End-of-life issues*
  Hospice
  Patient/family anger or grief
  Ethical and legal considerations
- *Late effects from treatment*
  Fertility
  Cognitive changes
  Genetic testing for other primary malignancy
  Secondary malignancies
- *Long-term survivorship implications*
  Access to care
  Ongoing surveillance
  Disability?
  Discrimination?

Table 6-3 Resources for Patients With Tumors of the Central Nervous System and Their Caregivers

Organization	Website
American Brain Tumor Association	www.braintumor.org
Brain Tumor Society	www.bts.org
Central Brain Tumor Registry of the United States	www.cbtrus.org
Epilepsy Foundation of America	www.efa.org
National Brain Tumor Foundation	www.braintumor.org
North American Brain Tumor Coalition	www.nabraintumor.org
Society of Neuro-Oncology	www.sno.org
Southeastern Brain Tumor Foundation	www.sbtf.org
Virtual Trials Clearinghouse	www.virtualtrials.com
TREATMENT CONSORTIA	
New Approaches to Brain Tumor Therapy	www.nabtt.org
North American Brain Tumor Coalition	www.nabtc.org

life. Support services, such as support groups, individual counseling, occupational, speech and physical therapy, and referral to social services should be considered (Table 6-3).

REFERENCES

1. Gurney JG, Kadan-Lottick N: Brain and other central nervous system tumors: rates, trends, and epidemiology, *Curr Opin Oncol* 13(3):160-166, 2001.
2. Thomas TL, Stolley PD, Stemhagen A et al: Brain tumor mortality risk among men with electrical and electronics jobs: a case-control study, *J Natl Cancer Inst* 79(2):233-238, 1987.
3. Thomas TL, Stolley PD, Fontham ETH et al: Occupational risk factors for brain tumors: a case-referent death-certificate analysis, *Scand J Work Environ Health* 12(2):121-127, 1986.
4. Ron E, Modan B, Boice JD et al: Tumors of the brain and nervous system after radiotherapy in childhood, *N Engl J Med* 319(16):1033-1039, 1988.
5. Mahaley MS Jr, Mettlin C, Natarajan N et al: National survey of patterns of care for brain-tumor patients, *J Neurosurg* 71(6):826-836, 1989.
6. Blatt J, Jaffe R, Deutsch M et al: Neurofibromatosis and childhood tumors, *Cancer* 57(6):1225-1229, 1986.
7. Lynch HT et al: Genetic epidemiology of breast cancer. In Hirayama T, editor: *Genetic epidemiology of cancer*, Boca Raton, 1989, CRC Press, pp 289-332.
8. Bondy ML, Wrensch MR: Epidemiology of primary malignant brain tumours, *Baillieres Clin Neurol* 5(2):251-270, 1996.

9. Gurney JG, van Wijngaarden E: Extremely low frequency electromagnetic fields (EMF) and brain cancer in adults and children: review and comment, *Neuro-oncol* 1(3): 212-220, 1999.
10. Wrensch M, Yost M, Miike R et al: Adult glioma in relation to residential power frequency electromagnetic field exposures in the San Francisco Bay area, *Epidemiology* 10(5):523-527, 1999.
11. Inskip PD, Tarone RE, Hatch EE et al: Cellular-telephone use and brain tumors, *N Engl J Med* 344(2):79-86, 2001.
12. Morgan RW, Kelsh MA, Zhao K et al: Radiofrequency exposure and mortality from cancer of the brain and lymphatic/hematopoietic systems, *Epidemiology* 11(2):118-127, 2000.
13. Armstrong T, Gilbert M: Glial neoplasms: classification, treatment, and pathways for the future, *Oncol Nurs Forum* 23(4):615-625, 1996.
14. Thomas DGT, McKeran RO: Clinical manifestations of brain tumors. In Thomas DGT, Graham DL, editors: *Neuro-oncology: primary malignant brain tumors*, Baltimore, 1990, Johns Hopkins Press, pp 94, 121.
15. Armstrong TS, Cohen MZ, Weinberg J et al: Imaging techniques in neuro-oncology, *Semin Oncol Nurs* 20(4): 231-239, 2004.
16. Healy ME et al: Increased detection of intracranial metastases with intravenous Gd-DTPA, *Radiology* 165(3):619-624, 1987.
17. Wen PYK, Koon TS, Black P: Clinical, imaging, and laboratory diagnosis of brain tumors. In Kaye A, editor: *Brain tumors*, New York, 2001, Jones and Bartlett, pp 24-50.
18. Ricci PE, Karis JP, Heiserman JE et al: Differentiating recurrent tumor from radiation necrosis: time for re-evaluation of positron emission tomography? *AJNR Am J Neuroradiol* 19(3):407-413, 1998.
19. Kaminogo M, Ishimaru H, Morikawa M et al: Diagnostic potential of short echo time MR spectroscopy of gliomas with single-voxel and point-resolved spatially localised proton spectroscopy of brain, *Neuroradiology* 43(5):353-363, 2001.
20. Chen CY, Lirng JF, Chan WP et al: Proton magnetic resonance spectroscopy-guided biopsy for cerebral glial tumors, *J Formos Med Assoc* 103(6):448-458, 2004.
21. Rock JP et al: Correlations between magnetic resonance spectroscopy and image-guided histopathology, with special attention to radiation necrosis, *Neurosurgery* 51(4):912-919; discussion 919-920, 2002.
22. Jackson RJ et al: Limitations of stereotactic biopsy in the initial management of gliomas, *Neuro-oncol* 3(3):193-200, 2001.
23. Lacroix M, Abi-Said D, Fourney DR et al: A multivariate analysis of 416 patients with glioblastoma multiforme: prognosis, extent of resection, and survival, *J Neurosurg* 95(2):190-198, 2001.
24. Kleihues P, Cavenee WK, editors: *Pathology and genetics of tumours of the nervous system, World Health Organization Classification of Tumours*, Lyon, France, 2000, International Agency for Research Cancer Press.
25. National Comprehensive Cancer Network: *Central nervous system practice guidelines*, 2005, Jenkintown, PA, National Comprehensive Cancer Network.
26. Nicolaou N: Radiation therapy treatment planning and delivery, *Semin Oncol Nurs* 15(4):260-269, 1998.
27. Borgardus CR: IMRT: an overview, *Oncol Issues* 12(2):5-7, 2003.
28. Welsh JS, Olivera GH, Mackie TR: Novel uses and applications of IMRT. In Mackie TR, editor: *Intensity-modulated radiation therapy: the state of the art*, Madison, Wis, 2003, Medical Physics Publishing, pp 875-882.
29. National Association of Proton Therapy: *Proton therapy*, 2004, Silver Spring, MD, The Association.
30. Bucholtz JD: Central nervous system tumors. In Hilderley LJ, editor: *Nursing care in radiation oncology*, Philadelphia, 1997, Saunders, pp 136-150.
31. Suh JH, Barner GH: Brachytherapy for brain tumors, *Hematol OncolClin North Am* 13(3):635-650, 1999.
32. Haas M, Keuhb EF: Brachytherapy. In Haas M, editor: *Outcomes in radiation therapy*, Sudbury, 2001, Jones and Bartlett, pp 67-72.
33. Martin CW, Whitehead T: Radiation modifiers chemical and thermal. In Haas M, editor: *Outcomes in radiation therapy*, Sudbury, 2001, Jones and Bartlett, pp 102-120.
34. Miyamoto C: Radiation therapy principles for high grade gliomas, *Principles Practice Radiat Oncol Updates* 1(3):2-16, 2000.
35. Stewart LA: Chemotherapy in adult high-grade glioma: a systematic review and meta-analysis of individual patient data from 12 randomised trials, *Lancet* 359(9311): 1011-1018, 2002.
36. Stupp R et al: *Concomitant and adjuvant temozolomide (TMZ) and radiotherapy (RT) for newly diagnosed glioblastoma multiforme (GBM): conclusive results of a randomized phase III trial by the EORTC Brain & RT Groups and NCIC Clinical Trials Group*, Proceedings of 23rd Meeting of American Society of Clinical Oncology, 2004, New Orleans, p 1.
37. Westphal M, Hilt DC, Bortey E et al: A phase 3 trial of local chemotherapy with biodegradable carmustine (BCNU) wafers (Gliadel wafers) in patients with primary malignant glioma, *Neuro-oncol* 5(2):79-88, 2003.
38. Brem H, Piantadosi S, Burger PC et al: Placebo-controlled trial of safety and efficacy of intraoperative controlled delivery by biodegradable polymers of chemotherapy for recurrent gliomas, the Polymer-brain Tumor Treatment Group, *Lancet* 345(8956):1008-1012, 1995.
39. Yung WK, Prados MD, Yaya-Tur R et al: Multicenter phase II trial of temozolomide in patients with anaplastic astrocytoma or anaplastic oligoastrocytoma at first relapse, Temodal Brain Tumor Group, *J Clin Oncol* 17(9):2762-2771, 1999.
40. Shaw EG, Tatter SB, Lesser GJ et al: Current controversies in the radiotherapeutic management of adult low-grade glioma, *Semin Oncol* 31(5):653-658, 2004.
41. Shaw EG, Wisoff JH: Prospective clinical trials of intracranial low-grade glioma in adults and children, *Neuro-oncol* 5(3):153-160, 2003.
42. Chinot O: Chemotherapy for the treatment of oligodendroglial tumors, *Semin Oncol* 28(4 Suppl 13):13-18, 2001.
43. Lesser GJ: Chemotherapy of low-grade gliomas, *Semin Radiat Oncol* 11(2):138-144, 2001.
44. Mason WP: Chemotherapy for low-grade gliomas, *Forum (Genova)* 10(2):95-104, 2000.
45. van den Bent MJ: Chemotherapy of oligodendroglial tumours: current developments *Forum (Genova)* 10(2):108-118, 2000.
46. Ino Y, Betensky RA, Zlatescu MC et al: Molecular subtypes of anaplastic oligodendroglioma: implications for patient management at diagnosis, *Clin Cancer Res* 7(4):839-845, 2001.
47. van den Bent, M, Chinot OL, Cairncross JG: Recent developments in the molecular characterization and

treatment of oligodendroglial tumors, *Neuro-oncol* 5(2): 128-138, 2003.
48. Levin VA: Chemotherapy for brain tumors of astrocytic and oligodendroglial lineage: the past decade and where we are heading, *Neuro-oncol* 1(1):69-80, 1999.
49. Armstrong TS, Gilbert MR: Metastatic brain tumors: diagnosis, treatment, and nursing interventions, *Clin J Oncol Nurs* 4(5):217-225, 2001.
50. Shrieve DC, Gutin PH, Larson DA: Central nervous system toxic effect of radiotherapy. In Wilson CB, editor: *The gliomas*, Philadelphia, 1999, Saunders, p 737.
51. Westbury C, Hines F, Hawkes E et al: Advice on hair and scalp care during cranial radiotherapy: a prospective randomized trial, *Radiother Oncol* 54(2):109-116, 1999.
52. Lovely MP, Miakowski C, Doss M: Relationship between fatigue and quality of life in patients with glioblastoma multiforme, *Oncol Nurs Forum* 26(5): 921-925, 1999.
53. Strohl RA: Radiation therapy in tumors of the central nervous system, *Semin Oncol Nurs* 14(1):26-33, 1998.

Chapter 7

Head and Neck Cancers

Elise Carper

The incidence of head and neck cancers in the United States is about 4% of all cancers, with an estimated 29,000 new cases and over 7400 deaths to occur in 2006.[1] Though a small proportion of all cancers, these malignancies cause effects that are extremely disturbing to patients, and treatment is quite difficult. Males contract head and neck cancers at a rate of 2:1 over females, although this ratio is decreasing as a result of increased smoking among women. The incidence of head and neck cancers peaks in the fifth and sixth decades of life. However, it can occur at any age.

The full etiology of upper aerodigestive tract cancers remains unknown, but it is clearly linked to exposure to tobacco and alcohol.[2] Tobacco exposure refers to cigarette smoke and chewing tobacco, pipe smoke, and cigars and includes not only direct exposure but also exposure from secondhand smoke. Oral irritants also may play a role in head and neck cancer as evidenced by the higher incidence of oral cavity and oral tongue cancers found among people from India and Southeast Asians who routinely chew betel nuts mixed with tobacco.

Two of the most common causes of head and neck cancers are thought to be mutations of the *p53* gene and exposure to mucosal irritants such as tobacco and alcohol. The effect of viral infection is also under investigation. Epstein-Barr virus (EBV) is specifically associated with nasopharynx cancers, and research on the effect of the human papilloma virus (HPV) has demonstrated a connection between HPV and oral cancers, especially tonsil carcinoma. Larynx cancers may be more common in persons with chronic gastroesophageal reflux because of the continuous irritation of the underside of the vocal cords by gastric acid.[3,4]

Environmental irritants to nasal, oral, and pharyngeal tissues are risk factors in head and neck cancers. Exposure to inhaled drugs, toxic dry-cleaning solvents or paint fumes, wood dust, and asbestos are considered risk factors for head and neck cancer. Irritation from ill-fitting dental obturators and dentures may be a risk factor for oral cavity and oral tongue cancers.[5]

More than 90% of head and neck cancers are squamous cell carcinomas (SCCs), arising from the mucosal surfaces of the upper aerodigestive tract. Other tissue types include mucoepidermoid, adenoid cystic carcinomas, and melanomas.[5] Head and neck lesions may be painful or painless, flat and endophytic, or bulky and exophytic, or a combination. Lesions may be easily observed or may never be clinically detected. In fact, head and neck cancers often present with a bulky neck mass without obvious primary tumor source.

Included in the descriptor, "head and neck cancers" are structures composing the face, nasal cavity and nasal sinuses, nasopharynx, oral cavity, oropharynx, hypopharynx, laryngeal structures, and the neck. The skin, soft tissues, muscles, and bones of the face and neck are considered part of this grouping as are the major and minor salivary glands. Given the wide variety of structures included in this body site, tumor behavior and patterns of spread are heterogeneous and dependent on the specific site of disease.

SPECIFIC SITES OF THE HEAD AND NECK

Nasal Cavity and Paranasal Sinus Tumors

Anatomy

The nasal cavity is the space connecting the nares to the nasopharynx. The septum forms the medial wall, and the bones of the maxilla, lacrimal process, ethmoid, and palatine fossa form the lateral wall. The roof of the nasal cavity is formed by the nasal, frontal, ethmoid, and sphenoid bones. The hard palate forms the floor of the mouth. The paranasal sinuses communicate with the nasal cavity through the various ostia and include the maxillary sinuses, the frontal sinuses, the ethmoid sinuses, and the sphenoid sinus.

Clinical Manifestations

Tumors of the nasal cavity and paranasal sinus complex may be asymptomatic until they reach late stages of growth. Over time nasal stuffiness, congestion, sinus headache, and epistaxis will occur. If aggressive, a maxillary sinus tumor may cause soft tissue and bony protrusion with resultant facial asymmetry, abnormal sensation, and pain. Regional metastasis may present as a neck mass.

Diagnostic Studies

Standard work-up for cancers of the nasal cavity and paranasal sinus complex include a thorough history with special attention to exposure to environmental irritants. The physical exam includes a full head and neck evaluation, and the use of a nasal speculum and fiberoptic endoscopy (if tumor mass allows) to determine the full extent of the lesion. Computed tomography (CT) and magnetic resonance imaging (MRI) with contrast of the primary lesion and a chest x ray to evaluate for distant metastasis are indicated. Histology is determined with a biopsy of the primary tumor, and if a neck mass is present, a fine-needle aspiration (FNA) of the neck is done.

Pathology and Patterns of Metastasis

Nasal cavity and paranasal sinus complex tumors are rare and are usually squamous cell carcinoma. Other histologies include minor salivary gland malignancies, adenocarcinomas, adenoid cystic carcinoma, mucoepidermoid carcinoma, and acinar cell carcinoma. Even rarer histologies include esthesioneuroblastoma, olfactory neuroblastoma, mucosal melanomas, and juvenile angiofibromas.[5]

Staging

Staging is available only for maxillary and ethmoid sinus tumors. A list of the stages is provided in Table 7-1.

Treatment

Cancers of the nasal cavity are usually treated with surgery and radiation therapy. Small lesions can be treated with either modality with near-equivalent results. Larger lesions and cancers of the sinuses necessitate a combined surgery and radiation therapy approach. For both ethmoid and maxillary sinus tumors, complete resection is the goal. Maxillectomy followed by postoperative radiation therapy is mainstay treatment for tumors in the maxillary sinus. Chemotherapy is given concomitantly with radiation therapy for T3 disease with adverse characteristics and for T4 inoperable tumors not suitable for a clinical trial.[6] Orbital exenteration may be necessary for tumors extending from the sinus to involve the orbital floor. This is followed by reconstructive surgery and postoperative radiation therapy. A craniofacial resection is used for tumors involving the skull base.

Radiation therapy is planned to maximize dose to the tumor and minimize injury to the normal tissues (Box 7-1). Injury to the eye or nerves innervating the eye that may occur while treating paranasal sinus tumors is a real concern. Postoperative radiation therapy (adjuvant treatment) using intensity-modulated radiation therapy (IMRT) may present a good option. Duthoy and colleagues[7] administered postoperative IMRT for sinonasal carcinoma, which resulted in good locoregional control with low acute toxicity and no radiation therapy–induced blindness.

Box 7-1 Nasal Cavity and Paranasal Sinus Radiation Therapy per NCCN Guidelines

DEFINITIVE RADIATION THERAPY

- Primary and gross adenopathy: ≥ 66 Gy (2.0 Gy/day)
  External-beam radiation therapy: ≥ 50 Gy + Brachytherapy
- Neck
  Low-risk nodal stations: ≥ 50 Gy (2.0 Gy/day)

ADJUVANT RADIATION THERAPY

- Primary: ≥ 60 Gy (2.0 Gy/day)
- Neck
  High-risk nodal stations: > 60 Gy (2.0 Gy/day)
  Low-risk nodal stations: ≥ 50 Gy (2.0 Gy/day)

Data from the National Comprehensive Cancer Network (NCCN): Practice Guidelines in Oncology—v.1.2005 Maxillary sinus tumors (website): www.nccn.org/professionals/physician_gls/PDF/head-and-neck.pdf. Accessed December 6, 2005.

Table 7-1 Staging Maxillary and Ethmoid Sinus Tumors

MAXILLARY SINUS PRIMARY TUMOR (T)	
TX	Primary tumor cannot be assessed
T0	No evidence of primary tumor
Tis	Carcinoma in situ
T1	Tumor limited to maxillary sinus mucosa with no erosion or destruction of bone
T2	Tumor causing bone erosion or destruction, including extension into the hard palate and/or middle nasal meatus, except extension to posterior wall of maxillary sinus and pterygoid plates
T3	Tumor invades any of the following: bone of the posterior wall of maxillary sinus, subcutaneous tissues, floor or medial wall of orbit, pterygoid fossa, ethmoid sinuses
T4a	Tumor invades anterior orbital contents, skin of cheek, pterygoid plates, infratemporal fossa, cribriform plate, sphenoid or frontal sinuses
T4b	Tumor invades any of the following: orbital apex, dura, brain, middle cranial fossa, cranial nerves other than (V_2), nasopharynx, or clivus
NASAL CAVITY AND ETHMOID SINUS PRIMARY TUMOR (T)	
T1	Tumor restricted to any one subsite, with or without bony invasion
T2	Tumor invading two subsites in a single region or extending to involve an adjacent region within the nasoethmoidal complex, with or without bony invasion
T3	Tumor extends to invade the medial wall or floor of the orbit, maxillary sinus, palate, or cribriform plate
T4a	Tumor invades any of the following: anterior orbital contents, skin of nose or cheek, minimal extension to anterior cranial fossa, pterygoid plates, sphenoid or frontal sinuses
T4b	Tumor invades any of the following: orbital apex, dura, brain, middle cranial fossa, cranial nerves other than (V_2), nasopharynx, or clivus
REGIONAL LYMPH NODES (N)	
NX	Regional lymph nodes cannot be assessed
N0	No regional lymph node metastasis
N1	Metastasis in a single ipsilateral lymph node, 3 cm or less in greatest dimension
N2	Metastasis in a single ipsilateral lymph node, more than 3 cm but not more than 6 cm in greatest dimension, or in bilateral or contralateral lymph nodes, none more than 6 cm in greatest dimension
N2a	Metastasis in a single ipsilateral lymph node, more than 3 cm but not more than 6 cm in greatest dimension
N2b	Metastasis in multiple ipsilateral lymph nodes, none more than 6 cm in greatest dimension
N2c	Metastasis in bilateral or contralateral lymph nodes, none more than 6 cm in greatest dimension
N3	Metastasis in a lymph node, more than 6 cm in greatest dimension
DISTANT METASTASIS (M)	
MX	Distant metastasis cannot be assessed
M0	No distant metastasis
M1	Distant metastasis

STAGE GROUPING: NASAL CAVITY AND PARANASAL SINUSES

Stage 0	Tis	N0	M0
Stage I	T1	N0	M0
Stage II	T2	N0	M0
Stage III	T3	N0	M0
	T1, T2, T3	N1	M0
Stage IVA	T4a	N0, N1	M0
	T1, T2, T3, T4a	N2	M0
Stage IVB	T4b	Any N	M0
	Any T	N3	M0
Stage IVC	Any T	Any N	M1

Used with the permission of the American Joint Committee on Cancer (AJCC), Chicago, Illinois. The original source for this material is the *AJCC Cancer Staging Manual, Sixth Edition* (2002), published by Springer-New York, www.springeronline.com.

Nasopharynx

Anatomy and Pathophysiology

The nasopharynx is an air-filled vault that extends from the posterior aspect of the nasal cavity to the posterior pharyngeal wall and laterally to include the eustachian tube openings. The superior aspect of the nasopharynx is the base of the skull itself, and the inferior border is the posterior pharynx at the level of the soft palate/uvula. The majority of these cancers are undifferentiated carcinomas, but typical keratinizing squamous cell carcinoma is also noted. Nasopharynx cancers are endemic in southeast China, especially in the Cantonese population. It is believed high dietary intake of salt-cured fish and meats are implicated in the higher rates of nasopharynx cancers among those from southeast China. It is found more often in men than women and in a younger population than other head and neck cancers, with peak incidence occurring in the fourth and fifth decades.

Clinical Manifestations

Presentation relates to the location of the tumor. Unilateral or bilateral hearing loss with or without tinnitus may be the main complaint with a tumor blocking one or both eustachian tubes. Congestion, sinus pressure, epistaxis occurs when tumor extends into the nasal cavity. If tumor invades the basilar foramen, foramen ovale, and/or cavernous sinus, cranial nerve (CN) symptoms are noted: dysphagia (CN XII), dysphonia (CN X), or difficulty moving the eye and eye symptoms such as pressure behind the eye, proptosis, or blurry vision (CN VI). Because of the proximity of the orbit and organs of sight, initial symptoms of disease may be changes in vision caused by direct pressure on the optic nerve or chiasm.

Diagnostic Studies

Evaluation of nasopharynx cancers includes a thorough history with special attention to genetic and environmental factors. Nasopharynx cancers are generally not associated with tobacco and alcohol use, but instead are associated with EBV virus and southern Chinese heritage. The physical exam includes a thorough neck evaluation, oral cavity examination, and fiberoptic endoscopy (if tumor mass allows) to determine the full extent of the lesion.

Extension of disease from the nasopharynx itself can be detected only with radiologic imaging. CT and/or MRI with contrast is done to reveal the extent of primary disease and the presence or absence of retropharyngeal lymphadenopathy and involvement of neck nodes. Chest x ray (CXR) and CT of the chest are indicated to evaluate distant metastasis. Combined imaging, if available, such as positron emission tomography/computed tomography (PET/CT), is an excellent way to evaluate both the extent of the primary and regional disease and verify any evidence of metastasis. Biopsy of the primary tumor is usually done intranasal, and an FNA is performed on any neck mass. A screening EBV titer is often obtained at presentation along with routine baseline serum chemistries and complete blood cell count.

Pathology and Patterns of Metastasis

The fossa of Rosenmüller located posterior to the eustachian tube opening is a common origin of nasopharynx disease. Tumors arise from the wall of the nasopharynx, expanding to fill the airspace of the nasopharynx and extending downward onto the posterior wall of the oropharynx or upwards toward the base of skull. Extension into the cranium via the foramen lacerum often leads to cranial nerve involvement and one in five patients will present with cranial nerve symptoms.[9]

The nasopharynx is rich in blood and lymph supply, leading to a high incidence of regional metastasis. Lymph nodes in the retropharyngeal space, spinal accessory, and jugular chains are readily accessible, and presentation with bilateral lymphadenopathy is seen in 9 of 10 patients with nasopharyngeal cancer. Unfortunately, the incidence of distant disease is higher in nasopharynx cancer than any other head and neck cancer, with bone, lung, and liver as primary metastatic sites.[9]

Staging

Staging of nasopharynx tumors is shown in Table 7-2.

Treatment

Because of the location of nasopharynx cancers and their radiosensitivity, radiation is almost always the treatment of choice for tumors without distant metastasis. These tumors often extend to the base of the skull and/or to the optic chiasm and involve the retropharyngeal lymph node chain, making it impossible to safely resect the entire

Table 7-2 Staging Nasopharynx Tumors

NASOPHARYNX TUMOR (T)	
TX	Primary tumor cannot be assessed
T0	No evidence of primary tumor
Tis	Carcinoma in situ
T1	Tumor confined to the nasopharynx
T2	Tumor extends to soft tissues
T2a	Tumor extends to the oropharynx and/or nasal cavity without parapharyngeal extension
T2b	Any tumor with parapharyngeal extension
T3	Tumor involves bony structures and/or paranasal sinuses
T4	Tumor with intracranial extension and/or involvement of cranial nerves, infratemporal fossa, hypopharynx, orbit, or masticator space
REGIONAL LYMPH NODES (N)	
NOTE: The distribution and the prognostic impact of regional lymph node spread from nasopharynx cancer, particularly of the undifferentiated type, are different from those of other head and neck mucosal cancers and justify the use of a different N classification scheme.	
NX	Regional lymph nodes cannot be assessed
N0	No regional lymph node metastasis
N1	Unilateral metastasis in lymph node(s), 6 cm or less in greatest dimension, above the supraclavicular fossa
N2	Bilateral metastasis in lymph node(s), 6 cm or less in greatest dimension, above the supraclavicular fossa
N3	Metastasis in a lymph node(s) more than 6 cm and/or to supraclavicular fossa
N3a	Greater than 6 cm in dimension
N3b	Extension to the supraclavicular fossa in greatest dimension
DISTANT METASTASIS (M)	
MX	Distant metastasis cannot be assessed
M0	No distant metastasis
M1	Distant metastasis

STAGE GROUPING: NASOPHARYNX

Stage 0	Tis	N0	M0
Stage I	T1	N0	M0
Stage IIA	T2a	N0	M0
Stage IIB	T1, T2	N1	M0
	T2a	N1	M0
	T2b	N0, N1	M0
Stage III	T1, T2a, T2b	N2	M0
	T3	N0, N1, N2	M0
Stage IVA	T4	N0, N1, N2	M0
Stage IVB	Any T	N3	M0
Stage IVC	Any T	Any N	M1

Used with the permission of the American Joint Committee on Cancer (AJCC), Chicago, Illinois. The original source for this material is the *AJCC Cancer Staging Manual, Sixth Edition* (2002), published by Springer-New York, www.springeronline.com.

tumor and obtain negative margins. Early stage nasopharynx tumors (T1 and small T2), without evidence of regional spread, are treated primarily with radiation therapy. Chemotherapy is used concurrently for bulky T2 to T4 tumors and tumors with any regional neck nodes. Cancers presenting with distant metastasis are given a platinum-based chemotherapy regimen for two to three cycles. If a complete response is elicited, this chemotherapy is followed by definitive radiation therapy to the primary site and neck.[10]

Radiation treatment is delivered with the patient in the supine, head neutral position. The majority of the treatment to the primary site of disease comes from two opposed lateral fields. An anterior field may be added if the tumor extends anteriorly or to better encompass an irregularly shaped tumor. Retropharyngeal lymph node involvement is treated with oblique fields. The lower neck is treated with a single anterior field, blocking the larynx/spinal cord after reaching the dose maximally tolerated by the spinal cord. Involved neck lymph nodes are treated using boost fields.[11]

Recent advances in radiation therapy have led to better treatment outcomes. In a study comparing the traditional shrinking opposed lateral fields with three-dimensional (3-D) plans comprised of lateral fields and a 3-D boost and IMRT plans, both the 3-D and the IMRT plans improved treatment parameters. IMRT plans provided the highest dose to the target and the lowest dose to normal structures. The dose to disease in the nasopharynx increased using IMRT to over 77 Gy, whereas the dose to the spinal cord, mandible, temporal lobes, and parotid glands all decreased below "typical" doses using opposed lateral fields.[12] IMRT may lead to better locoregional control while decreasing toxicity (Box 7-2).

Oral Cavity

Anatomy

The oral cavity involves the floor of the mouth, gingiva, lips, buccal mucosa, retromolar trigone, hard palate, and the anterior two thirds of the tongue. These structures are covered with a mucous membrane that is smooth and moist. The tongue is a muscle and contains taste buds composed of nervous tissue. Lymphatic drainage of the oral cavity structures is directed primarily to the submental, submandibular, and upper jugular-jugulodigastric nodal chains, with the exception of the oral tongue, which drains directly to the lower jugular lymph nodes. The oral tongue and floor of the mouth are the most common sites of disease in the oral cavity, and squamous cell carcinoma is the most common histology.

In the United States, oral cancers are 2 to 3 times more common in men than women and usually present in the fifth or sixth decade of life.[13] However, an increasing number of oral cancers are being diagnosed among those in their 20s through 40s.[14] Tumors of the oral cavity are significantly related to a history of smoking and alcohol. Oral irritation from poorly fitting dentures and chronic oral infections also may play a role in tumor development. Incidence of second primary cancers is high among patients with oral cancer. Malignancy occurs in the same oral cavity site or in other sites of the aerodigestive tract and is usually associated with continued smoking and alcohol use.

Clinical Manifestations

Oral cavity tumors are often visible to the eye and may present as an erythematous lesion or leukoplakia transformed into a malignant lesion. The lesion may have an ulcerative appearance, or it may be exophytic in nature. The lesion may be painless, or when perineural invasion is present, the lesion may be quite painful. Bleeding from an oral cavity lesion is considered highly predictive of malignancy and should always be investigated thoroughly. Occasionally pain is referred to the ear or posterior pharynx.

Diagnostic Studies

The history should include an in-depth review of cigarette and alcohol use and of dental hygiene. Any exposure to nicotine from smokeless tobacco should be noted, as well as history of oral irritation from poor-fitting dentures, orthodontia, and so on. The physical examination includes appropriate visualization of the oral cavity lesion and a thorough search for any synchronous lesions. A full neck examination including bimanual palpation of the floor of mouth to define any submental or submandibular lesions is required. Finally, fiberoptic endoscopy is done to rule out any other gross lesions of the aerodigestive tract. A contrast-enhanced CT scan and PET scan are used to delineate extent of primary disease and regional spread and to discover any distant metastasis.

Pathology and Patterns of Metastasis

More than 90% of oral cavity lesions are squamous cell carcinoma. Lesions are often locally invasive,

Box 7-2 Nasopharynx Radiation Therapy per NCCN Guidelines

DEFINITIVE RADIATION THERAPY

- Primary and gross adenopathy: ≥ 70 Gy (2.0 Gy/day)
  ± Brachytherapy
- Neck
  Low-risk nodal stations: ≥ 50 Gy (2.0 Gy/day)

Data from the National Comprehensive Cancer Network (NCCN): Practice Guidelines in Oncology—v.1.2005 Cancer of the nasopharynx (website): www.nccn.org/professionals/physician_gls/PDF/head-and-neck.pdf. Accessed December 6, 2005.

extending into adjacent mucosa and even adjacent bony structures. Floor-of-mouth and oral tongue cancers can invade muscles responsible for tongue movement. Tumors of the hard palate and maxillary gingiva may directly infiltrate the palatal bone and maxillary antrum. Cancers of the lower gingiva may invade the mandible via dental sockets. Therefore, extractions before surgery are strongly contraindicated so as to reduce the likelihood that tumor cells may extend into the mandibular canal.[15]

Spread of disease outside of the oral cavity depends on the site of the primary tumor (tongue and floor of mouth tend to spread to lymph nodes much more often than hard palate lesions) and to histological factors such as amount of cell differentiation and whether the lesion is endophytic or exophytic. The lymph nodes of the supraomohyoid triangle are most at risk, including submental and submandibular and levels I, II, and III anterior neck nodes (Figure 7-1). Distant metastasis to lung or bones is rare at time of presentation but does occur in late-stage disease.

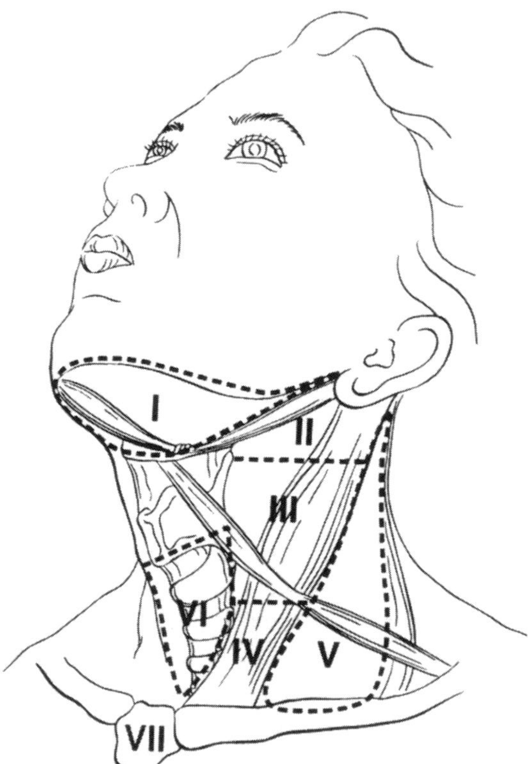

Figure 7-1 Lymph Nodes of the Neck, Levels I to VII. *Used with the permission of the American Joint Committee on Cancer (AJCC), Chicago, IL. The original source for this image is the* AJCC Cancer Staging Manual, Sixth Edition *(2002), published by Springer-New York, www.springeronline.com.*

Staging

Staging of oral cavity tumors is listed in Table 7-3.

Treatment

Early-stage and small, superficial lesions are treated with equal efficacy with either surgery alone or radiation therapy alone. The decision as to which modality is used depends on factors such as cosmesis, convenience, possible complications, and potential long-term effects. Functionality and form are important considerations and must be taken into account during the decision-making process.

T1 to T2, N0 tumors of the lip and oral cavity are treated either with surgery or radiation. Radiation for lip cancers can be given as external beam radiation therapy alone, brachytherapy alone, or a combination of external beam and brachytherapy. Radiation for the remaining structure of the oral cavity is either external beam alone or combined with brachytherapy. Surgery involves removal of the primary tumor alone. For larger tumors, (T3–4) or any oral cavity cancers with nodal involvement, selective or full-neck dissections are added. If surgery is chosen as the primary modality, the involved neck is dissected. If negative prognostic features are present (close/positive margins, perineural invasion, multiple positive nodes, extracapsular extension), postoperative chemo/radiation therapy is indicated. The presence of one positive node without adverse features might receive adjuvant radiation therapy alone.

If radiation is chosen as primary therapy, it will include external beam radiation therapy plus or minus brachytherapy. In lip cancer, when response at the primary site is complete, surgery is not indicated. If the primary site has only a partial response, salvage surgery is indicated. If response is complete in a patient with N1 disease, observation is indicated. If the response is less than complete or if the patient was originally diagnosed with N1 to N3 disease, a planned neck dissection of the involved side is done after completion of radiation therapy. For cancers other than lip, excision of the primary (and reconstruction) plus neck dissection is followed by postoperative radiation therapy alone or chemotherapy/radiation therapy. Stage IV tumors with bone involvement usually have primary

Table 7-3 Staging Oral Cavity Tumors

ORAL CAVITY TUMORS (T)			
TX	Primary tumor cannot be assessed		
T0	No evidence of primary tumor		
Tis	Carcinoma in situ		
T1	Tumor 2 cm or less in greatest dimension		
T2	Tumor more than 2 cm but not more than 4 cm in greatest dimension		
T3	Tumor more than 4 cm in greatest dimension		
T4	(lip) Tumor invades through cortical bone, inferior alveolar nerve, floor of mouth, or skin of face (i.e., chin or nose)		
T4a	(oral cavity) Tumor invades adjacent structures (e.g., through cortical bone, into deep muscle of tongue, maxillary sinus, skin of face)		
T4b	Tumor invades masticator space, pterygoid plates, or skull base and/or encases internal carotid artery		
REGIONAL LYMPH NODES (N)			
NX	Regional lymph nodes cannot be assessed		
N0	No regional lymph node metastasis		
N1	Metastasis in a single ipsilateral lymph node, 3 cm or less in greatest dimension		
N2	Metastasis in a single ipsilateral lymph node, more than 3 cm but not more than 6 cm in greatest dimension; or in multiple ipsilateral lymph nodes, none more than 6 cm in greatest dimension; or in bilateral or contralateral lymph nodes, none more than 6 cm in greatest dimension		
N2a	Metastasis in a single ipsilateral lymph node more than 3 cm but not more than 6 cm in greatest dimension		
N2b	Metastasis in multiple ipsilateral lymph nodes, none more than 6 cm in greatest dimension		
N2c	Metastasis in bilateral or contralateral lymph nodes, none more than 6 cm in greatest dimension		
N3	Metastasis in a lymph node, more than 6 cm in greatest dimension		
DISTANT METASTASIS (M)			
MX	Distant metastasis cannot be assessed		
M0	No distant metastasis		
M1	Distant metastasis		
STAGE GROUPING: ORAL CAVITY			
Stage 0	Tis	N0	M0
Stage I	T1	N0	M0
Stage II	T2	N0	M0
Stage III	T3	N0	M0
	T1, T2, T3	N1	M0
Stage IVA	T4a	N0, N1	M0
	T1, T2, T3, T4a	N2	M0
Stage IVB	Any T	N3	M0
	T4b	Any N	M0
Stage IVC	Any T	Any N	M1

Used with the permission of the American Joint Committee on Cancer (AJCC), Chicago, Illinois. The original source for this material is the *AJCC Cancer Staging Manual, Sixth Edition* (2002), published by Springer-New York, www.springeronline.com.

surgery followed by chemotherapy/radiation therapy. Those without bone involvement are treated with chemotherapy/radiation therapy, with surgery being used for tissue salvage (Box 7-3).

Oropharynx

Anatomy

The oropharynx encompasses the space between the nasopharynx superiorly and the hypopharynx inferiorly and is continuous with the oral cavity anteriorly. It includes the base of the tongue, the tonsilar fossa and pillars, the soft palate, and the lateral and posterior oropharyngeal walls. The part of the tongue considered the base extends upward from the valleculae or base of the epiglottis, to the circumvallate papilla located at the posterior aspect of the oral tongue. It is muscular and functions not only to propel the food bolus downward to the esophagus but also to work with the epiglottis to protect the airway.

Box 7-3 Oral Cavity Radiation Therapy per NCCN Guidelines

DEFINITIVE RADIATION THERAPY

- Primary and gross adenopathy: ≥ 70 Gy (2.0 Gy/day)
  External-beam radiation therapy: ≥ 50 Gy ± Brachytherapy
- Neck
  Low-risk nodal stations: ≥ 50 Gy (2.0 Gy/day)

ADJUVANT RADIATION THERAPY

- Primary: ≥ 60 Gy (2.0 Gy/day)
- Neck
  High-risk nodal stations: ≥ 60 Gy (2.0 Gy/day)
  Low-risk nodal stations: ≥ 50 Gy (2.0 Gy/day)

Data from the National Comprehensive Cancer Network (NCCN): Practice Guidelines in Oncology—v.1.2005 Cancer of the oral cavity (website): www.nccn.org/professionals/physician_gls/PDF/head-and-neck.pdf. Accessed December 6, 2005.

The soft palate forms both the "roof" of the oropharynx and the "floor" of the nasopharynx. It connects anteriorly to the hard palate and this junction forms the anterior border of the oropharynx. Laterally, it arises continuously from the vertical tonsilar pillars and meets at the midline to form the hanging uvula. It is important in preventing food from entering the nasopharynx and is important in phonation and enunciation of speech.

The tonsilar region is the posterolateral aspect of the oropharynx. Bilateral tonsillar fossae contain the actual palatine tonsils, which are lymphoid tissue in an oval shape. The pharyngeal wall begins at the most inferior aspect of the nasopharynx and extends inferiorly to the level of the epiglottis. It covers the lateral wall of the oropharynx to the tonsillar pillars bilaterally. Lymphatic flow from the oropharynx is primarily to the jugulodigastric lymph nodes, located in the upper neck. The tonsils, base of tongue, and parts of the pharyngeal soft palate also drain to the retropharyngeal and parapharyngeal nodes located in the parapharyngeal space.

Clinical Manifestations

Often tumors of the oropharynx are not discovered until quite advanced. Symptoms are usually mild and vague. A neck mass may not be the presenting symptom. Tumors of the tonsils and soft palate may be discovered during an open mouth exam by a primary care physician or dentist. Anterior tonsillar pillar cancers are the most common of the oropharynx cancers. Otalgia of the ear on the affected tonsillar side is a common presenting complaint. Lymphadenopathy is usually unilateral but may be bilateral and/or include retropharyngeal lymph nodes.

Base of tongue cancers are most often diagnosed at a late stage. The base of the tongue does not contain many pain receptors, and these tumors are often asymptomatic until quite large and metastatic. Complaints of "fullness" in the throat or a strange sensation during swallowing, without pain, are common. Occasionally speech is affected by tumor extension into the oral tongue, causing fixation and inability to extend the tongue normally. Tumor extension into the pterygoid muscles causes trismus, leading to weight loss and pain.

Diagnostic Studies

The history should include an in-depth review of cigarette and alcohol use and any co-morbidities. A baseline nutritional assessment is helpful in learning the effect of the lesion on normal swallowing. The physical examination includes a full head and neck examination including appropriate visualization of the area in question. Tumors of the base of the tongue can be difficult to visualize unless a flexible fiberoptic endoscopy is performed and, even then, may be quite difficult to locate. A contrast-enhanced CT scan and PET scan are used to delineate extent of primary disease and regional spread and to discover any distant metastasis.

Pathology and Patterns of Metastasis

Although malignant melanomas, minor salivary gland tumors, sarcomas, lymphomas, and other rare tumors may present in the oropharynx, the overwhelming majority of tumors in this area are squamous cell carcinomas. Non-Hodgkin's lymphoma comprises 5% of all tonsillar cancers but is never found in the base of the tongue. The ample lymphatic drainage from the base of tongue makes neck metastasis common, usually at level II, but also at levels III and IV (please refer to Figure 7-1). Tumors of the tongue are often midline, so bilateral lymphadenopathy may occur. Soft palate lesions often are found before regional spread, but again, bilateral lymphadenopathy can be seen with unilateral lesions. Anterior tonsillar pillar and tonsillar tumors tend to metastasize unilaterally. Tonsillar fossa tumors are more likely to have contralateral involvement and often present at a later stage.[13]

Staging

Staging of oropharynx tumors is listed in Table 7-4.

Treatment

Both surgery and radiation are used as sole modality therapies for early-stage lesions of the oropharynx. Radiation therapy often offers a better functional outcome, however, and so in recent years has become the treatment of choice for early lesions. In later-stage cancers, a combination of surgery and radiation is used. Chemotherapy is used in cases of advanced disease or for organ preservation.

In the case of soft palate cancers, radiation therapy is preferred. Treatment of the primary site is done using opposed lateral fields, which easily encompass the at-risk lymph nodes of the neck bilaterally. Late-staged soft palate lesions are treated with surgery and postoperative radiation therapy.

Table 7-4 Staging Oropharynx Tumors

OROPHARYNX TUMORS (T)	
TX	Primary tumor cannot be assessed
T0	No evidence of primary tumor
Tis	Carcinoma in situ
T1	Tumor 2 cm or less in greatest dimension
T2	Tumor more than 2 cm but not more than 4 cm in greatest dimension
T3	Tumor more than 4 cm in greatest dimension
T4a	Tumor invades the larynx, deep/extrinsic muscle of tongue, medial pterygoid, hard palate, or mandible
T4b	Tumor invades lateral pterygoid muscle, pterygoid plates, lateral nasopharynx, or skull base or encases the carotid artery
REGIONAL LYMPH NODES (N)	
NX	Regional lymph nodes cannot be assessed
N0	No regional lymph node metastasis
N1	Metastasis in a single ipsilateral lymph node, 3 cm or less in greatest dimension
N2	Metastasis in a single ipsilateral lymph node, more than 3 cm but not more than 6 cm in greatest dimension; or in multiple ipsilateral lymph nodes, none more than 6 cm in greatest dimension; or in bilateral or contralateral lymph nodes, none more than 6 cm in greatest dimension
N2a	Metastasis in a single ipsilateral lymph node more than 3 cm but not more than 6 cm in greatest dimension
N2b	Metastasis in multiple ipsilateral lymph nodes, none more than 6 cm in greatest dimension
N2c	Metastasis in bilateral or contralateral lymph nodes, none more than 6 cm in greatest dimension
N3	Metastasis in a lymph node, more than 6 cm in greatest dimension
DISTANT METASTASIS (M)	
MX	Distant metastasis cannot be assessed
M0	No distant metastasis
M1	Distant metastasis

STAGE GROUPING: OROPHARYNX			
Stage 0	Tis	N0	M0
Stage I	T1	N0	M0
Stage II	T2	N0	M0
Stage III	T3	N0	M0
	T1, T2, T3	N1	M0
Stage IVA	T4a	N0, N1	M0
	T1, T2, T3, T4a	N2	M0
Stage IVB	T4b	Any N	M0
	Any T	N3	M0
Stage IVC	Any T	Any N	M1

Used with the permission of the American Joint Committee on Cancer (AJCC), Chicago, Illinois. The original source for this material is the *AJCC Cancer Staging Manual, Sixth Edition* (2002), published by Springer-New York, www.springeronline.com.

Patients without palpable disease receive 50 Gy to 54 Gy. Any palpable lymph nodes will receive additional radiation to 60 Gy or more and may receive a neck dissection. Brachytherapy may be used in the setting of recurrent soft palate tumor when a full course of external beam radiation therapy was used, although these patients have higher rates of complication.[17]

Tonsillar lesions can be treated with either surgery or radiation therapy, but again, the functional outcome is better with radiation therapy, and it is used more commonly. Both the primary and the bilateral necks are within the opposed lateral portals, as are the at-risk retropharyngeal lymph nodes. Whenever possible, the contralateral parotid gland is spared to minimize xerostomia. If surgery is used, a transoral approach is preferred, although a mandibulotomy may be necessary if tumor approaches the mandible. A selective lymph node dissection is appropriate, for staging that warrants such an approach. Patients with node-positive disease receive postoperative radiation therapy.

Advanced tonsil lesions are usually treated with combined chemotherapy and radiation therapy, followed by planned neck dissection. Single-agent cisplatin is usually given on day 1 and day 22 of radiation therapy. Accelerated radiation is given using the delayed concomitant boost technique in which radiation is delivered daily for the first 4 weeks and twice a day during the last 2 weeks. Alternatively, radiation is given using a hyperfractionated technique that provides 2 times daily (b.i.d.) treatment throughout the entire course of radiation therapy.[15]

Early-stage pharyngeal wall tumors are usually treated with radiation therapy with portals including the site of primary disease and the bilateral necks. Surgery can be used, but leads to increased functional impairment. Advanced tumors are usually treated primarily with surgery followed by postoperative radiation therapy. Surgical options include pharyngectomy to a full pharyngolaryngoesophagectomy, requiring extensive reconstructive surgery to restore function and neck dissection. These patients should be referred for postoperative radiation therapy because a high incidence of retropharyngeal and cervical lymph node involvement is present. Planning for the treatment of these tumors is complicated by anatomy. Pharyngeal wall tumors are located near the spinal cord. The tumor requires radiation in excess of 60 Gy. However, spinal cord tolerance is 45 Gy or more,[17] and therefore precise measurements and field arrangements are necessary to provide adequate dose to the tumor and prevent injury to the spinal cord.

Base of tongue cancer treatment in the early stages is done with either surgery or radiation therapy. The survival and local control rates are equivalent with either modality, yet because of the functional morbidity of surgery, radiation therapy is the more common treatment choice. In advanced cancers, external beam radiation combined with brachytherapy is preferred. In both early- and late-stage cancers, the radiation-opposed lateral portals include the base of the tongue and a margin to include part of the oral tongue, vallecula, pharyngeal walls, epiglottis, and the bilateral regional and retropharyngeal lymph nodes.

In the combined external and brachytherapy approach, external beam radiation therapy is delivered daily, up to a dose of 54 Gy to the primary site, with involved neck nodes boosted to 60 Gy. Three weeks later an interstitial brachytherapy boost is given, using ^{192}Ir to a dose of 20 Gy to 30 Gy.[17] If neck nodes are involved, a planned neck dissection is done at the time of implant. If bilateral neck dissections are needed, the patient has staged surgeries; one side done at time of implant and the contralateral side done several weeks later.

Organ preservation and function preservation in the setting of advanced and/or unresectable disease is achieved by using combined chemotherapy and radiation therapy (Box 7-4). Cisplatin is the drug most often used, given at 100 mg/m^2 on days 1, 22, and 43 if the radiation treatments go into a seventh week.[17]

Hypopharynx and Cervical Esophagus

Anatomy

The hypopharynx extends from the lowest point of the oropharynx to the top of the esophagus. It surrounds the laryngeal structures, forming the posterior wall or postcricoid area, and includes the pyriform sinuses on either side of the larynx. The cervical esophagus extends from the lower edge of the cricoid cartilage to the thoracic inlet. The lymphatics draining from this subsite include the retropharyngeal and subdigastric and upper and midjugular nodes. The cervical esophagus drains to paratracheal nodes and upper mediastinal nodal groups. Squamous cell carcinoma is the most common histology, and the pyriform sinus is the most

Box 7-4 Oropharynx Radiation Therapy per NCCN Guidelines

CHEMORADIATION

- Conventional fractionation: ≥ 70 Gy (2.0 Gy/day)

DEFINITIVE RADIATION THERAPY (ALONE)

- T1-T2, N0
  - Conventional fractionation: ≥ 70 Gy (2.0 Gy/day) ± brachytherapy
- Selected T2, T3-T4, N1-3
  - Altered fractionation (preferred) Concomitant boost accelerated radiation therapy: 72 Gy/6 weeks (1.8 Gy/fraction, large field; 1.5 Gy boost as second daily fraction during last 12 treatment days) Hyperfractionation: 81.6 Gy/7 weeks (1.2 Gy/fraction b.i.d.)

ADJUVANT RADIATION THERAPY

- Primary: ≥ 60 Gy (2.0 Gy/day)
- Neck
  - High-risk nodal stations: ≥ 60 Gy (2.0 Gy/day)
  - Low-risk nodal stations: ≥ 50 Gy (2.0 Gy/day)

Data from the National Comprehensive Cancer Network (NCCN): Practice Guidelines in Oncology—v.1.2005 Cancer of the oropharynx (website): www.nccn.org/professionals/physician_gls/PDF/head-and-neck.pdf. Accessed December 6, 2005.

common site of disease within the hypopharynx. Tobacco and alcohol use are the major known risk factors, although a diet deficient in vitamin A may be a contributing factor.

Clinical Manifestations

Sore throat, dysphagia odynophasia, and referred otalgia are the most common symptoms of early-stage hypopharyngeal carcinomas. Hoarseness and severe dysphagia are indicative of advanced disease. A sensation of needing to clear the throat and difficulty swallowing even liquids are signs of lower hypopharynx and cervical esophagus tumors. The majority of patients with advanced tumors present with lymphadenopathy.

Diagnostic Studies

A careful history will include detailed nutritional and weight history. This may help elicit the degree of dysphagia present and the duration of symptoms. Physical examination requires flexible fiberoptic endoscopy in addition to a thorough head and neck exam. Evaluation of vocal cord movement may help reveal a small pyriform sinus tumor. Careful attention to the neck is needed because most hypopharynx tumors present with neck metastasis. CT scan of the neck with contrast is appropriate, along with baseline blood work that includes a complete blood count (CBC) with differential and a serum chemistry profile, and a CXR.

Pathology and Patterns of Metastasis

Hypopharynx and cervical esophageal tumors often metastasize via submucosal extension. It is common to find tumor extension greater than 10 mm beyond the original mass.[16] Esophageal tumors may grow around the circumference of the esophagus or may travel upward or downward along the esophagus and/or trachea. Pyriform sinus tumors often invade structures of the larynx, influencing function of the vocal cords. Occult nodal disease, often bilateral, is common, with up to 60% of patients with regional metastasis.[19]

Staging

Staging of the hypopharynx can be found in Table 7-5.

Treatment

Early stage (T1-2) hypopharynx lesions make up less than 20% of all hypopharyngeal cancers and are treated with either definitive radiation therapy, with or without neck dissection, or surgical excision. The surgery involves a partial laryngopharyngectomy plus selective neck dissection and is an attempt to maintain laryngeal function. Appropriate patient selection is very important in these cases. Patients must have excellent respiratory function (which is rare because many patients in this subset are smokers) and enthusiasm for rehabilitation in order to benefit. This surgery is then followed by postoperative radiation therapy to the primary site and bilateral neck fields. Primary radiation is given using opposed lateral fields and an anterior neck field that cover the primary site of disease and the cervical and mediastinal lymphatics at risk. Unfortunately, planned larynx-sparing surgeries often become total laryngectomy when the full extent of the tumor is exposed at time of surgery.

Combined modality treatment is necessary for advanced hypopharyngeal cancers and tumors

Table 7-5 Staging Hypopharynx Tumors

HYPOPHARYNX TUMORS (T)	
TX	Primary tumor cannot be assessed
T0	No evidence of primary tumor
Tis	Carcinoma in situ
T1	Tumor limited to one subsite of hypopharynx and 2 cm or less in greatest dimension
T2	Tumor invades more than one subsite of hypopharynx or an adjacent site, or measures more than 2 cm but not more than 4 cm in greatest diameter without fixation of hemilarynx
T3	Tumor more than 4 cm in greatest dimension or with fixation of hemilarynx
T4a	Tumor invades thyroid/cricoid cartilage, hyoid bone, thyroid gland, esophagus, or central compartment soft tissue
T4b	Tumor invades prevertebral fascia, encases carotid artery, or involves mediastinal structures
REGIONAL LYMPH NODES (N)	
NX	Regional lymph nodes cannot be assessed
N0	No regional lymph node metastasis
N1	Metastasis in a single ipsilateral lymph node, 3 cm or less in greatest dimension
N2	Metastasis in a single ipsilateral lymph node, more than 3 cm but not more than 6 cm in greatest dimension; or in multiple ipsilateral lymph nodes, none more than 6 cm in greatest dimension; or in bilateral or contralateral lymph nodes, none more than 6 cm in greatest dimension
N2a	Metastasis in a single ipsilateral lymph node more than 3 cm but not more than 6 cm in greatest dimension
N2b	Metastasis in multiple ipsilateral lymph nodes, none more than 6 cm in greatest dimension
N2c	Metastasis in bilateral or contralateral lymph nodes, none more than 6 cm in greatest dimension
N3	Metastasis in a lymph node, more than 6 cm in greatest dimension
DISTANT METASTASIS (M)	
MX	Distant metastasis cannot be assessed
M0	No distant metastasis
M1	Distant metastasis

STAGE GROUPING: HYPOPHARYNX			
Stage 0	Tis	N0	M0
Stage I	T1	N0	M0
Stage II	T2	N0	M0
Stage III	T3	N0	M0
	T1, T2, T3	N1	M0
Stage IVA	T4a	N0, N1	M0
	T1, T2, T3, T4a	N2	M0
Stage IVB	T4b	Any N	M0
	Any T	N3	M0
Stage IVC	Any T	Any N	M1

Used with the permission of the American Joint Committee on Cancer (AJCC), Chicago, Illinois. The original source for this material is the *AJCC Cancer Staging Manual, Sixth Edition* (2002), published by Springer-New York, www.springeronline.com.

of the cervical esophagus. Several options are currently being used. Patients may receive induction chemotherapy followed by surgery plus radiation or radiation plus neck dissection. Patients with hypopharyngeal tumors may have a laryngopharyngectomy with neck dissection followed by chemotherapy/radiation therapy. Patients with cervical esophageal tumors usually require a total laryngoesophagectomy because of submucosal extent of disease. Patients may receive concurrent chemoradiation on clinical trials, but it is unusual reserved for those with advanced-stage lesions (Box 7-5).[19]

Larynx

Anatomy

The glottis, supraglottic, and subglottic are the three components of the larynx. Each has a unique function and individual characteristics. The larynx is composed of the two true vocal cords and is responsible for airway protection during swallowing, coughing, and speech. The subglottis is the airway

Box 7-5 Hypopharynx Radiation Therapy per NCCN Guidelines

DEFINITIVE RADIATION THERAPY

- Primary and gross adenopathy: ≥ 70 Gy (2.0 Gy/day)
- Neck
  Low-risk nodal stations: ≥ 50 Gy (2.0 Gy/day)

ADJUVANT RADIATION THERAPY

- Primary: ≥ 60 Gy (2.0 Gy/day)
- Neck
  High-risk nodal stations: ≥ 60 Gy (2.0 Gy/day)
  Low-risk nodal stations: ≥ 50 Gy (2.0 Gy/day)

Data from the National Comprehensive Cancer Network (NCCN) Practice Guidelines in Oncology—v.1.2005 Cancer of the hypopharynx (website): www.nccn.org/professionals/physician_gls/PDF/head-and-neck.pdf. Accessed December 6, 2005.

found beneath the true vocal cords but superior to the trachea. The supraglottis runs from the inferior border of the hypopharynx and includes the false vocal cords, epiglottis, arytenoids, and aryepiglottic folds. The supraglottis protects the airway along with the true cords.

Clinical Manifestations

Early-stage glottic cancers are usually diagnosed early because of tell-tale changes in voice quality and volume. Hoarseness and changes in volume are noted in T1 lesions, allowing treatment at a very early stage. Supraglottic lesions do not affect the voice until they are quite large. Early signs of a supraglottic lesion are dysphagia and sore throat. Referred otalgia and neck metastasis are commonly seen at presentation. Advanced glottic and supraglottic lesions may present with hemoptysis and airway compromise that may ultimately lead to a tracheostomy.

Diagnostic Studies

A thorough history including tobacco and alcohol use and co-morbidities is essential. Larynx cancer is overwhelmingly a cancer of smokers, and treatment complications are increased in patients who continue to smoke.[21] Smoking cessation is vital, and patients may be motivated to quit at this time. An examination under anesthesia with biopsy is necessary to obtain histologic information. Physical examination with flexible endoscopy is the best way to confirm the presence of a laryngeal tumor. Imaging is not as useful in the staging of larynx cancers as in other cancers, but a CT with contrast helps delineate the depth and bulk of the tumor and any cartilage invasion, as well as the presence of metastatic disease in the neck. A CXR is indicated along with baseline blood work.

Pathology and Patterns of Metastasis

Greater than 95% of all larynx cancers are epithelial in origin. Other histologies include sarcomas, adenocarcinomas, and neuroendocrine tumors. Verrucous carcinomas are squamous cell carcinoma variants and are notoriously resistant to radiation therapy. Laryngeal carcinomas make up the largest group of cancers of the head and neck, and more than half of laryngeal cancers are localized to the glottis at presentation.[22]

The three parts of the larynx have individual patterns of spread and thus, separate staging systems. Most supraglottic larynx lesions arise from the epiglottis, but often extend into the tongue base via the preepiglottic space. Epiglottic lesions can also invade the true vocal cords and false cords, and can metastasize to the cervical lymph nodes in the neck.

Glottic cancers are fairly well differentiated but can infiltrate into the mucosa to affect motion of the vocal cord itself. Subglottic lesions are extremely rare, are poorly differentiated, and infiltrate freely. Cervical lymph node metastasis from all three sites is common in advanced stages, and cartilage invasion can occur.

Staging

Staging larynx cancer is listed in Table 7-6.

Treatment

Early-stage glottic tumors are often treated with surgery alone or radiation alone, and both provide excellent control. Surgery involves a partial laryngectomy that can lead to an impaired or suboptimal voice. Radiation is used more often, with surgery reserved for salvage treatment. Radiation is given using opposed lateral fields with very small portals to include only the larynx.[22]

Early supraglottic tumors can be treated primarily with conservation laryngeal surgeries that allow patients to maintain their ability to speak. Examples of this type of surgical approach include cordectomy, hemilaryngectomy or partial

Table 7-6 Staging Larynx Tumors

SUPRAGLOTTIS (T)	
TX	Primary tumor cannot be assessed
T0	No evidence of primary tumor
Tis	Carcinoma in situ
T1	Tumor limited to one subsite of supraglottis with normal vocal cord mobility
T2	Tumor invades mucosa of more than one adjacent subsite of supraglottis or glottis or region outside the supraglottis (e.g., mucosa of base of tongue, vallecula, medial wall of pyriform sinus) without fixation of the larynx
T3	Tumor limited to larynx with vocal cord fixation and/or invades any of the following: postcricoid area, preepiglottic tissues, paraglottic space, and/or minor thyroid cartilage erosion
T4a	Tumor invades through the thyroid cartilage and/or invades tissues beyond the larynx (e.g., trachea, soft tissues of neck including deep extrinsic muscle of the tongue, strap muscles, thyroid, or esophagus)
T4b	Tumor invades prevertebral space, encases carotid artery, or involves mediastinal structures
GLOTTIS (T)	
TX	Primary tumor cannot be assessed
T0	No evidence of primary tumor
Tis	Carcinoma in situ
T1	Tumor limited to vocal cord(s) with normal vocal cord mobility
T1a	Tumor limited to one vocal cord
T1b	Tumor involves both vocal cords
T2	Tumor extends to supraglottis and/or subglottis, and/or with impaired vocal cord mobility
T3	Tumor limited to larynx with vocal cord fixation and/or invades paraglottic space, and/or minor thyroid cartilage erosion
T4a	Tumor invades through the thyroid cartilage and/or invades tissues beyond the larynx (e.g., trachea, soft tissues of neck including deep extrinsic muscle of the tongue, strap muscles, thyroid, or esophagus)
T4b	Tumor invades prevertebral space, encases carotid artery, or involves mediastinal structures
SUBGLOTTIS (T)	
TX	Primary tumor cannot be assessed
T0	No evidence of primary tumor
Tis	Carcinoma in situ
T1	Tumor limited to subglottis
T2	Tumor extends to vocal cord(s) with normal or impaired vocal cord mobility
T3	Tumor limited to larynx with vocal cord fixation
T4a	Tumor invades cricoid or thyroid cartilage and/or invades tissues beyond the larynx (e.g., trachea, soft tissues of neck including deep extrinsic muscle of the tongue, strap muscles, thyroid, or esophagus)
T4b	Tumor invades prevertebral space, encases carotid artery, or involves mediastinal structures
REGIONAL LYMPH NODES (N)	
NX	Regional lymph nodes cannot be assessed
N0	No regional lymph node metastasis
N1	Metastasis in a single ipsilateral lymph node, 3 cm or less in greatest dimension
N2	Metastasis in a single ipsilateral lymph node, more than 3 cm but not more than 6 cm in greatest dimension; or in multiple ipsilateral lymph nodes, none more than 6 cm in greatest dimension; or in bilateral or contralateral lymph nodes, none more than 6 cm in greatest dimension
N2a	Metastasis in a single ipsilateral lymph node more than 3 cm but not more than 6 cm in greatest dimension
N2b	Metastasis in multiple ipsilateral lymph nodes, none more than 6 cm in greatest dimension
N2c	Metastasis in bilateral or contralateral lymph nodes, none more than 6 cm in greatest dimension
N3	Metastasis in a lymph node, more than 6 cm in greatest dimension
DISTANT METASTASIS (M)	
MX	Distant metastasis cannot be assessed
M0	No distant metastasis
M1	Distant metastasis

Table 7-6 Staging Larynx Tumors —cont'd

STAGE GROUPING: LARYNX			
Stage 0	Tis	N0	M0
Stage I	T1	N0	M0
Stage II	T2	N0	M0
Stage III	T3	N0	M0
	T1, T2, T3	N1	M0
Stage IVA	T4a	N0, N1	M0
	T1, T2, T3, T4a	N2	M0
Stage IVB	T4b	Any N	M0
	Any T	N3	M0
Stage IVC	Any T	Any N	M1

Used with the permission of the American Joint Committee on Cancer (AJCC), Chicago, Illinois. The original source for this material is the *AJCC Cancer Staging Manual, Sixth Edition* (2002), published by Springer-New York, www.springeronline.com.

laryngopharyngectomy. Another option is the use of definitive radiation therapy, with laryngeal surgery reserved for salvage treatment. Radiation portals include the primary tumor and the lymph nodes at risk for metastatic spread, including retropharyngeal and cervical lymph nodes.

Advanced supraglottic and glottic cancer treatment is influenced greatly by the desire to preserve voice function. Supraglottic tumors may be treated surgically with an extended supraglottic laryngectomy and neck dissection followed by postoperative radiation therapy. If there is vocal cord fixation or cartilage invasion, a total laryngectomy followed by radiation is indicated. Another option is concurrent chemoradiation with surgery for salvage treatment.

Historically, advanced T3 and T4 glottic cancers were managed by total laryngectomy with or without postoperative radiation therapy. Today larynx preservation is the goal of treatment, consisting of cisplatin cycled every 3 weeks, given concomitantly with radiation therapy. Radiation therapy is given using the delayed concomitant boost schedule; daily for the first 4 weeks and b.i.d. the last 2 weeks of treatment (Box 7-6). For T4, N2-3 cancers, total laryngectomy with neck dissection is still the preferred treatment, followed by radiation therapy plus or minus chemotherapy, depending on pathology findings.[23]

Salivary Gland

Anatomy

Salivary tissue consists of both major salivary glands; paired parotid, submandibular, and sublingual glands found on either side of the face; and minor salivary glands that are ubiquitous throughout the upper aerodigestive tract. The largest of the major glands is the parotid glands, located anterior and inferior to the ear between the mandibular ramus and mastoid bones, and is innervated by the multiple branches of the facial nerve. Lymphatics drain to intraglandular lymph nodes and to periparotid lymph nodes, as well as cervical, submandibular, and deep upper jugular nodes.

The submandibular gland is located inferior to the mandible, anterior to the parotid gland, and medially to the hyoglossus muscle. The marginal mandibular branch of the facial nerve, hypoglossal and lingual nerves, lie immediately adjacent to the gland. The submandibular gland lymphatics drain to submandibular lymph nodes and nodes of the deep jugular chain. The sublingual glands are small and are located next to the submandibular duct, next to the mandible and inferior to the oral mucosa of the floor of the mouth. Lymphatic drainage is directed to the submandibular and deep jugular lymph nodes.

Minor salivary glands are found throughout the upper aerodigestive tract, concentrated in the oral cavity and oropharynx. They are also found in the trachea, larynx, nasopharynx, paranasal sinuses, and nasal cavity.

Clinical Manifestations

Most salivary tissue malignancies occur in the parotid gland and present as a unilaterally enlarged parotid gland. Benign masses, pleomorphic adenoma in particular, can deteriorate into malignant tumors over time as evidenced by a rapid change in

Box 7-6 Larynx Radiation Therapy per NCCN Guidelines

CANCER OF THE GLOTTIC LARYNX*

Definitive radiation therapy

- Primary and gross adenopathy: ≥ 70 Gy (2.0 Gy/day)
  For early cancer of the glottic larynx, preferred dose is ≥ 2.0 Gy/day with total dose modification accordingly
- Neck
  Low-risk nodal stations: ≥ 50 Gy (2.0 Gy/day)

Adjuvant radiation therapy

- Primary: ≥ 60 Gy (2.0 Gy/day)
- Neck
  High-risk nodal stations: ≥ 60 Gy (2.0 Gy/day)
  Low-risk nodal stations: ≥ 50 Gy (2.0 Gy/day)

CANCER OF THE SUPRAGLOTTIC LARYNX†

Definitive radiation therapy

- Primary and gross adenopathy: ≥ 70 Gy (2.0 Gy/day)
- Neck
  Low-risk nodal stations: ≥ 50 Gy (2.0 Gy/day)

Adjuvant radiation therapy

- Primary: ≥ 60 Gy (2.0 Gy/day)
- Neck
  High-risk nodal stations: ≥ 60 Gy (2.0 Gy/day)
  Low-risk nodal stations: ≥ 50 Gy (2.0 Gy/day)

*Data from the National Comprehensive Cancer Network (NCCN) Practice Guidelines in Oncology—v.1.2005 Cancer of the glottic larynx (website): www.nccn.org/professionals/physician_gls/PDF/head-and-neck.pdf. Accessed December 6, 2005.

†Data from the National Comprehensive Cancer Network (NCCN) Practice Guidelines in Oncology—v.1.2005 Cancer of the supraglottic larynx (website): www.nccn.org/professionals/physician_gls/PDF/head-and-neck.pdf. Accessed December 6, 2005.

tumor size or addition of new symptoms such as pain or facial nerve sensitivity or paralysis. Submandibular tumors present with an asymptomatic mass and may have skin or deep tissue fixation. Both parotid and submandibular tumors tend to occur in the fifth and sixth decades, 10 to 15 years after most benign salivary tumors occur. Sublingual tumors present as asymptomatic floor of mouth swelling, usually discovered by dentists. Minor salivary gland tumors can present anywhere as a painless lesion, with histology determined at time of biopsy.

Diagnostic Studies

A full history including environmental factors and thorough examination of the head and neck is done. An FNA of the mass is usually done preoperatively to rule out malignancy. If not done preoperatively, then a frozen section pathology specimen at the time of surgery is done. Imaging is not usually done preoperatively because scans cannot differentiate malignant lesions from benign. After malignancy is proven, a CT scan with contrast and/or MRI is useful for determining extent of disease, both at the primary site and elsewhere in the neck region.

Pathology and Patterns of Metastasis

Fine-needle aspiration biopsy is commonly used in salivary lesions to determine histologic evidence of malignancy. Salivary gland tumors are divided into low-grade tumors: acinic cell carcinoma and low-grade mucoepidermoid carcinoma, and high-grade tumors: adenocarcinoma, adenoid cystic carcinoma, squamous cell carcinoma, high-grade mucoepidermoid carcinoma; and undifferentiated carcinoma. Salivary gland malignancies are not associated with alcohol use or smoking, and the etiology of these tumors is not well understood. Exposure to low-dose radiation and wood dust may be risk factors for this cancer. These tumors tend to extend into the immediate intraglandular and periglandular lymph nodes and less commonly to the jugular and cervical lymph nodes.[26]

Staging

Staging of salivary gland tumors is shown in Table 7-7.

Treatment

Parotidectomy with/without neck dissection, followed by external beam radiation therapy is the standard treatment for most parotid cancers unless they are T1-T2 and low grade. If the pathology reveals adenoid cystic carcinoma, or the neck dissection has negative features, the radiation fields must encompass the tumor bed and the facial nerves leading to the base of the skull. Chemoradiation may be used in situations where gross residual disease is left in the operative bed and no further surgery is possible. Similarly, submandibular gland cancers are excised, and if high-grade or T3-T4, postoperative radiation therapy is indicated.

Table 7-7 Staging Salivary Gland Tumors

SALIVARY GLAND TUMORS (T)			
TX	Primary tumor cannot be assessed		
T0	No evidence of primary tumor		
Tis	Carcinoma in situ		
T1	Tumor 2 cm or less in greatest dimension without extraparenchymal extension		
T2	Tumor more than 2 cm but not more than 4 cm in greatest dimension without extraparenchymal extension		
T3	Tumor more than 4 cm and/or tumor having extraparenchymal extension		
T4a	Tumor invades skin, mandible, ear canal, and/or facial nerve		
T4b	Tumor invades skull base, and/or pterygoid plates and/or encases the carotid artery		
REGIONAL LYMPH NODES (N)			
NX	Regional lymph nodes cannot be assessed		
N0	No regional lymph node metastasis		
N1	Metastasis in a single ipsilateral lymph node, 3 cm or less in greatest dimension		
N2	Metastasis in a single ipsilateral lymph node, more than 3 cm but not more than 6 cm in greatest dimension; or in multiple ipsilateral lymph nodes, none more than 6 cm in greatest dimension; or in bilateral or contralateral lymph nodes, none more than 6 cm in greatest dimension		
N2a	Metastasis in a single ipsilateral lymph node more than 3 cm but not more than 6 cm in greatest dimension		
N2b	Metastasis in multiple ipsilateral lymph nodes, none more than 6 cm in greatest dimension		
N2c	Metastasis in bilateral or contralateral lymph nodes, none more than 6 cm in greatest dimension		
N3	Metastasis in a lymph node, more than 6 cm in greatest dimension		
DISTANT METASTASIS (M)			
MX	Distant metastasis cannot be assessed		
M0	No distant metastasis		
M1	Distant metastasis		
STAGE GROUPING: SALIVARY GLAND TUMORS			
Stage 0	Tis	N0	M0
Stage I	T1	N0	M0
Stage II	T2	N0	M0
Stage III	T3	N0	M0
	T1, T2, T3	N1	M0
Stage IVA	T4a	N0, N1	M0
	T1, T2, T3, T4a	N2	M0
Stage IVB	T4b	Any N	M0
	Any T	N3	M0
Stage IVC	Any T	Any N	M1

Used with the permission of the American Joint Committee on Cancer (AJCC), Chicago, Illinois. The original source for this material is the *AJCC Cancer Staging Manual, Sixth Edition* (2002), published by Springer-New York, www.springeronline.com.

Radiation portals include the entire preoperative bed of the gland and a 2-cm margin. A wedged-field technique using multiple fields minimizes radiation to the contralateral gland, thereby minimizing xerostomia. The area of the deep lobe of the parotid must be included, as well as Stensen's duct. Care must be taken that posterior oblique fields, if used, do not exit the eye. When the histology is adenoid cystic, the portals must be enlarged to encompass the nerves traveling from the tumor bed to the base of the skull. Elective neck fields are added for T3 and T4 tumors that often involve neck lymph nodes.

Neutron beam radiation therapy is used as definitive treatment in a few selected cases and listed in the National Comprehensive Cancer Network (NCCN) guidelines as an appropriate treatment option (Box 7-7).[27] Although normal tissue injury, even necrosis, may be slightly increased with neutron beam treatment when compared to photon treatment, neutrons may be more effective on salivary tumors. Overall the treatment is usually well tolerated and should be considered a standard treatment choice when using radiation therapy alone for unresectable salivary gland malignancies.[26]

Box 7-7 Salivary Gland Radiation Therapy per NCCN Guidelines

DEFINITIVE RADIATION THERAPY

Unresectable disease or gross residual disease

- Photon/electron therapy or neutron therapy
- Dose
  - Primary and gross adenopathy: ≥ 70 Gy (1.8-2.0 Gy/day) or 19.2 nGy (1.2 nGy/day)

ADJUVANT RADIATION THERAPY

- Photon/electron therapy or neutron therapy
- Dose
  - Primary: ≥ 60 Gy (1.8-2.0 Gy/day)* or 18 nGy (1.2 nGy/day)
- Neck
  - 45 to 54 Gy (1.8-2.0 Gy/day)* or 13.2 nGy (1.2 nGy/day)

Data from the National Comprehensive Cancer Network (NCCN) Practice Guidelines in Oncology—v.1.2005 Salivary gland tumors (website): www.nccn.org/professionals/physician_gls/PDF/head-and-neck.pdf. Accessed December 6, 2005.

*Range based on grade/natural history of disease.

Thyroid

Anatomy

The thyroid is composed of glandular tissue and lies anterior to the thyroid cartilage immediately under the skin. It is composed of two lobes on either side of the trachea, joined by the thyroid isthmus. The thyroid lies quite close to the recurrent laryngeal nerve and the parathyroid glands. There is lymphatic drainage from both within and outside of the gland proper, leading to multifocal lesions. Prelaryngeal nodes, mediastinal nodes, tracheoesophageal nodes, and retropharyngeal nodes all drain the thyroid gland.

Clinical Manifestations

An enlarged thyroid nodule or mass, more than 1.0 cm in size, should be evaluated for malignancy. Thyroid nodularity itself is quite common, and enlargement may not be indicative of cancer. Some thyroid cancers are indolent, and incidental autopsy findings of asymptomatic thyroid carcinoma is fairly common. Thyroid nodules are more common in women than men; however, men are more likely to have malignant nodules. Occasionally thyroid cancer may present with hoarseness, a sign of late-stage malignancy, with impingement of the laryngeal nerves.

Diagnostic Studies

Most thyroid nodules are benign. Accordingly, the mere presence of a nodule does not indicate need for a biopsy, but instead appropriate studies to determine the cause of the nodule (ultrasound, lab studies). A thorough history and physical are, as always, important to work up for thyroid malignancy. An understanding of incidence is important here. Children are less likely to have thyroid nodules, but if present, the nodules are likely to be malignant in up to 50% of them. Likewise, being older than age 60 means a higher incidence of malignancy in nodules evaluated. Any history of irradiation that included the neck given in the early part of the twentieth century can lead to increased likelihood of malignancy in later years. Examples include radiation given for acne, tonsillitis, and impetigo. Medullary thyroid cancer may run in families. Thyroid function tests (T4, TSH) are usually normal, but should be part of the baseline work-up. Calcitonin levels can be elevated in medullary thyroid cancer, but also in benign disorders such as Hashimoto thyroiditis, hyperthyroidism, and goiter.

A chest x ray is useful to note any obvious lung metastasis and for visualizing trachea positioning and the presence or absence of calcifications within the thyroid gland (suggestive of medullary carcinoma). CT and MRI scans are helpful in determining the position of the tumor mass and presence/location of lymphadenopathy. A PET scan is very useful in imaging undifferentiated tumors and is helpful in monitoring response to treatment as well. Thyroid ultrasonography differentiates between solid and cystic lesions but is unable to determine presence of malignancy. It is commonly used to evaluate the progression of a thyroid lesion over time, response to treatment, or direct a FNA/biopsy of a suspicious lesion.

Pathology and Patterns of Metastasis

Most malignant thyroid cancers are differentiated (papillary or follicular), and papillary is the histology of 60% to 75% of all thyroid carcinomas. Other histologies include follicular, medullary, undifferentiated or anaplastic, squamous cell carcinomas, lymphomas, and sarcomas. Medullary carcinomas comprise 5% to 10%, and anaplastic carcinomas are rare, making up only 5% of all thyroid tumors.[28]

Most thyroid tumors (papillary and follicular) grow very slowly and spread within the thyroid itself or into the lymph nodes immediately adjacent to the gland; they cause few, if any, symptoms. Anaplastic thyroid disease is highly aggressive and is associated with death a few months or even weeks after diagnosis. Locoregional growth is fast and fatal. Enlarged thyroid nodules and regional lymph nodes are followed quickly by dysphagia, superior vena cava syndrome, and asphyxiation. Involvement of the jugular vein may lead to exsanguination as a cause of death.

Staging

Staging of thyroid tumors is listed in Table 7-8.

Treatment

If the lesion grows, an FNA is indicated, and if suspicious for cancer, surgical excision is recommended, except in the case of anaplastic carcinoma or lymphoma. The surgeries used for thyroid cancers vary, from a thyroid lumpectomy confined to just the area involved, to a near-total thyroidectomy. Ablative, radioactive ^{131}I is used to destroy any residual thyroid tissue left after surgery. Postsurgical morbidities may include hypothyroidism, hypocalcemia, and recurrent laryngeal nerve injury.

Patients with thyroid cancer are rarely treated with external beam radiation therapy, and the efficacy of treatment is not well documented when compared with other cancers of the head and neck. However, in cases of well-differentiated thyroid carcinoma, external beam radiaton therapy has been shown to enhance local control, especially in cases of gross residual disease after surgical resection.

Technically, treating thyroid cancers with radiation therapy is quite difficult because of the proximity of the spinal cord. Nutting and colleagues[29] reported a planning study done on patients with thyroid carcinoma, comparing three-dimensional conformal planning with inverse-planned IMRT. They found IMRT planning improved the coverage to the carcinoma and reduced the spinal cord dose as compared with conventional and 3-D planned

Table 7-8 Staging Thyroid Tumors

THYROID TUMORS (T)	
TX	Primary tumor cannot be assessed
T0	No evidence of primary tumor
Tis	Carcinoma in situ
T1	Tumor 2 cm or less in greatest dimension limited to the thyroid
T2	Tumor more than 2 cm but not more than 4 cm in greatest dimension limited to the thyroid
T3	Tumor more than 4 cm limited to the thyroid or any tumor with minimal extrathyroid extension
T4a	Tumor of any size extending beyond the thyroid capsule to invade subcutaneous soft tissues, larynx, trachea, esophagus, or recurrent laryngeal nerve
T4b	Tumor invades prevertebral fascia or encases the carotid artery or mediastinal vessels
All anaplastic carcinomas are considered T4 tumors	
T4a	Intrathyroidal anaplastic carcinoma—surgically resectable
T4b	Extrathyroidal anaplastic carcinoma—surgically unresectable
REGIONAL LYMPH NODES (N)	
Within the central compartment, lateral cervical and upper mediastinal lymph nodes	
NX	Regional lymph nodes cannot be assessed
N0	No regional lymph node metastasis
N1	Regional lymph node metastasis
N1a	Metastasis to level VI (pretracheal, paratracheal, and prelaryngeal/Delphian lymph nodes)
N1b	Metastasis to unilateral, bilateral, or contralateral cervical or superior mediastinal lymph nodes
DISTANT METASTASIS (M)	
MX	Distant metastasis cannot be assessed
M0	No distant metastasis
M1	Distant metastasis
STAGE GROUPING: THYROID	
Separate stage groupings are recommended for papillary or follicular, medullary and anaplastic (undifferentiated) carcinoma. See reference for details of each.	

Used with the permission of the American Joint Committee on Cancer (AJCC), Chicago, Illinois. The original source for this material is the *AJCC Cancer Staging Manual, Sixth Edition* (2002), published by Springer-New York, www.springeronline.com.

treatments, suggesting IMRT could reduce the risk of myelopathy and may allow increased doses to the malignancy.

Anaplastic thyroid carcinoma (ATC) is one of the most deadly of all cancers, with rapid local growth and spread of distant metastasis. Unfortunately, even with proper treatment, almost all patients with ATC succumb, with a median survival of only 2 to 6 months. Patients with anaplastic thyroid cancer are often treated with multimodality treatment, either preoperatively or adjuvantly. The chemotherapy agent doxorubicin appears to be somewhat effective and is given in combination with hyperfractionated radiation therapy, usually 1.6 Gy given twice daily, 3 to 5 times per week, to a preoperative dose of 46 Gy in 3 weeks.[30]

An analysis of 516 patients with anaplastic thyroid carcinoma treated over 27 years revealed patients who had surgical resection followed by external beam radiation therapy survived the longest.[31] Another study concluded that although overall prognosis of anaplastic thyroid cancer remains poor, complete macroscopic resection combined with adjuvant chemotherapy and radiation therapy did result in improved long-term survival.[32] Again, hyperfractionated radiation therapy was used, doses unspecified. There are no NCCN guidelines establishing radiation therapy guidelines or standard doses, but radiation therapy is recommended for treating skeletal metastases.[33]

NURSING INTERVENTIONS AND EDUCATION

Just as medical management of patients with head and neck cancer is often complex and challenging, so too is providing nursing care to this group of patients. Both the cancers themselves and the treatments used to cure or control the tumors have a huge impact on patients' appearance, function, and quality of life. Providing appropriate and effective symptom management during the actual treatment phase is necessary so as to minimize breaks in treatment, known to impact locoregional control and survival.[34–37] Supporting patients in accepting the long-term changes in form and function after treatment is an on-going responsibility and challenge for the radiation oncology team.

As discussed in the preceding site-specific sections, treatment of head and neck cancer nearly always involves multimodalities. Each of these produces acute and late effects specific to the modality used. When combined, surgery, chemotherapy, and radiation therapy side effects are modified and often exacerbated. Although this text is intended for nurses caring for patients receiving radiation therapy, the influence and impact of both surgical interventions and chemotherapy on radiation effects will be discussed.

This next section reviews acute side effects common to all patients treated for head and neck cancers and also some site-specific acute effects. Late effects, both temporary and permanent, are also described. This discussion is in no way exhaustive, but gives readers a broad overview of patient care and provides references for obtaining further information. Box 7-8 presents a listing of the most common acute toxicities and psychosocial concerns.

Common Acute Toxicities

Fatigue and Anemia

All patients receiving daily radiation therapy for head and neck cancer experience fatigue. This is true whether patients are treated for a T1N0 vocal cord lesion or for a bulky stage IV nasopharynx cancer. Although minimal bone marrow is exposed to the effects of radiation, the combination of

Box 7-8 Acute Toxicities and Psychosocial Issues

COMMON ACUTE TOXICITIES

Fatigue
Skin reaction
Xerostomia, taste changes
Mucositis
Pain
Nutritional deficit

SITE-SPECIFIC ACUTE TOXICITIES

Nasal congestion, epistaxis
Hearing deficit, eustachian tube changes
Scatter lesions
Laryngitis

PSYCHOSOCIAL ISSUES

Smoking cessation
Alcohol cessation
Detoxification
Depression
Anxiety
Social isolation

nutritional factors, anemia, self-care demands, and insomnia likely play a role in fatigue development. Fatigue is insidious and accumulates over the course of treatment, peaking 1 to 3 weeks after completion of treatment. Both the prevalence and the effect of fatigue on quality of life of cancer patients has been the subject of numerous papers and studies. Although defined differently by patients, caregivers, and healthcare professionals,[38] fatigue clearly has a negative impact on physical and social functioning, and interventions are needed to improve quality of life.[39]

Anemia related to cancer has been noted in up to 50% of cancer patients just before or while undergoing radiation therapy. A retrospective study reported in 2001 looked at 574 randomly selected patients undergoing radiation therapy; 12% receiving treatment for cancers of the head and neck. Sixteen percent of head and neck patients were mildly/moderately anemic (Hgb 10 to 12 g/dL) before beginning radiation therapy, and 32% became anemic during treatment (16% mild/moderate anemia, 16% severe (Hgb less than 9.9 g/dL).[40]

How anemia impacts efficacy of treatment was the purpose of a study reported in 2003. Patients with stages III and IV squamous cell carcinoma of the head and neck were randomized to receive either conventional or accelerated radiation therapy and were also grouped into those with normal hemoglobin and those considered anemic (13 g/dL or less in males, 12 g/dL or more in females). The impact of anemia was tested, and results showed significant reductions in locoregional control, disease-free survival, cause-specific survival, and overall survival in the presence of anemia.[41]

A more recent study by Henke et al.,[42] reported in Europe, has raised new concerns. A double-blind, placebo-controlled trial was conducted on 351 patients receiving curative radiation therapy for carcinoma of the oral cavity, oropharynx, hypopharynx, or larynx. Patients received either erythropoietin 300 IU/kg or placebo via subcutaneous injection 3 times per week. Erythropoietin, although effective in raising overall hemoglobin, did not improve cancer control and locoregional progression-free survival was poorer with epoetin-beta than with placebo. As a result of this study, many centers are no longer treating mild, asymptomatic anemia with erythropoietin.

Radiation Skin Reaction

A skin reaction from radiation therapy is a temporary expected part of the treatment process and is experienced by nearly everyone treated with radiation. The details of the radiation skin reaction; its etiology, presentation, and course are described in detail in Chapter 30. Effective nursing interventions and guidelines for patient education are also presented in that chapter.

Patients being treated for head and neck cancers develop a skin reaction beginning 3 to 4 weeks into treatment. If receiving concomitant chemotherapy, the reaction begins sooner and is more intense. Some areas of the head and neck are especially vulnerable to a severe reaction. Examples include thin-skinned areas (posterior neck), particularly sensitive areas (lips and eyelids), areas of skinfolds (ear lobes, nasal ala) and where fields overlap, such as at the shoulder where the parallel opposed lateral fields overlap with the low anterior neck field.

Because of the high visibility of their treatment portals, cosmetic considerations must be taken into account when recommending creams, ointments, or dressings. When necessary, dressings for skin in the head and neck area are extremely challenging to devise because of anatomic constraints. For moist desquamation, a tubular, meshlike dressing is sometimes useful to hold a nonstick dressing in place.

Xerostomia and Taste Changes

Xerostomia, the subjective experience of dryness in the mouth, is a common and often irreversible effect of head and neck irradiation.[43] The objective finding of hyposalivation is the result of radiation damage to the major and minor salivary glands during head and neck cancer treatment. Whether the salivary glands are the target of the radiation (as in parotid cancer) or not, it is rare that any patient treated for cancer of the head and neck does not complain of dry mouth and thickened saliva.

Normal function of salivary glands is governed by the nervous system. Gland stimulation occurs with the sight, smell, or taste of food.[44] Saliva has two parts, a thin serous component secreted primarily from the parotid glands when stimulated and a mucous component secreted near-continuously by the minor salivary glands found throughout the oral mucosa. The serous secretion is most affected by radiation therapy, and so patients' first complaint is often that their saliva is becoming thickened and sticky.

Low radiation doses can cause noticeable changes. A radiation dose of as little as 10 Gy or approximately 1 week of treatment causes salivary output decreases of 60% to 90%.[45] If the total dose to salivary tissue is 26 Gy or less, recovery of salivary function is possible; however, the typical total dose of 60 Gy or more used for head and neck cancers ensures permanent damage to salivary glands. Decrease in both quantity and quality of saliva leads acutely to mucositis, taste changes, dysphagia, and mouth discomfort or pain, all of which lead to increased risk of nutritional deficit and weight loss.

Loss of saliva's production and its protective properties leads to dental issues such as increased risk of dental caries, poor fit of dental appliances (dentures, obturators), and increased risk of candidiasis infection. Appropriate standardized oral self-care measures are important to initiate before treatment and to encourage throughout treatment.[46] Frequent and life-long dental evaluation and care is crucial for patients receiving radiation to the head and neck. Before beginning radiation therapy, repair of any existing caries and creation of fluoride trays for use nightly during treatment and after treatment is required (with the exception of edentulous patients). Pretreatment dental evaluation and care is especially important as studies have shown dental follow-up compliance is low among patients with head and neck cancers.[47,48]

Minimizing xerostomia is an area of great interest to radiation oncologists. IMRT and 3-D treatment planning are used to minimize normal tissue irradiation, including salivary tissue, particularly of the contralateral parotid gland. Use of the cytoprotectant amifostine may protect salivary tissue within the treatment portal.[49,50] Thorough discussion of this drug's chemical makeup, action, and longer term implications is beyond the scope of this chapter but can be obtained from its manufacturer.[51] Generally, amifostine is selectively taken up by specific organs of the body, including the salivary glands, and provides protection against the harmful effects of radiation therapy.

Amifostine is FDA-approved to be used in the postoperative setting to minimize xerostomia in patients receiving radiation therapy for head and neck cancer. It is administered either IV at a dose of 200 mg/m^2 or subcutaneously at 500 mg/m^2, daily before each radiation treatment. To allow time for the drug to arrive at the salivary glands, patients wait 15 to 30 minutes after IV administration, and if given subcutaneously, 30 to 45 minutes before receiving their radiation treatment. Common side effects include nausea and vomiting, hypotension, and allergic skin reaction. Antiemetics and preadministration hydration are needed, and a pretreatment antihistamine may be helpful.[52]

Cholinergic drugs such as cevimeline, bethanechol, and pilocarpine may be used to stimulate the salivary glands after radiation therapy.[53] A study reported by Gorsky and colleagues[54] showed minimal objective increases in stimulated saliva with either pilocarpine or bethanechol. However, resting saliva was increased with their study, and patients reported statistically significant improvement of "mouth wetness" using either drug. This may indicate that subjectively, the absence of resting saliva is most troublesome for patients.

Managing xerostomia involves increasing oral moisture, minimizing dental complications, and altering diet. Using a humidifier whenever possible, and especially at night, adds moisture to the environment, whereas minimizing the use of air conditioning and dry heat decreases their drying effect. Sipping water throughout the day and rinsing the mouth with water before eating to provide "immediate" moisture is helpful.[43] Some patients find relief with artificial saliva and other mouth moisturizers, and sour, sugarless gum or candies can stimulate salivary flow.

Studies examining acupuncture as a means to relieve xerostomia have been published. Although the administration techniques varied, response rates to acupuncture were high, and many patients reported improved taste and thinner saliva.[55–57]

Diet modification includes increasing moisture in foods by adding sauces, gravies, and condiments (butter, sour cream, etc.) to facilitate swallowing. Sensitivity of the tongue may make it difficult to eat spicy, sour, or salty foods, although taste changes are extremely unpredictable and vary from individual to individual. Rough-textured foods such as pretzels, toast, crackers and thick foods such as peanut butter should be avoided during treatment and eaten with caution after treatment.

Use of prescription-strength fluoride to prevent caries is a lifelong requirement. Thorough twice-yearly dental evaluations by a dentist familiar with the effects of radiation are important after treatment. Meticulous follow-up and close communication between radiation oncologist and dentist can lower the incidence of extractions and osteoradionecrosis.[58]

Mucositis and Pain

Although it may occur in any radiation patient receiving chemotherapy, mucositis is especially severe in patients receiving radiation to the head and neck because the majority of the oral and pharyngeal mucosa is directly in the path of the radiation beam. Pain and weight loss are inevitable, and management of these symptoms is of primary concern. Please refer to Chapters 31 and 32 for a full review of mucositis and pain in patients receiving radiation therapy.

Nutritional Deficits

Nutritional deficit in patients being treated for head and neck cancers is common and very challenging to manage. Weight loss can be quite severe because of the location of the tumor and the effects of surgery, chemotherapy and radiation therapy on normal tissues, as well as changes in metabolism brought on by cancer and its treatment (discussed in detail in Chapter 33). Unfortunately, these changes may continue even after completion of treatment and therefore affect survivorship.

Physiologic changes to the alimentary tract from the head and neck cancer itself or from surgical excision can be a primary cause of weight loss. The tumor may obstruct the nose and the olfactory apparatus, leading to diminished or changed sense of smell. Tongue cancers and tongue surgery may disrupt taste bud quantity and location, affecting the taste of food. Obstruction of muscles used to chew and swallow by tumor and/or postoperative physical changes can lead to difficulty with the swallowing process itself.

Partial or total glossectomy makes forming the food bolus and moving it to the back of the throat for swallowing extremely difficult. Larynx and hypopharynx surgeries can lead to impaired epiglottic function and food aspiration. The pain caused by tumors can lead to anorexia. Gross cosmetic disfigurement often leads to patient isolation and depression, indirectly impacting nutritional intake. Head and neck tumors and the treatment of the disease all contribute to a profound and significant risk of nutritional deficit.

Chemotherapy often causes anorexia, dysgeusia, fatigue, nausea, and emesis. Combined with radiation therapy, the fatigue and dysgeusia is heightened, leading to complete lack of desire to eat and food aversions. A metallic taste is common in patients receiving platinum-based chemotherapy. Antiemetics used to combat chemotherapy-induced emesis often lead to increased drowsiness and dry mouth, again, causing diminished desire for food.

Radiation therapy directed to the structures of the head and neck seems designed to negatively affect the nutritional status of patients. In all but the simplest of treatment designs, significant quantities of oral cavity, oropharynx, and pharynx mucosa are often within the treatment fields. Mucositis, xerostomia, and pain all contribute to patients' inability to maintain their nutritional status and weight.

Specific interventions for patients receiving head and neck cancer treatment center on careful assessment of nutritional status, supplementation of dietary calories and protein, and assisting patients with the physical ingestion of calories via a percutaneous endoscopically placed gastrostomy (PEG) tube or in rare instances, a nasogastric (NG) tube. If possible, an evaluation of patients' baseline nutritional status should be performed by a nutritionist before beginning treatment or during the first week of treatment. Daily weights are a basic nursing intervention that should be done on every patient treated for a head and neck cancer. Patient teaching and coaching is done as soon as a trend of weight loss is noted, to prevent further deterioration.

Changes in diet to increase protein and calories are encouraged from the very beginning of treatment. This often involves the use of commercial or patient-prepared nutritional supplements. The goal of supplementation is to "maximize calorie and protein intake for optimal tissue repair," leading to increased tolerance to radiation and fewer treatment breaks.[43]

Finally, all patients at high risk for severe mucositis, pain, and weight loss should have a PEG tube placed before beginning radiation therapy. This is especially important for patients receiving combined modality treatment (chemotherapy and radiation therapy) and for any patient with a baseline weight deficiency. It is the writer's own experience that instituting "up front" PEG tube placement in this group of patients has decreased treatment delays and treatment breaks. This may lead to better treatment outcomes, and patients seem more comfortable as they progress through treatment. However, some concern exists regarding indiscriminate use of PEG tubes in this patient population. PEG tube dependency may contribute to a lack of dedication to speech therapy, which ultimately is meant to improve and strengthen the action and muscles involved with swallowing. Therefore, some practitioners believe only high-risk patients should be considered for up-front PEG tube placement before radiation therapy.

Site-Specific Acute Toxicities

Some site-specific symptoms are commonly seen in patients receiving radiation for head and neck cancers. Although not experienced by all patients, the symptoms are significantly bothersome to patients and should be addressed. These symptoms and their management are excellent nursing research opportunities because they have not been explored. The following toxicities and interventions are experientially based and not based on the literature.

Patients receiving radiation to the nasopharynx, nasal cavity, and paranasal sinus complex often experience nasal congestion and occasional epistaxis. This often is upsetting to patients because these are the initial symptoms they experienced that led to their diagnosis. They fear a return of the cancer, or believe these nasal symptoms indicated "the treatment isn't working." It is important that patients and caregivers be reassured that such symptoms are normal sequelae of radiation therapy to these anatomic areas, primarily caused by dryness. Simple interventions such as use of a humidifier, application of a water-based lubricant into the nares, and use of commercially available normal saline nasal sprays usually alleviate these symptoms. Nasal decongestants are not recommended because of their drying effects.

Patients being treated for nasopharynx cancer also may experience "fullness" in their ears, similar to the air pressure change-related fullness experienced when traveling in an airplane or occupying an elevator moving rapidly upwards. They also may report decreased hearing towards the end of treatment. Because nasopharynx patients are often receiving concomitant therapy, they are at risk for permanent hearing loss resulting from cisplatin-based regimes. Cisplatin is a known ototoxic agent and is a commonly used drug in head and neck cancer. However, ear and hearing changes also can be precipitated by temporary radiation-induced factors.

The entire hearing apparatus and eustachian tubes are often in the pathway of the radiation beam. A study of otologic structures done by Ondrey and colleagues[59] demonstrated eustachian tube doses of least 4000cGy in a group of patients. Some temporary inflammation of this area is very common. This can be experienced as fullness or as a sensation of water in the ear. The external ear canal may become filled with increased amounts of hardened wax as the radiation dries the area, thereby impeding hearing. Patients receiving radiation therapy unilaterally (as in postoperative parotid therapy and for benign entities such as paraganglioma) will experience these symptoms unilaterally.

Symptom management again is relatively simple. Most patients adjust and tolerate the above sensations and resulting hearing loss when they understand their cause. Patients should be reassured that these symptoms are not dangerous or permanent. Antihistamines offer some relief of eustachian tube inflammation but also cause xerostomia, a side effect most patients find worse than the inflammation. Medications to soften wax and promote wax removal are sometimes useful if the skin of the external ear canal is intact. If desquamation is present, no ointment/medication should be used in the ear. The sensation of fullness usually is gone within 3 weeks of completing therapy. Otitis externa may be experienced throughout survivorship, and many patients see an otolaryngologist regularly for assistance in clearing the ear canal.[60,61]

Many patients receiving radiation therapy to the oral cavity experience a specific type of pain associated with their dental work. These are commonly called "scatter" lesions, the name referring to the cause of the lesion. When the radiation beam comes into contact with metalwork associated with fillings, crowns, for example, backscattering of radiation onto the mucous membranes in contact with the metalwork occurs. This leads to a bolus effect, resulting in an overdose of radiation therapy to either the buccal mucosa or lateral edge of the tongue. This readily demarcated area of mucositis is exquisitely painful and contributes to patients' inability to readily nourish themselves.

Prevention of these scatter lesions is the best management. Patients are instructed, whenever possible, to wear their fluoride trays (minus the fluoride) while receiving their treatment. This physically keeps the buccal and tongue mucosa away from the metalwork. A study by Reitemeier and colleagues[62] evaluated use of a 3-mm-thick "stent" placed over dental amalgam during treatment and found it quite effective in preventing backscatter of radiation.

Alternatively, water-soaked gauze may be placed between cheek and teeth, again, separating sensitive mucosa from dental appliances. Over-the-counter ointments designed for teething pain in infants are useful for providing pinpoint temporary anesthesia to painful areas. If multiple areas are affected, an oral rinse containing anesthetic may be more practical.

Patients with cancers of the larynx often present with hoarseness. Before beginning treatment, it is important these patients understand that changes in voice quality can be expected during and after radiation treatment. Tumor size may prevent normal movement, and function of the true vocal cords is the common cause of hoarseness at presentation. After 2 to 3 weeks of radiation therapy, tumors typically shrink rapidly, leading to a noticeable improvement in voice quality. Patients appropriately feel relieved and encouraged by this change. However, they will need support and education during the next phase of treatment. After 4 to 5 weeks of treatment to the larynx, the voice rapidly deteriorates and may lead to total laryngitis. This is caused by treatment-related vocal cord inflammation and is rarely due to tumor growth at this stage of treatment. However, unless thorough education is provided, patients often will become very worried and afraid the tumor has returned or is growing during treatment. Reassurance and teaching are crucial interventions at this point in the patients care.[63]

Finally, a review of symptom management in patients receiving radiation therapy isn't complete without a discussion of psychosocial interventions. These patients often require incredible amounts of time and patience from the radiation nursing team. They often come with multiple psychologic issues, financial worries, and preexisting addictions to tobacco, alcohol, or other addictive drugs. In some cases, these patients may have little in the way of a support system. As a result of alcoholism and/or drug abuse, patients with head and neck cancers often present with advanced disease and are underweight and malnourished because of inattention or neglect of their overall health.

An open, nonjudgmental attitude is required to create a professional and effective nurse-patient relationship. However, a "tough love" approach may be required when caring for these individuals. Actively drinking or drug-using patients must understand that continued abuse of alcohol and drugs interferes with their ability to withstand treatment and its effects and can threaten their survival as well.

At the time of consultation, patients should be given assistance for immediate smoking cessation. Referral to a formal cessation program (if available) or to other cessation supportive groups is helpful. Patients addicted to alcohol and drugs should be entered into a formal detoxification program and be fully detoxified before treatment initiation. Ongoing support of abstinence, via social work involvement, referral to support groups (Alcoholics Anonymous, Narcotics Anonymous) is important, as is daily support and encouragement by radiation nursing staff.

Depression is quite common in patients with head and neck cancer during and after surgery or radiation treatments. Changes in body appearance and function, and fears regarding the future lead to sadness, discouragement, and hopelessness.[64,65] Additional appearance and functional changes brought about by radiation treatment, as well as fatigue and pain medication, may intensify depression. Close observation, assessment, and quick interventions are important in managing depression. Referral to a social worker or a behavioral health specialist and support groups may be helpful. Additionally, the use of antidepressants may be indicated. This may be initiated by radiation oncology clinicians during treatment, but for long-term psychiatric management, patients should be monitored by a psychiatrist or primary care physician.

Patients receiving radiation therapy to the head and neck are usually immobilized by means of a face-fitted mask and being secured to the treatment table. If their shoulders need to be pulled downward, out of the treatment field, the mask may extend to include the shoulders, or patients' arms may be pulled downward and secured to their sides (Figures 7-2 and 7-3). These masks can feel constrictive and frightening. It is important to ascertain, during the consultation, whether patients have a history of claustrophobia. Asking a patient

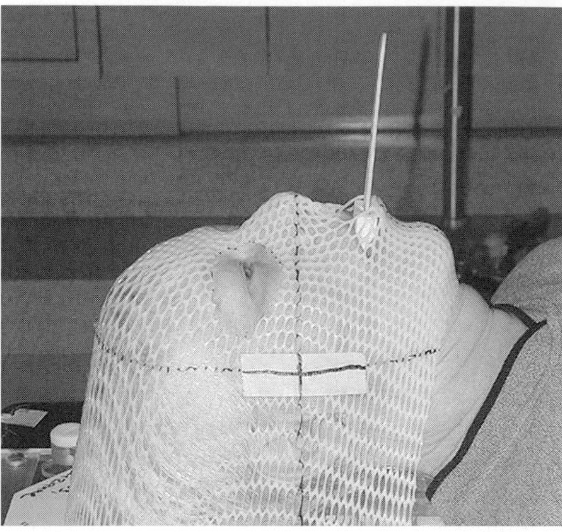

Figure 7-2 Immobilization Mask.
Photo courtesy of Louis Harrison, Beth Israel Medical Center, New York, NY.

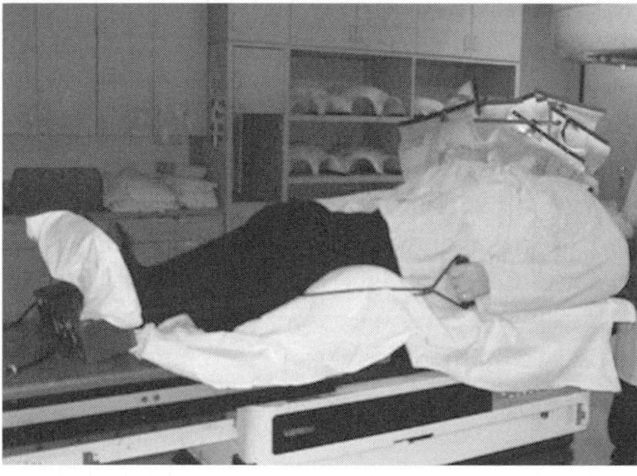

Figure 7-3 Shoulder Positioning.
Photo courtesy of Louis Harrison, Beth Israel Medical Center, New York, NY.

how they feel riding an extremely full elevator may be a way of eliciting this information. Claustrophobic patients may obtain relief from a constrictive treatment mask by cutting openings around the eyes and mouth.

Patients with a history of claustrophobia or panic disorder often require premedication with a mild antianxiolytic agent before undergoing simulation and treatment. This should be taken 1 hour before treatment, and patients should not drive for up to 4 hours after ingestion of the medication. Alternatively, or in addition, soft, soothing music during treatment is often helpful. If the claustrophobia is discovered at the time of simulation, the patient should be immediately freed from the immobilization device and administered an oral antianxiety medication.

Late Effects of Radiation Therapy

Late effects of treatment for head and neck cancers involve continued disfigurement and dysfunction and are primarily site-specific (Box 7-9). Disfigurement after surgical resection of cancers of the head and neck or disfigurement caused by growing, protruding tumors can be quite severe. Although reconstruction is a routine part of head and neck surgery, the significance of facial disfigurement cannot be overstated. The face and neck are our most prominent features and are integral to a positive body image, which affects our socialization and integration into society.[44]

Besides surgical deformities, permanent alopecia that may occur as a result of radiation therapy is often quite upsetting for patients. Hair loss directly behind the ear is common after postoperative radiation for parotid cancer. Hair loss in the back of the head, a result of nasopharynx or nasal sinus complex radiation, is usually temporary, but may be permanent, and is always disconcerting to patients because of the bizarre pattern of loss.

Bilateral facial hair loss is less of an issue than unilateral loss, but for patients who normally wear a beard, any change to hairlessness is upsetting. The loss of facial hair can be devastating for patients for whom a beard and forelock is a religious requirement. Fortunately, many centers that provide wigs for patients undergoing chemotherapy now also carry small beard and forelock prostheses to hide this hair loss.

The acute skin reaction usually fades by 3 to 4 weeks after completion of radiation therapy. In

Box 7-9 Possible Disfigurements and Dysfunctions

DISFIGUREMENT

Surgical defects
Alopecia
Pigmentation changes

DYSFUNCTION

Xerostomia, osteoradionecrosis
Hypothyroidism
Trismus
Dysphagia

dark-skinned patients, however, the fading of increased pigmentation may take up to a year, and in some cases, the treatment portals of radiation therapy are permanently visible. Many times these darkened areas can easily be covered up with makeup, or the unaffected areas can be darkened slightly to achieve a balanced look. It is important to educate patients about alopecia and skin coloration changes from the beginning of treatment. Offering practical assistance and psychologic support will make it easier for patients to adjust to these changes.

Patients should be instructed in the long-term use of sunscreens. The radiated skin should be protected from wind, sun, and extreme temperatures. Sunscreens with a sun protection factor of 30 (UVA/UVB protection) is recommended for irradiated skin.[66]

Xerostomia, which begins during the acute phase of radiation therapy, continues throughout the remainder of patients' lives. The degree of dryness is variable, but leads to an increased risk of cavities and bone damage after radiation treatment. Osteoradionecrosis (ORN) describes a condition of impaired healing and necrosis of the jawbone after radiation therapy. It can occur in 5% to 15% of patients receiving radiation therapy, and typically presents after a tooth extraction from the mandible.[67] Conservative treatment includes meticulous oral hygiene by patients and systemic antibiotics. Even with complete adherence to these measures, bone exposure may take 3 to 6 months to close.

Surgical management of osteoradionecrosis may be necessary. Resection of all necrotic tissue is followed by primary closure in most cases. Rarely, a bone graft is necessary to provide adequate bone for normal jaw function. Surgical treatment is prefaced by hyperbaric oxygen treatments given in 90-minute sessions. Twenty treatments are delivered, once daily, presurgery, and 10 additional treatments are delivered postoperatively. Antibiotics are given both preoperatively and post-operatively.[68]

Preventing ORN should be encouraged. Patients should apply fluoride to teeth nightly and see their dentist regularly, and foreseeable dental extractions should be done before beginning radiation therapy. If extractions must be done after radiation, again, hyperbaric oxygen should be used, 20 treatments, or "dives," preextraction and 10 more after the extraction. Providing high-pressure oxygen to the affected area before and after the trauma of an extraction may improve healing of radiated tissues.[67]

A late effect occurring in approximately 15% of patients treated for advanced head and neck cancers is hypothyroidism. This results from effects of radiation therapy on the thyroid gland itself. In a prospective trial reported by Sinard and colleagues,[69] hypothyroidism was most likely to occur in patients with tumors requiring total laryngectomy plus postoperative radiation therapy. In that group the incidence of hypothyroidism within a year of treatment was 61%. For patients not requiring laryngeal surgery, but who received radiation therapy, the incidence was 12%.[69]

Trismus is a late effect of radiation therapy seen commonly in patients treated for nasopharynx cancers, base of tongue, salivary gland, and tumors of the maxilla. It is defined as the contraction of the muscles of mastication, but commonly refers to any restriction in ability to open the mouth. Radiation doses greater than 60 Gy directed to the temporomandibular joint, pterygoid muscles, or the masseter muscles are most likely to cause injury leading to trismus. Usually, restriction is gradual, beginning after radiation is completed, and is slowly progressive.[70]

Trismus often goes unnoticed. Many patients are feeding tube–dependent and are not regularly opening their mouths. As they recover from therapy and begin to take oral nourishment, they notice difficulty opening their mouths and the unusual tightness of the jaw. Treatment of trismus should begin during radiation therapy, to minimize its severity and to promote a rapid return to normal jaw functioning. Patients should be instructed to continue to exercise their mouths despite lack of oral nourishment. They should open their mouths as widely as possible, hold this position a few seconds, close and repeat, multiple times throughout the day. Alternatively, they can use various devices to assist in this exercise.

Stacked tongue blades, approaching the widest diameter of mouth opening, can be inserted between the top and bottom teeth to assist in holding the mouth open. The mouth should be stretched, but not to the point of pain. A more elegant and expensive option is the use of the Therabite Jaw Motion Rehabilitation System.[71] This is a plastic device used to stretch the muscles of mastication.

Whatever method is used, the goal of treatment is to first prevent as much loss of function as possible and to repair damage done by regularly exercising the muscles affected.

Persistent dysphagia, or difficulty swallowing after treatment for head and neck cancers, negatively affects patients' quality of life. It is estimated that more than 25% of patients with nasopharyngeal carcinoma have significant dysphagia,[72] with endoscopically determined aspiration occurring during the act of swallowing. Other causes of dysphagia include tongue atrophy, vocal cord palsy, and pharyngeal constriction, and all are complicated by persistent xerostomia after radiation therapy.

A retrospective analysis of 73 patients complaining of dysphagia after primary radiation therapy, postoperative radiation therapy, or combined chemotherapy/radiation therapy was reported by Nguyen and colleagues.[73] Patients underwent a full swallowing evaluation including barium swallow to determine the severity and type of swallowing dysfunction and its impact on quality of life. The degree of dysphagia was moderate (requiring swallowing precautions) to severe (requiring enteral feeding support) in 45% of these patients, and the quality of life (QOL) scores were significantly decreased. Additionally, patients with the worst degree of dysphagia also had significantly increased anxiety and depression.

Recent research is directed toward identifying the structures that, when irradiated, most affect patient's ability to swallow without aspiration. Eisbruch and colleagues[74] used pre- and posttreatment evaluations of swallowing function on 26 patients receiving concomitant chemotherapy/radiation therapy. The pharyngeal constrictor muscles, the glottis, and the supraglottis were found to be the structures most likely to result in dysphagia if injured by the therapy. Dose sparing of these structures was achieved using specific IMRT planning versus standard 3-D radiation therapy. It is postulated that decreased dose to these critical structures may lead to decreased dysphagia although the clinical value of this has yet to be demonstrated.[74]

BRACHYTHERAPY FOR HEAD AND NECK CANCER

Brachytherapy is often used in the treatment of head and neck cancers. The ability to increase the total dose of radiation to the tumor and yet minimize the dose to normal tissues is especially important when treating these malignancies (Table 7-9). Anatomically, head and neck tumors often abut critical structures (optic chiasm, spinal cord, brainstem). These structures are unable to tolerate tumoricidal doses of radiation. Brachytherapy offers a means of delivering high doses of radiation to the tumor while adding dosage to these critical structures.

Many studies and reports are found in the literature to support the use of brachytherapy in patients with head and neck cancer. In treating the cancers of the oral cavity, brachytherapy alone offers efficacy equal to external beam radiation therapy plus brachytherapy boost and may cause less xerostomia.[75] High-dose-rate primary brachytherapy has been used for treating patients with early-stage oral tongue cancers with success. By using an

Table 7-9 Implants Types and Dose Rates

Head and neck site	Type of implant	Dose rate
Oral cavity		
Floor of mouth	Interstitial	HDR or LDR
Lip	Interstitial	Usually HDR
Oral tongue	Interstitial	Usually LDR
Oropharynx		
Base of tongue	Interstitial	HDR or LDR
Tonsil	Interstitial	HDR or LDR
Soft palate	Interstitial	HDR or LDR
Nasopharynx	Intracavitary	Usually HDR
Nasal cavity	Intracavitary	HDR
Paranasal sinus complex	Intracavitary	HDR or LDR

HDR, High-dose-rate; *LDR,* low-dose-rate.

interstitial tongue implant alone, xerostomia was minimized although mucositis lasted over 2 months.[76] Patients with tonsillar or soft palate cancers were treated either with surgery plus postoperative external beam radiation therapy or with primary external beam radiation therapy plus brachytherapy boost. Excellent locoregional control of disease was reported in both groups, and with use of highly conformal treatment techniques (IMRT), radiation exposure to salivary glands is minimized.[77]

Minimization of disfigurement is very important when treating patients with mid-face malignancies. Patients with nasal vestibule cancers are rarely treated with surgery because of the resulting unacceptable disfigurement. Patients with these cancers should be treated with an interstitial implant whenever possible. Local control rates from use of external beam radiation therapy alone is poor (less than 70%), but use of an implant alone for T1 lesions, or used in conjunction with external beam radiation therapy in more advanced tumors, increases locoregional control to above 95%.[78] As described previously, oropharyngeal cancers, especially cancers of the base of the tongue, are often treated with a combination of both external beam radiation therapy and interstitial brachytherapy boost in order to preserve function.[17]

Patients with recently diagnosed nasopharyngeal carcinoma and patients with recurrent disease can be treated with external beam radiation therapy plus a brachytherapy boost. Lee and colleagues[79] reported a 45-year experience using brachytherapy for nasopharyngeal carcinomas. Brachytherapy was delivered using balloon, ovoid, and ribbon applicators to patients with initial and recurrent disease. High-dose-rate delivery, (ranging from 5 Gy to 7 Gy), or low-dose-rate delivery, (ranging from 10 Gy to 54 Gy) was used after external beam radiation therapy. Intracavitary boost brachytherapy was reported to be effective and well tolerated.[79]

Use of brachytherapy for palliation in patients with head and neck cancer allows delivery of radiation in doses to provide local control, while shortening treatment time and avoiding daily trips to the radiation department (often burdensome for patients with end-stage disease). Proper patient selection is key, and strong support by the multidisciplinary team is important.[80,81] Brachytherapy is often used when patients have already received full doses of external beam radiation therapy, examples include instances of recurrent or residual disease. Glatzel and colleagues[82] reported use of high-dose-rate brachytherapy for both primary palliation and as a local boost to tumors persisting after standard treatment. Brachytherapy was found to be effective and was well tolerated.

Patients are challenged physically and emotionally during administration of brachytherapy. Not only are they going through a frightening cancer therapy involving radioactive materials, but the procedure for receiving the implant is quite stressful. It is important to understand the steps through which patients go during the implant procedure in order to implement thorough and appropriate teaching. Devine and Doyle[83] present an excellent case study of a patient's experience during hospitalization for a base of tongue implant. In addition to describing the brachytherapy process, they list some of the staff considerations as well. The following are some of the important teaching points for patients undergoing head and neck brachytherapy.

Surgery is necessary to provide a low-dose-rate base of tongue interstitial implant to a patient with base of tongue cancer. The patient is hospitalized, goes to surgery, receives anesthesia, and awakes to find catheters and buttons protruding from under his/her chin. The patient's face will be swollen, and his/her tongue, lips, and cheeks will be tender and bruised. The patient will have a temporary tracheotomy and must learn how to suction secretions, which is often the most frightening aspect of the brachytherapy procedure. The brachytherapy catheter exit sites are cared for by gentle cleansing, leaving open to air, and daily application of a triple antibiotic ointment. Although evidence regarding a specific ointment used in the care of brachytherapy catheters is not available, it is prudent to apply an antimicrobial ointment to minimize the risk of infection.

Several days after surgery, the patient will have localization films done in the radiation oncology department. Radiopaque "dummy" seeds attached to ribbons are threaded through the catheters and x rays are taken to demonstrate catheter position within the base of tongue. The physician and physicist create a plan and order the appropriate radioactive material for the implant. Iridium-192 is the radioactive source commonly used for low-dose-rate tongue implants, because it emits continuous local radiation over several days.

When the source arrives, the physician "loads" the implant by threading ribbons containing ^{192}Ir into the catheters at the bedside. This is not a painful procedure, but patients experience pulling sensations and are usually quite anxious. From this point until the ribbons are removed by the physician, the patient must remain isolated in a private room. Visitors are limited to just moments in the room and the staff must limit their time in the room as well. The patient is alone, providing much of his/her own care including suctioning, and is aware of being radioactive and having minimal exposure to others. This is an extremely stressful time for the patient. However, it is manageable if the patient has been properly educated regarding the implantation process. A laptop computer, video, or DVD player and books are helpful for distraction and to relieve boredom during the isolation period.

When the appropriate dose of radiation has been reached, the radiation oncologist removes the ribbons and then the catheters. During removal of the catheters, the patient experiences pulling and mild discomfort. Often an anxiolytic is given 30 minutes before catheter removal, and in some cases a pain medication may also be given. The tracheostomy is capped and usually removed within 24 hours. The patient is then subsequently discharged from the hospital.

Acute Effects of Brachytherapy and Nursing Interventions

Immediately after placement of the catheters, patients describe feelings of "fullness" in the mouth, because of the catheters and resulting edema. Mild skin irritation at catheter exit sites may be present, and most patients report mild discomfort. If a lymph node dissection was done at the time of catheter placement, patients usually report pain only at the dissection site.

The acute radiation effect is localized, involving only the area implanted. It peaks 10 to 24 days after implant removal and quickly subsides. This reaction is experienced as swelling and pain of the tissue implanted. Appropriate teaching is important so that patients are prepared for the abrupt onset of this reaction so long after the actual implant. Systemic and local pain medications will be needed and may include narcotic analgesics and local analgesic ointments such as lidocaine 2% or Benzocaine.[46]

Long-term effects of brachytherapy include soft-tissue injury or necrosis in as many as 15% to 30% of patients, with severe ulceration in 5%. Prevention of injury to radiated tissues is critical, and biopsies should be avoided whenever possible in the early post-implant period. Soft tissue ulcers heal slowly over 3 to 9 months, during which time patients must adhere to meticulous oral hygiene. Antibiotics and pain medications may be prescribed during this period and patients should be examined in follow-up frequently.[17]

In less than 5% of all brachytherapy cases, osteoradionecrosis results from an implant. Particularly at risk are patients who had brachytherapy treatment near the bones of the mandible or maxillae and for whom the implant was the sole form of radiation therapy delivered.[84] Osteoradionecrosis is a serious late effect and may require hyperbaric oxygen and surgical removal of necrotic bone. Please refer to the previous section on osteoradionecrosis for more details on management of this late effect.

SUMMARY

Although head and neck cancers account for a relatively small percent of all cancers diagnosed each year, patients with this disease are a tremendous challenge to the oncology clinician. In most cases, multimodality treatment is employed, thus exacerbating treatment morbidity. Increased morbidity often results in treatment breaks and may theoretically compromise overall treatment efficacy. Whether radiation treatments consist of external beam radiation therapy or brachytherapy, the side effect profile is similar. Although treatment can be difficult for most patients, aggressive nursing care and education can hopefully minimize side effects and decrease overall discomfort associated with treatment. It is hoped that with advanced treatment planning and the administration of IMRT, along with newer chemotherapeutic regimes, morbidity will be decreased and overall survival rates improved.

REFERENCES

1. American Cancer Society: *Cancer facts and figures, 2006 (website):* www.cancer.org/downloads/STT/CAFF2006PWSecured.pdf. Accessed December 12, 2006.
2. Spitz R, Trizna Z: Molecular epidemiology and genetic predisposition for head and neck cancer. In Harrison LB, Sessions RB, Hong WI, et al, editors: *Head and neck cancer:*

a multidisciplinary approach, ed 2, Philadelphia, 1999, Lippincott Williams & Wilkins, p 11.
3. Tsang NM, Chang KP, Lin SY et al: Detection of Epstein-Barr virus-derived latent membrane protein-1 gene in various head and neck cancers: is it specific for nasopharyngeal carcinoma? *Laryngoscope* 113(6): 1050-1054, 2003.
4. Gillison ML: Human papilloma virus-associated head and neck cancer is a distinct epidemiologic, clinical, and molecular entity, *Semin Oncol* 31(6):744-754, 2004.
5. Iwamoto RR: Cancers of the head and neck. In Dow K, Bucholtz JD, Iwamoto RI et al, editors: *Nursing care in radiation oncology,* ed 2, Philadelphia, 1997, Saunders, p 239.
6. Costantino PD, Murphy MR, Moche JA: Cancer of the nasal vestibule, nasal cavity, and paranasal sinus; surgical management. In Harrison LB, Sessions RB, Hong WI et al, editors: *Head and neck cancer: a multidisciplinary approach,* ed 2, Philadelphia, 2004, Lippincott Williams & Wilkins, p 458.
7. Duthoy W, Boterberg T, Claus F et al: Postoperative intensity-modulated radiotherapy in sinonasal carcinoma: clinical results in 39 patients, *Cancer* 104(1):71-82, 2005.
8. National Comprehensive Cancer Network: Practice Guidelines in Oncology—v.1.2005 Maxillary sinus tumors (website): www.nccn.org/professionals/physician_gls/PDF/head-and-neck.pdf. Accessed December 6, 2005.
9. BoPeters J, Rischin D, Corru J et al: Cancer of the nasopharynx. In Harrison LB, Sessions RB, Hong WI et al, editors: *Head and neck cancer: a multidisciplinary approach,* ed 2, Philadelphia, 2004, Lippincott Williams & Wilkins, p 533.
10. National Comprehensive Cancer Network Practice Guidelines in Oncology—v.1.2005 Cancer of the nasopharynx (website): www.nccn.org/professionals/physician_gls/PDF/head-and-neck.pdf. Accessed December 6, 2005.
11. Bourhis J, Cvitkovic E, Eschwege F et al: Nasopharyngeal carcinoma: cancer of the nasopharynx. In Harrison LB, Sessions RB, Hong WI, editors: *Head and neck cancer: a multidisciplinary approach,* Philadelphia, 1999 Lippincott Williams & Wilkins, p 646.
12. Hunt MA, Zelefsky MJ, Wolden S et al: Treatment planning and delivery of intensity-modulated radiation therapy for primary nasopharynx cancer, *Int J Radiat Oncol Biol Phys* 49(3):623-632, 2001.
13. Iwamoto RR: Cancers of the head and neck. In Dow K, Bucholtz JD, Iwamoto RI et al, editors: *Nursing care in radiation oncology,* ed 2, Philadelphia, 1997, Saunders, p 243.
14. Shiboski CH, Schmidt BL, Jordan RC: Tonsil and tongue carcinoma: increasing trends in the U.S. population ages 20-44 years, *Cancer* 103:1843-1849, 2005.
15. Shah JP, Zelefsky MJ: Cancer of the oral cavity. In Harrison LB, Sessions RB, Hong WI, editors: *Head and neck cancer: a multidisciplinary approach,* ed 2, Philadelphia, 2004, Lippincott Williams & Wilkins, p 273.
16. National Comprehensive Cancer Network: Practice Guidelines in Oncology—v.1.2005 Cancer of the oral cavity (website): www.nccn.org/professionals/physician_gls/PDF/head-and-neck.pdf. Accessed December 6, 2005.
17. Hu KS, Harrison LB, Culliney B et al: Cancer of the oropharynx. In Harrison LB, Sessions RB, Hong WI, editors: *Head and neck cancer: a multidisciplinary approach,* ed 2, Philadelphia, 2004, Lippincott Williams & Wilkins, pp 309, 312-315.
18. National Comprehensive Cancer Network: Practice Guidelines in Oncology—v.1.2005 Cancer of the oropharynx (website): www.nccn.org/professionals/physician_gls/PDF/head-and-neck.pdf. Accessed December 6, 2005.
19. Pfister DG, Hu KS, Lefebvre JL: Cancer of the hypopharynx and cervical esophagus. In Harrison LB, Sessions RB, Hong WI, editors: *Head and neck cancer: a multidisciplinary approach,* ed 2, Philadelphia, 2004, Lippincott Williams & Wilkins, pp 407-413.
20. National Comprehensive Cancer Network: Practice Guidelines in Oncology—v.1.2005 Cancer of the hypopharynx (website): www.nccn.org/professionals/physician_gls/PDF/head-and-neck.pdf. Accessed December 6, 2005.
21. van der Voet JC, Keus RB, Hart AA et al: The impact of treatment time and smoking on local control and complications in T1 glottic cancer, *Int J Radiat Oncol Biol Phys* 42(2):247-255, 1998.
22. Mendenhall WM, Sulica L, Sessions RB: Early stage cancer of the larynx. In Harrison LB, Sessions RB, Hong WI, editors: *Head and neck cancer: a multidisciplinary approach,* ed 2, Philadelphia, 2004, Lippincott Williams & Wilkins, pp 352-355.
23. Clayman GL, Frank DK, Garden AS et al: Advanced stage cancer of the larynx. In Harrison LB, Sessions RB, Hong WI, editors: *Head and neck cancer: a multidisciplinary approach,* ed 2, Philadelphia, 2004, Lippincott Williams & Wilkins, pp 383-386.
24. National Comprehensive Cancer Network: Practice Guidelines in Oncology—v.1.2005 Cancer of the glottic larynx (website): www.nccn.org/professionals/physician_gls/PDF/head-and-neck.pdf. Accessed December 6, 2005.
25. National Comprehensive Cancer Network: Practice Guidelines in Oncology—v.1.2005 Cancer of the supraglottic larynx (website): www.nccn.org/professionals/physician_gls/PDF/head-and-neck.pdf. Accessed December 6, 2005.
26. Eisele DW, Kleinberg LR. Management of malignant salivary gland tumors. In Harrison LB, Sessions RB, Hong WI, editors: *Head and neck cancer: a multidisciplinary approach,* ed 2, Philadelphia, 2004, Lippincott Williams & Wilkins, pp 631, 635.
27. National Comprehensive Cancer Network: Practice Guidelines in Oncology—v.1.2005 Salivary gland tumors (website): www.nccn.org/professionals/physician_gls/PDF/head-and-neck.pdf. Accessed December 6, 2005.
28. Sessions RB, Burman KD: Cancer of the thyroid gland. In Harrison LB, Sessions RB, Hong WI, editors: *Head and neck cancer: a multidisciplinary approach,* ed 2, Philadelphia, 2004, Lippincott Williams & Wilkins, p 723.
29. Nutting CM, Convery DJ, Cosgrove VP et al: Improvements in target coverage and reduced spinal cord irradiation using intensity-modulated radiotherapy (IMRT) in patients with carcinoma of the thyroid gland, *Radiother Oncol* 60(2): 173-180, 2004.
30. Schlumberger MJ: Anaplastic thyroid carcinoma. Orphanet Encyclopedia, 2004 (website): www.orpha.net/data/patho/GB/uk-ATC.pdf. Accessed December 1, 2005.

31. Kebebow E, Greenspan FS, Clark OH et al: Anaplastic thyroid carcinoma: treatment outcome and prognostic factors, *Cancer* 103(7):1330-1335, 2005.
32. Haigh PI, Ituarte PH, Wu HS et al: Completely resected anaplastic thyroid carcinoma combined with adjuvant chemotherapy and irradiation is associated with prolonged survival, *Cancer* 91(12):2335-2342, 2001.
33. National Comprehensive Cancer Network: Practice Guidelines in Oncology—v.1.2005 Thyroid carcinoma (website): www.nccn.org/professionals/physician_gls/PDF/head-and-neck.pdf. Accessed December 6, 2005.
34. Cox J D, Pajak RF, Marcial VA et al: Interruptions adversely affect local control and survival with hyperfractionated radiation therapy of carcinomas of the upper respiratory and digestive tracts: new evidence for accelerated proliferation from Radiation Therapy Oncology Group Protocol 8313, *Cancer* 69(11):2744-2748, 1992.
35. Suwinski R, Sowa A, Rutkowski T et al: Time factor in postoperative radiotherapy: a multivariate locoregional control analysis in 868 patients, *Int J Radiat Oncol Biol Phys* 56(2):399-412, 2003.
36. Robertson C, Robertson AG, Hendry JH et al: Similar decreases in local tumor control are calculated for treatment protraction and for interruptions in the radiotherapy of carcinoma of the larynx in four centers, *Int J Radiat Oncol Biol Phys*, 40(2):319-329, 1998.
37. Barton MB, Keane TJ, Gadalla T et al: The effect of treatment time and treatment interruption on tumour control following radical radiotherapy of laryngeal cancer, *Radiother Oncol* (3):137-143, 1992.
38. Stone P, Ream E, Richardson A et al: Cancer-related fatigue—a difference of opinion? Results of a multicentre survey of healthcare professionals, patients and caregivers, *Eur J Cancer Care (Engl)* 12(1):20-27, 2003.
39. Given B, Given CW, McCorkle R et al: Pain and fatigue management: results of a nursing randomized clinical trial, *Oncol Nurse Forum* 29(6): 949-956, 2002.
40. Harrison LB, Shasha D, Shiaova L et al: Prevalence of anemia in cancer patients undergoing radiation therapy, *Semin Oncol* 28:54-59, 2001.
41. Daly T, Poulesen MG, Denham JW et al: The effect of anaemia on efficacy and normal tissue toxicity following radiotherapy for locally advanced squamous cell carcinoma of the head and neck, *Radiother Oncol* 68(2):113-122, 2003.
42. Henke M, Laszig R, Rube C et al: Erythropoietin to treat head and neck cancer patients with anaemia undergoing radiotherapy: randomized, double-blind, placebo-controlled trial, *Lancet* 362(9392):1255-1260, 2003.
43. Carper E, Fleishman SB, McGuire M: Symptom management and supportive care for head and neck cancer patients. In Harrison LB, Sessions RB, Hong WI, editors: *Head and neck cancer: a multidisciplinary approach,* ed 2, Philadelphia, 2004, Lippincott Williams & Wilkins, p 144.
44. Bruce SD: Radiation-induced xerostomia: how dry is your patient? *Clin J Oncol Nursing* 8:1, 61, 2004.
45. Ship JA, Hu K: Radiotherapy-induced salivary dysfunction, *Semin Oncol* 31(suppl 18):29-36, 2004.
46. Shih A, Miaskowski C, Dodd MJ et al:. A research review of the current treatments for radiation-induced oral mucositis in patients with head and neck cancer, *Oncol Nurs Forum* 29(7):1063-1080, 2002.
47. Hancock PJ, Epstein JB, Sadler GR: Oral and dental management related to radiation therapy for head and neck cancer, *J Can Dent Assoc* 69(9):585-590, 2003.
48. Toljanic JA, Heshmati RH, Bedard JF: Dental follow-up compliance in a population of irradiated head and neck cancer patients, *Oral Surg Oral Med Oral Pathol Oral Radiol Endod* 93(1):35-38, 2002.
49. Mehta MP: Protection of normal tissues from the cytotoxic effects of radiation therapy: focus on amifostine, *Semin Radiat Oncol* 8(4 Suppl 1):14-16, 1998.
50. Werner-Wasik M: Future development of amifostine as a radioprotectant, *Semin Radiat Oncol* 26(2 Suppl 7): 129-134, 1999.
51. MedImmune Oncology, Inc: Amifostine [package insert], 2001 (website): www.medimmune.com/products/ethyol.asp. Accessed March 15, 2002.
52. Gosselin TK, Pavilonis H: Head and neck cancer: managing xerostomia and other treatment induced side effects, *ORL Head Neck Nurs* 20(4):15-22, 2002.
53. Nieuw Amerongen AV, Veerman EC: Current therapies for xerostomia and salivary gland hypofunction associated with cancer therapies, *Support Care Cancer* 11(4):226-231, 2003.
54. Gorsky M, Epstein JB, Parry J et al: The efficacy of pilocarpine and bethanechol upon saliva production in cancer patients with hyposalivation following radiation therapy, *Oral Surg Oral Med Oral Pathol Oral Radiol Endod* 97(2):190-195, 2004.
55. Johnstone P, Niemtzow R, Riffenburgh R: Acupuncture for xerostomia, *Cancer* 94:1151-1156, 2002.
56. Blom M, Dawidson I, Fernberg J et al: Acupuncture treatment of patients with radiation-induced xerostomia, *Eur J Cancer B Oral Oncol* 32B(3):182-190, 1996.
57. Blom M, Lunderberg T: Long-term follow-up of patients treated with acupuncture for xerostomia and the influence of additional treatment, *Oral Diseases* 6:15-24, 2000.
58. Sulaiman F, Huryn JM, Zlotolow IM: Dental extractions in the irradiated head and neck patient: a retrospective analysis of Memorial Sloan-Kettering Cancer Center protocols, criteria, and end results, *J Oral Maxillofac Surg* 61(10):1123-1131, 2003.
59. Ondrey FG, Greig JR, Herscher L: Radiation dose to otologic structures during head and neck cancer radiation therapy, *Laryngoscope* 110:217, 2000.
60. Robinson AC: Management of radiation-induced otitis externa, *J Laryngol Otol* 104(6):458-459, 1990.
61. Jereczek-Fossa BA, Zarowski A, Milani F et al: Radiotherapy-induced ear toxicity, *Cancer Treat Rev* 29(5):417-430, 2003.
62. Reitemeier B, Reitemeier G, Schmidt A et al: Evaluation of a device for attenuation of electron release from dental restorations in a therapeutic radiation field, *J Prosthet Dent* 87(3):323-327, 2002.
63. Haas M, Kuehn E: Head and neck cancers. In Watkins-Bruner D, Moore-Higgs GJ, Haas M, editors: *Outcomes in radiation therapy: multidisciplinary management,* Sudbery, Mass, 2001, Jones and Bartlett, pp 195-213.
64. Karnell LH, Funk GF, Christensen AJ et al: Persistent post-treatment depressive symptoms in patients with head and neck cancer, *Head Neck* 28(5):453-461, 2006.

65. Smets EM, Visser MR, Willems-Groot et al: Fatigue and radiotherapy: experience in patients undergoing treatment, *Brit J Cancer* 78:899-906, 1998.
66. Haas ML: Skin reaction. In Watkins-Bruner D, Haas ML, Gosselin-Acomb TK, editors: *Manual for radiation oncology nursing practice and education*, ed 3, Pittsburgh, 2005, Oncology Nursing Society, pp 49-52.
67. Viale PH, Lin A: Exposed bone in oral cavities, *Clin J Oncol Nurs* 9(3):355-357, 2005.
68. Jolly DE: Osteoradionecrosis, oral health and dental treatment, *Dent Assist* 73(2):4-7, 2004.
69. Sinard RJ, Tobin EJ, Mazaferri EL et al: Hypothyroidism after treatment for nonthyroid head and neck cancer, *Arch Otolaryngol Head Neck Surg* 126(5):652-657, 2000.
70. The Oral Cancer Foundation: *What is Trismus?* (website): www.oralcancerfoundation.org/dental/trismus.htm. Accessed January 14, 2006.
71. Atos Medical (website): www.atosmedical.com. Accessed January 14, 2006.
72. Wu CH, Hsiao TY, Ko JY et al: Dysphagia after radiotherapy: endoscopic examination of swallowing I patients with nasopharyngeal carcinoma, *Ann Otol Rhinol Laryngol* 109(3):320-325, 2000.
73. Nguyen NP, Frank C, Moltz CC et al: Impact of dysphagia on quality of life after treatment of head-and-neck cancer, *Int J Radiat Oncol Biol Phys* 61(3):772-778, 2005.
74. Eisbruch A, Schwartz M, Rasch C et al: Dysphagia and aspiration after chemoradiotherapy for head-and-neck cancer: which anatomic structures are affected and can they be spared by IMRT? *Int J Radiat Oncol Biol Phys* 60(5):1425-1439, 2004.
75. Lapeyre MB, Bollet MA, Racadot S et al: Postoperative brachytherapy alone and combined postoperative radiotherapy and brachytherapy boost for squamous cell carcinoma of the oral cavity, with positive or close margins, *Head Neck* 26(3):216-223, 2004.
76. Leung TW, Wong VY, Kwan KH et al: High dose rate brachytherapy for early stage oral tongue cancer, *Head Neck* 24(3):274-281, 2002.
77. Lenevdag P, Nijdam W, Noever I et al: Brachytherapy versus surgery in carcinoma of tonsillar fossa and/or soft palate: late adverse sequelae and performance status: can we be more selective and obtain better tissue sparing? *Int J Radiat Oncol Biol Phys* 59(3):713-724, 2004.
78. Parsons JT, Kies MS: Cancer of the nasal vestibule, nasal cavity and paranasal sinus. In Harrison LB, Sessions RB, Hong WI, editors: *Head and neck cancer: a multidisciplinary approach,* ed 2, 2004, Lippincott Williams & Wilkins, p 501.
79. Lee N, Hoffman R, Phillips TL et al: Managing nasopharyngeal carcinoma with intracavitary brachytherapy: one institution's 45-year experience, *Brachytherapy* 1(2): 74-82, 2002.
80. Shasha D, Harrison LB: The role of brachytherapy for palliation, *Semin Radiat Oncol* 10(3):222-239, 2000.
81. Quon H, Harrison LB: Brachytherapy in the treatment of head and neck cancer, *Oncology (Williston Park)* 16(10):1379-1393; discussion 1393, 1395-1396, 2002.
82. Glatzel M, Buntzel J, Schroder D et al: High-dose-rate brachytherapy in the treatment of recurrent and residual head and neck cancer, *Laryngoscope* 112(8 Pt 1):1366-1371, 2002.
83. Devine P, Doyle T: Brachytherapy for head and neck cancer: a case study, *Clin J Oncol Nurs* 5(2):55-57, 2001.
84. Gibbs IC, Le QT, Shah, RD et al: Long-term outcomes after external beam irradiation and brachytherapy boost for base-of-tongue cancers, *Int J Radiat Oncol Biol Phys* 57(2):489-494, 2003.

Chapter 8

Lung Cancer

Marilyn L. Haas

Before the twentieth century, lung cancer was uncommon. Today, however, lung cancer is the most significant health problem in the United States. In the United States, the American Cancer Society (ACS) reports lung cancer to be the second most common diagnosed cancer in men and women.[1] The ACS estimates there will be 186,370 new cases of lung cancer diagnosed in 2006, of whom 84,470 will be women. The mortality rates among males and females are high, with the ACS reporting lung cancer to be the most common cause of death in men and women.[1] In 1987, female deaths from lung cancer surpassed those from breast cancer; the margin is now growing progressively wider as time passes. Today, lung cancer kills more women each year than breast cancer, ovarian cancer, and uterine cancer combined, claiming an estimated 73,230 women in 2006.[1] The mortality figures for men in 2006 are estimated at 93,820. Although progress has been made in recent years in improving long-term survival in lung cancer patients, only small gains have been made in 5-year survival rates, which have reached 15% in all patients, regardless of stage at diagnosis.[2]

Although lung cancer is claiming many lives, it is referred to as the "unspoken" or ignored cancer.[3] Clear ribbons outlined in gold or yellow bracelets, worn by many individuals, are now the new symbols for lung cancer, which signify the almost invisible status of this devastating and stigmatized disease. Unlike many other types of cancer, social stigmas surround this disease. It is a well-known fact that tobacco products are the main contributor to the cause of lung cancer.[4,5] Other epidemiologic environmental factors include radon, occupational exposure (e.g., arsenic, asbestos, chromates), outdoor/indoor air pollutants (e.g., combustion-generated carcinogens, passive cigarette smoking, cooking stoves), and possibly socioeconomic factors such as age, race, gender, and class.[6]

Because bronchogenic carcinoma is a major oncologic problem, oncology nurses need to understand the pathophysiologic mechanisms that contribute to this disease. Nurses caring for lung cancer patients face significant challenges in dealing with different treatment modalities—surgery, radiation, chemotherapy, and/or biologic therapy—and with the natural progression of the disease.[7] Most patients who have lung cancer will receive radiation therapy at some point during the course of their disease. Radiation treatment strategies in this disease depend on its histopathologic type, extent (stage), and general well-being of the patient. Hence this chapter describes the current state of knowledge and some promising newer treatment options. Numerous clinical trials that are underway or have recently been completed may establish new approaches to radiation therapy and allow better integration with surgery and/or combined chemotherapy. Astute nursing skills and assessments and initiation of evidence-based interventions that can minimize the side effects of radiation therapy and thereby enhance an individual's quality of life are reviewed. Continuity of care issues provide a framework for acute and long-term planning, thus identifying potential problems for patients undergoing radiation therapy. Late effects of therapy are discussed because these must be anticipated so that appropriate interventions and follow-up can be determined. Finally, because nurses play a vital role throughout the process, educational information/resources are shared to help patients cope better while undergoing radiation therapy.

ANATOMY AND PATHOPHYSIOLOGY

To understand the complications of radiation therapy related to the pulmonary system, one must first have a basic understanding of normal anatomy and physiology.

Figure 8-1 illustrates the general anatomy of the thorax. The right lung consists of three lobes, the upper, middle, and lower. The oblique, or major, fissure separates the lower and the upper and middle lobes, and the horizontal, or minor, fissure divides the upper and middle lobes. The left lung consists of two lobes, upper and lower, divided by a single fissure. The trachea enters the mediastinum through the superior inlet of the thoracic cavity and bifurcates at the level of the fifth thoracic vertebrae. The hila of the lungs contain the bronchi, pulmonary arteries and veins, branches of the pulmonary plexus, bronchial arteries, veins, and lymphatics. The bronchi are lined with cilia to facilitate clearing foreign material from these tubes. This is accomplished by coughing and forcing air and foreign materials back up to the pharynx and out.

The respiratory unit consists of the bronchiole, alveolar ducts, atria, and alveoli. In the lungs there are approximately 300 million alveoli. Gaseous exchange occurs in the extremely thin alveolar walls, which consist almost entirely of capillaries. The alveolar gases being in close proximity to pulmonary blood allows the necessary diffusion to occur.[7]

The lungs have a rich lymphatic supply. The lymphatic vessels drain the interstitial connective tissue and empty into several groups of nodes: the intrapulmonary nodes (along the secondary bronchi), the bronchopulmonary (hilar) nodes, the mediastinal nodes, and the supraclavicular and scalene nodes. The intrapulmonary nodes are located peripherally along the segmental and subsegmental bronchi. The bronchopulmonary nodes consist of the interlobar nodes, found along the lobar bronchi, and the hilar nodes, which are adjacent to the main bronchi. The mediastinal lymph nodes are subdivided into superior and inferior groups; the superior mediastinal lymph nodes are located above the carina (bifurcation of trachea) and consist of the upper paratracheal, tracheal (azygos), and aortic nodes; the inferior group are those in the subcarinal and lower mediastinal areas: paraesophageal, subcarinal, and nodes in the pulmonary ligaments. These distinctions become significant when planning radiation treatment fields, because they must include all potentially involved nodes and spare noninvolved tissue.[7]

Guyton[8] divides the process of respiration into four major categories:

- Pulmonary ventilation—inflow and outflow of air between atmosphere and alveoli
- Diffusion of oxygen and carbon dioxide between alveoli and blood
- Transport of oxygen and carbon dioxide in blood and body fluids to cells
- Regulation of ventilation

MUSCLES OF BREATHING

Inflow and outflow of air is mediated by chest wall and diaphragmatic expansion and contraction. The movement of the diaphragm either lengthens or shortens the chest cavity, and the elevation or depression of the ribs regulates the anteroposterior chest cavity diameter. When the diaphragm contracts, the chest cavity is pulled downward, increasing its length; relaxation of the diaphragm allows it to move upward with the elastic recoil of the lungs. With labored breathing, the abdominal muscles are also used, and their contraction forces abdominal contents against the base of the diaphragm, supplementing this upward movement.

With expiration, the ribs are pulled downward via their posterior attachment to the spinal column. With inspiration, the sternum is lifted upward and the ribs extend more horizontally, increasing the anteroposterior diameter of the chest by approximately 20%. Normal breathing, however, is related almost entirely to the movement of the diaphragm. With dyspnea, the external intercostals, sternocleidomastoids, scapular elevators, scalene, and erectus muscles of the spine are used to supplement inspiration, and the abdominals, internal intercostals, and posterior inferior serratus muscles assist expiration.

PRESSURES IN THE LUNG

The compression and distention in the lungs caused by the respiratory muscles change the pressure in the alveoli. Negative pressure with respect to the atmosphere during inspiration causes air to flow into the lungs. During expiration, intraalveolar pressure rises and forces air out. The membranes of the intrapleural space absorb fluids and gas, thereby creating a partial vacuum. The negative pressure of fluid in the intrapleural space is generally 10 millimeters of mercury (mm Hg); this pressure allows the visceral pleura of the lungs to cling to the parietal pleura of the chest wall. The lungs are physically attached to the body only at the hila. As the chest cavity expands and contracts,

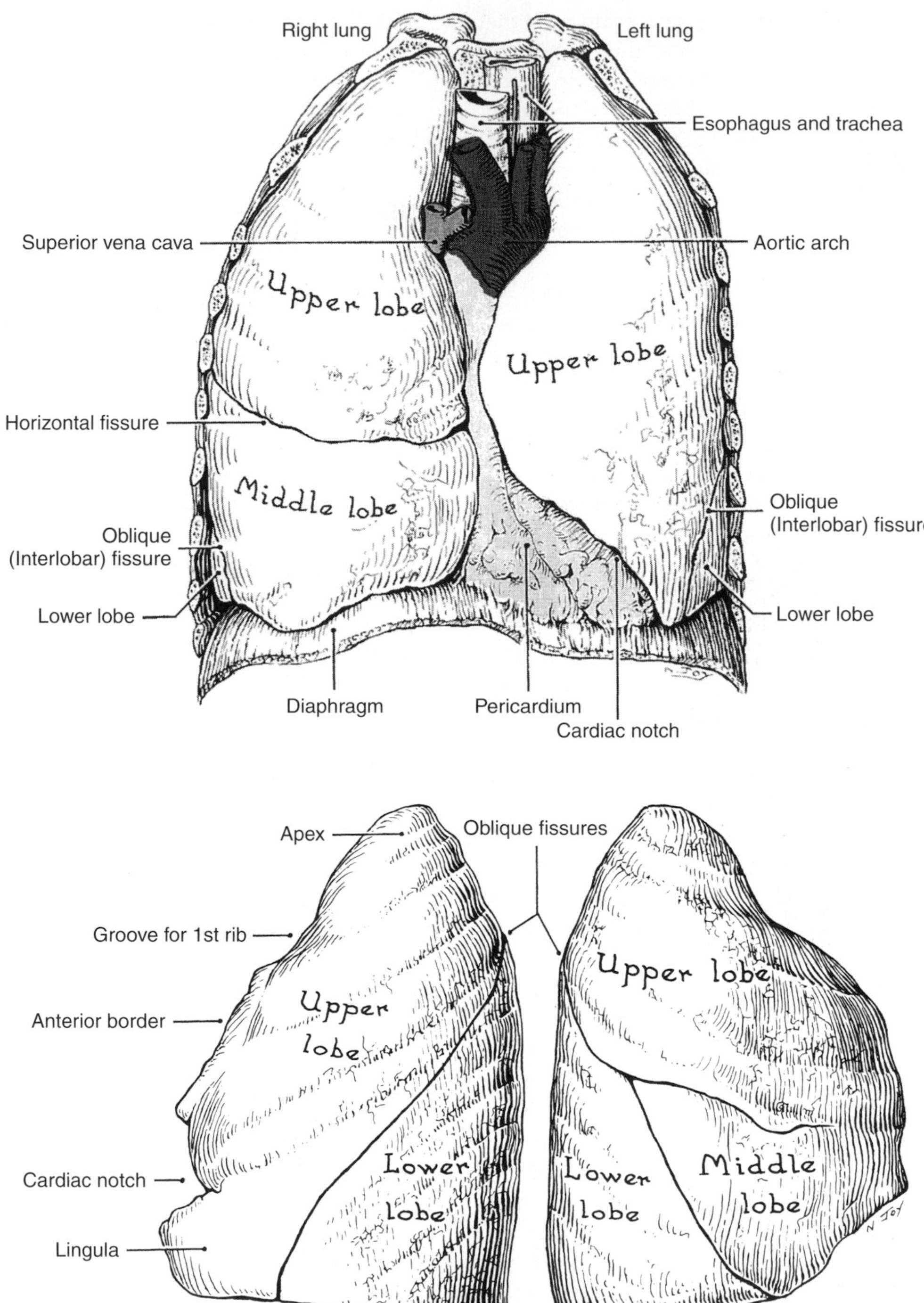

Figure 8-1 Anatomical Structures of the Lung.
From Grant J, Boileau C: Grant's atlas of anatomy, ed 6, Baltimore, 1972, Williams & Wilkins.

this adherence allows the lungs to expand and contract as well. A few millimeters of a mucopolysaccharide fluid are present in the intrapleural space, which permits the sliding of the visceral pleura over the partial pleura as the lungs move up and down in the chest cavity.[8]

LUNG RECOIL AND SURFACTANT

The lungs have a tendency to collapse based on their elastic properties and recoil away from the chest wall. Elastic fibers in the lung are stretched during inspiration and attempt to shorten. Alveoli also have a tendency to collapse as a result of the surface tension of fluid within them. Surfactant is a lipoprotein mixture secreted by alveolar type II pneumocytes in alveolar epithelium. The major component of surfactant is a detergent-like phospholipid known as phosphatidylcholine. This highly saturated phospholipid reduces surface tension within the alveoli and prevents alveolar collapse. Surfactant creates a layer between the fluid and air in the alveoli preventing the development of the high surface tension of a water-air interface.[8-10] Without surfactant, pressures as high as 20 to 30 mm Hg are necessary to maintain open alveoli because the contractile force created by water tension tends to cause collapse. As alveoli become smaller, they have an even greater proclivity for collapse. Surfactant can reduce this surface tension, and the pressure required to maintain open alveoli can be reduced to only 3 to 5 mm Hg. Surfactant also plays an important role in maintaining the size of alveoli: large alveoli develop higher surface tension and become smaller, whereas with surfactant, small alveoli become larger as their surface tension decreases. The effect of radiation on surfactant may result in the development of pneumonitis, as is discussed later.

Energy of Respiration

Normal breathing requires only 3.5% of the total energy expended by an individual. In pulmonary disease that alters compliance, increases airway resistance, or increases viscosity, as much as one third or more of total energy expended is devoted to respiration. This results in significant lifestyle changes for the individual.[8]

CLINICAL MANIFESTATIONS

The clinical manifestations of lung cancer depend on the location and extent of the tumor (Table 8-1). Although lung cancer can virtually remain undetected in the early stages, many individuals ignore the initial presenting symptoms until the tumor is large enough to interfere with normal lung functioning.

Patients with localized disease usually have symptoms related to airway obstruction, infiltration of the lung parenchyma, and/or invasion of the surrounding structures of the chest wall, major blood vessels, and viscera.[11] Cough is the most common presenting symptom of lung cancer, representing 75% of patients, and is severe in 40% of patients.[7,12] The underlining reasons relate to

Table 8-1 Signs and Symptoms of Lung Cancer at Presentation

Local-regional	Distant	Non-specific
Cough	Neurologic symptoms: (headaches, dizziness, nausea/vomiting)	Weight loss
Dyspnea	Bone pain	Fatigue
Shortness of breath	Hepatic/abdominal pain: (liver, kidney, pancreas, adrenal)	Anorexia
Febrile respiratory problems		
Hemoptysis		
Dysphagia (tumor compression)		
Chest/shoulder pain		
Hoarseness		
Nodal disease (neck/supraclavicular/hilar/mediastinal)		
SVC syndrome		
Horner syndrome		
Pancoast syndrome		

SVC, Superior vena cava.

smoking and other respiratory illnesses (e.g., chronic obstructive pulmonary disease [COPD] or upper respiratory infections). After a cough, dyspnea is the second most common manifestation, representing 40% to 60% of patients.[13] Typically, dyspnea is more prevalent in later stages because it is a direct result of airway obstruction. Wheezing or stridor, a severe wheeze, occurs when the airway becomes narrowed because of infection or bronchospasms or is blocked by the tumor itself. Hemoptysis results from the tumor eroding into surrounding tissues and blood vessels, occurring in 57% of patients, and presents as the first symptom in 4% of patients.[7,13] Patients describe hemoptysis in a range of severity from blood-streaked sputum, to expectorated blood clots, to frank bleeding. Chest pain occurs in 30% to 50% of patients.[13] The pain can be a result of chest wall or pleural invasion. Pancoast tumors can cause shoulder and arm pain as a result of brachial plexus compression. Also, patients can develop postobstructive pneumonia from partial or complete obstruction of the bronchus. Other nonspecific presenting symptoms occurring in 10% to 15% of patients are weight loss, weakness, anorexia, and/or malaise.[7]

Patients who have advance disease can present with any of the aforementioned symptoms, but usually have additional symptoms related to extrathoracic involvement or systemic disease signifying the cancer has spread to other parts of the body. Adenopathy, palpable cervical and/or supraclavicular lymph nodes, may be the first clue of nodal metastasis. Paresis or paralysis of the vocal cords can result in hoarseness. This occurs from the compression of the laryngeal nerve by central tumors or from mediastinal lymphadenopathy. Superior vena cava syndrome (SVC), depicted in Figures 8-2 and 8-3, is commonly referred to as SVC and occurs as a result of tumor compression of the superior vena cava. This phenomenon occurs in a small percentage of patients with lung cancer (0% to 4%).[12] Symptoms may include facial, neck, or upper extremity edema; headache, dizziness, drowsiness, visual distortion; and dilation of collateral veins on the upper chest, shoulders, and arms. Horner syndrome may occur as a result of apical tumors that invade the sympathetic ganglia, displayed by enophthalmos, ptosis, meiosis, and/or ipsilateral anhidrosis. Other symptoms of advanced disease that are considered oncologic emergencies include cardiac effusion and possibly tamponade, pleural effusion, or bone involvement possibly compressing the spinal cord. Paraneoplastic syndromes exhibit numerous signs and symptoms that are not well understood, but can include neuromuscular, skeletal, endocrine, and cutaneous problems.

DIAGNOSTIC STUDIES FOR WORK-UP

After a complete history, including risk factors and symptoms, and a physical examination, diagnostic

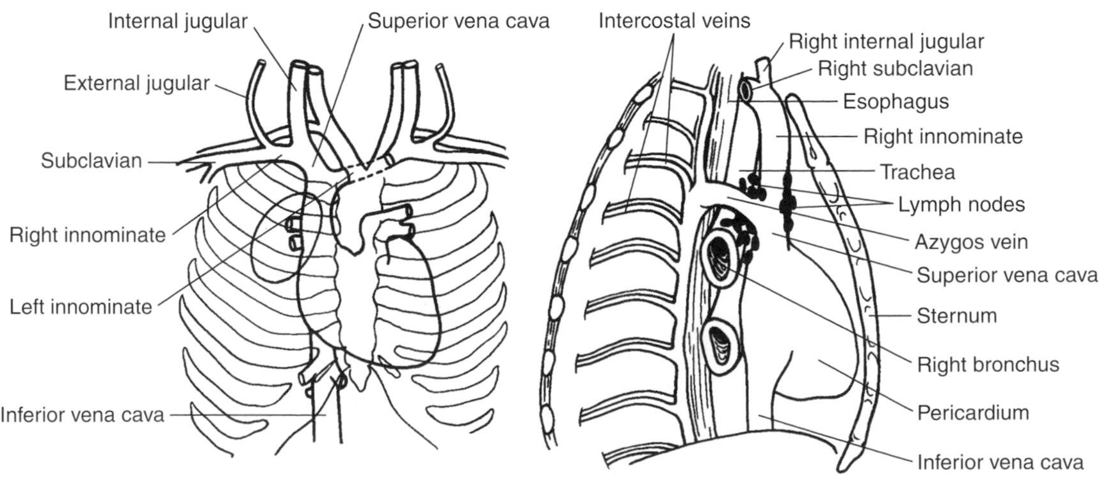

Figure 8-2 Superior Vena Cava Syndrome.
This schematic is a representation of the frontal (left) and sagittal (right) sections of the thorax.
Modified from Lokich J, Goodman R: JAMA 231:58-61, 1975.

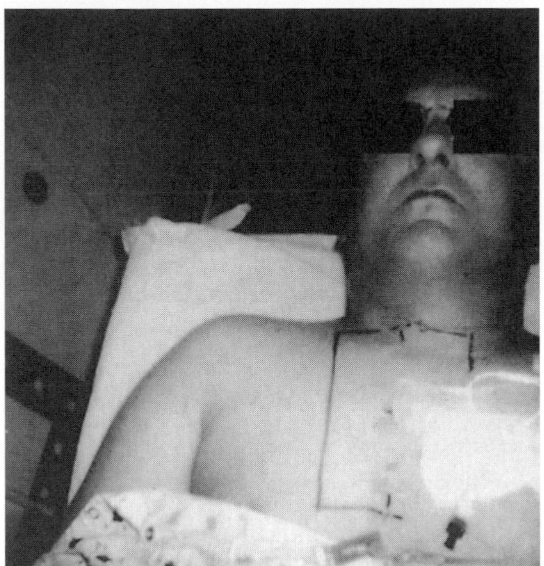

Figure 8-3 Clinical Manifestation of a Patient With SVC Syndrome.
From Dow KH, Bucholtz JD, Iwamoto R et al: Nursing Care in Radiation Oncology, ed. 2, Philadelphia, 1992, W.B. Saunders.

tests are ordered to assess the tumor and possible metastases. A chest radiograph is generally the first and probably the single most valuable tool in the diagnosis of lung cancer.[7] Except for the rare occult tumor, most lung cancers are detected by an abnormal chest x ray. Radiographs that include posteroanterior and lateral films can reveal peripheral nodules, a definitive mass, hilar and mediastinal changes suggestive of regional lymphadenopathy, and/or pleural effusions. Areas of segmental, lobar, or lung collapse suggest an endobronchial obstruction.[14]

Computed axial tomography (CAT or CT) of the thorax, which further determines the extent of the primary tumor and regional lymph node status, has become standard.[15] These chest CTs are typically used later in the radiation treatment planning phase. Addition of intravenous contrast further defines the mediastinal lymph nodes.[15] In addition, CT of the upper abdomen is valuable in the search for hepatic or adrenal metastasis. CT of the brain, to rule out brain metastasis at diagnosis, is usually performed in patients with small cell lung carcinomas (SCLC) and in patients with adenocarcinoma and large cell carcinoma. When a thorough clinical evaluation is completed, more than half of all patients with bronchogenic carcinoma are found to have distant metastasis.

Magnetic resonance imaging (MRI) is not routinely performed because of the cost, extensive time to perform the test, and the artifact that is caused by respiratory movement. However, MRIs may be ordered to evaluate the extent of tumor destruction, that is, brachial plexus, vertebral bodies, and/or spinal cord compression. In these cases, MRIs provide detailed information of the spinal cord, changes in the bone marrow, and invasion into surrounding tissues or vessels.[16] Patients presenting with non–small cell lung cancer (NSCLC), clinical stage II, the National Comprehensive Cancer Network (NCCN) currently recommends an MRI of the brain as inclusive of standard protocol.[17]

Positron emission tomography (PET) uses a radiopharmaceutical tracer called *F-2-deoxy-D-glucose (FDG)* that provides further information regarding tumor growth. Cancer cells metabolize the FDG faster than normal cells, thus allowing them to be visualized on the nuclear scan. PET scans can indicate whether lung tumors are growing or shrinking over progressive time intervals. PET scan cannot pinpoint exact locations and require anatomic correlations from the CT scans. Unfortunately, PET scans have limitations that can cause false positives, precipitated by conditions such as inflammation, rheumatoid arthritis, infections, pneumonia, abscess, histoplasmosis, aspergillosis, blastomycosis, active tuberculosis, granulomas, tumor necrosis, radiation pneumonitis, and airway inflammation.[18] False negatives also can occur, and tumors can be overlooked. Conditions that can lead to false negatives include hyperglycemia, microscopic tumor deposits, or indolent neoplasm.[15]

Bone scintigraphies, commonly referred to as *bone scans*, are not typically included in the routine work-up. These scans are ordered primarily when patients are complaining of persistent bone pain in the trunk or extremities. Because of the low sensitivity and specificity (50% and 92%, respectively), plain films are more helpful in determining abnormalities.[19]

Besides radiologic imaging, other noninvasive and invasive diagnostic tests are available to aid in staging and confirming a diagnosis. Pulmonary function tests are an example of special noninvasive procedures. These are important for assessing the patient's ability to withstand surgical resection or thoracic radiation treatments.[7] Invasive assessments includes either a needle biopsy or aspiration, bronchoscopy, and/or mediastinoscopy. Fine-needle biopsy, reporting an accuracy of 80% to 90%, helps diagnosis palpable lymph nodes, such as supraclavicular or cervical lymph nodes or peripheral lesions.[20] Needle aspirations, possibly guided by CT, are taken during various procedures and provide samples for histology or cytology diagnosis. Bronchoscopy can help visualize and obtain samples from centrally located masses.[14] Mediastinoscopy assists in staging and allowing for biopsies of the lymph nodes, when indicated.[21] Thoracoscopy and thoracentesis are reserved for patients who have pleural effusions and have the need for cytologic diagnosis to determine the extent of disease to provide optimum treatment options.[16]

Laboratory testing and molecular marker assays can be performed. Complete blood counts (CBC), platelet count, and chemistry profile including serum lactate dehydrogenase (LDH) helps to evaluate renal and liver disease. Molecular marker assays, such as *p-53* or *Ki-67* are currently under investigation to aid in diagnosing lung cancer early, to determine whether lung cancer has spread, and/or to monitor treatment response.[22]

Once the diagnostic tests are completed and tissue diagnosis is confirmed, staging is identified to guide treatment. The most widely used staging system for lung cancer is the TNM system adopted by the American Joint Committee for Cancer and the Union Internationale Contre le Cancer in 1996. In 1997, revisions were made to further separate patients with lung cancer into categories with similar survival rates and treatment options. The TNM international staging system is shown in Table 8-2. Significant changes were made in all stages. Stage I is divided into IA and IB because survival differences were shown in recent clinical trials. Stage II was similarly divided into IIA and IIB because of the same survival reasons. Stage IIIA remained the same except for tumors classified as T3, N0, M0. Survival was shown to be consistent with T2, N1, M0, therefore these two groups are classified as stage IIB. Stages IIIB and IV remain unchanged except for the T4 and M1 descriptors. Specifically, malignant pericardial effusion was added to the T4 description, the presence of satellite tumors within the lobe of the lung with the primary tumor is classified as T4, and an intrapulmonary ipsilateral distant metastasis is classified as M1.[21]

PATHOLOGY AND PATTERN OF METASTASIS

The World Health Organization (WHO) has divided lung cancer into two major classifications: non–small cell lung cancer (NSCLC) and small cell lung cancer (SCLC) (Table 8-3). The four major histologic types of bronchogenic tumors are squamous (epidermoid) carcinoma, adenocarcinoma, large cell carcinoma, and SCLC. The first three are usually classified as NSCLC. It is important to distinguish the different types, especially NSCLC from SCLC, because they have significant differences in presentation, natural history, and response to therapy. Both types of lung cancer most likely originate from a common pluripotent stem cell.[23]

Approximately 80% of patients with lung cancer will have NSCLC, and 20% will have SCLC.[1,2] Squamous cell cancers most often occur centrally near the mainstem bronchi and produce obstruction with associated pneumonitis. Because these cancers remain localized and are amenable to local resection, patients generally have longer survival rates than those with other cell types. Adenocarcinomas and large cell carcinomas are more often located peripherally to the bronchi. These tumors tend to metastasize widely and often spread to the brain, adrenals, and bone.[3]

Small cell tumors are usually located in the central regions of the lung, often at the hila, and are associated with early invasion of the surrounding structures, particularly the blood vessels. The rich supply of vessels and lymphatics in the lungs allows the disease to metastasize rapidly. Patients with SCLC usually have widespread disease at the time of diagnosis.[24] Metastases often will be found in regional lymph nodes, lung, abdominal lymph nodes, liver, adrenal gland, bone, central nervous system, and bone marrow.

TREATMENT

The appropriate treatment for bronchogenic cancer is based on consideration of several prognostic factors: histology, tumor extent, and the patient's physical condition. Surgery, radiation therapy, and chemotherapy are generally the considered treatment options, the first two of these having a long history of collaboration in the management of localized disease.

Table 8-2 AJCC Staging of Lung Cancer

PRIMARY TUMOR (T)

TX Primary tumor cannot be assessed, or tumor proven by presence of malignant cells in sputum or bronchial washings but not visualized by imaging or bronchoscopy

T0 No evidence of primary tumor

Tis Carcinoma in situ

T1 Tumor 3 cm or less in greatest dimension, surrounded by lung or visceral pleura, without bronchoscopic evidence of invasion more proximal than the lobar bronchus* (i.e., not in main bronchus)

T2 Tumor with any of the following features of size or extent:
More than 3 cm in greatest dimension
Involves main bronchus, 2 cm or more distal to the carina
Invades the visceral pleura
Associated with atelectasis or obstructive pneumonitis that extends to the hilar region but does not involve the entire lung

T3 Tumor of any size that directly invades any of the following: chest wall (including superior sulcus tumors), diaphragm, mediastinal pleura, parietal pericardium; or tumor in the main bronchus less than 2 cm distal to the carina but without involvement of the carina; or associated atelectasis of obstructive pneumonitis of the entire lung

T4 Tumor of any size that invades any of the following: mediastinum, heart, great vessels, trachea, esophagus, vertebral body, carina; separate tumor nodule(s) in the same lobe; or tumor with a malignant pleural effusion**

REGIONAL LYMPH NODES (N)

NX Regional lymph nodes cannot be assessed

N0 No regional lymph node metastasis

N1 Metastasis to ipsilateral peribronchial and/or ipsilateral hilar lymph nodes and intrapulmonary nodes involved by direct extension of the primary tumor

N2 Metastasis to ipsilateral mediastinal and/or subcarinal lymph node(s)

N3 Metastasis in contralateral mediastinal, contralateral hilar, ipsilateral or contralateral scalene, or supraclavicular lymph node(s)

DISTANT METASTASIS (M)

MX Distant metastasis cannot be assessed

M0 No distant metastasis

M1 Distant metastasis present (includes synchronous separate nodule(s) in a different lobe)

STAGE GROUPING

Stage grouping of the TNM subsets has been revised as follows:

Occult carcinoma	TX	N0	M0
Stage 0	Tis	N0	M0
Stage IA	T1	N0	M0
Stage IB	T2	N0	M0
Stage IIA	T1	N1	M0
Stage IIB	T2	N1	M0
	T3	N0	M0
Stage IIIA	T1	N2	M0
	T2	N2	M0
	T3	N1	M0
	T3	N2	M0
Stage IIIB	Any T	N3	M0
	T4	Any N	M0
Stage IV	Any T	Any N	M1

Used with the permission of the American Joint Committee on Cancer (AJCC), Chicago, Illinois. The original source for this material is the *AJCC Cancer Staging Manual, Sixth edition* (2002), published by Springer-New York, www.springeronline.com.

*The uncommon superficial tumor of any size with its invasive component limited to the bronchial wall, which may extend proximal to the main bronchus, is also classified T1.

**Most pleural effusions associated with lung cancer are due to tumor. However, there are a few patients in whom multiple cytopathologic examinations of pleural fluid are negative for tumor. In these cases, fluid is non-bloody and is not an exudate. Such patients may be further evaluated by videothoracoscopy (VATS) and direct pleural biopsies. When these elements and clinical judgment dictate that the effusion is not related to the tumor, the effusion should be excluded as a staging element and the patient should be stage T1, T2, or T3.

Table 8-3 Major Histopathologic Types of Lung Cancer

Non–small cell cancer	Small cell cancer
Squamous cell carcinoma	Pure small cell
Adenocarcinoma	Mixed small-cell carcinoma
Large-cell carcinoma	Combined small cell

Table 8-4 Acute and Late Effects of Thoracic Irradiation

Acute effects	Late effects
Cough	Lung fibrosis
Dyspnea	Pneumonitis
Pharyngitis	Esophageal problems (stenosis, ulceration, perforation and/or fistula formation)
Esophagitis	Cardiac sequelae
Radiodermatitis	Spinal cord myelopathy
Fatigue	Brachial plexopathy
Anorexia	
Radiation pneumonitis	
Lhermitte syndrome	

Most patients with lung cancer will receive radiation therapy. The overall poor prognosis in lung cancer creates difficulty in determining optimum treatment regimens and in evaluating acute and late effects of radiation (Table 8-4). Patients who are most often referred to radiation oncology departments for treatment of primary lung cancer are those with incomplete resections or whose conditions are inoperable as deemed by disease or performance status.

Large doses of radiation are required to eradicate lung cancers. Using Fletcher's technique to determine dose-response curves, it is believed that doses in the range of 80 Gy to 100 Gy are needed to sterilize 100% of bronchogenic carcinoma.[25] Most clinical trials report the use of doses ranging from 40 Gy to 65 Gy. This represents a compromise between tumor dose requirement and normal tissue tolerance.

The treatment is most commonly given using a pair of opposed anterior and posterior beams. By using CT scanning, treatment area and portal size can be established together with computerized dose planning for the tumor and spinal cord shielding. Treatment fields may need to be modified in cases where pulmonary function testing indicates severe COPD. In curative doses, the tumor dose exceeds the tolerance of the spinal cord, and part of the treatment is given with an alternate field arrangement that will spare the spinal cord. Coverage of a centrally placed tumor and mediastinum can be achieved by an arrangement of obliquely angled beams. This technique avoids the problem of under-dosing the mediastinum, which would otherwise result from employing a lead shield over the posterior beam to protect the spinal cord. A number of beam-modifying devices are often used to facilitate homogenous radiation of the tumor, such as shielding (layers of lead or metal alloys that absorb radiation to parts of the field that need not be treated), attenuators/compensators (thinner layers of lead that decrease the dose in selected parts of the field, such as the upper chest, where body thickness is least, and tissues at midplane that would otherwise receive an unintended high dose), and wedges (wedge-shaped attenuators). These planning techniques are important when the prescribed dose exceeds the tolerance of irradiated normal tissues.

The usual plan of treatment involves daily fractions in the range of 1.8 Gy to 2.0 Gy for a continuous 5- to 6-week treatment course.[7] Another regimen is the split-course higher-dose (3 Gy) fractionation, which involves 10 fractions over 2 weeks of daily therapy, then 2 plus weeks off, followed by an additional 7 or so fractions over $1^1/_2$ weeks for a total of 51 Gy.[7] This regimen allows for tumor regression during the hiatus. Smaller fields may be used after the break to decrease complications. No reported study has shown an increased survival with this approach, but several factors may necessitate its use. Extremely ill patients may find the continuous 5 to 6 weeks of conventional therapy difficult to manage. In addition, early discharge from the hospital has created tremendous transportation and home care problems that may make a split-course regimen more tolerable. Late effects of therapy are the same for both treatment approaches. Salazar and colleagues[26] report that acute reactions are minimized with the split-course technique approach. For the acutely ill individual, this plan of care may allow treatment to be completed.

Patients with locally advanced lesions have been treated with large doses on a once weekly basis. In this hypofractionated plan, patients receive 5 Gy per week for a total dose of 60 Gy in a 12-week-timeframe. The spinal cord is protected after 30 Gy. Although hypofractionation seems to promote much better acute tolerance and convenience, it can increase the potential for late complications such as pulmonary fibrosis and osteoradionecrosis of bone structures.[27] Radiobiologically, the use of larger than conventional doses is an approach to deal with hypoxic tumor cells that are less radiosensitive. In a large mass, large radiation fractions destroy more neoplastic cells, allowing better oxygenation of the tumor core and rendering it more radiosensitive for the next treatment. The treatment course of 12 weeks is long, but for the debilitated patient, being treated only once weekly is well tolerated. Late effects have been difficult to evaluate because of the generally poor prognosis of these patients.[28,29] Controversy does exist about hypofractionated therapy. However, Bradley and colleagues[7] report that in patients with inoperable tumors, 29% of those treated with conventional therapy were free of tumor at autopsy, compared with 18% of those treated once weekly. The best response (40% tumor-free) was achieved in a group receiving three large fractions of 4 Gy to 10 Gy followed by conventional daily fractions.

Multiple daily fractions delivered between a 4- to 6-hour interval have been advocated. Tumor cell kinetic studies have shown short potential doubling times in human NSCLCs. Accelerated radiation attempts to overcome this rapid cellular proliferation by shortening the overall treatment time, and thereby lessening the opportunity for tumor cell repopulation. CHART (continuous hyperfractionated accelerated radiation therapy) is being studied in numerous trials. The Radiation Therapy Oncology Group (RTOG) randomized phase 2 trial evaluated a dose range from 60 Gy to 80 Gy, with 70 Gy yielding the best 1-year survival rate of 58%.[30]

Many ongoing studies using doses greater than 60 Gy have shown that high doses can be administered safely with results and survival equivalent to trials of hyperfractionation or combined chemoradiotherapy. A review by Emami and colleagues[31] suggests that higher doses of radiation to the tumor may result in improved local control in inoperable NSCLC. These studies use new technology (CT planning using three-dimensional [3-D] displays), which allows for conforming the radiation dose more precisely to the shape of the tumor volume while minimizing the dose to critical normal tissues, such as the lungs, spinal cord, and heart.[32] The role for very high dose (greater than 60 Gy) hyperfractionation, including CHART, is currently being evaluated in ongoing studies.

NON–SMALL CELL LUNG CANCER

Surgery

Complete surgical resection offers the best chance for cure in patients with localized disease.[7,33,34] Unfortunately, only 20% to 25% of lung cancer patients qualify for curative surgery. Surgical candidates include those with localized NSCLC (stages I and II) and occasionally those with localized (stage IIIa) disease, particularly in instances of squamous cell tumors. The procedure of choice (lobectomy, pneumonectomy, segmental, or sleeve resection) is usually that which will excise all existing disease and provide maximum conservation of normal lung tissue.[34] The different surgical approaches are schematically shown in Figure 8-4. The presence of distant or extrathoracic metastasis indicates inoperability.

Preoperative CT scanning allows for the selection of appropriate surgical candidates. It is a useful way to avoid thoracotomy in selected patients who underwent this debilitating procedure in the past and were later found at surgery to be unresectable. When initial staging evaluation, including CT assessment, determines that the lesion is resectable, the patient also must be assessed for "operability." A high percentage of patients with lung cancer generally are chronic smokers and have significant cardiopulmonary compromise unrelated to the cancer.[35] There has been an increasing interest in limited surgical procedures such as segmented or wedge resection for patients with marginal pulmonary function. Small cell lung cancer is not considered a surgically treatable disease because of the high incidence of distant metastases.

The response and survival of surgically treated patients depend on their preoperative performance status and extent of disease. According to Mountain and colleagues,[36] if patients are clinically staged, surgery will control about 45% of patients with stage I, 25% of patients with stage II, and perhaps 10% of patients with stage IIIa disease. Patients having a complete resection (surgically complete responders) and who have squamous histology respond more favorably to treatment than those with nonsquamous histology. However, in many cases, surgical resection is limited because the primary tumor

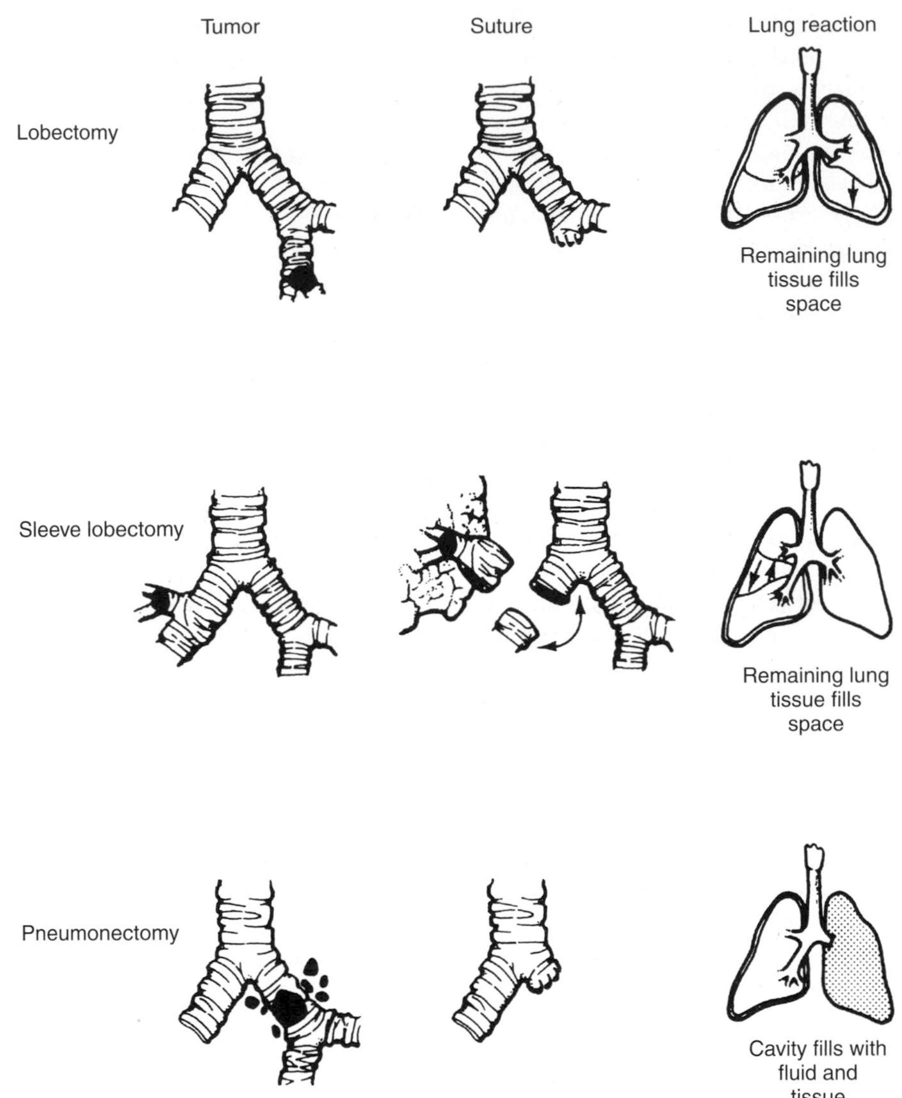

Figure 8-4 Different Approaches to Lung Resection.
From Elpern EH: Lung Cancer. In SL Gruenwald, MH Frogge, M Goodman et al, editors, Cancer Nursing, Principles and Practice, ed. 3, Boston, 1993, Jones and Bartlett.

invaded adjacent structures or organs or spread to mediastinal/supraclavicular lymph nodes.

Preoperative Radiation Therapy

As discussed, results for well-selected patients with early-stage disease who undergo surgery are good.[7] Patterns of treatment failure suggest good local control, which negates the benefit of additional therapy. Most studies failed to demonstrate that preoperative radiation therapy is beneficial on either operability or survival.[37,38] On the contrary, the number of postoperative complications and their severity generally increase. Similarly, a review of trials by Payne[39] found that postoperative radiation of early-stage disease showed no benefit.

Preoperative radiation may be used before complete surgical resection, particularly when tumors are located near a vital organ.[39] Likewise, preoperative radiation may be used for the treatment of surgically operable Pancoast tumors. Pancoast described the association of apical NSCLCs with the constellation of arm or shoulder pain, Horner syndrome, and rib erosion.[40] These tumors can involve not only the ribs but also the chest wall, brachplexus, vertebral bodies, and subclavian vessels. Radiation is given to the tumor and regional lymph nodes, either alone or in com-bination with chemotherapy. After a time inter-val, restaging is done and surgical treatment is undertaken if systemic metastatic involvement is not evident. Postoperative radiation also may be administered, because these tumors are often marginally resected.[41]

Lung cancer patients with limited pulmonary function or otherwise nonoperable early-stage disease may be candidates for curative treatment with radiation therapy. Because radiation toxicity may lead to serious compromise in pulmonary reserve, alternative beam arrangements may be used to spare the uninvolved lung parenchyma. When this is not possible, low-dose radiation may be used, but is unlikely to be curative. It is difficult to compare the results of patients treated with radiation versus surgery for early-stage lung cancer because of the different staging methods. One method is a clinical-radiologic schema usually without mediastinoscopy whereas the other is a surgical-pathologic one with accurate assessment of nodal involvement. It is known that tumors smaller than 4 cm to 6 cm are easier to eradicate than larger ones. Newer technical advances, such as portal imaging, 3-D treatment planning, and intensity-modulated radiation therapy (IMRT), may allow for reduction in normal tissue treated, thus allowing larger curative doses.[42,43]

Postoperative Radiation Therapy

In cases of complete resection of NSCLC with positive hilar and/or mediastinal nodes, postoperative radiation is known to decrease local recurrences. Daily dosing of 2 Gy at tumor doses of 60 Gy to 70 Gy is recommended.[7] An improvement in survival, however, has not been well established, although some retrospective studies have shown a survival benefit.[20] The Lung Cancer Study Group, in a 1986 prospective trial,[44] showed that although postoperative radiation decreased local relapses, no significant increase in overall survival was shown. A controversial report was later published by the PORT Meta-analysis Trialists Group,[45] which showed postoperative radiation therapy is detrimental to patients with early-stage, completely resected NSCLC, and therefore should not be recommended for this group. More prospective, case-controlled studies are needed to evaluate improvement in survival.

In cases of incomplete resection or regional lymph node metastasis, postoperative radiation is almost always recommended. It is usually given immediately after surgery rather than awaiting recurrence of disease.

Definitive Radiation Therapy

A significant number of lung cancers will be assessed as inoperable at presentation. Bradley and colleagues[7] reported that only 20% of new lung cancer cases are surgically curable. If disease is limited to the chest, radiation therapy is indicated. High doses (60 Gy to 70 Gy) are necessary for a reasonable probability of eradicating the primary tumor.[7] High-dose thoracic radiation is a prolonged treatment course with significant acute, subacute, and late side effects, a 30% risk of local relapse, and only 5% to 10% long-term survival rate.[42] Thus selection of therapy is often based on known prognostic factors such as good performance status and no evidence of weight loss. As in other areas of oncology, a clear and realistic goal of treatment, cure, or palliation, must be established at the outset.

When control is the goal of treatment, smaller radiation doses are used to lessen the treatment side effects. There is justification for treatment even without significant improvement in survival because the minimal morbidity associated with therapy may preclude or delay the development of the more debilitating sequelae of locally recurrent disease.[46] Airway obstruction, pneumonia, bleeding, fistula formation, and vocal cord paralysis may accompany recurrence. The improved quality of life achieved by preventing or delaying local recurrence justifies the treatment regimen. However, there is no clear benefit to altered fractionation.[7]

With the introduction of IMRT and dose escalation, the need to direct beams and assure accuracy becomes an issue. Some clinical studies are evaluating the respiratory gating system (RGS) to better improve patient positioning and organ movement during treatments, thus providing more accuracy.[47-49] The RGS uses an infrared camera to track a blocker that lays on the patient's chest or abdomen, which records the patient's normal breathing pattern (Figures 8-5, *A* and 8-5, *B*). The data is incorporated into the treatment plan, and the RGS can deliver radiation doses at the desired point in the respiratory cycle.

Pleural mesothelioma, a rarely curable neoplastic disease often caused by asbestos exposure, typically

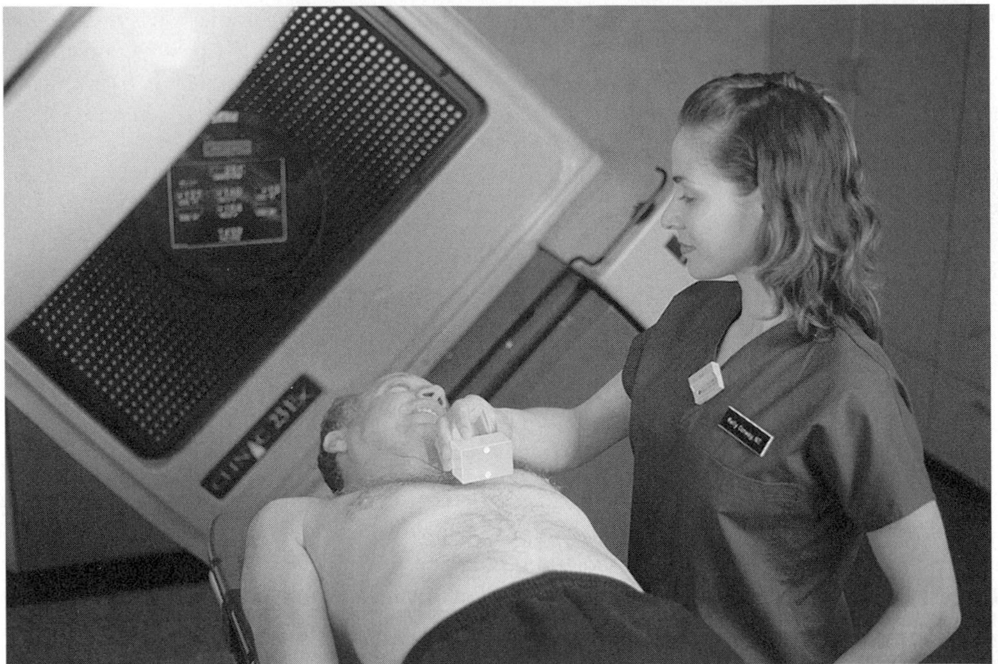

A

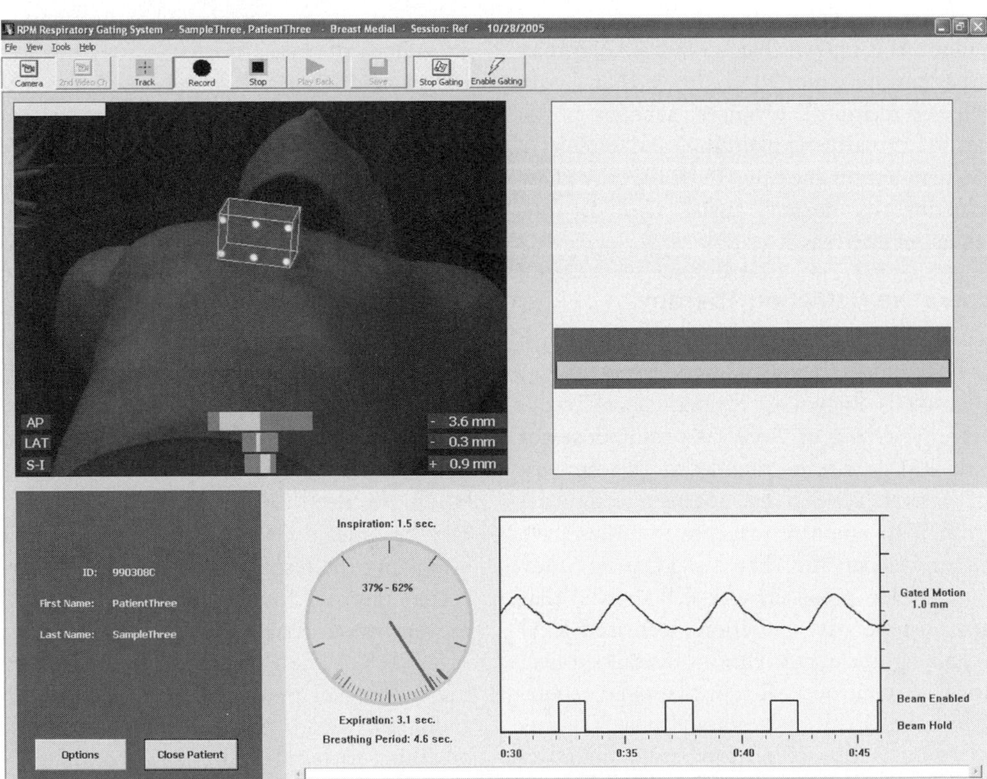

B

Figure 8-5 Respiratory Gating System.
A, Passive infrared-reflective marker block used to track chest wall motion. **B,** Resulting waveform.
Courtesy of Varian Medical Systems, Palo Alto, Calif.

causes dyspnea and nonpleuritic chest wall pain. The efficacy of radiation, like that of other treatments, is not clear in the definitive treatment of patients with pleural mesothelioma. The use of radioactive colloids such as phosphorus-32 in chromic phosphate instilled into the pleural space has been studied.[50] The exact response rate is unknown, but in one series, all six patients were alive at 12 months or longer after instillation of isotopes.

Palliative Radiation Therapy

Radiation therapy plays a larger role in treatment of problems caused by lung cancer, either by the tumor itself or its metastases, thus palliative treatments may become the goal of therapy. Common symptoms of the primary tumor are hemoptysis, cough; dyspnea, obstruction of major airways, chest pain, hoarseness caused by vocal cord palsy, and sometimes obstruction of the SVC or other major vessels. Localized metastases may produce bone pain. Mediastinal tumors may cause venous obstruction or esophageal compression. Brain involvement may produce neurologic deficits, and spinal cord compression may lead to paralysis. Radiation therapy often benefits patients with these grave symptomatic metastases, because it often can be delivered to the problem site without causing other untoward side effects. Palliative treatment is prescribed and generally given in a shorter time course.

Local progression of disease such as tumors involving the carina and/or trachea can affect the airways, causing a major problem. Patients generally receive maximal external beam radiation and are candidates for laser resection followed by endobronchial brachytherapy with the use of iridium-192. Although standard clinical indications and dosage schedules have not been established, endobronchial brachytherapy has been widely shown to effectively reduce symptoms of hemoptysis, dyspnea, and cough.[51]

Endobronchial brachytherapy can be delivered either by implanting or inserting a radioactive source into the patient's airway. Patient selection is described in Table 8-5. This criteria may vary from institution to institution. Generally speaking, high dose rate (HDR) brachytherapy has replaced low dose rate (LDR) brachytherapy primarily because HDR is delivered in a shorter timeframe, thereby reducing the overall source dwell time, thus decreasing the likelihood of catheter/radiation sources dislodgement, allowing for improved patient convenience (outpatient instead of inpatient procedure), and reduction of treatment cost.[52] During the HDR procedure, the pulmonologist assists the radiation oncologist by placing a flexible fiberoptic bronchoscope into the airway adjacent to the tumor/lesion. A polyethylene catheter is secured and its position verified, typically via fluoroscopy and with a chest x ray. Once confirmation is determined, the catheter is loaded with the radioactive source. The actual treatment time can range between 5 and 10 minutes depending on source strength and treatment prescription. Upon completion of the treatment, the catheter is removed. The patient is usually in the radiation department for

Table 8-5 Patient Selection for Endobronchial Tumors

Indications	Contraindications
• Biopsy-proven NSCLC or an extrathoracic malignancy metastatic to the lung • Inability to tolerate or failure to respond to potentially curative therapies or debulking of the tumor with laser or cryotherapy • Inability to tolerate external beam radiation because of poor pulmonary function • Symptoms due to malignant endobronchial lesions, e.g., dyspnea, postobstructive pneumonitis, hemoptysis, or intractable cough • Lesions that are accessible to placement of a brachytherapy catheter • Sufficient life expectancy (usually >3 months) to derive palliative benefit	• Presence of fistulas between bronchi and other structures • Endotracheal lesions already causing high-grade obstruction causing concern for postradiation tissue edema and complete airway obstruction • Bronchoscopy cannot be tolerated

Modified from Mathur P, Colt H: *Endobronchial brachytherapy,* 2005, UpToDate (website): www.utdol.com/application/topicTest.asp?file=lung_ca. Accessed August 12, 2005.
NSCLC, Non–small cell lung carcinoma.

Table 8-6 Nursing Assessments for Patients Receiving HDR Brachytherapy

Procedure timeline	Assessments
Preprocedure	• *Premedications:* Observe for possible hypotension, tachycardia, and arrhythmias, respiratory depression, agitation, allergic reaction, leading to anaphylactic reactions, nausea, and vomiting • *Topical anesthesia:* Observe for possible laryngospasms, bronchospasms, seizures, arrhythmias, cardiac arrest, nausea, and vomiting, both before and during procedure
During procedure	• Assess patient's vital signs and level of sedation. • Monitor pulse oximetry with supplemental oxygen available and electrocardiogram
Postprocedure	• Monitor patient for epistaxis (if nasal approach); laryngeal spasm, edema, or injury; hypoxemia; arrhythmias; fever, bacteremia, or infections • Assess vital signs until stable and patient regains consciousness and has a gag reflex

several hours preprocedure and postprocedure. HDR brachytherapy is generally administered in 1 to 4 fractions that are given 1 week apart.

The radiation oncology nurse plays a significant role in pre-procedure and post-procedure HDR brachytherapy. Specific nursing assessments are outlined in Table 8-6. The patient is not to eat or drink for 8 to 12 hours before the procedure. Vital signs are monitored and an intravenous (IV) line is started. The radiation oncology nurse prepares the patient for the insertion of a bronchoscope, which will be used to guide the catheter to the tumor area. Local anesthetic is used to numb the area, and the patient is lightly sedated. Nurses should follow the institution's conscious sedation policies. During the procedure additional medications may be given through the IV to help the patient relax or to decrease the gag reflex. Once the procedure is completed, the patient is monitored for several hours afterwards.

Managing Complications Related to Lung Cancer

Bone metastases from lung cancer are common and multiple. The main goals of irradiating bones are to relieve pain, prevent impending pathologic fractures, assist with orthopedic fixation in cases of impending or completed pathologic fractures, maintain activity and function, and prevent or alleviate compression syndromes, especially of the spinal cord. Further discussion can be found in Chapter 14.

Radiation remains the major treatment modality for most patients with SVC. Portals are designed after consideration of both the pathologic diagnosis and extent of disease. Mediastinal, hilar, and adjacent pulmonary parenchymal lesions are included in the treatment field. For solid tumors with an upper lobe lung lesion and mediastinal adenopathy, supraclavicular lymph nodes are usually treated. In patients with SVC, those with SCLC have a more rapid, complete response than patients with NSCLC, when treated with radiation therapy.[53] Patients with SCLC are usually treated with systemic chemotherapy and concomitant thoracic radiation if the disease is limited to the chest.[54] Current recommendations are that the radiation schedule include higher daily fractions of 3 Gy to 4 Gy for 2 to 4 days, followed by conventional daily dose fractions of 1.8 Gy to 2.0 Gy. Total dose is determined by the histologic features and the extent of disease. Patients with SCLC, which is a more radiosensitive cancer, generally receive a total dose of 20 Gy to 40 Gy. Less sensitive tumors such as squamous cell lung carcinoma or adenocarcinomas require a total dose of 50 Gy to 60 Gy.[55,56] Generally, corticosteroids have not been shown to contribute to an increase in a rapid relief of symptoms. With the addition of radiation therapy, 85% to 90% of patients have symptom relief within 3 weeks.

Chemotherapy Combined with Radiation

Persistent or recurrent intrathoracic disease and distant metastases are significant problems in locally advanced NSCLC treated with radiation. Over the years, various drugs, either as single agents or in combination, have been investigated. Response rates exceeding 50% are now commonly reported in selected studies of induction chemotherapy using cisplatin-based combinations in stages IIIa and IIIb disease. As a result, interest in evaluating multimodality programs in stage III NSCLC has increased. The use of neoadjuvant chemotherapy, in which two or three cycles of chemotherapy are given before radiation, is also being evaluated.[20] Advantages include enhancing reoxygenation of hypoxic cells, which in turn increases radiosensitivity. Drug complications, however, may interrupt the radiation therapy course.

It is clear that as the intensity of the concurrent chemotherapy/radiation regimens increase, treatment-related toxicity will be a major factor. Byhardt[57] suggests that decisions need to be made in regard to "acceptable" levels of acute and late toxicities. A recent phase I trial in regionally advanced, unresectable NSCLC patients compared (1) standard radiation therapy, (2) induction chemotherapy followed by standard radiation therapy, and (3) twice-daily radiation therapy.[58] One-year survival (percent) and median survival (months) were as follows: (1) standard radiation therapy—46%, 11.4 months; (2) chemotherapy plus radiation therapy—60%, 13.8 months; and (3) hyperfractionated radiation therapy—51%, 12.3 months. Tannock[59] suggests that even if small gains in survival are achieved, it is not certain whether they are of sufficient magnitude to recommend induction chemotherapy as routine clinical practice. He suggests the need for further research analyzing both the effects on quality of life of combined versus single modality treatment and the economic implications (expressed in cost per quality-adjusted life-year gained) for combined modality treatment. Newer cytotoxic agents such as docetaxel, paclitaxel, gemcitabine hydrochloride, vinorelbine tartrate, irinotecan hydrochloride, and topotecan hydrochloride, are being studied to improve local control and decrease distant metastasis.[60,61] More discussion on chemoradiotherapy can be found in Chapter 19.

Because of poor local control rates and the high rate of metastasis, recent trials have used radiosensitizers and the combination of radiation with chemotherapy. A review of study results done by Shaw and colleagues[41] failed to show that two radiosensitizers, misonidazole and levamisole, improved local control and survival in comparison to standard radiation therapy only. In addition, intraoperative radiation therapy failed to show benefit in local control or survival with either incompletely resected or unresectable NSCLC.

SMALL-CELL LUNG CANCER

The disseminated nature and chemoresponsiveness of SCLC makes the use of systemic chemotherapy a primary treatment for this type of lung cancer. However, local failure commonly occurs with chemotherapy alone. The role of thoracic radiation therapy in small cell carcinoma is predominantly that of consolidation. A review by Arriagada and colleagues[62] showed that chest radiation decreased the risk of thoracic recurrences and promised a gain in long-term survival of approximately 5% to 10% in patients with limited disease. In cases in which response has been limited or partial, radiation therapy often may convert this into a complete response.

Thoracic radiation is now standard treatment in limited SCLC and may benefit some patients with disseminated disease. However, the total radiation dose, volume fractionation, and method of integration with chemotherapy are all controversial and the subject of many studies. These treatment factors can clearly influence hematologic, pulmonary, and esophageal toxicities compared with the use of chemotherapy alone. The optimal radiation dose level, although not yet established, is thought to be at least 45 Gy to 50 Gy.[63] It is not clear, however, that a larger dose, by itself, will result in better survival or local control, particularly if the larger total dose is achieved at the price of interruption in treatment.

Prophylactic cranial radiation has been widely advocated in SCLC treatment because of the high incidence of central nervous system metastases (more than 50%). This concept is also being applied to both adenocarcinoma and large-cell anaplastic carcinomas. However, several studies have shown a reduction in brain metastasis but no effect on survival.[7,32] Neurotoxicities commonly associated with whole-brain radiation include impaired mentation, ataxic gait, and urinary incontinence. They typically occur 6 to 18 months after completing therapy.[64]

NURSING INTERVENTIONS AND EDUCATION

Pretreatment Teaching

Receiving radiation treatment may be a difficult experience for patients with lung cancer. Peck and Boland[65] reported that 4% of patients were concerned about being alone in the room. Even a large treatment room may seem claustrophobic to the individual who is short of breath. It is important to educate patients regarding the necessary amount of time they will be in the room for treatment and that they can be seen and heard during treatment. Reassuring patients about the length of remaining treatment time may be helpful. Extremely anxious individuals may benefit from bringing a tape recorder to the treatment room with them. Listening to recordings of their favorite music or relaxation tapes during treatment provides a time sense and endpoint for daily treatment.

Pretreatment Interventions

The necessity of lying flat for treatment also may be distressing for patients with dyspnea. Interruption of therapy may be necessary because some patients may have difficulty breathing in a fixed lying position, which is required for treatment. Allowing the patient to sit up at intervals during treatment might be required, especially in the initial phase of radiation treatment. Patients may actually need to start treatment in a sitting position if orthopnea is severe. Frequent reassurance may be required for the anxious, dyspneic individual. Although the role of oxygen in patients with COPD, lung cancer, and related dyspnea is not clear, Schwartzstein and colleagues[66] report that blowing oxygen on the face may have some effect in alleviating dyspnea. Humidified room air or a fan may be helpful in lessening air hunger as well.

Interventions During Radiation Therapy

The radiation oncology nurse plays a significant role in symptom management once the patient begins treatments. Specific nursing interventions for patients receiving thoracic irradiation are reviewed here and can be found in Table 8-7.

Table 8-7 Specific Nursing Interventions for Acute Side Effects of Thoracic Irradiation

Side effects	Interventions
Cough, shortness of breath, dyspnea	• Instruct patient to drink 2 to 3 liters per day unless contradicted • Instruct patient and family to keep the environment ventilated, free of smoke odors • Urge the patient to stay calm and to avoid crowds and people with infections • Teach use of oxygen at home, importance of humidification, amount, and safety techniques • Instruct in use of mediations as prescribed, including bronchodilators, expectorants, and steroids
Pharyngitis, esophagitis, anorexia	• Assess patient's nutritional status by frequent weighing and keeping dietary intake records • Instruct patient about protein-calorie packing of food and small frequent feedings of soft, nonirritating food • Advise patient to avoid tobacco, alcohol, and other irritants • Refer to dietitian as indicated • Provide analgesic and antacids as needed • Assess for symptoms of herpetic or fungal infections
Radiodermatitis	• Teach patient skin care guidelines including avoiding trauma to skin, avoiding sun exposure, and using skin care products as prescribed • Assess for dry/moist desquamation, topical fungal infections, and pruritic rashes; providing care as needed with use of topical agents and dressings to alleviate discomfort, manage drainage, and promote healing • Assess for use of chemotherapeutic agents or other drugs that may increase skin sensitivity
Fatigue	• Teach patient to alter daily schedule to allow for rest periods • Carefully monitor blood counts; when indicated give transfusions or growth factors

Data from Bradley J, Govindan R, Kimaki R: Lung. In Perez CA, Brady LW, Halperin EC, et al, editors: *Principles and practice of radiation oncology,* Philadelphia, 2003, Lippincott Williams & Wilkins and Watkins and Bruner D, Haas M, Gosselin-Acomb T: *Manual for radiation oncology nursing practice and education,* ed 3, Pittsburgh, 2005, Oncology Nursing Society (website): www.uptodate.com. Accessed February 9, 2006.

Cough and Dyspnea

Cough can be an extremely debilitating symptom that can lead to loss of appetite, sleep, and strength. As the cilia of the columnar epithelium and the mucus-secreting glands cease to function, the bronchial mucosa becomes edematous, hypervascular, dry, and irritated. Secretions turn thick and sticky and tend to accumulate distally because of narrowing of the edematous bronchi. A nonproductive cough can persist for many months after chest radiation. Increased hydration, humidification, and cough suppressants are all measures that may be helpful.[67] Observation of signs of respiratory infection or tumor lysis are an important part of the daily assessment of the patient.

Dyspnea, an unpleasant feeling of breathlessness, can be frightening and increase the person's fatigue. It can be caused by the tumor itself or aggravated by the treatments. Simple breathing exercises and positioning techniques may help focus the person and relieve dyspnea. Administration of oxygen can be ordered if saturation levels fall below 88% to 90%. Relaxation and coping strategies may be taught to alleviate anxiety. These measures may include meditation, music therapy or guided imagery. Pharmaceutical steroids or opioids given by nebulizers may allow the patient to breath easier, thereby allowing the patient to feel more relaxed and less anxious so they can complete the necessary treatment.[67] Teaching the patient to conserve energy may decrease the workload of the cardiopulmonary system.

Cough and dyspnea also can be aggravated by smoking. The issue of smoking in the individual with lung cancer is often a difficult topic to address. The patient may believe that because a cancer has developed, there is no reason to stop smoking. However, even patients with advanced disease may benefit from smoking cessation. Improved ventilation, appetite, and taste can enhance quality of life in advanced disease. Smoking during treatment will increase mucosal irritation. Respiratory compromise related to disease and treatment (acute and long-term effects) are exacerbated by the effects of tobacco. The focus of health care professionals should be on both prevention and reduction of smoking. Smoking cessation can be supported through the use of nicotine replacement, self-help "quit kits," and counseling. Educational tools are numerous and can be obtained through the American Lung Association, American Cancer Society (ACS), and the National Cancer Institute (NCI). The Great American Smoke-out, a well-known ACS event, encourages smokers to quit for 24 hours in hopes this will provoke continued smoking cessation. The increase in "no smoking" areas in public areas also discourages smoking and reduces exposure and risk of passive smoke.

Pharyngitis

The epithelial cells of the pharynx are highly radiosensitive and are frequently within the treatment area for lung cancer. Pharyngitis can occur approximately 2 to 3 weeks from the start of treatment or after 20 Gy to 30 Gy. For some patients, the pharyngitis spontaneously resolves after a few weeks, but for others it persists until the end of treatment. Patients may report a "lump" or "fullness" in their throats and have difficulty swallowing foods. It is common to hear patients say that although their throat is not painful, the food "just doesn't go down." Other patients may complain of a mild to severe sore throat.

Nursing interventions may include teaching the patient to gargle with warm saline before and after meals. Liquid narcotic-based analgesics are sometimes needed to control pain and should be taken 30 to 60 minutes before meals. Many patients may benefit from a local anesthetic antacid/antihistamine mixture. Dietary interventions include a soft, bland diet with the addition of commercially available high-caloric supplements. In general, patients find that thicker, soft foods and fluids are easier to swallow than clear fluids such as water or juice. Small frequent meals and snacks are advantageous, as is avoidance of irritants such as tobacco and alcohol.[67]

Esophagitis

Mediastinal radiation may lead to the inflammation and denudation of the surface epithelium of the esophagus. Dysphagia resulting from acute desquamation of the esophageal mucosa may develop as treatment progresses. Edema of the tissues can induce a stenosis observed several months after the treatment or a necrosis leading to fistula formation. The latter is a very rare complication in the absence of tumor progression, or prior surgery involving the esophagus.[68] Coarse foods and extremely hot or cold foods and/or liquids can further traumatize the mucosa. Patients may report epigastric pain or discomfort, esophageal reflux, and pain with swallowing certain foods. Esophagitis usually occurs approximately 2 to 3 weeks after the start of radiation therapy and may occur sooner if concurrent chemotherapy is administered. This symptom may last through the entire course of treatment and up to several weeks after completion of therapy.[67] Chronic esophagitis may indicate a herpetic or fungal infection, therefore should be investigated anytime during therapy.

Measures to relieve esophagitis include antacids before meals and as needed. Various recipes of *miracle mouthwash* can be a beneficial analgesic for patients as well and may reduce the incidence of candidiasis. Pain medications, immediate or long-term release, may be ordered to control the discomfort, allowing patients to eat and drink more easily. Dietary measures such as those discussed for pharyngitis will be helpful and should be included in patient teaching.[67] Cytoprotection agents, such as amifostine, has reduced the incidence of chemoradiation-induced esophagitis.[69-71] Several clinical trials have provided evidence that pretreatment with amifostine reduces the incidence of esophagitis without affecting antitumor efficacy of radiation treatment in lung cancer.[72]

Fatigue

For patients with lung cancer, fatigue is often associated with dyspnea and is known to be a common side effect during thoracic radiation. The actual mechanism has not been clearly defined, but appears to be related to the presence of excess toxic metabolites and waste products of cell destruction. Studies clearly show that increased levels of fatigue occur as radiation therapy progresses as the cumulative doses are increased.[73-75] Compounding factors may include anemia, pain, malnourishment, medications, chemotherapy, frequency of treatment visits, and depression.[76]

Fatigue that is directly related to radiation itself is usually self-limited. As noted by one study, however, it may take several months to completely recover. King and colleagues[75] found that during the first week of treatment, fatigue was experienced by 60% of patients. By the third week of therapy, 93% of patients reported fatigue, which persisted in 46% of patients 3 months after completion of treatment.

Anorexia

All of the above symptoms, cough, dyspnea, pharyngitis, esophagitis, and fatigue, as well as pain, contribute to anorexia. More than 50% of patients with lung cancer have been reported as experiencing some weight loss during the 6 months before diagnosis.[77] Anorexia has been reported in 60% of patients by the fourth week of treatment.[75] Brown[78] found that male gender, increased age, and current smoking status were positively associated with cancer-related weight loss 4 to 6 weeks post-radiation therapy. Interestingly, Larson and colleagues[79] found that patients over the age of 65 did not show any significant difference in caloric intake or in meeting their energy requirements. A review by Sarna and colleagues[80] found that, historically, variables predictive of treatment response and survival in adults with lung cancer are patients with high performance status, minimal symptom distress, and minimal weight loss. Patients need to be aware that preventing weight loss is important to maximize the benefit of lung cancer treatment.

Nursing management of anorexia includes helping the patient control other contributing factors such as fatigue, pain, and pharyngitis to minimize the detrimental effects on appetite.[81] Frequent, small meals rather than three large meals per day can be less overwhelming for the patient to consume. Nutrient-dense meals should be provided so that the patient will be able to obtain the necessary calories and proteins in a small volume of food. Commercial nutritional supplements can be used in the daily dietary plan to boost protein and calorie intake. The use of megestrol acetate has been shown to improve appetite and adequacy of food intake, which positively affected weight gain.[82] A dose of 800 mg in a single daily dose as an appetite stimulant is beneficial to many patients. If the patient has lost more than 5% to 10% of usual body weight and continues to experience nutritional problems, a dietitian should be consulted for expert advice and planning to meet the patient's individual nutritional needs.[61]

Radiodermatitis

Radiation may induce an acute skin reaction (erythema, dry or moist desquamation) or late damage (fibrosis, telangiectasia); however, these reactions are rarely observed for lung cancers treated with megavoltage equipment.[68] Chapter 30 describes measures for skin care.

Post-treatment/Follow-up

Given the low relative survival rates for lung cancer patients, follow-up visits are individualized and managed based on their symptomatology. However, evaluations should be performed every 3 months for the first 3 years, then every 6 to 12 months for the next 2 years, then annually.[11] Patient teaching and interventions are just as important in these follow-up visits.

Radiation Pneumonitis

The incidence and severity of radiation pneumonitis is directly related to the dose, fractionation, volume of lung irradiated, and whether the patient received concomitant chemotherapy. Symptoms can vary from dry cough to dyspnea and low-grade fevers. This can occur in 20% of patients and usually develops between 8 and 12 weeks after completing therapy.[83]

Symptoms are usually transient and do not require treatment. Reassurance is necessary for the patient to understand that the symptoms should resolve without undue intervention or treatment. Supportive care can include bed rest and nonsteroidals. Antibiotics are usually not recommended, unless evidence of infection is present.

Lung Fibrosis

Lung fibrosis develops during the regenerative phase and is generally considered to be a late effect. McDonald and colleagues[84] describe the progression to fibrosis, which typically takes 6 to 24 months to evolve, even though histologic and biochemical changes are evident sooner.[84,85] The slowly progressive arteriolar fibrosis and interstitial fibrosis contribute to a delayed parenchymal destruction, via both direct cellular effects and the effect of decreased circulation. Fibrosis can occur without previous pneumonitis, but once pneumonitis occurs, fibrosis is almost certain to follow next. The degree of blood flow impairment, preexisting vascular compromise, demand for collateral circulation, and capacity for vascular regeneration will determine the extent of fibrosis. In combined modality treatment, the late effects of thoracic radiation are exacerbated by the additional effects of chemotherapy. These late effects begin with swelling of small vessel endothelial cells leading to partial obstruction and decreased blood flow.

Radiation produces blistering of the capillary endothelial cells resulting in a generalized inflammatory response. With extensive lung damage, symptoms may develop from the resultant fibrosis. Abscess formation, infection, fever, chills, dyspnea, orthopnea, and clubbing may result. In an extreme case, progressive pulmonary capillary disease can lead to right-sided heart failure. Such severe cases are usually the result of large-field radiation.[84,85] Arteriovenous shunting may be a major cause of dyspnea and cyanosis. Treatment planning that avoids treating large volumes of normal lung tissue to a high dose obviates many of these severe sequelae.

Areas of fibrosis seen within the treated volume are generally asymptomatic.[86-89] The symptoms related to pulmonary fibrosis are proportional to the lung parenchyma involved and the patient's preexisting pulmonary reserves. A few patients will develop a picture of chronic debilitation caused by respiratory compromise. Clinical assessment should include evaluating for dyspnea, rales, cough, and decreased exercise tolerance. Regular chest films and pulmonary function tests can monitor for pulmonary insufficiency. Chest x rays may show linear streaking radiating from the area of previous pneumonitis, and that may extend outside the irradiated area, with concomitant regional contraction, pleural thickening, and tenting of the diaphragm.[85] Supportive care, such as with bronchodilators and oxygen, is warranted. Unless the symptoms are severe, it is preferable to avoid long-term use of corticosteroids with their potentially adverse effects.

Amifostine, a radioprotective agent, was found to protect against late effects in murine studies. Protection against radiation damage was greater for fibrosis than for pneumonitis but occurred for both late effects.[90,91] Komaki and colleagues[88] found amifostine reduced the severity and incidence of acute pulmonary toxicities, as well as esophageal and hematologic toxicities resulting from concurrent cisplatin-based chemotherapy and radiation therapy. Amifostine had no apparent effect on survival in these patients with unresectable non–small cell lung cancer, suggesting that it does not have a tumor-protective effect. Ongoing clinical trials are continuing to evaluate effects of patients receiving radiation alone or in combined therapies. For further details, refer to Chapter 22 for additional information on radioprotection.

SUMMARY

In the radiation oncology setting, the ultimate goal is to maximize the quality of life for persons with lung cancer using innovative treatment strategies and comfort measures. A major role of nursing is to help patients predict the sequelae of therapy and to manage the consequences of disease and treatment. Respiratory symptoms such as cough and dyspnea related to malignant disease and its treatment have the potential to disrupt the individual's life in a significant way. Nursing interventions that help the patient conserve energy and alleviate symptoms can assist the patient in maintaining quality of life. Clinicians caring for such patients must understand the etiology of these problems to make them comprehensible to the patient. As patient survival increases, the issues related to late effects will assume more importance. Education and support of patients and their families will provide them the knowledge and skills necessary to cope with treatment and its effects.

The need for more effective strategies for the prevention and early detection of lung cancer remains abundantly clear. The recent decrease in incidence of lung cancer in men is a positive trend, possibly indicating that programs to encourage smoking cessation are becoming effective, but more attention needs to be given to women. Nurses must

Table 8-8 Resources for the Lung Cancer Patient and Family

Organizations	Websites	Services
Alliance for Lung Cancer Advocacy (ALCASE)	www.alcase.org	Offers educational materials, telephone support, newsletter, and searches related to lung cancer
Lung Cancer Caring Ambassador Program (CAP)	http://lungcancercap.org	Offers patient advocacy by providing information and encouragement to people living with lung cancer and their loved ones.
With Every Breath: A Lung Cancer Guidebook	www.lungcancerguidebook.org	Written reference for health professionals and patients
American Lung Association (ALA)	www.cancer.org	Focuses on preventing lung cancer, sharing information on smoking cessation, environmental health issues effecting lung cancer
Lung Cancer On-Line	www.lungcanceronline.org	Provides comprehensive directory for patients and families
National Comprehensive Cancer Network (NCCN)	www.nccn.org	Provides evidenced-based clinical guidelines
SUPPORT GROUPS		
ALCASE		Toll-free buddy telephone system
American Cancer Society		National and local groups, cancer survivors network
Association of Cancer Online Resources		Online support groups
R.A. Bloch National Cancer Foundation		Patient-to-patient phone support
WRITTEN RESOURCES		
Lung Cancer		National Comprehensive Cancer Network/American Cancer Society
MEDICAL SEARCH RESOURCES		
PubMed	www.ncbi.nlm.nih.gov/PubMed	
Cochrane Collaboration	www.cochrane.org/index0.htm	
National Center For Biotechnology Information	www.ncbi.nlm.nih.gov/	
National Institute of Health Data Center	www.srv.net/~msdata/US_med-search.html#s10	
American Society for Therapeutic Radiology and Oncology	www.astro.org	

continue to play a leading role in the prevention and early detection of lung cancer by development of and involvement in smoking cessation programs and the education of the public in general.

RESOURCES

Making informed decisions is very important for patients and their families. Numerous materials are available to assist in making these critical decisions (Table 8-8). Guidelines are written for healthcare professionals and for the lay person.[17] Most of these can be located on the Internet for quick access. Also, both national and local support groups can help lung cancer patients.

REFERENCES

1. Jemal A, Siegel R, Ward E et al: Cancer statistics, 2006, *CA Cancer J Clin* 56:106-130, 2006.
2. *Cancer facts and figures,* Atlanta, 2004, American Cancer Society, pp 1-60.
3. Haas M: *Contemporary issues in lung cancer: a nursing perspective,* Sudbury, MA, 2003, Jones and Bartlett Publishers.
4. Chapple A, Ziebland S, McPherson A: Stigma, shame, and blame experienced by patients with lung cancer: qualitative study, *BMJ* 329:1470-1472, 2004.
5. Van Cleave J, Cooley M: Lung cancer. In Varricchio CG, Ades TB, Hinds PS et al, editors: *A cancer source book for nurses,* ed 8, Sudbury, MA, 2004, Jones and Bartlett Publishers, pp 215-228.
6. Davies M, Houlihan N, Joyce M: Lung cancer control. In Houlihan NG, editor: *Lung cancer,* Pittsburgh, 2004, Oncology Nursing Society, pp 17-34.
7. Bradley J, Govindan R, Komaki R: Lung. In Perez CA, Brady LW, Halperin, EC et al, editors: *Principles and practice of radiation oncology,* ed 4, Philadelphia, 2004, Lippincott Williams & Wilkins.
8. Guyton A: *Textbook of medical physiology,* ed 8, Philadelphia, 1991, WB Saunders.
9. Coultas PG, Ahier RG, Anderson RL: Altered turnover and synthesis rates of lung surfactant following thoracic radiation, *Int J Radiat Oncol Biol Phys* 13(2):233-237, 1987.
10. Shapiro LD, Finkelstein J, Rubin P: Radiation induced secretion of surfactant from cell cultures of type II pneumocytes: an in vitro model of radiation toxicity, *Int J Radiat Oncol Biol Phys* 10(3):375-378, 1984.
11. Moore-Higgs G, Strohl R, Suntharalingam M: Lung cancer. In Watkins-Bruner D, Moore-Higgs G, Haas M, editors: *Outcomes in radiation therapy: Multidisciplinary management,* Sudbury, MA, 2001, Jones and Bartlett Publishers, pp 251-276.
12. Knop S: Lung cancer. In Yarbro C, Frogge M, Goodman M, editors: *Cancer nursing: principles and practice,* ed 6, Sudbury, MA, 2005, Jones and Bartlett Publishers, pp 1379-1413.
13. Kraut M, Wozniak A: Clinical presentation. In Pass HI, Mitchell JB, Jonson DH et al., editors: *Lung cancer: principles and practice,* ed 2, Philadelphia, 2000, Lippincott Williams and Wilkins, pp 521-534.
14. Khuri F, Keller S, Wagner H: Non-small-cell lung cancer and mesothelioma. In Pazdur R, Hoskins WJ, editors: *Cancer management: a multidisciplinary approach,* ed 3, Melville, NY, PRR, 1999, pp 222-251.
15. MacDonald S, Hansell D: Staging of non-small cell lung cancer: imaging of intrathoracic disease, *Eur J Radiol* 45(1):18-30, 2003.
16. Maddus M, Ginsberg R: Clinical features, diagnosis, and staging of lung cancer. In Pearson FG, Cooper JD, Deslauriers J, et al., editors: *Thoracic surgery,* ed 2, New York, 2002, Churchill Livingstone, pp 813-836.
17. National Comprehensive Cancer Network: *Practice guidelines in oncology for non-small cell lung cancer,* V2.2005, 2005.
18. Lobrano M, Singha P: Positron emission tomography in oncology, *Clin J Oncol Nurs* 7(4):379-385, 2003.
19. Pope R, Hansell D: Extra-thoracic staging of lung cancer, *Eur J Radiol* 45(1):31-38, 2003.
20. Salazar A, Wescott J: The role of transthoracic needle biopsy for the diagnosis and staging of lung cancer, *Clin Chest Med* 14(1):99-110, 1993.
21. Detterbeck F, DeCamp M, Kohman L et al: Lung cancer: invasive staging: the guidelines, *Chest* 123(1 suppl): 167S-175S, 2003.
22. Valle R, Chavany C, Zhokov T et al: New approaches for biomarker discovery in lung cancer, *Expert Rev Mol Diagn* 3(1):55-57, 2003.
23. Feld R, Ginsberg RJ, Payne DG et al: Lung. In Abeloff MD, Armitage J, Lichter A et al., editors: *Clinical oncology,* New York, 1995, Churchill Livingstone, pp 1083-1152.
24. Glover J, Miaskowski C: Small cell lung cancer pathophysiologic mechanisms and nursing implications, *Oncol Nurs Forum* 21(1):87-97, 1994.
25. Fletcher GH: Clinical dose-response curves of human malignant epithelial tumors, *Br J Radiol* 46(541):1-12, 1973.
26. Salazar OM, Rubin P, Brown JC et al: The assessment of tumor response to radiation of lung cancer: continuous vs split-course regimens, *Int J Radiat Oncol Biol Phys* 1 (11-12):1107-1118, 1976.
27. Salazar OM, Van Houtte P, Rubin P: Lung cancer. In Rubin P: *Clinical oncology, a multidisciplinary approach for physicians and students,* ed 7, Philadelphia, WB Saunders, 1993.
28. Salazar OM, Van Houtte P, Rubin P: Once-a-week radiation for locally advanced lung cancer, *Int J Radiat Oncol Biol Phys* 9(6):923-930, 1983.
29. Salazar OM, Van Houtte P, Rubin P: Once-a-week radiation therapy for locally advanced lung cancer: final report, *Cancer* 54(4):719-725, 1984.
30. Cox JD, Azamia N, Byhardt RW et al: N2 (clinical) non-small cell carcinoma of the lung: prospective trials of radiation therapy with total doses 60 Gy by the Radiation Therapy Oncology Group, *Int J Radiat Oncol Biol Phys* 20(1):7-12, 1991.
31. Emami B, Graham MY, Purdy JA: Three-dimensional conformal radiotherapy in bronchogenic carcinoma:

considerations for implementation, *Lung Cancer* 11(suppl 3):S117-S128, 1994.
32. Hazuka MB, Turrisi AT: The evolving role of radiation therapy in the treatment of locally advanced lung cancer, *Semin Oncol* 20(2):173-184, 1993.
33. Scott WJ, Howington J, Movsas B: American College of Chest Physicians: Treatment of stage II non-small cell lung cancer, *Chest* 123(1 suppl):188S-201S, 2003.
34. Smythe WR, American College of Chest Physicians: Treatment of stage I non-small cell lung carcinoma, *Chest* 123(1 suppl):181S-187S, 2003.
35. Ruckdeschel JC: Carcinoma of the lung. In Ravel RE, editor: *Conn's Current Therapy*, Philadelphia, 2003, WB Saunders, pp 156-162.
36. Mountain CF, Lukeman JM, Hammar SP et al: Lung cancer classification: the relationship of disease extent and cell type to survival in a clinical trial population, *J Surg Oncol* 35(3):147-156, 1987.
37. Trakhtenberg A, Kiseleva E, Pitskhelauri V: Preoperative radiotherapy in the combined treatment of lung cancer patients, *Neoplasma* 35(4):459-465, 1988.
38. Damstrup L, Skovgaard-Poulssen H: Review of the curative role of radiotherapy in the treatment of non-small cell lung cancer, *Lung Cancer* 11(3-4):153-178, 1994.
39. Payne DG: Is preoperative or postoperative radiation therapy indicated in non-small cell cancer of the lung? *Lung Cancer* 10(suppl 1):S205-S212, 1994.
40. Pancoast HK: Superior pulmonary sulcus tumor, *JAMA* 99:1391-1396, 1932.
41. Shaw G, Bonner JA, Foote RL et al: Role of radiation therapy in the management of lung cancer, *Mayo Clin Proc* 68(6):593-602, 1993.
42. Bezjak A, Payne D: Radiotherapy in the management of non-small cell lung cancer, *World J Surg* 17(6):741-750, 1993.
43. Chang JY, Liu HH, Komaki R: Intensity modulated radiation therapy and proton radiotherapy for non-small cell lung cancer, *Curr Oncol Rep* 7(4):255-259, 2005.
44. Lung Cancer Study Group: Effects on postoperative mediastinal radiation on completely resected stage II and stage III epidermoid cancer of the lung, *N Engl J Med* 315(22):1377-1381, 1986.
45. PORT Meta-analysis Trialists Group: Postoperative radiotherapy in non-small cell lung cancer: systemic review and meta-analysis of individual patient data from nine randomized controlled trials, *Lancet* 352(9124):257-263, 1998.
46. Connell P, Martel M, Hellman S: Principles of radiation oncology. In DeVita V, Hellman S, Rosenberg S, editors. *Cancer principles and practice of oncology,* ed 7, Philadelphia: Lippincott Williams & Wilkins, pp 267-294.
47. Ramsey C, Scaperoth D, Arwood D et al: Clinical efficacy of respiratory gated conformal radiation therapy, *Med Dosimetry* 24(2):115-119, 1999.
48. Ford E, Mageras G, Yorke E et al: Respiration-correlated spiral CT: a method of measuring respiratory-induced anatomic motion for radiation treatment planning, *Med Phys* 30(1):88-97, 2003.
49. Chen Q, Weinhous M, Deibel F et al: Fluoroscopic study of tumor motion in breathing: facilitating precise radiation therapy for lung cancer patients, *Med Phys* 28(9):1850-1856, 2001.
50. Brady LW: Mesothelioma: the role for radiation, *Semin Oncol* 8(3):329-334, 1981.
51. Aygun MD, Blum JE: Treatment of unresectable lung cancer with brachytherapy, *World J Surg* 19(6):823-827, 1995.
52. Mathur P, Colt H: Endobronchial brachytherapy, *2005 UpToDate* (website): www.utdol.com/application/topic/topicTest.asp?file=lung_ca. Accessed August 12, 2005.
53. Perez CA, Presant CA, Van Amburg AL: Management of superior vena cava syndrome, *Semin Oncol* 5(2):123-134, 1978.
54. Komaki R, Cox JD: The lung and thymus. In Cox JD, editor: *Moss' radiation oncology rationale, technique, results,* ed 7, St Louis, 1995, Mosby, pp 122-135.
55. Carabell SC, Goodman RL: Superior vena caval syndrome. In DeVita VT, Hellman S, Rosenberg SA, editors: *Cancer: principles & practice of oncology,* ed 3, Philadelphia, 1985, Lippincott, pp 2273-2280.
56. Sculier JP, Evans WK, Feld R et al: Superior vena caval obstruction syndrome in small cell lung cancer, *Cancer* 57(4):847-851, 1986.
57. Byhardt RW: Turning up the heat on non-small cell lung cancer: is the toxicity of concurrent cisplatin-based chemotherapy and accelerated fractionation acceptable? *Int J Radiat Oncol Biol Phys* 31(2):431-433, 1995.
58. Sause WT, Scott C, Taylor S et al: Radiation Therapy Oncology Group (RTOG) 88-08 and Eastern Cooperative Oncology Group (ECOG) 4588: preliminary results of a phase III trial in regionally advanced, unresectable non-small cell lung cancer, *J Natl Cancer Inst* 87(3):198-205, 1995.
59. Tannock IF: New perspectives in combined radiotherapy and chemotherapy treatment, *Lung Cancer* 10(suppl 1): S29-S51, 1994.
60. Ornstein D, Nervi A, Rigas J: Docetaxel in combination chemotherapy and in association with thoracic radiotherapy for the treatment of nonsmall cell lung cancer, *Ann Oncol* 10(suppl 5):S35-S40, 1999.
61. Van Moorsel C, Peters G, Pinedo HG: Gemcitabine: future prospects of single-agent and combination studies, *Oncologist* 2(3):127-134, 1997.
62. Arriagada R, Pignon JP, Le Chevalier T: The role of chest radiation in small cell lung cancer, *Cancer Treat Res* 72:255-271, 1995.
63. Turrisi AT: Incorporation of radiotherapy fractionation in the combined-modality treatment of limited small cell lung cancer, *Chest* 103(4 suppl):418S-422S, 1993.
64. Abner A: Prophylactic cranial radiation in the treatment of small cell carcinoma of the lung, *Chest* 103(4 suppl): 445S-448S, 1993.
65. Peck A, Boland J: Emotional reactions to radiation treatment, *Cancer* 40(1):180-184, 1977.
66. Schwartzstein RM, Lahive K, Pope A et al: Cold facial stimulation reduces breathlessness induced in normal subjects, *Am Rev Respir Dis* 136(1):58-61, 1987.
67. Watkins Bruner D, Haas M, Gosselin-Acomb T: *Manual for radiation oncology nursing practice and education,* ed 3, Pittsburgh, 2005, Oncology Nursing Society.
68. VanHoutte P, Danhier S, Mornex F: Toxicity of combined radiation and chemotherapy in non-small cell lung cancer, *Lung Cancer* 10(suppl 1):S271-S280, 1994.
69. Leong SS, Tan EH, Fong KW et al: Randomized double-blind trial of combined modality treatment with or without

amifostine in unresectable stage III non-small cell lung cancer, *J Clin Oncol* 21(9):1767-1774, 2003.

70. Movsas B, Scott C, Langer C et al: Phase III study of amifostine in patients with locally advanced non-small cell lung cancer (NSCLS) receiving intensive chemo/hyperfractionated radiation, Radiation Therapy Oncology Group (RTOG 98-01). Proceedings at American Society of Clinical Oncology (ASCO Abstract #221814), 2003.
71. Antonadou D: Radiotherapy or chemotherapy followed by radiotherapy with or without amifostine in locally advanced lung cancer, *Semin Radiat Oncol* 12(1 suppl 1):50-58, 2002.
72. Antonadou D, Coliarakis N, Synodinou M et al, The Clinical Radiation Oncology Hellenic Group: Randomized phase III trial of radiation treatment ± amifostine in patients with advanced stage lung cancer, *Int J Radiat Oncol Biol Physics* 51(4):915-922, 2001.
73. Haylock JJ, Hart LK: Fatigue in patients receiving localized radiation, *Cancer Nurs* 2(6):461-469, 1979.
74. Kobashi-Schoot JA, Hanewald GJ, van Dam FS et al: Assessment of malaise in cancer patients treated with radiotherapy, *Cancer Nurs* 8(6):306-313, 1985.
75. King KB, Nail L, Kreamer K et al: Patients' descriptions of the experience of receiving radiation therapy, *Oncol Nurs Forum* 12(4):55-61, 1985.
76. Porock D, Spalding D: Surviving fatigue. In Haas M, editor: *Contemporary issues in lung cancer,* Sudbury, MA, 2002, Jones and Bartlett Publishers, pp 109-128.
77. DeWys WD, Begg C, Lavin PI: Prognostic effect of weight loss prior to chemotherapy in cancer patients, *Am J Med* 69(4):491-497, 1980.
78. Brown JK: Gender, age, usual weight, and tobacco use as predictors of weight loss in patients with lung cancer, *Oncol Nurs Forum* 20(3):466-472, 1993.
79. Larson PJ, Lindsey AM, Dodd MJ et al: Influence of age on problems experienced by patients with lung cancer undergoing radiation therapy, *Oncol Nurs Forum* 20(3): 473-480, 1993.
80. Sarna L, Lindsey AM, Dean H et al: Nutritional intake, weight change, symptom distress, and functional status over time in adults with lung cancer, *Oncol Nurs Forum* 20(3):481-489, 1993.
81. Tait N, Aisner J: Nutritional concerns in cancer patients, *Semin Oncol Nurs* 5(2 suppl 1):58-62, 1989.
82. Tchekmedyian N, Hickman M, Tiau J et al: Megestrolacetate in cancer anorexia and weight loss, *Cancer* 69(5): 1268-1274, 1992.
83. Robnett T, Machtay M, Vines E et al: Factors predicting severe radiation pneumonitis in patients receiving definitive chemoradiation for lung cancer, *Int J Radiat Oncol Biol Phys* 48(1):89-94, 2000.
84. McDonald S, Missaillidou D, Rubin P: Pulmonary complications. In Abeloff MD, Armitage J, Lichter A et al, editors: *Clinical oncology,* New York, 1995, Churchill Livingstone, pp 789-807.
85. McDonald S, Rubin P, Phillips TL et al: Injury to the lung from cancer therapy: clinical syndromes, measurable endpoints, and potential scoring systems, *Int J Radiat Oncol Biol Phys* 31(5):1187-1203, 1995.
86. Englestadt RB: Pulmonary lesions after roentgen and radium radiation, *Am J Roentgenol* 43:676-681, 1940.
87. Fryer CJ, Fitzpatrick PJ, Rider WD: Radiation pneumonitis: experience following a large single dose of radiation, *Int J Radiat Oncol Biol Phys* 4(11-12):931-936, 1978.
88. Komaki R, Lee JS, Milas L et al: Effects of amifostine on acute toxicity from concurrent chemotherapy and radiotherapy for inoperable non-small-cell lung cancer: report of a randomized comparative trial, *Int J Radiat Oncol Biol Phys* 58(5):1369-1377, 2004.
89. Rubin P: Late effects of chemotherapy and radiation therapy: a new hypothesis, *Int J Radiat Oncol Biol Phys* 10(1):5-34, 1984.
90. Travis EL, DeLuca AM: Protection of mouse lung by WR-2721 after fractionated doses of radiation, *Int J Radiat Oncol Biol Phys* 11(3):521-526, 1985.
91. Travis E, Parkins C, Holmes J et al: WR-2721 protection of pneumonitis and fibrosis in mouse lung after single doses of x-rays, *Int J Radiat Oncol Biol Phys* 10(2):243-251, 1984.

Chapter 9

Breast Cancer

Giselle J. Moore-Higgs

Radiation therapy plays an integral role in the management of breast cancer. The refinement of imaging technology, treatment planning techniques, and radiation delivery systems offer many options for the treatment of both early-stage disease and locally advanced and metastatic disease. This chapter reviews the role of radiation therapy in the treatment of breast cancer, including the indications for treatment, goals, and technical considerations.

Breast cancer is the second most common cancer overall worldwide and remains a major public health problem among women with more than 1.05 million new cases diagnosed each year.[1] It is the most common cancer in women in all developed countries other than Japan.[2] More than half of the cases are in industrialized countries, about 361,000 in Europe (27.3% of cancer in women) and 230,000 in North America (31.3%).[1] In part, the high incidence in the most affluent areas of the world is likely due to the availability of screening programs that detect early breast cancers, some of which would otherwise have been diagnosed at a later stage or not at all. In the United States, breast cancer is the most common malignancy in women, with an overall lifetime risk of developing the disease being 1 in 9 based on a life expectancy of 85 years.[3] After increasing about 3.7% per year between 1980 and 1987, the incidence of breast cancer increased by only 0.4% per year from 1987 to 2002.[4] Among women ages 40 to 49, the number of cases declined during this same period, and for women younger than 40 little change was noted.[4] The American Cancer Society (ACS) estimates 214,640 new cases of breast cancer will be diagnosed in 2006, which includes 1720 cases of male breast cancer.[5] The incidence of male breast cancer has increased by 1.1% a year from 1975 to 2002 for reasons that are unknown.[5]

Breast cancer is the fifth leading cause of death from cancer worldwide because of the relatively favorable prognosis,[1] and in the United States it will account for an estimated 41,430 deaths in 2006.[5] Although the overall death rate decreased by 2.3% annually from 1990 to 2002, death rates have declined by 3.3% a year among women younger than 50 and by 2.0% a year among women 50 or older.[4] The overall 5-year relative survival rate is estimated to be 88%, and the 10-year rate is estimated to be 80%.[5]

ANATOMY AND PHYSIOLOGY

The breast is a mammary gland that is located within the superficial fascia of the anterior thoracic wall (Figure 9-1). In the mature female, the breast extends inferiorly from the level of the second or third rib to the inframammary fold at approximately the level of the sixth or seventh rib and laterally from the lateral border of the sternum to the anterior or midaxillary line. The posterior surface rests on the pectoralis major, serratus anterior, and external abdominal oblique muscles and the upper extent of the rectus sheath.[6] The axillary tail (also known as the *tail of Spence*) refers to the axillary extension of breast tissue over the pectoralis major into the axilla.

The average adult female breast is composed of 80% fat and connective tissue and 20% glandular tissue.[7] The upper half of the breast, and particularly the upper outer quadrant, contains more glandular tissue than does the remainder of the breast.[6] The breast is composed of 15 to 20 lobes arranged in a radial fashion extending from the nipple. Each lobe has a terminal excretory or collecting duct. These ducts are 2 mm in diameter and converge into subareolar lactiferous sinuses or ducts that are 5 to 8 mm in diameter. Five to ten major ducts drain to the outside through the nipple. Each lobe consists of 20 to 40 lobules, each of which contains 10 to 100 alveoli. The alveoli are the secretory units of the breast.[7] The nipple contains sebaceous and apocrine sweat glands and

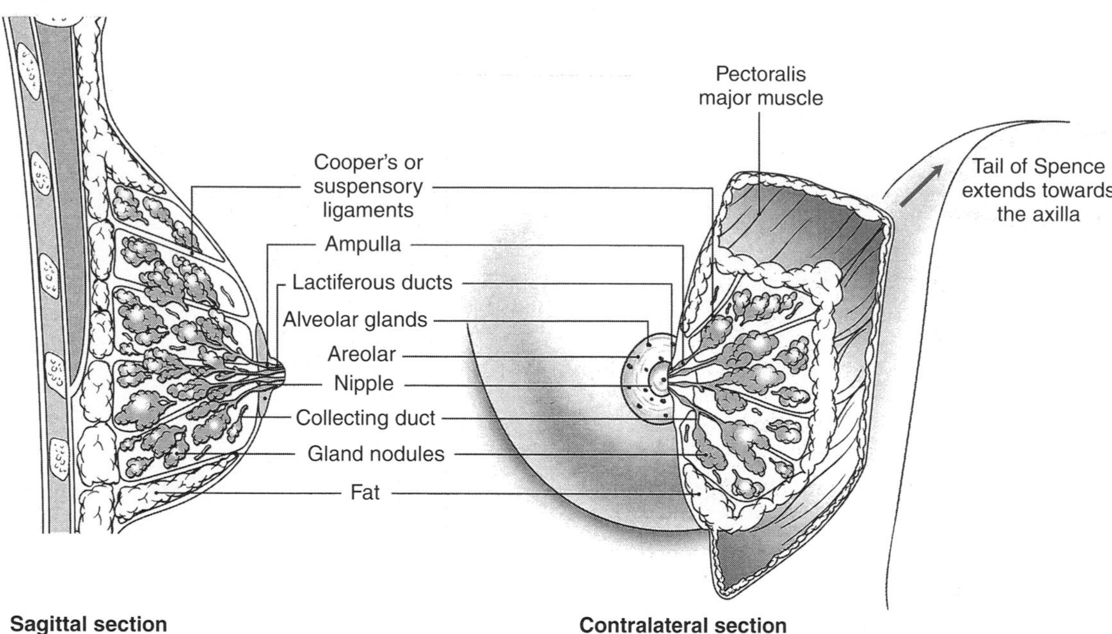

Figure 9-1 Anatomy of the Female Breast.
From Hall JA, Knaus JV: An atlas of breast disease, London, 2003, Parthenon Publishing Group, p 15.

nerve endings. The areola is the circular pigmented tissue around the nipple and contains the sebaceous glands of Montgomery, which are capable of secreting a milk-like substance.[7]

The vascular supply to the breast comes from the internal mammary artery and lateral thoracic artery. The internal mammary artery primarily supplies the medial and central portion of the breast whereas the lateral thoracic artery supplies the upper outer quadrant. The breast lymphatics drain by way of three major routes: axillary, transpectoral, and internal mammary. The primary route is through the axillary lymph nodes (75%).[7] The lymph nodes in the axilla are divided into three anatomic levels: level I nodes are lateral to the pectoralis minor muscle; level II nodes are beneath the pectoralis minor muscle, and level III nodes are medial to the pectoralis minor muscle (Figure 9-2). Rotter's nodes are found between the pectoralis major and minor muscles. Lymphatic drainage in general proceeds sequentially from levels I to III, a concept that is key to the success of sentinel lymph node mapping.

The female hormones estrogen and progesterone influence the configuration of the breast. They

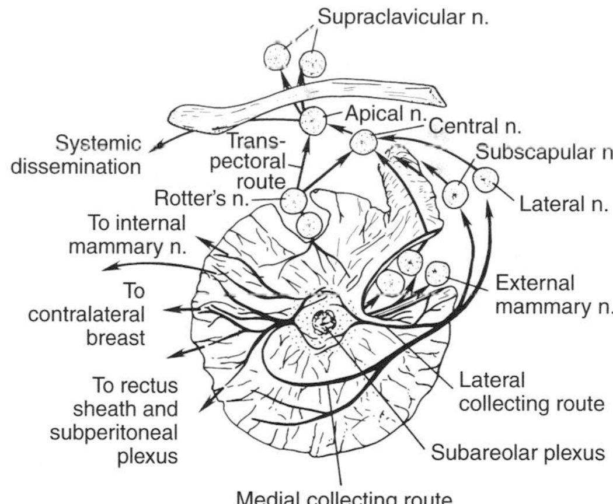

Figure 9-2 Lymphatic Drainage of the Breast.
From Romrell LJ, Bland KI: Anatomy of the breast, axilla, chest wall, and related metastatic sites. In Bland KI, Copeland EM, III, editors: The breast, ed 3, Philadelphia, 2004, Saunders, p 33.

cause an increase in the proportion of periductal connective tissue, fat deposition, ducts, lobes, and breast tissue. Age, familial tendency, and body size generally influence the size and shape of the adult female breast. At menopause, the fatty tissue begins to disappear and the breast slowly atrophies to a pendulous fold of skin. The primary physiologic function of the breast is lactation, but it is also associated with femininity and sexuality, especially in Western cultures.

ETIOLOGY AND EPIDEMIOLOGY

The etiology of breast cancer remains poorly understood, with known risk factors explaining only a small proportion of cases. Risk factors are variables that may be associated to some degree with increased potential for disease development and may be genetic or environmental. Based on hundreds of epidemiologic studies conducted on a wide variety of populations, well established and probable risk factors for breast cancer include age, geographic location, socioeconomic status, reproductive events, exogenous hormones, lifestyle risk factors, mammographic density, history of benign breast disease, ionizing radiation, bone density, height, IGF-1 and prolactin levels, chemopreventative agents, and genetic factors[8] (Table 9-1). However, estimating risk for the individual patient

Table 9-1 Factors That Increase and Decrease Breast Cancer Risk

	Breast cancer risk factors	Magnitude of risk
FACTORS THAT INCREASE BREAST CANCER RISK		
Well-confirmed factors	Increasing age	++
	Geographic region (USA and western countries)	++
	Family history of breast cancer	++
	Mutations in BRCA1 and BRCA2 genes	++
	Mutations in other high-penetrance genes (p53, ATM, NBS12, LKB1)	++
	Ionizing radiation exposure (in childhood)	++
	History of benign breast disease	++
	Late age of menopause (>54)	++
	Early age of menarche (<12)	++
	Nulliparity and older age at first birth	++
	High mammographic breast density	++
Probable factors	Hormonal replacement therapy	+
	Oral contraceptives, recent use	+
	Obesity in postmenopausal women	+
	Tall stature	+
	Alcohol consumption (~ drink/day)	+
	High insulin-like growth factor I (IGF-I) levels	++
	High prolactin levels	+
	High saturated fat and well-done meat intake	+
	Polymorphisms in low-penetrance genes	+
	High socioeconomic status	+
FACTORS THAT DECREASE BREAST CANCER RISK		
Well-confirmed factors	Geographic region (Asia and Africa)	– –
	Early age of first full-term pregnancy	– –
	High parity	– –
	Breastfeeding (longer duration)	– –
	Obesity in premenopausal women	–
Probable factors	Fruit and vegetable consumption	–
	Physical activity	–
	Chemopreventive agents	–
	Nonsteroidal antiinflammatory drugs	–
	Polymorphisms in low-penetrance genes	–

From Dumitrescu RG, Cotarla I: *J Cell Mol Med* 9(1):208-221, 2005.

++, Moderate to high increase in risk; +, low to moderate increase in risk; – –, moderate to high decrease in risk; –, low to moderate decrease in risk.

is difficult, and most breast cancers are not attributable to risk factors other than female gender and increased age.[3]

The National Comprehensive Cancer Network (NCCN) has identified four groups of individuals who are at an increased risk for developing breast cancer. They are (1) women who have previously received therapeutic thoracic irradiation or mantle irradiation; (2) women age 35 or older with a 5-year risk of invasive breast carcinoma greater than or equal to 1.7% on the modified Gail model risk assessment tool; (3) women with a strong family history or genetic predisposition; and (4) women with lobular carcinoma in situ (LCIS) or atypical ductal hyperplasia.[9]

Age

Age is the most important demographic risk factor for breast cancer.[10] The mean age at the time of diagnosis is 60 to 70 years. The risk increases steadily with age from about 100 cases per 100,000 at age 35 to almost 500 cases per 100,000 by age 75.[11]

Geographic Location

The large variation of breast cancer incidence among or within different regions of the world may be attributed to genetic differences among populations and/or differences in lifestyle, including diet and environmental exposures.[8] Women with a higher socioeconomic status or who are from urban communities have a slightly increased risk for breast cancer than women who have a lower socioeconomic status or come from rural communities.[12]

Family History

Family history is a complex risk factor that has a number of key variables including proximity of the relative, the relative's age at diagnosis, and whether the disease was bilateral. In a meta-analysis of 52 individual epidemiologic studies, 12% of women with breast cancer have one affected family member, and 1% have one or more relatives affected.[13] Approximately 5% of all women diagnosed with breast cancer may have a germ line mutation(s) in the BRCA1 gene localized to chromosome *17q21*. These mutations increase a woman's lifetime risk for breast cancer to 60% to 85%.[14,15] Women with first-degree relatives diagnosed with breast cancer have a two- to threefold increased risk of the disease as compared to women without a family history. First-degree relatives of premenopausal women with bilateral breast cancer have nearly 9 times the risk of women without a family history.[10] Specific mutations of the BRCA mutations are clustered among certain ethnic groups such as Ashkenazi Jews, in the Netherlands, Iceland, and Sweden.[16] An increased risk of male breast cancer has been reported in families in which the BRCA2 mutation on chromosome *13q* has been identified.[17,18]

Three screening criteria are commonly used to identify patients who may have a genetic predisposition for breast cancer and therefore be considered high risk (Box 9-1). If a woman is discovered to be at high risk, she should be referred to a cancer genetics professional for risk assessment, counseling, and discussion of genetic testing and for education on risk reduction methods.

Hormone Factors

The substantial body of experimental, clinical, and epidemiologic evidence on breast cancer indicates that a lifetime exposure to endogenous sex hormones may play a major role in the development of breast cancer. Reproductive factors such as early age at menarche, age at first full-term pregnancy, number of pregnancies, and age at menopause have all been studied in relation to breast cancer risk. Early age at menarche (younger than age 12 versus older than age 14) has been associated with an increase risk in breast cancer. Similarly, late age at menopause increases the risk of breast cancer.[8] Both of these factors prolong exposure of breast epithelium to estrogen and progesterone that may explain the higher risk.

Early age at first pregnancy appears to have a protective effect and has been associated with a

Box 9-1 Screening Criteria for Genetic Predisposition

- Family with more than two breast cancer cases and one or more cases of ovarian cancer diagnosed at any age.
- Family with more than three breast cancer cases diagnosed before the age of 50.
- Family with two or more sister pairs with two of the following cancers diagnosed before the age of 50:
  - Two breast cancers
  - Two ovarian cancers
  - One breast cancer and ovarian cancer

decreased risk. Both early age (less than 20 years versus more than 30 years) and higher parity decrease breast cancer risk to half of the risk of nulliparous women.[19] Early age at second pregnancy further reduces the risk.[19] Nulliparity or age at birth of first child after 30 has been associated with an increased risk for intraductal breast cancer.[20]

Other hormone-related risk factors include the use of oral contraceptives and hormone replacement therapy. The role of oral contraceptives as a risk for breast cancer has been controversial. An analysis of data from 54 studies found that women were at a small increased risk of having breast cancer diagnosed while taking combined oral contraceptives and in the first 10 years after stopping, with a relative risk in current users of 1.24 (95% confidence interval [CI] 1015-1.33).[21] Ten or more years after stopping oral contraceptives, there was no evidence of increased risk. The frequency of oral contraceptive use rather than duration of use appears to be more predictive of breast cancer. The effect of recent use was strongest among those women who first used oral contraceptives before age 20.

The role of hormone replacement therapy on breast cancer risk remains unclear. The basis of breast cancer risk associated with hormonal therapies may lie in the regulation of cell proliferation.[22] Estrogen is a well-known mitogen in human breast epithelium, but the action of progesterone is complex and incompletely understood, with some studies reporting a proliferative effect whereas others report an antiproliferative effect. Most studies that have evaluated long-term users of estrogen replacement therapy indicate a modest increase in risk of breast cancer among women who have used estrogen. In the United States, the reported breast cancer risk increases about 2.2% per year of use of a standard dose regimen of conjugated equine estrogen (0.625 mg/day).[10] This translates into increases in risk of 10% after 5 years, 20% after 10 years, and 40% after 15 years of use. Data from Women's Health Initiative (WHI) Randomized Controlled Trial and several other large studies have indicated that the addition of a progestin to estrogen regimen increases breast cancer risk after 5 years of use from 10% (estrogen alone) to 30% (combined HRT).[23] This is particularly true in continuous-combined regimens in which synthetic progestins are used rather than natural progesterone in cyclic regimens. In a recent review of progestins and progesterone in hormone replacement therapy, Campagnoli and colleagues (2005)[24] suggest that the increased breast cancer risk found with the addition of synthetic progestins to estrogen could be the result of the regimen and/or kind of progestin used. The "non-physiological" continuous-combined regimens inhibit the sloughing of lobular duct epithelium that occurs after progesterone withdrawal in a cyclic regimen. In addition, the progestins used are endowed with some non-progesterone-like effects that can potentiate the proliferative effect of estrogens on breast tissue and estrogen-sensitive cancer cells.

A synthetic estrogen, diethylstilbestrol (DES), was widely prescribed to pregnant women during the 1950s and 1960s, but was later discovered to be associated with an increased risk of clear-cell carcinoma of the vagina and cervix in female offspring. DES has not been linked to other cancers in female offspring, but studies of other prenatal factors such as twin gestation and preeclampsia have indicated that in-utero estrogen levels may influence breast cancer risk.[25] In a study of 4821 exposed women and 2095 unexposed women, the rate ratio for incidence of invasive breast cancer in exposed versus unexposed women was 1.4 (95% CI = 0.7–2.6). DES exposure was not associated with an increased risk of breast cancer in women under 40 years, but among women aged 40 and older, the rate ratio was 2.5 (95% CI = 1.0–6.3).

Dietary Factors

Epidemiologic studies have shown some beneficial and harmful effects of dietary components on breast cancer. Studies suggest that high intake of eicosapentaenoic acid (EPA) and docosahexaenoic acid (DHA) (abundant in fish), high intake of oleic acid (OA) (found in olive oil), and low intake of LA n-6 PFUA (linoleic acid polyunsaturated fatty acids) can reduce breast cancer risk.[26] Genistein (found in soy), enterolactone (derived from flax), DADS (diallyl disulfide) (found in garlic), perillyl alcohol (POH) (found in citrus fruits) and resveratrol (found in grapes) have also been shown to be protective.[26] Only a few consistent findings on individual foods or nutrients that influence breast cancer risk have emerged, including certain fatty acids and phytochemicals. The role of alcohol consumption as a risk factor is not clear. Longnecker (1994)[27] in a meta-analysis of 38 studies concluded that a modest, linear statistically significant dose-response relationship exists. In relation to nondrinkers, the breast cancer risks of women consuming one, two, and three alcoholic drinks daily were increased 11%, 24%, and 38% respectively.

Obesity

A number of large studies conducted in the United States and Europe have demonstrated that obesity and weight gain increase breast cancer risk among postmenopausal women, particularly among obese women who do not use hormone replacement therapy.[8] For each 5 kg of weight gain since the lowest adult weight, breast cancer risk increases by 8%.[28] The increased risk may be a result of higher levels of circulating endogenous estrogen that occur as a result of the conversion of the androgen precursor androstenedione to estrone in adipose tissue.

Other Factors

Other factors such as increased breast density, history of benign breast disease, increased bone density in postmenopausal women, tall stature, and high levels of IGF-I, or prolactin also have been associated with an increased breast cancer risk with different magnitudes. Environmental exposure to ionizing radiation in moderate to high doses has been found to increase the risk of breast cancer among women under age 40 at the time of exposure. Updated results from the Late Effects Study Group evaluating women who had been treated as a child for Hodgkin's disease with thoracic or mantle irradiation, showed a 56.7-fold increased risk of developing breast cancer, as compared with the general population.[29] The risk of developing breast cancer was elevated throughout the entire follow-up period, except for the interval between 5 and 10 years from diagnosis of Hodgkin's disease (HD). The cumulative incidence of developing breast cancer as a function of age of the cohort of female HD survivors who received mantle radiation was 13.9% at age 40 years and reached 20.1% (95% CI, 11.1% to 29.0%) at age 45 years.

Risk-Reduction Interventions

The development of effective strategies for the reduction of breast cancer incidence has been difficult, because few of the existing risk factors are modifiable and many of the potentially modifiable risk factors have social implications extending beyond concerns for breast cancer.[3] Estrogen-receptor modulators such as tamoxifen may reduce the risk of developing breast cancer. Results of a large chemoprevention trial, NSABP P-1, evaluated 13,366 high-risk premenopausal and postmenopausal women who took tamoxifen or placebo in a double-blind fashion for 5 years. Women who took tamoxifen for 5 years had a 50% decrease in invasive and noninvasive breast cancer, compared to women who took placebo.[30] However, tamoxifen is not without it's own health risks. The American Society of Clinical Oncology (ASCO) concluded in a technology assessment that for women with a defined 5-year projected breast cancer risk of 1.66% or higher, tamoxifen (at 20 mg/day for 5 years) may be offered to reduce their risk.[31] Risk/benefit models suggest that greatest clinical benefit with least side effects is derived from use of tamoxifen in younger (premenopausal) women (who are less likely to have thromboembolic sequelae and uterine cancer), women without a uterus, and women at higher breast cancer risk. Data do not yet suggest that tamoxifen provides an overall health benefit or increases survival. Use of tamoxifen combined with hormone replacement therapy or use of raloxifene, any aromatase inhibitor or inactivator, or fenretinide to lower the risk of developing breast cancer is not recommended outside of a clinical trial setting.[31]

DIAGNOSTIC EVALUATION

Early detection of breast cancer is critical for assuring the most favorable prognosis, and technology continues to evolve to improve the accuracy of screening techniques. Physical examination and x-ray film mammography of the breast are the recognized gold standard screening tests for breast cancer, together with breast self-examination.[2] Newer radiology modalities such as ultrasonography and magnetic resonance imaging (MRI) are currently used as adjuvant studies rather than screening studies for breast disease.

Mammography

The two types of mammogram imaging are screening and diagnostic. Screening is indicated for asymptomatic women, and two standard views are taken (craniocaudal and mediolateral oblique). Diagnostic mammography is performed for a specific indication (i.e., palpable mass or induration) and in addition to the standard views may include specialized imaging views (i.e., compression views of an area of abnormality).

Screening mammography is recommended for women aged 40 years and older and for women who are considered at high-risk for the development of breast cancer (Table 9-2). Efficacy of mammographic screening has been established by randomized controlled trials in which absolute mortality reduction has been achieved by the ability of the mammogram to find ductal carcinoma in situ and infiltrating cancers of a smaller size and earlier stage than in unscreened control groups.[32] Screening mammography reduces breast cancer mortality by about 20% to 35% in women ages 50 to 69 and slightly less in women ages 40 to 49 at 14 years of follow-up.[33] Approximately 95% of women with abnormalities on screening mammograms do not have breast cancer, with variability based on such factors as age of the woman and assessment category assigned by the radiologist.[33] Although studies have

Table 9-2 Screening Mammography Guidelines*

Patient demographic	Risk level	Screening recommendation
WOMEN AT NORMAL RISK		
	Ages 20 to 39	Clinical breast exam every 1 to 3 years with periodic breast self-examination (BSE) encouraged
	Age 40 years and older	Annual clinical breast examination and bilateral screening mammography with periodic BSE encouraged
WOMEN AT INCREASED RISK		
Women who have previously received thoracic or mantle irradiation	Women age 25 and older	• Clinical breast examination every 6 to 12 months • Annual bilateral screening mammogram • Initiate screening no later than 8 to 10 years after radiation exposure or at age 40 (whichever comes first) • Periodic BSE encouraged
	Women younger than age 25	• Annual clinical breast examination • Periodic BSE encouraged
Women of age 35 or older with a 5-year risk of invasive breast carcinoma greater than or equal to 1.7% (modified Gail Model)	Women age 35 or older	• Clinical breast examination every 6 to 12 months • Annual bilateral screening mammography • Periodic BSE encouraged. Consider risk reduction strategies
Women with a strong family history or genetic predisposition	Starting at age 25 for Hereditary Breast and Ovarian Cancer (HBOC) patients or 5–10 years prior to youngest breast cancer case for strong family history or other genetic predispositions	• Annual clinical breast examination • Annual bilateral screening mammography • Periodic BSE encouraged
	Women younger than age 25	• Annual clinical breast examination • Periodic BSE encouraged
Women with lobular carcinoma in situ (LCIS) or atypical hyperplasia		• Clinical breast examination every 6 to 12 months • Annual bilateral screening mammography • Periodic BSE encouraged. Consider risk reduction strategies

Data from National Comprehensive Cancer Network (NCCN): *Practice guidelines v.1.2006, Breast cancer screening and diagnosis,* Jenkinton, Penn, 20064, NCCN.

*Asymptomatic women with a negative clinical examination should be stratified based on risk factors for the purpose of screening recommendations.

shown a sensitivity range of 73% to 85%,[34-36] current imaging technology has improved significantly since these studies were published.

Screening in younger women has a small benefit, probably because of a lower incidence of breast cancer, more rapidly growing tumors, and greater radiographic density of the breast tissue in women less than 50 years of age. Greater density reduces the sensitivity of mammography.[37] In 2000, the U.S. Food and Drug Administration (FDA) approved the first full-field digital mammography unit for clinical use. Digital mammography, which was developed in part to address some of the limitations of film mammography, separates image acquisition and display allowing the optimization of both. Image processing of digital data allows the degree of contrast in the image to be manipulated, so that contrast can be increased in the dense areas of the breast with the lowest contrast.[37] This increases the ability of the radiologist to identify abnormalities within the dense breast tissue. Studies comparing full-field digital mammography to screen film have not shown statistically significant differences in cancer detection although the impact on recall rates (percentage of screening mammograms considered to have positive results) was unclear.

Ultrasound

Ultrasonography is primarily used as a diagnostic tool in the evaluation of a positive finding on screening mammography exam or in teens and young women who present with a palpable mass. The primary value of ultrasound is to help further characterize a mass (i.e., margins, internal echo patterns, and echogenicity). Because it does not involve the use of radiation, it is safe to use in teenagers, young women, and pregnant women who present with a breast mass.

Magnetic Resonance Imaging

MRI is a relatively recent diagnostic tool for the breast, and the role of MRI in breast cancer management is evolving. In addition to mammography and ultrasound, MRI can be a valuable addition to the evaluation of a breast abnormality or a biopsy-proven cancer.[38] It provides a three-dimensional view of the breast, and performs with high sensitivity in dense breast tissue without using ionizing radiation. However, it is expensive, variable in performance, and has only moderate specificity that in combination with high sensitivity often leads to unnecessary biopsies. The effect of the magnetic resonance imaging on breast cancer mortality is not known.

CLINICAL MANIFESTATIONS

Signs and Symptoms

Most early-stage breast cancers are found on physical examination or on screening mammogram and are asymptomatic. Patients may occasionally report slight tenderness, a feeling of fullness, or discomfort in an area of the breast during certain activities. Symptoms associated with locally advanced breast cancer include pain, nipple discharge, pruritus, shrinkage or enlargement of the breast, inflammation, skin changes, skin ulceration, and/or hand or arm swelling, heaviness, and pain.

Physical Examination

The initial evaluation should include a complete history and physical examination. The history should include all breast-related symptoms and personal and family history of breast disease. During the physical examination a careful visual inspection should be performed, looking for evidence of breast contour differences, skin changes including ulceration, rash, erythema, and peau d'orange (dimpled condition of the skin) and evidence of fullness of the chest wall or skin changes in nodal areas. The physical examination should include careful palpation of the breast and regional lymphatics (axilla, supraclavicular fossa, parasternal spaces, and infraclavicular area) and should be performed in the upright and supine positions. The size and position of the mass should be documented, and a detailed drawing or color photograph(s) provides additional documentation that may be useful for comparison later.

Biopsy

A biopsy of the suspicious mass or abnormality should be performed. Although complete removal of an abnormal breast lesion by excisional biopsy remains the gold standard in breast disease diagnosis, an array of less invasive techniques are available to determine the nature of the abnormality.[7] The choice of biopsy procedure depends on whether the abnormality is palpable and its characteristics. Several different available types of biopsies include fine-needle aspiration, Tru-Cut needle core biopsy, incisional biopsy, excisional biopsy, needle-localization excisional biopsy, and stereotactic core biopsy.

Fine-needle aspiration (FNA) may be performed in the office under local anesthetic. A fine needle is placed into the breast mass and a sample of tissue and/or fluid is aspirated. The diagnostic accuracy has been estimated at 80%.[39] Another simple technique is a biopsy using a Tru-Cut needle that incises a core of tissue. This method allows the practitioner to obtain more tissue in hopes of improving accuracy in an office setting. An incisional biopsy is performed by the surgeon, usually in the operating room. During this type of procedure, a portion of the suspicious mass is removed. This procedure is often performed in locally advanced breast cancer to provide histologic confirmation of diagnosis before initiation of neoadjuvant chemotherapy. The large amount of tissue provides the pathologist with enough tissue to perform specialized immunohistochemical studies, which may help define treatment.

An excisional biopsy is also performed in the operating room and removes the entire abnormality. A needle-localization excisional biopsy requires placement of a flexible hooked wire via a localizing needle under the guidance of ultrasonography or mammography before surgery. The wire provides the surgeon accurate localization of the abnormal tissue at the time of surgical excision. This is particularly useful when the abnormality is too small to feel or when only microcalcifications are present. A skin biopsy, either punch or incisional, should be performed if there is evidence of skin changes including erythema, peau d'orange, rash, or ulcerative lesion that may suggest inflammatory carcinoma. There may not be an underlying palpable mass. Radiologically there may be thickening of the skin of the breast. If nipple discharge is present, it may be collected onto a glass slide and submitted for cytologic evaluation.

Stereotactic core needle biopsy is now the preferred technique of choice in many institutions for the biopsy of breast masses and abnormal microcalcifications. This procedure is performed in the mammography suite with mammography, ultrasound, or MRI image guidance. It shortens the time from detection at mammography to diagnosis and permits appropriate discussion of treatment alternatives, reduces the positive margin rate and reexcision rate, and may represent a significant cost savings in the management of nonpalpable breast cancer.[40] A spring-loaded biopsy gun with a large-gauge needle allows multiple core biopsies to be obtained.

Staging System

Staging of breast cancer is helpful in predicting prognosis, selecting treatment, and facilitating comparisons between treatment regimens. The TNM staging system for breast cancer was developed by the American Joint Committee on Cancers (AJCC) and is used for both clinical and pathologic staging for in situ and invasive disease (Table 9-3). The sixth

Table 9-3 Staging Breast Cancer

PRIMARY TUMOR (T)		
TX		Primary tumor cannot be assessed
T0		No evidence of primary tumor
Tis		Carcinoma in situ; intraductal carcinoma, lobular carcinoma in situ, or Paget's disease of the nipple with no tumor
		NOTE: Paget's disease associated with a tumor is classified according to the size of the tumor.
T1		Tumor 2.0 cm or less in greatest dimension
	T1mic	Microinvasion 0.1 cm or less in greatest dimension
	T1a	Tumor more than 0.1 but not more than 0.5 cm in greatest dimension
	T1b	Tumor more than 0.5 cm but not more than 1.0 cm in greatest dimension
	T1c	Tumor more than 1.0 cm but not more than 2.0 cm in greatest dimension
T2		Tumor more than 2.0 cm but not more than 5.0 cm in greatest dimension
T3		Tumor more than 5.0 cm in greatest dimension
T4		Tumor of any size with direct extension to (a) chest wall or (b) skin, only as described below
	T4a	Extension to chest wall, not including pectoralis muscle
	T4b	Edema (including peau d'orange) or ulceration of the skin of the breast or satellite skin nodules confined to the same breast
	T4c	Both T4a and T4b
	T4d	Inflammatory carcinoma

Table 9-3 Staging Breast Cancer—cont'd

REGIONAL LYMPH NODES (N)		
NX		Regional lymph nodes cannot be assessed (e.g., previously removed)
N0		No regional lymph node metastasis
N1		Metastasis to movable ipsilateral axillary lymph node(s)
N2		Metastasis to ipsilateral axillary lymph node(s) fixed or matted, or in *clinically apparent** ipsilateral internal mammary nodes in the absence of clinically evident axillary lymph node metastasis
	N2a	Metastases in ipsilateral axillary lymph nodes fixed to one another (matted) or to other structures
	N2b	Metastasis only in clinically apparent ipsilateral internal mammary nodes and in the absence of clinically evident axillary lymph node metastasis
N3		Metastasis to ipsilateral infraclavicular lymph node(s) with or without axillary lymph node involvement, or in *clinically apparent** ipsilateral internal mammary lymph node(s) and in the presence of clinically evident axillary lymph node metastasis; or metastasis in ipsilateral supraclavicular lymph node(s) with or without axillary or internal mammary lymph node involvement
	N3a	Metastasis in ipsilateral infraclavicular lymph node(s)
	N3b	Metastasis in ipsilateral internal mammary lymph node(s) and axillary lymph node(s)
	N3c	Metastasis in ipsilateral supraclavicular lymph node(s)

**Clinically apparent* is defined as detected by imaging studies (excluding lymphoscintigraphy) or by clinical examination or grossly visible pathologically.

PATHOLOGIC CLASSIFICATION (pN)		
pNX		Regional lymph nodes cannot be assessed (e.g., previously removed, or not removed for pathologic study)
pN0		No regional lymph node metastasis histologically, no additional examination for isolated tumor cells (ITC)

NOTE: Isolated tumor cells (ITC) are defined as single tumor cells or small cell clusters not greater than 0.2 mm, usually detected only by immunohistochemical (IHC) or molecular methods, but which may be verified on H&E stains. ITCs do not usually show evidence of malignant activity, for example, proliferation or stromal reaction.

pN0(I–)		No regional lymph node metastasis histologically, negative IHC
pN0(I+)		No regional lymph node metastasis histologically, positive IHC, no IHC cluster greater than 0.2 mm
pN0(mol+)		No regional lymph node metastasis histologically, negative molecular findings (RT-PCR)
pN0(mol+)		No regional lymph node metastasis histologically, positive molecular findings (Rt-PCR)

NOTE: Classification is based on axillary lymph node dissection with or without sentinel lymph node dissection. Classification based solely on sentinel lymph node dissection without axillary node dissection is designated (sn) for sentinel node.

RT-PCR—REVERSE TRANSCRIPTASE/POLYMERASE CHAIN REACTION		
pN1		Metastasis to 1 to 3 axillary lymph nodes, and/or in internal mammary nodes with microscopic disease detected by sentinel lymph node dissection but not *clinically apparent*[†]
	PN1mi	Micrometastasis (greater than 0.2 mm, none greater than 2.0 mm)
	PN1a	Micrometastasis (greater than 0.2 mm, none greater than 2.0 mm)
	PN1b	Metastasis in internal mammary nodes with microscopic disease detected by sentinel lymph node dissection but not *clinically apparent*[†]
	PN1c	Metastasis in 1 to 3 axillary lymph nodes and in internal mammary nodes with microscopic disease detected by sentinel lymph node dissection but not *clinically apparent*[†] (If associated with greater than three positive axillary lymph nodes, the internal mammary nodes are classified as pN3b to reflect increased tumor burden)

Continued

Table 9-3 Staging Breast Cancer—cont'd

pN2		Metastasis in 4 to 9 axillary lymph nodes, or in *clinically apparent** internal mammary lymph nodes in the absence of axillary lymph node metastasis
	PN2a	Metastasis in 4 to 9 axillary lymph nodes (at least one tumor deposit greater than 2.0 mm)
	PN2b	Metastasis in *clinically apparent** internal mammary lymph nodes in the absence of axillary lymph node metastasis
pN3		Metastasis in 10 or more axillary lymph nodes, or in infraclavicular lymph nodes, or in *clinically apparent** ipsilateral internal mammary lymph nodes in the presence of 1 or more positive axillary lymph nodes; or in more than three axillary lymph nodes with *clinically negative* microscopic metastasis in internal mammary lymph nodes; or in ipsilateral supraclavicular lymph nodes
	PN3a	Metastasis in 10 or more axillary lymph nodes (at least one tumor deposit greater than 2.0 mm) or metastasis to the infraclavicular lymph nodes
	PN3b	Metastasis in *clinically apparent** ipsilateral internal mammary lymph nodes in the presence of one or more positive axillary lymph nodes; or in more than three axillary lymph nodes and in internal mammary lymph nodes with microscopic disease detected by sentinel lymph node dissection but *not clinically apparent*†
	PN3c	Metastasis in ipsilateral supraclavicular lymph nodes

**Clinically apparent* is defined as detected by imaging studies (excluding lymphoscintigraphy) or by clinical examination.
†*Not clinically apparent* is defined as not detected by imaging studies (excluding lymphoscintigraphy) or by clinical examination.

DISTANT METASTASIS (M)

MX	Presence of distant metastasis cannot be assessed
M0	No distant metastasis
M1	Distant metastasis present

AJCC STAGE GROUPINGS

Stage 0	Tis	N0	M0
Stage I	T1	N0	M0
Stage IIA	T0	N1	M0
	T1*	N1	M0
	T2	N0	M0
Stage IIB	T2	N1	M0
	T3	N0	M0
Stage IIIA	T0	N2	M0
	T1*	N2	M0
	T2	N2	M0
	T3	N1	M0
	T3	N2	M0
Stage IIIB	T4	N0	M0
	T4	N1	M0
	T4	N2	M0
Stage IIIC	Any T	N3	M0
Stage IV	Any T	Any N	M1
T1 includes T1mic			

Used with permission of the American Joint Committee on Cancer, Chicago, Illinois. The original source for this material is the *AJCC Cancer Staging Manual, Sixth Edition* (2002), published by Springer-New York www.springeronline.com. Also available from National Comprehensive Cancer Network (NCCN) at www.nccn.org/professionals/physician_gls/PDF/breast.pdf.

edition of the TNM staging manual reflects important changes and additions to the TNM staging system for breast cancer, which have been in effect since January 1, 2003. The clinical staging system is based on physical and radiologic examination findings. Pathologic staging includes histologic examination of the breast tissue and axillary specimen.

A bilateral mammogram should be performed to evaluate for evidence of synchronous disease, which is more common in infiltrating lobular cancer. Additional radiology studies that may be used for staging, particularly if clinical suspicion of locally advanced or metastatic disease exists, include chest x ray, bone scan, MRI, computerized tomography (CT) scans, or positron emission tomography (PET) scans. A complete blood count with chemistry studies to evaluate renal and liver function also should be performed.

Histopathology

The most widely used classification system for breast cancer is the World Health Organization histologic typing of breast tumors, second edition.[41] This classification scheme is based on the growth pattern and cytologic features of the invasive tumor cells and does not imply histogenesis or site of origin in the mammary duct system.[42] The most common histologic type of invasive breast cancer is invasive ductal carcinoma, followed by invasive lobular carcinoma (Table 9-4).[43] Other types include tubular, mucinous, medullary, invasive cribriform, invasive papillary, and metaplastic carcinoma.

Table 9-4 Histopathology of Breast Cancer

Cancer location	Histopathology
Ductal carcinoma, not otherwise specified (NOS)	Intraductal (in situ)
	Comedo
	Micropapillary
	Cribriform
	Invasive with predominant intraductal component
	Invasive, NOS
	Medullary with lymphocytic infiltrate
	Mucinous (colloid)
	Papillary
	Scirrhous
	Tubular
	Other
	Lobular
	In situ
	Invasive with predominant in situ component
	Invasive
Nipple	Paget's disease with intraductal carcinoma
	Paget's disease with invasive ductal carcinoma
	Paget's disease NOS
Other	Undifferentiated carcinoma
	Cystosarcoma phyllodes
	Angiosarcoma
	Primary lymphoma

In situ carcinomas have malignant changes within the ducts or lobules without invasion through the basement membrane into the surrounding tissue. Invasive breast cancer refers to a heterogeneous group of tumors that arise in the ducts of lobules and extend through the basement membrane into the adjacent tissue. Tumors also may be of mixed histology (i.e., invasive disease with a component of in-situ disease).

Prognostic Factors

A paradigm shift is occurring in the evaluation and treatment of breast cancer that is related to the significant advances that have been made in predicting tumor response to treatment. In the past, stage was one of the most important prognostic factors. However, with the ability to evaluate a tumor cell's response to therapy (i.e., gene-expression profiling studies), this may be changing. Currently the important prognostic factors include age, menopausal status, location of disease in the breast, stage of disease, number of involved axillary lymph nodes, pathologic characteristics of the primary tumor including the presence of tumor necrosis, estrogen and progesterone receptor levels, and measures of proliferative capacity. Other factors include DNA index, oncogene expression, and Karnofsky performance status (KPS). As the data from the basic science research arena and current clinical trials becomes available, these criteria may change to reflect the rapidly expanding knowledge base.

TREATMENT

The treatment of breast cancer is influenced by patient factors such as age, menopausal status, patient preference, and comorbid disease as well as by tumor factors including stage, histopathology, hormone receptor status, and other immunohistochemical studies. A multidisciplinary team approach to the treatment of breast cancer is important during the evaluation and treatment phases. The team should include a surgeon, medical oncologist, radiation oncologist, radiologist (specialty of mammography), pathologist, nurse, and social worker. Many institutions conduct a weekly conference to review new cases and make treatment recommendations.

Ductal Carcinoma In Situ

The frequency of ductal carcinoma in situ (DCIS) has increased dramatically because of the availability of screening and the improved sensitivity of mammography to detect clinically occult microcalcifications. DCIS, which is a preinvasive lesion, is also referred to as intraductal carcinoma and may be classified into several subtypes, based on histologic morphology: comedo, cribriform, papillary, micropapillary, and solid. Some lesions exhibit a mixture of these subtypes. DCIS may present as multicentric disease, but typically involves only a segment of the breast. Axillary lymph node metastasis is rare with DCIS. The natural history of DCIS and whether DCIS has the potential to progress to invasive cancer if left untreated are issues that are not completely understood.

Standard surgical treatment options include breast conservation therapy with lumpectomy followed by radiation therapy or mastectomy. The National Surgical Adjuvant Breast and Bowel Project (NSABP) Study B-17 randomized patients with localized intraductal carcinoma and negative margins after excision to breast irradiation or no further therapy.[44] At 8 years, the cumulative incidence of recurrent DCIS was reduced by the addition of postoperative radiation from 13.4% to 8.2% ($P = 0.007$), and the occurrence of invasive cancer decreased from 13.4% to 3.9% (P less than 0.001). Pathologic evaluation found that only the absence of clear tumor margins and moderate-to-marked comedo necrosis were independent predictors of ipsilateral tumor recurrence. Some single institution experiences with lumpectomy alone suggest that appropriately selected patients may do well with conservative surgery alone if margins are adequate (1 cm or more). Patients with persistent microscopic involvement of the margins after local excision or evidence of multicentric disease should be treated with mastectomy.

Radiation therapy to the breast may be given after complete excision of the area of abnormality with negative margins. The treatment usually consists of 50 Gy to the intact breast followed by a boost to the tumor bed of 10 Gy to 20 Gy depending on the adequacy of the surgical margins. Radiation may be offered after mastectomy if there is evidence of extensive or multicentric disease or close surgical margins. Endocrine therapy may be offered to lower subsequent risk of invasive carcinoma.

Lobular Carcinoma In Situ

Lobular carcinoma in situ (LCIS) is not associated with any mammographic or clinically apparent breast abnormalities. It is typically found incidentally during microscopic review of a biopsy for a benign breast problem and is characterized by proliferation of malignant cells within the lobules. It is an uncommon pathologic finding in the general female population and generally occurs more often in premenopausal women. LCIS has a tendency to be multicentric and is also likely to be found in the contralateral breast. Although it is clear that LCIS is not an obligate precursor to invasive lobular carcinoma, many studies have shown that a proportion of women with LCIS go on to develop invasive carcinoma, with a risk of 6.9 times to about 12 times that of women without LCIS.[45]

Careful radiographic evaluation of both breasts is necessary before initiating treatment. Treatment options include lumpectomy, segmental mastectomy, or mastectomy. The natural history of untreated LCIS suggests that the majority of patients do not develop invasive disease, and half of those who do develop it in the contralateral side. In NSABP Trial B-17, 182 patients who underwent excision alone for LCIS were evaluated at 5 years.[46] There was a 2.2% incidence of invasive ipsilateral tumor recurrence and a 1.1% incidence of contralateral breast tumor occurrence. Because of these findings, the most common management of LCIS is close surveillance only with bilateral prophylactic mastectomy occasionally offered. The options for postexcision management remain controversial.

Early Disease (Stages I and II)

Breast-conserving therapy (BCT) for early-stage breast cancer is now widely accepted as a safe and effective treatment. With more than 20 years of clinical data from a series of landmark clinical trials, breast-conserving surgery followed by radiation has been established as the preferable standard of care for the majority of women with early stage breast cancer (stages 0 to II).[47,48] Although strong evidence supports BCT as a safe alternative to mastectomy and as suitable treatment for as many as 75% of newly diagnosed breast cancer patients, BCT in the United States remains underutilized[49] and subject to wide geographic variation. Data from several studies have found that eligibility criteria for the procedure are not well understood in

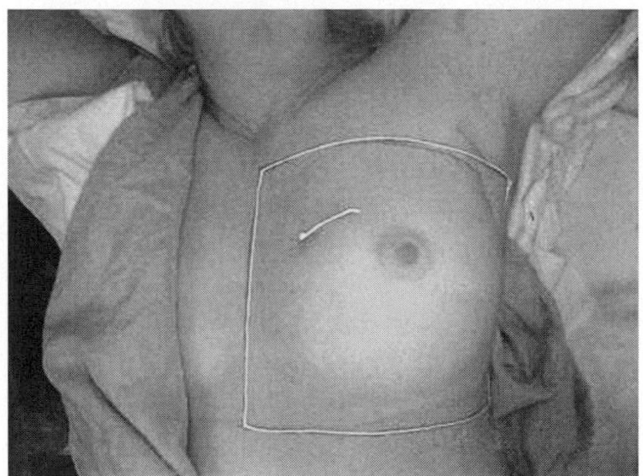

Figure 9-3 Field Borders for Patient With Early-stage Breast Cancer. Patient was receiving radiation to the breast after lumpectomy.

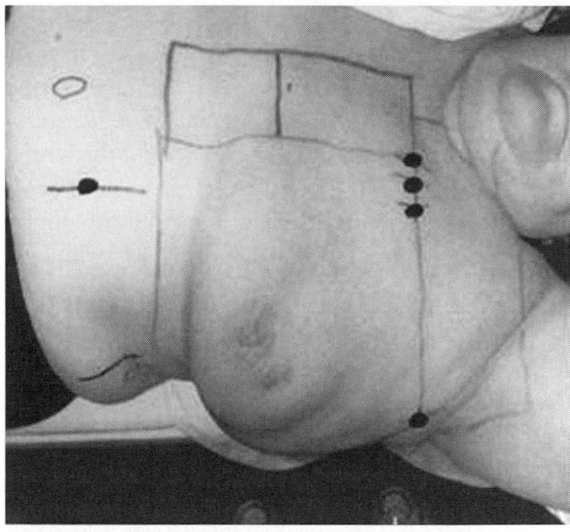

Figure 9-4 Field Borders for Patient With Stage II Breast Cancer. Patient was receiving radiation to the breast and regional lymph nodes after lumpectomy and axillary dissection.

the physician community and/or are not clearly communicated to patients.[49] In addition, selection bias due to age, comorbid disease, insurance coverage, convenience of radiation services, fear of radiation, and issues with sequencing adjuvant chemotherapy also have been reported. With that in mind, the last decade has seen the emergence of a new treatment paradigm for early breast cancer in the form of partial breast treatment with breast-conserving surgery and partial breast irradiation (PBI).[50] This treatment approach may provide an option that would allow more women to choose breast conservation, resolve the dilemmas regarding treatment sequencing and perhaps be more convenient and cost effective. Chapter 25 provides a complete review of the various techniques for PBI and accelerated PBI.

Surgery for early-stage breast cancer may include lumpectomy, segmental mastectomy, or modified radical mastectomy with axillary dissection. Six prospective randomized trials have demonstrated that survival after BCT is equal to survival after mastectomy.[51-56] In the largest trial (NSABP B-06), there was no difference in survival between the three treatment arms (modified radical mastectomy, lumpectomy plus axillary dissection followed by local breast radiation, or lumpectomy and axillary dissection alone) at a median follow-up of 12.5 years.[57] However, for all patients who received lumpectomy followed by irradiation, the rate of local recurrence in the breast was substantially lower than that of patients treated with lumpectomy alone (10% versus 35%, P less than 0.001). The rate of local control in the breast varies with surgical technique. Several contraindications exist for breast conservation procedures in early-stage disease:

- Large tumor size of more than 4 cm to 5 cm in small-breasted women
- Multicentric disease and/or diffuse indeterminate microcalcifications on mammography
- Positive surgical margins on reexcision
- Poor cosmetic outcome (breast to tumor ratio requires excision of large volume of breast tissue)
- Current first- or second-trimester pregnancy
- Previous history of radiation therapy to the chest or axilla
- History of collagen vascular disease

Axillary dissection (level I/II) has been the standard of care in early breast cancer. The rationale for dissection stems from two factors: (1) physical examination is an inadequate method of detecting axillary lymph node involvement, having a false-negative and false-positive rate of 30% in either case[58] and (2) lymph node status is the single best predictor of breast cancer prognosis.[59] Unfortunately, axillary lymph node dissection is associated with increased morbidity including axillary fibrosis, pain, decreased range of motion of the shoulder, and lymphedema. During the past decade, sentinel lymph node biopsy has been introduced into the care of early-stage breast cancer. This procedure is based on the rationale that the pathologic status of the sentinel lymph node that drains the tumor site will be reflective of the pathologic status of the remainder of the lymph nodes in the axilla. Currently, a number of trials are ongoing to evaluate the accuracy of the procedure, the minimal requirements for pathologic evaluation, as well as determining the criteria for selecting patients for the procedure.

Radiation therapy to the whole breast (WBRT) may be given following complete excision of the area of abnormality with negative margins. WBRT comprises of external beam irradiation delivered to the breast to a dose of approximately 50 Gy to 55 Gy in daily 1.8 Gy to 2 Gy doses over a 5- to 6-week period of time. See Figure 9-3 and 9-4 for examples of field sizes and set-up techniques for breast irradiation. This is often followed by a boost dose that is specifically directed to the area in the breast where the tumor was removed or where the surgical clips were placed at the time of surgery. This region is defined by a shell of tissue which may contain actual or potential tumor cells within a 10 mm margin. The boost technique may be altered to include an interstitial radioactive implant if there is evidence of close or positive surgical margins after excision. Radiation should be started as soon as possible after surgery, when the surgical wound has healed. The optimal sequencing of chemotherapy and radiation has not been clearly defined, but delays in radiation of 4 months or more have been associated with increased recurrence rates.[60]

Radiation therapy to the chest wall and regional lymphatics after mastectomy for early stage breast cancer has been used at many institutions to reduce the risk of local recurrence and distant metastasis and improve survival.[61,62] The popularity of postoperative chest wall and regional nodal radiation increased in response to data published in 1997. In a meta-analysis by the Early Breast Cancer Trialists' Collaborative Group (1995),[63] which analyzed all the randomized trials begun before 1985, a 67% reduction in rates of locoregional relapse (*P* less than 0.001) and a 6% reduction in mortality from breast cancer ($P = 0.03$) was found, but no improvement in overall survival. More recent studies have found that postmastectomy radiation therapy in premenopausal women with breast cancer reduces the rate of locoregional and systemic relapses and may improve overall survival.[61,62] Overgaard and colleagues (1997),[62] in a randomized trial of radiation therapy after mastectomy in high-risk premenopausal women, all of whom received systemic chemotherapy, found the frequency of locoregional recurrence alone or with distant metastases was 9% among the women who received radiation and chemotherapy as compared to 32% with chemotherapy alone (*P* less than 0.001). Overall survival at 10 years was 54% among those given radiation therapy and chemotherapy as compared to 45% among those who received chemotherapy alone (*P* less than 1.001). Therefore, postmastectomy radiation therapy is recommended for patients who are at high risk for local regional failure (stage T2 or higher, any N1, and any close surgical margin). Fields treated may include chest wall, supraclavicular fossa, axillary, and internal mammary fields. The treatment usually consists of 50 Gy in 1.8 Gy to 2.0 Gy fractions. The mastectomy scar may be boosted with an additional 10 Gy.

Adjuvant systemic therapy should be considered in tumors greater than 1 cm or with lymph node involvement. Unfavorable prognostic features include intramammary angiolymphatic invasion, high nuclear grade, high histologic grade, HER-2 overexpression or hormone receptor–negative status and should be taken into account along with age, menopausal status, and presence of comorbid disease. The appropriate adjuvant therapy also depends on the assessment of efficacy and toxicity of the treatment regimen. Currently, high-dose chemotherapy with bone marrow rescue is not standard practice. Adjuvant chemotherapy with anthracycline-based regimens has been shown to decrease the risk of relapse and cancer-related mortality in early-stage disease.[43] The protocols most commonly used include CMF (cyclophosphamide, methotrexate and 5-fluorouracil), AC (doxorubicin and cyclophosphamide), and CAF (cyclophosphamide, doxorubicin, and 5-fluorouracil). More recently, the taxanes (paclitaxel and docetaxel) have been incorporated into several adjuvant regimens and the available data does demonstrate a benefit in three-drug regimens such as doxorubicin, cyclophospahamide and docetaxeland AT (doxorubicin and taxanes).[43] In general, if adjuvant chemotherapy is indicated, it should be completed prior to initiating radiation therapy. Concurrent chemotherapy with radiation has been associated with an increase in local toxicity including skin reactions, tissue fibrosis and poor cosmetic outcomes. Targeted therapy, such as with trastuzumab for tumors that overexpress HER 2 have demonstrated a significant benefit in the adjuvant setting and should also be considered.[43]

Adjuvant endocrine therapy in estrogen or progesterone receptor-positive tumors should be considered. Tamoxifen is the most established therapy in both pre- and postmenopausal women and should be given for 5 years after completion of systemic chemotherapy and/or radiation therapy.[43] Recently, aromatase inhibitors have shown significant improvement in overall survival compared to tamoxifen alone in postmenopausal women.[43] The side effect profiles of these two agents are different and each woman should be evaluated for potential contraindications before initiating treatment.

In women over 70 years of age with stage I, estrogen receptor–positive breast cancer may be treated with breast conservation surgery plus tamoxifen or an aromatase inhibitor without breast irradiation.[43] Recent published data from an Intergroup (CALGB/RTOG/ECOG) study has shown a local-regional recurrence rate of 1% in the radiation plus tamoxifen arm and a 4% in the tamoxifen alone arm.[64] No differences were found in overall survival, disease-free survival, or need for mastectomy.

Advanced Disease (Stages III and IV) and Inflammatory Breast Cancer

Patients with advanced breast cancer should be carefully evaluated for evidence of metastatic disease before initiation of treatment. Patients who have locally advanced disease (stage IIIA) should receive systemic treatment, radiation, and surgery with the sequencing tailored to the individual patient and institution protocols. Surgery usually consists of a modified radical mastectomy with axillary lymph node dissection. Radiation therapy may be given preoperatively but is usually given after surgery. Chemotherapy may precede or follow surgery. A recent NSABP study comparing pre- and postoperative chemotherapy showed no survival difference related to the timing of the chemotherapy.[65] For patients with T0, T1, or T2 tumors, breast conservation may be an option. Patients with inoperable breast disease usually require neoadjuvant systemic treatment. If the disease responds sufficiently, mastectomy with axillary lymph node dissection may precede radiation therapy. If the tumor remains inoperable after chemotherapy, preoperative radiation maybe given in an attempt to render the tumor operable. Further systemic chemotherapy with or without endocrine therapy may be considered.

Breast Cancer and Pregnancy

Breast cancer diagnosed during pregnancy occurs in approximately 1 in 3000 pregnancies. The natural tenderness and engorgement of the pregnant breast may hinder detection of discrete masses and may delay diagnosis. Diagnostic procedures such as ultrasound and mammography may be used with adequate shielding of the fetus to evaluate dominant masses and occult carcinomas in the presence of other suspicious clinical findings.[66] Staging radiology studies should be limited because of potential risk to the fetus and should be used only when essential for making a treatment decision. Termination of pregnancy may be considered, based on the age of the fetus, if maternal options such as chemotherapy and radiation therapy are significantly limited by the continuation of the pregnancy.

NURSING INTERVENTIONS AND EDUCATION

Despite significant advances in the three primary modalities of treatment, survivors of breast cancer still face physiologic alterations to normal tissue and body functions that can have a negative impact on overall quality of life. Some of the most debilitating morbidity associated with the treatment of breast cancer is related to the treatment of the axilla with surgery and/or radiation therapy. Specifically, the types of problems and their frequency that have been described at 12 months posttreatment include reduced shoulder mobility (12% to 32%),[67-70] and lymphedema (9% to 30%).[67-72] These numbers probably underestimate the actual frequency of occurrence because of the subjective nature of many of the symptoms, the lack of reliable methods of clinical evaluation, and the inconsistent methods of documentation. This is particularly true with shoulder mobility and lymphedema. This section will review the most common acute and chronic toxicity's that occur with standard whole breast and chest wall irradiation. See Chapter 25 for toxicities related to partial breast and accelerated partial breast irradiation.

Fatigue is a common side effect of radiation therapy. In a study evaluating fatigue related to different treatment methods for breast cancer, women who received combination therapy (chemotherapy and radiation) had the highest fatigue scores; those who received only radiation therapy had the lowest fatigue scores.[73] Fatigue significantly increases over the course of treatment and is the highest during the last weeks of treatment. It usually returns to pretreatment levels by about 3 months after treatment and has been related to symptom distress, psychologic distress, and impairment of quality of life.[74]

Skin reactions commonly occur in women receiving radiation therapy for breast cancer. The severity of the reaction depends on radiation dose, energy used, and fields treated. The total effect for the dose schedule applied has been found to be the strongest factor for acute and late skin reactions.[75] In addition to radiation dose, weight, breast size, lymphocele aspiration, smoking, age, history of skin cancer, and tumor stage have been found to be important factors in predicting the severity of an acute radiation skin reaction in women with breast cancer.[76]

In breast irradiation, the breast will become gradually erythematous approximately 2 to 3 weeks after initiation of treatment. Patients may experience pruritus particularly in the upper medial area of the breast field associated with folliculitis. Areas of moist desquamation may occur in the inframammary fold and in the axilla. In chest wall irradiation, the chest wall skin will gradually become erythematous approximately 2 to 3 weeks into treatment. Areas of moist desquamation are common after 40 Gy both in the chest wall fields and in the axilla. Occasionally a treatment break maybe required. For nursing interventions specific to radiodermatitis, see Chapter 30.

Breast edema is common in women treated with breast conservation radiation therapy. Disruption of the draining lymphatics of the breast by surgery and/or radiation therapy increase the risk of breast edema. This is particularly true when the original site of disease is in the upper outer quadrant and in obese women. The onset of breast swelling is gradual, and continues until completion of treatment. It is associated with mild discomfort and breast tenderness, and the resolution is gradual. The majority of swelling disappears within the first 6 months in most women. However, in large-breasted women, the swelling may persist for a much longer period. In a prospective assessment of late changes in the breast, Moody and colleagues (1994)[76] found only 6% of women with small breasts developed moderate or severe late changes as compared with 22% of women with moderate size breasts, and 39% with large breasts (P less than 0.001). A significant correlation was found between breast size and dose inhomogeneity that may account for the marked changes in breast appearance in the larger breast.

Lymphedema is the buildup of lymph in the tissues, mainly in the fat just under the skin. The incidence of lymphedema of the upper extremity, a disabling complication of treatment, has been reported to range from 2% to 89%, depending on the type of surgery performed.[77,78] These data are similar to those occasionally included as part of the analysis of complications associated with therapeutic clinical trials. Lymphedema results from a disturbance of the equilibrium between the transport capacity of the clearing system and the amount of lymph fluid to be cleared.[79] It is associated with tightness, discomfort, hyperkeratosis, and Stemmer's sign (thickened skinfold at base of the second finger that cannot be lifted—only grasped as a lump of tissue). Prevention is key because lymphedema cannot be cured (Box 9-2). The primary aim of treatment is to achieve maximum improvement and long-term control.[79]

The earlier treatment is initiated, the better the result. There are three treatment approaches that may be recommended depending on the resources available in the patient's community. They are as follows:

- **Manual lymphatic massage/drainage (MLD).** This is a special form of very gentle, rhythmic,

Box 9-2 Lymphedema Prevention

- Avoid breaks in the skin of the affected limb.
- Treat evidence of cellulitis aggressively with antibiotic therapy.
- Avoid pressure on the involved extremity.
- Avoid constrictive clothing.
- Avoid vigorous activity with the limb.
- Use an electric razor under the affected arm.
- Avoid extremes of heat including sunbathing and hot tubs.
- Keep the skin in good condition.
- Maintain ideal weight.
- Avoid extended use of diuretics.
- Exercise regularly, but don't overdo.
- Choose a light prosthesis.
- Eat healthy foods. Avoid caffeine, alcohol, and excessive salt intake. Increase water consumption.
- Plan ahead when you travel. Avoid long airline flights. Take frequent rests breaks, and avoid lifting heavy luggage.

pumping massage movements that remove excess fluid and protein from an extremity. The treatment stimulates contraction of the skin lymphatics, which results in improvement of superficial drainage.[79]

- **Compression with vasopneumatic pumps.** This therapy is performed by placing the limb in an inflatable sleeve connected to a motor-driven air pump that inflates and deflates cyclically. Multichamber compression stimulates superficial lymph flow, decreases tissue fibrosis, and encourages fluid out of the limb. Compression should be performed for a total of 2 hours per day. The pressure of the machine should not exceed 60 mm Hg.[79]
- **Complete decongestive physiotherapy (CDP).** This therapy combines manual lymphatic drainage with compression bandaging. It has been found to be superior to pneumatic pumps and surgery in treating lymphedema.[79] Several methods are described in the literature: Lerner School,[80] Vodder School, and Casley Smith method. Boris and colleagues (1997)[81] found that patients who are compliant with treatment showed a significant reduction in lymphedema that was maintained for a minimum of 36 months.

Soft-tissue fibrosis is another common late effect. Mild atrophic and telangiectatic skin changes occur after radiation to the breast or chest wall. Patients describe the sensation of skin tightness or thickness. On exam, the skin may appear thickened and taut. Fibrosis may occur in the breast or chest wall and does affect cosmetic outcome. A number of variables have been studied in regards to fibrosis in breast tissue in regard to cosmetic outcome after BCT. Kramer and colleagues (1999)[82] found on univariate analysis of women receiving an interstitial implant as part of breast-conservation therapy that total excision volume and dose homogeneity index were significantly related to cosmetic outcome. In multivariate analysis, only the total excision volume remained significant. The mean total excision volume plus or minus standard deviation (± SD) in patients with excellent cosmetic outcome (81.8 cm^3 ± 84.0) was significantly less than that in patients with less than excellent cosmetic outcome (120 cm^3 ± 84). The probability of excellent cosmetic outcome linearly increased with an increase in the dose homogeneity index. Vrieling and colleagues (1999)[83] evaluated the influence of the boost and found that 86% of patients in the no-boost group had an excellent or good global result as compared to 71% of patients in the boost group (16 Gy) ($P = 0.0001$) at 3 years.

Radiation therapy also may cause fat necrosis, skin thickening, and other parenchymal distortion of the breast that can impact future radiographic interpretations (i.e., mammography). In addition to fibrosis, masses, fluid collections, scarring, edema, and calcifications are posttreatment findings that may mimic or mask local tumor recurrence.[84] Holli and colleagues (1998)[85] found that further diagnostic tests prompted by difficulties in interpreting mammograms were performed to the extent of 0.19 per mammography exam in those who had prior breast radiation as compared to 0.15 in those without radiation therapy (approximately 1.3 times more often).

Brachial plexopathy as a result of radiation is a rare complication. It is usually related to high total doses of radiation or nonstandard fractionation schemes.[86] Patients present with pain, arm edema,[87] and signs of upper trunk dysfunction (C-5 through C-7).[88] When associated with arm swelling, the symptoms of the brachial plexopathy may improve with aggressive lymphedema treatment.[89] Otherwise, treatment may involve nerve blocks, cordotomy, rhizotomy, or oral narcotic management for uncontrolled chronic pain (see Chapter 31).

Spontaneous rib fractures occur in approximately 10% of patients who receive radiation to the chest wall following mastectomy.[90] The fracture may be asymptomatic and found only on chest x ray or bone scan or they may be quite painful. Typically, the fractures heal spontaneously within 6 to 8 weeks. Overgaard (1988)[91] found that patients treated with a large dose per fraction had a significantly higher incidence of late bone damage (19%) than patients treated with a standard dose per fraction (6%). There was a clear dose-response relationship, especially in the 12-fraction regimen as compared to the 22-fraction regimen.

Radiation therapy for left-sided breast cancer has been associated with an increased risk of cardiac mortality and morbidity in early-stage breast cancer. The anterior left ventricle is frequently included in tangential chest wall fields and in en face fields treating the internal mammary nodes.[92] Cardiac mortality has been found to positively correlate with cardiac dose-volume.[92] Patients who receive high-dose volumes appear to have an increased mortality of ischemic heart disease, but not of myocardial infarction.[92] However, with modern technology, including CT simulation, it is possible to decrease the volume of heart in the irradiation of the left breast.

Pulmonary complications after radiation for breast cancer are related to radiation dose, technique, and volume of lung included in the treatment field. Depending on patient's anatomy and the treatment technique, a variable amount of lung is frequently irradiated when the breast, chest wall, and/or regional lymphatics are treated.[90] Acute pneumonitis is more likely when larger volumes of lung are irradiated. Acute pneumonitis is characterized by a dry hacking cough, shortness of breath, and occasionally febrile episodes. It may last 2 to 3 weeks or longer, but is usually self-limiting. In severe cases, steroids may be given to manage the acute symptoms. Asymptomatic pulmonary fibrosis limited to the treatment volume is often identified on chest x ray and CT imaging, including the apical region when the supraclavicular and/or axillary region is irradiated.

Range of motion of the shoulder may be limited after treatment. Sugden and colleagues (1998)[93] evaluated women at 18 months after surgery and postoperative radiation. Half of the patients reported that the function was reduced as compared with before treatment. Overall, 48% of the patients had measured limitation of at least one shoulder movement as compared to the other shoulder. Mastectomy patients had more problems than those patients with breast conservation (79% versus 35%). Patients who had axillary irradiation also had more problems (73% versus 35%). Patients with dysfunction of the shoulder movement before radiation therapy had a 60% chance of persistent movement problems at 18 months as compared with 24% of patients with normal postoperative function. Similar findings were reported by Hack and colleagues, 1999.[94] Seventy-two percent of women experienced arm/shoulder pain, weakness or numbness, and impaired range of motion of the impaired arm/shoulder. Pain severity correlated positively with the number of lymph nodes removed and treatment with chemotherapy, but was not significantly related to length of time since surgery or treatment with radiation therapy. Early physical therapy intervention can make a significant contribution to normal function without increasing the incidence of postoperative complications.[95]

With the introduction of estrogen suppression (endocrine therapy) as a treatment modality for breast cancer, premenopausal and perimenopausal women are experiencing menopausal symptoms and the consequences of estrogen deprivation much earlier than would naturally occur. The organ systems most commonly affected are the central nervous, cardiovascular, musculoskeletal, genitourinary, and integumentary systems. Sequelae include urogenital atrophy, vasomotor instability, osteoporosis, osteopenia, and diminished gender-related cardiovascular protection. Common vulvovaginal and urinary symptoms found in postmenopausal women include irritation, itching, burning, dyspareunia, and urinary difficulties. With these physiologic changes come changes in sexual health, with the dyspareunia due to vaginal dryness being the most common clinical symptom affecting sexual activity.[96]

Follow-Up Recommendations

A follow-up evaluation should be performed every 3 months for a minimum of 3 years, then every 6 to 12 months for the next 2 years, then annually.[97] The evaluation should include the following:

- History and physical examination.
- Careful visual inspection and physical examination of the breast and regional lymphatic bearing areas.
- Circumferential measurements of the midhand, wrist, forearm, and upper arm of both upper extremities for evidence of lymphedema.
- Appropriate radiographic studies. Women treated with breast-conserving therapy should have their first posttreatment mammogram approximately 6 months after completion of radiation therapy, then annually or as indicated for surveillance of abnormalities. If stability of mammographic findings is achieved, mammography can be performed yearly thereafter.[97] All women with a prior diagnosis of breast cancer should have yearly mammographic evaluation of the contralateral breast.
- Radiograph or laboratory studies as clinically indicated. There is insufficient data to suggest routine use of complete blood counts, automated chemistries, chest radiographs, bone scans, liver ultrasounds, CT scans, and carcinoembryonic antigen (CEA), CA-15-3, or CA 27.29 tumor markers for breast cancer surveillance.[97]

- Pelvic examination with appropriate Pap smear annually. If patient is on tamoxifen, ultrasonography examination or endometrial biopsy should be performed annually to evaluate for evidence of endometrial carcinoma.

Prognosis

The overall 5-year relative survival rate for 1995 to 2001 SEER data was 88.2%.[98] Five-year relative survival rates by race were 89.5% for Caucasian women and 75.9% for African-American women. Survival rates based on stage distribution were 97.9% for localized disease, 81.3% for regional disease, and 26.1% in women with distant disease at the time of diagnosis.

Quality of Life

Four key points can be abstracted from the data that describes breast cancer survivors. The first is that surviving breast cancer is a process of adjustment that occurs over time and may be influenced at any point by psychosocial and physical sequelae related to the diagnosis and treatment. Secondly, depression may be the most common emotional sequela after diagnosis and may continue or recur in response to treatment-related physical problems in the succeeding years. The third point is that there are insufficient data accurately describing the chronic physical effects of surgery and radiation therapy and their impact on quality of life. Finally, menopausal symptoms related to estrogen suppression after breast cancer may be responsible for a significant effect on a woman's sexual health, and ultimately on quality of life.

Data from several studies support the existence of one or more of these themes in long-term breast cancer survivors. A case-control comparison study by Craig and colleagues (1974)[99] revealed that quality of survival, as defined by physical and psychosocial criteria, was similar among 134 long-term breast cancer survivors (5 years or more) and 260 controls. Physical disability was reported by 19% of the women with breast cancer and 16% of the controls. The slight excess of disability among the breast cancer cases was attributed to surgical treatment. There was no evidence of increased psychosocial disability among the women with breast cancer.

Woods and Earp (1978)[100] explored the quality of survival of 49 women 4 years after mastectomy. They reported a positive association between the number of physical symptoms the women experienced and depressive symptoms. Many of these women continued to experience physical symptoms and depression 4 years after treatment. Although these two studies provided early evidence of chronic psychosocial and physical problems after treatment for breast cancer, they were conducted before the availability of many new surgical and radiation therapy techniques used today that alter the extent of surgical resection and physical disability. In addition, Woods' study did link the occurrence of physical disability with long-term psychosocial sequelae.

In 1996, Ganz and colleagues[101] reported one of the first prospective studies to specifically address quality of life, rehabilitation needs, and psychologic distress among breast cancer survivors. Furthermore, this study included repeat evaluations on a regular basis during the period of close surveillance. One hundred and thirty nine breast cancer survivors were interviewed on four occasions during the first year after primary therapy, and again at 2 or 3 years. They found that at 2 and 3 years after treatment, participants did not differ from each other on their prior assessments of quality of life. A significant decline in global quality of life, sexual functioning, and marital functioning occurred between the 1-year and 3-year evaluations. For the 2-year sample, only sexual functioning showed deterioration. These survivors reported a number of problems associated with physical and recreational activities, body image, sexual interest, and sexual functioning. The authors concluded that breast cancer survivors appear to plateau or reach maximum recovery from the physical and psychologic trauma of cancer treatment by 1 year after surgery, and decline in some areas in the following 2 years. Many physical, psychosocial and sexual functioning problems persist or even worsen over time. Physical problems include paresthesia, pain, skin sensitivity, changes in hair, changes in the irradiated breast, and endocrine problems. Psychosocial problems include a reduction in energy, changes in communication and affection with partner, body image, cognitive problems, a decreased interest in sexual activity, and feelings of decreased sexual attractiveness. They suggested that there were many hormone-related reasons why breast cancer patients experience profound menopausal symptomatology including hot flashes, sleep disturbances, vaginal dryness, and emotional lability, which may ultimately impact sexual health.

Table 9-5 Resources for the Breast Cancer Patient and Family

Resource	Types of services	Website
The Susan G. Komen Breast Cancer Foundation	Education materials Advocacy	www.komen.org
American Cancer Society	Education materials Local support groups Advocacy Financial support	www.cancer.org
National Cancer Institute	Education materials	www.cancer.gov
BreastCancer.org	Education Advocacy	www.breastcancer.org
Y-ME National Breast Cancer Organization	Education Local support groups Advocacy	www.y-me.org
National Lymphedema Network	Patient education Advocacy	www.lymphnet.org
Breast Cancer Research Foundation	Patient education	www.bcrfcure.org
National Breast Cancer Coalition	Patient education Advocacy	www.natlbcc.org
Team Survivor	Survivorship advocacy	www.teamsurvivor.org

SUMMARY

In summary, radiation plays an important role in the treatment of breast cancer, particularly in early-stage disease. Although it is associated with some acute and late toxicity, it is generally well tolerated and reduces the risk of local-regional recurrence. Patient education regarding the expected acute effects and long-term surveillance plan are key to patient satisfaction. Numerous resources are available to assist in the education of and support of patients and families (Table 9-5).

REFERENCES

1. Parkin DM, Bray F, Ferlay J et al: Global cancer statistics, 2002, *CA Cancer J Clin* 55(2):74-108, 2005.
2. Moss SM: Breast cancer. In Kramer B, Gohagen JK, Porock PC, editors: *Cancer screening: theory and practice*, New York, 1999, Marcel Dekker, p 78.
3. National Comprehensive Cancer Network: *NCCN clinical practice guidelines: breast cancer risk reduction,* V1.2005, Jenkintown, PA, 2005, National Comprehensive Cancer Network.
4. Edwards BK, Brown ML, Wingo PA et al: Annual report to the nation on the status of cancer, 1975-2002, featuring population-based trends in cancer treatment, *J Natl Cancer Inst* 97(19):1407-1427, 2005.
5. *Cancer facts and figures,* Atlanta, 2006, American Cancer Society.
6. Romrell LJ, Bland KI: Anatomy of the breast, axilla, chest wall and related metastatic sites. In Bland KI, Copeland EM, editors: *The breast: comprehensive management of benign and malignant disorders – Volume 1*, ed 3, St Louis, 2004, Mosby, pp 21-42.
7. Hall JA, Knaus JV: *An atlas of breast disease*, London, 2003, Parthenon Publishing Group, pp 15-20.
8. Dumitrescu RG, Cotarla I: Understanding breast cancer risk—where do we stand in 2005, *J Cell Mol Med* 9(1): 208-221, 2005.
9. National Comprehensive Cancer Network: *NCCN clinical practice guidelines: breast cancer screening and diagnosis,* V1.2004, Jenkintown, PA, 2004, National Comprehensive Cancer Network.
10. Bernstein L: The epidemiology of breast cancer, *Women Cancer* 1(suppl 1):7-13, 1998.
11. Offit KL: *Clinical cancer genetics*, New York, 1998, Wiley-Liss.
12. Collaborative Group on Hormonal Factors in Breast Cancer: Familial breast cancer: collaborative reanalysis of individual data from 52 epidemiological studies including 58,209 women with breast cancer and 101,986 women without the disease, *Lancet*, 358(9291):1389-1399, 2001.
13. Brose MS, Rebbeck TR, Calzone KA et al: Cancer risk estimates for BRCA1 mutation carriers identified in a risk evaluation program, *J Natl Cancer Inst* 94(18):1365-1372, 2002.
14. Thompson D, Easton DF: Cancer incidence in BRCA1 mutation carriers, *J Natl Cancer Inst* 94(18):1358-1365, 2002.
15. Nelson HD, Huffman LH, Fu R et al: Genetic risk assessment and BRCA mutation testing for breast and ovarian cancer susceptibility: systematic evidence review for the US Prevention Services Task Force, *Ann Intern Med* 134(5):362-379, 2005.
16. Wooster R, Bignell G, Lancaster J et al: Identification of the breast cancer susceptibility gene BRCA2, *Nature* 378(6559):789-792, 1995.

17. Thorlacius S, Tryggvadottir L, Olafsdottir GH et al: Linkage to BRCA2 region in hereditary male breast cancer, *Lancet* 346(9874):544-545, 1995.
18. Pathak DR, Osuch JR, He J: Breast carcinoma etiology: current knowledge and new insights into the effects of reproductive and hormonal risk factors in black and white populations, *Cancer* 88(5 suppl):1230-1238, 2000.
19. McPherson K, Steel CM, Dison JM: ABC of breast disease: breast cancer-epidemiology, risk factors, and genetics, *BMJ* 321(7261):624-628, 2000.
20. Kerlikowske K, Barclay J, Grady D et al: Comparison of risk factors for ductal carcinoma in situ, *J Natl Cancer Inst* 89(1):76-82, 1997.
21. Collaborative Group on Hormonal Factors in Breast Cancer: Breast cancer and hormonal contraceptives: collaborative reanalysis of individual data on 53,297 women with breast cancer and 100,239 women without breast cancer from 54 epidemiologic studies, *Lancet* 347(9017):1713-1727, 1996.
22. Preston-Martin S, Pike MC, Ross RK et al: Increased cell division as a cause of human cancer, *Cancer Res* 50(23):7415-7421, 1990.
23. Rossouw JE, Anderson GL, Prentice RL et al: Risks and benefits of estrogen plus progestin in healthy postmenopausal women: principal results from the Women's Health Initiative randomized controlled trial, *JAMA* 288(3):321-333, 2002.
24. Campagnoli C, Clavel-Chapelon F, Kaaks R et al: Progestins and progesterone in hormone replacement therapy and the risk of breast cancer, *J Steroid Biochem Mol Biol* 96(2):95-108, 2005.
25. Palmer JR, Hatch EE, Rosenberg CL et al: Risk of breast cancer in women exposed to diethylstilbestrol in utero: preliminary results (United States), *Cancer Causes Control* 13(8):753-758, 2002.
26. Tsubura A, Uehara N, Kiyozuka U et al: Dietary factors modifying breast cancer risk and relation to time of intake, *J Mammary Gland Biol Neoplasia* 10(1):87-100, 2005.
27. Longnecker MP: Alcoholic beverage consumption in relation to risk of breast cancer: meta-analysis and review, *Cancer Causes Control* 5(1):73-82, 1994.
28. Trentham-Dietz A, Newcomb PA, Egan KM: Weight change and risk of postmenopausal breast cancer (United States), *Cancer Causes Control* 11(6):533-542, 2000.
29. Bhatia S, Yasui Y, Robison LL, Late Study Group: High risk of subsequent neoplasms continues with extended follow-up of childhood Hodgkin's disease: report from the Late Effects Study Group, *J Clin Oncol* 21(23): 4386-4394, 2003.
30. Fisher B, Constantino JP, Wickerham DL et al: Tamoxifen for prevention of breast cancer: report of the National Surgical Adjuvant Breast and Bowel Project P-1 study, *J Natl Cancer Inst* 90(18):1371-1388, 1998.
31. Chlebowski RT, Col N, Winer EP et al: American Society of Clinical Oncology technology assessment of pharmacologic interventions for breast cancer risk reduction including tamoxifen, raloxifene, and aromatase inhibition, *J Clin Oncol* 20(15):3328-3343, 2002.
32. Berg WA: Rationale for a trial of screening breast ultrasound: American College of Radiology Imaging Network (ACRIN) 6666, *AJR* 180(5):1225-1228, 2003.
33. Elmore JG, Armstrong K, Lehman CD et al: Screening for breast cancer, *JAMA* 293(10):1245-1256, 2005.
34. Shapiro S, Venet W, Strax P et al: *Periodic screening for breast cancer: the Health Insurance Plan Project and its sequelae, 1963-1986,* Baltimore, 1988, Johns Hopkins University Press.
35. Tabar L, Fagerberg G, Duffy SW et al: The Swedish 2 county trial of mammographic screening for breast cancer: recent results and calculations of benefit, *J Epidemiol Community Health* 43(2):107-114, 1989.
36. Baines CJ, McFarlane DV, Miller AB: Sensitivity and specificity of the first screen mammography in 15 NBSS centers, *J Can Assoc Radiol* 39(4):273-276, 1988.
37. Pisano ED, Gatsonis C, Hendrick E et al: Diagnostic performance of digital versus film mammography for breast-cancer screening, *N Engl J Med* 353(17): 1773-1783, 2005.
38. Hylton N: Magnetic resonance imaging of the breast: opportunities to improve breast cancer management, *J Clin Oncol* 23(8):1678-1684, 2005.
39. Kline TS, Neal HS: Role of needle aspiration biopsy in diagnosis of carcinoma of the breast, *Obstet Gynecol* 46(1):89-92, 1975.
40. Lind DS, Minter R, Steinbach B et al: Stereotactic core biopsy reduces the re-excision rate and the cost of mammographically detected cancer, *J Surg Res* 78(1):23-26, 1998.
41. World Health Organization: The World Health Organization Histological Typing of Breast Tumors—Second Edition, *Am J Clin Pathol* 78(6):806-816, 1982.
42. Schnitt SJ, Guidi AJ: Pathology of invasive breast cancer. In Harris JR, Lippman ME, Morrow M, Osborne CK, editors: *Disease of the breast,* ed 3, Philadelphia, 2004, Lippincott Williams & Wilkins, pp 541-584.
43. National Comprehensive Cancer Network: *NCCN clinical practice guidelines: breast cancer,* V2.2006, Jenkintown, PA, 2006, National Comprehensive Cancer Network.
44. Fisher B, Dignam J, Wolmaker N et al: Lumpectomy and radiation therapy for the treatment of intraductal breast cancer: findings from the National Surgical Adjuvant Breast and Bowel Project B-17, *J Clin Onc* 16(2):441-452, 1998.
45. Haagensen CD, Lane N, Lattes R et al: Lobular neoplasia (so-called lobular carcinoma *in situ*) of the breast, *Cancer* 42(2):737-769, 1978.
46. Fisher B, Constantino J, Fisher B et al: Pathologic findings from the National Surgical Adjuvant Breast and Bowel Project (NSABP) Protocol B-17, *Cancer* 78(7): 1403-1416, 1996.
47. Fisher B, Jeong JH, Anderson S et al: Twenty-five-year follow-up of a randomized trial comparing radical mastectomy, total mastectomy, and total mastectomy followed by irradiation, *N Engl J Med* 347(8):567-575, 2002.
48. Veronesi U, Cascinelli N, Mariani L et al: Twenty-year follow-up of a randomized study comparing breast-conserving surgery with radical mastectomy for early breast cancer, *N Engl J Med* 347(16):1227-1232, 2002.
49. Morrow M, White J, Moughan J et al: Factors predicting the use of breast-conserving therapy in stage I and II breast carcinoma, *J Clin Oncol* 9(8):2254-2262, 2001.

50. Sarin R: Partial-breast treatment for early breast cancer: emergence of a new paradigm, *Nat Clin Pract Oncol* 2(1):40-47, 2005.
51. Fisher B, Redmond C, Poisson R et al: Eight-year results of a randomized clinical trial comparing total mastectomy and lumpectomy with or without irradiation in the treatment of breast cancer, *N Engl J Med* 320(13): 822-828, 1989.
52. Blichert-Toft M, Brinker H, Andersen JA et al: A Danish randomized trial comparing breast-preserving therapy with mastectomy in mammary carcinoma: preliminary results, *Acta Oncol* 27(6A):671-677, 1988.
53. Veronesi U, Banfi A, Salvadori B et al: Breast conservation is the treatment of choice in small breast cancer: long-term results of a randomized trial, *Eur J Cancer* 26(6): 668-670, 1990.
54. Sarrazin D, Le MG, Arriagada R et al: Ten-year results of a randomized trial comparing a conservative treatment to mastectomy in early breast cancer, *Radiother Oncol* 14(3):177-184, 1989.
55. Lichter AS, Fraass BA, Yanke B: Treatment techniques in the conservative management of breast cancer, *Semin Radiat Oncol* 2(2):94-106, 1992.
56. van Dongen JA, Bartelink H, Fentiman IS et al: Randomized clinical trial to assess the value of breast-conserving therapy in stage I and II breast cancer, EORTC 10801 trial, *J Natl Cancer Inst Monogr* 11:15-18, 1992.
57. Fisher B, Anderson S, Redmond CK et al: Reanalysis and results after 12 years of follow-up in a randomized clinical trial comparing total mastectomy with lumpectomy with or without irradiation in the treatment of breast cancer, *N Engl J Med* 333(22):1456-1461, 1995.
58. Harris JR, Hellman S: Natural history of breast cancer. In Harris JR, Lippman ME, Morrow M et al, editors: *Disease of the breast*, Philadelphia, 1996, Lippincott-Raven, pp 375-391.
59. Osuch JR: Surgical approaches to breast cancer, *LOWAC J* 1(suppl 1):22-28, 1999.
60. Dubey AK, Recht A, Come S et al: Why and how to combine chemotherapy and radiation therapy in breast cancer patients, *Recent Results Cancer Res* 152:247-254, 1998.
61. Ragaz J, Jackson SM, Le N et al: Adjuvant radiotherapy and chemotherapy in node-positive premenopausal women with breast cancer, *N Engl J Med* 337(14): 956-962, 1997.
62. Overgaard M, Hansen PS, Overgaard J et al: Postoperative radiotherapy in high-risk premenopausal women with breast cancer who receive adjuvant chemotherapy, *N Engl J Med* 337(14):949-955, 1997.
63. Early Breast Cancer Trialists' Collaborative Group: Effects of radiotherapy and surgery in early breast cancer: an overview of the randomized trials, *N Engl J Med* 333(22):1444-1455, 1995.
64. Hughes KS, Schnaper LA, Berry D et al: Lumpectomy plus tamoxifen with or without irradiation in women 70 years of age or older with early breast cancer, *N Engl J Med* 351(10):971-977, 2004.
65. Fisher B, Bryant J, Wolmark N et al: Effect of preoperative chemotherapy on the outcome of women with operable breast cancer, *J Clin Oncol* 16(8):2672-2685, 1998.
66. Barnavon Y, Wallack MK: Management of the pregnant patient with carcinoma of the breast, *Surg Gyn Obstet* 171(4):347-352, 1990.
67. Hladiuk M, Huchcroft S, Temple W et al: Arm function after axillary dissection for breast cancer: a pilot study to provide parameter estimates, *J Surg Oncol* 50(1):47-52, 1992.
68. Keramopoulos A, Tsionou C, Minaretzis D et al: Arm morbidity following treatment of breast cancer with total axillary dissection: a multivariate approach, *Oncology* 50(6): 445-449, 1993.
69. Kuehn T, Klauss W, Darsow M et al. Long-term morbidity following axillary dissection in breast cancer patients. Clinical assessment, significance for life quality and impact of demographic, oncologic and therapeutic factors. *Breast Cancer Res Treat* 64(3): 275-286, 2000.
70. Maunsell E, Brisson J, Deschenes L: Arm problems and psychological distress after surgery for breast cancer, *Can J Surg* 36(4):315-320, 1993.
71. Tasmuth T, von Smitten K, Hietanen P et al: Pain and other symptoms after different treatment modalities of breast cancer, *Ann Oncol* 6(5):453-459, 1995.
72. Kuehn T, Klauss W, Darsow M et al: Long-term morbidity following axillary dissection in breast cancer patients: clinical assessment, significance for life quality and impact of demographic, oncologic and therapeutic factors, *Breast Cancer Res Treat* 64(3):275-286, 2000.
73. Woo B, Dibble SL, Piper BF et al: Differences in fatigue by treatment methods in women with breast cancer, *Oncol Nurs Forum* 25(5):915-920, 1998.
74. Irvine DM, Vincent L, Graydon JE et al: Fatigue in women with breast cancer receiving radiation therapy, *Cancer Nurs* 21(2):127-135, 1998.
75. Turesson I, Nyman J, Holmberg E et al: Prognostic factors for acute and late skin reactions in radiotherapy patients, *Int J Radiat Oncol Biol Phys* 36(5):1065-1067, 1996.
76. Moody AM, Mayles WP, Bliss JM et al: The influence of breast size on late radiation effects and association with radiotherapy dose inhomogeneity, *Radiother Oncol* 33(2):106-112, 1994.
77. Hardy JR, Baum M: Lymphoedema—prevention rather than cure, *Ann Oncol* 2(8):532-533, 1991.
78. Segerstrom K, Bjerle P, Graffman S et al: Factors that influence the incidence of brachial oedema after treatment of breast cancer, *Scand J Plast Reconstr Surg Hand Surg* 26(2):223-227, 1992.
79. Twycross RG, Lack SA: *Therapeutics in terminal cancer*, ed 2, Edinburgh, 1990, Churchill Livingstone.
80. Lerner R: Complete decongestive physiotherapy and the Lerner Lymphedema Services Academy of Lymphatic Studies, *Cancer* 83:2861-2863, 1998.
81. Boris M, Weindorf S, Lasinkski S: Persistence of lymphedema reduction after noninvasive complex lymphedema therapy, *Oncology* 11(1):99-109, 1997.
82. Kramer BA, Arthur DW, Ulin K et al: Cosmetic outcome in patients receiving interstitial implant as part of breast-conservation therapy, *Radiology* 213(1):61-66, 1999.
83. Vrieling C, Collette L, Fourquet A et al: The influence of the boost in breast-conserving therapy on cosmetic outcome in the EORTC "boost versus no boost" trial: EORTC Radiotherapy and Breast Cancer Cooperative Groups, European Organization for Research and

Treatment of Cancer, *Int J Radiat Oncol Biol Phys* 45(3): 677-685, 1999.
84. Krishnamurthy R, Whitman GJ, Stelling CB et al: Mammographic findings after breast conservation therapy, *Radiographics* 19 Spec No:S53-S62, 1999.
85. Holli K, Saaristo R, Isola J et al: Effect of radiotherapy on the interpretation of routine follow-up mammography after conservative breast surgery: a randomized study, *Br J Cancer* 78(4):542-545, 1998.
86. Svensson H, Westling P, Larsson LG: Radiation-induced lesions of the brachial plexus correlated to the time-dose-fraction schedule, *Acta Radiol Ther Phys Biol* 14(3): 228-238, 1975.
87. Thomas JE, Colby MY: Radiation-induced or metastatic brachial plexopathy? A diagnostic dilemma, *JAMA* 222:1392-1395, 1972.
88. Kori SH, Foley KM, Posner LR: Brachial plexus lesions in patients with cancer: 100 cases, *Neurology* 31(1):45-50, 1981.
89. Ganel A, Engel J, Sela M et al: Nerve entrapments associated with postmastectomy lymphedema, *Cancer* 44(6):2254-2259, 1979.
90. Mendenhall NP, Fletcher GH, Million RR: Adjuvant radiation therapy following modified radical or radical mastectomy. In Bland KI, Copeland EM, editors: *The breast: comprehensive management of benign and malignant diseases*, Philadelphia, 1987, WB Saunders, pp 770-780.
91. Overgaard M: Spontaneous radiation-induced rib fractures in breast cancer patients treated with postmastectomy irradiation: a clinical radiobiological analysis of the influence of fraction size and dose-response relationships on late bone damage, *Acta Oncol* 27(2):117-122, 1988.
92. Gyenes G, Rutqvist LE, Liedberg A et al: Long-term cardiac morbidity and mortality in a randomized trial of pre- and postoperative radiation therapy versus surgery alone in primary breast cancer, *Radiother Oncol* 48(2):185-190, 1998.
93. Sugden EM, Rezvani M, Harrison JM et al: Shoulder movement after the treatment of early stage breast cancer, *Clin Oncol* 10(3):173-181, 1998.
94. Hack TF, Cohen L, Katz J et al: Physical and psychological morbidity after axillary lymph node dissection for breast cancer, *J Clin Oncol* 17(1):143-149, 1999.
95. Wingate L, Croghan I, Natarajan N et al: Rehabilitation of the mastectomy patient: a randomized, blind, prospective study, *Arch Phys Med Rehabil* 70(1):21-24, 1989.
96. Lamont JA: Sexuality. In Stewart SE, Robinson GE, editors: *A clinician's guide to menopause,* London, 1997, Health Press International, pp 63-76.
97. Smith TJ, Davidson NE, Schapira DV et al: American Society of Clinical Oncology 1998 update of recommended breast cancer surveillance guidelines, *J Clin Oncol* 17(3): 1080-1082, 1999.
98. Ries LAG, Eisner MP, Kosary CL et al, editors: *SEER Cancer Statistics Review, 1975-2002*, Bethesda, MD, 2004, National Cancer Institute.
99. Craig TJ, Comstock GW, Geiser PB: The quality of survival in breast cancer: a case-control comparison, *Cancer* 33(5):1451-1457, 1974.
100. Woods N, Earp JL: Women with cured breast cancer: a study of mastectomy patients in North Carolina, *Nurs Res* 27(5):279-285, 1978.
101. Ganz PA, Coscarelli A, Fred C et al: Breast cancer survivors: psychosocial concerns and quality of life, *Breast Cancer Res Treat* 38(2):183-199, 1996.

Chapter 10
Gastrointestinal Cancers

Jean C. Holland

Cancers of the gastrointestinal (GI) system account for an estimated 263,060 cases in the United States, with an estimated 136,180 deaths in 2006.[1] These cancers include cancers of the esophagus, stomach, small intestine, colon and rectum, anus, liver and bile duct, gallbladder, pancreas, and other digestive organs.[1] Cancer of the colon and rectum are the third most frequent cause of death in males, after lung and prostate cancers and in females after lung and breast cancers. The incidence and deaths of specific cancers are listed in Table 10-1. Cancers of the esophagus, stomach, pancreas, colon, rectum, and anus are discussed in this chapter.

ANATOMY AND PATHOPHYSIOLOGY OF THE GASTROINTESTINAL TRACT

The GI tract (Figure 10-1) extends from the esophagus through the anus, having the main functions of mechanically and chemically breaking down food and absorbing the nutrients. The esophagus extends about 23 cm to 25 cm from the pharynx to the gastroesophageal junction. It is in close proximity to the thoracic viscera, allowing dissemination of tumors of the esophagus into the posterior mediastinum.[2] The esophagus controls the movement of food from the pharynx to the stomach. The esophageal mucosa is composed of squamous epithelium, which affords protection from trauma, and a thick muscularis mucosa with mucous glands, which secrete mucus that aids in the passage of food. The lumen is surrounded by muscle; the upper third contains striated muscle, and the distal two thirds contain smooth muscle, as in the rest of the GI tract.[2,3]

The stomach breaks down food by mechanical and chemical mechanisms. It extends from left of the midline superiorly, where it joins with the esophagus, to the right of the midline inferiorly at the duodenum.[2] The mucosa is covered by glandular epithelium and is comprised of four anatomic regions as follows: Adjacent to the esophagus is (1) the cardia, which contains mucous secreting glands; (2) the fundus and (3) the body form the majority of the stomach, which secrete hydrochloric acid, pepsin, mucus, and intrinsic factor; (4) the pylorus/antrum region secretes mucus, gastrin, pepsin, somatostatin (which inhibits secretion of insulin and gastrin), and serotonin. The stomach contains three layers of involuntary muscles that physically break up food particles.

The pancreas is about 15 cm long in adults and consists of a head, body, and tail. The tail stretches to just in front of the spleen.[2] The pancreas is composed of exocrine and endocrine components. Most of the pancreas is made up of the exocrine segment, which produces and secretes the digestive enzymes lipases, peptidases, and amylases, which digest fats, proteins, and carbohydrates. The secretions are hormonally regulated, as is the discharge of bile from the gallbladder. The endocrine cells are located in the islets of Langerhans, which produce hormones, mainly insulin, glucaton, and somatostatin.[2,3]

The small intestine in adults is approximately 6 meters in length. The first section is the duodenum, which is located retroperitoneal and near the head of the pancreas. In this area, acid is neutralized and further digestion takes place. The jejunum is at the entry into the peritoneal cavity, the ileum enters the colon at the ileocecal valve. The mucosa is folded and consists of villi covered by epithelial lining cells, providing a large surface area available for absorption. Between the villi are crypts. Each villus has its own blood supply. Blood containing the digestive products goes to the liver via the hepatic portal system. The small intestine contains mucin-secreting cells, endocrine cells, and antimicrobial proteins.[2,3] A double muscle layer provides peristalsis.

The colon is divided into the cecum, the ascending, transverse, and descending colon. The right colon is subdivided into the cecum, peritoneally

Table 10-1 GI Cancers: Estimated Incidence and Mortality in the United States, 2006

Site	Estimated new cases	Estimated deaths
Colon*	106,680	55,170
Rectum	41,930	
Pancreas	33,730	32,300
Stomach	22,280	11,430
Liver, intrahepatic bile duct	18,510	16,200
Esophagus	14,550	13,770
Gallbladder, other biliary	8,570	3,260
Small intestine	6,170	1,070
Other digestive organs	5,980	2,320
Anus, anal canal, anorectum	4,660	660
Total digestive system	**263,060**	**136,180**

From American Cancer Society: *Cancer facts and figures 2006,* Atlanta, 2006, American Cancer Society.
*Estimated deaths from colon and rectal cancers are combined.
GI, Gastrointestinal.

located and about 6 cm to 9 cm long. The ascending colon is located retroperitoneally and is about 15 to 20 cm long. The descending colon is located retroperitoneally and is 10 cm to 15 cm long. The descending colon becomes the sigmoid colon at the origin of the mesosigmoid, and the sigmoid colon becomes the rectum at the termination of the mesosigmoid. The rectum is the distal large intestine beginning opposite the sacral promontory and ending at the anal canal. The mucosa of the large intestine contain tightly packed tubular glands and cells that absorb water, goblet cells that secrete mucus to aid in passage of feces, and lymphoid tissue (Peyer's patches) that provides local immunologic protection.[2,4,5]

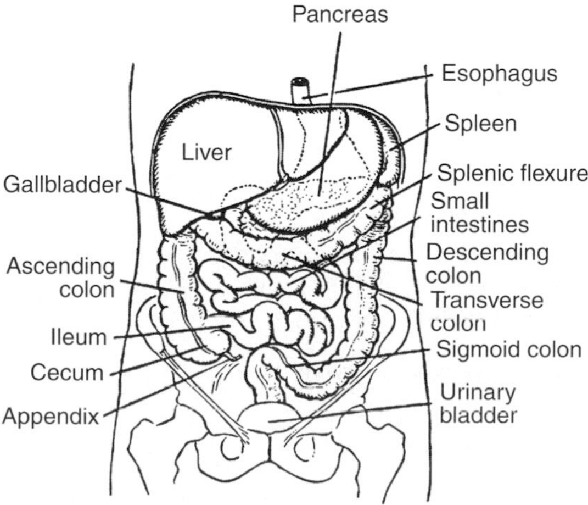

Figure 10-1 Structures of the Gastrointestinal Tract.

ESOPHAGEAL CANCER

Esophageal cancer, the eighth most common cancer worldwide, consists of two main types: squamous cell cancer, which is most prevalent in the developing world, and adenocarcinoma, which is more common in developed countries.[6] In the United States, the use of tobacco, moderate-to-heavy alcohol ingestion, infrequent consumption of raw fruits and vegetables, and low income account for most of the squamous cell cancers.[7] Patients with squamous cell carcinoma of the esophagus often have a history of prior head and neck carcinoma.[8] Declines in smoking and drinking and increased intake of fruits and vegetables may account for the declining incidence of squamous cell esophageal cancer in the United States.[7] The incidence of adenocarcinoma of the esophagus has increased 350% in the Western world.[9] Male gender and Caucasian race are risk factors.[10] Barrett's esophagus (also known as *Barrett's syndrome*), gastroesophageal reflux, and hiatal hernia are often associated with adenocarcinoma of the esophagus.[8] Barrett's metaplasia develops in 6% to 14% of individuals with gastroesophageal reflux. Approximately 0.5% to 1% of patients with Barrett's will develop adenocarcinoma. Obesity, which may be linked to the predisposition of reflux in these individuals, and smoking are weak risk factors.[10]

Clinical Manifestations

The most common presenting symptoms of esophageal cancer are dysphagia, weight loss, and pain. The dysphagia is typically progressive; the patient may have complete obstruction. Other symptoms may present as a result of complications of the tumor: cough or fever from a fistula, bleeding, hoarseness from laryngeal nerve involvement, or hiccups from phrenic nerve involvement. Malignant lymph nodes may be palpable in the supraclavicular fossa or axilla.[11]

Diagnostic Studies

Newly diagnosed patients should have an endoscopy of the entire upper GI tract. If the upper GI tract cannot be visualized, a double-contrast barium study of the upper GI tract should be done. A computed tomography (CT) scan of the chest and abdomen should be performed. If the carcinoma is located at or above the carina, bronchoscopy, including biopsy of any abnormality and cytology should be performed. If there is no evidence of metastatic disease, endoscopic ultrasonography (EUS) with fine-needle aspiration (FNA) if indicated, is recommended. EUS can provide nodal staging of esophageal cancer, and it can diagnose liver metastases. Positron-emission tomography (PET) scans may be useful. Additional tests are recommended for patients with locoregional disease. These may include pulmonary function studies, cardiac testing, and nutritional assessment. Laboratory studies include complete blood count, serum chemistry analysis, and coagulation studies.[8]

Pathology and Pattern of Metastasis

The American Joint Committee on Cancer (AJCC) TNM staging is used for esophageal cancer, (Table 10-2). At diagnosis, nearly 50% of patients have disease that extends beyond the definition of locoregional disease. Of those with locoregional disease, less than 60% can undergo curative resection. Nearly 70% to 80% of resected specimens have disease in the regional lymph nodes.[12] Patients whose tumors have a center that is 5 cm proximal or distal to the cardia are classified as having adenocarcinomas of the esophagogastric junction. These tumors are divided into type I, which infiltrates the gastroesophageal (GE) junction from above; type II, which arises from the GE junction, and type III, which infiltrates the GE junction from below.[13] Lymph nodes that may be involved include cervical, mediastinal, and celiac, as well as remote lymph nodes. The most common sites of distant metastases are the celiac lymph nodes and the liver. The brain, lung, bone, diaphragm, and adrenal glands are also sites of esophageal cancer that has spread.[14]

Definitive Treatment

Patients with stage I or II disease and who are candidates for resection have two options to consider: (1) surgery or (2) chemotherapy. Chemoradiotherapy is the preferred modality for cervical esophageal carcinoma, which requires more extensive surgery,[15] whereas esophagectomy is preferred for noncervical T1 disease.[6] Factors considered when selecting patients for surgery include patient status in regard to the ability to resect the cancer and the extent of disease. The surgical approach depends on several variables, including the following[16]:

- Location of the primary tumor
- Overall health status of the patient
- Extent of nodal resection
- Previous radiation and/or chemotherapy
- Prior thoracic surgery

Survival rates postoperatively depend on the stage of the disease. Stage I disease survival is approximately 60% to 70%, whereas those with stage III have only a 5% to 10% rate of survival.[15]

Postoperative chemoradiation is recommended for patients with lymph node involvement at the time of surgery.[15] Box 10-1 outlines chemotherapy agents

Box 10-1 Chemotherapy Agents Currently Used in Treatment of Esophageal Cancer

ESTABLISHED AGENTS

5-FU
Mitomycin
Bleomycin
Methotrexate
Mitoguazone
Doxorubicin
Vindesine

NEWER AGENTS

Paclitaxel
Docetaxel
Vinorelbine

COMBINATION AGENTS

Oxaliplatin, 5-FU
5-FU, cisplatin
Paclitaxel, 5-FU
Irinotecan, cisplatin

5-FU, 5-Fluorouracil.

Table 10-2 AJCC Staging of Esophageal Cancer

NCCN® Practice Guidelines in Oncology – v.1.2006

Esophageal Cancer

Staging

Table 1

American Joint Committee on Cancer (AJCC) TNM Classification of Carcinoma of the Esophagus*

Primary Tumor (T)

TX	Primary tumor cannot be assessed
T0	No evidence of primary tumor
Tis	Carcinoma in situ
T1	Tumor invades lamina propria or submucosa
T2	Tumor invades muscularis propria
T3	Tumor invades adventitia
T4	Tumor invades adjacent structures

Regional Lymph Nodes (N)

NX	Regional lymph nodes cannot be assessed
N0	No regional lymph node metastasis
N1	Regional lymph node metastasis

Distant metastasis (M)

MX	Distant metastasis cannot be assessed
M0	No distant metastasis
M1	Distant metastasis

Tumors of the lower thoracic esophagus:

M1a	Metastasis in celiac lymph nodes
M1b	Other distant metastasis

Tumors of the midthoracic esophagus:

M1a	Not applicable
M1b	Nonregional lymph nodes and/or other distant metastasis

Tumors of the upper thoracic esophagus:

M1a	Metastasis in cervical nodes
M1b	Other distant metastasis

Stage Grouping

Stage 0	Tis	N0	M0
Stage I	T1	N0	M0
Stage IIA	T2	N0	M0
	T3	N0	M0
Stage IIB	T1	N1	M0
	T2	N1	M0
Stage III	T3	N1	M0
	T4	Any N	M0
Stage IV	Any T	Any N	M1
Stage IVA	Any T	Any N	M1a
Stage IVB	Any T	Any N	M1b

Histologic Grade (G)

GX	Grade cannot be assessed
G1	Well differentiated
G2	Moderately differentiated
G3	Poorly differentiated
G4	Undifferentiated

*Used with permission of the American Joint Committee on Cancer (AJCC), Chicago, Illinois. The original and primary source for this information is the *AJCC Cancer Staging Manual*, Sixth Edition (2002) published by Springer-New York. (For more information, visit www.cancerstaging.net.) Any citation or quotation of this material must be credited to the AJCC as its primary source. The inclusion of this information herein does not authorize any reuse or further distribution without the expressed written permission of Springer-New York on behalf of the AJCC.

Modified from National Comprehensive Cancer Network (NCCN) Guidelines (website): www.nccn.org/professionals/physician_gls/PDF/anal.pdf. Used with the permission of the American Joint Committee on Cancer (AJCC), Chicago, Illinois. The original source is the *AJCC Cancer Staging Handbook, Sixth Edition* (2002), published by Springer-New York, www.springeronline.com.

used in treatment of esophageal cancer. Patients with stage IIA (T2, N0) disease may opt to be observed after surgery or receive chemotherapy/radiation. Patients considered to be at high risk are those with disease of the lower esophagus or GE junction, poorly differentiated histology, lymphovascular or neurovascular invasion, and young patients. Patients with adenocarcinoma of the distal esophagus or GE junction should receive postoperative adjuvant chemotherapy and radiation therapy.[8] Chemoradiotherapy includes 50 Gy to 50.4 Gy of radiation, plus concurrent chemotherapy with 5-fluorouracil (5-FU) plus cisplatin.[8] Concurrent chemoradiation is an alternative treatment to surgery. Patients who experience a complete response after chemoradiation can undergo an esophagectomy. This may be done with adenocarcinoma of the distal esophagus or GE junction, adenocarcinoma of the proximal or midesophagus, or any squamous cancer. In patients with a partial response, esophagectomy or palliative treatment is offered.[8] Radiation sensitivity and systemic disease is addressed by giving chemotherapy and radiation together.

Radiation Techniques

External-beam radiation therapy is usually given through ports that encompass the primary tumor with a 5-cm margin, proximally and distally, and provide a 3-cm to 5-cm margin in width to cover periesophageal lymph nodes. Irradiation is performed with anterior/posterior (A/P), posterior/anterior (P/A), lateral opposed fields, or with a four-field technique. Doses of 40 Gy to 70 Gy are given, with the spinal cord limited to 40 Gy to 45 Gy.[17] Intraluminal brachytherapy allows a high dose of radiation to the tumor while protecting the surrounding structures. Brachytherapy has been used as primary therapy and as a boost after external-beam radiation therapy. It can be delivered at high or low dose rates.

Palliative Treatment

Patients with unresectable, medically inoperable or metastatic cancer of the esophagus may be offered chemotherapy or supportive care.[8] Chemotherapy regimens may consist of 5-FU, cisplatin, or a taxane-based chemotherapy outside of a clinical trial.[8] Clinical trials of targeted therapies are currently being conducted for this disease state. In the community, 60% of patients will be treated with palliative therapy alone.[14] Relief of obstruction may be obtained with use of stenting, laser treatment, photodynamic therapy, external radiation or brachytherapy. Other endoscopic palliative methods to overcome dysphagia include balloon dilation, injection of alcohol or chemotherapeutic agents, and placement of a plastic or expandable metal prosthesis.[8] Relief of dysphagia may improve nutritional status, the feeling of well-being, and improved overall quality of life.

GASTRIC CANCER

Gastric cancer is the third most common GI cancer in the United States and the second most common worldwide.[18] Gastric cancer is the second leading cause of cancer death worldwide.[19] In recent years the incidence of gastric cancer has been reduced in the United States and globally as well,[20] possibly related to better refrigeration; reduced consumption of salted, smoked, and chemically preserved foods; an increased intake of fruits and vegetables; improved living standards; and a greater use of antibiotics with the subsequent reduction of *Helicobacter pylori* infection.[19] Studies support that the intake of dark green and yellow vegetables protects against adenocarcinoma of the distal stomach.[21,22] This decline in gastric cancer reflects a decrease in cancers in the distal stomach (body and antrum). Cancers of the proximal stomach and GE junction are increasing and are more common among higher socioeconomic classes.[20,23] Other risk factors for gastric cancer include age, sex, family history, inflammatory processes such as chronic atrophic gastritis with intestinal metaplasia, *H. pylori,* post-subtotal gastrectomy, gastric polyps, pernicious anemia, and Barrett's esophagus for gastric cancers arising in the proximal stomach.[18,24-26]

Clinical Manifestations

In the United States, most patients with gastric cancer present with advanced disease.[18,19] Weight loss and abdominal pain are the most common symptoms at initial diagnosis.[27] Weight loss is usually the result of anorexia, nausea, early satiety, dysphagia, or pain. The pain may be epigastric, substernal, or referred to the back. Relief of the pain may be obtained by taking antacids, H_2-receptor antagonists, proton pump inhibitors, or food. In some patients the pain is worse after eating. Anorexia and vomiting are associated with distal cancers causing pyloric obstruction. Dysphagia is a common symptom, with cancers arising in the gastric cardia or the GE junction. Acute and chronic GI bleeding may occur. Weakness and fatigue may be related to poor nutritional intake, and anemia is common. A palpable abdominal mass indicates advanced disease. Lymph nodes may be palpable in the left supraclavicular area and left neck.[18] Symptoms of the spread of gastric cancer may include jaundice, ascites, a rectal mass, and umbilical nodules. Metastases to the ovaries can occur.[18]

Diagnostic Studies

Upper GI endoscopy is the best overall method for diagnosing gastric cancer.[28] Any suspicious–appearing gastric ulcer should be biopsied. Biopsies from benign-appearing ulcers may afford early diagnosis. Barium upper GI series has a low sensitivity for diagnosing gastric cancer and may be as low as 14%.[29] CT scanning is used to evaluate gastric wall thickness, direct extension of tumor into adjacent organs, lymph node enlargement, ascites, and liver metastases.[30] EUS can show images of the gastric wall and its five layers, the degree of invasion, and regional lymph nodes, allowing an accurate assessment of tumor invasion.[31,32] Laparoscopic evaluation of the peritoneal cavity and liver may be used to assess for metastatic disease.[31] Additional studies include chest x ray, a complete blood count, serum chemistry analysis, coagulation studies, and in women, a pelvic CT scan or ultrasound.[33]

Pathology and Patterns of Metastasis

Adenocarcinoma accounts for approximately 95% of all gastric cancer. The AJCC TNM staging system is the system used in countries in the Western hemisphere,[33] as outlined in Table 10-3. At diagnosis, approximately 50% of patients have disease that extends beyond the locoregional area. Approximately 50% of patients with locoregional disease are unable to undergo a curative resection in Western countries.[34,35] Nearly 70% to 80% of resected gastric carcinoma specimens have metastases in the regional lymph nodes.[33] Early gastric carcinoma is defined as an invasive adenocarcinoma confined to the mucosa or submucosa with or without lymph node metastasis and has a favorable prognosis.[36] Gastric tumors that are bulky, involve the cardia, or have obviously spread to local lymph nodes on initial staging studies are considered to be locally advanced and unresectable. Poor prognostic factors include poor performance status, liver metastases, peritoneal metastases, and an alkaline phosphatase level above 100 units/L.[37] Proximal lesions are biologically more aggressive and have a worse prognosis.[27] Gastric cancers can spread by direct extension to the lesser and greater omentum, liver, diaphragm, spleen, pancreas, and transverse colon. Another mode of metastasis is through hematogenous spread to liver, lung, bone, brain, and peritoneal metastases.[38] Local, regional, and distant lymph node metastases can also occur.

Definitive Treatment

For gastric cancer, gastrectomy is the most widely used treatment approach. Total gastrectomy is usually performed for lesions in the upper third of the stomach and subtotal gastrectomy for lesions in the lower two-thirds.[39] A 5-cm margin is required. Fifteen or more lymph nodes should be obtained and examined.[33] After a gastrectomy, a Billroth I gastroduodenostomy or Billroth II gastrojejunostomy are performed for purposes of reconstruction.[38] Resection of extragastric organs may be required to control T4 disease.[38] Endoscopic mucosal resection (EMR) and laparoscopic wedge resection have been applied for treatment of early gastric cancer (T1, mucosal and submucosal). Indications for these modalities are well differentiated or moderately differentiated histology, tumor size less than 30 mm, absence of ulceration, and no evidence of invasive findings.[40] However, long-term and survival data are lacking for these procedures.[33]

Moderate-dose radiation therapy combined with 5-fluorouracil (5-FU) improves survival.[33] Neoadjuvant treatment may be done to convert an initially unresectable tumor to resectable status or may be used in advanced but resectable disease.[38] Preoperative induction chemotherapy, followed by chemoradiotherapy, is an approach that has some preliminary findings of increased survival time.[41,42] Because the 5-year survival rate after resection for cure is only between 30% and 40%,[38] adjuvant therapy is indicated. Patients for whom adjuvant treatment is recommended include those with stage IB (T2, N0) disease with risk features such as poorly differentiated or higher-grade cancer, lymphovascular and/or neural invasion, or patients younger than age 50. Patients who have negative margins but have a T3 or T4 cancer with positive nodes, as well as patients who have positive margins, should be offered adjuvant therapy. Adjuvant chemoradiotherapy has been shown to decrease

Table 10-3 AJCC Staging of Gastric Cancer

NCCN® Practice Guidelines in Oncology – v.1.2006

Gastric Cancer

Staging

Table 1

American Joint Committee on Cancer (AJCC) TNM Staging Classification for Carcinoma of the Stomach*

Primary Tumor (T)

TX	Primary tumor cannot be assessed
T0	No evidence of primary tumor
Tis	Carcinoma in situ: intraepithelial tumor without invasion of the lamina propria
T1	Tumor invades lamina propria or submucosa
T2	Tumor invades muscularis propria or subserosa†
T2a	Tumor invades muscularis propria
T2b	Tumor invades subserosa
T3	Tumor penetrates serosa (visceral peritoneum) without invasion of adjacent structures‡
T4	Tumor invades adjacent structures‡

Regional Lymph Nodes (N)

NX	Regional lymph node(s) cannot be assessed
N0	No regional lymph node metastasis§
N1	Metastasis in 1 to 6 regional lymph nodes
N2	Metastasis in 7 to 15 regional lymph nodes
N3	Metastasis in more than 15 regional lymph nodes

Distant Metastasis (M)

MX	Distant metastasis cannot be assessed
M0	No distant metastasis
M1	Distant metastasis

Histologic Grade (G)

GX	Grade cannot be assessed
G1	Well differentiated
G2	Moderately differentiated
G3	Poorly differentiated
G4	Undifferentiated

Stage Grouping

Stage 0	Tis	N0	M0
Stage IA	T1	N0	M0
Stage IB	T1	N1	M0
	T2a/b	N0	M0
Stage II	T1	N2	M0
	T2a/b	N1	M0
	T3	N0	M0
Stage IIIA	T2a/b	N2	M0
	T3	N1	M0
	T4	N0	M0
Stage IIIB	T3	N2	M0
Stage IV	T4	N1–3	M0
	T1–3	N3	M0
	Any T	Any N	M1

*Used with permission of the American Joint Committee on Cancer (AJCC), Chicago, Illinois. The original and primary source for this information is the *AJCC Cancer Staging Manual, Sixth Edition* (2002) published by Springer-New York. (For more information, visit www.cancerstaging.net.) Any citation or quotation of this material must be credited to the AJCC as its primary source. The inclusion of this information herein does not authorize any reuse or further distribution without the expressed written permission of Springer-New York on behalf of the AJCC.

†A tumor may penetrate the muscularis propria with extension into the gastrocolic or gastrohepatic ligaments, or into the greater or lesser omentum, without perforation of the visceral peritoneum covering these structures. In this case, the tumor is classified as T2. If there is perforation of the visceral peritoneum covering the gastric ligaments or the omentum, the tumor should be classified as T3.

‡The adjacent structures of the stomach include the spleen, transverse colon, liver, diaphragm, pancreas, abdominal wall, adrenal gland, kidney, small intestine, and retroperitoneum. Intramural extension to the duodenum or esophagus is classified by the depth of the greatest invasion in any of these sites, including the stomach.

§A designation of pN0 should be used if all examined lymph nodes are negative, regardless of the total number removed and examined.

Modified from National Comprehensive Cancer Network (NCCN) Guidelines (website): www.nccn.org/professionals/physician_gls/PDF/anal.pdf. Used with the permission of the American Joint Committee on Cancer (AJCC), Chicago, Illinois. The original source is the *AJCC Cancer Staging Handbook, Sixth Edition* (2002), published by Springer-New York, www.springeronline.com.

local failure, increase median survival, and even increase overall survival in some trials.[43,44] Radiation therapy, 45 Gy to 50.4 Gy, and treatment regimens consisting of a 5-FU–based radiosensitizer with or without leucovorin is recommended.[33] For patients with macroscopic disease after resection, chemoradiotherapy with 5-FU–based chemotherapy, chemotherapy alone, or supportive care are recommended.[33] Box 10-2 outlines chemotherapy used for gastric cancer.

Radiation Techniques

The radiation dose for gastric cancer is usually limited to 45 Gy. The critical organs to be considered when planning radiation therapy include the remaining stomach, liver, kidneys, small intestine, spinal cord, skin, and bone marrow. A multiple field technique allows for less small bowel in the field, though it may not always be advantageous if the tumor location will not spare the kidney or liver. Three-dimensional treatment planning helps to determine whether an AP/PA or multiple-field technique should be used.[45]

Box 10-2 Chemotherapy Agents Used for Gastric Cancer

SINGLE AGENT

5-FU
Mitomycin
Etoposide
Cisplatin
Paclitaxel
Docetaxel
Irinotecan

COMBINATION THERAPY

Combination therapy is more effective than a single agent. No combination is superior at this time.
FAM (5-FU, doxorubicin, mitomycin)
FAMTX (5-FU, adriamycin, methotrexate with leucovorin)
ECF (epirubicin, cisplatin, 5-FU)
ELF (etoposide, leucovorin, 5-FU)
UFT (uracil, tegafur)

NEW CATEGORIES OF AGENTS UNDER STUDY

Vaccines
Antireceptor agents
Antiangiogenic agents

5-FU, 5-Fluorouracil.

Palliative Treatment

The majority of patients with gastric adenocarcinoma will develop metastases at some point. Patients with advanced gastric cancer may require palliation for symptoms such as nausea, pain, bleeding, and obstruction. Tumors that are bulky, involve the cardia, or have obviously spread to local lymph nodes on initial staging studies, are considered unresectable.[45] Palliative treatment of local disease may include surgery, stent placement, laser surgery, photodynamic therapy, or radiation therapy to relieve obstruction. Palliative gastrectomy can provide symptomatic relief and prolong life.[46] External-beam radiation therapy is beneficial in the control of pain, bleeding, or obstruction. Chemotherapy enhances quality of life and prolongs survival when compared with best supportive care. Epirubicin plus cisplatin and 5-FU (ECF) probably has the strongest claim in treatment of advanced gastric cancer.[47] Chemotherapy for metastatic disease may include cisplatin or oxaliplatin, 5-FU, taxane, or irinotecan-based combination treatment.[33] Capecitabine has been shown to have a significant response in patients with advanced gastric cancer.[48,49] When indicated, enrollment in a clinical trial may offer the best available treatment option. Supportive care should be offered when a patient has a Karnofsky score less than 60 or an Eastern Cooperative Oncology Group (ECOG) score greater than 2.

PANCREATIC CANCER

Worldwide, more than 200,000 people die of pancreatic cancer each year. The incidence and mortality rate are highest in developed countries. Ductal adenocarcinoma accounts for 90% of pancreatic cancers. It is an increasing public health problem. In the United States, it is the fourth leading cause of cancer death. Pancreatic incidence and death rates are almost equal because of the high fatality rates.[50] The poor survival is the result of late diagnosis and low resection rates.[51] The incidence increases with advancing age and is rare before age 45. The incidence is highest in men and African Americans.[52] Environmental risk factors include tobacco smoking, exposure to the aromatic amines present in tobacco, and occupations such as petrochemical work, hairdressing, and working with rubber.[53] Other potential risk factors are obesity, inactivity, glucose intolerance, and hyperinsulinemia.[50,54] Chronic pancreatitis has been associated with pancreatic cancer, particularly in hereditary pancreatic cancer.[55] Relatives of patients with pancreatic cancer are at increased risk, especially those with at least three first-degree relatives who have been diagnosed.[56] Families with atypical multiple-mole melanoma and family history of ataxia-telangiectasia are at much higher risk,[57] and an increased risk has been identified in families with BRCA-2 mutations.[58] Diabetes mellitus may precede the appearance of pancreatic cancer, especially if it occurs during or beyond the sixth decade.[59] A diet with adequate quantities of fruits and vegetables and control of calories may help to prevent this cancer.[60]

Clinical Manifestations

Symptoms of pancreatic cancer usually occur late in the disease. Pain is the most common symptom, occurring in 80% of patients with late-stage disease. Painless jaundice is the most common symptom in potentially resectable disease[61] and occurs in about one-half of patients with advanced disease.[62] Weight loss may be severe and associated with anorexia, early satiety, diarrhea, or steatorrhea. Nausea and depression also may be present.[63] Tumors in the pancreatic body or tail usually present with pain and weight loss, and those in the head of the pancreas present with steatorrhea, weight loss, and jaundice.[64]

Diagnostic Studies

Several imaging studies are available. Spiral or helical CT scans provide definition of the tumor and surrounding structures and may be the only imaging study needed for advanced pancreatic cancer.[61] Other studies useful in visualizing the cancer are transabdominal ultrasonography, EUS, and endoscopic retrograde cholangiopancreatography (ERCP). Pancreatic ductal brushings or biopsies can be obtained at the time of ERCP. Laparoscopy can identify peritoneal implants or metastatic disease on the liver. A histologic diagnosis can be made using FNA biopsy.[63] PET scans may be useful in differentiating benign from malignant disease.[62] The tumor marker CA 19-9, although not tumor specific, may be useful in differentiating pancreatic adenocarcinoma from inflammatory conditions of the pancreas.[63]

Pathology and Patterns of Metastases

The AJCC has developed the TNM staging system for pancreatic cancer (Table 10-4). In addition, most clinical centers consider a staging system that is based on whether the disease is resectable or borderline resectable; locally advanced; or disseminated.[63] About two-thirds of ductal adenocarcinomas arise in the head of the pancreas, with the remainder in the body and tail. Metastases to regional nodes and the liver occur before distant metastases, which is usually to the lung. Local extension occurs along lymphatics and nerves in the region of the superior mesenteric artery. Direct extension into the walls of the portal vein and superior mesenteric artery may be present.[65]

Definitive Treatment

Surgical resection, which is resection of the tumor and the surrounding pancreatic tissue, is the only potentially curative treatment. Tumors of the body and tail are not commonly resectable, because symptoms usually do not occur until late in the disease.[63] Surgery for these patients is distal, extended distal, or total pancreatectomy. Patients with tumors of the head and body are treated with pancreaticduodenectomy (PD), the Whipple procedure. This involves resection of the distal third of the stomach, gallbladder, bile duct, duodenum and proximal 10 cm of jejunum, and the head of the pancreas and some of its neck, body, and surrounding lymph nodes. To alleviate symptoms of pruritus and cholangitis, preoperative biliary drainage for patients with obstructive jaundice may be done if surgery will be delayed.[63] Pylorus-preserving PD is an option, which may improve emptying and provide nutritional benefit. No consistent data have yet to show a benefit.[63] Anastomosis involves different options, with the goal of preventing leaks and fistulas. PD performed in hospitals with a higher number of procedures annually (more than five per year) has an improved outcome.[66] Survival after PD varies depending on tumor size, nodal status, vessel invasion, tumor differentiation, and completeness of resection.[67]

Preoperative chemoradiation is being used in selected patients with the goal of increasing the opportunity for resection and increasing the overall survival.[68,69] Postoperative chemoradiation may prolong the median survival of patients with 5-FU combined with radiation[70] by eliminating residual microscopic disease in the tumor bed and regional lymph nodes. Adjunctive therapy is recommended in almost all patients.[71] Postoperative radiation should be given at a dose of 45 Gy to 54 Gy to volumes based on the preoperative CT and/or surgical clips. The therapy should be given regardless of margin or nodal status.[63]

Table 10-4 Staging Pancreatic Cancer

NCCN® Practice Guidelines in Oncology – v.1.2006

Pancreatic Adenocarcinoma

Staging

Table 1

American Joint Committee on Cancer (AJCC) TNM Staging of Pancreatic Cancer (2002)

Because only a few patients with pancreatic cancer undergo surgical resection of the pancreas (and adjacent lymph nodes), a single TNM classification must apply to both clinical and pathologic staging.

Primary Tumor (T)

TX	Primary tumor cannot be assessed
T0	No evidence of primary tumor
Tis	Carcinoma in situ*
T1	Tumor limited to the pancreas, 2 cm or less in greatest dimension
T2	Tumor limited to the pancreas, more than 2 cm in greatest dimension
T3	Tumor extends beyond the pancreas but without involvement of the celiac axis or the superior mesenteric artery
T4	Tumor involves the celiac axis or the superior mesenteric artery (unresectable primary tumor)

*This also includes the "PanInIII" classification.

Regional Lymph Nodes (N)

NX	Regional lymph nodes cannot be assessed
N0	No regional lymph node metastasis
N1	Regional lymph node metastasis

Distant Metastasis (M)

MX	Distant metastasis cannot be assessed
M0	No distant metastasis
M1	Distant metastasis

Stage Grouping

Stage 0	Tis	N0	M0
Stage IA	T1	N0	M0
Stage IB	T2	N0	M0
Stage IIA	T3	N0	M0
Stage IIB	T1	N1	M0
	T2	N1	M0
	T3	N1	M0
Stage III	T4	Any N	M0
Stage IV	Any T	Any N	M1

Used with the permission of the American Joint Committee on Cancer (AJCC), Chicago, Illinois. The original and primary source for this information is the *AJCC Cancer Staging Manual, Sixth Edition* (2002) published by Springer-New York. (For more information, visit www.cancerstaging.net.) Any citation or quotation of this material must be credited to the AJCC as its primary source. The inclusion of this information herein does not authorize any reuse or further distribution without the expressed, written permission of Springer-New York, Inc., on behalf of the AJCC.

Modified from National Comprehensive Cancer Network (NCCN) Guidelines (website): www.nccn.org/professionals/physician_gls/PDF/anal.pdf. Used with the permission of the American Joint Committee on Cancer (AJCC), Chicago, Illinois. The original source is the *AJCC Cancer Staging Handbook, Sixth Edition* (2002), published by Springer-New York, www.springeronline.com.

Treatment of Locally Advanced Disease

Chemoradiation is a conventional option for treatment of unresectable locoregional pancreatic cancer. For primary definitive chemoradiation therapy, the recommended doses are 50 Gy to 60 Gy with concomitant 5-FU or other radiation sensitizers.[63] Agents under study as radiosensitizers include bromodeoxyuridine,[72] paclitaxel,[73] cisplatin,[74] and gemcitabine.[75] After combined 5-FU radiation, additional chemotherapy with a 5-FU–based regimen or gemcitabine is recommended.[63] Box 10-3 outlines chemotherapy used for pancreatic cancer.

Palliative Treatment

Chemotherapy in locally advanced or metastatic pancreatic cancer is of potential benefit to a small percentage of patients. Patients with poor performance status rarely benefit.[63] Gemcitabine has been shown to provide clinical benefit and some survival benefit over treatment with bolus 5-FU.[76] Gemcitabine reduces disease-related symptoms for many patients, reducing pain and nausea and improving performance status. Second-line therapy for patients who progress may be gemcitabine in patients who did not receive it, capecitabine, infusional 5-FU, or a clinical trial.[63] Other treatments for symptoms may be offered. Treatment of obstructive jaundice caused by bile duct obstruction is stenting, performed either percutaneously or endoscopically. Gastric outlet obstruction can be managed by gastrojejunostomy or by stenting. Patients with both gastric outlet obstruction and jaundice are treated with surgical gastric/biliary bypass.[77] Pain is managed by narcotic analgesics and celiac plexus block, which ablates the afferent nerve fibers that transmit pain from intraabdominal viscera. Radiation therapy also may be used to alleviate pain.[78]

Box 10-3 Chemotherapy Agents Used for Pancreatic Adenocarcinoma

FRONT LINE THERAPY

5-FU–based chemoradiation for locally advanced unresectable disease
Gemcitabine for locally advanced unresectable disease and metastatic disease

COMBINATIONS

Gemcitabine, cisplatin
Gemcitabine, oxaliplatin
Gemcitabine, irinotecan

SECOND-LINE THERAPY

Gemcitabine for patients not previously treated with the drug
Capecitabine
Infusional 5-FU

5-FU, 5-Fluorouracil.

COLON AND RECTAL CANCERS

Colorectal cancer accounts for approximately 10% of cancer deaths in the United States. It is second to lung cancer as a cause of cancer death and is the third in both frequency and cause of death in both men and women.[12] Age is a major risk factor for sporadic colorectal cancer. The highest incidence rates are in North America, Australia, and northern and western Europe.[79] The incidence rates for right-sided colon cancers has increased.[80] Five-year survival rates have improved for left and transverse colon cancers, but not for right-sided tumors.[81] Genetic disorders that are inherited in an autosomal dominant fashion are associated with a very high risk of developing colon cancer. Familial adenomatous polyposis (FAP) and hereditary nonpolyposis colorectal cancer (HNPCC) are the most common and account for less than 5% of cases.[82] Personal or family history of sporadic colorectal cancer or large adenomatous polyps with villous of tubulovillous histology are at increased risk.[83,84] Others at risk are people with inflammatory bowel disease,[85] diabetes mellitus, and insulin resistance.[86] Environmental factors include current smoking[87] and current moderate-to-heavy alcohol use, probably in combination with a diet low in micronutrients and underconsumption of energy (inactivity and excess body weight).[88] Protective factors include micronutrients in high-fiber foods, folate, aspirin, postmenopausal estrogens,[88] and calcium.[89]

Clinical Manifestations

Most patients with colorectal cancer present with symptoms, usually caused by luminal narrowing or blood vessel disruption. The most common symptoms are a change in bowel habits, rectal bleeding, abdominal pain, and weight loss.[90] Left-sided colon cancers generally cause constipation, diarrhea, abdominal pain, and obstructive symptoms such as nausea and vomiting. Right-sided cancers produce vague abdominal aching, anemia from chronic blood loss, weakness, and weight loss. An abdominal mass may also occur. Rectal cancers may cause a change in bowel movements, rectal fullness, urgency, tenesmus, or bleeding. Pelvic pain is a late symptom caused by local extension of the tumor to pelvic nerves.[91]

Diagnostic Studies

The best diagnostic test is a colonoscopy. It can localize lesions throughout the large bowel, allowing for biopsy of lesions and removal of polyps. A double-contrast barium enema can be used in patients for whom a colonoscopy is unsuccessful for technical reasons. Staging before surgery requires chest x ray; CT of the abdomen and pelvis, which can show regional tumor extension; regional lymphatic and distant metastases; and tumor-related complications, such as obstruction, perforation, and fistula formation. CBC and platelets, liver and renal function tests, and measurement of carcinoembryonic antigen (CEA) are the diagnostic lab tests.[91] EUS is used to stage the depth of transmural invasion and the presence of perirectal nodes for rectal cancers. PET scanning may be useful in staging.[92]

Staging of Colorectal Cancer

The TNM staging system, which is based on the depth of tumor invasion through the intestinal wall, lymph node involvement, and distant metastases is replacing the Duke's classification system (Tables 10-5 and 10-6). Adenocarcinomas constitute 90% to 95% of large-bowel cancers. Colorectal cancers tend to invade locally by circumferential growth and spread via lymph nodes, hematogenous, transperitoneal, and perineural. At the time of diagnosis, about 25% of cancers have extended through the bowel wall. Cancers of the rectum have extended through the wall in 50% to 70% and spread to lymph nodes in 50% to 60% of patients. The most common site of extralymphatic involvement is the liver, with the lung the most frequent organ outside of the abdomen. Other sites of hematogenous spread include the adrenal glands, bones, kidney, and brain.[91]

Definitive Treatment

The primary treatment for adenocarcinoma of the colon is surgical resection of the bowel section containing the tumor, the adjacent mesentery, and the draining lymph nodes. Resection of the involved segment with a 5-cm margin of normal bowel on either side is optimal. Emergency resection without bowel prep usually requires a temporary diverting colostomy to avoid infections with anastomotic breakdown and leakage. Most adenomas that contain early invasive carcinoma (the earliest form of colon cancer) can be removed endoscopically. Noninvasive lesions require no surgical therapy if the margins are free of cancer. Surgery for rectal cancer depends on tumor stage and the location of the cancer. Sphincter-sparing surgery using circular stapling devices and coloanal anastomosis and creation of intestinal pouches may be done. A tumor has to be high enough above the top of the anorectal ring to allow for an adequate margin, if sphincter preservation is to be achieved. Curative surgery for metastases of the liver and lung may be done in selected patients.[91,93]

Adjuvant treatment for colon cancer has the goal of eradicating micrometastases. Patients with T3 tumors with high risk of recurrence, including those with grade 3 to 4 lesions, lymphatic/vascular invasion, bowel obstruction, localized perforation, or indeterminate or positive margins and patients with T4 tumors may be given adjuvant chemotherapy.[94] Postoperative radiation therapy may be given to the tumor bed in patients with T4 tumors to prevent local recurrence.[91] For patients with rectal cancer, preoperative chemoradiation may be recommended for T3, T4, and any node-positive disease. Neoadjuvant therapy may be used to convert the surgery to a sphincter-preserving one.[95] Adjuvant therapy for rectal cancer is recommended for patients with T3 lesions and suspected or proven lymph node involvement. Patients with recurrent local disease should be considered for resection with or without radiation.[96] Preoperative radiation is preferred to increase respectability.[94] Box 10-4 outlines the chemotherapy used for colorectal cancer.

Radiation Techniques

Radiation therapy for colon cancer requires the fields to include the tumor bed, which should be defined by preoperative imaging or by surgical clips. Radiation doses should be 45 Gy to 50 Gy in 25 to 28 fractions, with small bowel doses limited to 45 Gy. 5-FU–based chemotherapy should be given concurrently with radiation. Intraoperative radiation therapy (IORT), if available, should be considered for patients with T4 or recurrent disease as a boost. If IORT is not available, low-dose external-beam therapy could be given before adjuvant chemotherapy.[94]

For radiation of rectal cancer, the radiation fields

Table 10-5 Staging Colon Cancer

NCCN® Practice Guidelines in Oncology – v.2.2006

Colon Cancer

Staging

Table 1

American Joint Committee on Cancer (AJCC) TNM Staging System for Colorectal Cancer*

Primary Tumor (T)

TX	Primary tumor cannot be assessed
TO	No evidence of primary tumor
Tis	Carcinoma in situ: intraepithelial or invasion of lamina propria[†]
T1	Tumor invades submucosa
T2	Tumor invades muscularis propria
T3	Tumor invades through the muscularis propria into the subserosa, or into non-peritonealized pericolic or perirectal tissues
T4	Tumor directly invades other organs or structures, and/or perforates visceral peritoneum[‡]

Regional Lymph Nodes (N)[§]

NX	Regional lymph nodes cannot be assessed
N0	No regional lymph node metastasis
N1	Metastasis in 1 to 3 regional lymph nodes
N2	Metastasis in 4 or more regional lymph nodes

Distant Metastasis (M)

MX	Distant metastasis cannot be assessed
M0	No distant metastasis
M1	Distant metastasis

Stage Grouping

Stage	T	N	M	Dukes[¶]	MAC[¶]
0	Tis	N0	M0	–	–
I	T1	N0	M0	A	A
	T2	N0	M0	A	B1
IIA	T3	N0	M0	B	B2
IIB	T4	N0	M0	B	B3
IIIA	T1–T2	N1	M0	C	C1
IIIB	T3–T4	N1	M0	C	C2/C3
IIIC	Any T	N2	M0	C	C1/C2/C3
IV	Any T	Any N	M1	–	D

Histologic Grade (G)

GX	Grade cannot be assessed
G1	Well differentiated
G2	Moderately differentiated
G3	Poorly differentiated
G4	Undifferentiated

*Used with the permission of the American Joint Committee on Cancer (AJCC), Chicago, Illinois. The original and primary source for this information is the *AJCC Cancer Staging Manual, Sixth Edition* (2002) published by Springer-New York. (For more information, visit www.cancerstaging.net.) Any citation or quotation of this material must be credited to the AJCC as its primary source. The inclusion of this information herein does not authorize any reuse or further distribution without the expressed, written permission of Springer-New York, Inc., on behalf of the AJCC.

[†]Tis includes cancer cells confined within the glandular basement membrane (intraepithelial) or lamina propria (intramucosal) with no extension through the muscularis mucosae into the submucosa.

[‡]Direct invasion in T4 includes invasion of other segments of the colorectum by way of the serosa; for example, invasion of the sigmoid colon by a carcinoma of the cecum. Tumor that is adherent to other organs or structures macroscopically is classified T4. However, if no tumor is present in the adhesion microscopically the classification should be pT3. The V and L substaging should be used to identify the presence or absence of vascular or lymphatic invasion.

[§]A tumor nodule in the pericolorectal adipose tissue of a primary carcinoma without histologic evidence of residual lymph node in the nodule is classified in the pN category as a regional lymph node metastasis if the nodule has the form and smooth contour of a lymph node. If the nodule has an irregular contour, it should be classified in the T category and also coded as V1 (microscopic venous invasion) or as V2 (if it was grossly evident), because there is a strong likelihood that it represents venous invasion.

[¶]Dukes B is a composite of better (T3 N0 M0) and worse (T4 N0 M0) prognostic groups, as is Dukes C (Any TN1 M0 and Any T N2 M0). MAC is the modified Astler-Coller classification.

NOTE: The y prefix is to be used for those cancers that are classified after pretreatment, whereas the r prefix is to be used for those cancers that have recurred.

Modified from National Comprehensive Cancer Network (NCCN) Guidelines (website): www.nccn.org/professionals/physician_gls/PDF/anal.pdf. Used with the permission of the American Joint Committee on Cancer (AJCC), Chicago, Illinois. The original source is the *AJCC Cancer Staging Handbook, Sixth Edition* (2002), published by Springer-New York, www.springeronline.com.

Table 10-6 Staging Rectal Cancer

NCCN® Practice Guidelines in Oncology – v.2.2006

Rectal Cancer

Staging

Table 1

American Joint Committee on Cancer (AJCC) TNM Staging System for Colorectal Cancer*

Primary Tumor (T)

TX	Primary tumor cannot be assessed
T0	No evidence of primary tumor
Tis	Carcinoma in situ: intraepithelial or invasion of lamina propria†
T1	Tumor invades submucosa
T2	Tumor invades muscularis propria
T3	Tumor invades through the muscularis propria into the subserosa, or into nonperitonealized pericolic or perirectal tissues
T4	Tumor directly invades other organs or structures, and/or perforates visceral peritoneum‡

Regional Lymph Nodes (N)§

NX	Regional lymph nodes cannot be assessed
N0	No regional lymph node metastasis
N1	Metastasis in 1 to 3 regional lymph nodes
N2	Metastasis in 4 or more regional lymph nodes

Distant Metastasis (M)

MX	Distant metastasis cannot be assessed
M0	No distant metastasis
M1	Distant metastasis

Stage Grouping

Stage	T	N	M	Dukes¶	MAC¶
0	Tis	N0	M0	–	–
I	T1	N0	M0	A	A
	T2	N0	M0	A	B1
IIA	T3	N0	M0	B	B2
IIB	T4	N0	M0	B	B3
IIIA	T1–T2	N1	M0	C	C1
IIIB	T3–T4	N1	M0	C	C2/C3
IIIC	Any T	N2	M0	C	C1/C2/C3
IV	Any T	Any N	M1	–	D

Histologic Grade (G)

GX	Grade cannot be assessed
G1	Well differentiated
G2	Moderately differentiated
G3	Poorly differentiated
G4	Undifferentiated

*Used with the permission of the American Joint Committee on Cancer (AJCC), Chicago, Illinois. The original and primary source for this information is the *AJCC Cancer Staging Manual, Sixth Edition* (2002) published by Springer-New York. (For more information, visit www.cancerstaging.net.) Any citation or quotation of this material must be credited to the AJCC as its primary source. The inclusion of this information herein does not authorize any reuse or further distribution without the expressed written permission of Springer-New York on behalf of the AJCC.

†Tis includes cancer cells confined within the glandular basement membrane (intraepithelial) or lamina propria (intramucosal) with no extension through the muscularis mucosae into the submucosa.

‡Direct invasion in T4 includes invasion of other segments of the colorectum by way of the serosa; for example, invasion of the sigmoid colon by a carcinoma of the cecum. Tumor that is adherent to other organs or structures, macroscopically, is classified T4. However, if no tumor is present in the adhesion, microscopically, the classification should be pT3. The V and L substaging should be used to identify the presence or absence of vascular or lymphatic invasion.

§A tumor nodule in the pericolorectal adipose tissue of a primary carcinoma without histologic evidence of residual lymph node in the nodule is classified in the pN category as a regional lymph node metastasis if the nodule has the form and smooth contour of a lymph node. If the nodule has an irregular contour, it should be classified in the T category and also coded as V1 (microscopic venous invasion) or as V2 (if it was grossly evident), because there is a strong likelihood that it represents venous invasion.

¶Dukes B is a composite of better (T3 N0 M0) and worse (T4 N0 M0) prognostic groups, as is Dukes C (Any TN1 M0 and Any T N2 M0). MAC is the modified Astler-Coller classification.

NOTE: The y prefix is to be used for those cancers that are classified after pretreatment, whereas the r prefix is to be used for those cancers that have recurred.

Modified from National Comprehensive Cancer Network (NCCN) Guidelines (website): www.nccn.org/professionals/physician_gls/PDF/anal.pdf. Used with the permission of the American Joint Committee on Cancer (AJCC), Chicago, Illinois. The original source is the *AJCC Cancer Staging Handbook, Sixth Edition* (2002), published by Springer-New York, www.springeronline.com.

Box 10-4 Chemotherapy Agents Used for Colorectal Cancer

COLORECTAL CANCER

5-FU/leucovorin
Capecitabine
FOLFOX 4 (leucovorin, 5-FU bolus followed by 22-hour infusion, oxaliplatin)
FOLFOX 6 (oxaliplatin 100 mg/m^2, leucovorin, 5-FU bolus, followed by 46-hour infusion)
MFOLFOX6 (oxaliplatin 85 mg/m^2, leucovorin, 5-FU bolus, followed by 46-hour infusion)
FOLFOX7 (oxaliplatin 130 mg/m^2, leucovorin, 5-FU 46-hour infusion)

METASTATIC COLORECTAL CANCER

First Line
FOLFOX (oxaliplatin, infusional 5-FU, leucovorin)
FOLFIRI (Irinotecan, infusional 5-FU, leucovorin)
Bevacizumab, 5-FU combinations

Second Line
Irinotecan, cetuximab
Irinotecan, cetuximab or FOLFAX

5-FU, 5-Fluorouracil.

should include the tumor with a 2-cm to 5-cm margin, the presacral nodes, and the internal iliac nodes. Multiple fields (usually a three- or four-field technique), with positioning to minimize small bowel in the field is recommended. Treatment with a full bladder and surgical clips for planning can limit small bowel in the treatment field. For postoperative patients, after abdominoperineal resection, the perineal wound should be included within the fields. Radiation doses of 45 Gy to 50 Gy in 25 to 28 fractions to the pelvis are recommended. For resectable cancers, a tumor bed boost with a 2-cm margin of 5.4 Gy in three fractions preoperatively and 5.4 Gy to 9 Gy in three to five fractions postoperatively are recommended. IORT, if available, can be given to patients with close or positive margins, especially patients with T4 or recurrent cancers. If IORT is not available, 10 Gy to 20 Gy external-beam therapy to a limited volume can be considered soon after surgery, before adjuvant chemotherapy. For unresectable rectal cancers, doses higher than 54 Gy may be required. 5-FU chemotherapy should be given concurrently with radiation.[96]

Palliative Treatment

Surgery is considered in unresectable patients if there is a risk for obstruction or if liver metastases are minimal. Generally, chemotherapy is the recommended treatment for advanced disease. A number of chemotherapy and biologic therapy regimens are available for these patients. Primary therapy for metastatic disease in a patient with good tolerance should be combination therapy of 5-FU or capecitabine and either irinotecan or oxaliplatin. Bevacizumab and cetuximab also may be used. Palliation of liver metastases can be done with ablative techniques.[94]

ANAL CANCER

Anal cancers compromise approximately 1.6% of GI cancers in the United States. They occur more often in women in the United States. More than 80% occur in people older than age 60. The incidence of anal cancer for single men is reported to be 6 times that of married men. An association has been found between men having anal sex and the HPV virus in those with anal cancer. A history of cervical, vulvar, or vaginal cancer and immunosuppression after organ transplant or immunosuppression related to human immunodeficiency virus (HIV) also can be associated with anal cancer.[91,97]

Clinical Manifestations

Most patients with anal cancer present with rectal bleeding. Thirty percent have pain or a sensation of a rectal mass. Diagnosis may be delayed because the symptoms are often attributed to hemorrhoids or anal fissure.[91]

Diagnostic Studies

Evaluation should include a digital rectal exam, endoscopic examination, inguinal lymph node evaluation by CT, biopsy or FNA if there are suspicious nodes, gynecological exam for women, and consideration of HIV testing.[97] The incidence of inguinal node metastases at diagnosis varies from 13% to 25% and is unusual with a tumor size less than 2 cm in diameter.[91]

Pathology and Patterns of Metastasis

The AJCC staging system for anal cancer is based on tumor size, lymph node status, and metastasis (Table 10-7). Most tumors arising in the canal, which extends from the anal verge to the rectal

Table 10-7 Staging Anal Cancer

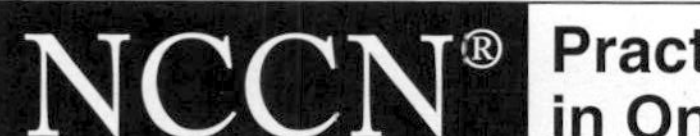

Practice Guidelines in Oncology – v.2.2006

Anal Carcinoma

Staging

Table 1

2002 American Joint Committee on Cancer (AJCC) Staging System for Anal Cancer*

Primary Tumor (T)

TX	Primary tumor cannot be assessed
T0	No evidence of primary tumor
Tis	Carcinoma in situ
T1	Tumor 2 cm or less in greatest dimension
T2	Tumor more than 2 cm but not more than 5 cm in greatest dimension
T3	Tumor more than 5 cm in greatest dimension
T4	Tumor of any size invades adjacent organ(s), e.g., vagina, urethra, bladder†

Regional Lymph Nodes (N)

NX	Regional lymph nodes cannot be assessed
N0	No regional lymph node metastasis
N1	Metastasis in perirectal lymph node(s)
N2	Metastasis in unilateral internal iliac and/or inguinal lymph node(s)
N3	Metastasis in perirectal and inguinal lymph nodes and/or bilateral internal iliac and/or inguinal lymph nodes

Distant Metastasis (M)

MX	Distant metastasis cannot be assessed
M0	No distant metastasis
M1	Distant metastasis

Stage Grouping

Stage 0	Tis	N0	M0
Stage I	T1	N0	M0
Stage II	T2	N0	M0
	T3	N0	M0
Stage IIIA	T1	N1	M0
	T2	N1	M0
	T3	N1	M0
	T4	N0	M0
Stage IIIB	T4	N1	M0
	Any T	N2	M0
	Any T	N3	M0
Stage IV	Any T	Any N	M1

Histologic Grade (G)

GX	Grade cannot be assessed
G1	Well differentiated
G2	Moderately differentiated
G3	Poorly differentiated
G4	Undifferentiated

*Used with the permission of the American Joint Committee on Cancer (AJCC), Chicago, Illinois. The original and primary source for this information is the *AJCC Cancer Staging Manual, Sixth Edition* (2002) published by Springer-New York. (For more information, visit www.cancerstaging.net.) Any citation or quotation of this material must be credited to the AJCC as its primary source. The inclusion of this information herein does not authorize any reuse or further distribution without the expressed written permission of Springer-New York on behalf of the AJCC.

†Direct invasion of the rectal wall, perirectal skin, subcutaneous tissue, or the sphincter muscle(s) is not classified as T4.

Modified from National Comprehensive Cancer Network (NCCN) Guidelines (website): www.nccn.org/professionals/physician_gls/PDF/anal.pdf. Used with the permission of the American Joint Committee on Cancer (AJCC), Chicago, Illinois. The original source is the *AJCC Cancer Staging Handbook, Sixth Edition* (2002), published by Springer-New York, www.springeronline.com.

mucosa, are squamous cell carcinomas. Anal cancers tend to spread by local extension, especially to the vagina in women. Local extension into the sphincter muscle is common at presentation. Anal cancers tend to spread via lymphatic and hematogenous routes. About 5% to 8% of patients develop liver metastases, and a small percentage develop lung and bone metastases. Approximately 50% of patients present with a superficial mass, and approximately 25% will have involvement of regional nodes.[98]

Definitive Treatment

In patients with small superficial tumors, local excision with adequate margins often achieves adequate local control and survival.[91,99] If margins are insufficient, reexcision is preferred or local radiation with or without 5-FU–based chemotherapy.[99] Historically, abdominoperineal resection (APR) was the treatment of choice for patients with invasive cancer, involving removal of the anorectum and a permanent colostomy, with local recurrences common.[91,98] Radiation alone for anal cancer, with external-beam therapy or brachytherapy for selected patients, gives local control and survival rates of 70% to 90%. However, late toxicity, such as anal ulcers, stenosis, and necrosis, can lead to colostomy.[100] Currently, chemoradiation is the treatment of choice for most patients with anal cancer. These patients would receive external-beam radiation therapy plus mitomycin/5-FU combination therapy. Newer combinations using cisplatin and 5-FU have been found so far to have equivalent results and less toxicity than mitomycin/5FU chemotherapy.[98]

If there is biopsy-proven disease after therapy, chemotherapy with 5-FU/cisplatin or APR is offered. Patients who develop inguinal node metastasis and who have not had resection could be considered for APR and groin dissection. Radiation therapy is recommended if no previous radiation to the groin was given for recurrent disease. Tumors no more than 2 cm in diameter are cured in 80% of cases and those of 5 cm or more are cured in less than 50% of cases.[99] Tolerance of therapy may be decreased in HIV-positive patients. Combination therapy can be effective, with decreased doses of radiation and chemotherapy.[98]

Radiation Techniques

Patients are typically treated with radiation fields encompassing the pelvis from the S1 to S2 level, the inguinal lymph nodes and the anus. After 30 Gy to 36 Gy, the fields are reduced to the low pelvis including the tumor.[100] The dose recommended for stages I and II disease (T1-2, N0 tumors) is 45 Gy to 59 Gy. If there is persistent disease, the dose should be increased to 55 Gy to 59 Gy. For stages II, III and IV disease (T3, T4, N0) or any node positive disease, the dose should be 55 Gy to 59 Gy.[99]

Palliative Treatment

Distant metastases are relatively low in anal cancer.[98,100] Cisplatin-based chemotherapy or a clinical trial are recommended for these patients.[99]

SIDE EFFECTS OF RADIATION THERAPY

The side effects of radiation occur because of the effects on cancer cells and normal cells in the area. Short-term effects are seen in renewing tissues such as the skin, mucosa, bone marrow, small intestine, and rectum. These rapidly proliferating tissues have less opportunity to repair radiation-induced DNA damage before reproducing and consequently may die. These effects heal with time. The long-term effects tend to be dose-limiting. These include necrosis, fibrosis, fistula formation, ulcers that fail to heal, and radiation-induced second cancers.[101]

Side effects of radiation therapy for GI cancers vary depending on the site, the volume of tissue treated, the dose and fractionation, and individual factors. The cells of the mucosa are rapidly dividing and are sensitive to radiation. Other areas have a slower cell turnover, are less sensitive to radiation, and may exhibit late-occurring side effects; an example of such an area is the pancreas.

Mucositis

Mucositis refers to injury to any mucosal surface, including the intestine. The reactions vary in different areas of the intestine because of different responses to radiation. Morphologic differences and differences in epithelial renewal also are found. Whereas the mucosa in the esophagus consists of stratified squamous epithelium, the intestinal mucosa consists of a layer of columnar epithelium, which is affected earlier in the treatment course. It is now thought that mucositis is the consequence of a series of biologic events. Initiation of mucositis occurs from DNA and non-DNA damage from direct cell death and reactive oxygen species. A number of central biologic control mechanisms are activated, with up-regulated genes controlling protein synthesis and cell signaling. Increased synthesis of the cytokines interleukin, IL6, and other enzymes trigger a variety of destructive processes. The production of proteins causes target cell injury and signaling and amplification of the process. In the case of fractionated radiation, there is continuous insult, with resultant constant acceleration and amplification of the biologic effects. Ulceration is the result, with macrophages and other inflammatory cells infiltrating the area, as well as angiogenesis. Healing is usually spontaneous.[102]

Esophagitis

The esophagus becomes inflamed during radiation therapy and the effect is greater with concurrent chemotherapy. The abnormalities include abnormal motility, mucosal edema, and ulceration.[103] Patients typically develop chest pain, dysphagia, and odynophagia shortly after the start of radiation therapy, usually within 2 to 3 weeks. Nursing assessment includes pain assessment, degree of difficulty in swallowing, and weight loss. Symptom management involves dietary changes and pain control. A soft, bland diet with elimination of hot, spicy, acidic, and coarse dry food and alcohol is recommended. As treatment progresses, eating with sauces and gravies and chewing well are helpful. Patients may require pureed foods or liquid supplements. Box 10-5 gives suggestions for soft, bland foods. Pain control can be local, as with a mixture of local anesthetic, antacid, and antihistamine. Antacids may decrease symptoms. Liquid preparations and/or H_2-receptor antagonists or proton pump inhibitors decrease symptoms of reflux. Systemic pain medications are usually required, such as liquid, time-release, or transdermal opioids. Prophylactic PEG tube or J tube placement may be recommended for chemoradiation regimens expected to cause significant esophagitis.[103] Box 10-6 lists nursing care that can help patients manage esophagitis side effects.

Box 10-5 Soft and Bland Foods That Help Lessen Effects of Dysphagia

PROTEIN

Custard, pudding, ice cream
Eggs soft cooked, scrambled, omelet
Quiche
Pasta dishes with cheese
Cheese strata
Cheese blintzes
Soufflés
Casseroles (mildly seasoned)
Yogurt

BREADS/CEREALS

Dry cereals soaked in milk
Cooked cereals
Mashed potatoes

FRUITS, VEGETABLES

Canned fruits
Cooked vegetables

MISCELLANEOUS FOODS

Blender combinations
Commercial supplements
Popsicles
Water ice
Sherbet
Slushies
Milk, milkshakes
Cookies soaked in milk
Cream soups
Instant Breakfast (powdered drink mix added to milk)

Box 10-6 Nursing Care for the Patient With Esophagitis

ASSESSMENT

Nutrition
Weight, height, percentage of weight loss
Dietary intake/24 hr
Dietary recall
Appetite changes
Pain with swallowing

Functional and social
Ability to prepare foods
Family support
Finances
Religious, cultural influences on food intake
Fatigue

INTERVENTIONS

Soft, bland diet
High-protein, high-calorie diet, supplements
Exercise to improve appetite
Referral to dietitian if needed
Medications if needed
- Megestrol acetate for anorexia
- H_2 blockers or proton pump inhibitors
- Local and systemic pain medications

Late effects include ulcer and stricture formation, fistula, and pseudodiverticulum. Fistula formation can occur when rapid tumor reduction as a result of radiation occurs and initial evidence of tracheal invasion is present.[103] Abnormal motility occurs as early as 1 week after chemoradiation and not until 4 to 6 weeks later with radiation alone. Ulcer and stricture formation may develop 4 to 8 months after therapy and occur in less than 5% of patients treated to doses to 63 Gy.[103,104] Referral to a gastroenterologist for dilation of strictures, cauterization of bleeding, or stent placement may be recommended.

Patient and family education involves teaching fundamentals of good nutrition and sources of nutritious calories and protein, with the patient and family being involved in the process of planning for nutrition during treatment and recovery. They should be taught how to complete food diaries and instructed regarding what symptoms to report that affect food intake.

Gastritis

Radiation to the abdomen causes anorexia, nausea, and vomiting. Sustained stimulation of GI receptors leads to early satiety and decreased appetite.[105] Activation of neurotransmittal receptors (serotonin, substance P, dopamine, neurokinin-1 [NK-1], and other receptors) stimulates the chemoreceptor trigger zone (CTZ) in the area postrema in the brain. Also, stimulation of enterochromaffin cells by abdominal radiation yields liberation of serotonin (5-HT), which binds to 5-HT_3 receptors on vagal terminals, which activates the CTZ.[106] Approximately 50% of people who receive radiation to the abdomen have onset of symptoms within 40 to 90 minutes of a treatment.[107] Patients at increased risk for nausea and vomiting are those who are at a younger age, female, have susceptibility to motion sickness, have had unsuccessful treatment of past nausea and vomiting, have anxiety, and are receiving concurrent chemotherapy. Other medications (e.g., opioids), infection, constipation, intestinal obstruction, hypercalcemia, and electrolyte abnormalities are also risk factors.[108] Anticipatory nausea may be present as well. Assessment of anorexia includes evaluation of preexisting conditions that contribute to anorexia, such as malignant symptoms, depression, infection, dyspnea, pain, and fatigue.[109] Socioeconomic conditions such as living alone and having a low income also need to be taken into consideration.[108,110] Nursing assessment includes obtaining weights at baseline and comparing this information on a weekly basis to the baseline; a weight loss of 2% to 5% is considered severe.[108] A 3-day diary of food intake that includes one weekend day[110] and physical findings such as weakness, loss of body fat and muscle mass, and decreased ability to care for oneself and maintain nutritional status are part of the nursing assessment of anorexia.[110] Assess nausea and vomiting, including the onset, frequency, intensity, and duration. Assess for symptoms of dehydration in a patient with nausea and vomiting, such as poor skin turgor, electrolyte imbalance, increased weakness or fatigue, concentrated urine, orthostatic hypotension, and oral cavity moisture. Box 10-7 outlines care of the patient with gastritis.

Chronic effects include gastric atrophy and ulceration, which may occur after doses of 45 Gy or more and may present months to years after cessation of treatment. A regimen of antacids or acid suppressive medications usually allows for healing of ulcers.[103]

Patient and family education to manage symptoms includes teaching patients at risk to self-administer antiemetics pretreatment on a daily basis. Instruct the patient and/or family to record nausea and vomiting in a diary, to check weight daily, and to report the weight loss or uncontrolled nausea or vomiting. They should be educated regarding the possible signs and symptoms of dehydration such as excessive thirst, dizziness, palpitations, concentrated urine, and fever. Dietary modifications that can be instituted such as consuming small, frequent meals and foods that are cool or at room temperature, avoiding fatty, spicy, salty, and sweet foods, and avoiding favorite foods (to prevent food aversions) may help the patient and family manage nutrition. Meals may be prepared by family members (or the patient when nausea is not present) and frozen. Education on pharmacologic and nonpharmacologic measures to alleviate nausea should be established.

Enteritis and Colitis

Radiation therapy mainly effects rapidly proliferating epithelial cells: those lining the small and large bowel. Crypt stem cells required for cellular replacement are affected, resulting in denudement and atrophy of villi in the small bowel and flattening of the epithelial surface in the large bowel.

Box 10-7 Nursing Care for the Patient Receiving Upper Abdominal Radiation

ASSESSMENT	INTERVENTIONS
Precipitating factors	**Pharmacologic**
Incidence, severity, precipitating factors of past nausea, vomiting (e.g., sea sickness, pregnancy)	Antiemetic medications before each radiation treatment and prn
Successful or unsuccessful treatment of past nausea, vomiting	5-HT_3 antagonists
Emetic potential of chemotherapy agents	Dopamine receptor antagonists
Medications that may cause nausea, such as opioids	Corticosteroids
Constipation	Benzodiazepines
Anxiety	Cannabinoid
	NK-1 antagonists for patients receiving chemotherapy
	IV fluids if necessary with electrolyte replacement
Present nausea, vomiting	**Nonpharmacologic**
Occurrence, frequency, intensity, onset, duration	Self-hypnosis
Use of diary, logs, journal	Biofeedback
Symptoms of dehydration	Relaxation
Skin turgor	Guided imagery
Oral mucous membranes	**Dietary**
Increased weakness, fatigue	Small, frequent meals
Concentrated urine	Foods at room temperature or cold
Orthostatic hypotension	Avoid favorite foods
CBC, electrolytes, creatinine	Avoid fatty, spicy, salty, sweet food

This results in loss of absorptive function with loss of water, electrolytes, protein, and blood and malabsorption of fat and vitamin B_{12}. Conjugated bile salts are not absorbed, and when they enter the colon, are deconjugated by bacterial flora, resulting in diarrhea. Decreased lactase causes accumulation of lactose.[111,112] Most patients undergoing radiation to the abdomen, pelvis, or rectum will show signs of acute enteritis.[111-113] The small intestine is particularly sensitive to radiation and is a dose-limiting structure. There is increased incidence of enteritis with a higher dose fraction, larger treatment volumes, concomitant chemoradiation, prior abdominal or pelvic surgery, history of colitis, ileitis and irritable bowel syndrome, and poor nutrition. The symptoms usually occur between 10 Gy and 30 Gy.[111,114] Acute symptoms may include nausea, vomiting, abdominal cramping, watery diarrhea, bleeding, and anemia. Symptoms usually resolve in 2 to 3 months.[112] Before starting radiation, the patient would be assessed for prior abdominal surgery, history or pelvic inflammatory disease or colitis, the usual pattern of elimination, the nutritional status of the patient, and usual eating habits such as the amount of fiber in the diet. In addition, the patient's lifestyle (daily routine, travel) is assessed because it may be impacted by diarrhea. During therapy, patients should be assessed, and changes in bowel pattern, including the onset, frequency, amount and character of stools, incontinence or noctural stool, blood in the stool,[115] and the presence of other symptoms such as flatus, nausea, vomiting, abdominal distension, abdominal pain, and cramping should be documented.[113] Patients are assessed for signs of dehydration: poor skin turgor for age, serum electrolyte imbalance, increased weakness, orthostatic hypotension, weight loss, fever, and altered mental status.[116] Also assess the patient's level of stress, affect of symptoms on the usual lifestyle, and coping patterns. Treatment of acute side effects involves dietary modification, adequate fluid intake and pharmacologic treatment for diarrhea. The diet for symptom management would include low-residue foods, potassium-rich foods, and avoidance of fried and fatty foods, lactose products, strong spices and herbs, caffeine, alcohol and tobacco. Patients also may need pain medication. Patients who have lost a significant amount of fluid and have indications of electrolyte imbalance should undergo fluid and electrolyte replacement.

Proctitis

Patients receiving radiation for rectal or anal cancer experience symptoms of proctitis, such as diarrhea, bowel urgency, or tenesmus and bleeding.[117] Assessment during therapy includes tracking the quantity and quality of bowel movements compared with the patient's pretreatment bowel function. Patients are assessed for bleeding and the amount of bleeding is documented. Pain assessment with exacerbating and alleviating factors and the relief obtained with pain interventions is paramount for the patient with proctitis. Interventions for these patients consist of treatment of these symptoms with pain management and pharmacologic measures such as Anusol or Anusol HC cream or suppositories, sitz baths and skin care for moist desquamation. The symptoms usually resolve within 2 to 6 months.[117]

Late effects of radiation to the colon or rectum have a median onset of 8 to 12 months to up to 15 years post-radiation, as a result of vascular insufficiency from damaged cells in blood vessels and connective tissue in the bowel wall.[111,112] These symptoms rarely occur with doses less than 55 Gy to 60 Gy.[101] Findings may include chronic bleeding, stricture, ulceration, obstruction, fistula formation, diarrhea, rectal pain, and urgency.[116] Diagnosis can be confirmed by colonoscopy or sigmoidoscopy. The mucosa appears pale with friability and with telangiectasias.[117] Barium studies are helpful in patients who are suspected of having fistulas and in patients with obstructive symptoms. Patients with mild symptoms may not require treatment, and bleeding may remit spontaneously.[117] Stool softeners for patients with mild obstructive symptoms resulting from strictures may help. Dilation procedures also may be used.[118] Relief of bleeding and pain may be obtained with use of enemas such as sucralfate (20 mL of a 10% sucralfate suspension in water twice daily) and/or corticosteroid enemas.[119,120]

Patient and family education for the patient experiencing enteritis and proctitis involves education about the expected side effects and management of diarrhea, including reporting the number and consistency of bowel movements, and when to seek medical attention for symptoms such as rectal spasms, excessive cramping, watery or bloody stools, and continued diarrhea not relieved by treatment.[111] In addition, teach the signs and symptoms of dehydration such as excessive thirst, fever, dizziness or lightheadedness and palpitations,[116] and instruct patients on dietary modifications, medications and how to take them. In follow-up, teach symptoms to report (change in stools, bleeding, and pain). Box 10-8 outlines care of the patient receiving radiation to the low abdomen and pelvis.

Cystitis

Symptoms of bladder irritation may occur if the bladder is in the radiation field, which sometimes occurs with patients treated for rectal or anal cancer. Symptoms are caused by inflammation and injury to the bladder mucosa and include urinary frequency, dysuria, nocturia, and urgency.[121] Assessment of the symptoms includes the frequency and pattern of voiding. Symptom relief can be obtained with a fluid intake of 2 to 3 liters a day unless contraindicated for medical reasons, avoidance of caffeine and spicy food and drinks, and pharmacologic treatment to decrease pain and spasms.

Sexual Effects

Some degree of sexual dysfunction occurs in most patients receiving radiation through the pelvis.[122] During radiation, patients may have reduced libido from disease symptoms or treatment side effects. Vaginal mucositis, an acute effect in women receiving radiation for rectal or anal cancer, causes pain. Chronically, the vaginal epithelium may appear thin, pale, and atrophic and may be traumatized by intercourse or masturbation. Vaginal dryness is a late effect of radiation. Men may have erectile dysfunction related to surgery in the pelvic area. Inability to have an orgasm affects about 50% of male and female patients with anal-rectal cancers after preoperative radiation therapy followed by surgery, 45% of patients after locally advanced primary cancer, and 57% of patients after locally recurrent rectal cancer treatments.[123] Assessment consists of a history of sexual function and medications that may affect sexual function. During treatment assess for symptoms that affect sexual function (pain, fatigue, vaginal discharge, and skin reactions). Treatment for these patients includes pain management, sitz baths, treatment of vaginal infections, and treatment of skin desquamation. After the treatment course, vaginal water-soluble lubricants, estrogen replacement systemically or locally, and trying different positions for intercourse can relieve symptoms of dyspareunia. Vaginal dilators may be

Box 10-8 Nursing Care for the Patient Receiving Radiation to the Lower Abdomen and Pelvis

ASSESSMENT

Prior abdominal surgery
History of intestinal inflammatory disease
Diabetes
Lactose intolerance
Usual pattern of elimination
Condition of peristomal, perineal areas

Nutritional status

Weight and height
Percentage of weight loss
Change in eating habits
Amount of residue in diet

Medications that may cause diarrhea

Laxatives
Antibiotics
Magnesium-containing medications
Promotility agents
Herbal supplements

INTERVENTIONS

Dietary modification

Low-residue diet
Low-fat diet
Low-lactose or lactose-free diet
Diet with foods that add consistence: rice, pectin-based foods.
Potassium-rich diet
Avoid strong spices, caffeine, alcohol, tobacco
Drink 3000 mL of fluid a day, including some with salt, sugar

Pharmacologic interventions

IV fluids if dehydrated
Bulk-forming agents
Loperamide
Diphenoxylate/atropine
Paregoric
Cholestyramine
Donnatal
Steroid foam for proctitis
Analgesics

Skin care for desquamation

Gentle cleaning
Skin moisturizers
Barrier products

recommended to prevent vaginal narrowing and adhesion formation.

Skin Reactions

Skin reactions with radiation for GI cancers vary with the site. The areas at risk are the supraclavicular area for some patients with esophageal cancer, the inguinal node areas, the groin, the perineal area, and stomal area for patients with a colostomy. Assessment of these areas weekly or more often is recommended. Patients who are experiencing diarrhea may have skin excoriation from the stool. Cleansing of the skin and anus after each bowel movement with mild soap and water or use of a peri-bottle or baby wipes is recommended. Barrier skin products to protect the skin from diarrheal stool is often helpful. Gently cleaning any thick skin product before a radiation treatment is recommended, while avoiding friction to radiated skin. Mild soap and water, patting the area dry or air drying, or a sitz bath for cleaning can accomplish this. Resources for patients and families are provided in Table 10-8.

Documentation is an essential component of patient care throughout all of the care of the patient. An initial assessment is recorded to document the patient's baseline status. This includes a medical, surgical, and psychiatric history along with the history of the present illness. Medications including nonprescription, herbal, and supplements are documented. A review of systems is recorded, including specific information about the GI function. This would include appetite, dyspepsia, nausea, vomiting, constipation, diarrhea, blood in stools, hemorrhoids, and pain. For the patient who has lost weight, documentation of dietary intake would be helpful. The initial assessment includes information about the patient's sexual function and, if of childbearing age, the desire to have more children and method of preventing pregnancy during treatment. The level of fatigue is documented, as is the sleep history. Other areas of importance to record are social habits and information about financial problems, work situation, with whom the patient lives, transportation problems, and spiritual issues. Patient and family teaching is documented at the initial visit and throughout the care of the patient. The evaluation of the patient's understanding of the information is essential to record, so additional

Table 10-8 Resources for Patients and Their Families

Name	Website and resource information
American Cancer Society	www.cancer.org 1-800-ACS-2345 Information about cancer and links to other sites
CancerSource	www.cancersource.com General cancer and treatment information, interactive opportunities such as live chats, support groups, and a cancer drug database
National Cancer Institute (NCI)	www.cancer.gov Cancer information, including prevention, screening, treatment, and research studies through its PDQ database
Cancer Information Service	http//cis.nci.nih.gov 1-800-4-CANCER (800-422-6237) NCI publications and live online assistance from NCI information specialists
Cancer Care	www.cancercare.org 1-800-813-HOPE (800-813-4673) Free professional help to people with all cancers through counseling, education, information and referral, and direct financial assistance
People Living With Cancer	www.plwc.org Patient information website of the American Society of Clinical Oncology Oncologist-reviewed and approved information, such as types of cancer, treatments, side effects, and support resources
Pancreatic Cancer Action Network	www.pancan.org 1-877-272-6226 Information and links to additional resources, support and clinical trial information for patients and caregivers
Colon Cancer Alliance	www.ccalliance.org 1-877-422-2030 Treatment information, research, advocacy, and support
Colorectal Cancer Network	www.colorectal-cancer.net 301-879-1500 Information and support
United Ostomy Associations of America	www.uoa.org 1-800-826-0826 Education, information, and support

teaching can be done. In addition to general information about radiation, teaching would consist of the side effects and their management. For the patient who will receive radiation to the abdomen and pelvis, the management of fatigue, pain, anorexia, nausea and vomiting, bowel and urinary management, perineal/vaginal care, skin care, and sexuality issues are taught. Documentation during radiation records the side effects with the severity, interventions for side effect management, and effectiveness of the interventions. Documentation of care during follow-up visits includes symptoms the patient may be experiencing, as mentioned above, nutritional status, and instructions about prevention measures such as smoking cessation and dietary factors.[124]

QUALITY OF LIFE AND GASTROINTESTINAL CANCER

Studies investigating quality of life in patients with GI cancers identify a range of symptoms from the cancer and treatment that decrease quality of life. Symptom distress, anxiety and depression, fatigue, pain, and weight loss are common at diagnosis.[125,126] Supportive care in addition to some chemotherapy agents may improve both survival and quality of life in patients with gastric and colorectal cancers.[127] Nutrition is also an important factor, with radiation patients receiving nutritional intervention being more satisfied than those without a specific intervention.[128] The scored Patient-Generated Subjective Global Assessment (PG-SGA) was found to identify malnutrition in ambulatory oncology patients receiving radiation therapy and can be used to predict change in quality of life.[129] Dysphagia from esophageal cancer affects all aspects of quality of life. Esophageal patients who received chemotherapy or chemoradiotherapy were impacted negatively on health-related quality of life.[130] The negative impact, however, was no longer evident in patients proceeding to surgery and recovery after esophagectomy was not impaired by neoadjuvant treatment.[131]

Patients with colorectal cancer had several areas of concern. Patients, especially those who were younger, had significant psychosocial and existential concerns, such as the value of life and how much longer they had to live.[132] Colorectal patients also have losses in professional and sexual identity and sexual confidence, dignity, privacy, independence, and ability to work, travel, and socialize. Quality of life for colorectal patients is also affected by fatigue, dyspnea, insomnia, constipation, diarrhea, and financial difficulties.[133,134] A study of older colorectal patients found overall satisfaction with their treatment, but many acknowledged difficulty coping with the side effects of treatment.[135] Patients receiving pelvic radiation therapy for rectal cancer were assessed. At the end of treatment, diarrhea, fatigue, appetite loss, physical function, social function, and global quality of life were significantly worse, but health-related quality of life scores had returned to pretreatment levels 4 to 6 weeks after radiation therapy.[136] Health-related quality of life in patients who received preoperative radiation therapy was affected by sexual dysfunction, and they had slower recovery of bowel function and impaired daily activity postoperatively; however, there was no serious affect on quality of life.[137] One year after combined treatment for locally advanced rectal cancer, improvement in some quality-of-life outcomes was shown, including global quality of life, although with a decrease in sexual function and

Table 10-9 Resources for Evidence-Based Research

Name	Website and resource information
Oncology Nursing Society	www.ons.org/research
Evidence-Based Practice Resource Area (EBP)	Assists in using research to change practice; includes evidence based summaries
Outcomes Resource Area (PEP)	Provides resources for oncology nursing-sensitive patient outcomes
Academic Center for Evidence-Based Nursing	www.acestar.uthscsa.edu The University of Texas Health Science Center at San Antonio
Evidence-Based Nursing Online	http://ebn.bmjjournals.com/ An online journal edited by Donna Ciliska, PhD, Nicky Cullum, PhD, RN, and Andrew Jull, MA, RN, faculty in the Department of Health Science at York University in Great Britain
The Joanna Briggs Institute	www.joannabriggs.edu.au/about/home.php An international research and development unit of Royal Adelaide Hospital, Australia, formed in response to the need for a collaborative approach to the evaluation of evidence derived from a diverse range of sources
Agency for Healthcare Research and Quality	www.ahrq.gov Fosters health care research that helps the American health care system provide access to high-quality, cost-effective services
Cochrane Collaboration	www.cochrane.org An international not-for-profit organization, providing up-to-date information about the effects of health care
Health Services Research & Development	www.hsrd.research.va.gov U.S. Department of Veterans Affairs website "Works to identify and evaluate innovative strategies that lead to accessible, high quality, cost-effective care"
National Comprehensive Cancer Network	www.nccn.org A comprehensive set of diagnostic, treatment, and supportive care guidelines

body image.[138] Rectal patients are shown to have a high quality of life, including stoma patients. A different study concluded that the quality of life for patients with rectal cancer was poorer than before the disease onset, but most could return to their former way of life without making too many compromises.[139] Spouses also are affected and have reported more emotional distress and less social support than patients. Women reported more distress and role problems and less marital satisfaction.[140,141] Both patients and spouses reported fear of the cancer's recurrence as their greatest concern. The studies on quality of life are significant in showing areas for nursing to impact patient care by addressing patient concerns and to have a positive effect on patients' well-being. Spouses should be included in health assessment and teaching. Information about the disease, the course of recovery, symptom management, and assistance with lifestyle changes will help patients and spouses.

The use of evidence-based nursing resources will guide the practitioner in caring for patients with GI cancers. Evidence-based practice uses the current best evidence in decision making about the care of patients. This involves the appraisal of the available research along with qualitative data and clinical judgment. Table 10-9 provides resources for exploring evidence-based research.

SUMMARY

Treatment for GI cancer typically has a large impact on the quality of life for patients. The side effects of treatment and the disease symptoms affect the patient's ability to eat, maintain adequate nutrition, and have normal bowel function. The patient may have pain and significant fatigue. These symptoms have an impact on the patient's ability to work and have a normal social life, on sexual function, and on performance of self-care. A major role of the nurse in the radiation setting is to maximize the patient's quality of life and help the patient finish the treatment course. Performing careful and complete assessment and providing education before, during, and after treatment and up-to-date symptom management helps the patient achieve these goals.

REFERENCES

1. Jaemal A, Murray T, Ward E et al: Cancer statistics, 2005, *CA Cancer J Clin* 55(1):10-30, 2005.
2. Crawford J: Principles of anatomy. In Rustgi A, Crawford J, editors: *Gastrointestinal cancers*, Philadelphia, 2003, Saunders, pp 121-131.
3. Silberg D, Wu G: Development of the alimentary tract, liver and pancreas. In Rustgi A, Crawford J, editors: *Gastrointestinal cancers*, Philadelphia, 2003, Saunders, pp 105-119.
4. Verma A, Mackay R, Taylor T: The virtual autopsy. In *Anatomy and physiology of the gastrointestinal system*, Leicester, England, 2001.
5. Compton C: Pathology and staging. In Willett CG, editor: *Cancer of the lower gastrointestinal tract*, Hamilton, Ontario, Canada, 2001, BC Decker, Inc, pp 53-81.
6. Hendricks D, Parker M: Esophageal cancer in Africa, *IUBMB Life* 53(4-5):263-268, 2002.
7. Brown L, Devesa S: Epidemiologic trends in esophageal and gastric cancer in the United States, *Surg Oncol Clin N Am* 11(2):235-256, 2002.
8. Ajani J, Burak W, D'Amico T: Esophageal cancer. In National Comprehensive Cancer Network (NCCN)—clinical practice guidelines in oncology, 2005, pp 1-27, at www.nccn.org.
9. Glenn TF: Esophageal cancer: facts, figures, and screening, *Gastroenterol Nurs* 24(6):271-273; quiz 274-275, 2001.
10. Reynolds JC, Rahimi P, Hirschl D: Barrett's esophagus: clinical characteristics, *Gastroenterol Clin North Am* 31(2):441-460, 2002.
11. Schmitt C, Brazer S: Clinical aspects of esophageal cancer. In Rustgi A, Crawford J, editors: *Gastrointestinal cancers*, Philadelphia, 2003, Saunders, pp 215-239.
12. Jaemal A, Tiwari RC, Murray T et al: Cancer statistics, 2004, *CA Cancer J Clin* 54(1):8-29, 2004.
13. Stein HJ, Feith M, Siewert JR: Cancer of the esophagogastric junction, *Surg Oncol* 9(1):35-41, 2000.
14. Dean D, Detterbeck F: Esophageal cancer: staging. In Kelsen D, Daly J, Dern S et al, editors: *Gastrointestinal oncology principles and practice*, Philadelphia, 2002, Lippincott Williams & Wilkins, pp 251-260.
15. Urba S: Combined modality therapy of esophageal cancer—standard of care? *Surg Oncol Clin N Am* 11(2): 377-386, 2002.
16. Marshall M, Kaiser L: Surgery of esophageal cancer. In Rustgi A, Crawford J, editors: *Gastrointestinal cancers*, Philadelphia, 2003, Saunders, pp 271-282.
17. Rich T: Chemotherapy and radiation therapy of esophageal cancer. In Rustgi A, Crawford J, editors: *Gastrointestinal cancers*, Philadelphia, 2003, Saunders, pp 283-289.
18. Kurtz R: Clinical aspects of gastric cancer. In Rustgi A, Crawford J, editors: *Gastrointestinal cancers*, Philadelphia, 2003, Saunders, pp 291-298.
19. Roder DM: The epidemiology of gastric cancer, *Gastric Cancer* 5(suppl 1):5-11, 2002.
20. Lambert R, Guilloux A, Oshima A et al: Incidence and mortality from stomach cancer in Japan, Slovenia and the USA, *Int J Cancer* 97(6):811-818, 2002.
21. Nomura A, Hankin J, Kolonel L et al: Case-controlled study of diet and other risk factors for gastric cancer in Hawaii (United States), *Cancer Causes Control* 14(6): 547-548, 2003.
22. Serafini M, Bellocco R, Wolk A et al: Total antioxidant potential of fruit and vegetables and risk of gastric cancer, *Gastroenterology* 123(4):985-991, 2002.

23. Devesa SS, Fraumeni JF Jr: The rising incidence of gastric cardia cancer, *J Natl Cancer Inst* 91(9):747-749, 1999.
24. Correa P: A human model of gastric carcinogenesis, *Cancer Res* 48(13):3554-3560, 1988.
25. Hsing AW, Hansson LE, McLaughlin JK et al: Pernicious anemia and subsequent cancer: a population-based cohort study, *Cancer* 71(3):745-750, 1993.
26. Drewitz DJ, Sampliner RE, Garewal HS: The incidence of adenocarcinoma in Barrett's esophagus: a prospective study of 170 patients followed 4.8 years, *Am J Gastroenterol* 92(2):212-215, 1997.
27. Wanebo HJ, Kennedy BJ, Chmiel J et al: Cancer of the stomach: a patient care study by the American College of Surgeons, *Ann Surg* 218(5):583-592, 1993.
28. Kurtz RC, Sherlock P: The diagnosis of gastric cancer, *Semin Oncol* 12(1):11-18, 1985.
29. Longo WE, Zucker KA, Zdon MJ et al: Detection of early gastric cancer in an aggressive endoscopy unit, *Am Surg* 55(2):100-104, 1989.
30. Sohn KM, Lee JM, Lee SY et al: Comparing MR imaging and CT in the staging of gastric carcinoma, *AJR Am J Roentgenol* 174(6):1551-1557, 2000.
31. Gerdes H, Markowitz A: Gastric cancer: staging systems and techniques. In Kelsen D, Kern S, editors: *Gastrointestinal oncology principles and practice*, Philadelphia, 2002, Lippincott Williams & Wilkins, pp 371-382.
32. Yanai H, Tada M, Karita M et al: Diagnostic utility of 20-megahertz linear endoscopic ultrasonography in early gastric cancer, *Gastrointest Endosc* 44(1):29-33, 1996.
33. Ajani J, Bekaii-Saab T, Boston B: Gastric cancer, *NCCN Prac Guidelines Oncol* 1:1-22, 2005.
34. Leichman L, Silberman H, Leichman CG et al: Preoperative systemic chemotherapy followed by adjuvant postoperative intraperitoneal therapy for gastric cancer: a University of Southern California pilot program, *J Clin Oncol* 10(12):1933-1942, 1992.
35. Ajani JA, Mayer RJ, Ota DM et al: Preoperative and postoperative combination chemotherapy for potentially resectable gastric carcinoma, *J Natl Cancer Inst* 85(22): 1839-1844, 1993.
36. Murakami T: Pathomorphological diagnosis: definition and gross classification of early gastric cancer, *Gann Monogr Cancer Res* 11:53, 1971.
37. Chau I, Norman AR, Cunningham D et al: Multivariate prognostic factor analysis in locally advanced and metastatic esophago-gastric cancer—pooled analysis from three multicenter, randomized, controlled trials using individual patient data, *J Clin Oncol* 22(12):2395-2403, 2004.
38. Bonin S, Coia L, Hoff P et al: Gastric cancer. In Pazdur R, Coia L, Hoskins W et al, editors: *Cancer management: a multidisciplinary approach*, Melville, NY, 2000, PRR Inc, pp 215-225.
39. Folli S, Dente M, Dell'Amore D et al: Early gastric cancer: prognostic factors in 223 patients, *Br J Surg* 82(7):952-956, 1995.
40. Ono H, Kondo H, Gotoda T et al: Endoscopic mucosal resection for treatment of early gastric cancer, *Gut* 48(2):225-229, 2001.
41. Ajani JA, Mansfield PF, Janjan N et al: Multi-institutional trial of preoperative chemoradiotherapy in patients with potentially resectable gastric carcinoma, *J Clin Oncol* 22(14):2774-2780, 2004.
42. Zhang ZX, Gu XZ, Yin WB et al: Randomized clinical trial on the combination of preoperative irradiation and surgery in the treatment of adenocarcinoma of gastric cardia (AGC)—report on 370 patients, *Int J Radiat Oncol Biol Phys* 42(5):929-934, 1998.
43. Moertel CG, Childs DS Jr, Reitemeier RJ et al: Combined 5-fluorouracil and supervoltage radiation therapy of locally unresectable gastrointestinal cancer, *Lancet* 2(1626): 865-867, 1969.
44. Smalley SR, Gunderson L, Tepper J et al: Gastric surgical adjuvant radiotherapy consensus report: rationale and treatment implementation, *Int J Radiat Oncol Biol Phys* 52(2):283-293, 2002.
45. Kulke M, Savarese D: Management of advanced gastric cancer. In Rose BD, editor: *UpToDate*, Wellesley, MA, 2005, UpToDate, pp 1-11.
46. Bozzetti F, Bonfanti G, Audisio RA et al: Prognosis of patients after palliative surgical procedures for carcinoma of the stomach, *Surg Gynecol Obstet* 164(2):151-154, 1987.
47. Alberts SR, Cervantes A, van de Velde CJ: Gastric cancer: epidemiology, pathology and treatment, *Ann Oncol* 14(suppl 2):ii31-ii36, 2003.
48. Hong YS, Song SY, Lee SI et al: A phase II trial of capecitabine in previously untreated patients with advanced and/or metastatic gastric cancer, *Ann Oncol* 15(9):1344-1347, 2004.
49. Koizumi W, Saigenji K, Ujiie S et al: A pilot phase II study of capecitabine in advanced or recurrent gastric cancer, *Oncology* 64(3):232-236, 2003.
50. Michaud DS: Epidemiology of pancreatic cancer, *Minerva Chir* 59(2):99-111, 2004.
51. Niederhuber JE, Brennan MF, Menck HR: The National Cancer Data Base report on pancreatic cancer, *Cancer* 76(9):1671-1677, 1995.
52. Ries L, Eisner M, Kosary C: *SEER cancer statistics review, 1973-1996,* 2000, National Cancer Institute.
53. Falk R, Pickle L, Fontham E: Occupation and pancreatic cancer risk in Louisiana, *Am J Industr Med* 18(5):565-576, 1990.
54. Michaud DS, Giovannucci E, Willett WC et al: Physical activity, obesity, height, and the risk of pancreatic cancer, *JAMA* 286(8):921-929, 2001.
55. Lowenfels AB, Maisonneuve P, DiMagno EP et al: Hereditary pancreatitis and the risk of pancreatic cancer: International Hereditary Pancreatitis Study Group, *J Natl Cancer Inst* 89(6):442-446, 1997.
56. Tersmette AC, Petersen GM, Offerhaus GJ et al: Increased risk of incident pancreatic cancer among first-degree relatives of patients with familial pancreatic cancer, *Clin Cancer Res* 7(3):738-744, 2001.
57. Krewski D: Epidemiology of pancreatic cancer: an overview, *Cancer Detect Prev* 27(2):87-93, 2003.
58. Hahn SA, Greenhalf B, Ellis I et al: BRCA2 germline mutations in familial pancreatic carcinoma, *J Natl Cancer Inst* 95(3):214-221, 2003.
59. Gullo L, Pezzilli R, Morselli-Labate AM: Diabetes and the risk of pancreatic cancer. Italian Pancreatic Cancer Study Group, *N Engl J Med* 331(2):81-84, 1994.
60. Lowenfels AB, Maisonneuve P: Epidemiology and prevention of pancreatic cancer, *Jpn J Clin Oncol* 34(5): 238-244, 2004.

61. Reiser M, Schmiegel W: Clinical aspects of pancreatic and ampullary cancers. In Rustgi A, Crawford J, editors: *Gastrointestinal cancers*, Philadelphia, 2003, Saunders, pp 507-518.
62. Kalser M, Barkin J, MacIntyre J: Pancreatic cancer: assessment of prognosis by clinical presentation, *Cancer* 56(2):397-402, 1985.
63. Tempero M, Behrman S, Benson A: Pancreatic adenocarcinoma. In *National Comprehensive Cancer Network (NCCN)—practice guidelines in oncology*, 2004, pp 1-41, at www.nccn.org.
64. Steer M: Clinical manifestations, diagnosis and surgical staging of exocrine pancreatic cancer. In Rose BD, editor: *UpToDate*, Wellesley, MA, 2005, UpToDate, pp 1-9.
65. Longnecker D: Pathology of pancreatic cancer. In Rustgi A, Crawford J, editors: *Gastrointestinal cancers*, Philadelphia, 2003, Saunders, pp 529-539.
66. Birkmeyer JD, Siewers AE, Finlayson EV et al: Hospital volume and surgical mortality in the United States, *N Engl J Med* 346(15):1128-1137, 2002.
67. Yeo CJ, Cameron JL, Lillemoe KD et al: Pancreaticoduodenectomy for cancer of the head of the pancreas: 201 patients, *Ann Surg* 221(6):721-731; discussion 731-733, 1995.
68. Spitz FR, Abbruzzese JL, Lee JE et al: Preoperative and postoperative chemoradiation strategies in patients treated with pancreaticoduodenectomy for adenocarcinoma of the pancreas, *J Clin Oncol* 15(3):928-937, 1997.
69. Breslin TM, Hess KR, Harbison DB et al: Neoadjuvant chemoradiotherapy for adenocarcinoma of the pancreas: treatment variables and survival duration, *Ann Surg Oncol* 8(2):123-132, 2001.
70. Kalser M, Ellenberg S: Pancreatic cancer: adjuvant combined radiation and chemotherapy following curative resection, *Arch Surg* 120(8):899-903, 1985.
71. Brower S, Menson A, Myerson R et al: Pancreatic, neuroendocrine GI and adrenal cancers. In Pazdur R, Coia L, Hoskins W et al, editors: *Cancer management: a multidisciplinary approach*, Melville, NY, 2000, PRR, pp 227-253.
72. Robertson JM, Ensminger WD, Walker S et al: A phase I trial of intravenous bromodeoxyuridine and radiation therapy for pancreatic cancer, *Int J Radiat Oncol Biol Phys* 37(2):331-335, 1997.
73. Safran H, King TP, Choy H et al: Paclitaxel and concurrent radiation for locally advanced pancreatic and gastric cancer: a phase I study, *J Clin Oncol* 15(3):901-907, 1997.
74. Boz G, De Paoli A, Roncadin M et al: Radiation therapy combined with chemotherapy for inoperable pancreatic carcinoma, *Tumori* 77(1):61-64, 1991.
75. Lawrence TS, Chang EY, Hahn TM et al: Radiosensitization of pancreatic cancer cells by 2',2'-difluoro-2'-deoxycytidine, *Int J Radiat Oncol Biol Phys* 34(4):867-872, 1996.
76. Burris HA 3rd, Moore MJ, Andersen J et al: Improvements in survival and clinical benefit with gemcitabine as first-line therapy for patients with advanced pancreas cancer: a randomized trial, *J Clin Oncol* 15(6):2403-2413, 1997.
77. Ryan D: Management of locally advanced pancreatic cancer. In Rose BD, editor: *UpToDate*, Wellesley, MA, 2005, UpToDate.
78. Fernandez-del Castillo F, Jimenez R: Pancreatic cancer: palliation of symptoms. In Rose BD, editor: *UpToDate*, Wellesley, MA, 2005, UpToDate.
79. Parkin DM, Pisani P, Ferlay J: Global cancer statistics, *CA Cancer J Clin* 49(1):33-64, 1999.
80. Weir HK, Thun MJ, Hankey BF et al: Annual report to the nation on the status of cancer, 1975-2000, featuring the use of surveillance data for cancer prevention and control, *J Natl Cancer Inst* 95(17):1276-1299, 2003.
81. Kawazuma Y, Tanaka H, Tsukuma H: Improvement of survival over time for colon cancer patients by anatomical sub-sites, *Jpn J Cancer Res* 90(7):705-710, 1999.
82. Burt RW, DiSario JA, Cannon-Albright L: Genetics of colon cancer: impact of inheritance on colon cancer risk, *Annu Rev Med* 46:371-379, 1995.
83. Atkin WS, Morson BC, Cuzick J: Long-term risk of colorectal cancer after excision of rectosigmoid adenomas, *N Engl J Med* 326(10):658-662, 1992.
84. Winawer SJ, Zauber AG, Gerdes H et al: Risk of colorectal cancer in the families of patients with adenomatous polyps. National Polyp Study Workgroup, *N Engl J Med* 334(2):82-87, 1996.
85. Ekbom A, Helmick C, Zack M et al: Ulcerative colitis and colorectal cancer: a population-based study, *N Engl J Med* 323(18):1228-1233, 1990.
86. Hu FB, Manson JE, Liu S et al: Prospective study of adult onset diabetes mellitus (type 2) and risk of colorectal cancer in women, *J Natl Cancer Inst* 91(6):542-547, 1999.
87. Colangelo LA, Gapstur SM, Gann PH et al: Cigarette smoking and colorectal carcinoma mortality in a cohort with long-term follow-up, *Cancer* 100(2):288-293, 2004.
88. Giovannucci E: Modifiable risk factors for colon cancer, *Gastroenterol Clin North Am* 31(4):925-943, 2002.
89. Giovannucci E: Diet, body weight, and colorectal cancer: a summary of the epidemiologic evidence, *J Womens Health (Larchmt)* 12(2):173-182, 2003.
90. Ahlquist D, Pasha T: Clinical aspects of sporadic colorectal cancer. In Rustgi A, Crawford J, editors: *Gastrointestinal cancers*, Philadelphia, 2003, Saunders. pp 379-405.
91. Coia L, Ellenhorn J, Ayoub J: Colorectal and anal cancers. In Pazdur R, Coia L, Hoskins W et al editors: *Cancer management: a multidisciplinary approach*, Melville, NY, 2000, PRR, pp 273-299.
92. Lawrence S, Ahnen D: Clinical manifestations, diagnosis and staging of colorectal cancer. In Rose BD, editor: *UpToDate*, Wellesley, MA, 2005, UpToDate, pp 1-11.
93. Ott M, Pierie J: Surgical management of primary colon cancer. In Rose BD, editor: *UpToDate*, Wellesley, MA, 2005, UpToDate, pp 1-12.
94. Engstrom P, Benson A, Chen Y et al: Colon cancer. In *National Comprehensive Cancer Network (NCCN) Practice Guidelines in Oncology*, 2005.
95. Allal AS, Bieri S, Pelloni A et al: Sphincter-sparing surgery after preoperative radiotherapy for low rectal cancers: feasibility, oncologic results and quality of life outcomes, *Br J Cancer* 82(6):1131-1137, 2000.
96. Engstrom P, Benson A, Chen Y et al: Rectal cancer. In *National Comprehensive Cancer Network (NCCN) Practice Guidelines in Oncology*, 2005, pp. 1-47.
97. Klencke BJ, Palefsky JM: Anal cancer: an HIV-associated cancer, *Hematol Oncol Clin North Am* 17(3):859-872, 2003.

98. Chawla A, Willett C: Cancer of the anal canal. In Rustgi A, Crawford J, editors: *Gastrointestinal cancers*, Philadelphia, 2003, Saunders, pp 491-505.
99. Engstrom P, Benson A, Chen Y: Anal canal cancer, In *National Comprehensive Cancer Network (NCCN) - Practice Guidelines In Oncology*, 2005, pp 1-12, at www.nccn.org.
100. Ryan D, Willett C: Anal cancer. In Gansler T, editor: *Cancer of the lower gastrointestinal tract*, Hamilton, Ontario, Canada, 2001, BC Decker Inc, pp 196-213.
101. Hellman S: Principles of cancer management. In DeVita V, Hellman S, Rosenberg S, editors: *Cancer: principles & practices of oncology*, Philadelphia, 2001, Lippincott Williams & Wilkins, pp 265-288.
102. Sonis ST: A biological approach to mucositis, *J Support Oncol* 2(1):21-32; discussion 35-6, 2004.
103. Coia L: Gastrointestinal cancer. In Coia L, Moylan D, editors: *Introduction to clinical radiation oncology*, Madison, WI, 1998, Medical Physics Publishing, pp 243-283.
104. Lepke RA, Libshitz HI: Radiation-induced injury of the esophagus, *Radiology* 148(2):375-378, 1983.
105. Hogan CM: Advances in the management of nausea and vomiting, *Nurs Clin North Am* 25(2):475-497, 1990.
106. Wickham R: Nausea and vomiting. In Yarbro C, Frogge M, Goodman M, editors: *Cancer symptom management*, Sudbury, MA, 2004, Jones and Bartlett Publishers, 187-212.
107. Pharmacists ASOHS: ASHP therapeutic guidelines on the pharmacologic management of nausea and vomiting in adult and pediatric patients receiving chemotherapy or radiation therapy or undergoing surgery, *Am J Health Syst Pharm* 56(8):729-764, 1999.
108. McMahon K, Brown JK: Nutritional screening and assessment, *Semin Oncol Nurs* 16(2):106-112, 2000.
109. Jacobsen PB, Andrykowski MA, Redd WH et al: Nonpharmacologic factors in the development of posttreatment nausea with adjuvant chemotherapy for breast cancer, *Cancer* 61(2):379-385, 1988.
110. Brown JK: A systematic review of the evidence on symptom management of cancer-related anorexia and cachexia, *Oncol Nurs Forum* 29(3):517-532, 2002.
111. Engelking C: Diarrhea. In Yarbro C, Frogge M, Goodman M, editors: *Cancer symptom management*, Sudbury, MA, 2004, Jones and Bartlett Publishers, pp 528-556.
112. Saclarides TJ: Radiation injuries of the gastrointestinal tract, *Surg Clin North Am* 77(1):261-268, 1997.
113. Engleking C, Sauerland C: Maintenance of normal elimination. In Bruner D, Moore-Higgs H, Haas M, editors: *Outcomes in radiation therapy: multidisciplinary management*, Sudbury, MA, 2000, Jones and Bartlett Publishers, pp 530-562.
114. Perez C, Brady L: *Principles and practice of radiation oncology*, ed 3, Philadelphia, 1998, Lippincott-Raven.
115. *Radiation enteritis (PDQ)* (website): www.cancer.gov, 2005, accessed April 18, 2005.
116. Hogan CM: The nurse's role in diarrhea management, *Oncol Nurs Forum* 25(5):879-886, 1998.
117. Schultheiss TE, Lee WR, Hunt MA et al: Late GI and GU complications in the treatment of prostate cancer, *Int J Radiat Oncol Biol Phys* 37(1):3-11, 1997.
118. Triadafilopoulos G, Sarkisian M: Dilation of radiation-induced sigmoid stricture using sequential Savaary-Gilliard dilators, *Dis Colon Rectum* 33(12):1065, 1990.
119. MacNaughton W: Review article: new insights into the pathogenesis of radiation-induced intestinal dysfunction, *Aliment Pharmacol Ther* 14(5):523-528, 2000.
120. Sher ME, Bauer J: Radiation-induced enteropathy, *Am J Gastroenterol* 85(2):121-128, 1990.
121. Marks LB, Carroll PR, Dugan TC et al: The response of the urinary bladder, urethra, and ureter to radiation and chemotherapy, *Int J Radiat Oncol Biol Phys* 31(5):1257-1280, 1995.
122. Bruner D: Maintenance of body image and sexual function. In Bruner D, Moore-Higgs H, Haas M, editors: *Outcomes in radiation therapy: multidisciplinary management*, Sudbury, MA, 2001, Jones and Bartlett Publishers, pp 611-636.
123. Mannaerts G, Schijven M, Hendrik A: Urologic and sexual morbidity following multimodality treatment for locally advanced primary and locally recurrent rectal cancer, *Eur J Surg Onc* 27(3):265-272, 2001.
124. Catlin-Huth C, Haas M, Pollock V: *Radiation therapy patient care record*, Pittsburgh, 2002, Oncology Nursing Society Publishing Division.
125. Yan H, Sellick K: Symptoms, psychological distress, social support, and quality of life of Chinese patients newly diagnosed with gastrointestinal cancer, *Cancer Nurs* 27(5):389-399, 2004.
126. Yan H, Sellick K: Quality of life of Chinese patients newly diagnosed with gastrointestinal cancer: a longitudinal study, *Int J Nurs Stud* 41(3):309-319, 2004.
127. Ahmed N, Ahmedzai S, Vora V et al: Supportive care for patients with gastrointestinal cancer, *Cochrane Database Syst Rev* 3:CD003445, 2004.
128. Isenring E, Capra S, Bauer J: Patient satisfaction is rated higher by radiation oncology outpatients receiving nutrition intervention compared with usual care, *J Hum Nutr Diet* 17(2):145-152, 2004.
129. Isenring E, Bauer J, Capra S: The scored Patient-generated Subjective Global Assessment (PG-SGA) and its association with quality of life in ambulatory patients receiving radiotherapy, *Eur J Clin Nutr* 57(2):305-309, 2003.
130. Watt E, Whyte F: The experience of dysphagia and its effect on the quality of life of patients with oesophageal cancer, *Eur J Cancer Care (Engl)* 12(2):183-193, 2003.
131. Blazeby JM, Sanford E, Falk SJ et al: Health-related quality of life during neoadjuvant treatment and surgery for localized esophageal carcinoma, *Cancer* 103(9):1791-1799, 2005.
132. Klemm P, Miller MA, Fernsler J: Demands of illness in people treated for colorectal cancer, *Oncol Nurs Forum* 27(4):633-639, 2000.
133. Arndt V, Merx H, Stegmaier C et al: Quality of life in patients with colorectal cancer 1 year after diagnosis compared with the general population: a population-based study, *J Clin Oncol* 22(23):4829-4836, 2004.
134. Kelly D: Patients with colorectal cancer expressed a loss of adulthood related to a loss of professional and sexual identity, dignity, privacy, independence, and ability to socialise, *Evid Based Nurs* 7(4):126, 2004.
135. Sabay T: A qualitative study of patient perspectives on colorectal cancer, *Cancer Pract Multidisciplinary J Cancer Care* 8(1):38-44, 2000.

136. Guren MG, Dueland S, Skovlund E et al: Quality of life during radiotherapy for rectal cancer, *Eur J Cancer* 39(5):587-594, 2003.
137. Marijnen CA, van de Velde CJ, Putter H et al: Impact of short-term preoperative radiotherapy on health-related quality of life and sexual functioning in primary rectal cancer: report of a multicenter randomized trial, *J Clin Oncol* 23(9):1847-1858, 2005.
138. Allal AS, Gervaz P, Gertsch P et al: Assessment of quality of life in patients with rectal cancer treated by preoperative radiotherapy: a longitudinal prospective study, *Int J Radiat Oncol Biol Phys* 61(4):1129-1135, 2005.
139. Harisi R, Bodoky G, Borsodi M et al: Rectal cancer therapy: decision making on basis of quality of life?, *Zentralbl Chir* 129(2):139-148, 2004.
140. Northouse LL, Mood D, Templin T et al: Couples' patterns of adjustment to colon cancer, *Soc Sci Med* 50(2):271-284, 2000.
141. Northouse LL, Schafer JA, Tipton J et al: The concerns of patients and spouses after the diagnosis of colon cancer: a qualitative analysis, *J Wound Ostomy Continence Nurs* 26(1):8-17, 1999.

Chapter 11 Urinary Cancers

Pamela Devine

Genitourinary malignancies, including the kidney, ureter, and bladder account for an estimated 565,000 malignancies worldwide each year.[1] The American Cancer Society (ACS) has estimated that in the United States approximately 102,740 new malignancies of the genitourinary system will be diagnosed in 2006, with an estimated 23,670 associated deaths.[2] Of this number, bladder cancer accounts for approximately 61,420 cases, kidney for 38,890 cases, and cancers of the ureter or other urinary organs for 2430 cases.[2]

This chapter discusses the evaluation and treatment of cancer of the kidney and bladder. The diagnostic recommendations and treatment approaches focus on the most common cancer histology in each site, namely renal cell carcinoma (RCC) of the kidney and transitional cell carcinoma (TCC) of the bladder.

ANATOMY AND PHYSIOLOGY

Kidney

The kidneys are bean-shaped organs situated in the posterior part of the abdomen, one on either side of the vertebral column, behind the peritoneum (Figure 11-1). They lie inferior to the diaphragm behind the floating ribs for protection and are surrounded by a layer of fat and fascia that hold them in place. The right kidney is usually positioned slightly lower than the left. Each kidney is about 11 cm long, 5 cm to 7.5 cm wide, and approximately 2.5 cm thick. The left kidney is slightly longer and narrower than the right. The blood supply comes from the renal arteries, which branch directly from the descending aorta to each kidney. The renal artery and vein meet at the kidney at the hilus. The lymphatics of the kidney and renal pelvis drain along the vessels in the renal hilum to the para-aortic, interaortacaval, and paracaval lymph nodes. Autonomic innervation of the kidney is both sympathetic and parasympathetic and is derived from the aorticorenal plexus.

Each kidney is composed of 1 to $1^1/_2$ million filtering units termed *nephrons* (Figure 11-2). The renal capsule is a layer of fibrous tissue that surrounds the kidney to maintain its structure and interior to the capsule is a double layer of renal fascia. The outer portions of the kidney comprise the renal cortex whereas the inner portions are the renal medulla. The renal medulla is organized into triangles called *renal pyramids* that house the nephrons. The renal pelvis receives urine produced by the nephrons, which is carried by the collecting ducts in the renal pyramids.

The function of the kidneys is to remove waste products from the bloodstream (e.g., urea, toxins, and drug metabolites) and regulate blood volume, blood pressure, and electrolyte composition of the blood plasma. In addition, the kidney contributes to glucogenesis and synthesis of the active form of vitamin D, secretion of erythropoietin, and helps to regulate the acid-base balance of blood plasma.

Ureter

The ureters are the two fibrous tubes that contain smooth muscle fibers that move urine from the hilum of each kidney to the bladder. As the ureter exits the kidney, it crosses the psoas muscles and external iliac arteries and travels posterior in the pelvis to join the bladder at the trigone.

Bladder

The urinary bladder is a hollow expandable musculomembranous organ that acts primarily as a reservoir for the urine; its size, position, and relations vary according to the amount of fluid it contains (Figure 11-3). It is triangular in shape and lies within the true pelvis when empty. The posterior surface, the base of the bladder, faces downward and backward. In the female, it is closely related to the anterior wall of the vagina. The critical adjacent structures in women include the uterus, ovaries, fallopian tubes, urethra, and pelvic

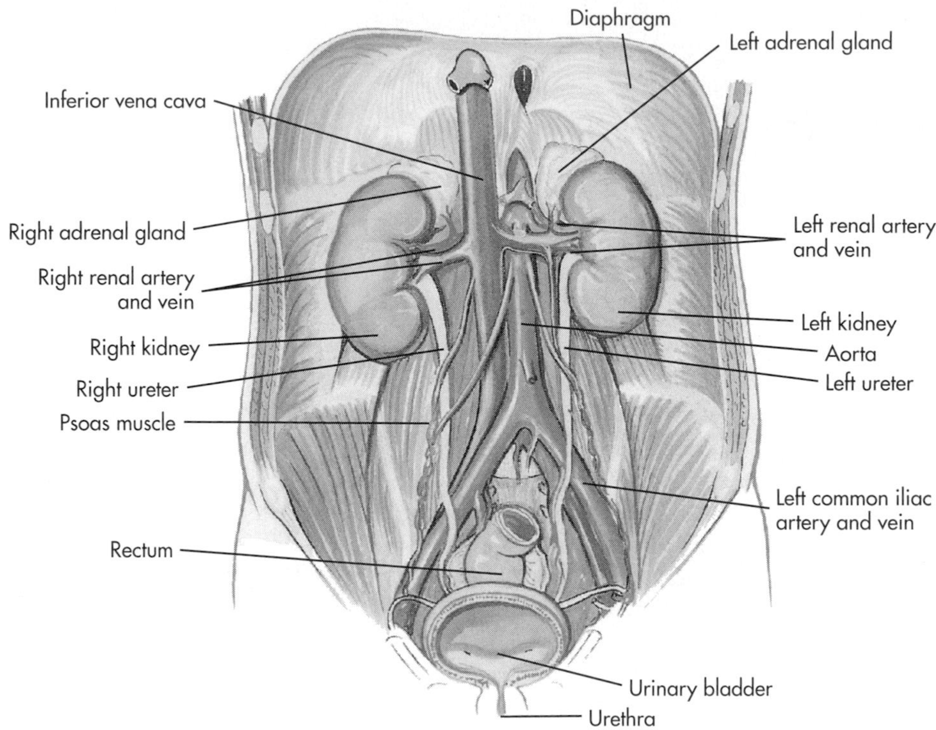

Figure 11-1 Structures of the Urinary System.
From Lewis SM, Heitkemper MM, Dirksen SR; Medical-Surgical Nursing, ed. 6, St. Louis, 2004, Mosby.

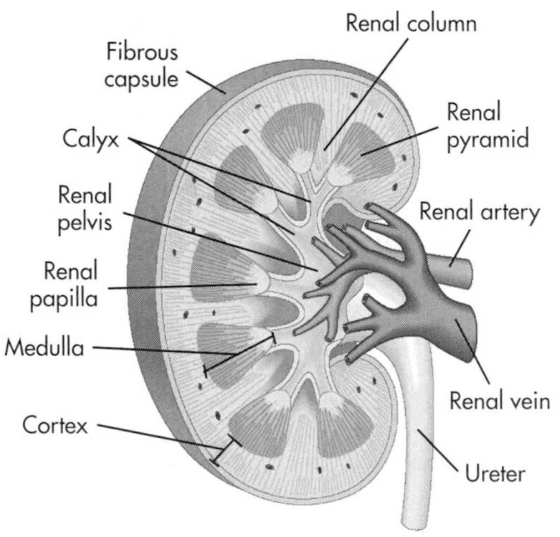

Figure 11-2 Structures of the Kidney.
From Lewis SM, Heitkemper MM, Dirksen SR; Medical-Surgical Nursing, ed. 6, St. Louis, 2004, Mosby.

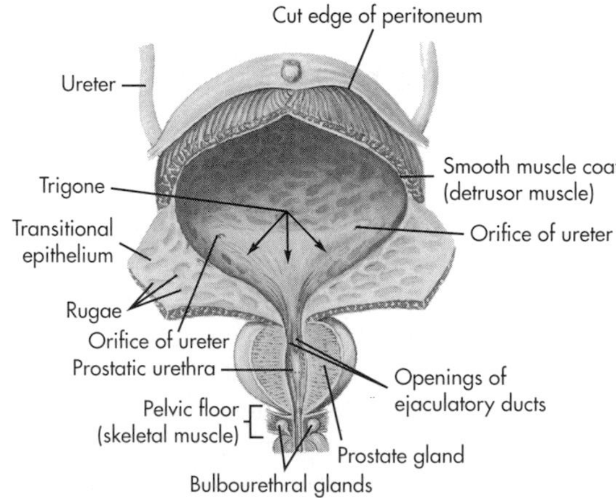

Figure 11-3 Structures of the Bladder.
From Lewis SM, Heitkemper MM, Dirksen SR; Medical-Surgical Nursing, ed. 6, St. Louis, 2004, Mosby.

lymph nodes. In the male, the upper part of the bladder is separated from the rectum by the rectovesical pouch. The lower part of the bladder is separated from the rectum by the seminal vesicles and the deferent duct. The critical adjacent structures in men include the prostate, seminal vesicles, urethra, and nerves at the base of the penis, as well as the pelvic lymph nodes.

The bladder wall is comprised of four distinct layers. The first is the epithelium (transitional epithelium or urothelium), which lines the bladder and is in direct contact with urine. The lamina propria is the second layer that lies under the epithelium. It is a layer of connective tissue and blood vessels. Within the lamina propria is a thin layer of smooth muscle called the muscularis mucosae. The third layer is the muscularis propria or detrusor muscle. This muscle layer consists of thick smooth-muscle bundles that form the wall of the bladder. The final layer is the outermost perivesical layer that consists of fat, fibrous tissue, and blood vessels.

The arterial blood supply to the bladder comes from the superior, middle, and inferior vesicle arteries, derived from the anterior trunk of the hypogastric artery. The obturator and inferior gluteal arteries also supply small visceral branches to the bladder, and in the female additional branches are derived from the uterine and vaginal arteries. The veins form a complicated plexus on the inferior surface, and fundus near the prostate, and end in the hypogastric veins. The lymphatic drainage is by the external and internal iliac and the presacral lymph nodes. The innervation of the bladder comes from fine medullated fibers from the third and fourth sacral nerves, and nonmedullated fibers from the hypogastric plexus. They are connected with ganglia in the outer and submucous coats and are finally distributed, all as nonmedullated fibers, to the muscular layer and epithelial lining of the viscus.

Urethra

The urethra is a tube of smooth muscle that exits the bladder and carries urine to the exterior of the body. In women, the urethra is short; in men, it is longer because it extends through the penis. A ring of skeletal muscle forms an external urethral sphincter that controls voluntary elimination.

EPIDEMIOLOGY

Cancer of the Kidney

Over the past 5 decades, the number of individuals diagnosed with RCC has dramatically increased. It is estimated that the prevalence in the United States has risen by 125% during this period.[3] The incidence of kidney cancer is approximately 2 times higher in men than in women (17.5 per 100,000 males versus 8.7 per 100,000 women).[4] The median age is approximately 65 years.[4] It appears to be equally distributed between Caucasians and African Americans in both men and women. The stage distribution based on historic stage shows that 54% of kidney and renal pelvis cancer cases are diagnosed while the cancer is still confined to the primary site, whereas 20% are diagnosed after the cancer has spread to regional lymph nodes or directly beyond the primary site.[4]

Cancer of the Bladder

The incidence of bladder cancer is approximately 4 times higher in men than women (37.0 per 100,000 men versus 9.3 per 100,000 women).[4] In addition, it is almost twice as common in Caucasian men (40.2 per 100,000) as in African-American men (19.8 per 100,000) or Hispanic men (19.9 per 100,000).[4] In the United States, bladder cancer is the fourth most common cancer in men and ninth most common in women.[2] Bladder cancer occurs most often in the sixth to eight decades of life; it is rare before age 40 and extremely rare in the first 2 decades of life.[4] Internationally the incidence of bladder cancer is higher in the United States than in Japan and Scandinavia.[1]

Risk Factors

Cancer of the Kidney

The diagnosis of hypertension, higher body mass index (BMI), and increasing pack-years of smoking appear to independently increase the risk of RCC.[5] Flaherty and colleagues[5] conducted an investigation using multivariate models including age, BMI, smoking, and hypertension. They found that higher BMI was a confirmed risk factor for women and smoking was a risk factor for men and women. Other studies have also found that exposure to gasoline, diesel, their exposure products, some metal and chemicals in shoe and leather works, and dry-cleaning products also may be associated with kidney cancer.[6]

Cancer of the Bladder

A number of risk factors have been associated with the development of bladder cancer. Tobacco smoking and occupational exposure to aromatic amines are the two major established environmental risk factors for bladder cancer.[7] Aromatic amines are often used in the synthetic textile industry, rubber industry, hair dyes, and paint pigments. There also appears to be an increased risk in occupations such as janitors, cleaners, mechanics, miners, and printers. Other risk factors include increasing age, previous exposure to radiation therapy (for pelvic malignancies), treatment with some chemotherapy agents (cyclophosphamide and ifosfamide), and chronic bladder inflammation related to long-term use of a urinary catheter (e.g., patients with paraplegia). Diet also may influence bladder carcinogenesis, because many compounds contained in foods—and their metabolites—are excreted through the urinary tract. Fruit and vegetable consumption has been inversely related with bladder cancer in many studies, but no consistent association has emerged between intake of related micronutrients and reduced risk of bladder cancer.[7] Other personal habits and dietary factors also have been investigated and not shown to increase risk. They include coffee consumption, artificial sweetener use, and exposure to frequent hair dye. Infections and stones in the urinary tract might cause chronic irritation of the bladder epithelium, and thus increase bladder cancer risk.[7]

Schistosomiasis (chronic parasitic infection) also has been associated with squamous cell carcinoma of the bladder in some parts of the developing world, especially North Africa. A family history of hereditary nonpolyposis colorectal cancer (HNPCC) also has been associated with an increased risk of a malignancy of the urinary system. First-degree relatives of bladder cancer patients have a 50% to 100% increased relative risk of developing the disease, a risk that could be even higher when the proband is diagnosed at an early age.[7]

CLINICAL MANIFESTATIONS

Cancer of the Kidney

Currently, there are no recommended guidelines for screening for cancer of the kidney. Presenting symptoms of RCC may include hematuria, flank mass, and/or flank pain. Other symptoms may include weight loss, fevers, or anemia.[8] Some patients may present with symptoms resulting from metastatic disease such as bone pain or adenopathy. In some patients (25% to 40%), the diagnosis is made after the incidental finding of a renal mass on an imaging study (e.g., ultrasound or computed tomography [CT] scan) performed for another condition.[8]

The initial evaluation should include a complete history and physical examination with Karnofsky performance status because many of these patients are elderly and have significant comorbidities. Care should be taken to evaluate for the presence of adenopathy (in particular supraclavicular), an abdominal mass, lower extremity edema, a varicocele, or subcutaneous nodules. Imaging studies should be ordered to determine the extent of disease; the studies would include a chest x ray to look for lung metastasis and a CT scan of abdomen and pelvis to evaluate the extent of disease in the kidney, find possible evidence of adenopathy, and look for spread of the disease away from the primary site.

RCC may spread by local infiltration through the renal capsule into the perinephritic fat and fascia.[9] It may grow directly along the venous channels to the renal vein or vena cava. RCC metastasizes mainly to the lung, bone, brain, liver, and adrenal gland. Additional radiographic studies such as magnetic resonance imaging (MRI) or positron imaging tomography (PET) scanning will depend on reported symptoms and physical examination findings. Initial laboratory studies may include a complete blood count with chemistry studies to look for evidence of renal and liver dysfunction. Additional studies may be warranted to assess overall medical condition, particularly when considering surgical resection or combined modality therapy.

RCC comprises 90% of all kidney malignancies, with 85% being clear cell tumors.[10] Other less common cell types include papillary, chromophobe, and Bellini duct (collecting duct) tumors.[10] Medullary renal carcinoma is a variant of collecting-duct renal carcinoma that has been described in patients who are sickle-cell trait positive. Collecting-duct carcinoma comprises less than 1% of kidney cancer cases.[8] A number of hereditary types of renal cell carcinoma are associated with different histological types of renal carcinoma including von Hippel-Lindau syndrome.

Prognosis is related to tumor grade and stage. The American Joint Committee on Cancer (AJCC) staging system is the primary method used to stage cancers of the kidney, (Table 11-1) and is the most important prognostic factor for RCC. Other factors include clinical signs and symptoms, performance status, laboratory values, tumor size, grade, histology, and ploidy. In the past 30 years, the overall prognosis of RCC appears to have improved,[11] but it remains the sixth leading cause of cancer death.[12] Patients with early, localized RCC have a good prognosis, but those with advanced disease do not respond to most tradi-

Table 11-1 AJCC Staging System for Kidney Cancer

Cancer stage	Clinical/pathologic findings
PRIMARY TUMOR (T)	
TX	Primary tumor cannot be assessed
T0	No evidence of primary tumor
T1	Tumor 7 cm or less in greatest dimension, l limited to the kidney
T1a	Tumor 4 cm or less in greatest dimension, limited to the kidney
T1b	Tumor more than 4 cm but not more than 7 cm in greatest dimension, limited to the kidney
T2	Tumor more than 7 cm in greatest dimension, limited to the kidney
T3	Tumor extends into the major veins or invades adrenal gland or perinephric tissues but not beyond Gerota's fascia
T3a	Tumor directly invades the adrenal gland or perirenal and/or renal sinus fat but not beyond Gerota's fascia
T3b	Tumor grossly extends into the renal vein or its segmental (muscle-containing) branches, or vena cava below the diaphragm
T3c	Tumor grossly extends into vena cava above diaphragm or invades the wall of the vena cava
T4	Tumor invades beyond Gerota's fascia
REGIONAL LYMPH NODES (N)*	
NX	Regional lymph nodes cannot be assessed
N0	No regional lymph node metastases
N1	Metastases in a single regional lymph node
N2	Metastases in more than one regional lymph node

* NOTE: Laterality does not affect the N classification.

NOTE: If a lymph node dissection is performed, then pathologic evaluation would ordinarily include at least eight nodes.

Cancer stage	Clinical/pathologic findings		
DISTANT METASTASIS (M)			
MX	Distant metastasis cannot be assessed		
M0	No distant metastasis		
M1	Distant metastasis		
STAGE GROUPING			
Stage I	T1	N0	M0
Stage II	T2	N0	M0
Stage III	T1	N1	M0
	T2	N1	M0
	T3	N0	M0
	T3	N1	M0
	T3a	N0	M0
	T3a	N1	M0
	T3b	N0	M0
	T3b	N1	M0
	T3c	N0	M0
	T3c	N1	M0
Stage IV	T4	N0	M0
	T4	N1	M0
	Any T	N2	M0
	Any T	Any N	M1

Reproduced with permission: Greene GL, Balch CM, Fleming ID, April F, & Page DL (2003). *AJCC Cancer Staging Manual*, (Sixth ed) (pp 323-328). New York: Springer-Verlag.

Used with the permission of the American Joint Committee on Cancer (AJCC), Chicago, Illinois. The original source for this material is the *AJCC Cancer Staging Manual, Sixth Edition* (2002), published by Springer-New York, www.springeronline.com.

tional regimens, and estimated median survival for late-stage disease is less than 1 year.[13]

Cancer of the Bladder

Currently, there are no recommended guidelines for screening for cancer of the bladder. Presenting symptoms may include painless hematuria. Other symptoms include irritative voiding symptoms (e.g., frequency, urgency, and/or hesitancy), reduced bladder capacity, pelvic pain, and urinary tract infection. Patients also may present with symptoms resulting from metastatic disease such as bone pain or adenopathy. In locally advanced cases, patients may present with voiding symptoms caused by bladder neck obstruction or with flank pain caused by hydronephrosis resulting from ureteral obstruction. Change in bowel habits or unexplained weight loss may be present in advanced cases.

The initial evaluation should include a complete history and physical examination along with determination of Karnofsky performance status because many of these patients are elderly and have significant comorbidities. The physical exam should include a bimanual exam under anesthesia to detect masses in the bladder. A cystoscopy with cytologies and transurethral resection of the bladder tumor (TURBT) is usually the first diagnostic test to confirm the diagnosis and determine the extend of disease. Other imaging studies may include a chest x ray to evaluate for pulmonary disease, an intravenous pyelogram (IVP), and a CT scan of the abdomen and pelvis. Whether to add radiographic studies such as MRI, bone scan, or PET scan as part of the work-up will depend on reported symptoms and physical examination findings. Initial laboratory studies may include a complete blood count with chemistry studies to look for evidence of renal and liver dysfunction. Additional studies may be warranted to assess overall medical condition, particularly when considering surgical resection or combined modality therapy.

Bladder cancer commonly spreads through direct extension and hematogenously. The disease may extend directly into other pelvic organs including the colon, prostate, uterus, or vagina. Hematogenous spread includes metastasis to bone, liver, or lung. Tumor can also spread rapidly through the regional lymph nodes including the obturator, hypogastric, external iliac, common iliac, hypergastric (or internal iliac), and paraaortic nodes.[14]

Urothelial (transitional cell) carcinomas are the most common histologic subtype in the United States and may develop anywhere there is transitional epithelium.[15] Within the category of transitional cell carcinomas, the cell types are further divided into carcinoma in situ (CIS), which is confined to the urothelial lining; papillary infiltrating; papillary noninfiltrating; and solid tumors. Urothelial tumors also may present with a mixture of histologic subtypes. Other types of bladder cancer include adenocarcinomas, small cell carcinomas, and sarcoma. Adenocarcinomas often occur in the dome of the bladder and in the periurethral tissues.[15] The AJCC staging system is the most commonly used system for bladder cancer (Table 11-2).

TREATMENT

Surgery is the mainstay of treatment for RCC, which, in general, is highly resistant to chemotherapy, hormone therapy, and radiation therapy. Immunotherapy medications are showing promising results in kidney cancer clinical trials.

Stage I or II Renal Cell Carcinoma of the Kidney

For localized tumors, surgery is the treatment of choice, and several options are available depending on the stage of disease and the patient's overall health and preference. When the tumor is small and confined to the top or bottom portion of the kidney, a partial nephrectomy may be performed. This procedure is useful for patients with RCC in both kidneys and for patients who have only one functioning kidney. Radical nephrectomy, the gold standard, involves removal of the entire kidney and the adrenal gland and may include removal of surrounding tissue and regional lymph nodes (regional lymphadenectomy). It is usually performed through a large abdominal incision (open radical nephrectomy) or may be performed using several small incisions (laparoscopic radical nephrectomy).

A nephron-sparing surgery known as *nephrectomy* may be indicated in select patients, including those with multiple primaries, patients in an uninephric state, patients with renal insufficiency, and select patients with small (less than 4 cm) unilateral tumors. Lymph node dissection is optional and the adrenal gland may be left if uninvolved and the tumor is not high risk based on size and location.[8]

Table 11-2 AJCC Staging System for Bladder Cancer

Cancer stage	Clinical/pathologic findings		
PRIMARY TUMOR (T)			
TX	Primary tumor cannot be assessed		
T0	No evidence of primary tumor		
Ta	Noninvasive papillary carcinoma		
Tis	Carcinoma in situ: "flat tumor"		
T1	Tumor invades subepithelial connective tissue		
T2	Tumor invades muscle		
T2a	Tumor invades superficial muscle (inner half)		
T2b	Tumor invades deep muscle (outer half)		
T3	Tumor invades perivesical tissue		
T3a	Microscopically		
T3b	Macroscopically (extravesical mass)		
T4	Tumor invades any of the following: prostate, uterus, vagina, pelvic wall, abdominal wall		
T4a	Tumor invades prostate, uterus, vagina		
T4b	Tumor invades pelvic wall, abdominal wall		
CLINICAL STAGING			
Primary tumor assessment includes bimanual examination under anesthesia before and after endoscopic surgery (biopsy or transurethral resection) and histologic verification of the presence or absence of tumor when indicated. Bimanual examination following endoscopic surgery is an indicator of clinical stage. The finding of bladder wall thickening, a mobile mass, or a fixed mass suggests the presence of T3a, T3b, and T4b disease, respectively. Appropriate imaging techniques for lymph node evaluation should be used. When indicated, evaluation for distant metastases includes imaging of the chest, biochemical studies, and isotopic studies to detect common metastatic sites.			
PATHOLOGIC STAGING			
Microscopic examination and confirmation of extent are required. Total cystectomy and lymph node dissection generally are required for this staging. Laterality does not affect the N classification.			
REGIONAL LYMPH NODES (N)			
Regional lymph nodes are those within the true pelvis: all others are distant lymph nodes.			
NX	Regional lymph nodes cannot be assessed		
N0	No regional lymph node metastasis		
N1	Metastasis in a single lymph node, 2 cm or less in greatest dimension		
N2	Metastasis in a single lymph node, more than 2 cm but not more than 5 cm in greatest dimension; or multiple lymph nodes, none more than 5 cm in greatest dimension		
N3	Metastasis in a lymph node more than 5 cm in greatest dimension		
DISTANT METASTASIS (M)			
MX	Distant metastasis cannot be assessed		
M0	No distant metastasis		
M1	Distant metastasis		
STAGE GROUPING			
Stage 0a	Ta	N0	M0
Stage 0is	Tis	N0	M0
Stage I	T1	N0	M0
Stage II	T2a	N0	M0
	T2b	N0	M0
Stage III	T3a	N0	M0
	T3b	N0	M0
	T4a	N0	M0
Stage IV	T4b	N0	M0
	Any T	N1	M0
	Any T	N2	M0
	Any T	N3	M0
	Any T	Any N	M1

Reproduced with permission: Greene, GL, Balch, CM, Fleming, ID, April, F, & Page, DL (2003). *AJCC Cancer Staging Manual*, (Sixth ed) (pp 335-340). New York: Springer-Verlag.

Used with the permission of the American Joint Committee on Cancer (AJCC), Chicago, Illinois. The original source for this material is the *AJCC Cancer Staging Manual, Sixth Edition* (2002), published by Springer-New York, www.springeronline.com.

Adjuvant chemotherapy, radiation therapy, or immunotherapy is usually not recommended after surgery. For patients with significant comorbid disease who may not be suitable candidates for surgery, treatment may include either cryoablation or arterial embolization. Radiation therapy has not been shown to be beneficial in the neoadjuvant setting, but may offer some benefit in the postoperative setting, particularly in patients with T3, N0 tumors.[9] Although postoperative irradiation maybe recommended in patients with incomplete resections, perinephric fat extension, adrenal gland invasion, or regional lymph node metastasis, further studies in phase III trials are needed to determine the exact benefit.[9] Postoperative radiation is usually given to doses of 45 Gy to 50 Gy in 1.8 Gy to 2.0 Gy daily fractions to the nephrectomy bed and regional lymph nodes with a boost (additional 10 Gy to 15 Gy) to small volumes of microscopic or gross residual disease (total dose of 50 Gy to 60 Gy).[9] Care should be taken to avoid excessive treatment to the contralateral kidney, liver, and spinal cord.

Stage III or IV RCC of the Kidney

Radical nephrectomy is the most common treatment for stage III RCC. For patients with metastatic RCC, treatment is individualized to the patient and usually involves palliative treatments to manage symptoms. Radical nephrectomy also may be used in palliative care, even if the disease has spread to other organs. Removing the diseased kidney may reduce symptoms and may improve short-term survival. Radiation therapy is often used to manage painful sites of disease in bone or soft-tissue by reducing the volume of disease. Short courses of treatment are often prescribed and well tolerated. Patients also may benefit from enrollment in a clinical trial.

Non-Muscle–Invasive Cancer of the Bladder (TIX, Ta, T1)

Superficial tumors comprise 70% of bladder cancer and are generally treated with some type of local treatment.[15] Only 10% to 20% will progress to a higher clinical stage over time.[16] Local therapies include transurethral resection of the bladder tumor (TURBT), laser photocoagulation, and intravesical therapy with agents such as bacillus Calmette-Guérin (BCG), mitomycin C, doxorubicin, thiotepa, or interferon. Although TURBT is typically the first step in treatment, adjuvant intravesical therapy has been found to be more effective than TURBT alone.[17] In patients with diffuse grade 3, T1 disease or involvement of the prostatic urethra or ducts are sometimes offered cystectomy.[9] The survival of patients with Ta tumors is 95% or more at 5 years, but decreases significantly in those with T1 lesions.[18]

Muscle-Invasive Cancer of the Bladder

Surgical treatment with radical cystectomy and creation of a urinary diversion is still the most effective local therapy in muscle-invasive bladder cancer. The surgery involves removal of the bladder, prostate, seminal vesicles, and proximal urethra. In females, the entire urethra, anterior vaginal wall, uterus, fallopian tubes, and ovaries are removed. Urinary diversions may include an ileal conduit or directing urine to an internal urinary reservoir, with drainage to the abdominal wall or the urethra. Radical cystectomy (without preoperative irradiation) is recommended for superficial disease (TIS, Ta, T1) when conservative management is unsuccessful. Cystectomy is also indicated for patients with clinical stage T2-3 disease and for recurrent tumors in patients with inadequate bladder capacity because of contracture caused by repeated transurethral resections (TURs) and intravesicular chemotherapy.[9]

Preoperative irradiation is recommended for large (4 cm or more) or deeply infiltrating (T3 and resectable T4) or high-grade lesions. Preoperative irradiation may be low-dose, 30 Gy in 10 fractions over 2 weeks, or 44 Gy in 22 fractions over 4.5 weeks. This is usually followed by surgery in 2 to 4 weeks.[9] In patients who have received higher-dose irradiation, lympyhadenectomy is not usually necessary.[9]

A partial cystectomy may be performed if the lesion is circumscribed in the dome of the bladder where a 1-cm to 2-cm margin can be obtained, or if a papillary transitional cell carcinoma is within a bladder diverticulum. In these circumstances, low-dose neoadjuvant radiation is usually performed to decrease the incidence of wound seeding with tumor during the surgical procedure.

The most effective nonsurgical treatment for bladder cancer remains radiation therapy. Patients who are not surgical candidates or refuse radical surgery may be offered radiation therapy. Patients treated with definitive irradiation ideally should have adequate bladder capacity without substantial voiding symptoms or incontinence.[9] A four-field box technique with the patient in a supine position is used most often. At the time of the simulation, the bladder should be empty and a small amount of contrast placed in the bladder and rectum to further define these structures on the images. The whole bladder is treated with 40 Gy to 55 Gy, followed by a boost to the bladder tumor of 64 Gy to 66 Gy (avoiding normal areas of the bladder if possible).[15] The regional lymph nodes are treated by including the bony pelvic side walls with approximately a 1.5-cm margin in the anterior and posterior portals.[9]

Both neoadjuvant and adjuvant therapy have been evaluated in patients with locally advanced bladder cancer. Combination cisplatin-based neoadjuvant chemotherapy may benefit patients with locally advanced bladder cancer. The presence of occult micrometastases at the time of radical cystectomy leads to both distant and local failure in patients with locally advanced transitional cell carcinoma of the bladder. Various regimens of combined chemotherapy and radiation also have been evaluated. Chemoradiation is feasible and effective in some patients, allowing bladder preservation with an acceptable risk of progression. Studies evaluating adjuvant chemotherapy have been limited by inadequate statistical power to detect meaningful clinical answers, as well as by experimental arms that use inadequate chemotherapy. This has led to the widespread use of gemcitabine/cisplatin as first-line chemotherapy for metastatic bladder cancer. The optimal agents and regimens for second-line chemotherapy remain undefined. Similarly, biologic and targeted therapies for advanced bladder cancer remain investigational. The optimal regimens for the medically unfit patient and second-line chemotherapy remain undefined. The development of targeted therapies, less toxic regimens, and improved cytotoxic agents are necessary to improve outcome. Two Radiation Therapy Oncology Group (RTOG) studies are currently evaluating the role of different systemic agents (chemotherapy and monoclonal antibodies) with radiation in the organ preservation setting (#0524 and #0233).[19]

A number of new approaches to treatment are on the horizon including particle beam therapy, new fractionation schemes with both hyperfractionated and hypofractionated radiation therapy, hypoxia modification using carbogen and nicotinamide, as well as some new systemic agents. Anti-EGFR agents and antiangiogenic agents also may show promise, as may the development of anti-apoptotic agents and gene therapy that may become a component of future multimodality therapy.

NURSING CARE AND EDUCATION

Acute and late toxicity associated with radiation therapy for genitourinary malignancies depends on the site of treatment, the volume of treatment included in the treatment fields, the technique used, the total dose given, and the presence of comorbid disease. In patients treated with abdominopelvic radiation, acute complications may include nausea, vomiting, diarrhea, frequency of urination, leukopenia, thrombocytopenia, transient hepatic enzyme elevation, and (on occasion) symptomatic basal pneumonitis.[20] Late toxicities may include bowel obstruction, enteritis, fistulae formation, proctitis, hemorrhagic cystitis, and infertility.

Patients who receive treatment directed to the pelvis may experience acute toxicities that are predominantly urinary or bowel related. These include urinary frequency, dysuria, nocturia, prostatism, vaginitis, tenesmus, rectal urgency, diarrhea, proctitis, nausea, and moist desquamation within skinfolds. Late toxicities may include bowel obstruction, hemorrhagic cystitis, urinary incontinence, urethral strictures, erectile dysfunction, chronic pelvic pain, vaginal stenosis, vesicovaginal fistula, rectovaginal fistula, enteritis, proctitis, pelvic nerve damage, and lower extremity edema. If the perineum is included in the treatment field, acute brisk erythema and moist desquamation will occur in the majority of patients. Infertility and menopause will be permanent in women treated with radiation therapy that involves the pelvis.

The key to successful management of these toxicities is patient education and accurate evaluation and documentation. Nurses play a significant role in patient education, including providing measures to reduce the risk of toxicities (e.g., diet modifications) and management of expected side effects during and after treatment. Table 11-3 provides a list of resources for both patient education material and nursing education support.

Accurate documentation of toxicity of treatment is the responsibility of the physician and nursing staff. Two instruments are available for grading the severity of acute effects. They are the National Cancer Institute's *Common Toxicity Criteria for Adverse Events* (CTCAE-v 3.0)[21] and the *Radiation Therapy Patient Care Record: A Tool for Documenting Nursing Care.*[22]

Table 11-3 Resources for the Patient and Family

Resource	Types of services	Website
American Cancer Society	Education materials Local support groups Advocacy Financial support	www.cancer.org
American Urological Association Foundation	Education Advocacy	www.auafoundation.org
Kidney Cancer Association	Education Advocacy	www.curekidneycancer.org
National Cancer Institute	Education materials	www.cancer.gov
National Lymphedema Network	Patient education Advocacy	www.lymphnet.org
Team Survivor	Survivorship advocacy	www.teamsurvivor.org
Urology Health	Patient education Advocacy	www.urologyhealth.org

Acute Toxicity

Skin reactions are usually confined to areas with skinfolds and the perineum. Treatment to the abdomen does not generally result in a skin reaction. Treatment to the pelvis may result in mild hyperpigmentation in the treatment fields and moist desquamation in folds of abdominal skin, in the groin, and between the buttocks. See Chapter 30 for skin care management recommendations.

Acute cystitis usually becomes symptomatic after 10 to 14 days of treatment and results in dysuria, increased frequency, urgency hesitancy, and increased nocturia. The symptoms usually resolve within 1 month of completing treatment. Adequate hydration and avoidance of food and beverages that may irritate the bladder will help. This includes beverages that contain caffeine and alcohol. Although infection is rare, a urine culture and sensitivity may be necessary if the patient's symptoms include cloudy urine samples or hematuria or if the patient becomes febrile. Urinary tract analgesics such as phenazopyridine hydrochloride and antispasmodics such as hyoscyamine sulfate and oxybutynin chloride may help with the symptoms.

Diarrhea (radiation-induced) results from a variety of different pathophysiologic mechanisms including malabsorption of bile salts and lactose, imbalances in local bacterial flora, and changes in the intestinal patterns of motility. Management options may be found in Chapter 34.

Nausea and vomiting may occur when patients are receiving treatment to the abdomen. Prophylactic antiemetics before radiation therapy often eliminate this problem. Occasionally patients receiving treatment only to the pelvis report mild nausea. Chapter 34 offers a variety of treatment approaches. If persistent nausea with vomiting occurs, evaluation for bowel obstruction may be warranted.

Vaginal mucositis usually occurs within the first 14 to 21 days of treatment. This occurs as a result of changes in the vaginal epithelium. Patients will report symptoms of discomfort and dyspareunia. If a foul-smelling or thin watery discharge begins, cultures should be obtained for infections such as *Candida albicans,* bacterial vaginosis, and chlamydia. Otherwise, patients may be treated symptomatically.

Fatigue is also common when patients are treated with pelvic or abdominal radiation therapy. The mechanisms that produce fatigue as a result of radiation are poorly understood. However, fatigue can significantly impact the patient's quality of life, ability to continue treatment, and tolerance of acute and late effects of treatment. Nursing education is key to reducing the impact of fatigue on the patient's ability to function. Adequate nutrition and hydration, adequate sleep and rest times, and a realistic approach to personal accomplishments and daily activities are three primary approaches to fatigue reduction. A comprehensive approach to management can be found in the NCCN Practice Guidelines in Oncology, *Cancer-Related Fatigue,* v.1.2006, available at www.nccn.org/professionals/physician_gls/PDF/fatigue.pdf

Late Toxicity

Radiation-induced intestinal injury (i.e., enteritis and proctitis) can result in local ischemia and fibrosis with the development of ulcers, strictures, and rectal bleeding. Symptoms may include rectal bleeding, painful bowel movements, and chronic or intermittent diarrhea. Occasionally, the rectal bleeding can be severe enough to result in anemia and transfusion dependency. Bleeding typically develops from 6 months to 1 year after completion of radiation therapy and is caused by friable mucosal angioectasias.

As might be expected because of the organs involved, sexual dysfunction and infertility may be reported among patients receiving treatment directed to the pelvis. The degree and nature of dysfunction will vary according to the type, length, and intensity of treatment. Management should be individualized depending on the patient's symptoms and reported interest in treatment options.

Obliterative endarteritis secondary to ionizing radiation may lead to tissue hypoxia, poor healing, and ultimately to fistulae formation. In patients who have had radiation therapy to the pelvis, fistulae may form between the bladder and vagina, vagina and rectum, bowel and vagina, or bowel and bladder. Patients may present with fecal material draining from the vagina, fecal material in the urine, or urine draining from the vagina. If the small bowel is involved, significant damage can occur to tissue exposed to the small bowel contents. Management of fistulae requires a multidisciplinary team of surgeons, wound care providers, and nutritional experts to design a program to divert the fecal matter or urine, and promote healing. Surgery may be necessary to create a diversion around the fistulae. Total parenteral nutrition may be necessary to reduce bowel content and provide adequate calories and protein for healing. Hyperbaric oxygen therapy has also been demonstrated to improve angiogenesis and promote healing in radiation-injured tissue.

A rare complication of radiation therapy to the pelvis (particularly when the groin area is included in the field) is necrosis and fracture of the femoral head/neck. Grigsby and colleagues[23] reported a 5% actuarial 5-year incidence of fractures in patients receiving doses of 50 Gy or greater.

Follow-Up Care

Cancer of the Kidney

A follow-up evaluation should be performed every 6 months for a minimum of 2 years, then annually for 5 years.[8] The evaluation should include a history and physical examination with complete metabolic profile and lactate dehydrogenase (LDH). A chest x ray should be performed annually. Every 4 to 6 months, a CT scan of the abdomen should be performed. Additional radiograph and laboratory studies should be performed based on reported symptoms and findings during the clinical exam.

The overall 5-year survival rate for years 1996 to 2002 from 17 Surveillance Epidemiology and End Result (SEER) geographic areas was 65.6%.[4] The corresponding 5-year relative survival rates were 90.4% for localized disease, 61.7% for regional disease, and 9.5% for patients with distant disease.[4]

Cancer of the Bladder

For patients with noninvasive bladder cancer, a follow-up evaluation should be performed every 3 months, with increasing intervals as appropriate.[15] The evaluation should include a history and physical examination with cystoscopy. Imaging studies of the upper tract collecting system should be performed every 1 to 2 years and may include IVP, CT urography, retrograde pyelogram, or MRI urogram. Additional radiograph and laboratory studies should be performed based on reported symptoms and findings during the clinical exam.

For patients with muscle-invasive disease, a follow-up evaluation should be performed every 3 months for a minimum of 2 years. A chest x ray should be performed every 6 to 12 months depending on risk of recurrence.[15] Additional studies may include comprehensive laboratory studies to evaluate liver and renal function. If the patient had a cystectomy, a CT scan of the pelvis should be performed every 3 to 6 months for 2 years and then as clinically indicated.[15] For patients who underwent bladder-sparing treatment, a cystoscopy with cytology (and biopsy of suspicious areas) should be performed every 3 months for the first year and then in increasing intervals.

The overall 5-year survival rate for years 1996 to 2002 from 17 SEER geographic areas was 80.8%.[4] The corresponding 5-year relative survival rates were: 93.7% for localized disease, 46.0% for regional disease, and 6.2% for patients with distant disease.[4]

REFERENCES

1. Ferlay J, Bray F, Pisani P et al: *GLOBOCAN 2002: Cancer incidence, mortality and prevalence worldwide. IARC cancer base no 5, version 2.0*, Lyon, France, 2004, IARC Press.
2. *Cancer facts and figures, 2006,* Atlanta, American Cancer Society, 2006.
3. Pantuck AJ, Zisman A, Belldegrun AS: The changing natural history of renal cell carcinoma, *J Urol* 166(5): 1611-1623, 2001.
4. Ries LAG, Eisner MP, Kosary CL et al, editors: *Seer cancer statistics review, 1975-2002*, Bethesda, MD, 2004, National Cancer Institute (website): http:/seer.coancr.gov/csr/1975-2002. Accessed June 9, 2006.
5. Flaherty KT, Fuchs CS, Colditz GA et al: A prospective study of body mass index, hypertension, and smoking and the risk of renal cell carcinoma (United States), *Cancer Causes Control* 16(9):1099-1106, 2005.
6. Ji J, Granstrom C, Hemminki K: Occupational risk factors for kidney cancer: a cohort study in Sweden, *World J Urol* 23(4):271-278, 2005.
7. Pelucchi C, Bosetti C, Nigri E et al: Mechanisms of disease: the epidemiology of bladder cancer, *Natl Clin Pract Urol* 3(6):327-340, 2006.
8. National Comprehensive Cancer Network: *Practice guidelines in oncology: kidney cancer,* V2.2006, Jenkintown, PA, 2006, National Comprehensive Cancer Network.
9. Chao KSC, Perez CA, Brady LW: *Radiation oncology: management decisions*, Philadelphia, 2002, Lippincott-Raven, p 431.
10. Motzer RJ, Bander NH, Nanus DM: Renal-cell carcinoma, *N Engl J Med* 335(12):865-875, 1996.
11. Drucker BJ: Renal cell carcinoma: current status and future prospects, *Cancer Treat Rev* 31(7):536-545, 2005.
12. Godely PA, Ataga KI: Renal cell carcinoma, *Curr Opin Oncol* 12(3):260-264, 2000.
13. Campbell SC, Flanigan RC, Clark JI: Nephrectomy in metastatic renal cell carcinoma, *Curr Treat Options Oncol* 4(5):363-372, 2003.
14. Brooks JD: Anatomy of the lower urinary tract. In Walsh P, Retik A, Vaughan E, Wein A, editors: *Campbell's Urology,* ed 7, Philadelphia, 1998, WB Saunders, pp 15-22.
15. National Comprehensive Cancer Network: *Practice guidelines in oncology: bladder cancer,* V1.2006, Jenkintown, PA, 2006, National Comprehensive Cancer Network.
16. Malkowicz S, Wein A: Adult genitourinary cancer. In Hanno P, Malkowicz SB, Wein A, editors: *Clinical manual of urology,* ed 3, New York, 2001, McGraw-Hill, pp 487-561.
17. Duque JL, Loughlin K: An overview of the treatment of superficial bladder cancer: intravesical chemotherapy, *Urol Clin North Am* 27(1):125-135, 2000.
18. Widmark A, Flodgren P, Damber J et al: A systematic overview of radiation therapy effects in bladder cancer, *Acta Oncol* 42(5):567-581, 2003.
19. Radiation Therapy Oncology Group: *Active protocols: genitourinary cancer* (website): www.rtog.org/members/active.html#genitourinary, 2006. Accessed June 19, 2006.
20. Fyles AW, Dembo AJ, Bush RS: Analysis of complications in patients treated with abdomino-pelvic radiation therapy for ovarian carcinoma, *Int J Radiat Oncol Biol Phys* 22(5):847-851, 1992.
21. *NCI common toxicity criteria for adverse events* (CTCAE v 3.0). Bethesda, MD, 2003, National Cancer Institute.
22. Radiation Therapy Special Interest Group Documentation Project Core Committee: *Radiation Therapy Patient*, Pittsburgh, Oncology Nursing Press, 2002.
23. Grigsby PW, Roberts HL, Perez CA: Femoral neck fracture following groin irradiation, *Int J Radiat Oncol Biol Phys* 32(1):63-67, 1995.

Chapter 12
Gynecologic Cancers

Giselle J. Moore-Higgs

Gynecologic malignancies are a major healthcare problem worldwide. In the most recent Globcon report, it was estimated that more than 900,000 women worldwide would be diagnosed with cervix, uterus, or ovarian cancer in the year 2000.[1] The vast majority of these cases (more than 490,000 cases) were cancers of the cervix.[1] In the United States, the American Cancer Society (ACS) estimates 77,250 new cases of female genital cancer will be diagnosed in 2006, with more than 28,000 associated deaths.[2]

This chapter discusses the evaluation and treatment of cancer of the vulva, vagina, cervix, uterus, ovary, and fallopian tube. The diagnostic recommendations and treatment approaches focus on the most common cancer histology in each site (i.e., squamous cell carcinoma of the vulva).

ANATOMY AND PHYSIOLOGY

The female genitalia are divided into separate organ sites for the diagnosis, staging, and treatment of cancer. Sites include the vulva, vagina, uterine cervix, uterine corpus, fallopian tube, and ovary. The organ-specific anatomy is as follows.

Vulva

The vulva includes those portions of the female genital tract that are externally visible in the perineal region, lying between the genitocrural folds laterally, the mons pubis anteriorly, and the anus posteriorly (Figure 12-1). This includes the vulvar vestibule, the clitoris, the labia minora, labia majora, and the mons pubis. The vulvar vestibule is the portion of the vulva that extends from the exterior surface of the hymen to the frenulum of the clitoris anteriorly, fourchette posteriorly, and laterally to Hart's line.[3] Hart's line is a distinctive mark on the vulva where the nonkeratinized squamous epithelium of the vestibule joins the more papillated-appearing keratinized epithelium of the lateral labia minora. The vestibule is composed of stratified, nonkeratinized squamous epithelium. Structures within the vestibule include the urethral orifice, vaginal introitus, openings of the Bartholin's gland ducts, and openings of the minor vestibular glands.[3]

The labia minora lie between the labia majora and are separated laterally from the labia majora by the intralabial sulcus. Anteriorly, the labia minora split, then fuse beneath the clitoris as the frenulum and above the clitoris to form the prepuce. They are thin folds of redundant connective tissue, composed of highly vascular erectile tissue, covered with stratified squamous epithelium that is not keratinized on the vestibular surface, and thinly keratinized on the lateral surface.

The labia majora are two longitudinal folds of skin that extend in an elliptical manner from the mons pubis, posteriorly to enclose the vulvar cleft. The labia majora are covered with stratified squamous epithelium, which is hair-bearing in the lateral and midportions of the labial surface and hairless on the medial surfaces. These hair shafts are associated with sebaceous glands and apocrine sweat glands. Both the sebaceous and apocrine glands are stimulated by sex hormones; however, the apocrine sweat glands are functional throughout life.[3] The labia minora are relatively prominent in children because the labia majora are not well developed until puberty. In some postmenopausal women, the labia majora tend to atrophy, and the labia minora again become prominent.

The mons pubis is the portion of the vulva presenting as the rounded, fleshy prominence over the symphysis pubis. The surface of the mons is composed of stratified squamous epithelium, similar to that of the labia majora with hair and sebaceous glands distributed throughout its substance. The underlying tissue of the mons is composed primarily of adipose tissue.

The blood supply to the vulva is abundant and comes from branches of the internal and external

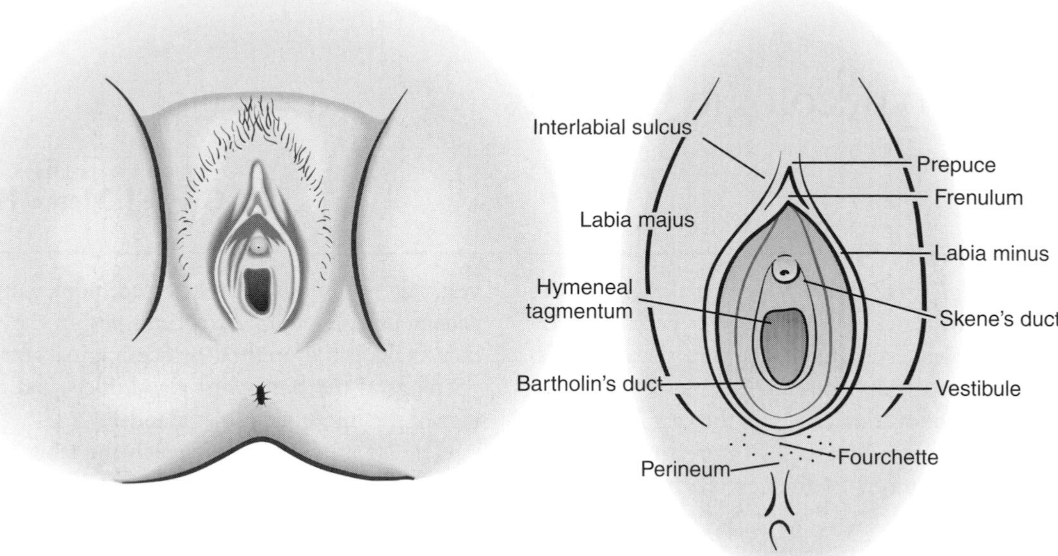

Figure 12-1 Anatomy of the Vulva.

pudendal artery. A network of lymphatics that terminate in the inguinal and femoral lymph nodes drain the vulva, the lower third of the vagina, and the perineum.

Vagina

The vagina is a thin-walled, muscular, dilatable tube, averaging 8 cm to 10 cm in length, that passes obliquely upward and backward at an angle of approximately 45 degrees from the introitus in the vestibule to the uterus. It attaches circumferentially to the uterine cervix, at a higher point on the posterior wall than on the anterior wall, forming a circular groove at the junction called the *fornix*. The base of the bladder is in direct contact with the upper one third of the anterior vaginal wall, the urethra is in contact with the lower two-thirds of the anterior vaginal wall, and the rectum lies directly below the posterior vaginal wall.

The vagina is composed of three layers of tissue. The lower part of the vagina is lined with a thick, nonkeratinizing, nonglandular, stratified, squamous epithelium. The upper two-thirds is derived initially from glandular tissue that undergoes a process of metaplasia in utero to form a "mucosa" of nonkeratinized stratified squamous epithelium extending onto the ectocervix. The mucosa forms many transverse folds called *rugae* and is lubricated by mucus emanating from the cervix and, during intercourse, from the Bartholin's glands. The muscularis layer is composed of smooth muscle fibers arranged circularly on the inner portion and longitudinally on the thicker outer portion. The adventitia is a thin, outer connective tissue layer that merges with that of adjacent organs. The vaginal sphincter at the introitus is formed by skeletal muscle.

The vagina is supplied with blood from branches of the internal iliac and uterine arteries. The lymphatic drainage of the upper vagina is shared by the cervix and includes the ureteral, hypogastric, obturator, external iliac, lateral sacral, and promontory lymph nodes in the pelvis. The lower third of the vagina has the same lymphatic drainage as the vulva.

Uterus

The uterus lies in between the bladder and the rectum (Figure 12-2). It is divided structurally and functionally into two parts, the corpus, or body, and the cervix, which are separated by a slight narrowing of the uterus known as the *isthmus*. The walls of the uterus are composed of muscular tissue called the myometrium. The epithelial membrane that lines the uterine corpus is called the *endometrium*. The principal ligaments of support for the uterus in the pelvis are the broad ligaments, the round ligaments, the uterosacral ligaments, and the cardinal ligaments.

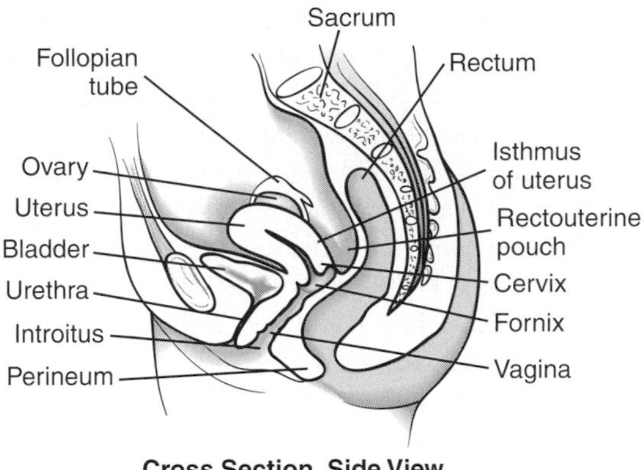

Figure 12-2 Anatomy of the Female Genital Tract.

Blood is supplied to the uterus by the uterine artery, which is a branch of the hypogastric or internal iliac artery, and enters the wall of the uterus at the isthmus. The lymphatics of the myometrium drain into the subserosal network of lymphatics, which coalesce into larger channels before leaving the uterus. Lymph flows from the fundus toward the adnexa and the infundibulopelvic ligaments. The lymph flow from the lower and middle thirds of the uterus tends to spread to the base of the broad ligaments towards the lateral pelvic sidewall.

Cervix

The cervix is the narrow, cylindrical segment of the uterus that extends from the isthmus of the uterus (narrow end of the corpus) to the vagina. Approximately one half of the cervix protrudes into the vagina through the anterior vaginal wall and lies, in most instances, at right angles to it. It measures approximately 2 cm to 4 cm in length. The anterior surface of the cervix is separated from the bladder by fatty tissue. The cervix is connected laterally to the pelvis by the broad ligaments and parametrium. The cervix receives its blood supply through the parametrium. The lower part of the cervix, called the *ectocervix*, projects into the vault of the vagina. On average, the ectocervix is 3 cm long and has a convex elliptical surface that is divided into the anterior and posterior lip. The endocervical canal is the passageway between the cervix's lower opening (the external os) and the upper opening (the internal os). It is lined with columnar epithelial cells. The ectocervix and the vagina are lined with squamous epithelial cells. The point at which these two types of epithelial cells meet is called the *squamocolumnar junction*, or *transformation zone*. The transformation zone is the usual site of cervical carcinoma.

The lymphatic drainage of the cervix flows along the uterine arteries and cardinal ligaments to the parametrial, external iliac, internal iliac, obturator, and presacral lymph nodes. From the pelvic lymph nodes, the drainage then proceeds to the para-aortic lymph nodes.

Ovaries and Fallopian Tubes

The ovaries are small, almond-shaped organs located lateral to the uterus, slightly posterior and caudal to the fallopian tubes. Before menopause, each ovary measures approximately 3.5 × 2.0 × 1.4 cm. They undergo significant changes in size, shape, position, and histology during a woman's lifetime and during each menstrual cycle as a result of hormone stimulation. Each ovary contains numerous Graafian follicles, egg-containing tubes that grow and develop between puberty, sexual maturation, and menopause, when the monthly menstrual cycle stops. The Graafian follicles are fixed in a network of supporting tissue (stroma) and blood vessels. They are covered by a clear, smooth, plasma-like membrane that develops from the peritoneum, which lines the abdominal cavity. The fallopian tubes are narrow muscular tubes 8 cm to 10 cm in length that connect the peritoneal cavity to the uterus. The end of the tube next to the ovary feathers out into fimbria that capture the ovum after ovulation and serve as a conduit to the uterus.

The blood supply to the ovary comes from the ovarian artery, which branches off the abdominal aorta immediately below the renal artery. The right ovarian vein enters the inferior vena cava below the renal vein; the left ovarian vein drains into the left renal vein. Lymphatic drainage flows into the periaortic lymph nodes near the kidney. There are three primary routes of lymphatic drainage into the retroperitoneal lymph nodes. The first route of drainage consists of a group of vessels that ascend bilaterally along the ovarian blood vessels to the lymph nodes between the renal arteries and the aortic bifurcation. The second route consists of vessels that travel toward the lateral and posterior pelvic wall and end in the high external and hypogastric lymph nodes. From there the drainage proceeds along the common iliac vessels into the periaortic lymph nodes. The third route of drainage is along the round ligament into the external iliac and inguinal lymph nodes.

EPIDEMIOLOGY

Cancer of the Vulva

Cancer of the vulva is a relatively rare malignancy accounting for approximately 3% to 5% of all female cancers,[4] although some reports have indicated a higher incidence of 8%.[5] In the United States, the ACS estimates 3740 new cases of cancer of the vulva will be diagnosed in 2006, with approximately 880 associated deaths.[2] According to the National Cancer Institute's (NCI) Surveillance Epidemiology and End Results (SEER) program data (1998–2002), the median age at diagnosis in the United States was 70 years.[6] The age-adjusted incidence rate was 2.2 per 100,000 women per year, primarily in Caucasian women (2.4 per 100,000 women) as compared with African-American women (1.7 per 100,000 women) and Hispanic women (1.7 per 100,000 women).[6] These numbers have been slowly rising over the past several decades. Two factors have been associated with this increase. The first factor is the rapid growth of the population of women living into their seventh and eighth decades of life. The second factor is the increasing number of women younger than age 65 diagnosed with human papilloma viral (HPV) infections and intraepithelial neoplasia of the vulva (VIN).

Cancer of the Vagina

Primary vaginal neoplasias are one of the rarest of the malignant processes in the human body and account for 1% to 3% of all female genital malignancies.[7] In the United States, the ACS estimates 2420 new cases of cancer of the vagina will be diagnosed in 2006, with 600 associated deaths.[2]

Cancer of the Cervix

Cancer of the cervix is the second most common cancer in women worldwide, accounting for approximately 493,000 new cases each year.[1] In most countries in North America and Western Europe, the incidence has been declining in part because of the availability of screening Pap smear examinations. In the United States, the ACS estimates 9710 new cases will be diagnosed in 2006, which is a decrease of approximately 3100 cases since 2000.[2] This decline has been found among women in all racial and ethnic populations. In many developing countries, cervix cancer is the most common cancer among women, and the incidence has not changed. According to the NCI's SEER data, the age adjusted incidence rate in the United States is approximately 8.9 per 100,000 women, with the highest incidence among Hispanic women (15.8 per 100,000 women) and African-American women (11.1 per 100,000).[6] Based on the rates from years 2000 to 2002, 1 in 135 women will be diagnosed with cancer of the cervix during their lifetime.[6]

The age-adjusted death rate is approximately 2.8 per 100,000 women per year.[6] Death rates are highest among African-American women (5.3 per 100,000), which continues to be almost twice that of Caucasians (2.5 per 100,000).[6]

Cancer of the Uterus

Cancer of the uterus is also described in the literature as cancer of the uterine corpus and/or endometrium. Worldwide, it is estimated that more than 190,000 new cases of uterine cancer are diagnosed annually, particularly in the more developed parts of the world.[1] Cancer of the uterus is the most common gynecologic malignancy and is the fourth most common malignancy in women in the United States.[2] It is estimated that 1 in 38 women will be diagnosed with cancer of the uterus during their lifetime.[6] The ACS estimates that 41,200 new cases will be diagnosed in 2006, with 7350 associated deaths.[2] Based on the NCI's SEER data (1998-2002), the age-adjusted incidence rate was 24.2 per 100,000 women per year, with the highest incidence among Caucasian women (25.7 per 100,000 women) followed by African-American women (19.0 per 100,000 women).[6]

The age-adjusted death rate was 4.1 per 100,000 women per year, with the median age at death of 73 years.[6] The death rate among African-American women (7.0 per 100,000 women) was significantly higher than that of Caucasian women (3.9 per 100,000 women) or Hispanic women (3.3 per 100,000 women).[6]

Cancer of the Ovary and Fallopian Tube

Cancer of the ovary is estimated to occur in approximately 204,000 women annually worldwide.[1] It is the fifth leading cause of cancer death in women in the United States and the most common cause of death from gynecologic malignancy.[8] The ACS estimates 20,180 new cases of ovarian cancer will be diagnosed in the United States in 2006, accounting for 4% of all cancers among American women, with an estimated 15,310 associated deaths.[2] According to the NCI's SEER data (1998–2002), the median age at diagnosis was 63 years of age.[6] The age-adjusted incidence rate was 13.9 per 100,000 women per year, with a higher incidence among Caucasian women (14.8 per 100,000 women) as compared with Hispanic (11.9 per 100,000 women) and African-American women (9.9 per 100,000).[6] The mean age at death was 71 years of age, with an age-adjusted rate of 8.9 per 100,000 women per year.[6] Based on rates from years 2000 to 2002, 1 in 68 women will be diagnosed with cancer of the ovary during their lifetime.[6]

Fallopian tube cancer is one of the rarest gynecologic malignancies, accounting for 0.1% to 0.8% of all female reproductive cancers.[9] Primary fallopian tube carcinoma (PFTC) is rare but may be underdiagnosed because it may be misdiagnosed as primary ovarian cancer because of the advanced nature of the disease at the time of surgery.

RISK FACTORS

Human papilloma viruses (HPVs) have been found to be an important factor in the development of many anogenital carcinomas. They are part of the taxonomic family *Papovaviridae*, and genital-infecting viruses are in the genus *Alpha-papillomavirus.*[10] HPVs can be broadly divided into those infecting cutaneous epithelium and those infecting mucosal epithelium, and further divided into high risk and low risk depending on their association with malignancy.[11] Of more than 118 different HPV types described, 40 infect the genital tract.[10] In a pooled analysis of 11 case-control studies from nine countries, HPV DNA was detected in 90.7% of the cancer cases and 13.4% of the controls.[12] HPV types 16, 18, 31, 33, 35, 39, 45, 51, 52, 58, 59, 68, 73, and 82 were found to be high-risk types and HPV types 26, 53 and 66 were found to be 'probable' high-risk types.[11]

Cancer of the Vulva

Historically, cancer of the vulva was associated with medical disorders such as obesity, hypertension, cardiovascular disease, diabetes, and syphilis. Over the past two decades, the focus has changed, and other risk factors have been identified. These include HPV infection, a personal history of cervical cancer, immunosuppression, and tobacco abuse. Recent studies support the concept that squamous cell cancer of the vulva represents at least two different entities. The first is the common keratinizing squamous cell cancer, which arises usually in a background of a nonneoplastic epithelial disorder such as lichen sclerosis or squamous cell hyperplasia and is not related to human papilloma virus (HPV) infection. The other is human papilloma virus–related warty or basaloid carcinoma, which arises usually in the corresponding warty or basaloid vulvar intraepithelial neoplasia (VIN).[13,14] A progression of disease from VIN, through carcinoma in situ, to invasive vulvar carcinoma has been identified. The intraepithelial disease may persist for long periods, with case data indicating 10 years or longer for the in situ phases.[15] The invasive disease tends to be slowly progressive in the early stages with acceleration occurring when the disease penetrates the epithelial basement membrane and lymphatic dissemination occurs

Immunosuppression also may be a potential risk factor. A review of tumor registries has shown a 100-fold increase in the incidence of vulvar cancer in transplant patients compared with the general population.[16] Similarly, HIV and AIDS-related immunosuppression and concomitant HPV infection of the lower genital tract may serve as a contributing factor to early development of vulvar cancer.[17] It also may be associated with the increasing incidence of invasive vulvar cancer in younger age groups.

Cancer of the Vagina

The exact etiology of vaginal cancer remains unknown. The proximity of the vagina to the cervix and the similarity of epithelium make it logical to assume that risk factors may be similar. The predominance of lesions in the upper third and on the posterior wall has led to speculation that an accumulation of irritating or macerating substances that pool in the posterior fornix produce a chronic irritation leading to malignant degeneration. Additional predisposing factors that have been postulated, but not validated, include use of a vaginal pessary, prolapse of the vaginal wall, leukorrhea, and leukoplakia. As with cancer of the cervix and vulva, HPV infection may be a significant etiologic factor. Intrauterine exposure to diethylstilbestrol (DES) has been associated with clear cell adenocarcinomas of the vagina.

Cancer of the Cervix

Cervix cancer is associated with 14 high-risk types of HPV; however, more than half are associated with HPV-16.[11] Persistent cervical infection with high-risk HPV types is an essential part of the multistep process leading to cervical cancer. Therefore, vaccination strategies to prevent HPV infection could have a major impact on the incidence of cervical cancer. Risk factors that increase risk of exposure to HPV place a woman at increased risk for the development of this disease. These behaviors include early age at first intercourse, multiple sexual partners, monogamous women whose husbands had multiple sexual partners, multiparous women, and those with a history of sexually transmitted diseases. Cervix cancer also has been associated with lower socioeconomic status and tobacco use. Nicotine and cotinine have been shown to exert mutagenic activity in the cervical mucus of smokers. Tobacco use also may produce a local immunosuppression in cervical epithelium, which may increase the likelihood of development of HPV-induced neoplastic transformation.[18] Women who are infected with human immunodeficiency virus (HIV) have been shown to have an increased risk of cervical dysplasia, as well as an increased risk of progression to higher-grade lesions.[19] Women who have never had a Pap smear are also at high risk of developing invasive cervix cancer.

Cancer of the Uterus

Uterine cancer can occur during both the reproductive and postmenopausal years but is more common in postmenopausal women, with a median age of 63 years.[20] It is widely accepted that prolonged endometrial exposure to estrogen increases the risk for hyperplastic endometrial disorders, including cancer, and is the basis for many of the identified risk factors. Unopposed estrogen replacement therapy in a woman with a uterus significantly increases the risk of endometrial cancer (relative risk of 2.3).[21] Obese women also have increased endogenous estrogen stimulation of the endometrium secondary to the peripheral conversion of ovarian and adrenal androgens to estrone by aromatase in adipose cells. The relative risk is positively associated with the number of pounds over ideal body weight or the body mass index.[21]

Other risk factors that have been identified include nulliparity, early menarche, longer days of menstrual flow, late menopause, diabetes mellitus, hyperthyroidism, and hypertension. Women on long-term tamoxifen have a 2 to 7.5 relative risk of endometrial cancer. The increased risk is thought to be caused by local estrogenic effects of tamoxifen on the endometrium.[20]

At least two distinct types of endometrial cancer have been recognized: an estrogen-dependent type that has a better prognosis and an estrogen-independent type.[20] The latter has been associated with genetic predisposition syndromes. Hereditary associations such as the Lynch II syndrome and hereditary nonpolyposis colorectal cancer (HNPCC) include a predisposition for endometrial cancer in which the lifetime risk is estimated to be 20%.[20]

Cancer of the Ovary and Fallopian Tube

A number of risk factors have been associated with ovarian cancer. They include advancing age, northern European descent, nulliparity, personal history of breast, colon, or endometrial cancer, and family history of ovarian cancer in a first-degree or second-degree relative. Women in the United States have a 1 in 68 lifetime risk of developing ovarian cancer that increases to 1 in 20 if the woman has a first-degree relative with ovarian cancer and to 7% if she has two first-degree relatives with ovarian cancer.[9] Hereditary associations such as the Lynch II syndrome, Li-Fraumeni syndrome, and HNPCC include a predisposition for ovarian cancer. Claus and colleagues[22] found that 10% of women with ovarian cancer carry a breast/ovarian cancer gene mutation. At least three different classes of genes confer increased risk for ovarian cancer, *BRCA1, BRCA2,* and *p53*. Factors also have been identified that may decrease ovarian cancer risk. They include reduction in incessant ovulation, use of oral contraceptives, and tubal ligation.

CLINICAL MANIFESTATIONS

Cancer of the Vulva

Currently, there are no recommended guidelines for screening for cancer of the vulva. However, age-appropriate guidelines for annual physical examination with pelvic exam and Pap smear should be applied. During these examinations, careful visual inspection of the vulva should be performed, and suspicious lesions or areas of abnormal pigmentation should be photographed and biopsied. Presenting symptoms of cancer of the vulva include a lump or mass, vulvar pruritus, bleeding, discharge, dysuria, dyspareunia, a lesion that will not heal, incontinence, or vulvar pain. Approximately two-thirds of patients present with a lesion involving the labia majora. The clitoris, labia minora, posterior fourchette, or perineum constitute the other one-third of sites.[23] Disease spreads via direct extension into the vagina, urethra, and anus. The superficial inguinofemoral lymph nodes are the first regional lymph nodes to become involved, followed by the deep inguinofemoral nodes and pelvic nodes. The overall incidence of lymph node involvement in cancer of the vulva is 30%.[24] Lung, liver, and bone are common sites of distant hematogenous metastasis.

The initial evaluation should include a complete history and physical examination with evaluation of Karnofsky performance status (KPS) because many of these women are elderly and have significant comorbidities. The physical examination should include a careful visual inspection of the vulva and vagina, colposcopy, and full-thickness biopsy of any suspicious lesions. A Pap smear of the cervix and vagina also should be obtained to evaluate for evidence of disease that may constitute a primary site other than the vulva. Imaging studies may be ordered to determine the extent of disease, particularly in a locally advanced cancer. The studies may include a chest x ray to look for evidence of lung metastasis and a computed tomography (CT) scan of the abdomen and pelvis to look for evidence of pelvic extension of disease and adenopathy. Additional radiographic studies such as magnetic resonance imaging (MRI) or positron imaging tomography (PET) scan will depend on reported symptoms and physical examination findings. Initial laboratory studies may include a complete blood count with chemistry studies to look for evidence of renal and liver dysfunction.

If there is clinical evidence of urethral involvement, a cystoscopy may be appropriate to document extent of disease. A proctosigmoidoscopy may be used if there is clinical evidence of anal involvement. Additional studies may be warranted to assess overall medical condition, particularly when considering surgical resection or combined modality therapy.

Most cancers of the vulva are squamous cell. Melanoma accounts for less than 5%, with Bartholin's gland adenocarcinoma, basal cell, verrucous carcinoma, and sarcoma comprising the rest. Important prognostic factors in cancer of the vulva include International Federation of Gynecology and Obstetrics (FIGO) stage and presence of clinically involved lymph nodes. Additional factors include tumor size and location, age, and KPS. Midline tumors tend to be more involved than lateral lesions.

The FIGO staging system is used in cancer of the vulva; this is a surgical staging system based on pathologic assessment of the tumor and lymph node specimens. Clinical staging (TNM) may be used in instances where the patient may not be a surgical candidate (Table 12-1). Approximately 63% of patients are diagnosed when the disease is still confined to the primary site; 28% are diagnosed after the cancer has spread to the regional lymph nodes or directly beyond the primary site; 3% are diagnosed after the disease has metastasized.[6]

Cancer of the Vagina

Currently, there are no recommended guidelines for screening for cancer of the vagina. However, the age-appropriate guidelines for annual physical examination with pelvic exam and Pap smear should be applied. During these examinations, careful visual inspection of the vaginal walls should be performed, and suspicious lesions or areas of abnormal pigmentation should be photographed and biopsied. The most common symptoms of cancer of the vagina are intermenstrual or postmenopausal bleeding, and/or vaginal discharge, urinary symptoms including dysuria or hematuria, and pelvic pain. Cancer of the vagina spreads by local invasion to the rest of the vagina, vulva, paravaginal tissues, and parametria. Lymphatic spread occurs in accordance with the site of the primary tumor in the vagina. The lymph nodes in the pelvis drain the upper two-thirds of the vagina and the inguinal nodes drain the lower one-third. Hematogenous spread is rare and occurs late in the disease process.

Initial evaluation should include a complete history and physical examination with documentation of the KPS. The physical examination should include a careful visual inspection of the vagina, vulva, and cervix with colposcopy and biopsy of any suspicious lesions. A Pap smear of the cervix also should be obtained to evaluate for evidence of disease that may constitute a primary site other than the vagina. Any suspicious lesions on the vulva also should be biopsied.

Radiographic studies should include a chest x ray to evaluate for evidence of metastatic disease and a CT scan or MRI of the abdomen and pelvis, looking for evidence of pelvic extension of disease and adenopathy. A transrectal or transvaginal ultrasound may help define the size and extent of the disease.

Table 12-1 FIGO Staging for Cancer of the Vulva

FIGO	TNM			Clinical/pathologic findings
Stage 0	Tis			Carcinoma in situ, intraepithelial carcinoma
Stage I	T1	N0	M0	Tumor confined to the vulva or perineum; < 2 cm in greatest dimension; nodes are negative
Stage IA				Invasion ≤ 1 mm*
Stage IB				Invasion > 1 mm
Stage II	T2	N0	M0	Tumor confined to the vulva and/or perineum; > 2 cm in greatest dimension; nodes are negative
Stage III	T1	N1	M0	Tumor of any size with:
	T2	N1	M0	1. Adjacent spread to the lower urethra and/or the vagina and/or anus
	T3	N0	M0	2. Unilateral regional lymph node metastasis
	T3	N1	M0	
Stage IVA	T1	N2	M0	Tumor invades any of the following: upper urethra, bladder mucosa, rectal mucosa, pelvic bone, and/or bilateral regional nodes
	T2	N2	M0	
	T3	N2	M0	
	T4	N0-2	M0	
Stage IVB	T1-4	N0-2	M1	Any distant metastases including pelvic lymph nodes

Reprinted from Benedet JL, Ngan HYS, Hacker NF, editors: FIGO staging classifications and clinical practice guidelines in management of gynaecologic cancers, *Int J Gynaecol Obstet* 70(2):209-262, 2000, with permission from the International Federation of Gynecology and Obstetrics.

*NOTE: The depth of invasion is defined as the measurement of the tumor from the epithelial-stromal junction of the adjacent most superficial dermal papilla to the deepest point of invasion.

FIGO, International Federation of Gynecology and Obstetrics.

Additional studies such as CT scans of other organs or PET scans should be ordered based on the clinical stage of disease and reported symptoms. A complete blood count with chemistry studies should be performed to evaluate renal and liver function.

An exam performed with the patient under anesthesia allows cystoscopy, proctosigmoidoscopy, and extensive clinical examination of the vagina in patients with extensive disease or those who cannot tolerate clinical pelvic examination. Additional studies may be warranted to assess overall medical condition, particularly when considering surgical resection or combined modality therapy.

Most cancers of the vagina are of squamous cell histology (90%). Melanoma, adenocarcinoma, and sarcoma comprise the rest. Cancer of the vagina is staged using the FIGO clinical staging system (Table 12-2). FIGO stage is the most important prognostic factor. Other prognostic factors are grade of tumor, depth of penetration, and presence of involved lymph nodes.

Cancer of the Cervix

Cytologic screening using the Pap smear with pelvic examination is the established method of screening for cancer of the cervix. The ACS recommends that all women begin cervical cancer screening about 3 years after they begin having vaginal intercourse, but no later than age 21.[25] Screening should be done every year with the regular Pap test or every 2 years using the newer liquid-based Pap test. Beginning at age 30, women who have had 3 normal Pap test results in a row may get screened every 2 to 3 years with either the conventional (regular) or liquid-based Pap test. Women who have certain risk factors such as diethylstilbestrol (DES) exposure before birth, HIV infection, or a weakened immune system resulting from organ transplant, chemotherapy, or chronic steroid use should continue to be screened annually as long as they are in good health. Another reasonable option for women over age 30 is that of being screened every 3 years (but not more frequently) with either the conventional or liquid-based Pap test, plus the HPV DNA test.[25]

Women age 70 and older who have had three or more normal Pap tests in a row and no abnormal Pap test results in the last 10 years may choose to stop having cervical cancer screening. Women who have had a total hysterectomy (removal of the

Table 12-2 FIGO Staging System for Cancer of the Vagina

FIGO	TNM			Clinical/pathologic findings
Stage 0	Tis	N0	M0	Carcinoma in situ, intraepithelial carcinoma
Stage I	T1	N0	M0	Tumor confined to the vaginal wall
Stage II	T2	N0	M0	Tumor invades paravaginal tissues, but not to the pelvic wall
Stage III	T1	N1	M0	Tumor extends to the pelvic wall
	T2	N1	M0	
	T3	N0	M0	
	T3	N1	M0	
Stage IVA	T4	N0-2	M0	Tumor invades mucosa of the bladder or rectum and/or extends beyond the true pelvis (Bullous edema is not sufficient evidence to classify a tumor as T4)
Stage IVB	T1-4	N0-2	M1	Distant metastases

Reprinted from Benedet JL, Ngan HYS, Hacker NF, editors: FIGO staging classifications and clinical practice guidelines in management of gynaecologic cancers, *Int J Gynaecol Obstet* 70(2):209-262, 2000, with permission from the International Federation of Gynecology and Obstetrics.
FIGO, International Federation of Gynecology and Obstetrics.

uterus and cervix) may also choose to stop having cervical cancer screening, unless the surgery was done as a treatment for cervical cancer or precancer. Women who have had a hysterectomy without removal of the cervix should continue to follow the standard guidelines for annual screening.[25]

The most common symptoms of cervical cancer are abnormal vaginal bleeding (postcoital, intermenstrual, or postmenopausal) and a malodorous discharge. Pain, urinary symptoms, including dysuria or hematuria, and pelvic or back pain are usually associated with advanced disease. Anemia secondary to vaginal bleeding may be present.

Cancer of the cervix spreads directly to the vaginal mucosa, endometrial cavity, parametrial tissues and ligaments, pelvic side wall, bladder, and rectum. Regional lymphatics at risk for metastases include the paracervical, internal iliac, obturator, external iliac, presacral, common iliac, and para-aortic lymph nodes. Hematogenous spread is usually late and may involve the lungs, bone, or liver.

Initial evaluation should include a complete history and physical examination with KPS. In early-stage disease, the cervical abnormality is usually discovered by Pap smear. Careful visual inspection of the cervix and vagina with colposcopy and a biopsy of any suspicious lesions usually follows an abnormal cytology result. Obvious cervical lesions may proceed directly to biopsy. Imaging studies may include a chest x ray to evaluate for metastatic disease and a CT scan or MRI of the abdomen and pelvis for evidence of pelvic extension of disease and adenopathy. A transvaginal ultrasound may help define the size and extent of the disease. Laboratory studies usually include a complete blood count to look for evidence of anemia and chemistry studies to evaluate renal and liver function. Tumor markers including CA-125, CA19-9, carcinoembryonic antigen (CEA), and squamous cell carcinoma (SCC) antigen have been shown to be elevated in cervical cancer. However, these are not specific markers for cervical cancer and therefore are not routinely used in clinical practice.

In some situations, exam under anesthesia may be performed to allow extensive clinical examination of the cervix, cystoscopy, and proctosigmoidoscopy. This may be necessary in patients who cannot tolerate a clinical examination or when there is evidence of locally progressive disease that may change the clinical stage. Additional metastatic evaluation studies will depend on reported symptoms and physical examination findings. Studies are currently ongoing to evaluate the role of laparoscopy, hysteroscopy, and retroperitoneal exploration in the clinical evaluation and staging of cervix cancer. Additional studies may be warranted to assess overall medical condition, particularly when considering surgical resection or combined modality therapy.

More than 90% of tumors of the cervix are squamous cell histology; approximately 7% to 10% are classified as adenocarcinoma, and 1% to 2% are clear cell, mesonephric type.[26] Important prognostic factors in cervical cancer include stage of disease, the tumor volume, lymph node metastasis, histology, and

Table 12-3 FIGO Staging of Cancer of the Cervix

FIGO	TNM			Clinical/pathologic findings
Stage 0	Tis	N0	M0	Carcinoma in situ, cervical intraepithelial neoplasia grade III
Stage I	T1	N0	M0	Cervical carcinoma confined to uterus
Stage IA	T1a	N0	M0	Invasive carcinoma diagnosed only by microscopy. All macroscopically visible lesions—even with superficial invasion—are T1b/IB. Stromal invasion with a maximal depth of 5.0 mm measured from the base of the epithelium and a horizontal spread of 7.0 mm or less. Vascular space involvement, either venous or lymphatic, does not affect classification.
Stage IA1	T1a1	N0	M0	Measured stromal invasion 3.0 mm or less in depth and 7.0 mm or less in horizontal spread
Stage IA2	T1a2	N0	M0	Measured stromal invasion more than 3.0 mm and not more than 5.0 mm with a horizontal spread 7.0 mm or less
Stage IB	T1b	N0	M0	Clinically visible lesion confined to the cervix or microscopic lesion greater than T1a/IA2
Stage IB1	T1b1	N0	M0	Clinically visible lesion 4.0 cm or less in greatest dimension
Stage IB2	T1b2	N0	M0	Clinically visible lesion more than 4.0 cm in greatest dimension
Stage II				Cervical carcinoma invades beyond uterus but not to pelvic wall or to the lower third of vagina
Stage IIA	T2a	N0	M0	Tumor without parametrial invasion
Stage IIB	T2b	N0	M0	Tumor with parametrial invasion
Stage III				Tumor extends to the pelvic wall, and/or involves the lower third of the vagina, and/or causes hydronephrosis or nonfunctioning kidney
Stage IIIA	T3a	N0	M0	Tumor involves lower third of the vagina, no extension to pelvic wall
Stage IIIB	T1	N1	M0	Tumor extends to the pelvic wall and/or causes hydronephrosis or nonfunctioning kidney
	T2	N1	M0	
	T3a	N1	M0	
	T3b	Any N	M0	
Stage IVA	T4	Any N	M0	Tumor invades mucosa of the bladder or rectum, and/or extends beyond the true pelvis (Bullous edema is not sufficient to classify a tumor as T4)
Stage IVB	T4	Any N	M1	Distant metastasis

Reprinted from Benedet JL, Ngan HYS, Hacker NF, editors: FIGO staging classifications and clinical practice guidelines in management of gynaecologic cancers, *Int J Gynaecol Obstet* 70(2):209-262, 2000, with permission from the International Federation of Gynecology and Obstetrics.

FIGO, International Federation of Gynecology and Obstetrics.

presence of vascular or lymphatic invasion. Host factors, such as anemia, also affect the prognosis.[26] Cervical cancer is staged using the FIGO staging system, a mainly clinical evaluation (Table 12-3). The imaging evaluation may include chest x ray, intravenous pyelography (IVP), and barium enema. MRI, CT scans, and lymphangiography are not accepted for staging. The FIGO surgical procedures for staging are limited to colposcopy, biopsy, conization of the cervix, cystoscopy, and proctosigmoidoscopy. Laparoscopy, hysteroscopy, and retroperitoneal exploration are not accepted.[27] Approximately 55% of patients are diagnosed while the cancer is still confined to the primary site; 32% are diagnosed with spread to the regional lymph nodes or directly beyond the primary site, and 8% are diagnosed with metastatic disease to a distant site.[6]

Cancer of the Uterus

Screening for endometrial cancer remains difficult. The ACS recommends that all women should be informed about the risks and symptoms of endometrial cancer. For women with or at high risk for HNPCC, annual screening should be offered for endometrial cancer with endometrial biopsy beginning at age 35.[25]

The American College of Obstetricians and Gynecologists (ACOG) recommendations state that screening techniques to detect endometrial cancer, including ultrasonography and endometrial sampling, have not demonstrated sufficient accuracy and cost effectiveness and therefore are not acceptable for general use.[28] Cervical cytology alone is not reliable. Therefore, endometrial biopsy should be used only as a diagnostic test for women with unexpected breakthrough bleeding during the perimenopausal period or while on estrogen replacement therapy, and in women with postmenopausal bleeding.

The most common presenting symptom is intermenstrual or postmenopausal vaginal bleeding. Additional symptoms in advanced disease include pelvic pain, back pain, and urinary symptoms (dysuria and frequency) secondary to uterine enlargement. Endometrial cancer may spread via direct extension into surrounding organs (cervix, vagina, bladder, rectum or parametria), lymphatic spread, and hematogenous spread. Lymph nodes at risk for metastasis include the pelvic and para-aortic nodes. Peritoneal seeding is common with endometrial cancer because an endometrial lesion may penetrate the uterine wall or seed transtubally.[26]

Initial evaluation should include a complete history and physical examination with KPS. An endometrial biopsy, aspiration curettage, or fractional dilation and curettage (D&C), are methods used to obtain tissue from the endometrium for histologic evaluation. Radiology studies may include a chest x ray to evaluate for evidence of metastatic disease and a CT scan or MRI of the abdomen and pelvis for evidence of pelvic extension of disease and adenopathy. Laboratory studies should include a complete blood count to evaluate for evidence of anemia and chemistry studies to evaluate renal and liver function.

An exam performed with the patient under anesthesia may be necessary if there is evidence of locally advanced disease. This exam allows extensive clinical examination of the pelvis, a cystoscopy and a proctosigmoidoscopy if necessary. Additional metastatic evaluation studies will depend on reported symptoms and physical examination findings. Additional studies may be warranted to assess overall medical condition, particularly when considering surgical resection or combined modality therapy.

The most common cancer of the endometrium is endometrioid adenocarcinoma.[26] This is further divided into four subtypes: papillary, secretory, ciliated cells, and adenocarcinoma with squamous differentiation. Other histologic types of tumors of the endometrium are rare and include papillary serous carcinoma, clear cell carcinoma, and sarcoma. Important prognostic factors include clinical or pathologic stage, histologic grade of the tumor, depth of myometrial invasion, presence of lymphovascular involvement, lymph node involvement, and age.

FIGO staging (based on surgical evaluation) is most commonly used (Table 12-4). Approximately 72% of patients are diagnosed with the disease confined to the primary site; 16% are diagnosed with disease that has spread to the regional lymph nodes or directly beyond the primary site, and 8% with disease in a distant site.[6]

Cancer of the Ovary and Fallopian Tube

Screening for cancer of the ovary and fallopian tube remains difficult because of the location of the ovaries deep in the pelvis among the viscera.[29] Routine screening of the general population is not recommended. Instead, definable populations of women who have an above average risk of ovarian cancer may benefit from screening. The CA-125 is a serum tumor marker that is elevated in 85% of women with advanced epithelial ovarian cancer, but only in 50% of women with early-stage disease.[29] Unfortunately, many other medical conditions may result in an elevated CA-125 including endometriosis, pelvic inflammatory disease, benign ovarian neoplasms, fibroids, liver disease, congestive heart failure, and a variety of other benign problems.[8] CA-125 appears to be more accurate for detecting ovarian cancer in postmenopausal women. Several new markers are currently under investigation for potential use with CA-125 as a panel for ovarian cancer screening. Two have shown particular promise including the macrophage–colony-stimulating factor (m-CSF), a hematopoietic cytokine, and a combination of various lysophosphatidic acids (LPA).[29] Other tumor markers including CA19-9, CEA, human chorionic gonadotropin, and alpha-fetoprotein may be used in nonepithelial tumors of the ovary.

Transvaginal and transabdominal ultrasound also have been studied as possible noninvasive screening

Table 12-4 FIGO Surgical Staging of Cancer of the Uterus

FIGO	Grade	TNM			Clinical/pathologic findings
	G123	Tis	N0	M0	Carcinoma in situ
Stage I					Tumor confined to the corpus uteri
Stage IA	G123	T1a	M0	M0	Tumor limited to endometrium
Stage IB	G123	T1b	N0	M0	Tumor invades up to or less than one-half of the myometrium
Stage IC	G123	T1c	N0	M0	Tumor invades to more than one-half of the myometrium
Stage II					Tumor invades cervix but does not extend beyond uterus
Stage IIA	G123	T2a	N0	M0	Endocervical glandular involvement only
Stage IIB	G123	T2b	N0	M0	Cervical stromal invasion
Stage III					Local and/or regional spread as specified in T#a, b, and/or N1 and FIGO IIIA, B, and C below
Stage IIIA	G123	T3a	N0	M0	Tumor involves serosa and/or adnexa (direct extension or metastasis) and/or cancer cells in ascites or peritoneal washings
Stage IIIB	G123	T3b	N0	M0	Vaginal involvement (direct extension or metastasis)
Stage IIIC	G123	T1	N1	M0	Metastasis to the pelvic and/or para-aortic lymph nodes
		T2	N1	M0	
		T3a	N1	M0	
		T3b	N1	M0	
Stage IVA	G123	T4	Any N	M0	Tumor invades bladder mucosa and/or bowel mucosa (Bullous edema is not sufficient to classify a tumor as T4)
Stage IVB		Any T	Any N	M1	Distant metastasis

Reprinted from Benedet JL, Ngan HYS, Hacker NF, editors: FIGO staging classifications and clinical practice guidelines in management of gynaecologic cancers, *Int J Gynaecol Obstet* 70(2):209-262, 2000, with permission from the International Federation of Gynecology and Obstetrics.

FIGO, International Federation of Gynecology and Obstetrics.

tools. Improvement in ultrasound technology has allowed three-dimensional (3-D) sonography and 3-D power Doppler imaging to become available, and both techniques are currently under evaluation in screening for ovarian cancer. Early studies show some hope when combining both techniques in stage I disease.[30]

The 1994 NIH Consensus Statement of Ovarian Cancer concluded that, at that time, there was no evidence available that the current screening modalities of CA-125 and transvaginal ultrasound could be used effectively for large-population screening to reduce the morality rate from ovarian cancer.[31] The statement said further that women with two first-degree relatives should have an annual physical examination with bimanual rectovaginal examination, CA-125 serum levels, and transvaginal ultrasound. At the conclusion of childbearing or at least by age 35 years, prophylactic bilateral oophorectomy may be appropriate.[31]

Symptoms associated with ovarian cancer usually do not occur until the disease is advanced. The symptoms include early satiety, abdominal distension, abdominal pain, nausea, and vomiting. Epithelial ovarian cancer arises from the ovarian surface epithelium and spreads through the peritoneal cavity. Lymphatic or hematogenous spread also may occur.

The initial evaluation of a patient with a suspected ovarian cancer should include a complete history and physical examination with KPS. Initial imaging studies include an ultrasound and/or CT scan of the abdomen and pelvis. A chest x ray should be performed to look for evidence of pleural effusion or lung mass. A complete blood count to assess for evidence of anemia, blood chemistry studies to evaluate renal and liver function, and serum CA-125 level should be performed.

A laparotomy with biopsy (usually associated with a cytoreductive surgery) will confirm the diagnosis and provide histologic confirmation. Additional metastatic evaluation studies depend on reported symptoms and physical examination findings. Additional studies may be warranted to assess overall medical condition, particularly when considering surgical resection or combined modality therapy.

Epithelial tumors arise from the germinal epithelium of the ovarian surface, and spread occurs via the transcoleomic, lymphatic, and/or hematogenous routes. They represent 85% to 90% of all malignant ovarian tumors.[26] The peritoneal surfaces are the most common sites of tumor implantation and growth. This includes surfaces of the bowel, liver, diaphragm, omentum, and spleen. The periaortic and pelvic lymph nodes are the most common nodal sites involved. The FIGO staging classification is the system used for cancer of the ovary and fallopian tube (Tables 12-5 and 12-6).

TREATMENT

Radiation therapy is a critical component in the management of cervical, vaginal, and uterine malignancies and also plays a role in the treatment of cancer of the vulva, ovary, and fallopian tube. With the advent of high-speed computers and new technology in radiology and radiation oncology, significant changes have impacted the treatment of gynecologic malignancies. In particular, the ability to carefully tailor treatment to the individual's body habitus and to reduce the dose to the normal surrounding structures in the pelvis. Three-dimensional conformal radiation therapy (3-D CRT), intensity modulated radiation therapy (IMRT), and proton beam therapy are examples of these new treatment approaches that may further improve the advantages of radiation therapy in these diseases. The focus of this discussion is on the most common types of cancer in each disease site.

Treatment of gynecologic cancers with radiation therapy is individualized to the disease site, histology, and stage of disease (Table 12-7). However, some

Table 12-5 FIGO Staging of Cancer of the Ovary

FIGO		TNM		Clinical/pathologic findings
Stage I				Tumor limited to ovaries (one or both).
Stage IA	T1a	N0	M0	Tumor limited to one ovary; capsule intact, no tumor on ovarian surface. No malignant cells in ascites or peritoneal washings.*
Stage IB	T1b	N0	M0	Tumor limited to both ovaries; capsule is intact, no tumor on ovarian surface. No malignant cells in ascites or peritoneal washings.*
Stage IC	T1c	N0	M0	Tumor limited to one or both ovaries with any of the following: capsule ruptured, tumor on ovarian surface, malignant cells in ascites or peritoneal washings.
Stage II	T2			Tumor involves one or both ovaries with pelvic extension.
Stage IIA	T2a	N0	M0	Extension and/or implants on uterus and/or tube(s). No malignant cells in ascites or peritoneal washings.
Stage IIB	T2b	N0	M0	Extension to other pelvic tissues. No malignant cells in ascites or peritoneal washings.
Stage IIC	T2c	N0	M0	Pelvic extension (2a or 2b) with malignant cells in ascites or peritoneal washings.
Stage III	T3			Tumor involves one or both ovaries with microscopically confirmed peritoneal metastasis outside the pelvis and/or regional lymph node metastasis.
Stage IIIA	T3a	N0	M0	Microscopic peritoneal metastasis beyond the pelvis.
Stage IIIB	T3b	N0	M0	Macroscopic peritoneal metastasis beyond pelvis 2 cm or less in greatest dimension.
Stage IIIC	T3c	N0	M0	Peritoneal metastasis beyond the pelvis more than 2 cm in greatest dimension and/or regional lymph node metastasis.
	Any T	N1	M0	
Stage IV	Any T	Any N	M1	Distant metastasis.

Reprinted from Benedet JL, Ngan HYS, Hacker NF, editors: FIGO staging classifications and clinical practice guidelines in management of gynaecologic cancers, *Int J Gynaecol Obstet* 70(2):209-262, 2000, with permission from the International Federation of Gynecology and Obstetrics.

*NOTE: The presence of nonmalignant ascites is not classified. The presence of ascites does not affect staging unless malignant cells are present.

FIGO, International Federation of Gynecology and Obstetrics.

Table 12-6 FIGO Staging of Cancer of the Fallopian Tube

FIGO	TNM			Clinical/pathologic findings
Stage I				Tumor limited to the fallopian tube(s)
Stage IA	T1a	N0	M0	Tumor limited to one tube without penetrating the serosal surface; no ascites
Stage IB	T1b	N0	M0	Tumor limited to both tubes, without penetrating the serosal surface; no ascites
Stage IC	T1c	N0	M0	Tumor limited to one or both tubes with extension onto or through the tubal serosa, or with malignant cells in ascites or peritoneal washings
Stage II	T2			Tumor involves one or both fallopian tubes with pelvic extension
Stage IIA	T2a	N0	M0	Extension and/or implants on uterus and/or ovaries
Stage IIB	T2b	N0	M0	Extension to other pelvic structures
Stage IIC	T2c	N0	M0	Pelvic extension with malignant cells in ascites or peritoneal washings
Stage III	T3			Tumor involves one or both fallopian tubes with peritoneal implants outside the pelvis and/or regional lymph node metastasis
Stage IIIA	T3a	N0	M0	Microscopic peritoneal metastasis beyond the pelvis
Stage IIIB	T3b	N0	M0	Macroscopic peritoneal metastasis beyond pelvis 2 cm or less in greatest dimension
Stage IIIC	T3c	N0	M0	Peritoneal metastasis beyond the pelvis more than 2 cm in
	Any T	N1	M0	greatest dimension and/or regional lymph node metastasis
Stage IV	Any T	Any N	M1	Distant metastasis

Reprinted from Benedet JL, Ngan HYS, Hacker NF, editors: FIGO staging classifications and clinical practice guidelines in management of gynaecologic cancers, *Int J Gynaecol Obstet* 70(2):209-262, 2000, with permission from the International Federation of Gynecology and Obstetrics.

FIGO, International Federation of Gynecology and Obstetrics.

Table 12-7 Radiation Therapy Treatment Fields for Gynecologic Malignancies

Disease site	Stage	Whole pelvis	Whole abdomen	Brachytherapy	Other
Cervix	IB	x		x	
	IIA, IIB, III, IVA	x		x	Periaortic field (PANS) Groin fields
Uterus	IA, IB	x		x	
	II, III, IV	x	x	x	1. Periaortic field 2. Groin fields
Vagina	I	x		x	
	IIA	x		x	
	IIB, III, IV	x		x	1. Additional fields to cover disease (e.g., inguinofemoral lymph nodes)
Vulva					1. Vulva 2. Inguinofemoral lymph nodes
Ovary			x	^{32}P Instillation	
Fallopian tube			x	^{32}P Instillation	

PANS, periaortic lymph node field.

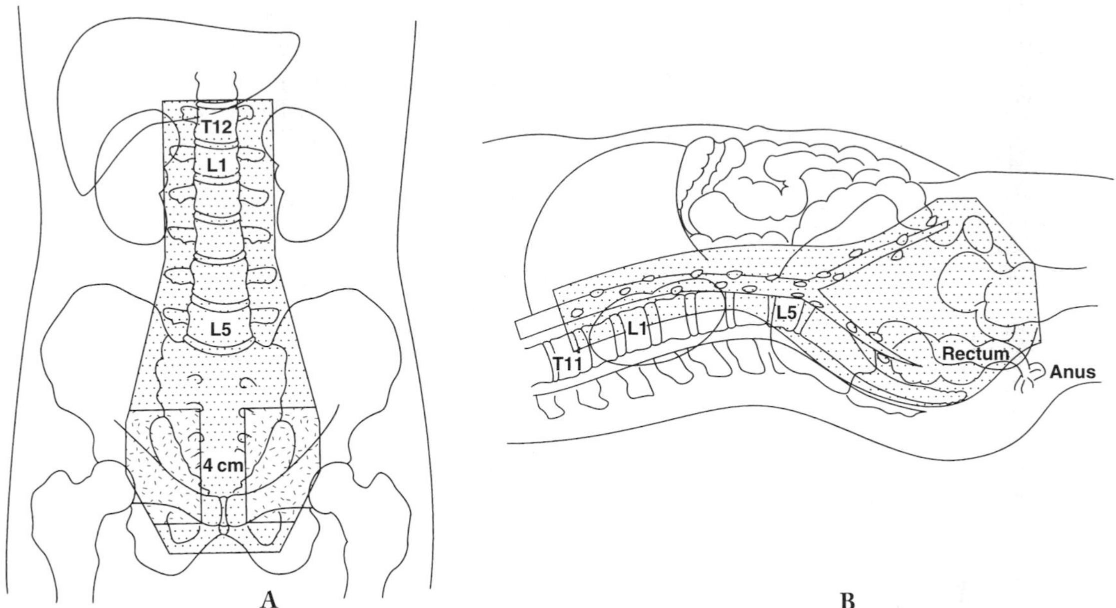

Figure 12-3 Whole-pelvis Irradiation Fields. **A,** *Anterior.* **B,** *Lateral.*
From Wang CC, editor: Clinical radiation oncology: indications, techniques, and results, ed. 2, 2000, John Wiley & Sons.

common descriptors of the treatment fields are used. They include whole pelvis irradiation, whole abdomen irradiation, periaortic irradiation, inguinofemoral field irradiation, and brachytherapy. The text that follows provides explanations of each term.

Whole-Pelvis Irradiation

Whole-pelvis irradiation is a four-field technique in which anterior and posterior (AP-PA) opposed fields and lateral opposed fields are used (Figure 12-3). The AP-PA fields usually measure approximately 15 cm × 15 cm at surface (16.5 cm at isocenter).[26] They maybe extended in more advanced disease (stages IIA, IIB, III, and IVA).

The superior border is a line that transverses the L 4-5 interspace to include all of the external iliac and hypogastric lymph nodes.[26] This margin must be extended to the L3-4 interspace if common iliac nodal coverage is indicated. The lateral border is placed 1 cm to 15 cm lateral to the widest true pelvic diameter.[26] The inferior border is a line that transverses below the obturator foramen and at least 4 cm beyond the vaginal cuff.[26] A radioopaque marker in the vagina to mark the vaginal cuff helps facilitate proper placement of the lower border. If there is vaginal involvement, the whole length of the vagina should be treated, all the way to the introitus. The lateral field superior border is usually identical to AP-PA fields.[26] The anterior border is placed at the cortex of the pubic symphysis and at least 1 cm anterior to common iliac nodes.[26] The posterior border is placed to cover at least 50% of the rectum in stage IB tumors and should extend to the sacral hollow in patients with more advanced disease.[26]

This treatment is usually given with the patient lying on her stomach or back. The typical daily dose to the pelvis is 1.8 Gy to 2.0 Gy. The total dose varies from institution to institution, but ranges from 40 Gy to 50 Gy.

Whole Abdomen Irradiation

The whole abdomen irradiation approach uses an open field treating the entire peritoneal cavity, including the periaortic, pelvic, and mesenteric lymph nodes along with the entire diaphragm (Figure 12-4).[26] The superior border of the field is approximately 2 cm above the domes of the diaphragm during quiet respiration.[26] The inferior border is the bottom of the obturator foramina, and the lateral borders extend 2 cm beyond the lateral peritoneum.[26] Parallel opposed fields (AP-PA) are preferred, with total doses being limited to 22.5 Gy to 30 Gy at 1.0 Gy to 1.5 Gy per daily fraction.[26] Kidney blocks may be used to protect the kidneys depending on the total dose and

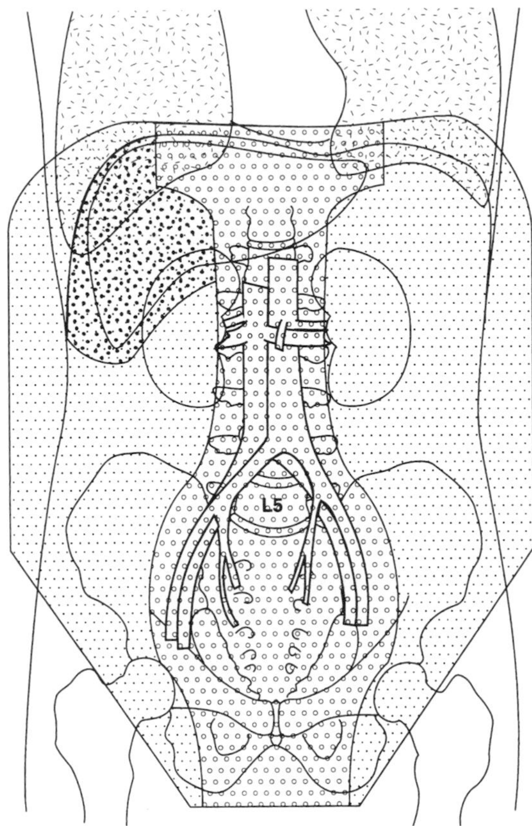

Figure 12-4 Whole-abdomen Irradiation Field.
From Wang CC, editor: Clinical radiation oncology: indications, techniques, and results, ed. 2, 2000, John Wiley & Sons.

fractionation scheme. Pelvic boost fields may be used with either AP-PA or four-field technique.

Periaortic Field

The periaortic lymph node field (PANS) is a field that incorporates the periaortic lymph nodes. The superior margin is placed at the T12 to L1 interspace, the width of the field is generally 9 cm to 10 cm wide, and the inferior border is determined by the placement of the whole pelvis port.[26]

Inguinofemoral Field

The inguinofemoral field encompasses the inguinal lymph nodes and the femoral lymph nodes while minimizing the dose to the femoral heads.

Brachytherapy

Brachytherapy is a form of radiation therapy in which radioactive sources are placed within or near the tumor. This therapy may be given alone or in conjunction with external beam radiation.[32] Combining brachytherapy with external beam radiation can not only treat bulky local disease but also improve local control. Various brachytherapy sequences and techniques can be used with comparable results, and institutions each have their own preferred approach for each disease site.[32] Both high-dose-rate brachytherapy and low-dose-rate brachytherapy techniques are used (see Chapter 2 for further discussion of dose rate).

Three different types of intracavitary applicators are used for gynecologic brachytherapy.[32] The first is the high-dose-rate cylinder that is used to treat cancers of the uterus and/or vagina (Figure 12-5). The second is the Syed template that is used to treated advanced cervical cancers and primary vaginal cancers and is typically placed in the patient in the operating room while the patient is under general or regional anesthesia (Figure 12-6). The third applicator is the tandem and ovoids or tandem and colpostat, which are used to treat cervical cancer and, in some situations, endometrial cancer (Figure 12-7). They are placed in the patient in the operating room while the patient is under general anesthesia or in the radiation oncology department with conscious sedation.

Once the applicator has been inserted, the radiation oncologist and physics staff calculate the dose prescription based on the patients diagnosis, stage, treatment plan, and anatomy. Point dose calculations are recommended for each brachytherapy insertion to

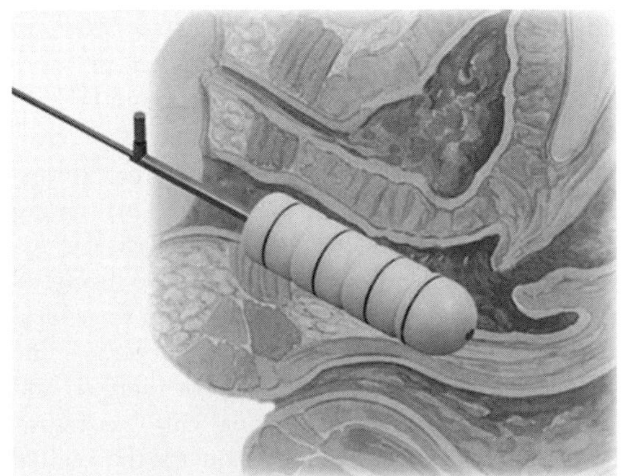

Figure 12-5 Vaginal Applicator.
Courtesy of Nucletron. Retrieved at www.nucletron.com/upload/applicators/big/084350vagina.jpg

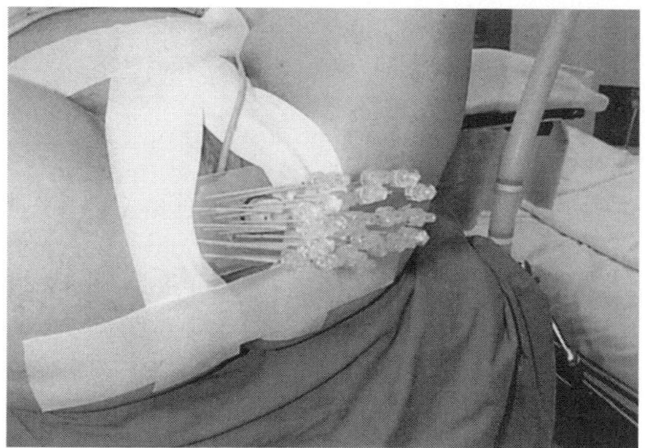

Figure 12-6 Syed Template.
Used with permission: Kushner, DM, Fleming, PA, Kennedy et al: High dose rate IR192 afterloading brachytherapy for cancer of the vagina. Br J Radiol, 76, page 720, Figure 1, 2003.

assess and document the dose to be given at dose specification points and at normal tissue points (i.e., rectum and bladder). Although these definitions vary from institution to institution, most attempt to quantify doses in the paracervical region (Point A), and at Point B, defined as 5 cm from the patient's midline at the same level as point A.[26] In addition, doses to the rectum and bladder are calculated.

Cancer of the Vulva

The combination of a better understanding of tumor biology and the consideration of different clinicopathologic factors that bear prognostic significance in therapeutic modalities have allowed individualization of treatment for cancer of the vulva. Although surgery remains the primary treatment of vulvar cancer, advances in imaging studies, surgical techniques, radiation technology, and chemotherapy have reduced surgical morbidity, resulting in fewer functional and psychosexual impairments without impairing survival. For patients with early-stage squamous cell cancer of the vulva, a conservative wide local excision with intentional macroscopic margins of at least 1 cm may be performed.[33] This is appropriate in stage I or II lesions and has been associated with decreased complications and 5-year overall survival and recurrence rate similar to those of radical vulvar surgery.[34] The procedure may include ipsilateral or bilateral inguinal and femoral lymphadenectomy using a triple incision technique if there is no clinical suspicion of nodal involvement. Radical vulvectomy and bilateral inguinofemoral lymphadenectomy is usually performed in advanced stage disease (stage III or IV).

Because inguinal lymph node status has been identified as one of the most important factors in predicting mortality in vulvar cancer, the appropriate method of evaluating the lymph nodes is currently under evaluation. Primary inguinofemoral lymphadenectomy has been the cornerstone of therapy but is associated with postoperative complications including wound infection, wound breakdown, and lymphedema. A number of minimally invasive and noninvasive studies are currently available that could reduce the morbidity of lymphadenectomy. Sentinel node identification (also described as mapping) using 99mTc appears to be the most promising test. Overall, this technique has a sensitivity rate of 97% and a negative LR 0.14.[35] However, further clarification is needed as to the exact population in whom this test is applicable. The Gynecologic Oncology Group (GOG) has a prospective study (GOG-17) to evaluate lymphatic mapping in patients with stage I or II vulvar cancer.

Elective primary radiation therapy to the groin nodes as an alternative to surgery is another area of current interest in early-stage disease. In 2002, van der Velden and Ansink[36] published a Cochrane review to compare primary groin irradiation versus primary groin surgery for early vulvar cancer. They concluded that primary radiation therapy to the groin resulted in less morbidity but also resulted in a higher number of groin recurrences compared to surgery.

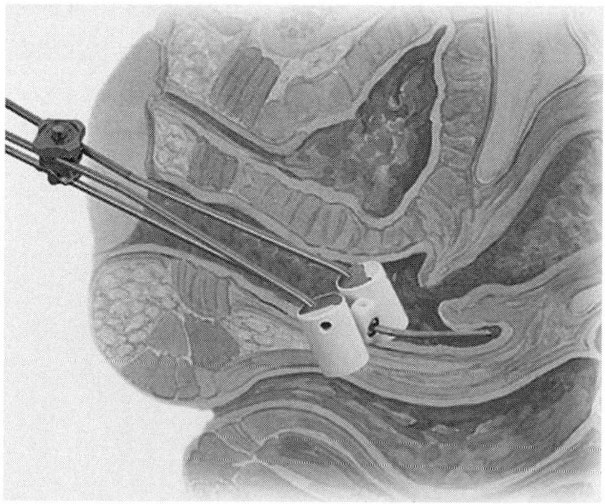

Figure 12-7 Fletcher-Williamson Applicator Set.
Courtesy of Nucletron. Retrieved at www.nucletron.com/upload/applicators/big/085230fletch.jpg

Prospective randomized studies are needed to further evaluate this approach and determine in which patient population it may be most appropriate.

Neoadjuvant radiation therapy to the vulva and groin may be used alone or adjuvantly with chemotherapy to reduce large volume disease in preparation for surgical resection. Postoperative radiation therapy may be given to the pelvic and inguinal areas for nodal metastasis. Unfortunately, the addition of radiation therapy to inguinofemoral lymphadenectomy can increase the already serious morbidity including wound breakdown and lymphedema. Radiation also has a role in the prevention of local recurrence in the vulva when there is a close or positive surgical margin. Radiation therapy also may be given alone or combined with chemotherapy for medically inoperable patients or used to palliate symptoms in advanced disease.

Chemotherapy use has been limited for cancer of the vulva, but may be given in the neoadjuvant setting for advanced disease either alone or in combination with radiation therapy (Table 12-8).

Cancer of the Vagina

Because cancer of the vagina is a rare disease, most of the data describing or comparing treatment techniques involve only a small number of patients. Therefore the basic treatment approach has not changed significantly over the past 20 years. Surgery is used primarily for very early stage I lesions when an adequate margin of tissue can be removed with the tumor. Radical hysterectomy with pelvic lymphadenectomy may be used for stage I lesions of the uppermost part of the vagina. Radiation therapy is the preferred method of treatment for most vaginal cancers. It may be given as a combination of external beam radiation with brachytherapy or brachytherapy alone depending on the position of the primary tumor in the vagina and the stage of the disease.

Cancer of the Cervix

Surgery is the primary therapy for very early stage squamous cell carcinoma of the cervix (CIS and stage IA). The surgical procedure may be tailored to the individual patient. The patient's desire to maintain fertility may result in a therapeutic conization or simple hysterectomy with or without a bilateral salpingo-oophorectomy. However, these patients must have very close follow-up with colposcopy to assure early recognition of recurrent disease.

Modified radical hysterectomy with or without bilateral salpingo-oophorectomy is the surgery of choice for stage IB1 and stage IIA (4 cm or less) cancers of the cervix (for patients who are surgical candidates). This procedure includes removal of the uterus, the upper one-third of the vagina, the broad ligament, the parametria, and biopsy of the pelvic lymph nodes. Radiation therapy is offered as an

Table 12-8 Chemotherapy Agents Used in Gynecologic Malignancies

Chemotherapy agents	Ovary and fallopian tube cancer	Uterine cancer	Cervical cancer	Vaginal cancer	Vulvar cancer
Carboplatin	x	x	x		
Cisplatin	x	x	x	x	x
Cyclophosphamide	x	x			
Doxorubicin HCL	x	x	x		
Ifosphamide	x	x	x		
Doxorubicin HCL liposome	x	x	x		
Epirubicin		(x)	(x)		
5-FU	(x)	(x)	(x)		
Gemcitabine	x				
Irinotecan			(x)		
Melphalan	(x)	(x)			
Mitomycin					(x)
Oxaliplatin	(x)				
Paclitaxel	x	x	x		
Topotecan HCL	x		x		
Vinorelbine			(x)		

x = Used in primary or recurrent disease; *(x)* = reported use in palliative setting.

alternative when patients are not candidates for surgery because of age or presence of significant comorbid disease or because of elderly status or obesity. Patients with stage IB2 or stage IIA (greater than 4 cm) cancers can be treated with either radical hysterectomy with pelvic lymph node dissection and para-aortic lymph node sampling or pelvic radiation therapy with concurrent cisplatin-containing chemotherapy and brachytherapy.[27] Some patients who receive radiation therapy may have an extrafascial hysterectomy after completion of radiation therapy.

In patients found during surgical staging to have positive pelvic lymph nodes, a positive surgical margin, disease extension into the parametrium and/or positive para-aortic lymph nodes may require adjuvant radiation therapy with or without concurrent cisplatin-containing radiation therapy.[27] The fields of treatment depend on the indicator(s) for treatment and may include external beam therapy to the pelvis and/or para-aortic lymph nodes and vaginal brachytherapy.

In advanced-stage disease, surgical resection is not an option because of the proximity of the cervix to the pelvis and the inability to obtain adequate margins. Over the past 5 years, the management has changed as the result of a number of studies that showed that the addition of concurrent chemotherapy to radiation improved the outcome in patients with stages IIB, III, IVA, bulky disease, or positive pelvic lymph nodes.[37-39] Keys and colleagues[37] found that adding weekly infusions of cisplatin to pelvic radiation therapy followed by hysterectomy significantly reduced the risk of disease recurrence and death in women with bulky stage IB cancers. The rates of both progression-free survival (*P* less than 0.001) and overall survival ($P = 0.008$) were significantly higher in the combined-therapy group at 4 years. Toxicities were higher in the combined group, particularly gastrointestinal effects and transient grade 3 and grade 4 hematologic effects. Morris and colleagues[39] reported on the effect of radiation therapy to the pelvis with concurrent 5-fluorouracil (5-FU) and cisplatin in women with advanced cancer (stages IIB to IVA, or stages IB or IIA with biopsy-proven pelvic lymph nodes or tumor size of at least 5 cm) versus radiation therapy alone to the pelvis and periaortic nodes. Estimated cumulative rates of survival at 5 years were 73% among patients treated with radiation therapy and chemotherapy and 58% among patients treated with radiation therapy alone ($P = 0.004$). Cumulative rates of disease-free survival at 5 years were 67% in the combined-therapy group and 40% among patients in the radiation therapy group (*P* less than 0.001). The rates of both distant metastasis and local-regional recurrence were significantly higher among patients treated with radiation therapy alone. The side effects were similar in both groups, with a higher rate of reversible hematologic effect in the combined-therapy group. Based on these data, the NCI issued a clinical announcement supporting the use of cisplatin alone or in combination with 5-FU or other agents (see Table 12-8) with radiation therapy for the treatment of cervical cancer.[40]

Surgery may be considered for patients who have a central recurrence after radiation therapy. In this setting, pelvic exenteration may be offered for a chance of cure in patients with limited disease. Chemotherapy and short courses of radiation therapy may be used to palliate patients with advanced disease who cannot tolerate aggressive therapy. Agents such as cisplatin, carboplatin and 5-FU have been used. Newer agents such as paclitaxel remain under study.

In patients with an unusual cervical cancer histology (i.e., neuroendocrine) the treatment is tailored to the tumor type, its sensitivity to radiation therapy and/or chemotherapy, the stage of disease, age of the patient, and presence of comorbid disease. Specific treatment guidelines may be found in the National Comprehensive Cancer Network Clinical Practice Guidelines for Cervical Cancer, v.1.2006.[27]

Cancer of the Uterus

Surgery is usually performed for patients with stage I to III adenocarcinoma of the uterus. The surgery includes a total abdominal hysterectomy with bilateral salpingo-oophorectomy (BSO), pelvic and para-aortic lymph node sampling, and peritoneal washings. If suspected or gross cervical involvement is present, radical abdominal hysterectomy with BSO, lymph node dissection (pelvic and para-aortic) and peritoneal washings, or primary radiation therapy may be offered.[41] In patients with suspected extrauterine disease in the abdomen (i.e., ascites, nodal, ovarian, peritoneal or omentum disease), a TAH/BSO, peritoneal washings, pelvic and para-aortic lymph node dissection, omentectomy, and debulking may be offered.[41] In extrauterine disease in the pelvis (i.e., vaginal, bladder, bowel, rectum, or parametrial disease), radiation therapy followed by surgery may be offered.[41]

Radiation therapy is given postoperatively to patients with pathologic findings that place them at risk for local-regional recurrence. Patients with stage I disease, but a more aggressive histology (grade 2 or 3) and/or more than 50% myometrial invasion may be offered adjuvant vaginal brachytherapy or pelvic radiation therapy with or without brachytherapy.[41] Patients with stage II disease with histologic grade 2 or 3 disease and/or more than 50% myometrial invasion should be offered adjuvant radiation therapy in the form of vaginal brachytherapy with or without external beam therapy. In patients with completely surgically staged IIIA disease, pelvic radiation therapy with or without brachytherapy or whole abdominopelvic radiation therapy with or without vaginal brachytherapy or chemotherapy with or without radiation therapy should be offered. Patients with stage IIIB, IIIC or IV disease may be offered individualized adjuvant radiation therapy that may include treatment to the pelvis, para-aortic lymph nodes and/or whole abdominopelvic radiation therapy alone or in combination with chemotherapy (see Table 12-8).

Radiation therapy also may be used alone for patients who are not surgical candidates. In some unusual pathologic types of endometrial cancer and in advanced stage disease, whole abdomen radiation therapy may be considered. Systemic therapy with chemotherapy or endocrine therapy has been used for patients with metastatic disease to provide palliation of symptoms and slow disease progression.

Treatment of rare uterine malignancies including sarcomas follow similar guidelines but are tailored to the individual and may include systemic chemotherapy. More specific guidelines are available in the National Comprehensive Cancer Network Clinical Practice Guidelines for Uterine Cancer, v.1.2006.[41]

Cancer of the Ovary and Fallopian Tube

The primary treatment approach for epithelial ovarian and fallopian tube cancer are surgical staging and cytoreduction followed by (when indicated) systemic chemotherapy. Laparotomy and surgical exploration are essential and should include peritoneal cytologic examination and sampling of surfaces of the pelvis, right and left paracolic gutters, and the undersurface of the right and left hemidiaphragms. All peritoneal surfaces should be inspected, and any suspicious areas should be biopsied. The para-aortic lymph nodes and pelvic lymph nodes should be sampled. An omentectomy, total abdominal hysterectomy, and bilateral salpingo-oophorectomy should be performed and maximal cytoreduction attempted.[42]

The role of radiation therapy in ovarian cancer remains controversial. Whole abdomen radiation and intraperitoneal ^{32}P have been used adjuvantly in an effort to improve survival after surgical resection and systemic chemotherapy (see Table 12-8). Currently, this is not standard practice and may be used on an individual basis or as part of a clinical trial.

Treatment of rare tumors of the ovary are individualized depending on the age of the patient, desire to maintain fertility, tumor type, stage, and presence of comorbidity. In general, surgery is the primary treatment. Specific guidelines are available in the National Comprehensive Cancer Network Clinical Practice Guidelines, v.1.2006.

NURSING CARE AND EDUCATION

Acute and late toxicity associated with radiation therapy for gynecologic malignancies depends on the site of treatment, the volume of treatment included in the treatment fields, the technique used (i.e., external beam vs. brachytherapy), the total dose given, and the presence of comorbid disease. In patients treated with abdominopelvic radiation, acute complications include nausea, vomiting, diarrhea, frequency of urination, leukopenia, thrombocytopenia, transient hepatic enzyme elevation, and (on occasion) symptomatic basal pneumonitis.[43] Late toxicities may include bowel obstruction, enteritis, proctitis, and hemorrhagic cystitis.

Patients receiving treatment to the pelvis may experience acute toxicities such as cystitis, diarrhea, proctitis, vaginal mucositis, nausea, and moist desquamation within skinfolds. Late toxicities may include bowel obstruction, hemorrhagic cystitis, vaginal stenosis, vesicovaginal fistula, rectovaginal fistula, enteritis, proctitis, pelvic nerve damage, and lower extremity edema. If the perineum is included in the treatment field, acute brisk erythema and moist desquamation will occur in the majority of patients. Infertility and menopause will be permanent in women treated with radiation therapy that involves the pelvis.

The key to successful management of these toxicities is patient education and accurate evaluation and documentation. Nurses play a significant role in patient education including measures to reduce

Table 12-9 Resources for Patients With Gynecologic Malignancies

Name of organization	Website	Type of information (patient and/or professional)
American Brachytherapy Society	www.americanbrachytherapy.org	Professional
American Cancer Society	www.cancer.org	Professional Patient
Cancersource.com	www.cancersource.com	Professional Patient
National Comprehensive Cancer Network	www.nccn.org	Professional Patient
National Ovarian Cancer Coalition	www.ovarian.org	Patient
Oncology Nursing Society	www.ons.org	Professional
Radiation Therapy Oncology Group	www.rtog.org	Professional Patient
Society of Gynecologic Nurse Oncologists	www.sgno.org	Professional
Gynecologic Cancer Foundation	www.thegcf.org	Professional Patient
Women's Cancer Network	www.wcn.org	Patient

risk of development of toxicities (e.g., diet modifications) and management of expected side effects during and after treatment. Table 12-9 provides a list of resources for both patient education material and nursing education support.

Accurate documentation of toxicity of treatment is the responsibility of the physician and nursing staff. Two instruments are available for grading the severity of acute effects. They are the National Cancer Institute's Common Toxicity Criteria for Adverse Events (CTCAE-v 3.0)[44] and the Radiation Therapy Patient Care Record: A Tool for Documenting Nursing Care.[45]

Acute Toxicity

Skin reactions are usually confined to areas with skin folds and the perineum. Treatment to the whole abdomen does not generally result in a skin reaction. Treatment to the pelvis may result in mild hyperpigmentation within the treatment fields, and moist desquamation in folds of abdominal skin, in the groin, and between the buttocks. Treatment to the perineum usually results in brisk erythema 10 to 14 days after treatment is initiated, with moist desquamation occurring shortly thereafter. The presence of numerous skinfolds and exposure to urine and fecal material increase the risk of skin breakdown. Wound dehiscence and soft tissue necrosis, particularly along suture lines is uncommon, but may occur in patients after recent radical vulvectomy. See Chapter 30 for skin care management.

Acute cystitis usually becomes symptomatic after 10 to 14 days of treatment and results in dysuria, increased frequency, urgency hesitancy, and increased nocturia. The symptoms usually resolve within 1 month of completing treatment. Adequate hydration and avoidance of food and beverages that may irritate the bladder will help. This includes beverages that contain caffeine and alcohol. Although infection is rare, a urine culture and sensitivity may be necessary if the patient's symptoms include cloudy urine samples, hematuria, or the patient becomes febrile. Urinary tract analgesics including phenazopyridine hydrochloride and antispasmodics such as hyoscyamine sulfate and oxybutynin chloride may help with the symptoms.

Diarrhea (radiation-induced) results from a variety of different pathophysiologic mechanisms including malabsorption of bile salts and lactose, imbalances in local bacterial flora, and changes in the intestinal patterns of motility. Wang and colleagues[46] found that patients with increased acute toxicity and diarrhea during radiation therapy for cervix cancer had significantly increased risk of late rectal injury, suggesting that early excessive damage of the acute-responding component of the rectal wall may play an important role in the initiation of rectal injury. A number of treatment approaches with antidiarrheal and diet interventions have been used with little research to evaluate efficacy. Henriksson and colleagues[47] reported on the use of sucralfate in preventing radiation-induced diarrhea and bowel discomfort. In a double-blind and placebo-controlled study of patients treated to the pelvis with radiation, frequency of defecation and stool consistency were significantly improved by sucralfate. One year later, the patients in the sucralfate group displayed significantly fewer problems with frequency of defecation, mucus, and blood in the stools compared with the placebo group. Other treatment options may be found in Chapter 36.

Nausea and vomiting may occur when patients are receiving treatment to the whole abdomen. Prophylactic antiemetics before radiation therapy often eliminate this problem. Occasionally patients receiving treatment only to the pelvis report mild nausea. Chapter 36 offers a variety of treatment approaches. If persistent nausea with vomiting occurs, evaluation for bowel obstruction may be warranted.

Vaginal mucositis usually occurs within the first 14 to 21 days of treatment. This occurs as a result of changes in the vaginal epithelium. Patients will report symptoms of discomfort and dyspareunia. If a foul-smelling or thin, watery discharge begins, cultures should be obtained for infectious agents such as *Candida albicans*, bacterial vaginosis, and chlamydia. Otherwise, patients may be treated symptomatically.

Bone marrow suppression may occur with whole abdomen radiation therapy. In addition, patients with active vaginal bleeding may develop anemia. Weekly or twice weekly laboratory studies including a complete blood count with differential should be performed. Management is individualized based on the severity of the symptoms and the laboratory results.

Fatigue is also common when patients are treated with pelvic or whole abdomen radiation therapy. The mechanisms that produce fatigue as a result of radiation are poorly understood. However, fatigue can significantly impact the patient's quality of life, ability to continue treatment, and tolerance of acute and late effects of treatment. Nursing education is key to reducing the impact of fatigue on the patient's ability to function. Adequate nutrition and hydration, adequate sleep and rest times, and a realistic approach to personal accomplishments and daily activities are three primary approaches to fatigue reduction. A comprehensive approach to management can be found in the NCCN Cancer-related Fatigue Clinical Practice Guidelines, v.1.2006.[48]

Late Toxicity

Radiation-induced intestinal (i.e., enteritis and proctitis) injury can result in local ischemia and fibrosis with the development of ulcers, strictures, and rectal bleeding. Montana and Fowler[49] identified a correlation between rectal dose and proctitis in patients receiving radiation therapy to the pelvis. The risk of proctitis increased as a function of rectal dose ranging from 2% for patients receiving 50 Gy or less to the rectum to 18% for patients receiving at least 80 Gy to the rectum. Symptoms may include rectal bleeding, painful bowel movements, and chronic or intermittent diarrhea. Occasionally, the rectal bleeding can be severe enough to result in anemia and transfusion dependency. Bleeding typically develops from 6 months to 1 year after completion of radiation therapy and is caused by friable mucosal angioectasias.[50] A number of treatment options have been described for rectal bleeding including the instillation of a variety of medications, endoscopic laser obliteration, diet modification, and surgery. See Chapter 34 for treatment options.

Hemorrhagic cystitis occurs in 1% to 2% of patients after pelvic radiation.[51] Montana and Fowler[49] found that the risk of cystitis increased as a function of bladder dose, ranging from 3% for patients receiving 50 Gy or less, to 12% in patients receiving at least 80 Gy to the bladder. Management includes endoscopy with obliteration, instillation of sodium pentosan polysulfate,[52] formalin instillation,[34] and hyperbaric oxygen therapy.[51]

As might be expected because of the organs involved, a high degree of sexual dysfunction is reported among gynecologic cancer survivors, with estimates ranging from 20% to 100%.[53] The degree and nature of sexual dysfunction vary according to the type, length, and intensity of treatment. Two surgical procedures, vulvectomy and exenteration result in the most dramatic anatomic changes. High-dose radiation to the pelvis may cause varying degrees of sexual dysfunction because of the effects on the ovaries and vagina. There may be a significant impact on vaginal function, with stenosis and loss of elasticity. Ovarian failure resulting in estrogen deprivation with induction of early menopause from oophorectomy or ovarian ablation aggravates other anatomic changes. Bruner and colleagues (1993)[54] evaluated the incidence and degree of vaginal stenosis, sexual activity, and satisfaction in women treated with intracavitary radiation therapy for cervical or endometrial cancer. They found that radiation at standard doses with or without hysterectomy can cause a decrease in vaginal length as compared to the normal vaginal length of 8 cm to 9 cm documented by Masters and Johnson. Women treated with intracavitary implants remained as sexually active post implant as preimplant. However, coital frequency and sexual satisfaction decreased and dyspareunia increased.

Vaginal dilators and sexual intercourse have been the standard recommendations to reduce the risk of vaginal stenosis. However, patient compliance has been a problem, motivating healthcare providers to look for alternatives. Topical estrogen products, which promote proliferation of the epithelium, may be prescribed to reduce vaginal dryness and dyspareunia. However, this may not be appropriate for patients with estrogen-sensitive tumors. For more specific treatment recommendations, see Chapter 35.

Obliterative endarteritis secondary to ionizing radiation may lead to tissue hypoxia, poor healing, and ultimately to fistulae formation. In women who had radiation therapy to the pelvis for a gynecologic malignancy, fistulae may form between the bladder and vagina, vagina and rectum, bowel and vagina, or bowel and bladder. Patients may present with fecal material draining from the vagina, fecal material in the urine, or urine draining from the vagina. If the small bowel is involved, significant damage can occur to tissue exposed to the small bowel contents. Management of fistulae requires a multidisciplinary team of surgeons, wound care providers, and nutritional experts to design a program to divert the fecal matter or urine, and promote healing. Surgery may be necessary to create a diversion around the fistulae. Total parenteral nutrition may be necessary to reduce bowel content and provide adequate calories and protein for healing. Hyperbaric oxygen therapy also has been demonstrated to improve angiogenesis and promote healing in radiation-injured tissue. Chronic lymphedema of the lower extremities may occur in response to surgical resection of or radiation to the groin and/or pelvic lymph nodes. Patient education regarding potential risk factors and early recognition are necessary to reduce the risk of permanent lymphedema, which can become painful and place the patient at risk for recurrent episodes of lymphangitis and cellulitis. Aggressive management with comprehensive decongestive therapy is important. Chapter 9 provides a review of lymphedema prevention and management approaches.

A rare complication of radiation therapy to the pelvis (particularly when the groin area is included in the field) is necrosis and fracture of the femoral head/neck. Grigsby and colleagues[55] reported a 5% actuarial 5-year incidence of fractures in patients receiving doses of 50 Gy or greater.

Quality of Life

The measurement of quality of life outcomes in women with gynecologic malignancies is sparse in the literature. In specific, only a few studies have been conducted on women receiving radiation therapy. Most studies on quality of life outcomes have focused on the physical domain, such as the development of a specific morbidity (such as fistulae development), and have not evaluated psychologic, spiritual, or social domains. Of the few studies that have focused on the other domains, the majority focused on psychologic adjustment to the diagnosis, on the treatment, and on the immediate sequelae—usually impact on sexuality. Unfortunately, evaluation of these studies is difficult because of the small populations included, the mixture of diagnoses and treatment approaches; and because of differences in design, outcome variability, and end results. However several key findings can be derived from the data.

Survivors of gynecologic malignancies face a number of issues in addition to those common in all cancer survivors. These issues include sexual and fertility issues, body image issues, and the impact of treatment-induced early menopause. Only one longitudinal prospective study has been conducted on the incidence and cause of major life difficulties for gynecologic cancer survivors.[56] Women with early-stage malignancies were assessed after their diagnosis but prior to treatment and then reassessed at 4, 8, and 12 months posttreatment. Two matched comparison groups (women diagnosed and treated for benign disease and healthy women) were also assessed. The emotional response to the life-threatening diagnosis and anticipation of treatment was characterized by depressed, anxious, and confused moods, whereas the response for women with benign disease was anxious mood only. In both cases, these responses were transitory and resolved posttreatment. There was no evidence for a higher incidence of relationship dissolution or impaired marital adjustment. However, women treated for disease (benign or malignant) reported posttreatment declines in intercourse frequency, a diminution of sexual excitement, and a less positive global evaluation of their sexual life. They also reported a three- to sixfold increase in incidence of sexual dysfunction diagnoses compared to healthy women. There was no evidence for impaired social adjustment. Women treated for cancer retained their employment and their occupations. However, their involvement (hours worked per week) was significantly reduced during recovery. The authors suggested that "islands" of significant life disruption after cancer do occur.

Sexual dysfunction has received more attention than any other aspect of quality of life research in this patient population. Anderson and colleagues[57] found that global sexual behavior changes in women did not occur, but frequency of intercourse declined for women with early-stage gynecologic cancer and those with benign disease. Of the women who had no sexual dysfunction before the diagnosis and treatment of cancer, approximately 50% eventually were diagnosed with at least one dysfunction during the year after treatment. Although some improved, others worsened, and by 12 months after treatment, approximately 30% of cancer patients had some sexual dysfunction. In relation to the sexual response cycle, diminution of sexual excitement was pronounced for women with benign disease, but was more severe and distressing for women with cancer, possibly due to significant coital and postcoital pain, premature menopause, treatment side effects, or a combination. Signs and symptoms of estrogen deficiency were significant in both the benign and malignant groups at 4 and 8 months but had resolved for the benign group by 12 months.

Regarding psychosocial issues, Auchincloss[58] found that gynecologic cancer survivors have difficulty in forming support groups to help deal with survivor problems and stresses, in part as the result of the relative rarity of each individual disease. This results in difficulties with depression, energy level, occupational functioning, relationships, and a sense of well-being.

In addition to evaluating long-term survivors of gynecologic cancer, it is important to evaluate the quality of life of patients with overall short life spans. Included in this population are women diagnosed with ovarian cancer. These women tend to have protracted courses of treatment, followed by short periods of disease control. The disease has a profound effect on physical function and social and psychosexual functioning. Studies of women with ovarian cancer have focused on descriptive information, assessment, or comparison of treatment alternatives, evaluation of programs or interventions, and facilitation of communication with patients.[59] Because radiation therapy is used in a limited number of patients, the impact of this therapy on quality of life has not been well documented.

Follow-Up Care

Cancer of the Vulva

A follow-up evaluation should be performed every 3 months for a minimum of 2 years. The evaluation should include a history and physical examination with careful visual inspection of the vulva and perineum. Colposcopy and biopsy should be performed if there are any suspicious lesions. A pelvic exam with Pap smear of the cervix should be performed annually. A chest x ray should be performed annually. Additional radiograph and laboratory studies should be performed based on reported symptoms and findings during the clinical exam. In addition to evaluating for recurrence during follow-up visits, patients should be evaluated for the development of a second primary cancer after vulva cancer. Sturgeon and colleagues[60] found an increased risk of all second cancers combined among women with cancer of the vulva (observed/expected in situ = 1.5; observed/expected invasive = 1.3). Most of the excess second cancers were smoking-related (including lung, head and neck sites, and esophagus), or related to infection with human papilloma virus (cervix, vagina, or anus).

The 5-year survival rate for patients with no lymph node spread is about 90% and is only marginally lower for patients with microscopic involvement of one node, providing there is no extracapsular tumor. Patients with two or three involved nodes have a survival rate of 66%, and those with more than three positive groin nodes have only a 30% survival rate.[61,62]

Cancer of the Vagina

A follow-up evaluation should be performed every 3 months for a minimum of 2 years. The evaluation should include history and physical examination with careful visual inspection of the vagina with colposcopy and biopsy of any suspicious lesions. A pelvic exam with Pap smear of the cervix and vagina should be performed every 3 to 6 months. A chest x ray should be performed annually. Additional radiograph or laboratory studies should be performed as clinically indicated. Patients with a history of vaginal squamous cell cancer are also at risk for the development of a second primary tumor in the same manner as patients with a history of vulva cancer and should be screened appropriately.

Because this is a rare malignancy, accurate survival rates are based on small series of patients. Kuçera and Vavra[63] reported the outcome of 434 patients with vaginal cancer. Five-year survival for patients with stage I disease was 77%, stage II disease was 45%, stage III disease was 31%, and stage IV was 18%.

Cancer of the Cervix

A follow-up evaluation should be performed every 3 months for a minimum of 1 year, then every 4 months for 1 year, then every 6 months for 3 years.[27] The evaluation should include history and physical examination with a pelvic exam with Pap smear each visit. Careful examination of the anus and anal canal should be performed. Women with primary invasive cervical cancer have been found to have a relative risk of 4.6 for subsequent invasive anal cancer.[64] A chest x ray should be performed annually. Additional radiograph or laboratory studies should be ordered as clinically indicated.

Five-year relative survival rates are 92% for local disease, 55% for regional disease, and 16% for patients that present with distant metastasis.[6]

Cancer of the Uterus

A follow-up evaluation should be performed every 3 to 6 months for a minimum of 2 years, then every 6 to 12 months. The evaluation should include history and physical examination with pelvic exam and Pap smear of the vaginal cuff every 6 months for 2 years and then annually. A chest x ray should be performed annually. Other radiograph or laboratory studies may be performed as clinically indicated. If the CA-125 was elevated initially, it maybe helpful to repeat it during each visit.[11] Five-year survival estimate for all stages is 84%.[6] Patients with disease confined to the uterus have a 96% chance of five-year survival. However, once the disease has extended beyond the uterus or involves regional lymphatics, survival decreases to 66%. Patients with distant metastasis have a five-year survival estimate of 25%.[6]

Cancer of the Ovary

A follow-up evaluation should be performed every 2 to 4 months for 2 years, then every 6 months for 3 years, then annually. The evaluation should include a history and physical examination including pelvic exam. A complete blood count should be performed annually. A CA-125 assay should be performed at each visit if level was elevated before initial cytoreduction surgery. Ozols[65] reported that the median time for clinical relapse after a rising CA-125 is 2 to 6 months. Radiograph or laboratory studies should be performed as clinically indicated. No role has been established for routine CT scans of the abdomen or pelvis.[65]

Despite advances in surgical technology and chemotherapy agents, the prognosis for ovarian and fallopian tube cancer remains poor. The 5-year survival rate for all stages is only 50%.[6] Survival of disease confined to the ovary is 95%, but decreases to 68.1% for patients with local-regional disease, and to 29% for patients with stage III or stage IV disease.[6]

REFERENCES

1. Ferlay J, Bray F, Pisani P et al: *GLOBOCAN 2002. Cancer incidence, mortality and prevalence worldwide. IARC cancer base no 5, version 2.0*, Lyon, France, 2004, IARC Press.
2. American Cancer Society: *Cancer facts and figures, 2006*, Atlanta, American Cancer Society, 2006.
3. Wilkinson EW, Stone IK: *Atlas of vulvar disease*, Baltimore, MD, 1995, Williams & Wilkins, pp 1-13.
4. Beller U, Sideri M, Maisonneuve P et al: Carcinoma of the vulva, *J Epidemiol Biostat* 6(1):155-173, 2001.
5. Keys H: Gynecologic Oncology Group randomized trials of combined therapy for vulvar cancer, *Cancer* 71(4 suppl):1691-1696, 1993.
6. Ries LAG, Eisner MP, Kosary CL et al, editors: *Seer cancer statistics review, 1975-2002*, Bethesda, MD, 2004, National Cancer Institute (website): http://seer.cancer.gov/csr/1975_2002. Accessed February 10, 2006.
7. Creasman WT: Vaginal cancers, *Curr Opin Obstet Gynecol* 17(1):71-76, 2005.
8. Seltzer VL: Ovarian cancer. In Kramer BS, Gohagan JK, Prorock PC, editors: *Cancer screening: theory and practice*, New York, 1999, Marcel Dekker, pp 431-440.
9. Nordin AJ: Primary carcinoma of the fallopian tube: a 20-year literature review, *Obstet Gynecol Surv*, 49(5): 349-361, 1994.
10. deVilliers E, Fauquet C, Broker TR et al: Classification of papillomaviruses, *Virology* 324(1):17-27, 2004.
11. Williamson AL, Passmore JA, Rybicki EP: Strategies for prevention of cervical cancer by human papilloma virus vaccination, *Best Pract Res Clin Obstet Gynaecol* 19(4): 531-544, 2005.

12. Munoz N, Bosch FX, deSanjoee S et al: Epidemiologic classification of human papilloma virus types associated with cervical cancer, *N Engl J Med* 348(6):518-527, 2003.
13. Trimble CL, Hildesheim A, Brinton LA et al: Heterogeneous etiology of squamous carcinoma of the vulva, *Obstet Gynecol* 87(1):59-64, 1996.
14. Jones RW, Baranyai J, Stables S: Trends in squamous cell carcinoma of the vulva: the influence of vulvar intraepithelial neoplasia, *Obstet Gynecol* 90(3):448-452, 1997.
15. van Seters M, van Beurden M, de Craen AJ: Is the assumed natural history of vulvar intraepithelial neoplasia III based on enough evidence? A systematic review of 3322 published patients, *Gynecol Oncol* 97(2):645-651, 2005.
16. Penn I: Cancers of the anogenital region in renal transplant recipients, *Cancer* 58(3):611-616, 1986.
17. Brown JE, Sunborg MJ, Kost E et al: Vulvar cancer in human immunodeficiency virus-seropositive premenopausal women: a case series and review of the literature, *J Low Genit Tract Dis* 9(1):7-10, 2005.
18. Barton SE, Maddox PH, Jenkins D et al: Effect of smoking on cervical epithelial-immunity: a mechanism for neoplastic change (letter), *Lancet* 2(8612):652-654, 1988.
19. Holcomb K, Maiman M, Dimaio T et al: Rapid progression to invasive cervix cancer in a woman infected with the human immunodeficiency virus, *Obstet Gynecol* 91(5 Pt 2):848-850, 1998.
20. Walker JL, Nunez ER: Endometrial cancer. In Kramer BS, Gohagan JK, Prorock PC, editors: *Cancer Screening*, New York, 1999, Marcel Dekker, pp 531-556.
21. Grady D, Gebretsadik T, Kerlikowske K et al: Hormone replacement therapy and endometrial cancer risk: a meta-analysis, *Obstet Gynecol,* 85(2):304-313, 1995.
22. Claus EB, Schildkraut JM, Thompson WD et al: The genetic attributable risk of breast and ovarian cancer, *Cancer* 77(11):2318-2324, 1996.
23. Blake P, Lambert H, Crawford R: *Gynecological oncology: a guide to clinical management,* Oxford, England, 1998, Oxford University Press, pp 98-121.
24. Figge DC, Tamimi HK, Greer BE: Lymphatic spread in carcinoma of the vulva, *Am J Obstet* 152(4):387-394, 1985.
25. Smith RA, Cokkinides V, Eyre HJ: American Cancer Society guidelines for early detection of cancer, *CA Cancer J Clin* 53(1):41-52, 2004.
26. Chao KSC, Perez CA, Brady LW: *Radiation oncology: management decisions*, Philadelphia, 2002, Lippincott-Raven, pp 489-519.
27. National Comprehensive Cancer Network: *Cervical cancer clinical practice guidelines,* V1.2006. Jenkintown, PA, 2006, National Comprehensive Cancer Network.
28. American College of Obstetrics and Gynecology (ACOG): ACOG practice bulletin, clinical management guidelines for obstetrician-gynecologists number 65: management of endometrial cancer, *Obstet Gynecol* 106(2):413-425, 2005.
29. Fields MM, Chevlen E: Ovarian cancer screening: a look at the evidence, *Clin J Oncol Nurs* 10(1):77-81, 2006.
30. Kurjak A, Kupesic S, Sparac V et al: The detection of stage I ovarian cancer by three-dimensional sonography and power Doppler, *Gynecol Oncol* 90(2):258-264, 2003.
31. National Institutes of Health Consensus Conference: Ovarian cancer: screening, treatment, and follow-up, *JAMA* 273(6):491-497, 1995.
32. Gosselin TK, Waring JS: Nursing management of patients receiving brachytherapy for gynecologic malignancies, *Clin J Oncol Nurs* 5(2):59-61, 2001.
33. Hullu JA, Oonk MHM, van der Zee AGJ: Modern management of vulvar cancer, *Curr Opin Obstet Gynecol* 16(1):65-72, 2004.
34. Magrina JF, Gonzalez-Bosquet J, Weaver AL et al: Primary squamous cell cancer of the vulva: radical versus modified radical vulvar surgery, *Gynecol Oncol* 71(1):116-121, 1998.
35. Selman TJ, Luesley DM, Acheson N et al: A systematic review of the accuracy of diagnostic tests for inguinal lymph node status in vulvar cancer, *Gynecol Oncol* 99(1):206-214, 2005.
36. van der Velden J, Ansink A: Primary groin irradiation vs primary groin surgery for early vulvar cancer, *Cochrane Database Syst Rev* (3):CD002224, 2000.
37. Keys HM, Bundy BN, Stehman FB et al: Cisplatin, radiation, and adjuvant hysterectomy compared with radiation and adjuvant hysterectomy for bulky stage IB cervical carcinoma, *N Engl J Med* 340(15):1154-1161, 1999.
38. Rose PG, Bundy BN, Watkins EB et al: Concurrent cisplatin-based chemoradiation improves progression-free and overall survival in advanced cervical cancer: results of a randomized Gynecologic Oncology Group study, *N Engl J Med* 34(15):1144-1153, 1999.
39. Morris M, Eifel PJ, Lu J et al: Pelvic radiation with concurrent chemotherapy compared with pelvic and para-aortic radiation for high-risk cervical cancer, *N Engl J Med* 340(15):1198-2000, 1999.
40. National Cancer Institute: *NCI issues clinical announcement on cervical cancer chemotherapy plus radiation improves survival,* 1999 (website): www.cancer.gov/newscenter/cervicalcancer. Accessed March 28, 2006.
41. National Comprehensive Cancer Network: *Uterine cancer clinical practice guidelines,* V1.2006, Jenkintown, PA, 2006, National Comprehensive Cancer Network.
42. National Comprehensive Cancer Network: *Ovarian cancer clinical practice guidelines,* V1.2006, Jenkintown, PA, 2005, National Comprehensive Cancer Network.
43. Fyles AW, Dembo AJ, Bush RS: Analysis of complications in patients treated with abdomino-pelvic radiation therapy for ovarian carcinoma, *Int J Radiat Oncol Biol Phys* 22(5):847-851, 1992.
44. National Cancer Institute: *NCI common toxicity criteria for adverse events (CTCAE v 3.0).* Bethesda, MD, 2003, National Cancer Institute.
45. Oncology Nursing Society Radiation Therapy Special Interest Group Documentation Project Core Committee: *Radiation Therapy Patient Care Record: A Tool for Documenting Nursing Care,* Pittsburgh, 2002, Oncology Nursing Press.
46. Wang CJ, Leung SW, Chen HC et al: The correlation of acute toxicity and late rectal injury in radiotherapy for cervical carcinoma: evidence suggestive of consequential late effect (CQLE). *Int J Radiat Oncol Biol Phys* 40(1): 85-91, 1998.
47. Henriksson R, Franzen L, Littbrand B: Effects of sucralfate on acute and late bowel discomfort following radiotherapy of pelvic cancer, *J Clin Oncol* 10(6):969-975, 1992.
48. National Comprehensive Cancer Network: *NCCN Clinical Practice Guidelines in Oncology: Cancer Related Fatigue,*

V1.2006. Jenkintown, PA: National Comprehensive Cancer Network.

49. Montana GS, Fowler WC: Carcinoma of the cervix: analysis of bladder and rectal radiation dose and complications, *Int J Radiat Oncol Biol Phys* 16(1):95-100, 1989.
50. Swaroop VS, Gostout CJ: Endoscopic treatment of chronic radiation proctopathy, *J Clin Gastroenterol* 27(1):36-40, 1998.
51. Mathews R, Rajan N, Josefson L: Hyperbaric oxygen therapy for radiation induced hemorrhagic cystitis, *J Urol* 161(2):435-437, 1999.
52. Parsons GL: Successful management of radiation cystitis with sodium pentasanpolysulfate, *J Urol* 136(4):813-814, 1986.
53. Anderson B, Lutgendorf S: Quality of life in gynecologic cancer survivors, *CA Cancer J Clin* 47(4):218-225, 1997.
54. Bruner DW, Lanciano R, Keegan M et al: Vaginal stenosis and sexual function following intracavitary radiation for the treatment of cervical and endometrial carcinoma, *Int J Radiat Oncol Biol Phys* 27(4):825-830, 1993.
55. Grigsby PW, Roberts HL, Perez CA: Femoral neck fracture following groin irradiation, *Int J Radiat Oncol Biol Phys* 32(1):63-67, 1995.
56. Anderson BL, Anderson B, deProsse C: Controlled prospective longitudinal study of women with cancer. II. Psychological outcomes, *J Consult Clin Psych* 57(6):692-697, 1989.
57. Anderson BL, Anderson B, deProsse C: Controlled prospective longitudinal study of women with cancer. I. Sexual functioning outcomes, *J Consult Clin Psych* 57(6):683-691, 1989.
58. Auchincloss SS: After treatment: psychosocial issues in gynecologic cancer survivorship, *Cancer* 76(10 suppl): 2117-2124, 1995.
59. Bezjak A: Quality of life in women with cancer. In Kavanagh JJ, Singletary SE, Einhorn N, DePetrillo AD, editors: *Cancer in women*, Malden, MA, 1998, Blackwell Science.
60. Sturgeon SR, Curtis RE, Johnson K et al: Second primary cancers after vulvar and vaginal cancers, *Am J Obstet Gynecol* 174(3):929-933, 1996.
61. Burger MP, Hollema H, Emanuels AG et al: The importance of the groin node status for the survival of T1 and T2 vulva carcinoma patients, *Gynecol Oncol* 57(3): 327-334, 1995.
62. Origoni M, Sideri M, Garsia S et al: Prognostic value of pathological patterns of lymph node positivity in squamous cell carcinoma of the vulva: stage III and IVA FIGO, *Gynecol Oncol* 45(3):313-316, 1992.
63. Kuçera H, Vavra N: Primary carcinoma of the vagina: clinical and histopathological variables associated with survival, *Gynecol Oncol* 40(1):12-16, 1991.
64. Rabkin CS, Biggar RJ, Melbye M et al: Second primary cancers following anal and cervical carcinoma: evidence of shared etiologic factors, *Am J Epidemiol* 136(1):54-58, 1992.
65. Ozols RF: Update of NCCN ovarian cancer practice guidelines, *Oncology* 11(11A):95-105, 1997.

Chapter 13

Male Genitourinary Cancers

William P. Hogle

This chapter examines the realm of male genitourinary cancers. Specifically, the areas addressed include prostate, penile, male urethral, and testicular cancers. In addition to the clinical manifestation, diagnosis, and pathologic features of each site, an extensive review of treatment options is provided. Further, particular attention is placed on the radiation treatment techniques, associated side effects of radiation, and nursing interventions aimed at alleviating side effects.

PROSTATE CANCER

Regardless of the radiation setting in which one works, the number of patients treated for prostate cancer is likely to be a significant portion of a cancer center's total patient population. Prostate cancer rates have continually increased from 180,400 in 2000 to an estimated 230,110 in 2004, and an estimated 234,460 men will be diagnosed in 2006.[1-3] It is the most common non–skin-related cancer diagnosed in men today and is a leading cause of cancer deaths among men, second only to lung cancer.[2] Conservative estimates suggest that as baby boomers age, incidence and prevalence rates of prostate cancer will continue to rise. By 2015, the number of newly diagnosed prostate cancer cases will increase to over 300,000 annually and peak at 400,000 cases per year by 2035.[4] It stands to reason that mortality rates from this disease will also continue to rise. An estimated 27,350 attributable deaths are expected in 2006, with up to 50,000 in 2020, and rates are estimated to peak eventually at 80,000 per year in 2030.[4]

Incidence rates for prostate cancer in the United States range from 51.2 per 100,000 among American Indians/Alaskan Natives to 271.3 per 100,000 among African-American males. Five-year relative survival rates are also lower for African-American males than for Caucasian males diagnosed with prostate cancer.[5] Theories as to the reason for these disparities range from inequalities in access to health care, to whether quality health care is received, to associated comorbidities. However, some research suggests that when African-American males receive cancer treatment and medical care similar to that provided to Caucasian males, disease outcomes are similar.[3,6]

Risk factors for developing prostate cancer include ethnicity, age, and family history. African-American males whose father or brother was diagnosed with prostate cancer at an early age appear to have an even greater risk of developing the disease.[7] To date, the exact etiology of prostate cancer is unclear. It is believed that molecular and biologic factors exist as causative agents. Prostate intraepithelial neoplasia (PIN), insulin-like growth factor I (IGF-I), and vascular endothelial growth factor (VEGF) have been shown to have a role in prostate cancer. The cancer itself is the result of cumulative changes in the genetic code of cells in the prostate gland that may cause uncontrolled cellular proliferation, altered differentiation, and metastatic spread.[8,9]

Other considerations that have been examined for a possible link to prostate cancer include occupational/chemical exposure, hormonal exposure, nutritional deficiencies, body mass index, and issues surrounding male sexuality (i.e., sexual frequency, vasectomy, and human papilloma virus [HPV] exposure).[10,11] However, little supportive evidence exists to indicate a strong relationship between these factors and prostate cancer.

Anatomy

The prostate is a small, firm, walnut-shaped gland that lies in the pelvis below the urinary bladder; it surrounds the neck of the bladder and a portion of the urethra. It also lies adjacent to the rectum, which allows for easy palpation of a portion of the gland by means of a digital rectal exam (DRE).

The gland's primary function is to secrete fluids that act as a vehicle for sperm during ejaculation. Just prior to ejaculation, seminal fluid mixes with sperm in the prostate gland. At the point of orgasm, the bladder neck closes and semen is propelled through the penis.

The gland is essentially divided into four zones. The inner most region, known as the *transitional zone*, surrounds the urethra adjacent to the ejaculatory ducts. *The central zone* surrounds the ejaculatory ducts and projects beneath the base of the bladder. The *peripheral zone* encircles the central zone and typically contains 75% of the overall glandular tissue. Not surprisingly, it is here that 75% of all prostate tumors originate.[12] The outer most zone is referred to as the *anterior fibromuscular zone*, which consists mostly of smooth muscle.

Pathophysiology

Carcinogenesis results from an accumulation of mutagenic changes in the cells of the prostate gland that occur over a period of time. Cells that are partially transformed could potentially result in PIN, which is considered a precancerous condition and a significant precursor of prostate cancer.[13] PIN is classified as low or high grade with high-grade lesions being associated with prostate cancer. Patients with high-grade PIN and negative biopsy results should be followed closely for up to 2 years.[14] PIN may be present for up to 10 years before cancer is diagnosed.[15]

It is theorized that all prostate cancers arise from glandular epithelial cells.[16] Approximately 95% of all cancers that develop in the prostate are adenocarcinomas. The remaining 5% predominantly consist of transitional cell, squamous cell, and small cell carcinomas. The minority (5%) of prostate neoplasms generally metastasize quickly and are difficult to treat using conventional systemic means. Very rarely is the diagnosis of primary prostate carcinosarcoma or prostate lymphoma made.[8,9,11]

The most widely used pathologic grading system for prostate cancer is the Gleason score. Developed by Donald Gleason, MD, in 1974, this subjective method of histologic evaluation examines the cellular architecture present in a biopsy specimen or series of specimens.[17] The Gleason score essentially incorporates five histologic patterns based on the degree of cellular differentiation and assigns a numeric value from 1 to 5. A classification of 1 represents well-differentiated cells and 5 represents poorly differentiated cells. Approximately 50% of tumors found in the prostate demonstrate more than one histologic pattern. As a result, the total Gleason score is obtained by adding the assigned numbers that represent the two most dominant cell patterns within the obtained specimen. Therefore, a total possible score will range from 2 to 10.[18] Tumors with a lower combined Gleason score (2 to 6) are generally viewed as less aggressive.

In general, prostate cancers are slow growing. However, more aggressive tumors are more likely to spread outside the initial area of involvement and may exhibit perineural invasion or involvement of the seminal vesicles or urinary bladder. Area lymph node involvement can occur and occasional locoregional lymph node sampling may be indicated. Prostate cancer cells can metastasize to distant organs/structures if they gain access to the vascular system through the Batson plexus, a collection of presacral veins.[19] After regional lymph nodes, areas most likely to develop metastatic disease include bone (lumbar spine, pelvis, femur, or skull) followed by lungs, bladder, liver, and brain.[11]

The staging of prostate cancer by means of the American Joint Committee on Cancer staging manual can be viewed in Table 13-1.[20]

Diagnostic Studies and Clinical Manifestations

In addition to family history, it is important to determine the patient's personal history, specifically inquiring about any changes in normal bowel or bladder function (dysuria, frequency, nocturia, hematuria, or signs of bladder outlet obstruction). It also may be helpful to determine a patient's American Urological Association (AUA) score upon initial evaluation and during subsequent follow-up appointments, as well as during follow-up exams after intervention. The present AUA scoring system is derived from an index of seven questions to which patients respond by providing answers in the form of a numeric value (Table 13-2).[21] When the AUA system is used, symptoms should be classified as mild (0 to 7), moderate (8 to 19), or severe (20 to 35). Originally derived from a more extensive survey to determine the degree of bothersome urinary symptoms experienced by patients with benign prostatic hypertrophy (BPH), the AUA index has demonstrated high internal consistency (Cronbach's alpha = 0.86) and high test-retest

Table 13-1 AJCC Staging of Prostate Cancer

Cancer stage	Clinical/pathologic findings
PRIMARY TUMOR (T)	
TX	Primary tumor cannot be assessed
T0	No evidence of primary tumor
T1	Clinically unapparent tumor neither palpable nor visible by imaging
T1a	Tumor incidental histologic finding in 5% or less of tissue resected
T1b	Tumor incidental histologic finding in more than 5% of tissue resected
T1c	Tumor identified by needle biopsy (e.g., because of elevated PSA)
T2	Tumor confined within the prostate*
T2a	Tumor involves one-half of one lobe or less
T2b	Tumor involves more than one-half of one lobe but not both lobes
T2c	Tumor involves both lobes
T3	Tumor extends through the prostatic capsule†
T3a	Extracapsular extension (unilateral or bilateral)
T3b	Tumor invades the seminal vesicle(s)
T4	Tumor is fixed or invades adjacent structures other than seminal vesicles; bladder neck, external sphincter, rectum, levator muscles, and/or pelvic wall

*NOTE: Tumor found in one or both lobes by needle biopsy, but not palpable or reliably visible by imaging, is classified as T1c.
†NOTE: Invasion into the prostatic apex or into (but not beyond) the prostatic capsule is not classified as T3, but as T2.

Cancer stage	Clinical/pathologic findings
PATHOLOGIC (PT)	
pT2*	Organ confined
pT2a	Unilateral, involving one-half of one lobe or less
pT2b	Unilateral, involving more than one-half of one lobe but not both lobes
pT2c	Bilateral disease
pT3	Extraprostatic extension
pT3a	Extraprostatic extension†
pT3b	Seminal vesicle invasion
pT4	Invasion of bladder, rectum

*NOTE: There is no pathologic T1 classification.
†NOTE: Positive surgical margin should be indicated by an R1 descriptor (residual microscopic disease).

Cancer stage	Clinical/pathologic findings
REGIONAL LYMPH NODES (N)	
NX	Regional lymph nodes were not assessed
N0	No regional lymph node metastasis
N1	Metastasis in regional lymph nodes(s)
PNX	Regional lymph nodes not sampled
pN0	No positive regional nodes
pN1	Metastases in regional node(s)
DISTANT METASTASES (M*)	
MX	Distant metastasis cannot be assessed (not evaluated by any modality)
M0	No distant metastasis
M1	Distant metastasis
M1a	Non-regional lymph node(s)
M1b	Bone(s)
M1c	Other site(s) with or without bone disease

*NOTE: When more than one site of metastasis is present, the most advanced category is used. pMIc is most advanced.
Used with the permission of the American Joint Committee on Cancer (AJCC), Chicago, Illinois. The original source for this material is the *AJCC Cancer Staging Handbook, Sixth Edition* (2002), published by Springer-New York, www.springeronline.com.

Table 13-2 American Urological Association Scoring System

Patient name: Date:	Not at all	Less than 1 time in 5	Less than half the time	About half the time	More than half the time	Almost always
1. Over the past month, how often have you had a sensation of not emptying your bladder completely after you finished urinating?	0	1	2	3	4	5
2. Over the past month, how often have you had to urinate again less than 2 hours after you finished urinating?	0	1	2	3	4	5
3. Over the past month, how often have you found you stopped and started again several times when you urinate?	0	1	2	3	4	5
4. Over the past month, how often have you found it difficult to postpone urination?	0	1	2	3	4	5
5. Over the past month, how often have you had a weak urinary stream?	0	1	2	3	4	5
6. Over the past month, how often have you had to push or strain to begin urinating?	0	1	2	3	4	5
	None	1 time	2 times	3 times	4 times	5 times
7. Over the past month, how many times did you most typically get up to urinate from the time you went to bed at night until the time you got up in the morning?	0	1	2	3	4	5
Sum of seven circled numbers:						
		Scoring	Mild:	0-7		
			Moderate:	8-19		
			Severe:	20-35		

Data from the American Urological Association website, www.urologyhealth.org. Accessed 1/4/07.

reliability ($r = 0.92$).[22] It is believed that patients with a higher pretreatment AUA score, may have a higher degree of urinary morbidity secondary to radiation/intervention.

Actually few, if any, symptoms may be present during a physical examination in early-stage prostate cancer. If a patient presents with advanced disease, however, symptoms such as bowel or bladder incontinence, motor weakness, hematospermia, peripheral neuropathy, or leg edema may be present.[23,24] One important aspect of the physical examination is the DRE. The American Cancer Society (ACS) recommends yearly DREs along with serum prostate-specific antigen (PSA) levels yearly beginning at age 50, to men who have at least a 10-year life expectancy. Men at high risk should begin screening at age 45. Men at even higher risk could begin screening at age 40. Depending on results of the initial screening, men in their early 40s may require no further testing until age 45.[25]

An irregular DRE reflective of asymmetry, induration, or firmness should warrant further work-up including serum PSA level and biopsy. A serum PSA level, usually obtained before biopsy, is helpful in the patient's initial assessment. PSA levels are also monitored at predetermined intervals to determine the overall effectiveness of a particular treatment. PSA levels are often indicative of the extent of disease a patient may have.[26] However, not all prostate cancers produce PSA. In these cases, diagnostic imaging studies such as a magnetic resonance imaging (MRI), computed tomography (CT) scans, bone scan, or prostascint scan may be necessary to determine extent of disease. Further, several other factors exist that can cause changes in serum total PSA levels (Table 13-3).[27]

Table 13-3 Factors That Can Alter Serum Total PSA Level

Factors	Elevates PSA level	Depresses PSA level
Benign prostatic hypertrophy	X	
Prostate cancer	X	
Prostatitis	X	
Physical manipulations of the prostate gland	X	
Urine retention	X	
Ejaculation	X	
Pelvic trauma	X	
Prostatic needle biopsy	X	
Prostate volume	X	
African-American race	X	
Relief of urine retention		X
Finasteride		X

PSA, Prostate-specific antigen.

Patients with a normal DRE and a slightly elevated PSA have historically presented a unique challenge to clinicians. Most of the present literature supports a normal total PSA range of 0 to 4.0 ng/mL regardless of age. Although some consideration has been given to age-specific PSA ranges. In 1994, a major prospective study, along with other subsequent studies, has confirmed that a PSA threshold of 4.0 ng/mL is associated with optimal sensitivity and specificity for the detection of prostate cancer.[28] Thus a PSA level of 4.0 ng/mL has long been recognized as the lower limit for biopsy consideration. This is assuming the patient presents with a normal DRE and is otherwise asymptomatic.

When used to evaluate prostate cancer, MRIs are helpful in evaluating nodal involvement in the inguinal, abdominal, and pelvic areas. CT scans also may be helpful in obtaining similar information. Some clinicians may perform a cystogram to visually inspect the urinary bladder for involvement. A bone scan may be obtained to evaluate the potential for metastatic prostate cancer to the skeletal system. Such scans are usually negative when the PSA level is less than 20[29] but may be indicated when the Gleason score is greater than 7 or the patient voices complaints of new or significant bone pain.[30] Transrectal ultrasound may be helpful in evaluating the extent of localized disease.[31] A prostascint scan is the use of a radiolabeled monoclonal antibody directed against the glycoprotein prostate-specific membrane antigen (PSMA). The use of this tool is somewhat controversial, and studies seem to indicate its effectiveness is limited to patients with localized disease.[32] Current use of positron emission tomography (PET) scans in prostate cancer is limited because prostate cancer cells are typically slow growing and do not readily uptake the ^{18}F-fluorodeoxyglucose (FDG) tracer used in this exam.

The ultimate diagnostic exam is an actual prostate biopsy. An ultrasound-guided needle biopsy of the prostate gland is considered minimally invasive and is often performed in the physician's office. It is customary to obtain multiple core biopsies from each zone and from each side of the gland. Pathologic confirmation of malignancy is necessary before proceeding with any type of treatment plan.

Treatment

Improved treatment and overall management of localized prostate cancer has lead to cure rates of over 70%.[33] Unlike many neoplasms, a number of treatment options are available to patients diagnosed with prostate cancer. Issues such as general anesthesia, overall surgical risk, impotency, incontinence, self-esteem, and bowel and bladder injury are often considered by patients when choosing a treatment modality. In addition, clinicians must consider the patient's expected survival, comorbid conditions, tumor staging and pathologic features, PSA levels, potential side effects, and the patient's treatment preference.[34]

Watchful Waiting

The incidence rate of prostate cancer significantly exceeds the death rate from the disease. Thus more men die with prostate cancer but not as a direct result of the neoplasm itself. In addition, because of the slow-growing nature of most prostate tumors and associated side effects of more invasive therapy, watchful waiting is a viable option for some men with early-stage disease. In terms of overall survival, patients who present with T1 to T2 disease do not significantly benefit by having a radical prostatectomy versus watchful waiting.[35]

Watchful waiting, also known as *observation, expectant management*, and *surveillance therapy*, is defined as initial surveillance followed by active treatment when tumor progression results in bothersome side effects. Watchful waiting should not imply deferred care or ignoring the patient. Integral components of this treatment option include regularly scheduled DREs and PSA testing. However, no firm standard of care exists for the management of patients undergoing watchful waiting. Clinicians often follow personal ideals of best practice and use subjective clinical judgement.[36,37]

Treatment is usually initiated after watchful waiting when the patient decides to execute a more aggressive treatment option, side effects of the disease become bothersome, or in some cases, PSA doubling time and stage/disease progression become apparent. The amount of time a patient can remain on a watchful waiting regimen varies widely. It is important that these patients be followed regularly and be supported in their decision to use watchful waiting. In addition to clinical indicators of disease progression, the patient's quality of life and increased side effects during watchful waiting must be considered when deciding to discontinue this treatment option. Patients require educational and psychosocial support before pursuing watchful waiting and during the time they are actively on watchful waiting.[38]

Hormone Therapy

Androgen deprivation therapy (ADT) has been the cornerstone of systemic treatment for patients with locally advanced or metastatic prostate cancer since the 1940s. Essentially, three different prostate cell populations are consistently found in the prostate gland: androgen-dependent, androgen-sensitive, and androgen-independent cells. Hormone therapy is aimed at reducing the level of circulating androgens to castration levels, resulting in death of androgen-dependent cells and growth suppression of androgen-sensitive cells.[11] This usually results in a significant reduction of tumor size and, subsequently, overall prostate volume. Therapeutic approaches that interrupt the actions of testosterone include bilateral orchiectomy, suppression of luteinizing hormone-releasing hormone (LHRH) by the pituitary gland, inhibiting 5-alpha reductase conversion of testosterone to dihydrotestosterone (DHT) in the prostate, and blocking binding of DHT to androgen receptors in the prostate. These strategies may be employed individually or in combination.[39]

Bilateral orchiectomy is the oldest method of inducing androgen blockade. By removing the testicular source of androgen production, approximately 90% of circulating testosterone is eliminated and serum testosterone levels remain low thereafter. Side effects associated with orchiectomy include hot flashes, decreased libido, erectile dysfunction, fatigue, osteoporosis, weight gain, decreased muscle mass, anemia, and a decline in cognitive function.[40]

The administration of LHRH agonists is effective at achieving significant reduction in testosterone levels, essentially causing a medically induced castration. The initial response to most LHRH agonists causes a "flare" of testosterone production, which may exacerbate symptoms in patients within weeks of initiating therapy. Pain and bladder outlet problems are typically seen during a flare reaction. Patients should be notified of this potential, and such symptoms may require prompt medical intervention.[11,40] A list of presently available LHRH agonists along with dosing schedules is shown in Table 13-4.[40]

In order to eliminate the flare caused by LHRH agonists, antiandrogens may be administered. Studies have shown that antiandrogens minimize symptoms associated with the early testosterone surge.[41-43] The use of antiandrogen agents with LHRH agonists beyond the flare period has been evaluated only in patients with metastatic prostate cancer, showing some improvement in overall survival.[41,44-46] It is unclear whether this extended combined approach is beneficial to patients who present with early-stage disease. Table 13-5 lists the available nonsteroidal antiandrogens and their dosing schedules.[39]

Some clinicians have employed an approach known as *intermittent ADT* in an attempt to improve the efficacy of LHRH agonists. This approach also provides patients with a therapeutic break allowing for a temporary reduction in side effects. By periodically stopping treatment, the suppressed androgen-dependent cells are allowed to

Table 13-4 LHRH Agonists and Dosing Schedules

Agent	Form	Dosage schedule
Leuprolide	Eligard	7.5 mg IM q 1 month
	Lupron depot	22.5 mg IM q 3 months
		30 mg IM q 4 months
		7.5 mg IM q 1 month
	Lupron injection	22.5 mg IM q 3 months
	Viadur implant	30 mg IM q 4 months
		1 mg SQ qd
		65 mg SQ q 12 months
Goserelin	Zoladex	3.6 mg SQ q 28 days (abdominal wall)
		10.8 mg SQ q 3 months
Triptorelin	Trelstar depot	3.75 mg IM q 1 month
	Trelstar LA	11.25 mg IM q 3 months
Abarelix	Plenaxis	100 mg IM on days 1, 15, 29, and every 4 weeks thereafter

Data from Gleave ME, Small EJ: *Androgen deprivation for prostate cancer. Report to the Nation on prostate cancer 2004.* Medscape (website): www.medscape.com/viewprogram/3440_pnt. Accessed November 6, 2005.

Table 13-5 Nonsteroidal Antiandrogens and Dosing Schedules

Agent	Form	Dosage schedule
Bicalutamide	Casodex	50 mg PO once daily
Flutamide	Eulexin	250 mg PO every 8 hours
Nilutamide	Nilandron	300 mg PO once daily for 30 days then 150 mg PO daily

Adapted with permission from Gleave ME, Small EJ. *Androgen deprivation for prostate cancer.* In: Carroll PR, Nelson WG, eds. *Report to the Nation on Prostate Cancer; 2004.* Santa Monica, Calif: Prostate Cancer Foundation; 2004. Chapter 3. Retrieved on 11/06/2005 from www.medscape.com/prostatecancer. © Prostate Cancer Foundation.

repopulate. Thus the time period to androgen independence is prolonged.[47] Patients remain on LHRH agonist monotherapy for 6 to 12 months until a low PSA level is maintained, at which time treatment is stopped. As serum PSA levels rise, growth of androgen-dependent cells resume. Hormone therapy is resumed when PSA levels rise to 4 to 10 ng/mL or to 50% of the initial PSA level.[48] Currently clinical trials are underway comparing the efficacy of intermittent ADT versus continuous ADT.[49,50]

The use of ADT prior to and during other forms of treatment has been examined. Neoadjuvant ADT for 3 months before prostatectomy was shown to decrease the rate of positive surgical margins but showed no long-term benefit in biochemical recurrence rates.[51] However, ADT used with primary radiation therapy does provide a benefit.[52,53] The use of neoadjuvant ADT in patients undergoing primary radiation therapy has shown mixed results.[54,55]

Patients receiving hormonal therapy will show beneficial results 70% to 80% of the time, with responses lasting anywhere from several months to several years.[56] Disease progression is traditionally managed by second-line hormonal manipulation or palliative radiation therapy.

The side effects of long-term hormonal manipulation are similar to those in patients who undergo surgical castration. Of recent concern is osteoporosis in men on ADT.[57,58] Bone mineral density studies obtained at baseline and at periodic intervals are helpful in evaluating the overall effect of ADT on these patients. Along with dietary counseling, the administration of bisphosphonates has been shown to reduce skeletal-related events in patients with metastatic prostate cancer.[59] No evidence exists to indicate whether bisphosphonates can prevent osteoporosis or bone metastasis.

The optional use and timing of ADT in the treatment of prostate cancer continues to evolve. Hormonal therapy offers patients improved outcomes in various adjuvant settings and slows progression of metastatic disease. Ongoing clinical trials will hopefully yield additional information on the optional use of hormone therapy for patients with prostate cancer.

Chemotherapy

Historically, chemotherapy has demonstrated little success in improving overall cure rates in prostate cancer. Patients who benefit from systemic chemotherapy include those who become hormone refractory. Despite an initial response to ADT, most patients with advanced prostate neoplasms experience disease progression, and most become refractory to hormone manipulation within 18 to 24 months. When this occurs, median survival time ranges between 12 and 16 months.[60]

Chemotherapy in this setting is not curative. Only recently have certain agents, and combination of agents, been shown to prolong life. When initiating chemotherapy, it is generally understood that its use is for palliation with endpoint goals being a slowing of disease progression, as evidenced by PSA values and bone scan studies, or decreased levels of pain and improved quality of life.

In 1996, Tannock and colleagues[61] demonstrated significant palliative responses in patients with advanced prostate cancer who received mitoxantrone 12 mg/m^2 every 3 weeks plus prednisone 5 mg twice daily over patients who received only prednisone 10 mg daily. Kantoff and colleagues[62] yielded similar results using mitoxantrone 14 mg/m^2 every 3 weeks and 10 mg of hydrocortisone twice daily over those who received hydrocortisone 30 mg in the morning and 10 mg in the afternoon. These studies established chemotherapy as a viable option for palliative treatment in patients with hormone-refractory prostate cancer.

More recently, docetaxel-based chemotherapy has proven effective when used with estramustine over subjects who received mitoxantrone and prednisone.[63] A 20% reduction in risk of death was noted among patients treated with docetaxel/estramustine. This group also yielded a superior median time to disease progression and significantly lower post-therapy PSA levels. Docetaxel, in combination with agents such as calcitriol, thalidomide, bevacizumab, and ixabepilone is in various stages of clinical trials.[64-68]

Most patients with localized prostate cancer are adequately treated with conventional modalities such as radical prostatectomy or radiation therapy. However, a small subset of patients do fail hormonal and conventional therapies. Trials are underway to examine the proper sequencing and initial administration of chemotherapy for the treatment of prostate cancer. Because of the recent success of docetaxel-based agents, the role of chemotherapy in this setting is being reexamined and exists as a viable option for advanced cases of the disease.

Surgery

Surgical removal of the prostate gland has long been a mainstay in the treatment of prostate cancer. The surgical techniques used in radical prostatectomy continue to evolve as technological advances are introduced and refined.[69] Radical prostatectomy involves the removal of the entire prostate, prostate capsule, seminal vesicles, and a portion of the bladder neck. Radical prostatectomy has traditionally been performed by way of a retropubic or perineal surgical approach. The approach used is usually dependent on surgeon preference and expertise.

A nerve-sparing surgical technique may be used, but its success is highly dependent on patient selection. Recovery of sexual function depends on age, preoperative sexual function, stage of disease, and whether unilateral or bilateral nerve presentation exists. Bilateral nerve-sparing potency rates have ranged from 31% to 76%. Unilateral nerve-sparing potency rates have ranged between 13% and 56%.[70,71]

In recent years, laparoscopic radical prostatectomy (LRP), either by transperitoneal or extraperitoneal approach, has gained increased attention. Continence and potency rates have varied compared to nonlaparoscopic radical prostatectomy, although shorter hospital stays, lower rates of margin positivity, and decrease in operative blood loss have been reported.[72,73] The surgeon's level of experience with LRP is a significant limitation in this approach, because a steep learning curve for procedural skill exists.[69]

As with most of the treatment modalities available for prostate cancer, patient selection is very important when considering radical prostatectomy. Generally, men with localized disease (T1 to T2, PSA less than 10 ng/mL, and Gleason score less than 7) who are age 70 or younger with few or no comorbidities and a life expectancy of 10 to 20 years are considered for radical prostatectomy. Patients who undergo radical prostatectomy are considered cured if there are no signs and symptoms of recurrence 5 years after surgery. Patients with recurrence after surgery may undergo further treatment at some point in the future.

Another surgical technique, cryoablation, or cryosurgery, of the prostate gland has been used since the 1960s. Recent improvements in surgical instrumentation and transrectal ultrasonography have made this a viable option for some men with prostate cancer. Probes that are inserted into the prostate and the prostatic capsule, deliver a gaseous substance that freezes the tissue in an attempt to kill cancer cells. The freezing is typically done over two cycles to optimize tumor cell kill. Cryoablation is being used to treat clinically localized prostate cancer (T1 to T3), as salvage therapy for local failures of primary treatment, and to debulk large primary tumors.[74,75]

Radiation Therapy

The use of radiation therapy has long been a standard treatment modality for patients with prostate cancer. Radiation is typically administered via linear accelerator or via brachytherapy. A combination approach using both modalities is available to a subset of patients. Radiation for prostate cancer has several advantages over radical prostatectomy.[76] Bleeding, transfusion-related events, and risks associated with anesthesia are avoided with external beam radiation therapy (EBRT). Further, radiation therapy offers a low risk of urinary incontinence and stricture formation. Additionally, radiation offers short-term preservation of erectile function, especially with the use of CT-based treatment planning.

Disadvantages of EBRT include prolonged treatment course, usually 7 to 8 weeks; temporary bowel and bladder morbidity; and lastly, the risk of developing erectile dysfunction increases over time. In the event of recurrence, surgical intervention following EBRT is associated with significant complication rates. Most radiation oncologists consider the following to be contraindications for radiation therapy in prostate cancer: prior pelvic irradiation, active inflammatory disease of the bowel or rectum, permanent indwelling urinary catheter, and morbid obesity. Other considerations when deciding on the appropriateness of radiation are the existence of chronic diarrhea, urinary bladder outlet obstruction, and inactive ulcerative colitis.

Variation exists within both academic and community hospital centers as to the treatment technique and dosage range used to treat prostate cancer. The National Comprehensive Cancer Network (NCCN) has established practice guidelines so as to standardize treatment as much as possible (Table 13-6).[77]

Earlier EBRT treatment techniques for prostate cancer were rather simplistic and employed a four-field "box technique" that essentially treated a square- or rectangular-shaped field that encompassed the majority of the pelvis. Beam-blocking techniques were limited, and patients were treated by way of anterior/posterior (AP) and posterior/anterior (PA) fields. Morbidity rates associated with these treatment techniques were high. The use of box-field techniques for prostate cancer still exists. However, CT-guided imagery has greatly enhanced and improved treatment techniques and resulted in more complex treatment plans for prostate cancer. CT scans should be used if the patient is to receive radiation to nearby lymph nodes. A four-field box technique with lateral portals can be used if lymph nodes are to be treated. Using this approach, a typical treatment field consists of the upper border at midsacral level and the lower border determined by the inferior-most aspect of the prostate. The lateral margins of the inferior field are 1.5 to 2.0 cm from the lateral pelvic wall. For the lateral field, the anterior margin is 1 cm posterior to the projection of the anterior cortex of the pubic symphysis. The posterior border is generally at the posterior ischium, and the posterior rectum should be appropriately shielded. Barium can be used to define the rectum, urethra, or urinary bladder.[78]

Recent advances in computer software and diagnostic imaging capabilities have allowed the introduction of three dimensional (3-D) conformal radiation therapy and intensity-modulated radiation therapy (IMRT). CT images are necessary for 3-D treatment planning in which multiple beams are used to help decrease the dose to any nearby organs while maximizing tumor dose. Such images allow for a clear delineation of prostatic tissue, thereby reducing the volume of normal tissue in the treatment field. It is theorized that lower radiation doses to normal tissue may result in fewer bowel- and bladder-related side effects.

In 3-D and IMRT treatment planning, computer software enables the planning CT to be reconstructed in three dimensions. The prostate, seminal vesicles, and other surrounding tissues can be anatomically defined and outlined on each CT slice. Treatment margins are usually dependent on prescribed dose, setup, and internal organ motion.

Table 13-6 NCCN Practice Guidelines for Prostate Cancer

Treatment modality	Description and guidelines
EXTERNAL BEAM RADIOTHERAPY	• 3-D conformal or IMRT techniques should be employed. • Doses of 70 Gy to 75 Gy in 35–41 fractions to the prostate (± seminal vesicles for part of the therapy) appear to be appropriate for patients with low-risk cancers. For patients with intermediate- or high-risk disease, doses between 75 Gy and 80 Gy appear to provide improved PSA-assessed disease control. • Patients with high-risk cancers are candidates for pelvic lymph node irradiation and the addition of neoadjuvant ± adjuvant androgen deprivation therapy for a total of 2–3 y or 4–6 mo if they have only a single high risk adverse factor. • Patients with intermediate risk cancer may be considered for pelvic lymph node irradiation and 4–6 mo neoadjuvant ± adjuvant ADT. • Patients with low risk cancer should not receive pelvic lymph node irradiation or ADT. • If target (PTV) margins are reduced, such as for doses above 75 Gy, extra attention to daily prostate localization, with techniques such as ultrasound, implanted fiducials, or an endorectal balloon, is indicated.
BRACHYTHERAPY	• Permanent brachytherapy as monotherapy is indicated for patients with low-risk cancers. For intermediate-risk cancers, consider combining brachytherapy with EBRT (40 Gy to 50 Gy) ± neoadjuvant androgen deprivation therapy. Patients with high-risk cancers are generally considered poor candidates for permanent brachytherapy; however, with the addition of EBRT and androgen deprivation therapy, it may be effective in select patients. • Patients with a large prostate (> 60 m) or small prostate (< 15–20 gm), symptoms of bladder outlet obstruction (IPSS score > 15), or a previous transurethral resection of the prostate (TURP) are not appropriate candidates because of increased risk of urinary morbidity. Neoadjuvant androgen deprivation therapy may be used to shrink the prostate to an acceptable size. • Post-implant dosimetry should be performed to document the quality of the implant. • The recommended prescribed doses for monotherapy are 145 Gy for 125-Iodine and 125 Gy for 103-Palladium. The corresponding boost doses after 40 Gy to 50 Gy EBRT are 110 Gy and 100 Gy, respectively.

From National Comprehensive Cancer Network (NCCN): NCCN Clinical Practice Guidelines in Oncology: Prostate Cancer v. 2 2005, www.nccn.org/professionals/physician_gls/PDF/prostate.pdf. Accessed February 5, 2007.

NCCN, National Comprehensive Cancer Network; *IMRT,* intensity-modulated radiotherapy; *PSA,* prostate-specific antigen; *PTV,* planning target volume; *ERBT,* external beam radiation therapy; *IPSS,* International Prostate Symptom Score; *TURP,* transurethral resection of the prostate.

Attempts to control setup and organ motion are done through external immobilization devices and the use of implanted fiducial markers, rectal balloons, or transabdominal ultrasound. Margins on the clinical target volume usually range from 0.75 to 1.5 cm for standard conformal techniques and doses in the 70-Gy to 72-Gy range. The use of specialized treatment techniques, such as IMRT and transabdominal ultrasound, allow a decrease in margin size to .5 cm to 1.0 cm.

In this setting, a common treatment plan will consist of a right and left lateral pair and two parallel-opposed oblique pairs 45 degrees from the lateral pair angles. An anterior beam may be used, usually for the purpose of portal imaging. This may be referred to as a *seven-field arrangement.* If lymph nodes are to be treated, a four-field box technique followed by a six-field technique may be combined. Beam shaping, so as to conform to tumor or normal tissue borders, is achieved through the use of cerrobend blocks or multileaf collimator (MLC) settings. Pelvic lymph node dose is approximately 50 Gy with 54 Gy to 56 Gy directed to the seminal vesicles. Prostate doses can range between 70 Gy and 80 Gy.[78,79]

IMRT is a more advanced treatment technique and often considered a form of 3-D conformal radiation therapy. IMRT allows for the specification of the prescribed dose to the tumor volume as well as acceptable dose levels for surrounding structures inclusive of the rectum, urethra, urinary bladder, and femoral heads. IMRT also allows for variance in the intensity of the radiation beam across the target area. Up to 10 or more beam angles can be used in IMRT treatments. During beam delivery, MLC settings can continually change, thus shielding critical structures a portion of the time and treating the tumor to a higher dose than surrounding organs that may have a lower tolerance for radiation. IMRT allows radiation therapy doses in the 85 Gy or more range to be delivered. Dose volume histograms must be closely analyzed to determine the volume of critical organs receiving high doses of radiation. Researchers have found that patients treated with IMRT, when compared to those treated with conventional or 3-D radiation, have demonstrated increased disease-free survival (8- to 12-year follow-up) and also experienced an 80% decrease in overall toxicity score.[79,80]

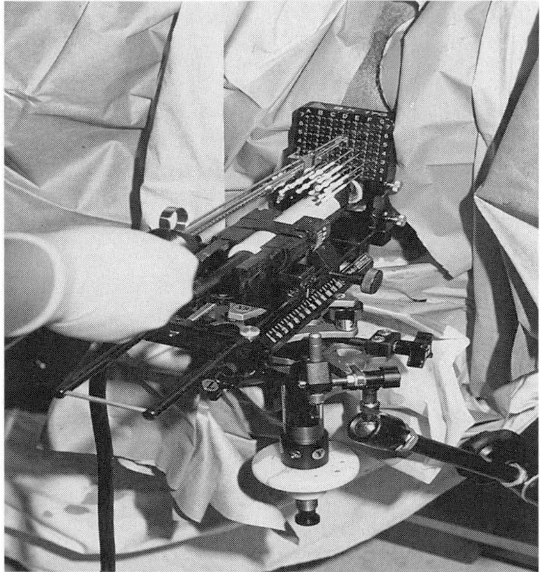

Figure 13-1 Low-dose-rate Permanent Prostate Brachytherapy. Low-dose-rate permanent prostate brachytherapy needles inserted through perineal template just above transrectal ultrasound.
Courtesy of Alex Chen, MD, UPMC Cancer Centers, Pittsburgh, Pa.

Brachytherapy

Prostate brachytherapy has evolved over the past century from crudely placed radium sources placed through a urinary catheter; to the placement of needles into the prostate by a "free-hand" method using gold and iodine seeds; to the present day use of transrectal ultrasound and perineal template that assists in multiple needle placement directly into the gland. Because of its relatively low cost, patient convenience, and short recovery time, prostate brachytherapy is a widely used modality for treatment of early-stage prostate cancer.

Prostate brachytherapy can be used as monotherapy for patients with low-risk disease (T1 to T2, Gleason score 6 or less, PSA level less than 10 ng/mL) or in combination with external beam radiation for patients with moderate- to high-risk disease (advanced T2 or greater lesions, Gleason score 7 or above, PSA level above 10 ng/mL).

The radioactive sources used most often in permanent prostate brachytherapy, also known as low dose rate (LDR) are iodine-125 (^{125}I) and palladium-103 (^{103}Pd). Although no clinical data exists that demonstrate an advantage of one permanent source over another, differences in half-life and dose rate suggest ^{125}I is better suited for slow-growing, low-grade tumors, whereas ^{103}Pd may be better suited for high-grade disease. The half-life of ^{125}I is 60 days, and ^{103}Pd has a half-life of 17 days. Limited long-term data examining biochemical relapse-free survival rates for patients who receive brachytherapy as primary treatment has yielded 85% to 94% for low-risk disease, 77% to 84% for intermediate disease, and 45% to 54% for high-risk disease.[81-84]

Placement of the radioactive source is performed in the operating room under general or spinal anesthesia. The patient is placed in a dorsal lithotomy position and a grid or template is placed against the perineum. A transrectal ultrasound probe is inserted into the rectum to allow visualization of needle placement on a video monitor. Brachytherapy needles are placed through the template and into the prostate gland (Figure 13-1). The needles are either preloaded or attached to a Mick applicator that deposits the radioactive seeds into the gland. Dosimetry planning, done either at the time of implant or days to weeks before, dictates the exact placement of the seeds. Typically, seeds are distributed throughout the prostate, approximately 1 cm apart. Total number of seeds inserted depends on overall prostate volume. In general, the number ranges between 80 and 100. The usual prescribed dose for implant alone with ^{125}I is 145 Gy and ^{103}Pd is 125 Gy.[77,79,85]

In patients with higher-grade prostate tumors, brachytherapy alone is not sufficient to deliver a high enough total dose to the prostate and surrounding tissues. Higher-grade tumors require a higher total dose. Combining EBRT and brachytherapy offers an effective approach for patients with high-grade disease. Various combinations of EBRT and brachytherapy are used. When receiving combined treatment, the patient generally receives 45 Gy to 50 Gy of EBRT to the prostate gland followed by a low-dose boost of 90 Gy if using ^{103}Pd and 110 Gy if using ^{125}I. There is no clinical evidence to support the use of EBRT before or after seed implant nor is there evidence supporting the use of ^{125}I over ^{103}Pd in this setting. Further, EBRT following permanent seed implant has not been shown to significantly increase overall morbidity versus EBRT alone.[79]

An iridium isotope is used for high dose rate (HDR) prostate brachytherapy treatments. This modality also can be administered as primary treatment or in combination with EBRT. Similar to permanent seed implantation, needles are placed into the prostate gland under anesthesia and with the use of ultrasound-guided imagery. Either the needles or plastic catheters are left behind to act as a vessel for the iridium source (Figure 13-2). After CT-based treatment planning, several high-dose fractions ranging from 4 Gy to 6 Gy are administered over an interval of 24 to 36 hours. The radioactive source is then removed. This modality may be followed by EBRT to a dose of 45 Gy to 50.4 Gy. Some clinicians have performed prostate HDR treatments throughout the course of EBRT and have examined the efficacy of dose escalation per fraction of HDR treatments. Improved outcomes were observed compared with outcomes using lower dose levels.[86,87]

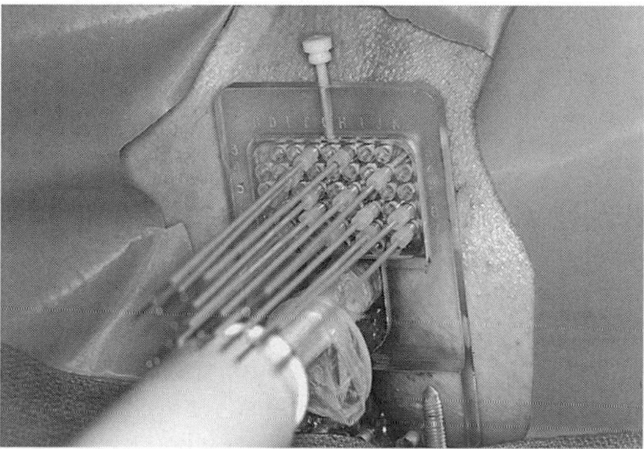

Figure 13-2 High-dose-rate Brachytherapy. High-dose-rate brachytherapy catheters placed through perineal template just above transrectal ultrasound. *Courtesy of Mountain Radiation Oncology, Asheville, N.C.*

The decision to use HDR or LDR ultimately rests with the physician. Training and personal preference are factors that often determine physician choice of one type of brachytherapy over another. Some argue that an HDR after-loading approach allows for the limiting of underdosed areas within the gland. Another consideration is decreased exposure to clinicians with the use of HDR. HDR also offers a higher rate of tumor cell kill, which can be advantageous in patients with bulky tumors or adverse prognostic features.[79]

Side Effects of Radiation and Nursing Interventions

As in other sites, side effects of radiation therapy to the prostate can be categorized into acute and late toxicities. Acute toxicities are considered to be those that occur within 90 days from the initiation of treatment. Late or delayed effects are considered to occur after 90 days and may occur years after treatment. Side effects are site specific and are related to total dose, treatment field, and individual tolerance. Radiation-induced side effects are similar, be they from EBRT or brachytherapy. The major difference is that patients who undergo brachytherapy may develop a more rapid onset of side effects and have additional side effects related to anesthesia or surgical intervention.

Skin Effects and Edema

Skin tolerance to radiation is dose dependent, and morbidity results from a loss of cells in the epidermis, dermis, and microvascular endothelium.[88] Skin reactions such as erythema, pain, or dry or moist desquamation may develop in the perineum, groin, or intragluteal folds. Reactions in these areas are intensified when skin folds are in the treatment area, because of the uneven radiation dose distribution.[89] For pathophysiology of erythema and desquamation and specific nursing interventions for these effects, see Chapter 30.

Edema of the leg, scrotum, and penis can occur but is rare in patients treated with radiation alone. It is more often associated with prior lymphadenectomy and is not seen with brachytherapy or small fields of EBRT.

Urinary Effects

Genitourinary symptoms such as dysuria, nocturia, urgency, frequency, hesitancy, and outlet obstruction are not uncommon during EBRT or immediately after brachytherapy. These symptoms can continue to be problematic for some patients well after 90 days from treatment. Radiation causes edema, irritation, inflammation, and vascular changes of the urinary bladder, urothelium, vasculature, and smooth muscle. Reduced bladder capacity may result from functional and anatomic changes caused by vascular damage with fibroblast and collagen deposits in the bladder's smooth muscle. These changes can lead to the previously described urinary side effects.[89] If the bladder remains inflamed, hematuria, be it microscopic or gross in nature, can occur for months to years after treatment.

Though rare, urinary infection must be ruled out when symptoms begin to be problematic. Noninfectious cystitis can be mild and intermittent and usually presents itself after 3 to 5 weeks of EBRT.[90] Patients with enlarged prostates are at increased risk for outlet obstruction symptoms because of edema of the gland, which can occur at any point throughout treatment.[91] For incidence rates of urinary symptoms for conventional, 3-D conformal, and IMRT, see Table 13-7.

Evidence-based nursing interventions for the relief of urinary symptoms in patients undergoing radiation are limited. Table 13-8 lists interventions for both acute and late effects of treatment. For most patients, urinary symptoms subside 2 to 8 weeks after treatment completion.

Bowel Effects

Bowel-related morbidity is one of the most common acute manifestations of radiation therapy to the abdomen and pelvis. For a detailed description of the pathophysiology and nursing interventions for the management of diarrhea secondary to radiation therapy, see Chapter 34. Table 13-9 lists incidence rates of bowel toxicity using 3-D conformal and IMRT treatment techniques.

In addition to diarrhea, proctitis can occur during or after radiation therapy secondary to the radiation itself or from increased bowel movements/diarrhea. See Table 13-10 for medication commonly administered for the management of proctitis and other interventions to try if medications are not effective. Additionally, proctitis and rectal discomfort may be alleviated by warm sitz baths several times a day.[92] In some cases, consultation with a gastroenterologist/proctologist may become necessary. Laser treatments may be indicated to cauterize bleeding vessels within the rectum, or the instillation of formalin may be applied for patients experiencing chronic hemorrhagic proctitis.[93,94]

Sexual Dysfunction

Rates of impotence among this patient population have a wide degree of variance, ranging from 6% to 84%.[95] A recent review by Inrocci and colleagues[95] details potency rates for patients who underwent EBRT and brachytherapy (Table 13-11). Specific pathophysiology and management of sexual dysfunction as it relates to radiation therapy is discussed in Chapter 35. Though radiation-induced impotence is multifactorial, a high percentage of men who undergo radiation for prostate cancer will experience some degree of impotence at some point after treatment. Erectile dysfunction can significantly affect the quality of life of many patients undergoing radiation therapy for prostate cancer. The administration of sildenafil has shown significant improvement in erectile function.[96] Other phosphodiesterase-5 inhibitors such as tadalafil or vardenafil also may be helpful. Vasoactive agents such as intracavernosal injections and intraurethral suppositories also may provide benefit for patients suffering from erectile dysfunction, as may vacuum devices or penile prosthesis. The long-term effects of erectile dysfunction can be problematic to patients and their sexual partners. The importance of professional counseling regarding the physical and psychologic effects of sexual dysfunction in men with prostate cancer should not be overlooked.[97]

Fatigue

Complaints of mild to moderate fatigue are common during radiation therapy. Studies have suggested that increased levels of fatigue occur as cumulative radiation doses are increased.[98-100] Incidence rates range from 65% to 100% and most often occur during the fourth week of treatment;[101] differences in incidence and severity are affected by age, gender, stage of disease, and functional ability. For most patients, fatigue resolves within 1 month of completing therapy.[91] The underlying mechanism of fatigue in patients who receive radiation therapy is inconclusive; theories include alterations in serum interleukin levels, anemia, decreased nutritional status, and alterations in cytokine and prostaglandin levels.[11,102,103]

Table 13-7 Incidence of Urinary Symptoms for Conventional, 3-D Conformal Treatment, and IMRT

Tumor grade	Criteria	Conventional and 3-D conformal treatment (%)	IMRT (%)
ACUTE			
Grade 0	No change	38–62	33
Grade 1	Frequency of urination or nocturia twice pretreatment habit/dysuria, urgency not requiring medication	53–59	38
Grade 2	Frequency of urination or nocturia that is less than every hour; dysuria, urgency, or bladder spasm requiring local anesthetic	20–23	28–34
Grade 3	Frequency with urination and nocturia hourly or more frequently or dysuria, pelvis pain, or bladder spasm requiring regular/frequent, gross hematuria with or without clot passage	1–3	Less than 0.5
Grade 4	Hematuria requiring transfusion, acute bladder obstruction not secondary to clot passage, ulceration, or necrosis	—	—
LATE			
Grade 0	None		74
Grade 1	Slight epithelial atrophy, minor telangiectasia (microscopic hematuria)	83*	16
Grade 2	Moderate frequency, generalized telangiectasia, intermittent macroscopic hematuria	5–37	9.5
Grade 3	Severe frequency and dysuria, severe generalized telangiectasia (often with petechiae), frequent hematuria, reduction in bladder capacity (< 150 mL)	0.1–2	0.5
Grade 4	Necrosis/contracted bladder, capacity < 100 mL, severe hemorrhagic cystitis	—	
Grade 5	Death related to radiation	—	

Data from:

Chism DB, Horwitz EM, Hanlon AL et al: Late morbidity profiles in prostate cancer patients treated to 79-84 Gy by a simple four-field coplanar beam arrangement. *Int J Radiat Oncol Biol Phys* 55(1):71-77, 2003.

Dearnaley DP, Khoo VS, Norman AR et al: Comparison of radiation side effects of conformal and conventional radiotherapy in prostate cancer: a randomised trial, *Lancet* 353(9149):267-272, 1999.

Michalski JM, Purdy JA, Winter K et al: Preliminary report of toxicity following 3D radiation therapy for prostate cancer on 3DOG/RTOG 9406. *Int J Radiat Oncol Biol Phys* 46(2):391-402, 2000.

Shu HK, Lee TT, Viqneauly E et al: Toxicity following high dose three-dimensional conformal and intensity modulated radiation therapy for clinically localized prostate cancer. *Urology* 57(1):102-107, 2001.

Zelefsky MJ, Cowen D, Fuks Z et al: Long term tolerance of high dose three-dimensional conformal radiotherapy in patients with localized prostate carcinoma, *Cancer* 85(11):2460-2468, 1999.

Zelefsky MJ, Fuks Z, Hunt M et al: High dose intensity modulated radiation therapy for prostate cancer: early toxicity and biochemical outcome in 772 patients. *Int J Radiat Oncol Biol Phys* 53(5):1111-1116, 2002.

Zelefsky MJ, Wallner KE, Ling CC et al: Comparison of the five-year outcome and morbidity of three-dimensional conformal radiotherapy versus transperineal permanent iodine 125 implantation for early stage prostatic cancer. *J Clin Oncol* 17(2): 517-522, 1999.

*Grade 0 and 1 combined.

3-D, Three-dimensional; *IMRT,* intensity-modulated radiotherapy.

Management of fatigue should be directed at the suspected causative agent. Anemia should be treated with iron or folic acid supplementation; administration of human erythropoietin if hemoglobin drops below 10 g/dL,[104] or by way of blood transfusion. Other interventions aimed at supplementing nutritional intake, decreasing sleep disturbance patterns, or treating clinical/subclinical depression may warrant consideration.

Myelosuppression

Myelosuppression can be experienced in varying degrees by patients who receive treatment to the pelvic area for prostate cancer. Approximately 40%

Table 13-8 Nursing Interventions for Urinary Morbidity Secondary to Radiation Therapy

Acute effects	Late effects
Maintain hydration. Drink 1–2 liters during the day. Decrease intake in the evening to minimize nocturia.[1,2] Avoid alcohol and caffeine.[3,4,5] Administer appropriate medication[2]: Ibuprofen Oxybutynin chloride Phenazopyridine Tamsulosin hydrochloride Terazosin hydrochloride Doxazosin mesylate Treatment break may be indicated.	Generally managed by long-term administration of urinary analgesics, antispasmotics, or alpha-1 receptor-blocking agents listed under acute effects. If decreased bladder capacity or urinary outlet obstruction persist, endoscopic evaluation with possible urethral dilation may be indicated.

Data from:

Abel LJ, Blatt HJ, Stipetich RL et al: Nursing management of patients receiving brachytherapy for early stage prostate cancer, *Clin J Oncol Nurs* 3(1):7-15, 1999.

Albertsen PC: Urologic nuisances: How to work up and relieve men's symptoms, *Geriatrics* 52(2):46-50, 1997.

Gray M: Caffeine and urinary continence, *J Wound Ostomy Continence Nurs* 28(2):66-69, 2001.

Hogle WP: Male pelvis. In Bruner DW, Haas ML, Gosselin-Acomb TK, editors: *Manual for radiation oncology nursing practice and education,* ed 3, Pittsburgh, 2005, Oncology Nursing Society, pp 132-141.

Iwamoto RR, Maher KE: Radiation therapy for prostate cancer, *Semin Oncol Nurs* 17(20):90-100, 2001.

of active bone marrow is located within the pelvis. Despite this significant percentage, patients rarely have myelosuppression of significance that requires a treatment break.[102] However, 80% to 90% of patients who receive a combination of radiation and androgen suppression show decreased hemoglobin levels up to 4 g/dL.[105] Aside from monitoring blood work, nurses should inquire as to fatigue levels and presence of dyspnea, chest pain, or parasthesias.[106] These patients may require a treatment break or may benefit from administration of human erythropoietin.[104]

Education

Nursing education for patients undergoing radiation for prostate cancer begins at the initial consultation, continues throughout treatment, and is reinforced during follow-up care. Patients should be instructed in the simulation, treatment planning, and treatment administration processes. During the initial consultation, it may be helpful to take the patient on a tour through the department and introduce the patient to staff members who will be participating in his care. Demonstration of any immobilization devices that will be used during simulation and treatment may be done at this time. The number of treatments to be given, length of time for each treatment, and anticipated side effects should be extensively reviewed with the patient and his significant other. If medications are prescribed during the course of treatment, the side effect profile should be reviewed as well as potential interactions with foods or other concurrently prescribed medications. The purpose of the on-treatment-visit should be explained, and the patient should be encouraged to report any noticeable side effects, regardless of severity.

When instructing the patient, the nurse should consider several factors. These include the patient's readiness to learn; the patient's learning style, which is defined by the way one perceives and processes information; and the patient's literacy level.[107]

Education for patients undergoing prostate brachytherapy is slightly more inclusive. In addition to the teaching points for EBRT, see Table 13-12 for a list of items that should be reviewed with patients who plan to undergo prostate brachytherapy. See Table 13-13 for a list of resources (pamphlets, books, and Internet sites) available to patients seeking more information about prostate cancer and the existing treatment options.

CANCER OF THE PENIS AND MALE URETHRA

Carcinoma of the penis is very rare in the United States. An estimated 1530 cases of penile and other male genital cancer (exclusive of testicular and

Table 13-9 Incidence of Bowel Toxicity Using 3-D Conformal Treatment and IMRT

Tumor grade	Criteria	Conventional and 3-D conformal treatment (%)	IMRT (%)
ACUTE			
Grade 0	No change	45–62	—
Grade 1	Increased frequency or change in quality of bowel habits not requiring medication Rectal discomfort not requiring medication	21–31	—
Grade 2	Diarrhea requiring parasympatholytic drugs, mucinous discharge not necessitating sanitary pads Rectal or abdominal pain requiring analgesics	16–24	4.5
Grade 3	Diarrhea requiring parenteral support Severe mucous or bloody discharge necessitating sanitary pads Abdominal distention (flat plate yields distended bowel loops)	0–1	0
Grade 4	Acute or subacute obstruction, fistula, or perforation; GI bleeding requiring transfusion Abdominal pain or tenesmus requiring tube decompression or bowel diversion	0	0
LATE			
Grade 0	None		—
Grade 1	Mild diarrhea, mild abdominal cramping, bowel movement 5 times daily, slight rectal discharge or bleeding	90*	—
Grade 2	Moderate diarrhea and colic bowel movement more than 5 times daily Excessive rectal mucus or intermittent bleeding	9–14	1.5
Grade 3	Obstruction or bleeding requiring surgery	0.75–3	0.1
Grade 4	Necrosis/perforation/fistula	0	0

Data from:

Chism DB, Horwitz EM, Hanlon AL et al: Late morbidity profiles in prostate cancer patients treated to 79-84 Gy by a simple four-field coplanar beam arrangement, *Int J Radiat Oncol Biol Phys* 55(1):71-77, 2003.

Michalski JM, Purdy JA, Winter K et al: Preliminary report of toxicity following 3D radiation therapy for prostate cancer on 3DOG/RTOG 9406, *Int J Radiat Oncol Biol Phys* 46(2):391-402, 2000.

Zelefsky MJ, Cowen D, Fuks Z et al: Long term tolerance of high dose three-dimensional conformal radiotherapy in patients with localized prostate carcinoma, *Cancer* 85(11):2460-2468, 1999.

Zelefsky MJ, Wallner KE, Ling CC et al: Comparison of the five-year outcome and morbidity of three-dimensional conformal radiotherapy versus transperineal permanent iodine 125 implantation for early stage prostatic cancer, *J Clin Oncol* 17(2): 517-522, 1999.

Zelefsky MJ et al: High dose intensity modulated radiation therapy for prostate cancer: Early toxicity and biochemical outcome in 772 patients, *Int J Radiat Oncol Biol Phys* 53(5):1111-1116, 2002.

*Grade 0 and 1 combined.

3-D, Three-dimensional; *IMRT,* intensity-modulated radiotherapy.

prostate cancer) will be diagnosed in 2006.[3] Annual incidence of penile cancer is estimated to be one in 100,000 males, accounting for less than 1% of all cancers in men. Circumcision performed early in life seems to have a preventive effect in the development of cancer of the penis.[108] Circumcision performed in adulthood does not seem to have the same beneficial results.[109] The incidence of penile cancer is higher in countries that do not routinely practice neonatal circumcision such as Asia, Africa, and South America. Phimosis, which is a narrowing of the opening of the prepuce, is common in men with penile cancer. Smegma, a white secretion that collects under the prepuce of the foreskin, is carcinogenic in animals, although the exact component of smegma responsible for its carcinogenic effect is not known. Other etiologic factors such as viruses and sexually transmitted diseases (STDs)

Table 13-10 Pharmacologic Management of Proctitis Secondary to Radiation Therapy*

Drug	Form available	Use
Hydrocortisone	Cream Ointment Suppositories Foam	May be used up to 4 times daily
Topical lidocaine		Apply as needed, not to exceed 30 g/day
Aluminum acetate	Powder Tablets	Dissolve in tepid water and apply soaks 3–4 times daily for 1 week
Sucralfate	Tablets Enema	1 g 4 times daily by mouth or dissolve in tepid water and use as enema
Mesalamine	Suppositories Enema	Administer rectally at night; may cause diarrhea

Data from:

Blot E, Escande MC, Besson D et al: Outbreak of clostridium difficile-related diarrhea in an adult oncology unit: risk factors and microbiological characteristics, *J Hospital Infection* 53:187-192, 2003.

Boyd EL, Berardi R: Anorectal disorders. In Berardi EM et al, editors: *Handbook of nonprescription drugs,* ed 13, Washington, DC, 2002, American Pharmaceutical Association.

Deglin JH, Vallerand AH: *Davis's drug handbook for nurses,* ed 8, Philadelphia, 2003, FA Davis.

Donjon RP, Goeckner BJ: *Mosby's OTC drugs*, St Louis, 1999, Mosby.

Goldstein F, DiMarino AJ Jr: Diarrhea as a side effect of mesalamine treatment for inflammatory bowel disease, *J Clin Gastroenterology* 31(1):60-62, 2000.

Hogle WP: Male pelvis. In Bruner DW, Haas ML, Gosselin-Acomb TK, editors: *Manual for radiation oncology nursing practice and education,* ed 3, Pittsburgh, 2005, Oncology Nursing Society, pp 132-141.

Holland J: Gastrointestinal/abdomen. In Bruner DW, Haas ML, Gosselin-Acomb TK, editors: *Manual for radiation oncology nursing practice and education,* ed 3, Pittsburgh, 2005, Oncology Nursing Society, pp 116-126.

Melko GP, Turco TF, Phelan TF et al: Treatment of radiation-induced proctitis with sucralfate enemas, *Ann Pharmacotherapy* 33(12):1274-1276, 1999.

Sasai T, Hiraishi H, Suzuki Y et al: Treatment of chronic post-radiation proctitis with oral administration of sucralfate, *Am J Gastroenterol* 93(9):1593-1595, 1998.

*If no response to pharmacologic interventions, consider that proctitis may result from *Clostridium difficile* toxin (send stool sample). Consult a gastroenterologist or proctologist. Patient may need treatment breaks.

Table 13-11 Impotence After EBRT and Brachytherapy

Researcher	Treatment	Sample size	Follow-up (months)	Erectile dysfunction incidence
Mameghan et al.	EBRT	42	55	45% at 2 years
Roach et al.	EBRT	60	21	38%
Crook et al.	EBRT	158	33	35%
Mantz et al.	EBRT	68	18	25% at 2 years
Zelefsky et al.	EBRT	544	42	39%
Pilepich et al.	EBRT	230	54	72%
Blasko et al.	BRACHY	469	38	< age 70: 15% > age 70: 50%
Stock et al.	BRACHY	65	18	21%
Zelefsky et al.	BRACHY	221	48	29%
Merrick et al.	BRACHY	209	40	61% at 6 years

Data from Inrocci L, Slob AK, Levendag PC: Sexual (dys)function after radiotherapy for prostate cancer: a review. *Int J Radiat Oncol Biol Phys* 52(2):681-693, 2002.

EBRT, External beam radiation therapy.

have been implicated in the development of penile cancer, although evidence remains inconclusive.[110]

Carcinoma of the male urethra is also rare. There is no correlation with recognized racial or geographic predisposing factors. Despite an unknown etiology, some correlation seems to exist between male urethral cancer and infection, STDs, and urethral strictures. The area of the urethra covered by

Table 13-12 Education for Patients Undergoing Prostate Brachytherapy

Surgical procedure	• Usually outpatient unless complications • General or spinal anesthesia • Postanesthesia nausea, sore throat • Perineal bruising/tenderness after surgery • Urinary catheter may remain in place for a few days after procedure
Side effects	• Similar to EBRT[1] and somewhat dependent on half-life of source used • Consider use of medication for urinary- and bowel-related side effects (see Tables 13-8 and 13-10) and sildenafil for impotency • Instruct patient in side effect profile and potential interactions with other drugs/dietary intake[1]
Dietary modifications	• Avoid caffeine; doing so may decrease urinary symptoms[2,3] • Maintain hydration with 1–2 liters/day; decrease at night to avoid excessive nocturia[1,4] • Consider bulking agents if loose stools are present
Sexual activity	• A condom should be worn for 2 months post-implant with LDR sources • Seeds may appear in ejaculate[1] • Blood may appear in ejaculate for 2–3 months postprocedure
Exposure to public	• Controversy exists as to whether LDR brachytherapy patients should limit exposure to children and pregnant women • Smathers et al.[5] concurred that such precautions are unnecessary • Exposure precautions are usually institution specific
Seed migration	• Inform patient of potential for seed migration with LDR brachytherapy • Migration can occur to any part of the body • 20% of patients will develop pulmonary seed migration[6,7]
Expulsion of seed(s)	• If seed is passed during urination, ejaculation, or nocturnal emission, it should be placed in a container with a lid and stored away from people • Patient should notify radiation oncology and await further instructions

Data from:

Abel LJ, Blatt HJ, Stipetich RL et al: Nursing management of patients receiving brachytherapy for early stage prostate cancer, *Clin J Oncol Nurs* 3(1):7-15, 1999.

Ankem MK, DeCarvalho VS, Harangozo AM et al: Implications of radioactive seed migration to the lungs after prostate brachytherapy, *Urology* 59(4):555-559, 2002.

Dafoe-Lambie JC, Abel LJ, Blatt HJ et al: Radioactive seed embolization to the lung following prostate brachytherapy, *The W V Med J* 96(1):357-360, 2000.

Gray M: Caffeine and urinary continence, *J Wound Ostomy Continence Nurs* 28(2):66-69, 2001.

Hogle WP: Male pelvis. In Bruner DW, Haas ML, Gosselin Acomb TK, editors: *Manual for radiation oncology nursing practice and education,* ed 3, Pittsburgh, 2005, Oncology Nursing Society, pp 132-141.

Iwamoto RR, Maher KE: Radiation therapy for prostate cancer, *Semin Oncol Nurs* 17(2):90-100, 2001.

Smathers S, Wallner K, Simpson C et al: Patient perception of local anesthesia for prostate brachytherapy, *Semin Urologic Oncol* 18(2):142-146, 2000.

EBRT, External beam radiation therapy; *LDR,* low dose rate.

transitional epithelium may be susceptible to the same carcinogenic factors that affect the bladder and upper urinary tract. The average patient who presents with urethral cancer is between ages 58 and 60, although 10% occur in men younger than age 40.[111,112]

Anatomy and Pathophysiology

The basic structural components of the penis include the corpora cavernosa and the corpus spongiosum. These are encased in a dense fascia, which is separated from the skin by a layer of loose connective tissue. Distally, the corpus spongiosum expands into the glans penis, which is covered by a skinfold known as the *prepuce.*

The male urethra is composed of mucous membrane and submucosa. It extends from the bladder neck to the urethral meatus. The posterior urethra is subdivided into the membranous urethra and the prostatic urethra. The anterior urethra is divided into fossa navicularis or glanular (a widening of the glans), the penile urethra, and the bulbous urethra (Figure 13-3).

Most penile tumors are well-differentiated squamous cell cancers. No significant correlation between the histologic grade and survival time has

Table 13-13 Resources for Patients With Prostate Cancer

Title	Author/resource
BOOKS	
ABC's of Advanced Prostate Cancer	Moyad, Mark & Pienta, Kenneth, MD
ABC's of Prostate Cancer: The Book That Could Save Your Life	Oesterling, Joseph E
ACS's Complete Guide to Prostate Cancer	Bostwick, et al
Dr. Patrick Walsh's Guide to Surviving Prostate Cancer	Walsh, Patrick, MD
Hard Bargain: Life-Lessons from Prostate Cancer	Bringhan, Kenneth, MD
He Said You Have Prostate Cancer	Sadage, Stanley
Humanizing Prostate Cancer	Oliver, Alex and Schultz, Roger E
In Sickness and in Health: A Love Story	Propp, Karen
Lovin' Ain't Over	Alterowitz, Ralph & Barbara
Man to Man	Korda, Michael
Men's Club: How to Lose Your Prostate Without … Sense of Humor	Gottlieb, Bert & Mawn, Thomas
Men, Women, and Prostate Cancer: A Medical & Psychological Guide for Women and The Men They Love	Barbara Rubin, EdD, & Sandra Haber, PhD
No Such Thing as a Bad Day	Jordan, Hamilton
Oh No, Not Me: Prostate Cancer	Lintzerich, Joseph
Prostate & Cancer: A Family Guide to Diagnosis, Treatment & Survival	Marks, Sheldon
Prostate Cancer: A Doctor's Personal Triumph	Fine, Robert, MD, & Fine, Saralee
Prostate Cancer For Dummies: A Reference for the Rest of Us!	Lange, Paul, MD, & Adamec, Christine
100 Questions and Answers about Prostate Cancer	Ellsworth, P, et al.
Seeds of Hope: A Physician's Personal Triumph over Prostate Cancer	D'orso, Michael A
You Can't Make Love If You're Dead: Curing Prostate Cancer and …	Prochnik, Leon
Prostate Cancer Treatment Book	Grimm, P, et al.
PAMPHLETS	
After Diagnosis: Prostate Cancer	American Cancer Society
American Cancer Society's Guidelines for the Early Detection of Prostate Cancer	American Cancer Society
Erectile Dysfunction	American Cancer Society
Facts on Prostate Cancer	Prostate Health Council
For Men Only: What You Should Know About Prostate Cancer	American Cancer Society
Hormonal Therapy for Prostate Cancer	National Cancer Institute/Us Too!
Know Your Options: Understanding Treatment Choices for Prostate Cancer	Krames Communication/Staywell
Let's Talk About It: Questions and Answers about Prostate Cancer	National Cancer Institute/Us Too!
Living with Prostate Cancer: Is Radiation Treatment Right For You?	American Cancer Society
Man To Man—Prostate Cancer	Cancer Care
Managing Incontinence After Treatment For Prostate Cancer	American Cancer Society
Prostate Cancer: Treatment Guidelines for Patients	American Cancer Society
Should I Be Tested for Prostate Cancer?	Astra Zeneca Pharmaceuticals
Treatment Choices For Localized Prostate Cancer	Bristol-Myers Squibb
Understanding Prostate Cancer: A Guide to Treatment and Support	American Cancer Society

Table 13-13 Resources for Patients With Prostate Cancer—cont'd

Title	Author/resource
PAMPHLETS—cont'd	
Understanding Prostate Changes: A Health Guide for All Men	National Cancer Institute (NIH)
Understanding Treatment Choices for Prostate Cancer	National Cancer Institute (NIH)
What You Need to Know About: Prostate Cancer	Schering Oncology Biotech
What You Should Know About Prostate Cancer	National Cancer Institute (NIH)
INTERNET SITES	
American Cancer Society	www.cancer.org
American Urologic Association	www.afud.org
CancerNews Prostate Cancer	www.cancernews.com/male.htm
National Cancer Institute: Prostate Cancer	www.nci.nih.gov/cancertopics/types/prostate
Prostate Cancer Education Council	www.pcaw.com
Prostate Cancer Foundation	www.prostatecancerfoundation.org
Prostate Cancer Research Foundation of Canada	www.prostatecancer.ca/english
Prostate Health	www.prostatehealth.com
Us Too International!	www.ustoo.com

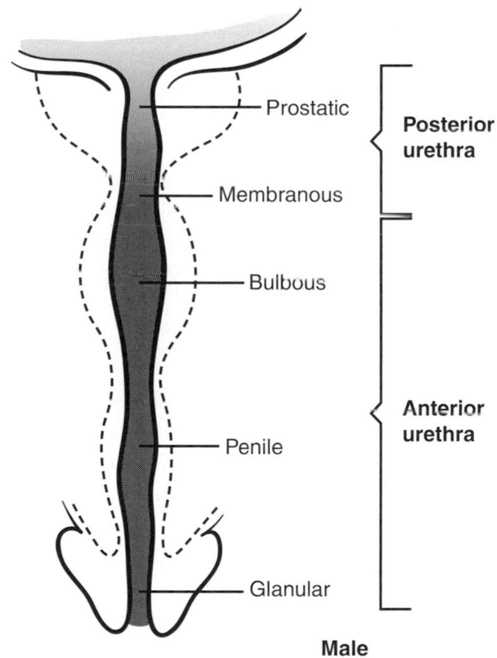

Figure 13-3 Urethra Staging Diagram. *Copyright @ 2006. BC Cancer Agency. All Rights Reserved. Accessed August 14, 2006 from www.bccancer.bc.ca/HPI/CancerManagementGuidelines/Genitourinary/MiscellaneousGenitourinaryTumours/UrethraStaging.htm*

been found.[113,114] Penile cancers typically begin as small lesions on the glans or prepuce. They grow laterally along the surface, covering the entire glans and prepuce and invading the corpora and the shaft of the penis. If untreated, penile autoamputation can occur.

Bowen's disease is squamous cell cancer in situ that may involve the shaft of the penis and the hairy skin of the inguinal and suprapubic area. Clinically, this lesion is solitary with areas of dry or moist desquamation.[115]

Erythroplasia of Queyrat (EOQ) is an epidermoid carcinoma in situ that involves the mucosal or mucocutaneous areas of the prepuce or glans.[116] Clinically, it appears as a raised, reddened, or ulcerated lesion. EOQ is not associated with other internal malignancies as often as is Bowen's disease.[117]

Basal cell carcinoma is rare and accounts for 1% to 2% of all cases of penile cancer.[118]

Soft tissue tumors are also rare, and many of these are benign; these may include angiomatous, neurogenous myogenous, fibrous, and lymphoreticular tumors.[119,120] Most soft tissue tumors occur on the shaft of the penis.[115]

Primary lymphoma of the penis is rare and has been reported in only one patient with Peyronie's disease. The literature does, however, report five cases of secondary involvement by lymphoma.[121]

Cancers that metastasize to the penis are rare and usually represent late, advanced carcinomatosis when they occur. These metastatic tumors are usually from the genitourinary system, followed by gastrointestinal system and respiratory system.[115]

Approximately 95% of urethral cancers in males are well or moderately differentiated squamous cell cancer.[122] Others include transitional cell cancer, adenocarcinoma, and undifferentiated or mixed. Tables 13-14 and 13-15 reflect the AJCC staging system for penile and male urethral cancers, respectively.

Clinical Manifestations

Carcinoma of the penis typically presents as an infiltrative, ulcerative, or exophytic papillary lesion. The growth rates of the papillary and ulcerative lesions are similar, but the flat ulcerative lesions have a tendency to metastasize to the lymph nodes earlier and are therefore associated with a lower 5-year survival rate. One report demonstrated the glans and prepuce as the predominant sites of penile cancer.[123] The presence of phimosis may visually obscure the primary lesion. Secondary infection with or without a foul odor is not unusual. Most penile cancers do not display urethral obstructions. However, the most common presenting symptom is a mass with pain or itching, bleeding, groin mass, and urinary symptoms.[114,115,124] Inguinal lymph nodes may not be palpable at presentation. If palpable, they are associated either with spread of the disease or secondary infection.[115]

Patients with urethral cancer typically present with urinary outlet obstruction, mass, bleeding (gross or occult), tenderness, discharge, abscess or irritative symptoms. Occasionally, urethral stricture or urethritis may precede the diagnosis of urethral cancer. The majority of urethral carcinomas occur in the posterior region (61%) and have a worse prognosis compared to those that arise from the anterior urethra.[112]

Most carcinomas of the penis spread locally to the abdominal wall or inguinal lymph nodes, which are the most common site of spread. About 20% of patients with clinically nonpalpable inguinal lymph nodes have micrometastases. Distant metastasis is uncommon.[125]

Tumors of the urethra also spread locally and involve the inguinal or pelvic lymph nodes.

Diagnostic Studies

Penile lesions are usually first seen or palpated, then biopsied to confirm the diagnosis of cancer. Urethral lesions are evaluated by urethroscopy and cystoscopy. CT scans are useful in the evaluation of enlarged pelvic and para-aortic lymph nodes. Although these scans are limited when evaluating inguinal nodes in penile cancer patients because many present with a secondary infectious process. In urethral cancer, the inflammatory changes in the regional lymph nodes are less problematic, and these patients may benefit from a lymphangiogram.

Table 13-14 AJCC Staging for Penile Cancer

Tumor stage	Clincal/pathologic findings
PRIMARY TUMOR (T)	
TX	Primary tumor cannot be assessed
T0	No evidence of primary tumor
Tis	Carcinoma in situ
Ta	Noninvasive verrucous carcinoma
T1	Tumor invades subepithelial connective tissue
T2	Tumor invades corpus spongiosum or cavernosum
T3	Tumor invades urethra and prostate
T4	Tumor invades other adjacent structures
REGIONAL LYMPH NODES (N)	
NX	Regional lymph nodes cannot be assessed
N0	No regional lymph node metastasis
N1	Metastasis in a single superficial, inguinal lymph node
N2	Metastasis in multiple or bilateral superficial inguinal lymph nodes
N3	Metastasis in deep inguinal or pelvic lymph node(s) unilateral or bilateral
DISTANT METASTASES (M)	
MX	Distant metastasis cannot be assessed
M0	No distant metastasis
M1	Distant metastasis

Treatment

Penile Cancer

Surgical intervention for penile cancer includes local excision or laser surgery and partial or total penectomy. In severe advanced proximal tumors, surgical excision may include the entire penis, scrotum, testes, bladder, or prostate as indicated. Although total penectomy is quite effective in treating most cases, it is not always acceptable to sexually active patients.[115] Surgery is usually performed first, followed by treatment of regional lymph node chains with either radiation or radical

Table 13-15 AJCC Staging for Urethral Cancer

Cancer stage	Clinical/pathologic findings
PRIMARY TUMOR (T)	
TX	Primary tumor cannot be assessed
T0	No evidence of primary tumor
Tis	Carcinoma in situ
Ta	Noninvasive verrucous carcinoma
T1	Tumor invades subepithelial connective tissue
T2	Tumor invades corpus spongiosum, prostate, or periurethral muscle
T3	Tumor invades corpus cavernosum, beyond prostatic capsule, or bladder neck
T4	Tumor invades other adjacent structures
REGIONAL LYMPH NODES (N)	
NX	Regional lymph nodes cannot be assessed
N0	No regional lymph node metastasis
N1	Metastasis in a single lymph node 2 cm or less in greatest dimension
N2	Metastasis in a single node more than 2 cm in greatest dimension, or in multiple nodes
DISTANT METASTASES (M)	
MX	Distant metastasis cannot be assessed
M0	No distant metastasis
M1	Distant metastasis

Used with the permission of the American Joint Committee on Cancer (AJCC), Chicago, Illinois. The original source of this material is the *AJCC Cancer Staging Handbook, Sixth Edition* (2002), published by Springer-New York, www.springeronline.com.

lymphadenectomy. Ideally, patients and physicians seek a surgical procedure that removes the lesion with adequate margins while preserving sexual and urinary function. Depending on extent of disease, this is not always possible.

Bowen's disease and EOQ can be treated with topical 5-FU (5% cream), a local excision, or superficial radiation to 45 Gy to 50 Gy. The principal advantage of radiation therapy in the management of primary penile lesions is organ preservation. A variety of external beam treatment techniques, doses, and fractionation schemes are reported in the literature.[122,126] Often, custom moldings and bolus techniques are necessary for adequate treatment of the penis. A significant association exists between large fraction size and late tissue damage. Most series report daily fractions of 2.5 Gy to 3.5 Gy for a total dose of 50 Gy to 55 Gy, although a smaller daily fraction size of 1.8 Gy to 2.0 Gy and a higher total dose are preferable. A total dose of 65 Gy to 70 Gy with the last 5 Gy to 10 Gy delivered to a reduced portal is believed to decrease the incidence of late fibrosis.[78]

Regional lymph nodes can be treated with EBRT and include bilateral inguinal and pelvic nodes. If there is no evidence of pelvic nodal involvement, dosage can be limited to 50 Gy. If clinically evident nodes exist, doses of 65 Gy to 70 Gy in 7 to 8 weeks (1.8 Gy to 2.0 Gy/day) with decreased field size after 50 Gy are advised.[78]

Brachytherapy to the penis is technically difficult but can be offered as an alternative to penectomy. Iridium-loaded needles or wires, with or without a custom mold, are surgically placed through the penis. Depending on the exact techniques used, dose ranges from 60 Gy to 70 Gy and is administered over a period of 5 to 7 days. Crook and colleagues[127] reported overall results for 49 patients who received 60 Gy of radiation via various brachytherapy techniques between 1983 and 2003. All had squamous cell carcinoma, and at 5 years, actuarial overall survival rate was 78.3% and cause-specific survival was 90%. Four men died of penile cancer and six died of other causes with no evidence of recurrence.[127]

Practice guidelines from the NCCN for the treatment of penile and male urethral cancers with radiation therapy do not presently exist.

The use of chemotherapy for penile cancer is limited at best. Agents such as bleomycin, 5-FU, and methotrexate have demonstrated limited activity.[128] In most cases, systemic treatment is reserved for metastatic or recurrent disease or lesions that are so advanced that cure is likely impossible by other means.

Urethral Cancer

As in penile cancer, the primary treatment for male urethral cancer is surgery. Noninvasive carcinoma of the proximal urethra can be treated with transurethral resection. In lesions of the distal urethra, treatment is either penectomy or radiation therapy. Most patients, unfortunately, present with advanced invasive disease, which tends to be more difficult to manage by any means. Involved regional lymph nodes are treated with lymphadenectomy.[115]

Chemotherapy can be given alone or in conjunction with radiation therapy. Regimens consist of 5-FU and mitomycin C, 5-FU and cisplatin, or methotrexate, vinblastine, adriamycin, and cisplatin depending on cell type and presentation. EBRT to 30 Gy in 15 fractions with a boost of 20 Gy showed positive results in a small number of patients.[129] In the preoperative setting, a total dose of approximately 45 Gy is indicated.

Radiation treatment techniques for male urethral cancer are similar to those used for penile cancer.

Side Effects of Radiation and Nursing Interventions

Most patients who receive radiation to the penis develop a brisk erythema, dry or moist desquamation, and some degree of swelling of the subcutaneous tissue of the penile shaft. These reactions are considered to be acute in nature and usually subside within a few weeks. Late effects include hyperpigmentation, telangiectasia, urethral strictures, ulceration, necrosis of the glans, or necrosis of the skin of the shaft. The latter being extremely rare.[130] Lymphedema of the legs of varying degrees has been reported; however, the role of radiation in this complication remains controversial.[115] Psychosocially, cancer of the penis can cause feelings of shame or embarrassment that have significant psychologic impact.

Nursing interventions for skin-related morbidity are found in Chapter 30. When applying these measures to the penis, it is important to maintain aggressive hygiene, as infections in this patient population are common. This area can be especially challenging when trying to maintain a dry and clean skin surface area. Patients with outlet obstruction problems should be referred to a urologist for urethral dilation. If urinary morbidity occurs during or after radiation, nursing interventions for such are outlined in the prostate section of this chapter and can be applied to this patient population as well. Given the risk of sexual dysfunction, both psychologically and physically, referral to behavioral medicine or a sex therapist/counselor is encouraged. Other evidence-based interventions for sexual dysfunction are outlined in Chapter 35. Bowel-related side effects may occur when treating the penis or male urethra with radiation therapy. Interventions for diarrhea are found in Chapter 34.

Education

Aside from being informed as to the radiation course and expected side effects, patients should be instructed on the potential for sexual dysfunction related to both the disease and the treatment.[131] Changes in sexual practice or routines may be necessary to accommodate physical or psychologic barriers that were not problematic before diagnosis.[132] Patients should be informed that seeking the assistance of a sex counselor/therapist ought not be viewed as a sign of weakness. Rather, it is a healthy response in an attempt to improve a difficult situation. The radiation oncology nurse should assure patients that referral to behavioral medicine or sex therapist/counselor is available at any time during the continuum of care.[133] Table 13-16 lists appropriate resources.

TESTICULAR CANCER

It is estimated that 8250 newly diagnosed cases of testicular cancer and 370 deaths from the disease will occur in 2006.[3] A great majority of testicular malignancies (98%) are of germ cell origin. Approximately 95% of patients with newly diagnosed germ cell tumors (GCTs) will be cured through optimal management involving multiple disciplines. Testicular cancer is the most common solid tumor malignancy in men ages 15 to 35, but most often it affects men ages 20 to 34. It is less common in adolescents, but increased rates of incidence seem to occur at age 40 and after age 60. Worldwide incidence of these tumors has more than doubled in the past 40 years.[3,134] Incidence rates are lowest among Asians, Africans, Puerto Ricans, and men of African-American descent. Higher rates are reported among Caucasians in the United States, the United Kingdom, and Denmark.[78]

Table 13-16 Resources: Cancer of the Penis or Urethra

Resource	Website
American Cancer Society	www.cancer.org
American Urologic Association	www.afud.org
National Cancer Institute	www.cancer.gov/cancerinfo/pdq/treatment/penile www.cancer.gov/cancertopics/types/urethral

The exact cause of testicular carcinoma is unknown, although several risk factors have been suggested as a possible link to this disease. Such risk factors include a personal history of testicular cancer, cryptorchism, genetics, family history, Klinefelter's syndrome, environmental factors, and hormones. A large cohort failed to link vasectomies to an increased risk in testicular cancer. Environmental factors such as exposure to diethylstilbestrol (DES) and polyvinyl chloride have been weakly correlated with testicular cancer.[135]

Anatomy and Pathophysiology

The testes are located in the scrotum and are suspended by the spermatic cord. The left testis normally descends lower than the right. Three membrane-like layers known as the *tunica vaginalis, tunica albuginea,* and *tunica vasculosa* surround each testis. The function of the testes are to produce and store spermatozoa in various stages of development, and they are responsible for testosterone production. The epididymis is coiled on the outer surface of the testis and is the endpoint of a vast network of tubules that originate in the testis itself. The vas deferens is a muscular tube that extends from the epididymis along the medial side of the testis to become part of the spermatic cord. The seminal vesicle is a convoluted sac-like structure that is attached to the vas deferens near the base of the bladder. The seminal vesicle secretes nutrients so as to provide energy to the sperm cells and contains prostaglandins, which assist the sperm cell's movement through the female anatomy toward the unfertilized egg. At the time of ejaculation, the contents of the seminal vesicles are emptied into the ejaculatory duct, thereby greatly increasing the volume of semen discharged from the vas deferens.

Clinical Manifestations

The most common presenting symptom of testicular cancer is a painless swelling or nodular lesion in the scrotum. This is usually noticed by the patient himself or by a sexual partner. Occasionally, patients will complain of a dull ache, heaviness, or pulling sensation in the scrotum or an aching sensation in the lower abdomen. At times the mass or discomfort may be attributed to recent trauma. In many cases, however, this turns out to be an incidental finding. On rare occasions, patients do present with signs of metastatic disease such as distant nodal enlargement, respiratory symptoms, or low-back pain. Gynecomastia occurs in approximately 5% of patients with testicular germ cell tumors.[78]

The most common site of metastasis for GCTs is the lung. When painful scrotum enlargement is present, epididymitis or torsion of the testis must be ruled out because they appear more often than testicular carcinoma.[134]

Diagnostic Studies

In many cases, the initial diagnostic test performed is a testicular ultrasound. This study can differentiate tissues in the scrotum with accuracy and reliability. Seminomatous masses will be hypoechoic in nature when compared to nearby tissue. Nonseminomatous masses can be hypoechoic, hyperechoic, or isoechoic in nature. Another important diagnostic test in the staging process is a CT scan, which will rule out pulmonary involvement and provide information regarding retroperitoneal and pelvic disease. A chest x ray may be performed but has limited value in revealing subcentimeter lymph nodes that may be involved with metastatic disease. Bone scans, which involve the injection of a radioactive isotope, are useful in the detection of metastatic testicular cancer. Magnetic resonance imaging and PET scans have been used more often in the follow-up setting to determine the presence of recurrent disease. However, PET scans have not been proven to be more successful in this setting when compared to other more conventional radiologic imaging.[134,136]

Serum tumor markers are important diagnostic tools in testicular cancer. Alpha-fetoprotein (AFP) and beta human chorionic gonadotropin (HCG) are elevated in approximately 85% of nonseminomatous tumors. Lactate dehydrogenase isoenzyme (LDH) is often elevated in patients with advanced disease. Tumor markers should be obtained at baseline, during interventional therapy, and during follow-up after intervention has taken place. Teratomas are benign tumors that do not secrete markers. Table 13-17 lists tumor markers that are most often associated with specific types of testicular cancer.

Pathology and Metastatic Patterns

Testicular tumors are most often (98%) germ cell in nature, thus the name *germ cell tumors.* GCTs are composed of seminomatous and nonseminomatous cell types. Seminomatous tumors are classified as anaplastic and spermatocytic. Nonseminomatous tumors are classified into four types: teratomas, embryonal tumors, choriocarcinoma, and yolk sac tumors. The other major classifications of testicular tumors are either stromal cell tumors or secondary tumors resulting from metastasis from another site of the body.

The routes of metastasis are similar for both seminomatous and nonseminomatous tumors. Pure seminoma, however, has a greater tendency to remain localized or involve only nearby lymph nodes. Nonseminomatous germ cell tumors are more often spread by the surrounding vascular system. Seminoma spreads in an orderly fashion, initially to the retroperitoneal lymph nodes, followed by the mediastinal and supraclavicular nodal chains. Only in rare cases do pure seminomas spread to the lungs, bone, liver, or brain. Less than 5% of patients with pure seminoma present with stage III or IV disease.[78]

When nonseminomatous tumors spread, they typically follow a similar pattern in terms of nodal involvement, but usually spread to the lungs and liver.

There are numerous staging systems used for testicular cancer. As with most malignancies, staging is based on tumor size and lymph node involvement. In addition, testicular cancer is also staged by the status of tumor markers. Table 13-18 details the version put forth by the AJCC.

Treatment

Nonseminoma

The standard of care for most testicular cancers has long been, and continues to be, surgery. Whether it is employed as primary treatment or in the neoadjuvant setting depends on the stage at presentation and, to a lesser degree, the exact cell type of the testicular tumor itself. Early stage I nonseminomas are most often treated by orchiectomy and a retroperitoneal lymph node dissection (RPLND). Increasingly, this subset of patients is being offered a second approach, which consists of orchiectomy and surveillance. The RPLND is omitted if the patient chooses this approach. Surgery alone provides cure in about 70% of pathologic stage II testicular cancer, with a less than 1% chance of local recurrence.[137]

RPLND can be performed laparoscopically or during an open operative procedure. Both techniques can employ a nerve-sparing approach, but success in this area depends largely on surgical skill. Surgery followed by RPLND offers a 99% survival rate in patients with stage I disease.[138] If the patient has stage I disease and is considered at high risk for recurrence, chemotherapy is often recommended.

Patients who present with disease later than stage I are typically offered chemotherapy consisting of cisplatin, vinblastine, bleomycin (PVB) or bleomycin, etoposide, cisplatin (BEP). The number of courses of chemotherapy may vary depending on actual clinical and pathologic staging and whether the patient is enrolled in a clinical trial, or on physician preference. Upon completion of chemotherapy, one-third of patients have a residual mass detected by imaging studies. Generally, these masses should be excised because 40% are teratomas and 10% to 15% are carcinomas. Unresectable teratomas may lead to later relapse. Radiation therapy has little role in the management of patients with disseminated nonseminomas with the exception of palliative cases.[78,138]

Table 13-17 Tumor Markers for Testicular Cancer

Serum tumor marker	Tumor type
Alpha-fetoprotein (AFP)	Nonseminomous germ cell tumor
Beta-human chorionic gonadotropin (B-hCG)	Choriocarcinoma
	Embryonal tumor
	Pure seminoma
Lactic acid dehydrogenase (LDH) isoenzyme	Advanced or large-volume disease
	Advanced pure seminoma
Placental alkaline phosphatase (PLAP)	Nonseminomous germ cell tumor
Germ cell–specific alkaline (GCAP)	Seminoma
Inhibin-alpha	Leydig cell tumor

Data from Lee, Hamid, Arya, Patel et al, *Hosp Med* 63(10), 615-620.

Table 13-18 AJCC Staging System for Testicular Cancer

Cancer stage	Clinical/pathologic findings
PRIMARY TUMOR (PT)	
The extent of primary tumor is usually classified after radical orchiectomy, and for this reason, a *pathologic* stage is assigned.	
pTX*	Primary tumor cannot be assessed
pT0	No evidence of primary tumor (e.g., histologic scar in testis)
pTis	Intratubular germ-cell neoplasia (carcinoma in situ)
pT1	Tumor limited to the testis and epididymis without vascular/lymphatic invasion; tumor may invade into the tunica albuginea but not the tunica vaginalis
pT2	Tumor limited to the testis and epididymis with vascular/lymphatic invasion, or tumor extending through the tunica albuginea with involvement of the tunica vaginalis
pT3	Tumor invades the spermatic cord with or without vascular/lymphatic invasion
pT4	Tumor invades the scrotum with or without vascular/lymphatic invasion

*NOTE: Except for pTis and pT4, extent of primary tumor is classified by radical orchiectomy. TX may be used for other categories in the absence of radical orchiectomy.

Cancer stage	Clinical/pathologic findings
REGIONAL LYMPH NODES (N)	
NX	Regional lymph nodes cannot be assessed
N0	No regional lymph node metastasis
N1	Metastasis with a lymph node mass 2 cm or less in greatest dimension; or multiple lymph nodes, none more than 2 cm in greatest dimension.
N2	Metastasis with a lymph node mass, more than 2 cm but not more than 5 cm in greatest dimension; or multiple lymph nodes, any one mass greater than 2 cm but not more than 5 cm in greatest dimension
N3	Metastasis with a lymph node mass more than 5 cm in greatest dimension
PATHOLOGIC (PN)	
pNX	Regional lymph nodes cannot be assessed
pN0	No regional lymph node metastasis
pN1	Metastasis with a lymph node mass, 2 cm or less in greatest dimension and less than or equal to 5 nodes positive, none more than 2 cm in greatest dimension
pN2	Metastasis with a lymph node mass more than 2 cm but not more than 5 cm in greatest dimension; or evidence of extranodal extension of tumor
pN3	Metastasis with a lymph node mass more than 5 cm in greatest dimension
DISTANT METASTASES (M)	
MX	Distant metastasis cannot be assessed
M0	No distant metastasis
M1	Distant metastasis cannot be assessed
M1a	Nonregional nodal or pulmonary metastasis
M1b	Distant metastasis other than to nonregional lymph nodes and lungs
SERUM TUMOR MARKERS (S)	
SX	Marker studies not available or not performed
S0	Marker study levels within normal limits
S1	LDH less than 1.5 × N† AND hCG (mlu/mL) less than 5000 AND AFP (ng/ml) less than 1000
S2	LDH 1.5–10 × N OR hCG (mlu/mL) 5000–50,000 OR AFP (ng/mL) 1000–10,000
S3	LDH more than 10 × N OR hCG (mlu/mL) more than 50,000 OR AFP (ng/mL) more than 10,000

†N indicates the upper limit of normal for the LDH assay.

Used with the permission of the American Joint Committee on Cancer (AJCC), Chicago, Illinois. The original source for this material is the *AJCC Cancer Staging Handbook, Sixth Edition* (2002), published by Springer-New York, www. springeronline.com.

Mlu, Million international units.

Seminoma

Treatment outcome from all available therapies depends on stage and extent of disease at presentation. With the use of chemotherapy and radiation therapy, the overall cure rate for all stages of seminoma exceeds 90%.[139] Seminoma is particularly sensitive to radiation therapy and is used to treat stages I, IIA, and IIB disease. More advanced stages are treated with chemotherapy regimens consisting of cisplatin. Regimens that use additional agents vary as does the practice of administering three or four cycles.[78,138]

After surgical resection of the involved testis and spermatic cord, most patients with early- to mid-stage seminoma should receive radiation therapy to the para-aortic and ipsilateral pelvic lymph nodes. The top of the field borders should be at the T9 to T10 interface, and the inferior border should be at the bottom of L5 or at the top of the obturator foramen, depending whether pelvic nodes will be included in the treatment plan. The lateral border should include the para-aortic lymph nodes and ipsilateral renal hilum. A shaped field with 2-cm margins should be designed to include the ipsilateral pelvic lymph nodes. If the patient is concerned about preserving fertility, testicular shielding should be applied to decrease primary and scatter radiation doses to the unaffected testicle.[138]

The recommended dose to retroperitoneal lymph and pelvic lymph nodes for patients with stage I and IIA seminoma is 25 Gy in fractions of 1.6 Gy to 1.8 Gy with AP/PA fields given 5 days per week and both fields treated daily. For stage IIB and IIC disease, the treatment fields are essentially the same as those in stages I and II. However, exact field sizes should be modified to cover the known mass with an adequate margin. The initial 25 Gy to 30 Gy delivered to the entire nodal field should be administered in fractions of 1.6 to 1.8 Gy. A boost of 5 Gy to 10 Gy in 1.8-Gy to 2.0-Gy fractions is given to a reduced field that is inclusive of the known mass with a margin of 2 cm.[78]

The NCCN guidelines for treating seminoma with radiation therapy are as follows: Patients with stage IA, IB, or IS disease should receive infradiaphramatic or para-aortic radiation to a dose of 25 Gy to 30 Gy, stage IIA or IIB disease should receive infradiaphramatic radiation inclusive of the para-aortic and ipsilateral iliac nodes to a dose of 35 Gy to 40 Gy.[140]

Care should be taken during the treatment planning phase to minimize exposure of the kidney. At least two-thirds of the kidney should be spared from receiving doses higher than 18 Gy. Field size reductions may be necessary to accomplish this goal because larger masses shrink. The liver dose should be reviewed because doses greater than 30 Gy to a significant portion should be avoided.

Radiation to the inguinal nodes, scrotum, and mediastinum has fallen out of favor by most radiation oncologists. Morbidity and data collected from various reports have caused many to abandon this practice.[141-143]

Nursing Interventions

Acute Effects

For the radiation oncology nurse, interventions are directed at both the physical manifestations of treatment and the psychosexual aspects of the disease. Side effects most commonly dealt with include gastrointestinal symptoms, myelosuppression, and aspects surrounding fertility/sexuality issues. Table 13-19 lists acute and late effects of radiation for testicular carcinoma.

In general, para-aortic and pelvic radiation is well tolerated. Interventions for the management of nausea and diarrhea can be found in Chapter 34. However, it should be mentioned that nausea and vomiting can occur very early in the treatment course of para-aortic irradiation. It is not unusual for patients to experience this after the first or second treatment. Therefore, antiemetics should be prescribed and taken at least 1 hour before radiation.[144]

Interventions for skin reactions, although rare in this patient population because radiation doses range from 25 Gy to 40 Gy, can be found in Chapter 30.

Interventions for fatigue are similar to those for patients receiving radiation therapy to the prostate gland as described earlier in this chapter.

Dyspepsia or peptic ulcers occur in 3% to 5% of irradiated patients.[145] Gastric ulcerations can occur at doses between 40 Gy and 45 Gy and may present months to years after treatment has been completed.[144] Proton pump inhibitors can be helpful in the management of some patients with functional dyspepsia and duodenal acid hypersensitivity.[145]

Radiation to the para-aortic lymph node chain and pelvis can cause varying degrees of myelosuppression. Weekly blood counts with differential should be performed to monitor the patient's ab-

67. Bok RA, Halabi S, Fei DT et al: Vascular endothelial growth factor and basic fibroblast growth factor urine levels as predictors of outcome in hormone-refractory prostate cancer patients: a cancer and leukemia group B study, *Cancer Res* 61(6):2533-2536, 2001.
68. Hussain M, Faulkner J, Vaishampayan U et al: Epithilone B analogue BMS-247550 (NSC #710428) administered every 21 days in patients with hormone refractory prostate cancer: a Southwest Oncology Group Study (S0111), Program and abstracts of the 40th Annual Meeting of the American Society of Clinical Oncology; June 5-8, 2004; New Orleans, Louisiana (abstract 4510).
69. Klein EA, Roach M: Management of localized prostate cancer. In *Report to the Nation on Prostate Cancer 2004* (website): www.medscape.com/viewprogram/3440_pnt. Accessed on November 6, 2005.
70. Talcott JA, Rieker P, Clark JA et al: Patient-reported symptoms after primary therapy for early prostate cancer: results of a prospective cohort study, *J Clin Oncol* 16(1):275-283, 1998.
71. Van Erps P, Van Den Weyngaert D, Denis L: Surgery or radiation: is there really a choice for early prostate cancer? *Crit Rev Oncol Hematol* 27(1):11-27, 1998.
72. Gettman MT, Hoznek A, Salomon L et al: Laparoscopic radical prostatectomy: description of the extraperitoneal approach using the da Vinci robotic system, *J Urol* 170 (2 pt 1):416-419, 2003.
73. Roumeguere T, Bollens R, Vanden Bossche M et al: Radical prostatectomy: a prospective comparison of oncological and functional results between open and laparoscopic approaches, *World J Urol* 20(6):360-366, 2003.
74. Schmidt JD, Doyle J, Larison S: Prostate cryoablation: update 1998, *CA Cancer J Clin* 48(4):239-253, 1998.
75. Zippe CD: Cryosurgery of the prostate techniques and pitfalls, *Urol Clin North Am* 23(1):147-163, 1996.
76. Potosky AL, Cavis WW, Hoffman RM et al: Five-year outcomes after prostatectomy or radiotherapy for prostate cancer: the prostate cancer outcomes study, *J Natl Cancer Inst* 96(18):1358-1367, 2004.
77. National Comprehensive Cancer Network: *Practice guidelines in oncology for prostate cancer,* V.2.2005, 2005, at www.nccn.org/professionals/physician_gls/PDF/prostate.pdf, accessed November 26, 2005.
78. Kuban DA: Male reproductive and genitourinary tumors. In Washington CM, Leaver D: *Principles and practice of radiation therapy,* ed 2, St Louis, 2004, Mosby, pp 799-842.
79. Zelefsky MJ, Valicenti RK, Goodman K et al: Male genitourinary tumors. In Perez CA, Brady LW, Halperin EC, Schmidt-Ullrich RK, editors: *Principles and practice of radiation oncology,* ed 4, Philadelphia, 2004, Lippincott Williams & Wilkins, pp 1692-1762.
80. Zelefsky MJ, Fuks Z, Hunt M et al: High dose intensity modulated radiation therapy for prostate cancer: early toxicity and biochemical outcome in 772 patients, *Int J Radiat Oncol Biol Phys* 53(5):1111-1116, 2002.
81. Blasko JC, Grimm PD et al: The role of external beam radiotherapy with 1-125/Pd103 brachytherapy for prostate carcinoma, *Radiother Oncol* 57(3):273-278, 2000.
82. Sylvester JE, Blasko JC, Grimm PD et al: Ten-year biochemical relapse-free survival after external beam radiation and brachytherapy for localized prostate cancer: the Seattle experience, *Int J Radiat Oncol Biol Phys* 57(4):944-952, 2003.
83. Kollmeier MA, Stock RG, Stone N: Biochemical outcomes after prostate brachytherapy with 5-year minimal follow-up: importance of patient selection and implant quality, *Int J Radiat Oncol Biol Phys* 57(3):645-653, 2003.
84. Grimm PD, Blasko JC, Sylvester JE et al: 10-year biochemical (prostate-specific antigen) control of prostate cancer with 125-I brachytherapy, *Int J Radiat Oncol Biol Phys* 51(1):31-40, 2001.
85. Beyer D, Nath R, Butler W et al: American brachytherapy society recommendations for clinical implementation of NIST-1999 standards for 103 palladium, *Int J Radiat Oncol Biol Phys* 47(2):273-275, 2000.
86. Kestin LL, Martinez AA, Stromberg JS et al: Matched-pair analysis of conformal high-dose rate brachytherapy boost versus external beam radiation therapy alone for locally advanced prostate cancer, *J Clin Oncol* 18(15):2869-2880, 2000.
87. Martinez A: High dose rate brachytherapy for prostate cancer. In Greco C, Zelefsky MJ, editors: *Radiotherapy for prostate cancer,* Amsterdam, 2000, Harwood Academic, pp 279-286.
88. Haas ML: Skin reaction. In Bruner DW, Haas ML, Gosselin-Acomb TK, editors: *Manual for radiation oncology nursing practice and education,* ed 3, Pittsburgh, 2005, Oncology Nursing Society; pp 49-52.
89. Volpe HM: Radiation therapy. In Held-Warmkessel J, editor: *Contemporary issues in prostate cancer: a nursing perspective,* Sudbury, MA, Jones and Bartlett, 2000.
90. Bruner DW, Bucholtz JD, Iwamoto R et al: *Manual for radiation oncology nursing practice and education,* Pittsburgh, 1998, Oncology Nursing Society.
91. Forman JD, Keole S, Bolton S et al: Association of prostate size with urinary morbidity following mixed conformal neutron and photon irradiation, *Int J Radiat Oncol Biol Phys* 45(4):871-875, 1999.
92. Anton ML: Female pelvis. In Bruner DW, Haas ML Gosselin-Acomb TK, editors: *Manual for radiation oncology nursing practice and education,* ed 3, Pittsburgh, 2005, Oncology Nursing Society.
93. Kaassis M, Oberti E, Burtin P et al: Argon plasma coagulation for the treatment of hemorrhagic radiation proctitis, *Endoscopy* 32(9):673-676, 2000.
94. Counter SF, Froese DP, Hart MJ: Prospective evaluation of formalin therapy for radiation proctitis, *Am J Surg* 177(5):396-398, 1999.
95. Inrocci L, Slob AK, Levendag PC: Sexual (dys)function after radiotherapy for prostate cancer: a review, *Int J Radiat Oncol Biol Phys* 52(3):681-693, 2002.
96. Valicenti RK, Choi E, Chen C et al: Sildenafil citrate effectively reverses sexual dysfunction induced by three-dimensional conformal radiation therapy, *Urology* 57(4):769-773, 2001.
97. Hogle WP: Male pelvis. In Bruner DW, Haas ML, Gosselin-Acomb TK, editors: *Manual for radiation oncology nursing practice and education,* ed 3, Pittsburgh, 2005, Oncology Nursing Society, pp 132-141.
98. Haylock JJ, Hart LK: Fatigue in patients receiving localized radiation, *Cancer Nurs* 2(6): 461-469, 1979.
99. Kobashi-Schoot JA, Hanewald GJ, van Dam FS et al:

Table 13-19 Acute and Late Effects of Radiation for Testicular Carcinoma

Acute effects	Late effects
Fatigue	Peptic ulcers
Skin irritation	Low sperm count
Nausea/vomiting	Infertility
Diarrhea	Secondary malignancy
Dyspepsia/peptic ulcers	
Myelosuppression	

solute neutrophil count and platelet count. If these blood counts drop to dangerous levels, patients should be instructed about neutropenic and bleeding precautions.

Late Effects

Education regarding low sperm count and the need for sperm cryopreservation are important aspects of care for these patients. If the patient is interested in maintaining fertility, baseline sperm analysis should be performed; such studies evaluate sperm count, motility, and overall viability of sperm. Once obtained and stored, cryopreserved sperm samples can be obtained at a later date and potentially used for the purpose of artificial insemination. Sperm cryopreservation has invigorated and encouraged cancer survivors and alleviated fears about the future regarding fertility and family planning.[146,147]

In some cases, a testicular prosthesis may be indicated if the patient is relatively young or if he has a negative self-image after orchiectomy and cancer therapy. Other psychosocial or psychosexual problems may require intervention from a trained behavioral medicine specialist or sex therapist/counselor. Referral to such practitioners should be considered on an individual basis.

Patients treated for testicular malignancies are at a higher risk for developing a second primary malignancy. One large study by Travis and colleagues[148] examined the occurrence of second malignancies among almost 29,000 men after treatment for testicular cancer. The median follow-up was 10 years and more than 1400 second primary cancers were detected. The risk for development of a second malignancy, excluding contralateral testicular involvement, was 15.7% and 22.6% at 25 and 30 years, respectively. These are considered significant because the corresponding population expected risks were 9.3% and 13.1%.[148]

Therefore, it is imperative that these patients are informed of the importance of follow-up care with a primary care practitioner and a urologist. Additionally, they should be informed of the ACS guidelines/recommendations for screening and early detection of the most common malignancies, available at the organization's website at www.cancer.org/docroot/PED/content/PED_2_3X_ACS_Cancer_Detection_Guidelines_36.asp?sitearea=PED. Table 13-20 lists additional resources.

Table 13-20 Resources: Testicular Cancer

Title	Author/resource
BOOKS	
Its Not About the Bike	Armstrong, Lance
Landing it: My Life on and Off The Ice	Hamilton, Scott with Benet, Lorenzo
PAMPHLETS	
Facts on Testicular Cancer	American Cancer Society
For Men Only—Testicular Cancer & How to Do TSE (Testicular Self Exam)	American Cancer Society
Get Smart About Testicular Cancer—General Cancer Facts for Young Men	American Cancer Society
INTERNET RESOURCES	
American Cancer Society	www.cancer.org
American Urologic Association	www.afud.org
National Cancer Institute: Testicular Cancer	www.nci.nih.gov/cancertopics/types/testicular
The Testicular Cancer Resource Center	www.tcrc.acor.org

REFERENCES

1. American Cancer Society: *Cancer facts & figures 2003* (website): www.cancer.org/downloads/STT/Caff2003 PWSecured.pdf. Accessed June 17, 2004.
2. American Cancer Society: *Cancer prevention & early detection facts & figures 2000* (website): www.cancer.org/downloads/STT/CPED2000PWSecured.pdf. Accessed June 17, 2004.
3. Jemal A, Murray T, Ward E et al: Cancer statistics 2005, *CA Cancer J Clin* 55(1):10-30, 2005.
4. Carroll PR, Nelson WG, Scardino PT et al: *Optimal strategies for the multidisciplinary management of prostate cancer* (archived web conference): www.medscape.com/viewprogram/3398_pnt. Accessed December 1, 2005.
5. Ries LAG, Eisner MP, Kosary CL et al, editors: *Seer cancer statistics review, 1975-2002*, Bethesda, MD, 2004, National Cancer Institute (website): http://seer.coancr.gov/csr/1975-2002. Accessed February 10, 2006.
6. Bach PB, Scrag D, Brawley OW et al: Survival of blacks and whites after a cancer diagnosis, *JAMA* 287(16):2106-2112, 2002.
7. National Cancer Institute: *Understanding prostate changes: a health guide for men*, (website): www.cancer.gov/cancertopics/understanding-prostate-changes. Accessed June 17, 2004.
8. Bostwick DG: Evaluating prostate needle biopsy: therapeutic and prognostic importance, *CA Cancer J Clin* 47(5):297-319, 1997.
9. Carroll PR, Lee KL, Fuks ZY et al: Cancer of the prostate. In Devita VT, Hellman S, Rosenberg SA, editors: *Cancer: principles and practice of oncology*, ed 6, Philadelphia, 2001, Lippincott-Raven, pp 1418-1479.
10. Esper P: Epidemiology, risk factors and prevention strategies. In Held-Warmkessel J, editor: *Contemporary issues in prostate cancer*, Sudbury, MA, 2000, Jones and Bartlett, pp 1-23.
11. Held-Warmkessel J: Prostate cancer. In Henke-Yarbro C, Hansen-Frogge M, Goodman M, editors: *Cancer nursing*, ed 6, Boston, 2005, Jones and Bartlett, pp 1552-1580.
12. Applewhite JC, Matlaga BR, McCullough DL et al: Transrectal ultrasound and biopsy in the early diagnosis of prostate cancer, *Cancer Control* 8(2):141-150, 2001.
13. Sakr WA, Partin AW: Histological markers of risk and the role of high-grade prostatic intraepithelial neoplasia, *Urology* 57(4 suppl 1):115-120, 2001.
14. Bostwick DG: High grade prostatic intraepithelial neoplasia: the most likely precursor of prostate cancer, *Cancer* 75(suppl):1823-1836, 1995.
15. Sakr WA, Haas GP, Cassin BF et al: The frequency of carcinoma and intraepithelial neoplasia of the prostate in young male patients, *J Urol* 150(2 pt 1):379-385, 1993.
16. Bostwick DG, Junqu J, Schlesinger C: Contemporary pathology of prostate cancer, *Urol Clin North Am* 30(2):181-207, 2003.
17. Gleason D: Classification of prostate carcinomas, *Cancer Chemother Rep* 50(3):125-128, 1966.
18. Cash J: Cellular characteristics, pathophysiology, and disease manifestations. In Held-Warmkessel J, editor: *Contemporary issues in prostate cancer*, Sudbury, MA, 2000, Jones and Bartlett, pp 36-48.
19. Kadmon D, Weinberg AD, Williams RH et al: Pitfalls in interpreting prostate specific antigen velocity, *J Urol* 155(5):1655-1657, 1996.
20. *AJCC cancer staging manual*, ed 5, Philadelphia, 1997, Lippincott-Raven.
21. Nitti V, Kim Y, Combs AJ: Correlation of the AUA symptom index with urodynamics in patients with suspected benign prostatic hyperplasia, *Neurourol Urodyn* 13(5):521-529, 1994.
22. Barry MJ, Fowler FJ, O'Leary MP et al: The American Urological Association symptom index for benign prostatic hyperplasia: the measurement committee of the American Urological Association, *J Urol* 148(5):1549-1557, 1992.
23. Kim ED, Grayhack, JT: Clinical symptoms and signs of prostate cancer. In Vogelzang NJ, Scardino PT, Shipley WU et al, editors: *Comprehensive textbook of genitourinary oncology*, ed 2, Philadelphia, 2000, Lippincott Williams & Wilkins, pp 525-532.
24. Wilkes GM: Spinal cord compression. In Yarbro CH, Frogge MH, Goodman M, editors: *Cancer symptom management*, ed 3, Sudbury, MA, 2004, Jones and Bartlett, 359-371.
25. American Cancer Society: *American Cancer Society updates prostate cancer screening guidelines* (website): www.cancer.org/docroot/MED/content/MED_2_1X_American_Cancer_Society_Updates_Prostate_Cancer_Screening_Guidelines.asp. Accessed November 26, 2005.
26. Partin AW, Mangold LA, Lamm DM et al: Contemporary update of prostate cancer staging nomograms (Partin tables) for the new millennium, *Urology* 56(5):843-848, 2000.
27. Carter HB, DeMarzo A, Lilja H: Detection, diagnosis, and prognosis of prostate cancer. In *Report to the Nation on Prostate Cancer 2004* (website): www.medscape.com/viewprogram/3440_pnt. Accessed November 6, 2005.
28. Catalona WJ, Richie JP, Ahmann FR et al: Comparison of digital rectal examination and serum prostate specific antigen in the early detection of prostate cancer: results of a multicenter clinical trial of 6,630 men, *J Urol* 151(5):1283-1290, 1994.
29. Lin K, Szabo Z, Chin BB et al: The value of a baseline bone scan in patients with newly diagnosed prostate cancer, *Clin Nucl Med* 24(8):579-582, 1999.
30. Lee N, Fawaaz R, Olsson CA et al: Which patients with newly diagnosed prostate cancer need a radionuclide bone scan? An analysis based on 631 patients, *Int J Radiat Oncol Biol Phys* 48(5):1443-1446, 2000.
31. Hanson KA: Diagnostic tests and tools in the evaluation of urologic disease, part II: *Urol Nurs* 23(6):405-414, 2003.
32. Sodee DB, Malguria N, Faulhaber P et al: Multicenter ProstaScint imaging findings in 2154 patients with prostate cancer. The ProstaScint Imaging Centers, *Urology* 56(6):988-993, 2000.
33. Kupelian PA, Elshaikh M, Reddy CA et al: Comparison of the efficacy of local therapies for localized prostate cancer in the PSA era: large single institution experience with radical prostatectomy and external beam radiotherapy, *J Clin Oncol* 20(16):3376-3385, 2002.
34. Tester W, Brouch MD: Treatment decision making. In Held-Warmkessel J, editor: *Contemporary issues in prostate cancer*, Sudbury, MA, 2000, Jones and Bartlett, pp 81-101.
35. Holmberg L, Bill-Axelson A, Helgeson F et al: A randomized trial comparing radical prostatectomy with watchful waiting in early prostate cancer, *N Engl J Med* 347(11):781-789, 2002.
36. Adolfsson J: Deferred treatment for clinically localized prostate cancer, *Eur J Surg Oncol* 21(4):333-336, 1995.
37. Palmer JS, Chodak G: Defining the role of surveillance in the management of localized prostate cancer, *Urol Clin North Am* 23(4):551-556, 1996.
38. Wallace M: Uncertainty and quality of life of older men who undergo watchful waiting for prostate cancer, *Oncol Nurs Forum* 30(2):303-309, 2003.
39. Gleave ME, Small EJ: Androgen deprivation for prostate cancer. In *Report to the nation on prostate cancer 2004* (website): www.medscape.com/viewprogram/3440_pnt. Accessed November 6, 2005.
40. See WA: Adjuvant hormone therapy after radiation or surgery for localized or locally advanced prostate cancer, *Curr Treat Options Oncol* 4(5):351-362, 2003.
41. Crawford ED, Eisenberger MA, McLeod DG et al: A controlled trial of leuprolide with and without flutamide in prostatic carcinoma, *N Engl J Med* 321(7):419-424, 1989.
42. Labrie F, Dupont A, Belanger A et al: Flutamide eliminates the risk of disease flare in prostatic cancer patients treated with a luteinizing hormone-releasing hormone agonist, *J Urol* 138(4):804-806, 1987.
43. Kuhn JM, Billebaud T, Navratil H et al: Prevention of the transient adverse effects of a gonadotropin-releasing hormone analogue (buserelin) in metastatic prostatic carcinoma by administration of an antiandrogen (nilutamide), *N Engl J Med* 321(7):413-418, 1989.
44. Denis LJ, Keuppens F, Smith PH et al: Maximal androgen blockade: final analysis of EORTC phase III trial 30853. EORTC genitourinary tract cancer cooperative group and the EORTC data center, *Eur Urol* 33(2):144-151, 1998.
45. Prostate Cancer Trialists' Collaborative Group: Maximum androgen blockade in advanced prostate cancer: an overview of the randomised trials, *Lancet* 355(9214):1491-1498, 2000.
46. Caubet JF, Tosteson TD, Dong EW et al: Maximum androgen blockade in advanced prostate cancer: a meta-analysis of published randomized controlled trials using nonsteroidal antiandrogens, *Urology* 49(1):71-78, 1997.
47. Gleave M, Bruchovsky N, Goldenberg SL et al: Intermittent androgen suppression for prostate cancer: rationale and clinical experience, *Eur Urol* 34(suppl 3):37-41, 1998.
48. Goldenberg SL, Bruchovsky N, Gleave ME et al: Intermittent androgen suppression in the treatment of prostate cancer: a preliminary report, *Urology* 45(5):839-845, 1995.
49. *Hormone therapy in treating men with stage IV prostate cancer* (website): www.clinicaltrials.gov/ct/show/NCT00002651?amp;order=24. Accessed July 18, 2004.
50. *Hormone therapy in treating patients with rising PSA levels following radiation therapy for prostate cancer* (website): www.clinicaltrials.gov/ct/show/NCT00003653?amp;order=34. Accessed July 18, 2004.
51. Soloway MS, Pareek K, Sharifi R et al: Neoadjuvant androgen ablation before radical prostatectomy in cT2bNxM0 prostate cancer: 5-year results, *J Urol* 167(1):112-116, 2002.
52. Bolla M, Gonzalez D, Warde P et al: Improved survival in patients with locally advanced prostate cancer treated with radiotherapy and goserelin, *N Engl J Med* 337(5):295-300, 1997.
53. Pilepich MV, Caplan R, Byhardt RW et al: Phase III trial of androgen suppression using goserelin in unfavorable-prognosis carcinoma of the prostate treated with definitiv radiotherapy: report of Radiation Therapy Oncology Grou Protocol 85-31, *J Clin Oncol* 15(3):1013-1021, 1997.
54. Galalae RM, Martinez A, Mate T et al: Long-ter outcome by risk factors using conformal high-dose-ra brachytherapy (HDR-BT) boost with or without neoa juvant androgen suppression for localized prostate canc *Int J Radiat Oncol Biol Phys* 58(4):1048-1055, 2004.
55. Potters L, Torre T, Ashley R et al: Examining the role neoadjuvant androgen deprivation in patients underg ing prostate brachytherapy, *J Clin Oncol* 18(6):1187-11 2000.
56. Kirby RS, Christmas TJ, Brawer MK: *Prostate cancer*, e London, 2001, Mosby.
57. Berruti A, Dogliotti L, Tucci M et al: Metabolic b disease induced by prostate cancer: rationale for us bisphosphonates, *J Urol* 166(6):2023-2031, 2001.
58. Townsend MF, Sanders WH, Northway RO et al: B fractures associated with luteinizing hormone-relea hormone agonists used in the treatment of prostate c noma, *Cancer* 79(3):545-550, 1997.
59. Smith MR: Bisphosphonates to prevent skeletal c plications in men with metastatic prostate cancer, *J* 170(6 pt 2):S55-S58, 2003.
60. Martel CL, Gumerlock PH, Meyers FJ e Current strategies in the management of hor refractory prostate cancer, *Cancer Treat Rev* 2 171-187, 2003.
61. Tannock IF, Osobo D, Stockler MR et al: Chemoth with mitoxantrone plus prednisone or prednisone for symptomatic hormone-resistant prostate can Canadian randomized trial with palliative end *J Clin Oncol* 14(6):1756-1764, 1996.
62. Kantoff PW, Halabi S, Conaway M et al: Hydroco with or without mitoxantrone in men with hor refractory prostate cancer: results of the Canc Leukemia Group B 9182 Study, *J Clin Oncol* 2506-2513, 1999.
63. Petrylak DP, Tangen C, Hussain M et al: SWOG- randomized phase III trial of docetaxel (D)/estra (E) versus mitoxantrone (M)/prednisone (p) in m androgen-independent prostate cancer (AIPCA *Am Soc Clin Oncol* 23:2, 2004 (abstract 3).
64. Beer TM, Eilers KM, Garzotto M et al: Weekly hi calcitriol and docetaxel in metastatic androgen-inde prostate cancer, *J Clin Oncol* 21(1):123-128, 2003.
65. Salimichokami M: Combining angiogenesis wit toxic chemotherapy enhances PSA response in h refractory prostate cancer (HRPC): a randomize of weekly docetaxel alone or in combination w lidomide, *Proc Am Soc Clin Oncol* 22:429, 2003 (1725).
66. George DJ, Halabi S, Shepard TF et al: Progno nificance of plasma vascular endothelial growt levels in patients with hormone-refractory prost cer treated on Cancer and Leukemia Group B 9 *Cancer Res* 7(7):1932-1936, 2001.

Assessment of malaise in cancer patients treated with radiotherapy, *Cancer Nurs* 8(6):306-313, 1985.

100. King KB, Nail L, Kreamer K et al: Patients' descriptions of the experience of receiving radiation therapy, *Oncol Nurs Forum* 12(4):55-61, 1985.
101. Monga U, Kerrigan AJ, Thornby J et al: Prospective study of fatigue in localized prostate cancer patients undergoing radiotherapy, *Radiat Oncol Investig* 7(3): 178-185, 1999.
102. Volpe HM: Radiation therapy. In Held-Warmkessel J, editor: *Contemporary issues in prostate cancer*, Sudbury, MA, 2000, Jones and Bartlett, pp 137-169.
103. Schwartz AL, Nail LM, Chen S et al: Fatigue patterns observed in patients receiving chemotherapy and radiotherapy, *CA Invest* 18(1):11-19, 2000.
104. Magnan MA, Mood DW: The effects of health state, hemoglobin, global symptom distress, mood disturbance, and treatment site on fatigue onset, duration, and distress in patients receiving radiation therapy, *Oncol Nurs Forum* 30(2):E33-E39, 2003.
105. Asbell SO, Leon SA, Tester WJ et al: Development of anemia and recovery in prostate cancer patients treated with combined androgen blockade and radiotherapy, *Prostate* 29(4):243-248, 1996.
106. Lynch MP, Jacobs LA: The assessment and diagnosis of anemia in the patient with cancer. In *Anemia and fatigue in cancer patients: nursing care management*, Newtown, PA, 1998, Associates in Medical Marketing, pp 10-17.
107. Moss VA: Assessing learning abilities, readiness for education, *Semin Perioper Nurs* 3(3):113-120, 1994.
108. Schoen EJ, Oehrli M, Colby CJ et al: The highly protective effect of newborn circumcision against invasive penile cancer, *Pediatrics* 105(3):E36, 2000.
109. Schrek R, Lenowitz H: Etiologic factors in carcinoma of the penis. *Cancer Res* 7:180-187, 1947.
110. Crawford ED, Dawkins CA: Cancer of the penis, In Skinner DG, Lieskovsky G, editors: *Diagnosis and management of genitourinary cancer,* Philadelphia, 1988, WB Saunders, pp 549-563.
111. Dalbagni G, Zhang Z-F, LaCombe L et al: Male urethra carcinoma: analysis of treatment outcome, *Urology* 53(6): 1126-1132, 1999.
112. Kaplan GW, Buckley GJ, Grayhack JT: Carcinoma of the male urethra, *J Urol* 98(3):365-371, 1967.
113. Barnes RD, Sarembock LA, Abratt RP et al: Carcinoma of the penis: the Groot Schuur Hospital experience, *J R Coll Surg Edinb* 34(1):44-46, 1989.
114. Hardner GJ, Bhanalaph T, Murphy GP et al: Carcinoma of the penis: an analysis of therapy in 100 consecutive cases, *J Urol* 108(3):428-430, 1972.
115. Mansur DB, Clifford Choa KS: Penis and male urethra. In Perez CA, Brady LW, Halperin EC et al, editors: *Principles and practice of radiation oncology,* ed 4, Philadelphia, 2004, Lippincott Williams & Wilkins, pp 1785-1799.
116. Graham JH, Helwig EB: Erythroplasia of Queyrat: a clinicopathologic and histochemical study, *Cancer* 32(6): 1396-1414, 1973.
117. Nichols P: Pathology of cancer of penis. In Skinner DG, Lieskovsky G, editors: *Diagnosis and management of genitourinary cancer*, Philadelphia, 1988, WB Saunders, pp 207-214.
118. Greenbaum SS, Krull EA, Simmons EB: Basal cell carcinoma at the base of the penis in a black patient, *J Am Acad Dermatol* 20:317-319, 1989.
119. Derakhshani P, Neubauer S, Braun M et al: Results and 10 year follow up in patients with squamous cell carcinoma of the penis, *Urol Int* 62(4):238-244, 1999.
120. Malcaluso JN Jr, Sullivan JW, Tomberlin S: Glomus tumor of glans penis, *Urology* 25(4):409-410, 1985.
121. Yu GSM, Nseyo UO, Carson JW: Primary penile lymphoma in a patient with Peyronie's disease, *J Urol* 142(4):1076-1077, 1989.
122. Grossman H: Premalignant carcinomas of the penis and scrotum, *Urol Clin North Am* 19(2):221, 1992.
123. Rozan R, Albuisson E, Giraud B et al: Interstitial brachytherapy for penile carcinoma: a multicentric survey (259 patients), *Radiother Oncol* 36(2):83-93, 1995.
124. Haddad F: Re: Cavernosography in diagnosis of metastatic tumors of the penis: 5 new cases and a review of the literature, *J Urol* 141(4):959-960, 1989 (letter).
125. de Kernion JB, Tynberg P, Persky L et al: Proceedings: carcinoma of the penis, *Cancer* 32(5):1256-1262, 1973.
126. Ekstrom T, Edsmyr F: Cancer of the penis: a clinical study of 229 cases, *Acta Chir Scand* 115(1-2):25-45, 1958.
127. Crook JM, Jezioranski J, Grimard L et al: Penile brachytherapy: results for 49 patients, *Int J Radiat Oncol Biol Phys* 62(2):460-467, 2005.
128. Eisenberger MA: Chemotherapy for prostate cancer, *NCI Monogr* (7):151-163, 1988.
129. Licht MR, Klein EA, Bukowski R et al: Combination radiation and chemotherapy for the treatment of squamous cell carcinoma of the male and female urethra, *J Urol* 153(6):1918-1920, 1995.
130. Chaudhary AJ, Ghosh S, Bhalavat RL et al: Interstitial brachytherapy in carcinoma of the penis, *Strahlenther Onkol* 175(1):17-20, 1999.
131. Shover LR: Counseling cancer patients about changes in sexual function, *Oncology* 13(11):1585-1591, 1999.
132. Bruner DW, Berk L: Altered body image and sexual health. In Yarbro CH, Frogge MH, Goodman M, editors: *Cancer symptom management,* ed 3, Sudbury, MA, 2004, Jones and Bartlett, pp 596-603.
133. Bruner DW: Sexual dysfunction. In Bruner DW, Haas ML, Gosselin-Acomb TK, editors: *Manual for radiation oncology nursing practice and education,* ed 3, Pittsburgh, 2005, Oncology Nursing Society, pp 61-66.
134. Zack E: Testicular germ cell cancer. In Henke-Yarbro C, Hansen-Frogge M, Goodman M, editors: *Cancer nursing,* ed 6, Boston, 2005, Jones and Bartlett; pp 1630-1646.
135. Moller H, Knudsen LB, Lynge E: Risk of testicular cancer after vasectomy: cohort study of over 73,000 men, *BMJ* 309(6950):295-299, 1994.
136. Hofer C, Kubler H, Hartung R et al: Diagnosis and monitoring of urological tumors using positron emission tomography, *Eur Urol* 40(5):481-487, 2001.
137. Poirier S, Rawl S: Testicular germ cell cancer. In Yarbro CH, Frogge MH, Goodman M, editors: *Cancer nursing practice and principles,* ed 5, Sudbury, MA, 2000, Jones and Bartlett, pp 1494-1510.
138. Morton GC, Thomas GM: Testis. In Perez CA, Brady LW, Halperin EC et al, editors: *Principles and practice of radiation oncology,* ed 4, Philadelphia, 2004, Lippincott Williams & Wilkins, pp 1763-1784.

139. Banduceau O, Souleau B, Le-Moulec S et al: Radiotherapy in stage I testicular seminoma: retrospective study and review of literature, *Cancer Radiother* 7(6):386-394, 2003.
140. National Comprehensive Cancer Network: *NCCN clinical practice guidelines in oncology: testicular cancer,* V.1.2007 (website): www.nccn.org/professionals/physician_gls/PDF/testicular.pdf. Accessed on December 1, 2005.
141. Sagerman RH, Kotlove DJ, Regine WF: Stage II seminoma: results of postorchiectomy irradiation, *Radiology* 172(2):565-568, 1989.
142. Thomas G, Jones W, VanOosterom A et al: Consensus statement on the investigation and management of testicular seminoma, *EORTC Genitourinary Group Monogr* 7:285-294, 1990.
143. Fossa SD, Aass N, Kaalhus O: Radiotherapy for testicular seminoma stage I: treatment results and long-term post-irradiation morbidity in 365 patients, *Int J Radiat Oncol Biol Phys* 16(2):383-388; 1989.
144. Holland J: Gastrointestinal/abdomen. In Bruner DW, Haas ML, Gosselin-Acomb TK, editors: *Manual for radiation oncology nursing practice and education,* ed 3, Pittsburgh, 2005, Oncology Nursing Society, pp 116-126.
145. Tack J, Lee KJ: Pathophysiology and treatment of functional dyspepsia, *J Clin Gastroenterol* 39(5 suppl): S211-S216, 2005.
146. Huddart RA, Norman A, Moynihan C et al: Fertility, gonadal and sexual function in survivors of testicular cancer, *Br J Cancer* 93(2):200-207, 2005.
147. Saito K, Suzuki K, Iwasaki A: Sperm cryopreservation before cancer chemotherapy helps in the emotional battle against cancer, *Cancer* 104(3):521-524, 2005.
148. Travis LB, Fossa SD, Schonfeld SJ et al: Second cancers among 40,576 testicular cancer patients: focus on long-term survivors, *J Natl Cancer Inst* 97(18):1354-1365, 2005.

Chapter 14

Spinal Cord and Bone Metastases

Diane Williams and Kathryn Burrows

Bone metastases are common and cause significant morbidity in cancer patients,[1,2] with 80% of patients with advanced cancer experiencing pain.[3] Cancers that have a greater propensity for bone metastases include breast, prostate, and lung.[3-5] Bone metastases occur in up to 75% of breast cancers; 68% of prostate cancers, and 30% to 40% of lung, renal, and thyroid cancers.[2] Cancers of the bladder, uterine, cervix, testis, colorectal, melanoma, lymphoma, and sarcoma metastasize to bone less commonly.[5-9]

People are living longer with metastatic bone disease. Survival depends on the type of primary cancer and areas of involvement.[2,3] Besides logistical and homecare considerations, these patients have the opportunity to develop more symptomatic metastases. Although the average survival time is 2 to 4 years for patients with secondary metastases to the bone resulting from breast, prostate, thyroid, and myeloma, for patients with lung and renal malignancies, the prognosis is 1 year or less.[3]

Because people are living longer with metastatic bone disease,[2] increased vigilance is required to detect new metastases. Adequate pain management is essential, as is awareness of additional potential problems such as hypercalcemia, pathologic fractures, bone marrow infiltration, impaired mobility, and spinal cord and nerve root compression.[1-3] Spinal cord compression is one of the most devastating complications of bone metastases because of its potential to induce paralysis if not treated in a timely manner. Unfortunately, as many as 10% of cancer patients experience spinal cord compression.[7,10-12] Therefore, it is essential that clinicians be aware of patients who are at high risk for spinal cord compression, as well as the sign's and symptoms. Early detection of spinal cord compression is crucial because time is of the essence in alerting physicians to changes with patients' conditions so as to decrease the risk of potential complications such as irreversible paralysis.

ANATOMY/PATHOPHYSIOLOGY

Bone

Living bone is a specific connective tissue that consists of bone cells that play a part in bone formation and maintenance and of an organic matrix that is made up of collagen fibers, proteins, and mineral elements such as calcium and phosphate. The minerals crystallize amongst the collagen fibers to give the bone its typical hardness and strength. Cells consist of osteoblasts that form bone. Osteoclasts are destructive or lytic cells whose function is to remove (resorb) bone during the process of growth and repair and to help with mineral homeostasis. Osteoblasts stimulate the resorptive activity of the osteoclasts. Osteocytes are osteoblasts that maintain the bone matrix. Hormones and local factors, such as weight bearing, muscle contractions, and stress, control the function of the osteoblasts and osteoclasts and determine the scaffold structure of bone. Both types of cells are involved in bone remodeling. This is undertaken to replace any bone matrix that has developed defects from normal use; bone remodeling also plays a role in mineral homeostasis. At any given time, only 10% of the skeleton is undergoing active remodeling.[4,13,14]

Bone is composed of two forms of bony tissue—compact bone and spongy bone. Compact bone is solid, strong, and highly organized. The haversian system is the basic structural unit. It is composed of the haversian canal, channels in the bone that contain blood vessels and nerves and run throughout the long axis of the bone. The blood vessels within the canal communicate with the periosteum (a connective tissue that covers all the bones) and the marrow cavity. They transport nutrients and waste to and from the osteocytes contained in the lacunae, which are tiny spaces that each contain one osteocyte. These lacunae are found throughout the concentric layers of the crystallized matrix, called *lamellae*. Small canals called *canaliculi* connect the lacunae.[14] Spongy bone also has lamellae; however, these are arranged irregularly in plates or bars called *trabeculae* that branch and unite to establish an irregular meshwork. Red bone marrow fills the trabeculae spaces. The lacunae that contain osteocytes are dispersed between the trabeculae and connected by the canaliculi. Capillaries passing through the marrow nourish the osteocytes.[14]

The Vertebral Column and Spinal Cord

The vertebral column is composed of 33 vertebrae supported by ligaments and muscles. There are 7 cervical, 12 thoracic, 5 lumbar, 5 sacral, and 5 coccygeal vertebrae. The sacral and coccygeal vertebrae are fused into the sacrum and coccyx in that order.[7] The spinal cord is approximately 10 inches shorter than the vertebral column and stops at L1-L2, where it expands to form the conus medullary from where the lumbar and sacral spinal nerve roots exit. These long nerve roots resemble a horse's tail hair. They are known as the *caudal equine*.[5]

Thirty-one pairs of spinal nerves exit the spinal cord. Each spinal nerve is made up of the dorsal root, which conducts sensory or afferent impulses, and the ventral root, which transmits sensory information from the body to the spinal cord. Motor, or efferent, stimuli, as well as autonomic impulses, exit the spinal cord through a spinal nerve ventral root, transmitting the impulse from the spinal cord back to the body.[5] The impulses that go back and forth from the brain travel in both the ascending and descending tracts, which stretch the span of the spinal cord. Impulses that originate from the spinal cord going to the brain are transmitted via the anterior spinothalamic tracts. Impulses returning from the brain bound for the spinal cord are transmitted by means of the lateral corticospinal tract. Any injury sustained by either the spinal nerves or cord, can result in a sensory-motor and autonomic impairment.[5] The bony spinal column surrounds the spinal cord to provide mechanical protection. The spinal cord additionally has three protective membranes called *meninges,* or *leptomeninges*. The outer layer is the dura mater, the middle layer is the arachnoid membrane, and the inner most layer is the pia mater (Figure 14-1).[7,15] These membranes are continuous with the coverings of the brain.

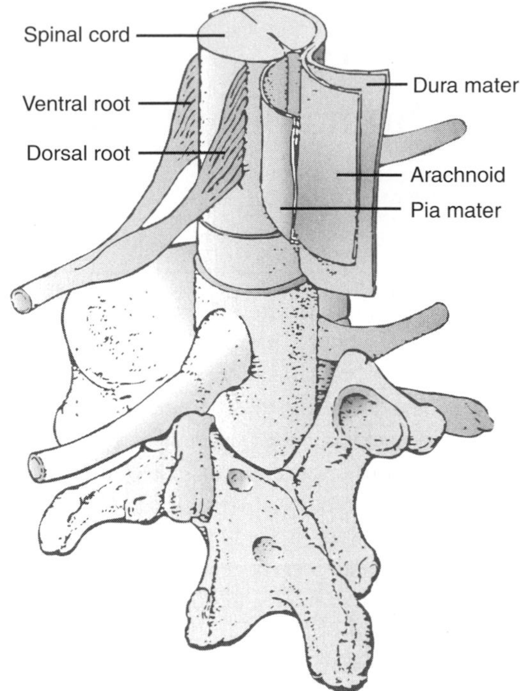

Figure 14-1 Diagram of the Meninges.
From Hickey JV: The clinical practice of neurological and neurosurgical nursing, ed. 3, Philadelphia, Lippincott, 1992.

The epidural or extradural space lies between the vertebral column bony walls and the external surface of the dura mater (Figure 14-2). The subdural space is present between the inner layer of the dura and the arachnoid membrane. The subarachnoid space, which contains cerebrospinal fluid, lies between the arachnoid membrane and the pia mater.[7]

CLINICAL MANIFESTATIONS

Pain from bone metastases can develop over time and becomes progressively worse. There are many descriptions of bone pain. It can be depicted as aching, deep, constant, dull, and stabbing in nature. Patients may have referred pain or neuropathic pain, especially with nerve root involvement. The pain is usually localized to a specific area. It may be worse during the night and may be exacerbated with weight-bearing activity.[4,5,9,16]

Patients with spinal cord compression (SCC) may present with back pain that may predate the onset of neurologic deficits by days or even months. Fast-growing tumors can progress swiftly and

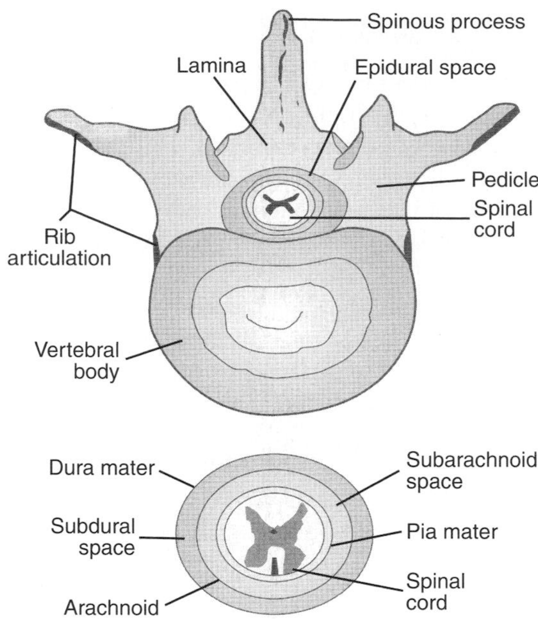

Figure 14-2 Cross Section of the Spinal Cord and Vertebrae
From Myers J: Oncologic complications—spinal cord compression. In Otto S, editor: Oncology nursing, ed 4, St Louis, 2001, Mosby, pp 513-518.

compress the blood supply to the spinal cord to the point that irreversible paraplegia can occur in just hours or days after the initial onset of a neurologic deficit.[7,9] The cardinal signs of SCC are pain, motor weakness, sensory deficit, and autonomic dysfunction.[5,7,15] Pain in the region of the back is the most common presenting complaint. Pain is either localized or has a radicular component depending on the level of spine that is involved. It may involve dermatomes and may be made worse by activity such as sneezing, coughing, lying down, or straight-leg raises. Patients may complain of feeling a band-like sensation or constriction around their chest or abdomen.[5,7,9,15,17]

Motor weakness may be a minor complaint. Myers[7] noted that on initial examination, between 75% and 86% of patients will have subtle motor defects. Patients may complain of a stiffness or heaviness in one or both of the extremities, or difficulty climbing stairs. They may have problems with walking, experiencing ataxia, unsteady gait, or may drag or favor the affected limbs.[5,7,15] With regard to sensory loss, patients may complain of numbness, tingling, paresthesia, and a loss of thermal sensation. Progressive sensory loss ultimately results in a loss of proprioception, deep pressure, and vibration sensation. Autonomic dysfunction emerges as the compression progresses. Urinary symptoms of hesitancy and retention are followed with overflow incontinence. Bowel dysfunction presents as the lack of urge to defecate and inability to bear down, which results in constipation, incontinence, and spurious diarrhea. Loss of control of the anal sphincter is a sign of poor prognosis.[5,7,9,15]

DIAGNOSIS/DIAGNOSTIC STUDIES

Before any diagnostic tests are undertaken, it is essential that a thorough history and physical examination be undertaken. Complaints of changes in mobility, or back/neck pain warrant a comprehensive neurologic examination, especially if SCC is suspected. Physical findings can reveal an irregularity of the spinal curvature and tenderness at the level of the bone metastases, and neurologic examination may reveal a sensory defect level. Radicular pain increases with spinal movement and when straight-leg raises are performed. Motor and sensory involvement exhibits signs such as positive Babinski signs, hyperactive reflexes, and variable spastic weakness in addition to bilateral sensory loss, which occurs below the level of the cord compression. Bladder and bowel problems also may be detected, such as urinary incontinence or retention, the inability to bear down resulting in constipation, and the lack of urge to defecate.[5,7]

Radiographic evaluation for bone metastases and potential SCC usually begins with plain x rays, bone scan, myelogram, magnetic resonance imaging (MRI), or computerized tomography (CT) scan.

Plain X Rays

X rays will reveal epidural metastatic sites indirectly in 83% to 85% of cases as being osteolytic or osteoblastic lesions, vertebral body collapse, or erosion of pedicles (Figure 14-3).[7,15] However, x rays will be positive only if over half of the bone volume is affected by metastases.[5,9,15] Additionally, tumors could be present for 6 months without obvious changes on the x ray, and paraspinal masses with transforminal extension may go undetected.[7,12]

Bone Scan

Bone scan is a sensitive diagnostic tool for detecting bone metastases. It can reveal bone metastases as small as 2 mm in size[9] and may identify metastases

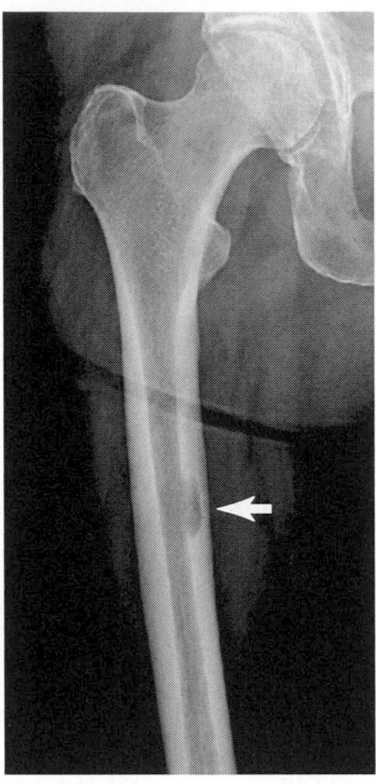

Figure 14-3 X Ray of a Lytic Lesion of the Femur. *Courtesy of Princess Margaret Hospital, University Health Network, Toronto, Ontario, Canada.*

6 months before a conventional x ray.[7] However, bone scans are not helpful in diagnosing possible areas of SCC. The scan can identify the bone changes but cannot identify the level of bony destruction or degree of epidural cord compression (Figure 14-4). False positives can occur because a bone scan can highlight osteoblastic activity associated with diseases such as arthritis and Paget's disease and with trauma. It also can have false-negative results in some lytic lesions, (e.g., myeloma).[9,15]

Magnetic Resonance Imaging

Magnetic resonance imaging (MRI) has now emerged as the preferred diagnostic test to rule out SCC. It is noninvasive and can identify cord compression, soft tissue masses, lesions in the cord, and bone metastases (Figure 14-5). It can also differentiate between extradural, extramedullary, and intradural lesions. MRIs are usually performed both with and without gadolinium, because leptomeningeal disease, paravertebral masses, and intramedullary tumors are visualized better.[7,8,12,15] However, there are some drawbacks, as listed below:

- If the patient suffers from claustrophobia, he may not be able to tolerate the procedure. This may be alleviated by the patient having the MRI performed at a center with an "open" MRI machine.[15]
- If the patient has a lot of pain, he may not be able to lie still in the same position for the duration of the test (estimated length of a study can be between 30 and 45 minutes).
- If the patient has mechanical valves, pacemakers, or other metal implants, MRI cannot be undertaken.[7,8]
- The machine tends to produce a lot of noise during the procedure. If the patient has a low tolerance for noise, the patient must be informed of this before treatment.

Computerized Tomography

Computerized tomography (CT) is superior to MRI in evaluating bone destruction and vertebral instability but not in evaluating epidural disease (Figure 14-6). It also can delineate paraspinal tumors that could extend into the epidural space and can help distinguish osteoporosis from tumor.[7]

Myelogram With CT

Myelogram with computerized axial tomography gives information that is comparable to that of an MRI. During this study, contrast media is injected via lumbar puncture into the subarachnoid space, and the fluid column is then observed for flow defects and filling. One advantage of this study is that cerebral spinal fluid, which is withdrawn before injecting the contrast medium, can be analyzed for the presence of meningeal carcinomatosis. However, some risks are associated with this procedure. It is invasive and there is risk of infection and bleeding.[7,15] Adequate blood supply coagulation and renal function must be present (to ensure elimination of the contrast dye).

PATHOLOGY AND PATTERNS OF METASTASES

Cancer cells disengage/separate from the primary malignancy and enter the blood circulation. After surviving the immune system, they transplant themselves to distant bony sites where they start to grow. The tumor cells cause bone destruction by stimulating osteoclasts. A variety of substances are produced, such as transforming growth factors, prostaglandins, parathyroid hormone–related protein, and other cytokines. These substances act either directly on the osteoclast to stimulate

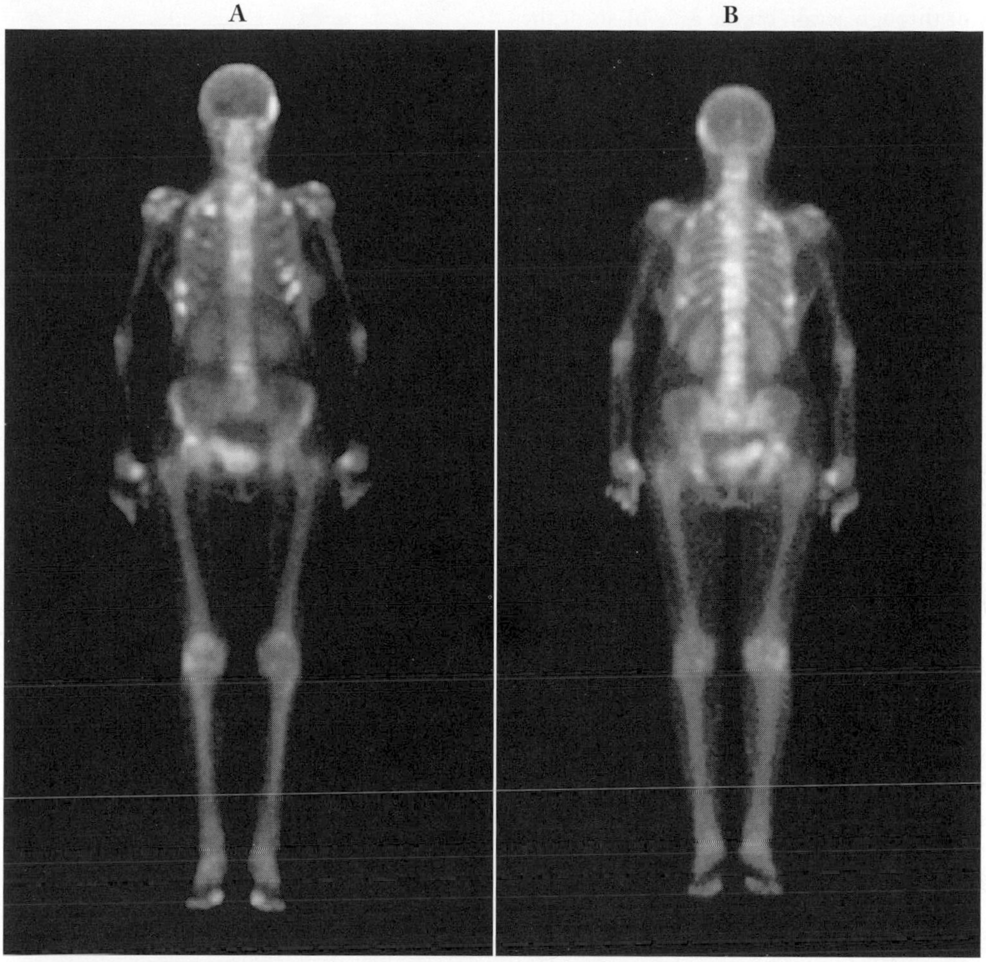

A B

Figure 14-4 Bone Metastases. **A,** Anterior bone scan highlighting bone metastases. **B,** Posterior bone scan highlighting bone metastases.
Courtesy of Princess Margaret Hospital, University Health Network, Toronto, Ontario, Canada.

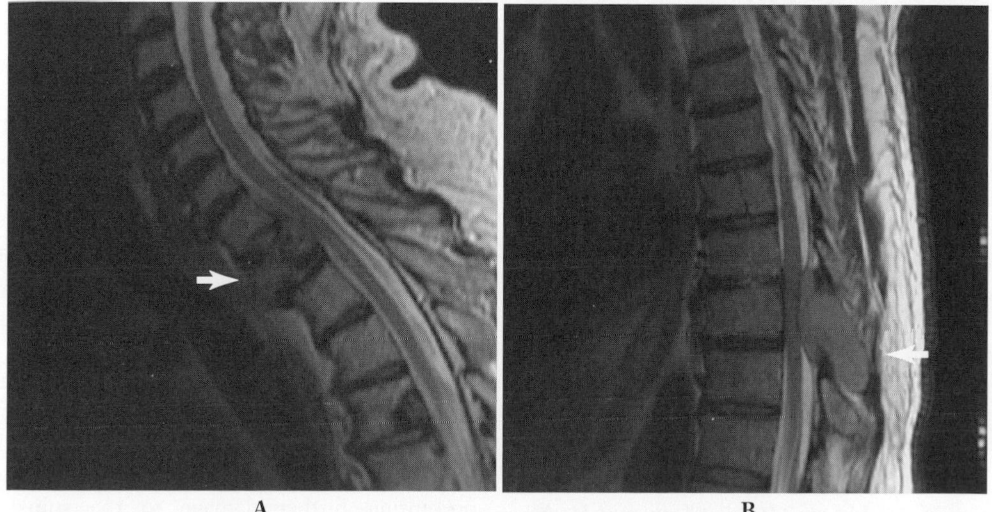

A B

Figure 14-5 Spinal Cord Compression. **A** and **B,** MRIs of spinal cord compression.
Courtesy of Princess Margaret Hospital, University Health Network, Toronto, Ontario, Canada.

activity or through action on the osteoblasts or the immune cells.[4,9,14,16]

Metastases to the bone are known by the terms *lytic, blastic,* or *mixed* depending on the appearance of the bones on x-ray film. Where bone resorption is prevalent, bone destruction occurs, and the lesion has the appearance of being lytic. These lesions have a higher risk of fracture. They are common in myeloma patients.[3,4] If increased osteoblastic activity occurs, then the lesions are sclerotic and appear as composite deposition on the bone. For example, patients who have prostate cancer can present with sclerotic bone metastases caused by the increasing osteoblastic activity. As a result, the serum alkaline phosphates will be elevated. The unstable bone matrix results in a risk of fracture. Metastases from breast cancer can have mixed lesions presenting with both sclerotic and lytic metastases.[4,9]

The most common site of skeletal metastases is the vertebral column—the thoracic spine being the most commonly affected (70%), followed by lumbar spine (20%), and the cervical spine (10%) (Figure 14-7).[10] Extradural or epidural metastases are the most common causes of SCC and arise from direct extension of the metastases within the vertebral body into the epidural space. The spinal cord can be compressed when a pathologic fracture involving the vertebral body is infiltrated by tumor. This can result in a cord injury caused by pressure from bone fragments or instability of the spine.

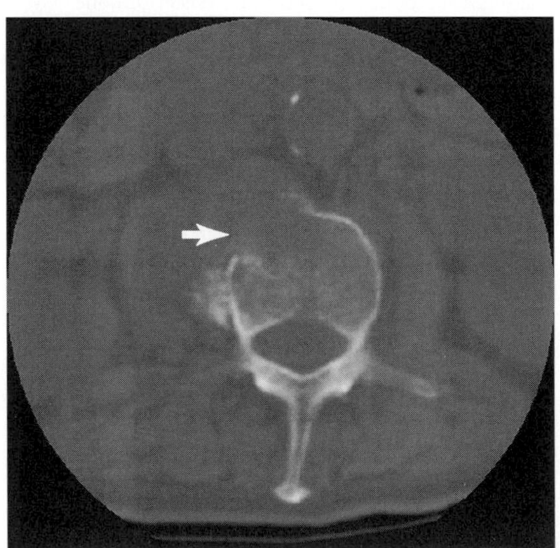

Figure 14-6 CT Scan Showing L-Spine Metastases. *Courtesy of Princess Margaret Hospital, University Health Network, Toronto, Ontario, Canada.*

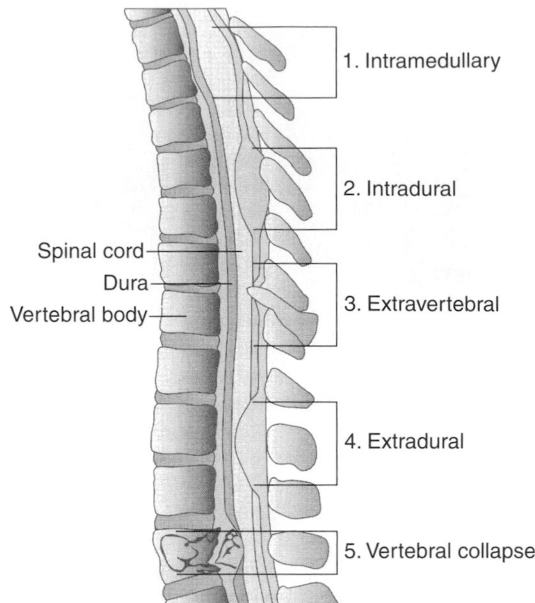

Figure 14-7 Malignant Invasion of the Spinal Cord. *From Myers J: Oncologic complications—spinal cord compression. In Otto S, editor: Oncology nursing, ed 4, St Louis, 2001, Mosby, pp 513-518.*

Paraspinal tumors can cause cord compression as they grow in the intervertebral foramen. Tumors that develop in the spinal cord are called *intramedullary*. Intradural tumors occur in the meninges or nerve roots. Both types are less common.[5,7,12,15,17]

TREATMENT

Pain Management

Pain and symptom management are major concerns.[18] In clinical practice, the incidence of pain in patients related to bone metastases is high.[3,19] Pain management strategies need to be the first priority of care.[20-23] Aggressive pain management does not prevent detection of the underlying problem. Providing pain relief and symptom control will contribute significantly to an increase in patients' quality of life.

Steroids

Corticosteroids are prescribed for patients with spinal cord compression (SCC) and severe unrelieved pain from bone metastases. The steroids help with pain management by reducing spinal cord edema, preventing further damage to the spinal cord, and improving neurologic function. Steroids are prescribed for the acute management of SCC and should be instituted immediately if SCC is suspected until more definitive therapy is initiated. The customary dosing for the dexamethasone (Decadron) is 10 mg intravenously as a bolus followed by 4 mg PO every 6 hours. If steroids are given for severe pain without the complication of SCC, the dose is usually lower, such as 4 mg Decadron daily. Heimdal et al[24] evaluated high-dose dexamethasone (96 mg IV bolus, which was tapered down to 0 by 14 days) for patients with SCC. Because of serious side effects, standardized therapy of 16 mg of dexamethasone daily was implemented. Improved neurologic recovery was not evident in daily dosages above 16 mg. However, a randomized single-blind trial by Sorensen et al[25] of high-dose dexamethasone in addition to treatment with radiation in patients with SCC found that the high-dose steroids improved neurologic and pain outcomes. Few severe side effects were observed with the shortened course of higher-dose dexamethasone. It was noted that if dexamethasone was used longer than 3 weeks, the toxicity level increased 76%.[25] Consequently, tapering with a plan to discontinue the medication should be commenced if the patient's neurologic condition has improved or stabilized. If during the medication taper the patient's symptoms become worse, the dose of dexamethasone should be increased until the patient is restabilized. A slower taper should be initiated because the long-term use of high-dose steroids results in an increased risk of hyperglycemia, gastric ulceration, hallucinations, oral candidiasis, proximal myopathy, psychosis, and weight gain.[12,15,24,25]

Bisphosphonates

Bisphosphonates are bone resorption inhibitors used in the treatment of malignancy-induced hypercalcemia. In addition to hypercalcemia, bisphosphonates also reduce the incidence of skeletal events such pathologic fractures and bone pain. However, they are not used in the acute management of patients with SCC. Bisphosphonates can be used orally daily or intravenously every 3 to 4 weeks (Table 14-1).[12,15,26-29]

Percutaneous Vertebroplasty

Percutaneous vertebroplasty is a relatively new interventional procedure where a percutaneous injection of acrylic cement or polymethylmethacrylate (PMMA) is injected into a vertebral body with the aid of either fluoroscopy or computed tomography.[30] The PMMA is an acrylic polymer that is activated by a liquid monomer and barium sulfate for opacification,[31] which is then injected into a diseased, collapsed vertebra. PMMA has exceptional compressive strength; after the vertebral body is filled, it hardens like a cement.[31] It provides mechanical stabilization within the vertebral body and also provides pain relief.[31] A study undertaken by Chow et al[31] looked at 15 cancer patients who had procedures performed for pain despite palliative radiation therapy for spinal metastases or for osteoporotic compression fractures. The study demonstrated that the procedure significantly lessened pain and improved mobility and quality of life. However, it was a small study, and further research needs to be performed in a variety of patients to establish guidelines for use.

Table 14-1 Current Bisphosphonates and Recommended Treatment Schedules

Bisphosphonate	Dosage	Schedule
Pamidronate (Aredia)	90 mg IV	Q 3–4 weeks
Zoledronic acid (Zometa)	4 mg IV	Q 3–4 weeks
Clodronate (Bonefos)	1600 mg PO	Daily
Ibandronate (Bondronat)	6 mg IV	Q 3–4 weeks
Ibandronate (Bondronat)	50 mg PO	Daily

Data from Pavlakis N, Stockler M: Bisphosphonates for breast cancer, *Cochrane Database Syst Rev* (Online) (1):CD003474; Saad F, Karakiewicz P, Perrotte P: *World J Urol* 23(1):14-18, 2005.

Chemotherapy/Hormonal Therapy

In SCC, chemotherapy may be an effective treatment in exceptionally chemosensitive tumors such as non-Hodgkin's lymphoma.[12,15] However, for the majority of patients, chemotherapy and hormone therapy are used primarily as adjuvant treatment. Caution must be exercised if chemotherapy is given along with radiation because it may increase acute side effects, particularly with anthrocycline derivatives such as taxanes, doxorubicin, and mitoxantrone that induce radiosensitization.[19] Hormone therapy such as estrogen suppression may be a treatment option for patients with breast and prostate cancers.[15]

Radiation Treatment

Radiation treatment is an effective form of therapy for patients with bone metastases because it can palliate symptoms and prevent complications. A number of indications have been reported, including the following[3,32,33]:

- To relieve pain related to either single or multiple bone metastases
- To prevent pathologic fracture in bones that are weight bearing (e.g., femur)
- To prevent SCC and neurologic dysfunction
- To prevent progression of metastases at sites where surgery has been recently performed to treat pathologic fractures and SCC

The dose and fractionation schedules vary widely. They can range from 8 Gy in 1 fraction to 20 Gy in 5 fractions and 30 Gy in 10 fractions. More radical doses such as 40 Gy in 20 fractions also have been employed.[15,33] Practice guidelines produced by Cancer Care Ontario[34] recommended that a single dose of 8 Gy should be administered for uncomplicated bone metastases. The recommendation does not apply to bone metastases in the skull or in the hands or feet or to lesions causing pathologic fractures or cord caudal equina compression. van den Hout and colleagues[35] investigated multiple versus single fractionation schedules for painful bone metastases and found that a single fraction provided equal palliation with regard to pain management; side effects of treatment and quality of life were similar as compared with multiple fraction. However, with single fraction treatment, there was a greater need for retreatment. Hartsell et al.[36] investigated single fraction (8 Gy) versus 30 Gy in 10 fractions and concluded that both were equivalent with regard to pain management. However, as with van den Hout et al.,[35] there were more retreatments in patient's who had a single fraction. A meta-analysis[37] of clinical trials looking at the dose fractionation with regard to pain response for patients with painful bone metastases found differences between single versus multiple fractions with regard to pain relief and side effects of therapy, but confirmed the higher pain relapse rate. Currently, the National Cancer Institute of Canada Clinical Trials Group is conducting a phase III international, randomized clinical trial investigating re-irradiation of painful bone metastases using single versus multiple fractions.[38] The National Cancer Institute at present has a supportive care clinical trial comparing ibandronate (Boniva) with a single dose of local radiation therapy in patient's with localized metastatic bone pain.[39] Additionally, a phase I/II study is looking at radiofrequency ablation in treating patients with bone metastases.[40]

The conventional treatment for patients with SCC is external-beam radiation therapy (EBRT). The treatment volume extends one to two vertebral bodies above and below the site of metastases or cord compression to encompass the epidural tumor extent.[7,15] Standard treatments include 20 Gy, in 5 fractions, 30 Gy in 10 fractions, or 40 Gy in 20 fraction.[12,15,33] Palliative radiation is preferred over surgical decompression if the patient:

- Has a radiosensitive tumor such as myeloma, breast cancer, prostate cancer, lymphoma, or small cell lung cancer
- Is not a candidate for surgical intervention because of general debility or additional comorbid conditions
- Has a limited life expectancy in the range of a few days or few weeks
- Has extensive metastases of the vertebrae or epidural region that would thwart surgical stabilization
- Presents with a long-standing, established, neurologic loss of function but has constant pain in the region of the SCC.[33,41]

The most significant prediction of neurologic outcome after radiation for SCC is ambulatory status at time of therapy. Kirkbride and Bezjak[41] note that 89% of patients who were ambulatory continue to be so after treatment and 53% of patients with weakness were able to walk again after treatment. However, only 10% of paraplegic patients regained mobility after therapy. Side effects of treatment (such as nausea, vomiting, and increases in the pain for 24 to 48 hours after radiation therapy) depend on the volume of radiation and can be anticipated in advance and are usually minimal.

If a patient develops recurrent pain as a result of bone metastases in an area previously treated, retreatment is often possible. Factors to be considered are the interval since the last course of radiation therapy, previous dose and fractionation schedule, the specific region treated, and the anticipated long-term effects if treatment is repeated. If a patient has had previous treatment to the spine and develops a SCC, additional radiation therapy may be provided. However, smaller fraction sizes to prevent long-term complications such as myelopathy need to be considered. Radiation oncologists should not dismiss lightly the risk of paralysis. The risks of treatment versus the possible benefits should be weighed carefully.[15,41]

For patients with multiple bone metastases, hemibody irradiation or systematically administered bone-seeking radiopharmaceuticals such as strontium-89 are an option. Hemibody involves radiation therapy to a large volume of the body, either the upper or lower half. Treatment is given as a single fraction. However, the incidence of toxic side effects is much higher with this treatment. Therefore it is usually held in reserve for patients who require prompt relief for widespread painful metastatic bone disease.[32,42,43]

Radioisotopes commonly used for alleviating pain as a result of metastatic disease to the bone are strontium-89 or samarium-153. Silberstein[19] notes that radioisotopes can diminish or eliminate the pain caused by osteoblastic metastases by 55% to 80%. Side effects of therapy include pain flare-ups and myelosuppression. The pain management effect of radiation is not permanent (it can last weeks or months), therefore, treatment may need to be repeated.[3,19,43]

Spinal Surgery

Improvements in the quality of imaging with MRI and the introduction of new surgical techniques allow an increasing role for surgery, which can be employed earlier in the management of SCC. The aim of surgery is to achieve decompression of the spinal cord by tumor resection, followed by reconstruction and stabilization of the vertebral column.

Surgery is indicated under the following conditions[7,10,15]:

- If spinal instability or vertebral collapse results in significant neural compromise
- If there is no pathologic diagnosis and tissue is required for histology
- If rapid neurologic deterioration is noted in a patient on steroids
- If prior radiation has been given to the spine and the patient is unable to have further treatment (due to the maximum tissue tolerance)
- If the tumor is radioresistant
- If a solitary recurrence is found in the spinal cord
- If intractable pain is unresponsive to other therapies

Although patients may satisfy the above criteria, it is necessary to determine whether they are fit for surgery; their expected life expectancy also should be considered.[10] Surgery is usually followed by radiation therapy with the aim of eradicating any tumor that remained in the surgical bed. Flaherty[15] suggests that an appropriate time interval between surgery and radiation is 4 weeks.

NURSING INTERVENTIONS AND EDUCATION

The life expectancy of patients with spinal cord compression is generally short and measured in months. Certain patients, especially those with breast and prostate primaries, can live longer in the absence of metastatic disease.[44] Patients needing treatment may originate from Hospice programs, general or oncology hospital settings, or as an ambulatory care patient living at home. Therefore, nursing interventions and education must be a collaborative approach between a number of healthcare providers, the patient, and the family. At initial assessment, the clinician needs to undertake a comprehensive holistic assessment. Early detection by clinicians of patients at risk for SCC can prevent devastating problems such as paralysis leading to immobility and bowel and bladder dysfunction. The goal of monitoring and treating patients is to preserve or improve quality of life. Thus the nursing assessment focuses on the physical well-being of the patient—psychological well-being, social well-being, and spiritual well-being.[45] The symptoms and functional aspects that are of specific relevance to patients with bone metastases and/or SCC are described below in more detail.

Pain

Pain is the most common problem associated with bone metastases and SCC. Oncology clinicians require extensive knowledge regarding pain management and ways of ameliorating medication side effects such as drowsiness, nausea/vomiting, constipation, or hallucinations. Complementary therapies such as massage also may be beneficial.[15] Optimal management of pain should improve patients quality of life and functioning. Patients and families need to be educated about the possibility of pain flare (increase in pain) related to radiation therapy, and the use of breakthrough analgesics. The effectiveness of pain management must be reassessed approximately 2 to 4 weeks after radiation so as to reduce analgesia if there has been a response to radiation therapy. Many patients require a combination of opioids and co-analgesics such as nonsteroidal antiinflammatory drugs, steroids, or medications for neuropathic pain.[15] Please refer to Chapter 31 for further information regarding pain management.

Mobility

Paralysis/paresis is one of the most dreaded complications of SCC. It greatly impacts on patients' quality of life and leads to life-threatening complications (e.g., deep vein thrombosis (DVTs) or infections). Patients with impaired mobility should be referred to a physical/occupational therapist for assessment because they may require equipment/devices to help maintain stability, spinal alignment, strength, range of motion, and mobility. The establishment of a physician-recommended, patient-specific activity regimen is also important. The patient may require assistance with transfer and ambulation, and an antiembolic stocking may be required. It is important to encourage patients to perform activities of daily living if they are able to do so. In addition, home assessment in regard to equipment and environmental mobility concerns is important as well.[7,15] If the patient is at risk of injury because of paralysis, safety must be a high priority at all times. It may be necessary to assess the patient and reorganize the environment to prevent thermal, physical, and chemical hazards from becoming a problem.[7,15]

Respiratory Problems

If the level of cord compression is in a region that affects breathing, monitoring of vital signs and respiratory status is of monumental importance. If necessary, mechanical respiratory support may have to be implemented. It is also necessary to reposition the patient every 2 hours and encourage deep breathing exercises and coughing. If necessary, discuss with a physician more aggressive measures such as physiotherapy to chest and incentive spirometry.[7]

Bladder Dysfunction

Patients may develop bladder dysfunction as one of the signs of cord compression. Symptoms and signs to watch for are urinary incontinence, retention, or frequency. Even in patients with incontinence or frequency, the bladder often will be distended and palpable as a suprapubic mass. Percussion above the symphysis pubis reveals dullness rather than the usual hollow (tympanic sound). Urinary catheterization should be done after an attempt to void. Residual of 400 mL indicates urinary retention. In such a case, an indwelling catheter may be required to empty the bladder and maintain continence. Patients should be observed for early signs of urinary tract infection and treated accordingly. Fluid intake and output must be monitored. The use of cranberry juice can be given to maintain the acidity of the urine. After completion of treatment, patients may require bladder training and assessment concerning the possibility of removing the catheter. In addition, it is important to maintain perineal care.[7,15]

Bowel Dysfunction

Bowel disturbances can occur as a result of both autonomic dysfunction and the use of opioids. They may range from slowing of the transit tissue to constipation to fecal incontinence. It is essential to preserve regular bowel elimination so as to avoid ileus and constipation. Patients require a combination of stool softeners such as docusate, laxatives such as senna or milk of magnesium, and suppositories or enemas if no bowel movement occurs for 4 to 5 days. Patient diets require high fiber such as fresh fruit and vegetables and high-fiber bread and cereals, in addition to adequate amounts of fluid. Perineal hygiene also must be maintained.[7,15]

Radiation-Induced Side Effects and Radiopharmaceuticals

Radiation side effects of therapy depend on the area treated. For example, radiation to the cervical and upper to mid thoracic spine can cause esophagitis because the esophagus is immediately anterior to the vertebral column, whereas radiation to the lower thoracic and lumber spine can cause nausea and vomiting because of the proximity of stomach and bowel. Additionally, treatment to the lumbar-sacral and pelvic region can produce diarrhea. Nausea and vomiting are typically seen on the day of treatment, whereas esophagitis and diarrhea occur 5 to 8 days after start of treatment. Nausea, vomiting, and diarrhea are addressed in more detail in Chapter 34.

Esophagitis after palliative radiation treatment is usually short lived, typically 5 to 7 days in duration. Patients may require instruction regarding eating small, frequent meals of nonirritating soft food, particularly avoiding high-acid and spicy food. Patients also may require instruction regarding the use of protein-rich food, commercial food supplements, an increase in oral fluids, and the avoidance of alcohol and tobacco. One should be vigilant for presence of infections because they may add to dysphagia and prolong the course of symptoms. Referral to a dietician may be helpful. Analgesics, antacids, sucralfate suspension, and Xylocaine-containing mouthwashes may provide symptomatic relief.

Treatment by radiopharmaceuticals, such as strontium and samarium, are undertaken in either a nuclear medicine or radiation oncology outpatient department and follows appropriate nuclear regulatory measures. The entire procedure takes less than an hour.[46,47] The radiopharmaceutical infusion, administered with a freely running intravenous line, takes approximately 1 to 3 minutes. During treatment, facial flushing can occur and may be minimized by injecting the radiopharmaceutical over a longer period of time.[46-47] Although monitoring is not necessary, a patient may be discharged after a short observation period. Patients need to be informed of the purpose of the therapy and the potential side effects of the treatment, such as myelosuppression (predominantly thrombocytopenia and leukopenia) and flare up of pain.[46-48]

The posttreatment therapy response may be dramatic (i.e., within days), although it averages 1 to 4 weeks.[46,48] Response duration is typically 2 to 12 months, with a median of 3 to 4 months.[49,50] Treatment may be repeated within 3 to 6 months and administered multiple times presuming there are no contraindications such as disseminated intravascular coagulation, compromised bone marrow from disease infiltration, or previous therapy. Caution is also required in patients with renal insufficiency. Treatment is not indicated for patients with SCC, pathologic fractures, or patients who are pregnant.[46] A platelet count of no less than 60,000/mL and a white blood count of at least 2400/mL is also required.[46,47]

The risk to nursing staff is minimal while monitoring patients posttreatment. However, nursing staff need to adhere to universal precautions when dealing with bodily fluids. Patients should be instructed to flush the toilet and wash their hands twice after voiding and defecation. Spilled urine or stool needs to be wiped up immediately. Incontinent patients should be catheterized. Caregivers who handle urine and stool need to wear gloves. Soiled linens and clothes should be washed separately. Precautions need to be observed for a period of at least 2 weeks for strontium and 24 hours for samarium-153 lexidronam.[46,47,50]

Analgesic adjustments are required for the treatment of pain flare-up. Additionally, the assessment and tapering of analgesics is required once the radiopharmaceutical takes effect. Clinicians also need to ensure that blood counts are monitored biweekly until there is an acceptable bone marrow recovery. For the most part, it is rare that treatment-induced myelosuppression will lead to life-threatening thrombocytopenia or leukopenia.[19,46-48,50]

Skin Integrity

Skin care at the site of radiation and integrity issues resulting from immobility are a concern. During radiation, the treatment site can be washed gently with either water or water and mild soap. Skin should be patted dry.[51] Cancer Care Ontario guidelines for the management of acute skin reactions related to radiation could not support or refute the use of topical agents.[51] Flaherty[15] suggests a water-soluble lotion such as Aquafor. However, aloe vera gel may be applied on an as-needed basis to the affected area 3 to 4 times a day.[52] With shorter fractionation doses, typically the reaction is the equivalent to a mild sunburn with redness and slight discomfort. If a patient is immobilized because of SCC, skin integrity must be observed for breakdown, particularly areas over bony prominences. The appropriate skin care protocols should be implemented, as well as the use of a pressure-reducing mattress and frequent repositioning.[7,15] For additional measures to treat radiodermatitis, refer to Chapter 30.

Mutually Agreed Plan of Care

The plan of care must be mutually developed with the patient and family, evaluated and adjusted according to changes in patients' clinical condition.[53,54] Patients need to understand why the radiation treatment is being given. Studies by Chow et al.[55] and Koller et al.[56] investigating patient expectations of radiation therapy found that patients possessed both misconceptions regarding their illness and unrealistic expectations regarding treatment. Clinicians must evaluate and acknowledge the caregiver needs in addition

Table 14-2 Resources for Patients and Their Caregivers

Organization	Contact information
American Academy of Hospice and Palliative Medicine	www.aahpm.org
American Cancer Society	www.cancer.org
Canadian Hospice Palliative Care Association	www.chpca.net
Caring To The End of Life. Princess Margaret Hospital	www.caringtotheend.ca
Bone Metastases Clinic, Toronto Sunnybrook Regional Cancer Centre: Helping You to Help Yourself: An educational binder for patients and families to help them understand, live and cope with bone metastases, 2004	Diane Dilnot, Toronto Sunnybrook Regional Cancer Centre, 2075 Bayview Avenue, Toronto M4N 3M5; fax: 416-480-4180
Willow Breast Cancer Support Canada: Living With Metastatic Cancer:	www.willow.org/info/prs1.asp
National Hospice and Palliative Care Organization	www.nhpco.org
Palliative Care	www.palliativecarenursing.net

to the needs of the patients. Patient caregivers face the emotional, financial, and physical stress of caring for an ill family member in addition to the pressure of meeting their own needs and responsibilities.[22,53,54,57,58]

An interdisciplinary approach that includes nurses, physicians, radiation therapists, dieticians, social workers, pastoral caregivers, pharmacists, psychologists, family, and volunteers is of utmost importance.[54,59] Information regarding radiation treatment, its potential side effects, and posttreatment issues should be communicated among all individuals, because effective communication and continuity of care among all members of the interdisciplinary teams and within each healthcare setting and institution is needed (Table 14-2).

After completion of radiation therapy, it is important to conduct a follow-up telephone call because there is the potential for issues such as pain flare-up or esophagitis to arise. As a result, the patient or caregiver may become anxious and require reassurance or further treatment or medication education. In addition, it also ensures that the patient has a follow-up appointment with a healthcare team.

REFERENCES

1. Coleman R, Rubens R: Bone metastases. In Abelhoff M, Armitage J, Niederhuber J et al, editors: *Clinical oncology,* ed 3, Philadelphia, 2004, Elsevier–Churchill Livingstone, pp 1091-1128.
2. Manoso M, Healey J: Metastatic cancer to the bone. In DeVita Jr V, Hellman S, Rosenberg, SA, editors: *Cancer principles and practice of oncology,* ed 7, Philadelphia, 2005, Lippincott Williams & Wilkins, pp 2368-2381.
3. Saarto T, Janes R, Tenhunen M et al: Palliative radiotherapy in the treatment of skeletal metastases, *Eur J Pain* 6: 323-330, 2002.
4. Maxwell T, Givant E, Kowalski MO: Exploring the management of bone metastasis according to the Roy Adaptation Model, *Oncol Nurs Forum* 28:1173-1181, 2001.
5. Flounders JA, Ott BB: Oncology emergency modules: spinal cord compression, *Oncol Nurs Forum* 30:E17-E23, 2003.
6. Hawkins R: Mastering the intricate maze of metastasis, *Oncol Nurs Forum* 28:959-965, 2001.
7. Myers J: Oncologic complications—spinal cord compression. In Otto S, editor: *Oncology nursing,* ed 4, St Louis, 2001, Mosby, pp 513-518.
8. Yalamanchili M, Lesser GJ: Malignant spinal cord compression, *Curr Treat Options Oncol* 4:509-516, 2003.
9. Woodruff R: Musculoskeletal. In *Palliative medicine: symptomatic and supportive care for patients with advanced cancer and AIDS,* ed 3, Melbourne, 1999, Oxford University Press, pp 235-242.
10. Klimo Jr P, Schmidt MH: Surgical management of spinal metastases, *Oncologist* 9:188-196, 2004.
11. Loblaw DA, Laperriere NJ: Emergency treatment of malignant extradural spinal cord compression: an evidence-based guideline. *J Clin Oncol* 16:1613-1624, 1998.
12. Baehring JM: Spinal cord compression. In DeVita V, Hellman Jr S, Rosenberg S, editors: *Cancer principles and practice of oncology,* ed 7, Philadelphia, 2005, Lippincott Williams & Wilkins, pp 2287-2292.
13. Wickham R: Hypercalcemia. In Yarbro C, Goodman M, Frogge M et al, editors: *Cancer nursing principles and practice,* ed 5, Sudbury, Mass, 2000, Jones & Bartlett, pp 776-791.
14. Mourad LA: Structure and function of the musculoskeletal system. In McCance K, Huether S, editors: *Pathophysiology: the biologic basis for disease in adults and children,* ed 3, St Louis, 1998, Mosby, pp 1405-1434.
15. Flaherty AM: Spinal cord compression. In Yarbro C, Goodman M, Frogge MG, editors: *Cancer nursing principles and practice,* ed 5, Sudbury, Mass, 2000, Jones & Bartlett, pp 887-899.

16. Hoskin P, Makin W: Bone metastases. In *Oncology for palliative medicine,* Oxford, 1998, Oxford University Press, pp 168-178.
17. Caraceni A, Matini C: Neurological problems. In *Palliative medicine,* ed 2, Oxford, 2001, Oxford University Press; pp 727-749.
18. American Health Decisions. The quest to die with dignity: An analysis of American's values, opinions and attitudes concerning end-of-life care; 1997.
19. Silberstein EB: Systemic radiopharmaceutical therapy of painful osteoblastic metastases, *Semin Radiat Oncol* 10:240-249, 2000.
20. Abraham JL: Promoting symptom control in palliative care, *Semin Oncol Nurs* 14:95-109, 1998.
21. Cleary JF: Cancer pain management, *Cancer Control* 7:120-131, 2000.
22. Miller RD, Walsh TD: Psychosocial aspects of palliative care in advanced cancer, *J Pain Symptom Manage* 6:24-29, 1991.
23. Perron V, Schonwetter RS: Assessment and management of pain in palliative care patients, *Cancer Control* 8:15-24, 2001.
24. Heimdal K, Hirschberg H, Slettebo H et al: High incidence of serious side effects of high-dose dexamethasone treatment in patients with epidural spinal cord compression, *J Neurooncol* 12:141-144, 1992.
25. Sorensen S, Helweg-Larsen S, Mouridsen H et al: Effect of high-dose dexamethasone in carcinomatous metastatic spinal cord compression treated with radiotherapy: a randomised trial, *Eur J Cancer* 30A:22-27, 1994.
26. Coleman RE: Metastatic bone disease: clinical features, pathophysiology and treatment strategies, *Cancer Treat Rev* 27:165-176, 2001.
27. Berry S, Waldron T, Winquist E et al, and the Members of the Genitourinary Cancer Disease Site Group: The Use of Bisphosphonates in Men with Hormone-Refractory Prostate Cancer. Practice Guideline Report #3-14. Toronto, 2005, Cancer Care Ontario, pp 1-39.
28. Warr D, Johnston M, and the Members of the Genitourinary Cancer Disease Site Group: Use of Bisphosphonates in Women with Breast Cancer. Practice Guideline Report #1-11 (Version 2.2002). Toronto, 2004, Cancer Care Ontario, pp 1-39.
29. Wong R, Wiffen P: Bisphosphonates for the relief of pain secondary to bone metastases, *Cochrane Database Syst Rev* 2, 2005.
30. Gugliemli G, Andreula C, Muto M et al: Percutaneous vertebroplasty: indications, contradictions, technique and complications, *Acta Radiologica* 46:256-268, 2005.
31. Chow E, Holden L, Danjoux C et al: Successful salvage using percutaneous vertebroplasty in cancer patients with painful spinal metastases or osteoporotic compression fractures, *Radiother Oncol* 70:265-267, 2004.
32. Anderson PR, Coia LR: Fractionation and outcomes with palliative radiation therapy, *Semin Radiat Oncol* 10:191-199, 2000.
33. Ferris FD, Bezjak A, Rosenthal SG: The palliative uses of radiation therapy in surgical oncology patients. *Surg Oncol Clin North Am* 10:185-201, 2001.
34. Wu J, Wong R, Johnston M et al, and Members of The Supportive Care Guidelines Group: Radiotherapy fractionation for the palliation of uncomplicated painful bone metastases. In *Practice guideline, No. 13-2,* Toronto, 2003, Cancer Care Ontario, pp 1-4.
35. van den Hout WB, van der Linden YM, Steenland E et al: Single- versus multiple-fraction radiotherapy in patients with painful bone metastases: cost-utility analysis based on a randomized trial, *J Nat Cancer Inst* 95:222-229, 2003.
36. Hartsell WF, Scott CB, Bruner DW et al: Randomized trial of short- versus long-course radiotherapy for palliation of painful bone metastases, *J Nat Cancer Inst* 97:798-804, 2005.
37. Wu JS, Wong R, Johnston M et al: Meta-analysis of dose-fractionation radiotherapy trials for the palliation of painful bone metastases, *Int J Radiat Oncol Biol Phys* 55:594-605, 2003.
38. National Cancer Institute of Canada Clinical Trials Group: A phase III international randomized trial of single versus multiple fractions for re-irradiation of painful bone metastases; 2003.
39. National Cancer Institute, United States National Institutes of Health: Supportive care clinical trial comparing ibandronate with a single dose of local radiation in patients with localized metastatic bone pain; 2004.
40. National Cancer Institute, United States National Institutes of Health: Supportive care clinical trial (phase I, phase II) study looking at radiofrequency ablation in treating patients with bone metastases; 2001.
41. Kirkbride P, Bezjak A: Palliative radiation therapy. In Berger A, Portenoy RK, Weissman DE, editors: *Principles and practice of palliative care and supportive oncology,* Philadelphia, 2002, Lippincott Williams & Wilkins, pp 685-697.
42. Ciezki JP, Komurcu S, Macklis RM: Palliative radiotherapy, *Semin Oncol* 27:90-93, 2000.
43. Barton R, Kirkbride P: Special techniques in palliative radiation oncology, *J Palliat Med* 3:75-83, 2000.
44. Hoskin PJ, Grover A, Bhana R: Metastatic spinal cord compression: radiotherapy outcome and dose fractionation, *Radiother Oncol* 68:175-180, 2003.
45. Ferrell B: The impact of pain on quality of life, *Nurs Clin North Am* 30:609-624, 1995.
46. Reisfield GM, Silberstein EB, Wilson GR: Radiopharmaceuticals for the palliation of painful bone metastases, *Am J Hospice Palliat Med* 22:41-46, 2005.
47. Altman GB, Lee CA: Strontium-89 for treatment of painful bone metastasis from prostate cancer, *Oncol Nurs Forum* 23:523-527, 1996.
48. Mertens WC, Filipczak LA, Ben-Joseph E et al: Systemic bone-seeking radionuclides for palliation of painful osseous metastases: current concepts, *CA Cancer J Clin* 48:361-374, 1998.
49. Roque M, Marinez MJ, Alonso-Colle P et al: Radioisotopes for metastatic bone cancer, *Cochrane Database Syst Rev* CD003347; 2003.
50. Otto S: Radiopharmaceuticals (strontium 89) and radiosensitizers(idoxuridine): innovative therapies for pain management and cancer care. *Intraven Nurs Soc* 21:335-337, 1998.
51. Bolderston A, Lloyd N, Wong R et al: The prevention and management of acute skin reactions related to radiation therapy. *Practice Guideline Report #13-7.* Toronto, 2005, Cancer Care Ontario, pp 1-39.

52. Radiation Medicine Program: Radiation skin reaction guidelines. Toronto, 2004, Princess Margaret Hospital; pp 1-12.
53. Cherny NI, Coyle N, Foley KM: Guidelines in the care of the dying cancer patient, *Hematol Oncol Clin North Am* 10:261-286, 1996.
54. Scanlon C: Public policy and end-of-life care: the nurse's role. In Ferrel B, Coyle N, editors: *Textbook of palliative nursing,* New York, 2001, Oxford University Press; pp 682-689.
55. Chow E, Andersson L, Wong R et al: Patients with advanced cancer: a survey of the understanding of their illness and expectations from palliative radiotherapy for symptomatic metastases, *Clin Oncol (R Coll Radiol)* 13:204-208, 2001.
56. Koller M, Lorenz W, Wagner K et al: Expectations and quality of life of cancer patients undergoing radiotherapy, *J R Soc Med* 93:621-628, 2000.
57. Weitzner MA, McMillan SC, Jacobsen PB: Family caregiver quality of life: differences between curative and palliative cancer treatment settings, *J Pain Symptom Manage* 17:418-428, 1999.
58. Covinsky KE, Goldman L, Cook EF et al: The impact of serious illness on patients' families. SUPPORT Investigators: Study to understand prognoses and preferences for outcomes and risks of treatment, *JAMA* 272:1839-1844, 1994.
59. Bascom PB, Tolle SW: Care of the family when the patient is dying, *West J Med* 163:292-296, 1995.

Chapter 15
Skin Cancers

William P. Hogle

The skin is the largest and most visible organ of the human body. It is subject to a myriad of environmental agents that could potentially inflict injury or discoloration. The skin performs a number of important functions including temperature regulation, maintaining homeostasis, prevention of infection, and prevention of internal injury. Like internal organ systems, the skin is subject to mutagenicity and carcinomatosis. This chapter discusses the most common forms of skin cancer and methods used to treat them. Specific attention is placed on the role of radiation therapy in the treatment of skin cancer and nursing interventions aimed at treating acute and late effects of radiation.

The term *skin cancer* is used often to describe several different malignancies that occur on the surface or within the layers of the skin. Skin neoplasms are essentially divided into two different categories: nonmelanoma skin cancer (NMSC) and malignant melanoma (MM). NMSCs include many premalignant skin conditions and a nonexclusive list that includes basal cell carcinoma (BCC), squamous cell carcinoma (SCC), Bowen's disease, erythroplasia of Queyrat (EOQ), keratoacanthoma, verrucous carcinoma, and cutaneous T-cell lymphoma. Specific attention is given to BCC, SCC, and malignant melanoma (MM). For information regarding T-cell lymphoma and its treatment, refer to Chapter 16.

Numerous factors contribute to the etiology of skin cancer.[1] Heredity factors such as race and family history play an important role in the likelihood of whether one will develop skin cancer. The epidermis of individuals of African descent have a natural skin protection factor (SPF) of 13.4, thereby allowing twice the filtration rate of ultraviolet B (UVB) rays than Caucasions.[2] Congenital skin conditions such as xeroderma pigmentosa, albinism, phenylketonuria, Gorlin's syndrome, melanocytic nevi, and dysplastic nevi appear to correlate with higher incidence rates of MM. Environmental factors, predominantly ultraviolet radiation (UVR), are associated with higher incidence rates of BCC, SCC, and MM. Chemical exposure from tar, arsenic, topical nitrogen mustard, and ionizing radiation, human papilloma virus (HPV), and immunosuppression also have been associated with skin cancer.

The incidence of skin cancer continues to grow throughout the world. In the United States alone, the American Cancer Society (ACS) estimates that 1 billion cases of BCC and SCC will be detected annually. It is theorized that many cases of BCC go unreported because they are often removed during routine visits to a primary physician office. BCCs predominate over SCCs by approximately 5:1 in males and 10:1 in females. Skin cancers account for approximately one-third of all cancer diagnoses. The annual incidence of MM also continues to rise. The ACS estimates that 62,190 new cases will be diagnosed in 2006. For men, the relative risk of developing MM is 1 in 55; for women, the relative risk is 1 in 82. The mortality rate from BCC and SCC is roughly 2000 persons per year. An estimated 7770 person die annually from MM.[3,4]

ANATOMY

The skin, which is the primary component of the integumentary system, is divided into three layers: the epidermis, the dermis, and the subcutaneous tissue (Figure 15-1). The epidermis is the outermost part of the skin and is considered stratified squamous epithelium. The thickness of the epidermis ranges from 0.05 millimeters (mm) on the eyelids to 1.5 mm on the palms and soles. The inner most layer of the epidermis consists of a single row of columnar cells called *basal cells*. Basal cells divide and develop into keratinocytes, which comprise the spinous layer. The keratinocytes synthesize insoluble protein. As these cells continue to migrate toward the surface, they flatten and their

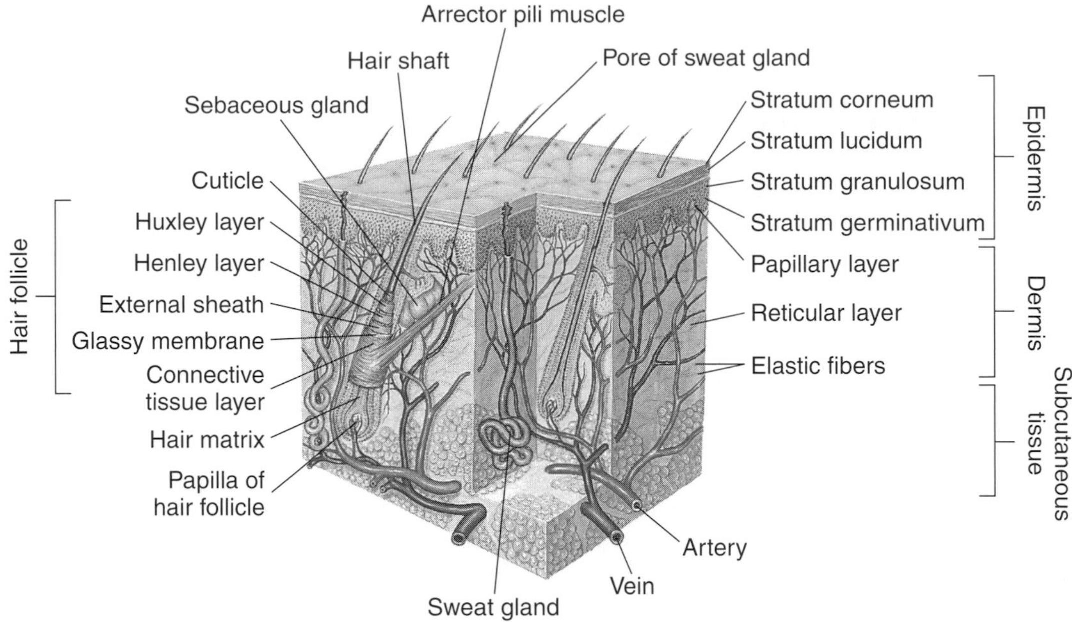

Figure 15-1 Skin Anatomy.
From Seidel HM, Ball JW, Dains JE, et al: Mosby's guide to physical examination, ed. 6, St. Louis, 2006, Mosby.

cytoplasm appear granular (stratum granulosum). Eventually these cells die as they reach the surface to form the stratum corneum. The three types of branched cells in the epidermis are (1) the melanocyte, which synthesizes pigment (melanin); (2) Langerhans' cell, which is active in the immune process; and (3) Merkel's cell, the function of which is not clearly understood.[5]

The dermis varies in thickness from 0.3 mm on the eyelid to 3.0 mm on the back. It is composed of three types of connective tissue: collagen, elastic tissue, and reticular fibers. The dermis is divided into two layers: the upper layer, also known as the *papillary layer,* is composed of thin collagen fibers; the thicker lower layer, also known as the *reticular layer,* extends from the base of the papillary layer to the subcutaneous tissue and is composed of thick collagen fibers that are arranged parallel to the surface of the skin.[5]

The autonomic nervous system supplies the motor innervation of the skin. Adrenergic fibers innervate the blood vessels, hair erector muscles, and apocrine glands. The sebaceous glands are regulated by the endocrine system and are not innervated by autonomic nerve fibers.

PATHOPHYSIOLOGY

Basal Cell Skin Cancer

BCCs arise from basal keratinocytes of the epidermis. When removed from dermal tissue, BCCs do not survive.[6] This may explain why these cells are not capable of metastasizing through blood vessels or lymphatics, because it appears they need the surrounding stroma to remain viable. The course of BCC is unpredictable. They can occur at the site of previous trauma or thermal burns. BCCs also can occur years later at sites previously treated with ionizing radiation. The cells that constitute BCC resemble those of the basal layer of the epidermis. They are basophylic and have a large nucleus. The five major histologic patterns of BCC are shown in Table 15-1.[7]

Squamous Cell Skin Cancer

Atypical squamous cells originate in the epidermis from keratinocytes and proliferate indefinitely. A flat, scaly lesion becomes an indurated SCC when cells penetrate the epidermal basement membrane and proliferate into the dermis. SCC can occur anywhere on the skin or mucous membranes and

Table 15-1 Histologic Patterns of Basal Cell Carcinomas

Histology	Frequency	Description
Nodular	21%	A rounded mass of neoplastic cells with well-defined peripheral contours
Superficial	17%	Contains buds of atypical basal cells extending from the basal layer of the epidermis
Micronodular	15%	Small, rounded nodules of tumor about the size of hair bulbs; tumor islands are rounded, well demarcated, and demonstrate peripheral palisading
Infiltrative	7%	Tumor islands vary in size and show a jagged configuration
Morpheaform	1%	Numerous small, elongated islands containing a few cells that appear as strands or cords in a fibrous stroma

Data from Sexton M, Jones DB, Maloney ME: *J Am Acad Dermatol* 23(6 Pt 1):1118-1126, 1990.
NOTE: A mixed pattern of two or more major histologic patterns is present in 38.5% of cases.

Table 15-2 Subtypes and Frequency of Malignant Melanomas

Subtype	Frequency	Description
Superficial spreading melanoma	70%	Irregular asymmetric borders Begins as flat or elevated brown lesion
Nodular melanoma	15%–20%	Rapid growth, ulcerates and bleeds
Lentigo malignant melanoma	4%–15%	Precursor lesion present, slow growth Raised blue-black nodules
Acral lentiginous melanoma	2%–8% in Caucasians 30%–75% in African Americans, Asians, Hispanics	Appears on palms, soles, and nail plates

Data from Habif TP: *Clinical dermatology: a color guide to diagnosis and therapy,* ed 4, St Louis, 2004, Mosby, pp 773-813.

essentially anywhere squamous epithelium exists. These lesions are usually seen on the scalp, backs of the hands, and superior surface of the external ear. SCCs are often separated into two major groups based on the malignant potential. Those arising from areas of prior irradiation or thermal injury, in a chronically draining sinus, and in chronic ulcers are usually aggressive and have a high rate of metastasis. SCCs originating from UVR are generally less aggressive and less likely to metastasize. The potential for an SCC to metastasize is related to its size, location, degree of differentiation, histologic evidence of perineural involvement, immunologic status, and depth of invasion.[8,9] In the majority of cases, SCC first metastasizes to regional lymph nodes[10] and has the potential to travel to distant sites.

Malignant Melanoma

Melanomas consist of malignant pigment cells (melanocytes) that grow and extend through the epidermis and into the dermis. This unrestricted growth produces a lesion, which can very in size, shape, color, and surface characteristics. See Table 15-2 for a breakdown of the four major subtypes and frequency with which they occur.[11] Most MMs display two growth phases: radial and vertical. In the radial phase, cells grow in a radial fashion from the original tumor site and do not metastasize.[12] Eventually the MM cells enter a vertical growth phase in which the cells invade down through the dermis and have the potential to metastasize. In general, MM tends to recur or metastasize in an orderly process of local recurrence, regional metastasis, followed by distant metastasis.[12,13] Distant metastasis more commonly involves nonvisceral sites including the skin, subcutaneous tissue, and distant lymph nodes. Other common sites of metastasis include lungs, liver, brain, bone, and small intestine.

CLINICAL MANIFESTATIONS

Skin cancers vary greatly in clinical presentation and symptomatology. Distinguishing one type of malignancy from another can be difficult and is best left to a dermatologist. BCC usually presents as a pearly white or pink dome-shaped papule. The mass extends peripherally and may remain flat. Telangiectactic vessels appear and become more recognizable as the epidermis thins and the lesion grows. The center of the mass usually ulcerates and bleeds and subsequently accumulates crust and scale. The ulcerated areas eventually heal, which results in scarring. Patients may assume the lesion is healing. In fact, the growth-ulceration-healing cycle continues, resulting in a larger, deeper mass.

SCCs tend to arise more often from precursor lesions as compared with BCCs.[14] Table 15-3 contains lesions that may precede a diagnosis of SCC. In general, SCCs tend to have a scaly, crusty, slightly elevated lesion that may develop a cutaneous horn. Approximately 80% of ultraviolet-induced SCCs develop on the arms, head, and neck.[15] A physician should evaluate any skin ulceration that takes longer than 3 weeks to heal for possible BCC, SCC, or a precancerous lesion.

Approximately 70% of melanomas occur as the result of a change in a preexisting nevus. The other 30% arise from de novo melanomas, which are growths not associated with previously observed nevi.[16] Malignant melanoma often present on the lower extremities in women and on the trunk in men.[1] The classic signs in a preexisting nevus include darkening or irregular color, increase in size, nodularity, ulceration, pruritus, and bleeding. The ACS has released the ABCD rules for early detection of melanoma (Table 15-4).[17]

DIAGNOSTIC STUDIES

Diagnosing a cancerous lesion of the skin can be difficult for the non-dermatologist. A history of the disease; noting duration, rate of onset, location, symptoms, family history, allergies, occupation, and previous treatment are necessary.

A thorough physical exam is also necessary in the diagnosis of skin cancer. Patients should disrobe completely so that the extent and severity of the eruption can be assessed. Some clinicians may use a hand lens or some other type of visual aid to magnify and study skin lesions. To the naked eye, some lesions are difficult to define as malignant or nonmalignant. One method of enhanced skin visualization is epiluminescence microscopy (ELM) or dermatoscopy (Figure 15-2). ELM is a noninvasive

Table 15-3 Precursor Lesions of Squamous Cell Carcinomas

Precancerous lesions	Description
Actinic (solar) keratoses	Warty lesions or areas of red, scaly patches occurring on the sun-exposed skin of the face or hands
Arsenical keratoses	Multiple, hard, cornlike masses on palms and soles from long-term arsenic ingestion
Bowen's disease	Precancerous dermatosis or carcinoma in situ Appear as pink or brown papules covered with a thickened horny layer
Keratoacanthoma	Rapid-growing dome-shaped mass on a sun-exposed area; may resolve themselves if left untreated

Table 15-4 American Cancer Society Early Signs of Skin Melanomas

ABCD signs	Descriptions
Asymmetry	One half of the mole does not match the other half
Border	The edges of the mole are irregular, ragged, blurred, or notched
Color	The color over the mole is not the same. There may be differing shades of tan, brown, or black, and sometimes patches of red, blue, or white
Diameter	The mole is larger than 6 mm (about 1/4 inch, or about the size of a pencil eraser), although in recent years doctors are finding more melanomas between 3 mm and 6 mm

From American Cancer Society: The ABCD rule for early detection of melanoma. Retrieved on 12/17/2005 from www.cancer.org/docroot/SPC/content/SPC_1_ABCD_Mole_Check_Tips.asp.

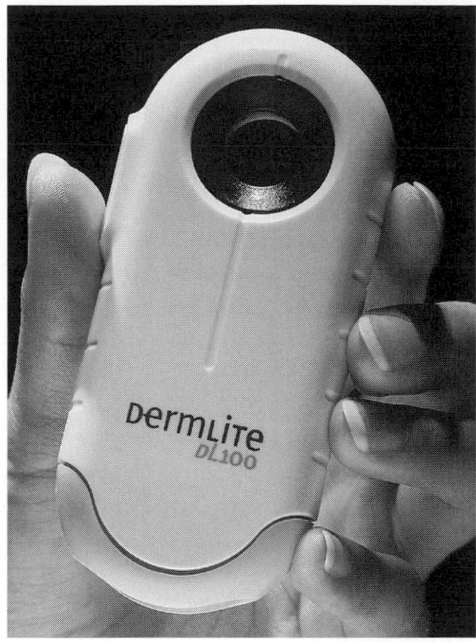

Figure 15-2 Dermatoscope.
From Habif TP: Clinical dermatology, ed. 4, St Louis, 2004, Mosby.

procedure that allows physicians to differentiate between benign and malignant lesions while they are in the early phases of development. ELM images can be digitally transmitted via telephone for analysis and interpretation by specialists, thus enabling the patient's primary care physician (PCP) to more actively screen for skin malignancies.

If an advanced SCC or MM is suspected, a work-up for staging and metastasis should be conducted. In addition to a history and physical exam, such a work-up should include a chest x ray to rule out lung involvement; serum liver function studies to rule out liver involvement; serum alkaline phosphatase levels and bone scan if bone pain exists; and complete blood counts to detect anemia potentially caused by an invasive bleeding lesion. If metastatic disease is suspected, magnetic resonance imaging (MRI) or computer tomography (CT) scans are indicated. Full body CT scans are necessary when initially staging advanced melanomas.

The ultimate diagnostic tool is a biopsy. Biopsies can be accomplished using various techniques such as punch, shave, saucerization, and incisional or excisional techniques. Although BCCs may be biopsied using any of these techniques, SCCs and lesions suspected for MM should be biopsied only using methods that remove the necessary tissue for pathologic examination so as to allow for accurate diagnosis and staging. Potential complications from biopsies include infection, bleeding, hyperpigmentation, hypopigmentation, adhesions, scarring, and problems with wound healing.[1]

STAGING

Nonmelanoma Skin Cancer

Pathologic staging is accomplished by the examination of completely resected tumors and lymph nodes. If a pathologist is unsure or unfamiliar about a skin specimen, it should be sent for consultation to a specialist trained in dermatopathology. The TNM staging categories for both clinical and pathologic classifications of nonmelanoma skin cancer (NMSC) are the same and are grouped as stages I to IV (Table 15-5). Histologically, the grade of the specimen is described as grades 1 to 4. Grade 1 is well-differentiated tumor, grade 2 is moderately differentiated, grade 3 is poorly differentiated, and grade 4 is an undifferentiated tumor. Grade X indicates that the grade cannot be assessed.[18]

Malignant Melanoma

Clinical staging of MM is based on biopsy interpretation, clinical exam, and radiologic staging. Biopsied lesions can be described using one of two systems: Clark's level or Breslow's measurement. Drs. Wallace Clark and Alexander Breslow developed the main microstaging systems for melanomas. Both systems rely on measures of tumor volume. Clark's system categorizes melanomas based on their level of invasion through the epidermis and layers of the dermis. Clark's levels (Figure 15-3) may indicate the potential for metastasis because the access of tumor cells to nearby lymphatic and vascular channels can be assessed. Additionally, the extent of invasion may indicate the tumor's progression from relatively harmless radial growth to more aggressive vertical growth.[19] Table 15-6 details Clark's levels of microstaging. Breslow's system categorizes melanoma based on tumor thickness from the top of the granular layer of the epidermis, or the ulcerated surface, to the deepest identifiable melanoma cell as measured by an ocular micrometer (Figure 15-4). Table 15-7 details Breslow's microstaging system.

The American Joint Committee on Cancer (AJCC) revised the MM staging system in 2002

Table 15-5 AJCC Staging for Nonmelanoma Skin Cancers

Cancer stage	Clinical/pathologic findings		
PRIMARY TUMOR (T)			
TX	Primary tumor cannot be assessed		
T0	No evidence of primary tumor		
Tis	Carcinoma in situ		
T1	Tumor 2 cm or less in greatest dimension		
T2	Tumor more than 2 cm, but not more than 5 cm, in greatest dimension		
T3	Tumor more than 5 cm in greatest dimension		
T4	Tumor invades deep extradermal structures (i.e., cartilage, skeletal muscle, or bone)		
REGIONAL LYMPH NODES (N)			
NX	Regional lymph nodes cannot be assessed		
N0	No regional lymph node metastasis		
N1	Regional lymph node metastasis		
DISTANT METASTASIS (M)			
MX	Distant metastasis cannot be assessed		
M0	No distant metastasis		
M1	Distant metastasis		
STAGE GROUPING			
Stage 0	Tis	N0	M0
Stage I	T1	N0	M0
Stage II	T2	N0	M0
	T3	N0	M0
Stage III	T4	N0	M0
	Any T	N1	M0
Stage IV	Any T	Any N	M1

Used with the permission of the American Joint Committee on Cancer (AJCC), Chicago, Illinois. The original source for this material is the *AJCC Cancer Staging Manual, Sixth Edition* (2002), published by Springer-New York, www.springeronline.com.
NOTE: Definitions for clinical (cTNM) and pathologic (pTNM) classifications are the same.

to incorporate research-proven prognostic factors and to organize subsets of patients by expected outcomes.[20] This system for staging MM assesses primary tumor thickness, regional node status, and distant metastasis (Table 15-8). The T category of the melanoma is classified primarily by measuring the thickness of the melanoma as defined by Breslow's system. The level of invasion, as defined by Clark's system, is used to define subcategories of T1 melanomas but not for thicker melanomas (i.e., T2, T3, or T4).[21]

Table 15-6 Clark's Classification System

Level	Description
Level 1	Confinement to the epidermis above the basement membrane
Level 2	Invasion through the basement membrane to the papillary dermis
Level 3	Presence of tumor cells at the papillary-reticular junction of the dermis
Level 4	Invasion into the reticular dermis
Level 5	Invasion into subcutaneous fat

Washington CM, Lever D, editors: *Principles and practice of radiation therapy,* ed. 2, St. Louis, 2004, Mosby.

Table 15-7 Breslow's Classification System

Level	Description
Level 1	Melanoma in situ, limited to the epidermis
Level 2	< 0.75 mm
Level 3	0.76-1.5 mm
Level 4	1.51-4 mm
Level 5	> 4 mm

Washington CM, Lever D, editors: *Principles and practice of radiation therapy,* ed. 2, St. Louis, 2004, Mosby.

TREATMENT

Nonmelanoma Skin Cancer

Skin cancers usually begin as small, locally invasive lesions that can be easily removed through a variety of methods with minimal morbidity.[22] Surgery is the primary treatment of choice in almost all cases of skin cancer. Complete removal of the lesion, including tumor free margins, is the goal of surgery. On occasion, the lesion may be small enough so that the excisional boundaries are similar to those of a biopsy. In such circumstances, the diagnosis and treatment phases may be completed in one step.[1] If the lesion is larger or more invasive, treatment is likely to include surgical excision along with chemotherapy or radiation therapy. Table 15-9 shows the types of surgical procedures available for the removal of NMSCs.

Chemotherapeutic agents such as topical and intralesional 5-FU (5-fluorouracil) has been used to effectively treat BCC. Application of 5-FU 1 to 2 times daily for several weeks can cause irritation and inflammation but does not usually result in

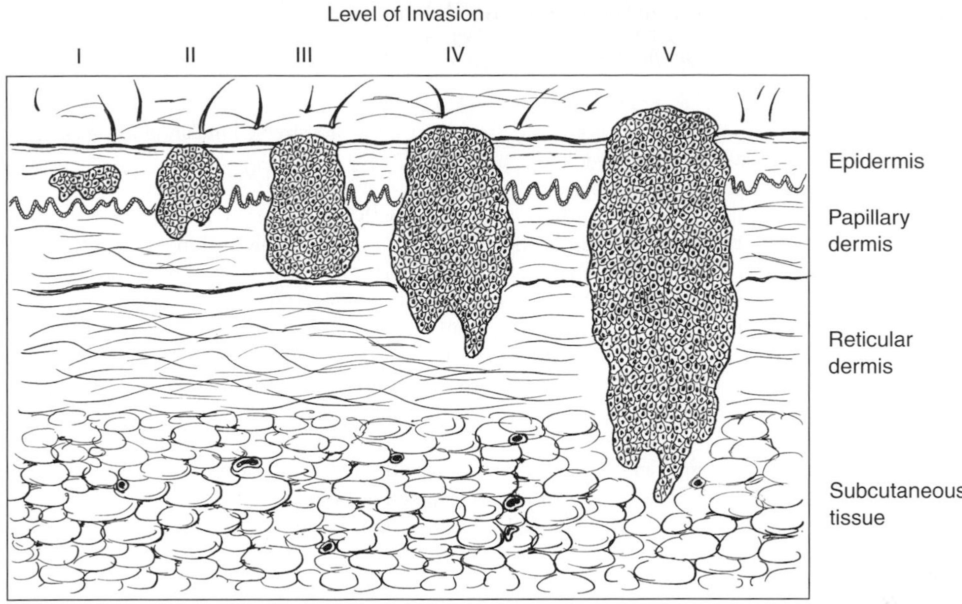

Figure 15-3 Clark's Microstaging.
From Washington CM, Leaver DT: Principles and practice of radiation therapy, ed. 2, St Louis, 2004, Mosby.

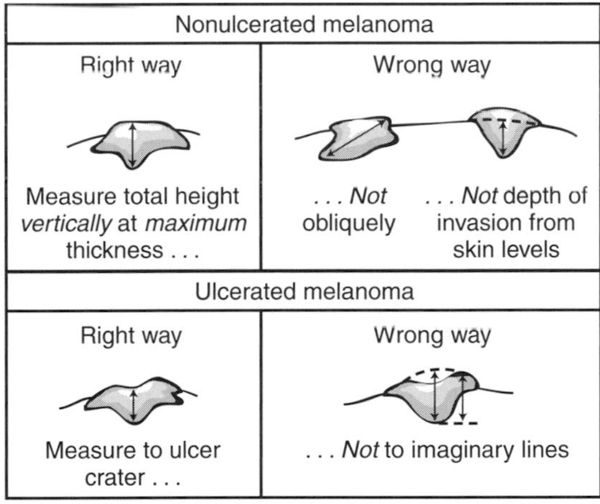

Figure 15-4 Breslow's Measurement Process.
From Washington CM, Leaver DT: Principles and practice of radiation therapy, ed. 2, St Louis, 2004, Mosby.

permanent scarring.[23] Topical chemotherapy is a viable alternative for patients who cannot tolerate other forms of treatment. Other investigational therapies for NMSCs include photodynamic therapy (PDT),[23] immunotherapy, using intralesional interferon alpha,[15] and an oral retinoid known as *isotretinoin*.[24]

Radiation therapy is effective in the treatment of NMSC and is often used to treat lesions on the lips, nose, eyelids, face, and ears because these areas are highly visible and cosmetic results are usually rather favorable. Because most skin lesions tend to be superficial in nature, electrons and kilovoltage x rays are often used in their treatment. Megavoltage x rays are rarely employed but may be used with or without electrons for special circumstances such as scalp lesions or tumors that are deeply infiltrating.[25] Radiation fields should include a 2-cm margin completely surrounding the tumor so as to cover possible microscopic extension.[14] A 1-cm margin may be adequate for small superficial BCCs.[14] Tumors and their full margins should receive a majority of the dose with a boost field encompassing the clinical tumor. Bolus may be used with electron therapy to fill in the gaps on uneven surfaces, maximize the surface dose, or reduce the underlying tissue dose. Various beam-blocking or shielding techniques may be used to spare nearby structures of the face and the lens of the eye. Prescribed total dosage of radiation therapy varies according to size and depth of the tumor and often differs from institution to institution. In general, both tumor types are treated to a total dose between 40 Gy and 66 Gy.[26] Table 15-10 out-lines the National Comprehensive Cancer Network (NCCN) practice guidelines for radiation therapy for the treatment of BCCs and SCCs.

Table 15-8 AJCC Staging System for Malignant Melanoma

Cancer stage	Clinical/pathologic findings		
PRIMARY TUMOR (T)			
TX	Primary tumor cannot be assessed (e.g., shave biopsy or regressed melanoma)		
T0	No evidence of primary tumor		
Tis	Melanoma in situ		
T1	Melanoma 1.0 mm or less in thickness, with or without ulceration		
T1a	Melanoma 1.0 mm or less in thickness and level II or III, no ulceration		
T1b	Melanoma 1.0 mm or less in thickness and level IV or V, or with ulceration		
T2	Melanoma 1.01–2.0 mm in thickness, with or without ulceration		
T2a	Melanoma 1.01–2.0 mm in thickness, no ulceration		
T2b	Melanoma 1.01–2.0 mm in thickness, with ulceration		
T3	Melanoma 2.01–4.0 mm in thickness, with or without ulceration		
T3a	Melanoma 2.01–4.0 mm in thickness, no ulceration		
T3b	Melanoma 2.01–4.0 mm in thickness, with ulceration		
T4	Melanoma greater than 4.0 mm in thickness, with or without ulceration		
T4a	Melanoma greater than 4.0 mm in thickness, no ulceration		
T4b	Melanoma greater than 4.0 mm in thickness, with ulceration		
REGIONAL LYMPH NODES (N)			
NX	Regional lymph nodes cannot be assessed		
N0	No regional lymph node metastasis		
N1	Metastasis in one lymph node		
N1a	Clinically occult (microscopic) disease		
N1b	Clinically apparent (macroscopic) metastasis		
N2	Metastasis in two to three regional lymph nodes or intralymphatic regional metastasis without nodal melanoma		
N2a	Clinically occult (microscopic) disease		
N2b	Clinically apparent (macroscopic) metastasis		
N2c	Satellite or in-transit metastasis without nodal metastasis		
N3	Metastasis in four or more regional nodes, or in-transit metastasis or satellite(s) with metastasis in regional lymph nodes		
DISTANT METASTASIS (M)			
MX	Distant metastasis cannot be assessed		
M0	No distant metastasis		
M1	Distant metastasis		
M1a	Metastasis to skin, subcutaneous tissues, or distant lymph nodes		
M1b	Metastasis to lung		
M1c	Metastasis to all other visceral sites or distant metastasis at any site associated with an elevated serum lactic dehydrogenase (LDH)		
CLINICAL STAGE GROUPING			
Stage 0	Tis	N0	M0
Stage IA	T1a	N0	M0
Stage IB	T1b	N0	M0
	T2a	N0	M0
Stage IIA	T2b	N0	M0
	T3a	N0	M0
Stage IIB	T3b	N0	M0
	T4a	N0	M0
Stage IIC	T4b	N0	M0
Stage III	Any T	N1	M0
	Any T	N2	M0
	Any T	N3	M0
Stage IV	Any T	Any N	M1

Used with the permission of the American Joint Committee on Cancer (AJCC), Chicago, Illinois. The original source for this material is the *AJCC Cancer Staging Manual, Sixth Edition* (2002), published by Springer-New York, www.springeronline.com.

Table 15-9 Surgical Procedures for Nonmelanoma Skin Cancers

Procedure	Description
Surgical excision	Surgical procedure that usually requires local sedation; treatment of choice for squamous cell cancer (SCC) overlying bone and cartilage and for SCC occurring in scars, ulcers, and sinuses Margins of 4 mm around visible tumors and 6 mm for tumors greater than 3 mm
Electrosurgery	Involves the use of heat to cut involved tissue; is useful in the removal of basal cell carcinomas (BCC) and smaller, less invasive SCC
Mohs micrographic surgery	Used for tumors that are recurrent, are large, have distinct margins, and are in a location where excision with wide margins of healthy skin removal would be surgically or cosmetically unacceptable The tumor is excised under local anesthesia using horizontal frozen sections that are microscopically examined during the surgery Can be repeated until margins are clear; offers 95%–99% chance for complete removal without recurrence
Cryosurgery	The use of freezing temperatures to destroy tissue; chemical elements are either swabbed or sprayed on the lesion in question; in some cases, cryoprobes are used Effectiveness depends on the tumor reaching -50° Celsius

Table 15-10 NCCN Practice Guidelines for Radiation Therapy Treating Basal and Squamous Cell Carcinomas

Tumor size	Margin	Orthovoltage dose and fractions
< 20 mm	5–10 mm	Total of 45 Gy–50 Gy in 2.5–3 Gy fractions
> 20 mm	15–20 mm	Total of 60 Gy–66 Gy in 2 Gy fractions or total 50 Gy–60 Gy in 2.5 Gy fractions

From National Comprehensive Cancer Network: *Clinical practice guidelines on oncology Version 1. 2006, Basal Cell and Squamous Cell Skin Cancer* (website): www.nccn.org/professionals/physician_gls/PDF/nmsc.pdf. Accessed December 1, 2005.

NOTE: Varying energies of orthovoltage or electron-beam equipment should be available.

Add 10% to 15% to total and daily doses if using electron beam and add bolus for low-energy electrons.

Maximize fractions to maximize cosmesis.

Radiation therapy is contraindicated in genetic conditions predisposing to skin cancer (e.g., nevoid basal cell carcinoma, xeroderma pigmentosum), connective tissue diseases (e.g., lupus, scleroderma), and verrucous carcinomas.

Brachytherapy using iridium-192 or cesium-136 has produced good curative and cosmetic results. However, brachytherapy does not possess any significant advantage over external beam radiation therapy (EBRT). There are, in fact, disadvantages to brachytherapy that should be considered: cost, trauma, possible infection, possible inpatient hospitalization, questionable dose distribution, and risks associated with anesthesia.[27]

Malignant Melanoma

The treatment for MM is based on its location, appearance, and extent of disease. Patient comorbidities also should be taken into consideration. Initial treatment consists of complete surgical excision of the primary lesion and attaining disease-free margin status. Adequate size of disease-free margins varies between 0.5 cm and 3 cm, depending on size of primary lesion (in situ of 4 mm or more). Excision of lesions greater than 4 mm should include skin and underlying adipose tissue. No improvements have been noted from wider excisions through muscle and fascia.[28]

Patients with proven lymph node metastasis should undergo complete excision of regional lymph nodes, removing as much of the soft tissue and its associated lymphatics as possible between the site of the primary lesion and the regional lymph nodes. Despite lymphadenectomy in patients with known nodal involvement, the risk of distant metastasis is high.[29]

Chemotherapy has been successful in producing remissions in some patients, but its use in the treatment of MM is palliative. Historically, dacarbazine

(DTIC) has been the standard used in single-agent treatment for MM. Complete remissions are rare and response rates of only 20%[30,31] have been documented with median duration of response lasting only 4 to 6 months.[29,32] Temozolomide, nitrosoureas, vinca-alkaloids, cisplatin, paclitaxel, and docetaxel also have been used as single-agent therapy for MM. Combination regimes have shown some improvement in response but have not significantly improved long-term survival.

One method of using regional chemotherapy and hyperthermia treatment has been used when MM is confined to a particular area, usually one extremity. This type of treatment, known as isolated limb perfusion (ILP) prevents blood from getting to a limb by means of a tourniquet while the blood in the limb circulates through a machine that pumps, oxygenates, and heats it. Because the blood supply is cut off from the rest of the body, larger doses of chemotherapy can be administered and circulated throughout the limb. Melphalan or cisplatin are the drugs most often used during ILP. The heating action during ILP aids in tumor cell kill because melanoma cells cannot survive above 105.8° F. After approximately 1 hour of treatment, the process is stopped, allowing normal blood supply to return to the limb. Overall response rates for ILP have been as high as 65%, with complete remission rates of 44%.[33]

Immunotherapy is another approach to treating MMs. The fact that MMs have a history of spontaneous regression[30,34] has lead to the notion that immunotherapy may play a vital role in a successful treatment regime. Several agents, given alone or in combination with chemotherapy, have been used.

Alpha-interferon (α-IFN) is a nonspecific immunotherapy agent that acts to stimulate the patient's entire immune system. Historically, α-IFN has been used to treat MM since the 1970s. In one study, intravenous α-IFN (20 MU/M^2/day) was administered to patients for 1 month, followed by subcutaneous α-IFN (10 MU/M^2) 3 times a week for 11 months. Although dose reductions and significant toxicity were reported, an increase in relapse-free survival and increased overall survival was observed.[35]

Interleukin-2 (IL-2) acts to stimulate a number of aspects related to the immune system. IL-2 has been administered as single-agent therapy and in combination with lymphokine-activated killer (LAK) cells and with tumor-infiltrating lymphocytes (TIL). A synergistic affect is believed to exist when IL-2 is given with α-IFN or with certain chemotherapeutic agents.[1] Clinical trials of IL-2 have examined the effectiveness of a number of different dosages and routes of administration.

A third example of nonspecific immunotherapy is bacille Calmette-Guérin (BCG). This agent is administered locally (intralesionally or epilesional scarification) so as to create a local inflammatory reaction, which is thought to be the primary method of killing tumor cells. The immune response also causes cytokine production and lymphocyte activation to occur, resulting in further tumor cell death. Injection of BCG into MM lesions has resulted in regression at regional and distant sites of disease.[36]

Examples of specific immunotherapy agents include monoclonal antibodies and vaccines. Monoclonal antibodies can be administered systematically, intralesionally, intrathecally, and intravascularly during ILP.[33,37] They may be conjugated with chemotherapeutic agents, toxins, or radionuclides to increase their overall cytotoxic effects.[1] MM vaccines may inhibit metastasis and are most effective for patients who have undergone complete resection of all known tumor sites.[30] Several phase III studies are examining the overall effectiveness of vaccine therapy for MM.

Side effects of chemotherapy and immunotherapy vary depending on the agents used and the route of administration. When administered locally, patients can expect a local inflammatory reaction and, in some cases, a local hypersensitivity reaction that may potentially lead to a systemic reaction. With systemic administration, side effects may include bone marrow suppression, fatigue, nausea, hypotension, sepsis, respiratory distress, and systemic hypersensitivity or anaphylaxis. These side effects can potentially occur with each cycle of chemotherapy administered.

Radiation therapy is not used as primary treatment for MM because it has traditionally been considered a radioresistant tumor. Recently, however, larger doses per fraction have been examined as a means to overcome the known radioresistance. Megavoltage x rays are used as deeper levels of tissue become involved or major organs become affected. Dose fractions of at least 5 Gy should be used to treat cutaneous, subcutaneous, lymph node, or visceral metastases. If potential late effects are deemed undesirable, lower daily doses of 2 Gy to 4 Gy may be used up to normal tissue tolerance or hyperfraction may be used 1.15 Gy twice daily to a total dose of 35 Gy to 40 Gy.[14,38] Specific NCCN treatment guidelines outlining the use of radiation therapy for the treatment of MM do not currently exist.

Theoretically, melanoma can occur wherever melanocytes are present. When MM presents in the choroids or ciliary body of the eye, brachytherapy is a viable treatment option. Modern brachytherapy techniques used for ocular melanoma have resulted in survival rates at least as good as enucleation.[39] Radioactive eye plaque application, using isotopes such as Cobalt-60 (CO-60), Ruthenium-106 (Ru-106), and Iodine-125 (I-125) have achieved local control rates in the range of 88% to 98% at 5 years.[40-43] Plaque brachytherapy with I-125 is currently the most common treatment modality for ocular melanoma in the United States. Despite favorable results, patients often experience eventual decline in visual acuity, cataract formation, and other ocular morbidity over the subsequent 1 to 3 years. However, brachytherapy does have some advantages over enucleation, such as delay or reduction of vision loss and a more favorable cosmetic result.[44]

In most cases of MM, however, radiation therapy serves as an adjunct to surgery for patients with high-risk disease, presence of positive surgical margins, primary lesions greater than 4 mm, or positive nodal involvement. Radiation is used in the palliative treatment of metastatic melanoma. Patients who demonstrate signs of spinal cord metastasis, brain involvement, or experience bowel obstruction or significant bone pain from metastatic disease may benefit from palliative radiation treatments.

NURSING INTERVENTIONS AND EDUCATION

Morbidity associated with radiation therapy can be divided into acute and late effects. The severity of the reaction depends on volume of tissue treated, dose, and intensity of treatment received. High doses to large volumes in a short amount of time result in more severe reactions than lower doses to small volumes over longer periods of time.[14] Table 15-11 outlines acute and late effects of radiation therapy for skin cancer. Specific evi-

Table 15-11 Acute and Late Skin Effects From Radiation Therapy

Skin reactions	Radiation effects
ACUTE	
Erythema	Usually the first signs of the effects of radiation Can occur after one fraction and continue throughout the course of treatment
Dry desquamation	Shedding of the epidermis at intermediate levels of radiation
Moist desquamation	Appears at higher dose levels and is the result of an absence of cells from the germinal layer that replaces cells in the epidermis; seen as exposed dermis that oozes a serous substance
LATE	
Pigmentation changes	Caused by the increased or decreased production of melanin
Telangiectasia	Capillaries become dilated and fewer in number; epithelial layer becomes thinned
Fibrosis	Damage to the dermis results in thicker, firmer skin
Necrosis	Can occur in patients who receive large doses in short amounts of time
ACUTE OR LATE	
Alopecia	Appears as moderate doses of radiation are achieved Can be permanent at doses of 45 Gy or higher
Decreased sweating	Sebaceous (oil) and sudoriferous (sweat) glands may show decreased or absent function when subjected to moderate to high doses of radiation therapy

Data from:

Haas ML: Skin reaction. In Bruner DW, Haas ML, Gosselin-Acomb TK, editors: *Manual for radiation oncology nursing practice and education,* ed 3, Pittsburgh, 2005, Oncology Nursing Society, pp 49-52.

Solan MJ, Brady, LW: Skin cancer. In: Perez CA, Brady LW, Halperin EC, et al, editors: *Principles and practice of radiation oncology,* ed 4, Philadelphia, 2004, Lippincott Williams & Wilkins, pp 757-775.

Washington CM, Blobe TA: Skin and melanoma. In Washington CM, Lever D, editors: *Principles and practice of radiation therapy,* ed 2, St Louis, 2004, Mosby, pp 893-918.

dence-based nursing interventions aimed at treating skin reactions can be found in Chapter 30. Other than treating the obvious skin-related side effects of radiation therapy, nursing interventions should focus on education regarding prevention and follow-up care.

In terms of receiving daily radiation treatments, patients should be informed of acute and late side effects and the expected duration of each. Patients should be told that receiving a treatment is very similar to receiving a regular x ray. If bolus material is to be used, inform the patient as to its purpose and the anticipated feeling of coolness on the skin from the bolus material itself. In patients receiving I-125 plaque brachytherapy for ocular melanoma, the surgical risks should be reviewed, as should the side effects of cataract formation and eventual decreased visual acuity and the possibility that enucleation may still be necessary.

Educating individuals about skin cancer prevention is not limited to just those who have received radiation therapy. Such interventions are applicable to most members of the general public, and oncology clinicians should take every opportunity to remind people regarding the ways one can minimize his or her risk of developing skin cancer from UVR. Skin cancer is one of the few malignancies in which the causes are known and preventable. Approximately 90% of skin cancer can be avoided if individuals take appropriate precautions to minimize skin exposure. Damage to melanocytes after radiation therapy results in hypopigmentation and increased sensitivity to the sun's UVRs. Therefore, decreasing the risks associated with sun exposure is crucial for patients having been treated for skin cancer and the general population as a whole. Measures one should undertake to minimize UV exposure include wearing long-sleeved shirts and long pants, wearing hats and visors, and covering unprotected skin with sunscreen. Most clothing offers an SPF of 2 to 6.5, although clothing that offers SPF protection of up to 30 does exist. Protection of the eyes and lips are also important. Patients should be instructed to obtain sunglasses that block UVRs.[45,46]

Chemical sunscreens are classified according to their level of SPF. Sunscreens generally offer protection from UVB rays and, to a lesser extent, UVA rays. Agents that block both types of rays are referred to as broad-spectrum sunscreens. It is recommended that patients use a chemical sunscreen with an SPF of at least 15 but preferably 30.[47] To permit maximum absorption, sunscreens need to be applied 15 to 30 minutes before sun exposure. Liberal amounts of sunscreen should be evenly applied and allowed to dry. Reapplication should occur every 90 minutes or after one has been submersed in water. Patients should be instructed that sunscreens do not eliminate the risk of developing skin cancer and that sunscreen should be used as an adjunct to an overall UVR reduction lifestyle.[1,48,49]

Certain types of medication, such as antibiotics and diuretics and some chemotherapy agents and porfimer sodium, can increase one's sensitivity to the sun. Side effect profiles of the patient's medication should be reviewed to evaluate his or her risk for increased sun sensitivity.

Patients also should be encouraged to take part in a yearly skin screening program in which a board-certified dermatologist provides an overall skin examination for suspicious, precancerous, or cancerous lesions. In programs with trained skin cancer screening specialists, reports suggest an overall sensitivity of 84%, a specificity of 99%, and a positive predictive value of 73% for the detection of MM.[50]

Patients also need to be informed of the importance of follow-up examinations after radiation therapy. The risk of developing a second BCC after initial treatment is estimated to be 45%.[51,52] The risk of recurrence of MM is related to tumor thickness and overall aggressiveness. The risk of a second primary MM is estimated to occur in 5% of persons previously diagnosed with the disease.[4,53,54] Patients with previously diagnosed skin cancers need to be informed of their risk for developing recurrence or a second primary site. Resources for patients having been treated for skin cancer can be found in Table 15-12.

REFERENCES

1. Mahon SM, Yackzan SG: Skin cancer. In Yarbro CH, Frogge MH, Goodman M, editors: *Cancer nursing*, ed 6, Boston, 2005, Jones & Bartlett, pp 1581-1616.
2. Halder RM, Bridgeman-Shah S: Skin cancer in African Americans, *Cancer* 75:667-673, 1995.
3. *Facts and figures 2006,* Atlanta, American Cancer Society, 2005.
4. Ries LAG, Kosary CL, Hankey BF et al: *SEER Cancer statistics review, 1973-1995,* Bethesda MD, National Cancer Institute, 1998.

Table 15-12 Resources for Patients With Skin Cancer

Resources	Locations	Publication dates
PAMPHLETS		
Many Faces of Malignant Melanoma	Skin Cancer Foundation	1996
Facts on Skin Cancer	American Cancer Society	1996
Take Action Against Skin Cancer	Skin Cancer Foundation	1996
The ABCD's of Melanoma	Skin Cancer Foundation	1996
Understanding Melanoma	Schering Oncology Biotech	1997
Why You Should Know About Melanoma	American Cancer Society	1997
What You Should Know About Melanoma	American Cancer Society	1997
Things You Should Know About Melanoma (fact sheet)	Schering Corporation	1997
Melanoma: Know Your Treatment Options	Schering Oncology Biotech	1998
Actinic Keratosis: What You Should Know About This Common Precancer	Skin Cancer Foundation	1999
Basal cell carcinoma	Skin Cancer Foundation	1999
Sun Safety Quiz—Has Your Skin Been Touched by Melanoma?	Schering Oncology Biotech	2000
The Many Faces of Malignant Melanoma	Chiron Biopharmaceuticals	2000
If You Are Concerned About Melanoma/ Information About Dx and Rx	Schering Oncology Biotech	2000
Face the facts about skin cancer	Schering Oncology Biotech	2001
What You Need to Know About: Melanoma	National Cancer Institute/NIH	2002
What You Need to Know About: Moles & Dysplastic Nevi	National Cancer Institute/NIH	2002
Prevention and early diagnosis of melanoma	Chiron biopharmaceuticals	2003
Staging and Treatment of Melanoma	Chiron biopharmaceuticals	2003
Melanoma Treatment Guidelines for Patients	American Cancer Society/National Comprehensive Cancer Network	2004
BOOKS		
100 Q & A About Melanoma and Other Skin Cancer	McClay E, McClay M, Smith J	2003
Melanoma Prevention, Detection and Treatment	Poole CM	1998
Melanoma Treatment Guidelines for Patients, version ii	ACS/NCCN	
Sun Sense	Robins P	1990
The Official Patient's Sourcebook on Melanoma	Icon Health Publications	2002
There's a Flying Squirrel in My Coffee: Overcoming Cancer	Goss W, Lt. Commander, USN (ret)	2002
Understanding Melanoma: What You Need to Know	Robins P, Perez M	1996
What You Really Need to Know About Moles and Melanoma	Schofield J, Robinson W	2000
INTERNET		
The Skin Cancer Foundation	www.skincancer.org	
Skin Cancer—Medline Plus	www.nlm.nih.gov/medlineplus/skincancer.html	
American Academy of Dermatology	www.aad.org	
American Cancer Society	www.cancer.org	
Cancer Index: the Skin Cancer Resources Directory	www.cancerindex.org/clinks2s.htm	
Cancer Prevention and Control	www.cdc.gov/cancer/nscpep/skin.htm	
Melanoma: the ABCs	www.melanoma.com/melanoma/index.jsp	
National Cancer Institute	www.cancer.gov/cancertopics/types/skin	

5. Habif TM: Principles of diagnosis and anatomy. In *Clinical dermatology* ed 4, Philadelphia, 2004, Mosby, pp 1-22.
6. Leffell DL, Fitzgerald DA: Basal cell carcinoma. In Freedberg IM, Eisen AZ, Wolff K et al, editors: *Dermatology in general medicine, vol 1,* ed 5, New York, 1999, McGraw-Hill, pp 857-864.
7. Sexton M, Jones DB, Maloney ME: Histologic pattern analysis of basal cell carcinoma: study of a series of 1039 consecutive neoplasms, *J Am Acad Dermatol* 23:1118-1126, 1990.
8. Rowe DE, Carroll RJ, Day CL Jr: Prognostic factors for local recurrence, metastasis, and survival rates in squamous cell carcinoma of the skin, ear, and lip: implications for treatment modality selection, *J Am Acad Dermatol* 26:976-990, 1992.
9. Dinehart SM, Pollack SV: Metastases from squamous cell carcinoma of the skin and lip: an analysis of twenty-seven cases, *J Am Acad Dermatol* 2:241-248, 1989.
10. Habif TM: Premalignant and malignant nonmelanoma skin tumors. In *Clinical dermatology,* ed 4, Philadelphia, 2004, Mosby, pp 724-772.
11. Habif TM: Nevi and malignant melanoma. In *Clinical dermatology,* ed 4, Philadelphia, 2004, Mosby, pp 773-813.
12. Morton DL, Essner R, Kirkwood JM et al: Malignant melanoma. In Holland JF, Bast Jr RC, Morton DL et al, editors: *Cancer medicine, vol 2,* ed 4, Baltimore, 1997, Williams and Wilkins, pp 2467-2499.
13. Langley R, Barnhill RL, Mihm MC et al: Neoplasms: cutaneous melanoma. In Freedberg IM, Eisen AZ, Wolff K et al, editors: *Dermatology in general medicine, vol 1,* ed 5, New York, 1999, McGraw-Hill, pp 1080-1116.
14. Washington CM, Blobe TA: Skin and melanoma. In Washington CM, Lever D, editors: *Principles and practice of radiation therapy,* ed 2, St Louis, 2004, Mosby, pp 893-918.
15. Preston DS, Stern RS: Nonmelanoma cancers of the skin, *N Engl J Med* 327:1649-1662, 1992.
16. Casciato DA, Lowitz BB: *Manual of clinical oncology*, ed 4, Philadelphia, 2000, Lippincott Williams & Wilkins.
17. American Cancer Society: *The ABCD rule for early detection of melanoma.* Retrieved on 12/17/2005 from www.cancer.org/docroot/SPC/content/SPC_1_ABCD_Mole_Check_Tips.asp
18. Otto SE: *Oncology nursing,* ed 3, St Louis, 1997, Mosby.
19. Morton DL et al: Multivariate analysis of the relationship between survival and the microstage of primary melanoma by Clark level and Breslow thickness, *Cancer* 71:3737-3743, 1993.
20. Balch CM, Buzaid AC, Soong SJ et al: Final version of the American Joint Committee on Cancer staging system for cutaneous melanoma, *J Clin Oncol* 19:3635-3648, 2001.
21. *AJCC cancer staging manual,* ed 5, Philadelphia, 1997, Lippincott-Raven.
22. Fleming ID, Amonette R, Monaghan T et al: Principles of management of basal and squamous cell carcinoma of the skin, *Cancer* 75:699-704, 1995.
23. *Research report: skin cancers: basal cell and squamous cell carcinomas.* National Institutes of Health publication No. 91-2977, Bethesda, MD, 1990, National Cancer Institute.
24. Neel VA, Sober AJ: Other skin cancers. In Kufe DW, Pollock RE, Weichselbaum RR et al, editors: *Cancer medicine, vol 2,* ed 5, Baltimore, 2003, BC Decker, pp 1997-2013.
25. Mendenhall WM et al: T2-T4 carcinoma of the skin of the head and neck treated with radical irradiation, *Int J Radiat Oncol Biol Phys* 13:975-981, 1987.
26. National Comprehensive Cancer Network: Clinical practice guidelines on oncology, Version 1. *Basal cell and squamous cell skin cancer.* Retrieved on 12/01/2005 from www.nccn.org/professionals/physician_gls/PDF/nmsc.pdf
27. Moss WT, Cox JD: *Radiation oncology rationale, technique, results,* ed 6, St Louis, 1989, Mosby.
28. Essner R: Surgical treatment of malignant melanoma, *Surg Clin North Am* 83:109-156, 2003.
29. Fink DJ, Holleb AI, Murphy GP: *American Cancer Society textbook of clinical oncology,* Atlanta, 1991, American Cancer Society.
30. Morton DL, Barth A: Vaccine therapy for malignant melanoma, *CA Cancer J Clin* 46:225-244, 1996.
31. Tong AKF, Fitzpatrick TB: Neoplasms of the skin. In Holland JF, Bast Jr RC, Morton DL et al, editors: *Cancer medicine, vol 2,* ed 4, Baltimore, 1997, Williams & Wilkins, pp 2433-2464.
32. Cocconi G, Bella M, Calabresi F et al: Treatment of metastatic malignant melanoma with dacarbazine plus tamoxifen, *N Engl J Med* 327:516-523, 1992.
33. Nathan FE, Berd D, Mastrangelo MJ: Chemotherapy of melanoma. In Perry M, editor: *The chemotherapy source book,* ed 2, Baltimore, 1996, Williams & Wilkins, pp 1043-1069.
34. Kadison AS, Morton DL: Immunotherapy of malignant melanoma, *Surg Clin North Am* 83:343-370, 2003.
35. Kirkwood JM, Strawderman MH, Ernstoff MS et al: Interferon alpha-2b adjuvant therapy of high-risk resected cutaneous melanoma: the Eastern Cooperative Oncology Group trial EST1684, *J Clin Oncol* 14:7-17, 1996.
36. Balch CM, Atkins MB, Sober AJ: Cutaneous melanoma. In Devita VT, Hellman S, Rosenberg SA, editors: *Cancer principles and practice of oncology,* ed 7, Philadelphia, 2005, Lippincott Williams & Wilkins, pp 1754-1808.
37. Ang KK, Byers RM, Peters LJ et al: Regional radiotherapy as adjuvant treatment for head and neck malignant melanoma, *Arch Otolaryngol Head Neck Surg* 116:169-172, 1990.
38. Pyrhonen SO, Kajanti MJ: The use of large fractions in radiotherapy for malignant melanoma, *Radiother Oncol* 24:195-197, 1992.
39. Munzenrider JE: Uveal melanomas: conservative treatment, *Hematol Oncol Clin North Am* 15:389-402, 2001.
40. Karlsson UL, Augsburger JJ, Shields JA et al: Recurrence of posterior uveal melanoma after CO60 episcleral plaque therapy, *Ophthalmology* 96:382-388, 1989.
41. Wilson MW, Hungerford JL, St Bartholomew's Hospital: Comparison of episcleral plaque and proton beam radiation therapy for the treatment of choroidal melanoma, *Ophthalmology* 106:1579-1587, 1999.
42. Char DH, Kroll S, Phillips TL et al: Late radiation failures after iodine 125 brachytherapy for uveal melanoma compared with charged-particle (proton or helium ion) therapy, *Ophthalmology* 109:1850-1854, 2002.
43. Robertson DM: Changing concepts in the management of choroidal melanoma, *Am J Ophthalmol* 136:161-170, 2003.
44. Jensen AW, Petersen IA, Kline RW et al: Radiation complications and tumor control after 125I plaque brachytherapy for ocular melanoma, *Int J Radiat Oncol Biol Phys* 63:101-108, 2005.

45. Hill L, Ferrini RL: Skin cancer prevention and screening: summary of the American College of Preventive Medicine's practice policy statements, *CA Cancer J Clin* 48:232-235, 1998.
46. Koh HK: Sunbathing habits and sunscreen use among white adults: results of a national survey. *Am J Public Health* 87:1214-1217, 1997.
47. Oliveria SA, Christos PJ, Marghoob AA et al: Skin cancer screening and prevention in the primary care setting: National Ambulatory Care Medical Survey 1997, *J Gen Intern Med* 16:297-301, 2001.
48. Lamberg L: Sunscreen, in office dispensing, surgery debated at annual dermatology meeting, *JAMA* 281:1363-1364, 1999.
49. Vainio H, Miller AB, Bianchini F: An international evaluation of the cancer-preventive potential of sunscreens, *Int J Cancer* 88: 838-842, 2000.
50. Mackie RM, Koh HK, Geller P: Skin cancer and melanoma. In Reintgen DS, Clark RA, editors: *Cancer screening,* St Louis, 1996, Mosby, pp 168-195.
51. Easton D: The role of atypical mole syndrome and cutaneous naevi in the development of melanoma, *Cancer Surv* 26:237-249, 1996.
52. Marghoob A, Slade J, Salopek TG et al: Basal cell and squamous cell carcinomas are important risk factors for cutaneous malignant melanoma screening implications, *Cancer* 75:704-714, 1995.
53. Albert RA, Weinstock MA: Keratinocyte carcinoma, *CA Cancer J Clin* 53:292-302, 2003.
54. Rigel DS: Malignant melanoma: incidence issues and their effect on diagnosis and treatment in the 1990s, *Mayo Clin Proc* 72:367-371, 1997.

Chapter 16

Hodgkin's Disease and Non-Hodgkin's Lymphoma

Heather Lynn Brumbaugh

Non-Hodgkin's lymphoma (NHL) is a diverse group of blood-borne neoplasms that arise from uncontrolled growth of lymphocytes, whereas Hodgkin's disease is a very distinct and predictable type of lymphoma. Approximately 4% of all cancer diagnoses in 2006 will be NHL. The estimated number of new cases in 2006 for lymphoma is 66,670, with 58,870 being NHL and 7800 Hodgkin's disease. In 2006 it is estimated that there will be 18,840 deaths from NHL and 1490 from Hodgkin's disease. The incidence of NHL increases with age, with the peak around age 60. Hodgkin's disease has a bimodal peak with a peak between ages 15 and 34 and a second peak in older adults over the age of 50.[1-3]

From 1970 to 2000 the incidence of NHL nearly doubled. This is thought to be due to several factors including earlier detection, the aging population, and wider use of scanning techniques, but other factors also have an influence.[4] Immunodeficiency and immunosuppression are known to play a role in the development of NHL. This includes not only people with HIV but also patients who have undergone organ transplantation and individuals with collagen vascular or autoimmune disorders who have altered immune systems. Chemical exposure and radiation are known risk factors for NHL. Some unique subtypes of NHL are specifically caused by bacteria or viruses. For example, *Helicobacter pylori* is the cause of most gastric lymphomas and is treated with antibiotics alone. Epstein-Barr virus has been implicated in some subtypes of NHL and in Hodgkin's disease. As more is learned about NHL, evidence suggests that chromosomal abnormalities may contribute to the development of the disease.[5]

ANATOMY AND PATHOPHYSIOLOGY

Hodgkin's disease and NHL are neoplasms of the immune system caused by uncontrolled growth of lymphocytes. There are two types of lymphocytes—B cells and T cells. These cells are characterized by their function and surface proteins, which are markers on the cell surface called *CD* (cluster of differentiation) molecules that are recognized by specific sets of antibodies. Based on the CD molecules present, the cell can be identified as a B cell or T cell, and the stage of differentiation and activity of the cell also can be determined. The B cells function as "workers" and produce antibodies. The T cells function as "supervisors" and regulate the immune system by controlling the B cells. The lymphocytes live in lymph nodes until they are needed to respond to an insult or injury to the body. The normal lymph node is divided into different sections. Each subtype of lymphocyte has a specific place in which it normally resides within a lymph node. The normal lymph node architecture consists of paracortex, mantle zone, follicular center, and medullary cords.[5] The immune system is a tightly regulated system in which cells have a designated role and life span. When lymphoma develops, it is the result of an alteration in the immune system resulting in an accumulation of lymphocytes caused by overproduction or an abnormal extension of the lymphocyte's existing life cycle.

CLINICAL MANIFESTATIONS

Hodgkin's disease typically presents as enlarged, painless, firm, freely movable lymph nodes. Hodgkin's disease has a predictable pattern of spread, moving from one lymph node group contiguously to the next. The most common areas involved are the cervical, axillary, and mediastinal nodes. Approximately 30% of patients present with B symptoms, so named because staging for Hodgkin's disease and NHL includes both a number (I-IV) and a letter (A or B). "A" indicates absence of symptoms, while "B" indicates they are present. B symptoms include fever, night sweats, weight loss (more than 10% of body weight in the last 6 months), and pruritus.[3]

NHL also typically presents with enlarged lymph nodes. Depending on the subtype, the patient can be asymptomatic or very sick. Extranodal presentation occurs in approximately 30% of cases, involving sites such as gastrointestinal (GI) tract, skin, spleen, pharyngeal tissue, salivary glands, thymus, testis, central nervous system (CNS), bone, and lung.[2] In low-grade lymphomas, the patient often reports a history of lymph nodes that have waxed and waned before further evaluation was sought. Bone marrow involvement is common, and cytopenias can be seen. Splenomegaly also can occur. Because of immune dysregulation, some patients present with infections, hemolytic anemia, or skin rashes. In intermediate- or high-grade lymphomas, the presentation can involve B symptoms and even tumor lysis.

DIAGNOSTIC STUDIES

Hodgkin's Disease

Hodgkin's disease requires an excisional biopsy to make an adequate diagnosis and confirmation of disease subtype. According to National Comprehensive Cancer Network (NCCN) guidelines, a fine-needle aspirate (FNA) is inadequate to diagnose Hodgkin's disease. Immunohistochemical stains are recommended to include CD15, CD30, CD3, CD20 and CD45 in classical Hodgkin's disease.[3] Once a diagnosis of Hodgkin's disease has been confirmed, additional studies are needed to determine the extent of the disease so a curative treatment plan can be prescribed. A history and physical should include evaluation for palpable adenopathy, B symptoms, and performance status. Laboratory studies should include: complete blood count (CBC), inclusive of a differential and platelet count, erythrocyte sedimentation rate (ESR), serum lactate dehydrogenase (LDH), and liver and renal panels. Computed tomography (CT) scan of the chest, abdomen, and pelvis and a bone marrow exam are needed to evaluate extent of disease. A functional study such as a gallium or positive emission tomography (PET) scan is recommended as part of disease staging. Functional studies help distinguish between scarring, fibrosis, or active disease. It is helpful to obtain a functional study at baseline and at the end of treatment, typically 3 to 4 weeks after the completion of chemotherapy. PET scans have become the study of choice because of convenience and efficacy over gallium scans (half-day study vs. 3 days for gallium).

Non-Hodgkin's Lymphoma

NHL also requires an excisional biopsy for initial diagnosis to evaluate the lymph node architecture and determine the histologic subtype.[6] Flow cytometry on the lymph node is helpful to assess surface proteins on the lymphocytes, which is necessary to determine the disease subtype. Immunohistochemical stains also can be used to evaluate for specific markers. A CD20 marker study is positive in the majority of B-cell lymphomas and is the target of the monoclonal antibody rituximab. A CD10 marker study may help distinguish follicular lymphoma versus other lymphoma subtypes, and CD5 is positive in small lymphocytic lymphoma and mantle cell lymphoma.[2] A history and physical exam is needed to evaluate for palpable nodes, hepatosplenomegaly, B symptoms, and performance status. Laboratory studies should include CBC, differential, platelets, ESR, LDH, liver and renal function panels, and immune studies (serum protein electrophoresis and quantitative immunoglobulins). Additional laboratory studies that may be of benefit include beta-2-microglobulin, direct Coombs, and reticulocyte count. Diagnostic studies such as CT scan of the chest, abdomen, and pelvis, and a bone marrow biopsy are needed to determine the extent of the disease. A PET scan may be of benefit in intermediate- and high-grade subtypes.

PATHOLOGY

Hodgkin's Disease

A lymph node involved with Hodgkin's disease usually contains a small number of malignant cells, with the majority of cells being inflammatory or reactive cells. The classical finding on pathology is the Reed-Sternberg cell, which is a large binuclear cell that has markers for CD30 and CD15. The most common subtype of Hodgkin's disease is nodular sclerosis characterized by prominent fibrosis, mature lymphocytes, and Reed-Sternberg cells (RSCs).[3] Mixed cellularity subtype has less fibrosis and more RSCs.[3] Lymphocyte depleted subtype is rare and has numerous RCSs but a sparse background of other cells.[3] Lymphocyte predominant is the fourth subtype and is characterized by a vague nodular pattern that is rich in lymphocytes. This subtype has recently been noted to resemble a low-grade NHL because it is CD20 positive and CD15 negative and it has an indolent course with late relapses after treatment.[3]

Non-Hodgkin's Lymphoma

NHL has over 30 subtypes. Several different classification systems have been used over the years and continue to change and evolve as understanding of immunologic, cytogenetic, and molecular studies increases. The *working formulation,* proposed in 1982, is based on morphologic criteria and describes the subtypes based on their natural history while providing a framework that is clinically relevant. Because NHL is a spectrum of diseases, the terms low-grade, intermediate-grade, and high-grade are helpful in determining treatment and the expected outcomes.

In 1994, the REAL (revised European-American lymphoma) classification was developed in an attempt to define the disease by morphologic, immunologic, and genetic criteria. In 2001 the World Health Organization (WHO) classification (Table 16-1) modified the REAL classification based on more current data and is now becoming the standard.[7] Morphology remains the basis on which a diagnosis is made because it looks at the appearance and the pattern of the cells in the lymph node. Immunohistochemical stains, flow cytometry, cytogenetics, and molecular studies then help to further classify and define the subtype.

The most common types of NHL are diffuse, large B-cell lymphoma (31%), follicular lymphoma (22%), small lymphocytic lymphoma (6%), mantle cell lymphoma (6%), peripheral T-cell lymphoma (6%), and marginal zone B–cell (mucosa-associated lymphoid tissue, MALT) (5%). Marginal-zone lymphoma includes gastric MALT, nongastric MALT, nodal marginal-zone lymphoma, and splenic marginal-zone lymphoma. The remaining subtypes occur in less than 2% of cases of NHL.[8]

The staging system for both NHL and Hodgkin's disease is the Ann Arbor staging system

Table 16-1 WHO Classification of Lymphoid Neoplasms

B-cell neoplasms	T-cell and NK-cell neoplasms
Precursor B-cell neoplasm	Precursor T-cell neoplasm
Precursor B-lymphoblastic leukemia/lymphoma	Precursor T-lymphoblastic leukemia/lymphoma
Mature (peripheral) B-cell neoplasms	*Mature (peripheral) T-cell neoplasms*
B-cell chronic lymphocytic leukemia/small lymphocytic lymphoma	T-cell prolymphocytic leukemia
B-cell prolymphocytic lymphoma	T-cell granular lymphocytic leukemia
Lymphoplasmacytic lymphoma	Aggressive NK-cell leukemia
Splenic marginal zone B-cell lymphoma (± villous lymphocytes)	Adult T-cell lymphoma/leukemia (HTLV1+)
Hairy cell leukemia	Extranodal NK/T cell lymphoma
Plasma cell myeloma/plasmacytoma	Enteropathy-type T-cell lymphoma
Extranodal marginal zone B-cell lymphoma of MALT type	Hepatosplenic gamma-delta T-cell lymphoma
Nodal marginal zone B-cell lymphoma	Subcutaneous panniculitis-like T-cell lymphoma
Follicular lymphoma	Mycosis fungoides/Sézary syndrome
Mantle cell lymphoma	Anaplastic large-cell lymphoma primary cutaneous or systemic
Diffuse large B-cell lymphoma	Peripheral T-cell lymphoma
Burkitt's lymphoma/Burkitt cell leukemia	Angioimmunoblastic T-cell lymphoma

Data from:

Armitage JO, Weisenburger DD: New approach to classifying non-Hodgkin's lymphomas: clinical features of the major histologic subtypes. Non-Hodgkin's Lymphoma Classification Project, *J Clin Oncol* 16:2780–2795, 1998.

Harris NL, Jaffe ES, Diebold J et al: The World Health Organization classification of neoplastic diseases of the hematopoietic and lymphoid tissues. Report of the clinical advisory committee meeting, Airlie House, Va, November 1997, *Ann Oncol* 10:1419–1432, 1999.

WHO, World Health Organization; *MALT,* mucosa-associated lymphoid tissue.

Box 16-1 Ann Arbor Staging System

Stage I—Limited to one lymph node area
Stage II—More than one lymph node area but on the same side of the diaphragm
Stage III—Lymph nodes above and below the diaphragm
Stage IV—Diffuse disease, bone marrow involvement
- "A"—No systemic symptoms
- "B"—Systemic symptoms
- Weight loss more than 10% in past 6 months, fever, drenching night sweats, pruritus.

Data From Rosen ST, Winter JN, Gordon LI et al: Non-Hodgkin's lymphoma. In Pazdur R, editor: Cancer management: a multidisciplinary approach, Manhasset, NY, 2005, CMP.

Box 16-2 International Prognostic Index

RISK FACTORS
- Age (>60)
- LDH (lactate dehydrogenase) level (elevated)
- Performance status (2-4)
- Ann Arbor stage (stage III or IV)
- Extranodal involvement (> one site)

One point is assigned for each risk factor and then totaled.

Risk	Points
Low	0 or 1
Low intermediate	2
High intermediate	3
High	4 or 5

Data From Rosen ST, Winter JN, Gordon LI et al: Non-Hodgkin's lymphoma. In Pazdur R, editor: Cancer management: a multidisciplinary approach, Manhasset, NY, 2005, CMP.

(Box 16-1). This system is a shorthand way to describe where the disease is located, but unlike staging in solid tumors, stage IV does not indicate a poor prognosis. In NHL the subtype is most important in determining expected outcomes. Because stage is not helpful in predicting prognosis, the international prognostic index (IPI) was developed to predict the aggressiveness of the disease and then was used in treatment planning (Box 16-2). The IPI includes five factors: age, Ann Arbor stage, serum LDH level, number of extranodal sites, and performance status. A point is assigned for each unfavorable factor and then totaled. Based on the number of points, a patient is considered low risk, low-intermediate risk, high-intermediate risk or high risk.

Table 16-2 Chemotherapy Regimens for Hodgkin's Disease

Medication	Dose
ABVD	
Doxorubicin	25 mg/m^2 on days 1 and 15
Bleomycin	10 U/m^2 on days 1 and 15
Vinblastine	6 mg/m^2 on days 1 and 15
Dacarbazine	375 mg/m^2 on days 1 and 15, repeated every 28 days
Stanford V	
Doxorubicin	25 mg/m^2 on days 1 and 15
Vinblastine	6 mg/m^2 on days 1 and 15
Mechlorethamine	6 mg/m^2 on day 1
Vincristine	1.4 mg/m^2 on days 8 and 22 (max 2 mg)
Bleomycin	5 U/m^2 on days 8 and 22
Etoposide	60 mg/m^2 on days 15 and 16
Prednisone	40 mg/m^2 qod, repeated every 28 days
MOPP	
Mechlorethamine	6 mg/m^2 on days 1 and 8
Vincristine	1.4 mg/m^2 on days 1 and 8 (max 2 mg)
Procarbazine	100 mg/m^2 on days 1–14
Prednisone	40 mg/m^2 on days 1–14, repeated every 28 days

qod, Every other day.

TREATMENT

Hodgkin's Disease

The treatment for Hodgkin's disease is designed to cure the patient with the least amount of therapy needed to prevent or minimize long-term complications. Treatment includes chemotherapy alone, radiation therapy alone, or combined modality treatment. Recent studies show that a combination approach to treatment allows for less of each modality while still enabling a cure.[9]

The most common chemotherapy regimens used to treat Hodgkin's disease are doxorubicin, bleomycin, vinblastine, and dacarbazine (ABVD) and Stanford V (Table 16-2). Mechlorethamine, vincristine, procarbazine, and prednisone (MOPP) was previously used but resulted in an increase in secondary leukemia and is now used only in select settings. Radiation also has evolved over time. Previously, patients received mantle field radiation, which included bilateral cervical/supraclavicular, axillary, mediastinal, and bilateral hilar nodes. An inverted Y field, which encompassed bilateral pelvic nodes and para-aortic/spleen fields, was also standard treatment. The current standard, however, has become radiation to involved field only—treating the areas where disease was present at diagnosis only. Radiation, when used, is delivered daily in fractions of 1.5 GY to 1.8 Gy with opposed anterior and posterior fields. Cumulative radiation dose is determined by the extent of the disease.[10]

For stage I to II Hodgkin's disease, the standard treatment is now four cycles of ABVD followed by consolidative radiation. If radiation is not given, six cycles of chemotherapy is standard. If Stanford V is used, two cycles are given in nonbulky stage I to II disease and three cycles in bulky stage I to II disease followed by consolidative radiation. The dose of radiation used in combined modality therapy is 20 Gy to 30 Gy to involved field only.[11] If radiation is contraindicated, then a full course of chemotherapy is given. Conversely, in patients that cannot tolerate chemotherapy who have stage I to IIA disease, subtotal lymph node (mantle and para-aortic/spleen) radiation can be used.[11]

Stage III to IV disease is treated with six to eight cycles of ABVD with restaging after four to six cycles so that two additional cycles can be given once a complete response is obtained. Consolidative radiation is then given to areas of bulk disease with 20 Gy to 36 Gy. If Stanford V is used, then three cycles (12 weeks) of therapy is given followed by consolidative radiation.[11]

Relapse, if it occurs, is most common in the first 2 years. A repeat biopsy is recommended followed by treatment with salvage chemotherapy (Table 16-3). Typically, a couple of cycles of standard therapy are given, and then the patient is treated with high-dose chemotherapy with stem cell support for curative intent. Radiation also can be used at relapse but may be limited depending on previous dose and treatment fields.[12]

Table 16-3 Salvage Chemotherapy Regimens for Hodgkin's Disease and NHL

Medication	Dose
ICE	
Ifosfamide	2 g/m^2 day 1–3
Carboplatin	350 mg/m^2 day 1
Etoposide	75 mg/m^2 days 1–3, repeated every 21-28 days
DHAP	
Dexamethasone	40 mg days 1–4
Cisplatin	100 mg/m^2 day 1
Cytarabine	2 g/m^2 over 3 hr every 12 hr for 2 doses on day 2, repeated every 21–28 days
ESHAP	
Etoposide	60 mg/m^2 days 1–4
Methylprednisolone	500 mg/m^2 days 1–5
Cytarabine (Ara-C)	2 g/m^2 over 2 hr on day 5 following completion of cisplatin
Cisplatin (Platinol)	25 mg/m^2 continuous infusion on days 1–4, repeated every 21–28 days

Non-Hodgkin's Lymphoma

NHL has a variety of treatment options, as would be expected with the numerous disease subtypes. This chapter addresses the most common subtypes: diffuse large cell lymphoma, small lymphocytic lymphoma, follicular lymphoma and gastric MALT, and cutaneous T-cell lymphoma in which radiation therapy has a unique role.

Diffuse large B-cell lymphoma is typically treated with combined modality therapy (Table 16-4). The goal of treatment is cure and over 50% are cured with standard therapy.[2] Clinical trials are ongoing, especially in high-risk disease, to evaluate improved treatment outcomes. Standard treatment is cyclophosphamide, doxorubicin, vincristine and prednisone

Table 16-4 Chemotherapy Regimens for Diffuse Large B-Cell Lymphoma

Medication	Dose
CHOP ± RITUXIMAB	
Cyclophosphamide	750 mg/m^2 day 1
Doxorubicin	50 mg/m^2 day 1
Vincristine (Oncovin)	1.4 mg/m^2 day 1 (max 2 mg)
Prednisone	100 mg daily days 1–5
Rituximab	375 mg/m^2 day 1, repeat every 21 days
MINE	
Mesna	1330 mg/m^2 with ifosfamide
Ifosfamide	1330 mg/m^2 days 1–3
Mitoxantrone (Novantrone)	8 mg/m^2 day 1
Etoposide	65 mg/m^2 days 1-3, repeat every 21 days
ICE	See Table 16-3 for doses
DHAP	See Table 16-3 for doses
ESHAP	See Table 16-3 for doses

(CHOP) chemotherapy along with the monoclonal antibody rituximab.[13] As in Hodgkin's disease, low-risk stage I or II disease is treated with chemotherapy for four cycles and followed by involved field radiation therapy. In high-risk stage I or II disease or stage III or IV disease, six to eight cycles of chemotherapy is given. Radiation can be considered in these patients for consolidation but is not standard. When used, radiation is given to the areas of bulk disease because those are the most likely sites of relapse. If a patient has heart disease that contraindicates the use of doxorubicin, then alternative treatment is used that does not contain an anthracycline, such as ESHAP (methylprednisolone, etoposide, cytarabine and cisplatin). If relapse occurs, salvage chemotherapy is used, and once a response is seen, patients are treated with high-dose chemotherapy with stem cell support with curative intent.[13]

Small lymphocytic lymphoma is the nodal manifestation of chronic lymphocytic leukemia. These two diseases have the same surface markers, one of which circulates in the bloodstream and the other involves the nodes. Both diseases are essentially treated in the same manner. Because it is a low-grade/chronic process, watchful waiting is often the initial approach. Indications for treatment include eligibility for clinical trial, autoimmune cytopenia, recurrent infections, symptoms, threatened end-organ damage, cytopenias, bulky disease, steady progression, patient preference, or histologic transformation.[13] Multiple chemotherapeutic options are available for treatment (Table 16-5). Radiation is used only for palliation in this disease subtype.

The subtype of follicular lymphoma is further subdivided into grades. Grades 1 and 2 are

Table 16-5 Chemotherapy Regimens for Small Lymphocytic Lymphoma/Chronic Lymphocytic Leukemia

Medication	Dose
Fludarabine ± Rituximab	
Fludarabine	25 mg/m^2 days 1-5
Rituximab	375 mg/m^2 day 1
Chlorambucil ± Prednisone	
Chlorambucil	4-6 mg daily for 6–18 months or pulse
Prednisone	40 mg/m^2 to 80 mg/m^2 days 1–5
Cyclophosphamide ± Prednisone	
Cyclophosphamide	50–100 mg daily for 6–18 months
Prednisone	40 mg/m^2 to 80 mg/m^2 days 1–5
CVP ± Rituximab	
Cyclophosphamide	300 mg/m^2 PO days 1–3
Vincristine	1.4 mg/m^2 on day 1 (max 2 mg)
Prednisone	40 mg/m^2 on days 1–5, repeat every 21 days
COP ± Rituximab	
Cyclophosphamide	800 mg/m^2 IV day 1
Vincristine (Oncovin)	1.4 mg/m^2 on day 1 (max 2 mg)
Prednisone	60 mg/m^2 on days 1–5, repeat every 14 days
FCR	
Fludarabine	25 mg/m^2 days 1–3
Cyclophosphamide	250 mg/m^2 days 1–3
Rituximab	375 mg/m^2 day 1 cycle 1
	500 mg/m^2 day of subsequent cycles over 1 hour, repeat every 28 days
Alemtuzumab (CAMPATH)	
Alemtuzumab	3 mg on day 1
	10 mg on day 3
	30 mg on day 5
	Then 30 mg M/W/F, given for 6–12 weeks
	Requires supportive medications to prevent PRP and HSV

IV, Intravenous; *PCP, Pneumocystis jiroveci* (historically indentified as *Pneumocystis carinii*) pneumonia; *HSV,* herpes simplex virus.

indolent/low-grade processes, whereas grade 3 is more aggressive and treated like diffuse large B-cell lymphoma. The grade is determined by pathology and is based on the appearance of the actual cells. The grade is assigned by the proportion of large cells seen per high-power field under the microscope. Grade 1 is mostly small cells, grade 2 is mixed small and large cells, and grade 3 is mostly all large cells, but the lymph node has still retained its normal structure so it is called *follicular*. If there is any area of diffuse involvement in which the nodal structure is changed, transformation to diffuse large-cell lymphoma has likely occurred.[7]

Follicular lymphoma often presents with bone marrow involvement.[2] A bilateral bone marrow biopsy is performed in this population because it increases the diagnostic yield. If a patient is found to have nonbulky localized disease (stage I or II), then a PET scan can be used to look for occult disease. In nonbulky localized disease, radiation therapy to a dose of 30 Gy to 36 Gy is used to attempt cure.[13] The addition of chemotherapy or extended-field radiation has not shown improvement in overall survival although it can improve one's length of response.[13]

For the majority of patients with stage III or IV NHL, multiple treatment options exist. Unfortunately, none are curative with the current state of knowledge. Therefore these patients are encouraged to participate in clinical trials. Watchful waiting is an option in patients that have small-volume disease, are asymptomatic, and are mentally able to deal with no treatment. Indications for treatment are similar to those in small lymphocytic lymphoma, including eligibility for clinical trial, symptoms, threatened end-organ damage, cytopenia secondary to the lymphoma, massive bulky disease at presentation, steady progression over at least 6 months, or patient preference.[13] When treatment is indicated, factors in choosing a regimen include age, comorbidities, and future treatment possibilities.[13] Chemotherapy and monoclonal antibodies are used in combinations or as single agents as outlined in Box 16-3. Radiation is used as palliation except for radioimmunotherapy.

Because follicular lymphoma is not curative, the expectation of relapse exists. Depending on the length of time from last treatment, the same regimen may be repeated or an altogether different regimen may be prescribed. Radioimmunotherapy is currently approved for relapsed or refractory disease but is being studied in clinical trials as front line therapy. Two agents are available: ibritumomab tiuxetan (Zevalin) and tositumomab (Bexxar).[14,15] Both agents require a multidisciplinary approach because the patient receives a "cold" dose of antibody to clear the peripheral blood of CD20+ cells followed by a "hot" dose of the radiolabeled antibody for treatment of the disease. In some settings this is done in nuclear medicine and in others it is given in the radiation oncology department. Both drugs have a small "test" dose given to evaluate uptake and determine the dose for tositumomab. This is followed approximately 1 week later by the therapeutic dose.

Box 16-3 Chemotherapy Regimens for Follicular Lymphoma Grade 1 or 2

Single-agent rituximab
Chlorambucil
Cyclophosphamide
CVP or COP
Fludarabine ± rituximab
Radioimmunotherapy with iodine-131 and tositumomab (Bexxar) or ibritumomab tiuxetan (Zevalin)

CVP, Cyclophosphamide, vincristine, and prednisone; *COP,* cyclophosphamide, Oncovin (vincristine), and prednisone.

Clinical trials continue to look for better treatment outcomes for follicular lymphoma. Ongoing studies include radioimmunotherapy after chemotherapy as first line treatment and chemotherapy followed by an idiotypic vaccine.

Gastric MALT is a unique subtype of NHL that is caused by a bacterium, *H. pylori*. Initial treatment, if it is localized to the stomach, includes antibiotic administration in conjunction with a gastric proton pump inhibitor. A follow-up endoscopy is performed at 3 months to assess whether bacteria has been eradicated and to evaluate response/improvement of the lymphoma. Serial endoscopies, performed every 3 months, are performed to evaluate for continued improvement over the next 12 to 18 months.[13] As long as continued improvement is seen, the patient can continue without cytotoxic treatment. If the lymphoma worsens or does not resolve, radiation therapy is initially used to treat the disease. Over two-thirds of patients respond to the antibiotic therapy alone.

Cutaneous T-cell lymphoma is a subtype that is characterized by erythematous skin patches and plaque-like lesions. It can wax and wane over many years and is often difficult to diagnosis initially. It is responsive to multiple treatments including topical creams, ultraviolet light treatments, interferon, oral chemotherapeutic agents, and IV chemotherapy.[2] Unfortunately, over time the duration of therapeutic response becomes shorter and shorter. Total skin electron beam therapy has proven useful in these patients and is addressed in Chapter 29 of this book. This remains a difficult subtype to treat, and these patients require a great deal of support.

As would be expected with a disease that has over 30 subtypes, multiple treatment options and approaches are available. When treating the patient with NHL, it is important to keep in mind the natural history of the disease subtype and the goal of therapy. In the subtypes that are not curable, caution must be exercised so as not to cause long-term complications from therapy.

NURSING INTERVENTIONS AND EDUCATION

The diagnosis of cancer is overwhelming to the patient and family; then treatment begins and they have to learn a whole new language. The clinician is critical to ensuring that patients and their families understand what to expect and what to report to the health-care team. There are many acute and long-term side effects from therapy, some of these are noted in Box 16-4. Hodgkin's and NHL can present anywhere in the body. When radiation therapy is used, side effects are usually localized to that specific area. For nursing interventions for side effects to specific regions of the body, refer to the table of contents of this book. Unfortunately, Hodgkin's disease and NHL are not unusual diseases within the realm of pediatric oncology. Caring for pediatric oncology patients and their families creates a unique set of challenges. The Pediatric Considerations box on page 304 lists issues to consider when caring for this patient population.

Many chemotherapy treatment regimens contain corticosteroids, as part of the regimen itself or as part of the antiemetic regimen. Steroid-induced diabetes can be a problem in this patient population. If the patient already has diabetes, corticosteroids can make the disease more difficult to manage. The clinician can help by educating the patient to monitor for signs of hyperglycemia.[16,17]

Box 16-4 Physical Toxicities and Complications of Therapy

TREATMENT-RELATED

Infusion reactions
Depression
Anemia
Neutropenia
Fatigue
Decreased QOL
Nausea/vomiting
Constipation/diarrhea
Weight gain or loss
Diabetes—steroid induced

LONG-TERM

Pulmonary toxicity
Cardiac toxicity
Cataracts
Infertility
Secondary cancer
Lymphedema
Pain/neuropathy
Weight gain
Sleep disorders

QOL, Quality of life.

Corticosteroids irritate the lining of the GI tract. Administration of H_2 antagonists or a gastric proton-pump inhibitor can decrease gastric irritation from corticosteroids. Oral candidiasis, or thrush, is common in patients on high-dose steroids and can result in oral or throat discomfort and taste alterations. These symptoms can be avoided by treating the patient with an antifungal agent while on steroids.[18]

Constipation also can be a problem, particularly in older patients receiving vincristine.[19] Again, the clinician can help by being proactive and educating the patient in the use of stool softeners or laxatives to decrease this problem. If the patient is on narcotics for pain control, the degree of constipation can be exacerbated and will require aggressive management.[20]

Radioimmunotherapy is a fairly new modality of treatment that has unique educational needs for the patient and family, as well as unique nursing implications. Clinicians must educate the patient and family on radiation safety precautions and on the treatment protocol/schedule. The radionuclide used in Zevalin is yttrium-90, which emits beta particles only and has a half-life of 2.7 days.[21]

Therefore patients treated with Zevalin should observe universal precautions in regard to body fluids but do not need any additional safety measures. Bexxar's radionuclide is iodine-131, which emits both beta and gamma photons.[22] The gamma emission allows for dosimetry measurements for patient-specific dosing but also requires additional radiation safety measures. The principles of time, distance, and shielding apply to these patients.[22] Treatment protocols are similar for both agents. The patient receives a small dose on day 1, for biodistribution evaluation in Zevalin and dosimetry in Bexxar.[21,22] Scans are obtained on day 1, with two additional scans between days 2 and 7 postadministration. The therapeutic dose is then administered within a week after completion of the scans. Another unique aspect of Bexxar is the need for a thyroid protectant 24 hours before the start of therapy and for 14 days after the therapeutic dose to prevent absorption of radioactive iodine by the thyroid gland.[22] Clinicians need to be aware that hematologic toxicity is seen with these agents and that it is different from chemotherapy, the onset is later, and it lasts longer. A decrease in blood counts is seen 5 to 7 weeks after treatment and recovery occurs in 8 to 10 weeks.[22] The degree and length of bone marrow suppression will vary depending on previous treatments the patient has received.

Patients with NHL and Hodgkin's disease can have oncologic emergencies, and it is important to be aware of these so they can be recognized early and treated or prevented if possible. Patients that have large mediastinal adenopathy can develop superior vena cava syndrome. This resolves with treatment but sometimes is treated with several doses of radiation up front, depending on the severity.[23] Patients with bulky disease or high-grade disease are at risk for tumor lysis and should be treated with allopurinol and have their electrolytes and serum and urine uric acid levels closely monitored.[24] NHL, specifically diffuse large cell, can cause hypercalcemia due to marrow involvement resulting in increased calcium release from the bone.[25] Patients also can develop spinal cord compression caused by adenopathy/soft tissue masses along the spinal column.[26]

The other area to be aware of in this patient population is long-term complications because most Hodgkin's disease patients are cured, as are many intermediate- and high-grade NHL patients. The lower-grade NHL population also can develop long-term complications from treatment because the natural history of the disease is long. Therapy given early on in the course may cause complications years later. As noted in the treatment section, the standard therapy in these diseases is changing to a combined modality approach, so that less chemotherapy and radiation are used in hopes that there will be fewer long-term complications, specifically secondary malignancies.[27,28] MOPP chemotherapy is known

Pediatric Considerations

- Does child require anesthesia for treatment?
  Conscious sedation policy
  Adequately trained staff
  Availability of adequate staffing
- Role of child life therapist
  Family-focused care
  Parent and sibling guilt/grieving
  Sibling alienation
  Access to care
  Medical bills
- Role of dietitian
  Nutritional screening
  Considerations related to age, growth and development, disease process
- Care coordination across the continuum
  Ongoing quality-of-life assessment
  Transition from pediatric to young adult to adult practitioners
- Age-specific milestones
  Growth and development
  Attainment of independence
  Social skills
  Peer acceptance
  Self image
- End-of-life issues
  Hospice
  Patient/family anger or grief
  Ethical and legal considerations
- Late effects from treatment
  Fertility
  Cognitive changes
  Genetic testing for other primary malignancy
  Secondary malignancies
- Long-term survivorship implications
  Access to care
  Ongoing surveillance
  Disability?
  Discrimination?

to be associated with an increased risk of developing acute leukemia or myelodysplasia.[3] There is also an increased risk of solid tumors and NHL in survivors of Hodgkin's disease. The increased risk of breast cancer is directly related to the dose of radiation, with higher doses resulting in higher risk and younger age having a higher risk.[3] Lung cancer risk is associated with alkylating agents and radiation.[27] NHL survivors also have an increased risk of acute myelogenous leukemia, melanoma, Hodgkin's disease, lung cancer, kidney cancer, brain tumors, and bladder cancer.[2]

It is important that these patients have primary and secondary prevention. Primary prevention efforts such as smoking cessation and exercise are important.[29,30] General guidelines for secondary prevention (screening) include physical examinations, yearly skin examinations, screening colonoscopy, and routine mammograms. In female Hodgkin's disease survivors that have received radiation, mammography should begin yearly at age 40 if not earlier.[31]

Pulmonary toxicity also can be seen in patients that have received bleomycin and/or radiation therapy.[32] The likelihood of developing this toxicity may be increased in patients who receive high dose chemotherapy with stem cell support. The key is close monitoring and early detection so that the causative agent can be discontinued. Early symptoms can be subtle, so it is important to question patients about their breathing. Asking specific questions such as "Have you noticed any change in your breathing or ability to take a deep breath?" can alert to early changes. Intervention with steroids can reduce symptoms, and over time, pulmonary function can improve. Patients that have this complication need to be aware so as to avoid further exposure to other pulmonary irritants. Clinicians need to remember that oxygen is a drug and high doses are damaging to patients with lung toxicity.[33]

Cardiac toxicity is also seen in patients treated for Hodgkin's and NHL. Cardiomyopathy is a known side effect of doxorubicin requiring total cumulative dose to be monitored so as to keep the lifetime dose below 400 mg/m^2.[3] Unfortunately patients can still have complications even at lower doses. Studies have also shown that Hodgkin's disease survivors often have cardiovascular abnormalities, particularly those who received mediastinal radiation at a young age.[34-38] These patients should be monitored and encouraged to follow a heart-healthy lifestyle (blood pressure control, lipid control, and weight control).[29]

Another long-term complication from combination chemotherapy is infertility. In males the risk of infertility with ABVD is estimated to be 15% to 25% and is significantly higher with MOPP.[3] Counseling regarding sperm banking is recommended for all men who want to potentially have children after chemotherapy. The overall rate of primary ovarian failure is 50%, the risk is less in women 25 and younger (25%–30%) and increases to 80% to 100% in women over 25.[3] Premature menopause also can be a problem for women who have maintained ovarian function during chemotherapy. These women will need counseling regarding osteoporosis prevention.[31,39] Treatment also can have an impact on sexuality, which is addressed in Chapter 35.

SUMMARY

The treatment of Hodgkin's and NHL has changed and evolved over the years. As it continues to change with increasing treatment options, it is important that clinicians keep up to date so they can continue to provide support and education to the patient (Table 16-6). A final issue to keep in mind when helping the patient deal with therapy is the actual completion of therapy. Clinicians can be proactive and help patients cope with the changes that occur when therapy finishes. Often, the patient has been coping with the diagnosis of cancer by focusing on getting through the therapy. Once therapy stops, the patient may suddenly begin to face the reality of what has happened. The patient's life will never be the same, and he or she may then view things differently. Survivors have to adapt to a new "normal" because their life will always be impacted by what they have been through.[31] During treatment they will have seen healthcare professionals regularly who have reassured them that they are doing well. Once treatment ends, patients are on their own, often not returning for a follow-up visit for several months. The clinician can help patients by educating them about this change and reassuring them that it is normal to feel insecure and uncertain. Often, just knowing is enough to help the patient cope.

Table 16-6 Resources for Patients with Hodgkin's and Non-Hodgkin's Lymphoma

Organization	Website	Description
National Comprehensive Cancer Network (NCCN)	www.nccn.org	Resource for the *NCCN Clinical Practice Guidelines in Oncology* and *Treatment Guidelines for Patients*.
People living with cancer	www.peoplelivingwithcancer.org	Patient information website designed by ASCO (American Society of Clinical Oncology); helps patients and families make informed healthcare decisions. Provides information on more than 85 types of cancer, clinical trials, coping, side effects, a Find an Oncologist database, message boards, patient support organizations, and more.
Lymphoma Research Foundation	www.lymphoma.org	Provides education, patient support, advocacy, professional information, and more.
Leukemia and Lymphoma Society	www.leukemia.org	Has patient services, disease information, advocacy, professional information, and more.
Oncology Nursing Society's Cancer-Symptoms.org	www.cancersymptoms.org	Designed for patients and caregivers to provide information on learning about and managing each of eight common cancer treatment symptoms: fatigue, anorexia, pain, depression, neutropenia, cognitive dysfunction, dyspnea, and sexual dysfunction.

REFERENCES

1. American Cancer Society: *Cancer facts and figures 2006*, Atlanta, 2006, American Cancer Society.
2. Rosen ST, Winter JN, Gordon LI et al: Non-Hodgkin's lymphoma. In Pazdur R, editor: *Cancer management: a multidisciplinary approach*, Manhasset, NY, 2005, CMP.
3. Yahalom J, Strauss D: Hodgkin's disease. In Pazdur R, editor: *Cancer management: a multidisciplinary approach*, Manhasset, NY, 2005, CMP.
4. Groves FD, Linet MS, Diebold J et al: Cancer surveillance series: non-Hodgkin's disease lymphoma incidence by histologic subtype in the United States from 1978 through 1995, *J Natl Cancer Inst* 92:1240-1251, 2000.
5. Hillman RS, Ault KA: Non-Hodgkin's lymphomas. In *Hematology in clinical practice*, NY, NY 1998, McGraw-Hill.
6. Hehn ST, Grogan TM, Miller TP: Utility of fine-needle aspiration as a diagnostic technique in lymphoma, *J Clin Oncol* 22:3046-3052, 2004.
7. Harris NL, Jaffe ES, Diebold J et al: The world health organization classification of neoplastic diseases of the hematopoietic and lymphoid tissues. Report of the clinical advisory committee meeting, Airlie House, Va, November 1997, *Ann Oncol* 10:1419-1432, 1999.
8. Armitage JO, Weisenburger DD: New approach to classifying non-Hodgkin's lymphomas: clinical features of the major histologic subtypes. Non-Hodgkin's lymphoma classification project, *J Clin Oncol* 16:2780-2795, 1998.
9. Engert A, Schiller P, Josting A et al: Involved-field radiotherapy is equally effective and less toxic compared with extended-field radiotherapy after four cycles of chemotherapy in patients with early-stage unfavorable Hodgkin's lymphoma: results of the HD8 trial of the German Hodgkin's lymphoma study group, *J Clin Oncol* 21:3601-3608, 2003.
10. Koontz BF, Kirkpatrick JP, Clough RW et al: Combined-modality therapy versus radiotherapy alone for treatment of early-stage Hodgkin's disease: cure balanced against complications, *J Clin Oncol* 24:605-611, 2006.
11. *NCCN clinical practice guidelines in oncology: Hodgkin's lymphoma*, Version 1; 2005.
12. Josting A, Nogova L, Franklin J et al: Salvage radiotherapy in patients with relapsed and refractory Hodgkin's lymphoma: a retrospective analysis from the German Hodgkin's lymphoma study group, *J Clin Oncol* 23:1522-1529, 2005.
13. *NCCN clinical practice guidelines in oncology: non-Hodgkin's disease*, Version 1; 2005.
14. Kaminski MS, Zelenetz AD, Press OW et al: Pivotal study of iodine 131 tositumomab for chemotherapy-refractory low-grade or transformed low-grade B-cell non-Hodgkin's lymphomas, *J Clin Oncol* 19:3918-3928, 2001.
15. Witzig TE, Gordon LI, Cabanillas F et al: Treatment with ibritumomab tiuxetan radioimmunotherapy in patients with rituximab-refractory follicular non-Hodgkin's lymphoma, *J Clin Oncol* 20:3262-3269, 2002.
16. Gurwitz JH, Bohn RL, Glynn RJ et al: Glucocorticoids and the risk for initiation of hypoglycemic therapy, *Arch Intern Med* 10:97-101, 1994.
17. Feld, S: AACE diabetes guidelines, *Endocr Pract* 8:40-82, 2002.
18. Pappas PG, Rex JH, Sobel JD et al: Guidelines for the treatment of candidiasis, *Clin Infect Dis* 38:161-189, 2004.

19. Cope DG: Management of chemotherapy-induced diarrhea and constipation. *Nurs Clin North Am* 36:695-707, 2001.
20. Robinson CB, Fritch M, Hullett L et al: Development of a protocol to prevent opioid-induced constipation in patients with cancer: a research utilization project, *Clin J Oncol Nurs* 4:79-84, 2000.
21. Byar K: Educating patients about radioimmunotherapy with yttrium 90 ibritumomab (Zevalin), *Semin Oncol Nurs* 20:20-25, 2004.
22. Estes JM, Clapp KJ: Radioimmunotherapy with tositumomab and iodine-131 for low-grade non-Hodgkin lymphoma: nursing implications, *Oncol Nurs Forum* 31:1119-1126, 2004.
23. Flounders JA: Oncology emergency modules: superior vena cava syndrome, [Online exclusive], *Oncol Nurs Forum* 30:E84-E88, 2003.
24. Hogan DK, Rosenthal LD: Oncologic emergencies in the patient with lymphoma, *Semin Oncol Nurs* 14:312-320, 1998.
25. Shuey KM: Hypercalcemia of malignancy: Part I, *Clin J Oncol Nurs* 8:209-210, 2004.
26. Flounders JA, Ott BB: Oncology emergency modules: spinal cord compression, [Online exclusive], *Oncol Nurs Forum* 30:E17-E21, 2003.
27. Dores GM, Metayer C, Curtis RE et al: Second malignant neoplasms among long-term survivors of Hodgkin's disease: a population-based evaluation over 25 years, *J Clin Oncol* 20:3484-3494, 2002.
28. Prosnitz LR: Reducing treatment-related morbidity and mortality in early-stage Hodgkin's disease and why the recent southwest oncology group trial is not the way to go, *J Clin Oncol* 20:2225-2228, 2002.
29. Hengstler P, Battegay E, Cornuz J et al: Evidence for prevention and screening: recommendations for adults, *Swiss Med Wkly* 132:363-373, 2002.
30. Champion VL, Rawl SM, Menon U: Population-based cancer screening, *Oncol Nurs Forum* 29:853-861, 2002.
31. Ganz PA: Late effects of cancer and its treatment, *Semin Oncol Nurs* 17:241-248, 2001.
32. Jackson RM: Pulmonary oxygen toxicity, *Chest* 88: 900-905, 1985.
33. Toledo CH, Ross WE, Hood CI et al: Potentiation of bleomycin toxicity by oxygen, *Cancer Treat Rep* 66: 359-362, 1982.
34. Adams MJ, Lipsitz SR, Colan SD et al: Cardiovascular status in long-term survivors of Hodgkin's disease treated with chest radiotherapy, *J Clin Oncol* 22:3139-3148, 2004.
35. Greving DM, Santacroce SJ: Cardiovascular late effects, *J Pediatr Oncol Nurs* 22:38-47, 2005.
36. Gustavsson A, Eskilsson J, Landberg T et al: Late cardiac effects after mantle radiation in patients with Hodgkin's disease, *Ann Oncol* 1:355-363, 1990.
37. Lund MB, Ihlen H, Voss BM et al: Increased risk of heart valve regurgitation after mediastinal radiation for Hodgkin's disease: an echocardiographic study, *Heart* 75:591-595, 1996.
38. Piovaccari G, Ferretti RM, Prati F et al: Cardiac disease after chest irradiation for Hodgkin's disease: incidence in 108 patients with long follow up, *Int J Cardiol* 49:39-43, 1995.
39. Pfeilschifter IJ: Osteoporosis due to cancer treatment: pathogenesis and management, *J Clin Oncol* 18: 1570-1593, 2000.

Chapter 17

Soft Tissue Sarcomas

Kellie L. Ritari

Soft tissue sarcomas (STSs) are malignant tumors that can develop within any musculoskeletal connective tissue of the body including fat, muscle, nerve sheath, joint spaces, blood vessels, or deep fibrous connective tissue. Relatively rare, STS accounts for less than 1% of all adult malignancies.[1] In 2006, approximately 9530 new cases are expected in the United States, with approximately 3500 deaths predicted.[2] This chapter focuses on adults with STS in the extremity and retroperitoneum, the modalities used to treat them, and the nursing interventions aimed at decreasing or alleviating radiation-induced toxicity.

EPIDEMIOLOGY AND ETIOLOGY

Because of the uncommon nature of these tumors, little is known about the epidemiology of the disease. In general, STS does not seem to result from malignant changes or dedifferentiation of benign soft tissue tumors.[3] Almost half of all cases are found in adults older than age 60 (51.7%), with 27.6% found in adults ages 40 to 60, and 20.7% in adults younger than age 40. Incidence is only slightly higher in males.[4] Studies in large cohorts of patients demonstrate that the race distribution of soft tissue sarcomas mirrors that of the United States population: 86% Caucasian, 10% African American, 1% Asian, 3% other.[4] There is a similar distribution and incidence worldwide, with studies suggesting there is an increased incidence and mortality in New Zealand.[4]

A number of risk factors have been identified as being high risk for the development of sarcomas, although no specific etiologic agent has been identified. A family history of certain inherited conditions increases a person's risk of developing STS (Box 17-1). Data suggests that genetic mutations in pluripotent mesenchymal stem cells give rise to malignant clones that differentiate along pathways that resemble normal histogenesis. Alterations in the *RB-1* and *p53* genes are detected in a substantial proportion of sarcomas.[5]

Exposure to various chemicals in specific occupations or situations has been linked with the development of STS. Such chemicals include the phenoxyacetic acids (forestry and agricultural workers), chlorophenols (sawmill workers), Thorotrast (diagnostic x-ray workers), vinyl chloride workers, and arsenic (vineyard workers).[4] In an evaluation of occupational risks, Hoppin and colleagues[6] associated herbicide use, chlorophenol exposure, and cutting oil exposure with malignant fibrohistiocytic sarcoma. Their analysis also suggested that occupational risk factors for STS are not uniform across all histologic subtypes. STS also has been reported after previous exposure to alkylating chemotherapy agents (such as cyclophosphamide, melphan, procarbazine, nitrosoureas, and chlorambucil). The relative risk appears to increase with cumulative drug exposure.[4]

No clear causal relationship has been found between tissue injury and the development of sarcoma. Most often, trauma to a specific area precedes the diagnosis of STS. Rare examples of soft tissue sarcomas have arisen in postsurgical scar tissue, thermal or acid burns, at fracture sites, and in the vicinity of plastic or metal implants, usually after a latent period of several years.[7] Sarcomas can develop in parts of the body where lymphatic drainage has been disrupted congenitally or by surgery or radiation. One example of this process is Stewart-Treves syndrome, or chronic lymphedema after axillary lymph node dissection associated with radical or modified radical mastectomy.

Radiation exposure has been related to the development of STS. However, considering the frequency in which radiation therapy is administered, radiation-induced STSs are still rare, and the benefit of radiation in the treatment of malignant neoplasms outweighs the risk of developing a secondary STS. The incidence of postradiation sarcoma is difficult to

Box 17-1 Genetic Predisposition to Soft Tissue Sarcomas

- Carney's triad
- Gardner's syndrome
- Gorlin's syndrome
- Li-Fraumeni syndrome
- Neurofibromatosis type 1
- Retinoblastoma
- Tuberous sclerosis
- Werner's syndrome

Modified from Brennan M, Alektiar K, Maki R: *Sarcomas of the soft tissue and bone: cancer principles and practice of oncology*, ed 6, Philadelphia, 2001, Lippincott.

estimate, but reports generally range from 0.03% to 0.8%.[7] Radiation-induced sarcomas rarely arise sooner than 3 years after radiation therapy and most often develop decades later.[4]

ANATOMY, PATHOPHYSIOLOGY, AND HISTOLOGY

Sarcomas are a heterogeneous group of tumors that arise predominantly from the embryonic mesoderm. STS can occur within any organ or anatomic location within the body, but most originate in an extremity (59%), the trunk (19%), the retroperitoneum (15%), or the head and neck (9%).[3] They are histologically diverse with more than 100 types described in the Who Health Organization (WHO) classification.[8] Some examples include the following:

- *Malignant fibrous histiocytoma* (MFH) arises from fibrohistiocytic tissue. It is the most common malignant soft tissue sarcoma found in the arms or legs. This sarcoma is most common in older adults. It also can occur in the retroperitoneum.
- *Angiosarcomas* are malignant tumors that can develop either from blood vessels (hemangiosarcomas) or from lymph vessels (lymphangiosarcomas).
- *Fibrosarcoma* is cancer of the fibrous tissue, usually occurring in the arms, legs, or trunk.
- *Hemangiopericytoma* is a sarcoma of the perivascular tissue. Perivascular cells help control the amount of blood flowing through the veins. It most often develops in the legs, pelvis, and retroperitoneum.
- *Leiomyosarcoma* is a malignant tumor of involuntary muscle tissue. It is therefore most common in the retroperitoneum, but also may develop in the deep soft tissues of the extremities.
- *Malignant peripheral nerve sheath tumors* are malignant tumors of the cells that surround a nerve. They are also called *malignant schwannomas*, *neurofibrosarcomas*, or *neurogenic sarcomas*.
- *Rhabdomyosarcoma* is a malignant tumor of skeletal muscle and is most common in the extremities. Although it is more common in children, it does affect adults and therefore is included here.
- *Synovial sarcoma* is a malignant tumor of the soft tissue around a joint, not actually arising from the synovium or joint space. It is most common in young adults.

CLINICAL MANIFESTATIONS

Signs and symptoms depend largely on the location from which the soft tissue mass arises. Because the majority of STSs present in an extremity or superficial trunk, the initial presentation may be an enlarging painless mass, although one-third of patients may report discomfort. Tumors in the distal extremities are often small when discovered, whereas tumors in the proximal extremities can be quite large before they become apparent. STSs grow in a centrifugal fashion and compress surrounding normal structures, but rarely does impingement on bone or neurovascular bundles produce pain, edema, and swelling.[3] Sarcomas arising in the retroperitoneum may initially present with nonspecific symptoms that are not clear indicators of a STS diagnosis. As the size of the mass increases, surrounding organs become affected. Complaints of pain, signs of bowel obstruction, or internal bleeding may eventually lead to the discovery of an impinging mass. STS found in the region of the head and neck often present as the tumor begins to compress surrounding critical structures, usually impacting the patient's vision, swallowing, or breathing. Of course, close examination for patients with any of the aforementioned risk factors is critical to early diagnosis of sarcoma.

DIAGNOSTIC STUDIES

The *National Comprehensive Cancer Network (NCCN) Sarcoma Practice Guidelines* (2006) recommend that the first consideration for patients who are suspected of having STS is an evaluation by a multidisciplinary team before diagnostic testing.[9] The team should include a diagnostic radiologist, surgical and/or orthopedic oncologist, medical oncologist, and radiation oncologist, all of whom should be skilled in the evaluation and management of STS. Another critical member is a pathologist skilled in accurately identifying the histology and grading of rare STS subtypes, a key factor in providing appropriate treatment recommendations. It is not unusual to obtain a second pathologic opinion because numerous histologies exist and appropriate treatment depends on accurate diagnosis.

Initial evaluation should include a complete medical history and physical exam. This is essential to gather information on presenting symptoms, risk factors, and other medical conditions. The palpable mass should be evaluated for size, mobility, depth, and involvement of other structures such as bone, nerves, and organs.

Radiographic evaluation should include imaging studies to evaluate the size of the tumor and its relationship to surrounding tissues. To date, magnetic resonance imaging (MRI) has been considered the imaging study of choice in the evaluation of a soft tissue mass in an extremity or superficial trunk because of the enhanced contrast between the tumor and muscle tissue and between tumor and adjacent neurovascular structures. However, a large study performed by the Radiology Diagnostic Group (1997)[10] showed no advantage of MRI over computerized axial tomography (CAT or CT) imaging. For retroperitoneal sarcomas, a CT scan is usually sufficient. However, for tumors that invade the intestinal tract or midline vascular structures, an MRI may add critical information.[5]

Overall, at diagnosis, approximately 10% of patients present with demonstrable metastatic disease.[11] There is a high propensity for STS of the extremity to metastasize to the lungs. Therefore, a plain radiograph of the chest (x ray) or CT scan of the chest should be performed to complete the staging work-up. The decision on which chest study to perform is usually based on the size of the lesion. Patients with lesions smaller than 5 cm are at low risk of pulmonary metastasis so a chest x ray is sufficient for staging. Patients presenting with a high-grade tumor over 5 cm are at more risk and would benefit from a more thorough evaluation with CT. The majority of soft tissue sarcomas do present with masses larger than 5 cm.[5] The liver is the most common site of metastasis from sarcomas of the retroperitoneum. The imaging study selected to evaluate the primary site also can be used to determine liver involvement.

Blood work including a complete blood cell count and chemistry should be performed. These are beneficial as baseline studies or for the diagnosis of a potential anemia secondary to these highly vascular tumors.

Currently, positron emission tomographic (PET) scanning is the primary means by which unsuspected sites of metastasis are identified in patients with recurrent high-grade tumors.[5] This is possible because PET depicts the increased metabolism in abnormal tissues, enabling visualization and quantification in vivo.[12]

Suspected soft tissue tumors of the extremities require a carefully planned biopsy to confirm the diagnosis of sarcoma. Several forms of biopsy may be performed depending on the location and size of the mass. These include a fine-needle aspiration (FNA) biopsy, core-needle biopsy, and incisional biopsy. An FNA is diagnostically accurate in 60% to 96% of cases.[3] The success of this technique is determined by the skill of the cytopathologist in collecting an accurate and adequate sample and interpreting the results. A core-needle biopsy can be combined with CT or ultrasonography to yield more tissue, which can be submitted for a wider variety of diagnostic tests. The diagnostic accuracy of core-needle biopsy is 93%, with a less than 1% complication rate.[3] An incisional biopsy is usually performed only when FNA or core-needle biopsies yield nondiagnostic findings. The incisional biopsy must always be performed in the direction of the muscle compartment (i.e., the long axis of the extremity), never in a transverse orientation. This allows for a subsequent wide local excision that encompasses the biopsy site, scar, and tumor en bloc. A poorly oriented biopsy incision can result in an excessively large surgical defect from a wide local excision, which in turn necessitates a larger postoperative radiation therapy field. Adequate hemostasis is also critical at time of biopsy to prevent tumor seeding.[3] The routine use of an excisional biopsy is to be discouraged because of the possibility of local tumor spread.

PATHOLOGY

Pathologic classification of the biopsy should include histologic subtyping and grading, precise location of the origin of the tumor, size of primary lesion, regional lymph node involvement, and distant metastases. The histologic grade of an STS remains the most important prognostic factor. The features that define the grade are the degree of cellularity, differentiation, pleomorphism, and necrosis, as well as the number of mitoses.[3] STSs are graded as grade 1, well differentiated; grade 2, moderately differentiated; grade 3, poorly differentiated; and grade 4, undifferentiated. Grades 1 and 2 are considered low-grade, and grades 3 and 4 are high-grade. Sarcomas may be misdiagnosed or misclassified by the general pathologist in up to 25% to 40% of cases; therefore it is strongly recommended that cases be reviewed by experts in sarcoma pathology before therapy is begun.[3]

There are two recognized staging systems for STS: the American Joint Committee on Cancer (AJCC) system and the Enneking system. The AJCC uses the histologic grade, the tumor size and depth, and the presence of distal or nodal metastases (Table 17-1). The size of an STS is classified into two groups: lesions that are 5 cm or smaller (T1) and lesions that are larger than 5 cm (T2). The larger lesion size carries a decrease in 5-year survival rate. STSs are shown to have nodal spread in less than 5% of cases. STSs of the extremities most commonly metastasize to the lung, but other potential sites are to bone, the brain, and liver. Retroperitoneal sarcomas tend to metastasize to the liver and peritoneum.[3]

The Enneking system, which is recognized by the Musculoskeletal Tumor Society (MSTS) and

Table 17-1 AJCC Staging System for Soft Tissue Sarcomas

PRIMARY TUMOR					
Tx	Primary tumor cannot be assessed				
T0	No evidence of primary tumor				
T1	Tumor 5 cm or less in greatest dimension				
T1a	Superficial tumor				
T1b	Deep tumor				
T2	Tumor more than 5 cm in greater dimension				
T2a	Superficial tumor				
T2b	Deep tumor				
REGIONAL LYMPH NODES					
Nx	Regional lymph nodes cannot be assessed				
N0	No regional lymph node metastasis				
N1	Regional lymph node metastasis				
DISTANT METASTASIS					
Mx	Distant metastasis cannot be assessed				
M0	No distant metastasis				
M1	Distant metastasis				
HISTOPATHOLOGIC GRADE					
Gx	Grade cannot be assessed				
G1	Well differentiated				
G2	Moderately differentiated				
G3	Poorly differentiated				
G4	Undifferentiated				
STAGE I					
T1a, 1b, 2a, 2b	N0	M0	G1-2	G1	Low
STAGE II					
T1a, 1b, 2a	N0	M0	G3-4	G2-3	High
STAGE III					
T2b	N0	M0	G3-4	G2-3	High
STAGE IV					
Any T	N1	M0	Any G	Any G	High or Low
Any T	N0	M1	Any G	Any G	High or Low

Used with the permission of the American Joint Committee on Cancer (AJCC), Chicago, Illinois. The original source is the *AJCC Cancer Staging Manual, Sixth Edition* (2002), published by Springer-New York, www.springeronline.com.

shown in Table 17-2. The MSTS system includes grade (G), site (T), and metastasis (M). The main focus of this system is whether the tumor is intracompartmental, confined within the boundaries of well-defined anatomic structures, or extracompartmental, involving extrafascial spaces or planes that have no natural anatomic barriers to extension.[13] Grade is defined as low grade (G1) or high grade (G2). Site is defined as intracompartmental lesion (T1) or extracompartmental lesion (T2). No regional or distant metastasis is designated M0, and the identification of regional or distant metastasis is M1.

Both of these staging systems serve as a valuable guide to therapy and provide useful prognostic information. The AJCC system is applicable to STS at any site, whereas the Enneking system, with its emphasis on compartmentalization, is best suited for well-documented sarcomas arising in the extremities. It does not include the type, size, or depth of the tumor as separate parameters, and its two-tier grading system is probably too narrow for the wide biologic range of STS. Because of the need for adequately defining compartmentalization, the system does not lend itself to retrospective staging. On the other hand, one drawback of the AJCC system is its greater complexity (four stages with two subclassifications for each stage).[13]

TREATMENT

Surgery is a potential first treatment choice for tumors at stage I. Radiation therapy is beneficial at this stage in two instances. Preoperative radiation can be used to reduce tumor volume and increase the success of removing a previously unresectable lesion. Postoperative radiation therapy can be used if adequate margins could not be obtained during surgical resection. Radiation can be considered an alternative to surgery if the tumor is considered inoperable because of involvement of critical structures or if the patient cannot tolerate the surgical procedure because of other health conditions. Radiation therapy alone is most often not effective for cure of soft tissue sarcoma.

In patients with stage II disease, preoperative radiation therapy should strongly be considered to facilitate complete surgical resection. Otherwise, postoperative radiation therapy may be required.

In stage III disease, surgery is required with a need for radiation therapy either pre- or postoperatively because of the increased chance of tumor recurrence with surgery alone. Chemotherapy may be considered at this stage.

Metastasis to distant sites (stage IV) is the limiting factor affecting treatment outcomes at this stage. Surgery to remove the primary tumor plus radiation therapy is the treatment of choice. Amputation may be required if complete surgical removal is not possible. Surgical removal of all metastases should be done, if possible. If surgery is unable to accomplish complete removal of the primary tumor and all metastases, palliative radiation and/or chemotherapy is recommended.

Surgical resection is the mainstay of treatment for soft tissue sarcoma and should be attempted in virtually every case. Radiation is often used in an attempt to reduce the risk of local recurrence. Chemotherapy can be used in cases where the patient is felt to be at high risk of developing systemic disease.[14] The goal of surgery is to obtain optimal margins for local control while maximizing function, ideally sparing the limb. Changes in patterns of treatment have been identified, with wide local excision increasing threefold over a 5-year period to 45.2% of patients by 1993, whereas amputation had decreased from 35.5% to 11.1% of patients.[15] Intralesional excision, marginal excision, wide local excision, radical excision, and amputation are the types of surgical procedures used. Limb salvage has been achieved with sarcoma by means of compartmental resection, soft-tissue reconstruction, and adjuvant therapy without increased rates of local recurrence, metastasis, or mortality.[16] Limb salvage procedures have encouraged the development of composite, one-stage reconstructions that employ microvascular surgical techniques with a combination of autologous tissues, bone allografts, and endoprosthetic devices in an effort to improve functional outcome. The

Table 17-2 Enneking System for Surgical Staging of Soft Tissue Sarcomas

Stage	Grade	Site	Metastasis
IA	G1	T1	M0
IB	G2	T2	M0
IIA	G2	T1	M0
III	G1 or G2	T1 or T2	M1

From Enneking WF, Spanier SS, Goodman MA: A system for the surgical staging of musculoskeletal sarcoma, *Clin Orthop Relat Res* Nov-Dec (153):106-120, 1980.

complications of limb salvage continue to decrease while the durability of the reconstructions continues to increase.[17]

The inclusion of adjuvant radiation therapy in the treatment of sarcomas is primarily for high-grade lesions in an attempt to improve functional and cosmetic outcomes and to reduce the risk of late complications of high-dose radiation therapy alone.[8] Two types of adjuvant radiation therapy are available to treat sarcomas: external beam and brachytherapy. Rosenberg and colleagues[18] established the use of radiation in a National Cancer Institute (NCI) prospective randomized trial of amputation alone versus wide local excision plus external-beam radiation. The trial showed that high rates of local control could be achieved, thus avoiding amputation. Yang and colleagues,[19] in a study of limb-sparing surgery with or without postoperative external beam radiation, found a highly significant decrease (P = 0.0028) in the probability of local recurrence with radiation, but no difference in overall survival. In low-grade lesions, there was also a lower probability of local failure (P = 0.016) in patients receiving radiation, without a difference in overall survival. For extremity sarcomas, typically a total dose of 50 Gy to 74 Gy is delivered to the site using fractions of 1.2 Gy twice daily or 1.8 Gy to 2.0 Gy once daily. For retroperitoneal sarcomas, the total dose is restricted to 45 Gy to 54 Gy because of the tolerance limits of sensitive abdominal organs.

Brachytherapy is the use of a radioactive source to deliver radiation to a specific site inside a patient. It has the advantages of treating complex areas (with less exposure to normal tissues and organs) and of reducing the time commitment to treatment. This procedure generally requires intraoperative placement of the radioactive sources. Ideal patients are those with intermediate- or high-grade tumors amenable to en bloc resection.[20] Harrison and colleagues[21] compared surgery alone versus surgery plus brachytherapy for either high- or low-grade sarcomas. They found that high-grade tumors treated with brachytherapy had 5-year local control rates of 90% compared with rates of 60% to 70% with resection alone. The systemic administration of chemotherapeutic agents allows for treatment of disease that has spread to distant sites or for locally advanced unresectable tumors. Contemporary data clearly indicates that multidrug chemotherapy regimens combined with radiation therapy have a significant impact on improving local control and ultimate outcome.[8] Only three drugs—doxorubicin, dacarbazine, and ifosfamide—are consistently associated with response rates of 20% or more in patients with advanced STS.[3] However, many combination regimens are under investigation (Box 17-2).

SURVEILLANCE

Follow-up evaluation by the treatment team is recommended every 3 to 4 months for 2 to 3 years, then every 6 months for 5 years, then on an annual or as needed basis.[11] Follow-up is to evaluate for local recurrence and distant metastasis and to monitor side effects of treatment. Recurrence is most common in the first 2 to 3 years after treatment, hence close follow-up is crucial. A complete history and physical examination and a chest x ray every 6 to 12 months (or CT scan) because of the high risk of pulmonary metastasis should be performed. In 75% of patients with primary tumors of an extremity, the predominant site of first

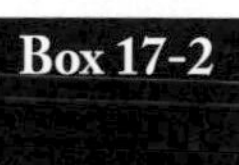

Box 17-2 Generally Accepted Chemotherapy Agents and Regimens for Soft Tissue Sarcoma

COMBINATION REGIMENS

AIM: doxorubicin, ifosfamide, mesna
MAID: mesna, doxorubicin, ifosfamide, dacarbazine
AD: doxorubicin, dacarbazine
Gemcitabine and docetaxel

SINGLE AGENTS

Dacarbazine
Doxorubicin
Gemcitabine
Ifosfamide
Liposomal doxorubicin

SPECIAL SITUATIONS

Rhabdomyosarcoma second-line therapy
- Irinotecan
- Cyclophosphamide and topotecan

Angiosarcoma
- Taxanes
- Interferon
- Vinorelbine

From Chao K, Perez C, Brady L: *Radiation oncology: management decisions,* Philadelphia, 1999, Lippincott.

recurrence is the lung.[11,13] Whooley and colleagues[22] found that chest x-ray imaging was a cost-effective strategy for follow-up of patients with high-grade extremity soft tissue sarcomas. Primary site imaging with CT scan or MRI on an annual basis was found to be an ineffective strategy for detecting recurrence. However, certain patient characteristics such as body habitus, previous radiation therapy, and location of the primary tumor site may require the use of imaging for adequate clinical assessment.[22] Of note, laboratory blood studies have been found to be ineffective strategies for detecting recurrence.[22]

One tool that can be useful for grading the severity of acute effects of radiation therapy in all sites is the NCI Common Toxicity Criteria (CTC) Version 2 with the Radiation Therapy Oncology Group (RTOG) and European Organization for Research and Treatment of Cancer (EORTC) Acute Effects Criteria instrument. It provides a scale for many different organ systems and some symptoms.[23] Also, the Radiation Therapy Patient Care Record: A Tool for Documenting Nursing Care provides a tool for weekly assessment and grading of severity of acute effects of radiation therapy in all sites.[24]

PROGNOSIS AND RECURRENCE

Improvements have taken place in STS patient survivorship and quality of life over the past 20 years, with overall 5-year survival currently at approximately 50%.[15] Many factors must be considered in the survival data, including histology, grade of tumor, stage of disease, and treatment approaches. A key factor in determining overall patient survival is whether distant metastasis has occurred by the time of presentation. At diagnosis, approximately 10% of patients have demonstrable disease.[11] In patients with sarcomas of the extremity, about 90% of treatment failures are ultimately the result of pulmonary metastasis. In patients with truncal or retroperitoneal sarcomas, 50% fail at the local site.[11]

NURSING INTERVENTIONS AND EDUCATION

The patient can experience side effects based on the type of treatment and location of the tumor. Surgery carries the risk of infection, scarring, nerve damage, pain, bleeding, and edema. Chemotherapy has systemic effects such as nausea/vomiting, weight loss, alopecia, fatigue, neuropathy, or organ toxicity. Radiation therapy has effects that are confined to the local treatment area and progress slowly throughout the course of treatment. Outcomes of radiation therapy can be divided into acute side effects and late/chronic side effects. Management options for these symptoms follow.

Acute Toxicities of Treatment

Pain

Patients who begin treatment with pain from previous surgery or injury or pain secondary to the tumor compressing nearby structures (primarily the neurovascular bundles), can be successfully managed with medications. Patients often report general aching and muscle spasms in the treatment field secondary to tissue inflammation as the treatment progresses. This can be managed with the use of nonsteroidal antiinflammatory drugs (NSAIDs), muscle relaxants, anticonvulsants, which act on neurogenic pain, or short- or long-acting narcotic analgesics. Refer to Chapter 31 on pain for further recommendations.

Skin Reactions

The skin will gradually develop a dry desquamation and pigment changes at 3 weeks (27 Gy to 30 Gy) after the start of radiation therapy.[25] Initial skin care includes the use of a moisturizer after daily treatments. Products available range from over-the-counter aloe to prescription radiodermatitis treatments. See Chapter 30 for a detailed discussion of options. Skin changes may progress to erythema or moist desquamation depending on the area being treated. Although the entire treatment area is at risk, special care needs to be paid when the field includes a skinfold (such as the groin or behind the knee) or a healing incision. These areas carry a higher risk of skin breakdown and difficulty healing.

Edema

Nurses should educate patients to monitor treated extremities for swelling, especially in the postoperative setting. Drainage of the extremity might be compromised secondary to surgery or damage to lymph vessels. Edema also can be exacerbated by radiation and will contribute to the discomfort a patient feels. It is recommended that the patient be referred to a therapist certified in combined decongestive therapy (CDT) for education on techniques to improve drainage such as elevation of the extremity, massage, or the use of a compression stocking.

Neuropathy

Neuropathy may exist as a consequence of the location of the tumor in relation to nerve structure or as a side effect of surgery or chemotherapy. It may be aggravated by the inflammation from radiation and needs to be monitored closely.

Fatigue

An estimated 90% of cancer patients receiving treatments such as radiation therapy or chemotherapy have fatigue.[26] Cancer-related fatigue is defined as a persistent and subjective sense of tiredness that can occur with cancer or cancer treatment. Although the exact cause is unknown, it is recognized that in addition to the effects of the tumor burden and treatment, five primary conditions also can be attributing factors for fatigue and need to be evaluated. These are anemia, pain, emotional distress, sleep problems, and altered thyroid function.[26] Acute effects of fatigue from radiation occur between 2 and 3 weeks after the start of radiation and may last for months after completion. Thirty percent to seventy-five percent of cancer survivors have reported fatigue continuing for months or years after completing active treatment.[26] Patient limitations as a result of fatigue can range form mild to severe. Monitoring and intervention are necessary to minimize negative effects on patient's quality of life and to promote compliance with treatment.

The first step in managing fatigue is to detect and correct underlying conditions that may be contributing to one's level of fatigue. Patient and family education is critical so an understanding of the nature and course of fatigue may be achieved. Patients should be educated to promote sleep by limiting sleep disruptions (family, medication administration), avoiding stimulants before sleep, using behavioral techniques such as relaxation and imagery, assuring good sleep hygiene (a clean bed, usual bedtime routine, dim lighting), and by the use of sedative/hypnotics as appropriate.[27] Energy conservation during the day is also important. Patients need to prioritize, delegate, and pace activities. Encourage short rest periods after major activities, encourage rest periods of 30 to 45 minutes during the day, suggest patients develop a plan that encourages activities during the time of day when they have the least fatigue.[28] Consider consulting a physical or occupational therapist to help identify alternate ways of performing desired activities or to start an exercise/rehabilitation program appropriate to the patient's status.[27,28]

Anorexia

Patients who receive radiation to the abdomen for a retroperitoneal mass can experience a loss of appetite. Close monitoring of weight at least weekly during treatment is recommended. Immediate dietary counseling should be instituted for patients with weight loss of 10% of their usual body weight.[29] Interventions for anorexia and malnutrition can be found in Chapter 33.

Nausea and Vomiting

Patients receiving radiation therapy to the abdomen often experience nausea and vomiting. These side effects can occur after the first treatment, be intermittent, or continuous and can last several days after the completion of therapy. Management with antiemetics should be instituted 1 hour before the first radiation treatment and monitored closely for effectiveness. The goal is to prevent weight loss, dehydration, and interruption of treatment. Collaboration with the dietary team is crucial, especially for patients already compromised, again see Chapter 33 for appropriate interventions.

Gastrointestinal Effects

Disruption of bowel function is an expected short-term side effect of radiation to the abdomen and pelvis. Patients may have constipation from narcotic use and need to be regulated with an appropriate stool softener or laxative. If the radiation treatment field includes the pelvis, then generally about the third week of treatment, diarrhea can be an expected side effect. Patients should be monitored for frequency and consistency of stools, rectal discomfort, rectal bleeding, pain, and signs of dehydration. Management with dietary modifications and antidiarrheals should be initiated and monitored. Additional nursing interventions for diarrhea can be found in Chapter 34.

Acute Bladder Symptoms

Acute bladder symptoms may begin between the second and third weeks of treatment to the pelvis and can include pain or burning with urination, increased frequency of urination, hesitancy, urgency, or increased nocturia. Management includes urinary tract analgesics, antispasmodics, and bladder agents such as tamsulosin, alfuzosin HCl, tolterodine tartrate, or oxybutynin to improve urine flow and decrease symptoms.

Late and Chronic Toxicities

Fibrosis

The formation of scar tissue can occur secondary to surgery with or without radiation or with radiation therapy alone. Fibrosis may cause discomfort in the treatment site and permanent loss of range of motion (ROM) of an extremity. Encouraging patients to begin a regular daily stretching program immediately after surgery and during and after the course of radiation is vital to maximizing the patient's functional status. A physical therapist should be consulted when initiating such a program.

Edema

Damage to lymph vessels may compromise drainage from an extremity and lead to chronic edema. Such chronic states can increase risk of infection, cause pain, alter body image, and decrease ROM. Treatment of lymphedema is complex and a referral should be made to a therapy program specializing in CDT and patient education.

Bone Fracture

Bones may be damaged because of original tumor destruction or as a result of resection of bone or the periosteum or secondary to radiation. Bones may have a greater risk of fracture because of limited healing capacity and may have increased risk of infection.

Skin Reactions

Late skin reactions are classified as occurring 6 or more months after radiation is completed and includes fibrosis, atrophy, ulceration, pigment changes, thinning, and telangiectasia.

Resources

Following the completion of treatment, patients and families should be encouraged to participate in an ongoing support group or outreach program. Although such resources are limited for this patient population, Table 17-3 provides a list of organizations that may be helpful.

QUALITY OF LIFE

Currently no tool is available to specifically evaluate a patient's quality of life after treatment for sarcoma with multimodality therapy. However, several studies have recently reported functional outcome results after multimodality therapy for soft tissue sarcomas of the limb. Although these data are focused on surgical intervention, they give some insight into the complications that occur.

Amputation Versus Limb-Sparing Multimodality Therapy

In one of the earliest evaluations of quality of life in patients with soft tissue sarcoma, Sugarbaker and colleagues[30] found minimal differences between a group of individuals treated with amputation and a group treated with limb-sparing surgery and postoperative radiation with or without chemotherapy. Sexual function was significantly decreased in patients who underwent limb-sparing multimodality therapy, probably related to a protracted course of treatment.

In a matched case-controlled study, Davis and colleagues[31] evaluated the differences in physical disability and handicap experienced by patients with lower extremity sarcoma who required amputation

Table 17-3 Resources for Patients with Sarcoma and Their Caregivers

Organization	Website
American Cancer Society	www.cancer.org
Association of Cancer Online Resources	www.acor.org
CancerBackUp	www.cancerbackup.org.uk/Cancertype/Softtissuesarcomas
National Cancer Institute	www.cancer.gov/cancertopics/types/soft-tissue-sarcoma
National Coalition for Cancer Survivorship	www.canceradvocacy.org
National Comprehensive Cancer Network	www.nccn.org
National Lymphedema Network	www.lymphnet.org
People Living with Cancer	www.plwc.org
Sarcoma Foundation of America	www.curesarcoma.org
Sarcoma Alliance	www.sarcomaalliance.org

for the primary tumor compared with those treated with limb-sparing surgery. They found a trend toward increased disability for those in the amputation group, with significantly higher levels of handicap.

Limb-Sparing Procedures With Reconstruction

Zunino and Johnson[32] evaluated the functional and subjective condition of individuals during a 2-year postoperative period, evaluating the nature and frequency of complications after surgical procedures. They found that during the first 6 months, most patients have a poor functional and subjective condition that progressively improves throughout the first and second years. There was a high rate of complications during this period (46%), most often related to proximal femur and proximal tibia sites and were primarily mechanical dysfunction of the reconstructive system.

Similar findings were reported by Ham and colleagues[33] in an evaluation of 32 patients with primary bone sarcomas of the femur or proximal tibia who had undergone endoprosthetic procedures. They found that these reconstructions gave satisfying functional results in most patients after long-term survival (median survival = 10 years). Endoprosthetic-related complications occurred in 41%; most complications were mechanical failures. Proximal tibial and distal femoral endoprosthesis were found to be particularly at risk for complications requiring additional surgical procedures.

Serletti and colleagues[16] evaluated the functional outcome of 20 patients with sarcoma after soft-tissue reconstruction for limb salvage. Patients were examined for range of motion, deformity, stability, pain level, strength, functional activity, and emotional acceptance. Using the Musculoskeletal Tumor Society Scale (MSTSS), 45% achieved an overall rating of excellent, 25% a rating of good, and 30% a rating of fair.[34] There were no differences in the results obtained comparing upper versus lower extremity, immediate versus delayed reconstruction, or reconstructions performed with a free flap versus a pedicle flap.

Radiation Therapy With Limb-Sparing Procedures

Yang and colleagues[19] evaluated quality of life in a randomized prospective study assessing postoperative radiation therapy after limb-sparing resection of extremity sarcomas. They found that radiation therapy resulted in significantly worse limb strength, edema, and range of motion, but these deficits were often transient and had few measurable effects on activities of daily living or global quality of life. Similar findings were identified by Robinson and colleagues.[35] Doses in excess of 60 Gy resulted in increased fibrosis and a worse functional outcome.

Karasek and colleagues[36] evaluated the functional outcome of patients treated with surgery and irradiation. They found a positive relationship between volume irradiated to at least 55 Gy and functional score, strength, fibrosis, and skin changes. Total dose independent of volume was significantly associated with skin changes. Increasing peak dose was associated with fibrosis and skin changes. In patients in whom a portion of the joint was included in the treatment field, neither range of motion nor functional score was correlated with joint dose. Edema and functional score were not related to either the volume or percent of limb spared.

Several instruments are available to measure quality of life and functional outcomes in this population. The Functional Assessment of Cancer Therapy (FACT-G) is a 33-item self-report scale of quality-of-life for people with cancer.[37] The general version has been validated in English and has been used extensively in the United States. The European Organization for Research and Treatment of Cancer (EORTC) QLQ-C30 is a 36-item questionnaire for assessing the quality-of-life of cancer patients participating in international clinical trials.[38] It has been validated and used extensively in a wide range of cancer clinical trials in Europe and around the world. The Toronto Extremity Salvage Score (TESS) is a measure of functional status for patients with lower extremity sarcoma.[39,40] It recently has been found to be a reliable and efficient measure for evaluating patients.[40] The MSTSS is a standardized system of reporting end results of various surgical alternatives after limb-salvage and ablative procedures for musculoskeletal tumors.[34]

REFERENCES

1. Khatri V, Goodnight J: Extremity soft tissue sarcoma: controversial management issues, *Surg Oncol* 14:2, 2005.
2. *American Cancer Society 2006 facts and figures* (website):. www.cancer.org/downloads/STT/CAFF2006PWSecured.pdf. Accessed April 30, 2006.
3. Cormier JN, Pollack RE: Soft tissue sarcomas, *CA Cancer J Clin* 54(2):94-109, 2004.

4. Pisters P, Casper E, Mann G et al, editors: *Cancer management: a multidisciplinary approach: medical, surgical, and radiation oncology,* ed 9, Darian, CT, 2005, CMP Medica.
5. Brennan M, Alektiar K, Maki R: *Sarcomas of the soft tissue and bone: cancer principles and practice of oncology,* ed 6, Philadelphia, 2001, Lippincott.
6. Hoppin J, Tolbert P, Flanders W et al: Occupational risk factors for sarcoma subtypes, *Epidemiology* 10(3):300-306.
7. Weiss S, Goldblum J: *Enzinger and Weiss's soft tissue tumors,* ed 4, St Louis, 2001, Mosby.
8. Chao K, Perez C, Brady L: *Radiation oncology: management decisions,* Philadelphia, 1999, Lippincott.
9. Demetri G, Baker L, Beech D et al: *NCCN soft tissue sarcoma: clinical practice guidelines in oncology,* vol 1, 2006.
10. Panicek D, Gatsonis C, Rosenthal D et al: CT and MRI imaging in the local staging of primary malignant musculoskeletal neoplasms: report of the Radiology Diagnostic Oncology group, *Radiology* 202:237-246, 1997.
11. Demetri G, Pollock R, Baker L et al: NCCN sarcoma practice guidelines, *Oncology* 12(7A):183-218.
12. Bastiannet E, Groen H, Jager PL et al: The value of FDG-PET in the detection, grading and response to therapy of soft tissue and bone sarcomas: a systemic review and meta-analysis, *Cancer Treat Rev* 30:83-101, 2004.
13. Enzinger FM, Weiss SW: *Soft tissue sarcomas,* ed 3, St Louis, 1995, Mosby.
14. Clarkson P, Ferguson P: Management of the soft tissue sarcomas of the extremities, *Expert Rev Anticancer Ther* 4(2):237-246, 2004.
15. Pollock RE, Karnell LH, Menck HR et al: The National Cancer Data Base report on soft tissue sarcoma, *Cancer* 78(10):2247-2257, 1996.
16. Serletti JM, Carras, AJ, O'Keefe RJ et al: Functional outcome after soft-tissue reconstruction for limb salvage after sarcoma surgery, *Plastic Reconstr Surg* 102(5):1576-1583, 1998.
17. Terek RM: Sarcoma of bone, *Med Health Rhode Island* 80:19-25, 1997.
18. Rosenberg SA, Tepper J, Glatstein E et al: The treatment of soft-tissue sarcomas of the extremities: prospective randomized evaluations of (1) limb-sparing surgery plus radiation therapy compared with amputation and (2) the role of adjuvant chemotherapy, *Ann Surg* 196(3):305-315, 1982.
19. Yang JC, Chang AE, Baker AR et al: Randomized prospective benefit of adjuvant radiation therapy in the treatment of soft tissue sarcomas of the extremity, *J Clin Oncol* 16(1):197-203, 1998.
20. Crownover RL, Marks KE: Adjuvant brachytherapy in the treatment of soft-tissue sarcomas, *Hematol/Oncol Clin North Am* 13(3):595-607, 1999.
21. Harrison LB, Franzese F, Gaynor JJ et al: Long-term results of a prospective randomized trial of adjuvant brachytherapy in the management of completely resected soft tissue sarcomas of the extremity and superficial trunk, *Int J Radiat Oncol Biol Phys* 27(2):259-265, 1993.
22. Whooley BP, Mooney MM, Gibbs JF et al: Effective follow-up strategies in soft tissue sarcoma, *Semin Surg Oncol* 17(1):83-87, 1999.
23. National Cancer Institute: 1999 NCI Common Toxicity Criteria (CTC), Version 2, with the Radiation Therapy Oncology Group (RTOG) and the European Organization for Research and Treatment of Cancer (EROTC) acute effects criteria, Bethesda, Md, 1999, National Cancer Institute.
24. Oncology Nursing Society–Radiation Therapy Special Interest Group, Documentation Project Core Committee: *Radiation therapy patient care record: a tool for documenting nursing care,* Pittsburgh, 1994, Oncology Nursing Society.
25. Maher KE: Radiation therapy: toxicities and management. In Yarbro CH, Frogge MH, Goodman M, editors: *Cancer Nursing Principles and Practice,* ed 6, Sudbury, MA, 2005, Jones and Bartlett, pp 283-314.
26. *NCCN website 2006.* Downloaded on 4/30/06 from http://www.nccn.org/patients/patient_gls/_english/_fatigue/contents.asp
27. Nail L: *Fatigue: Clinical Manual for the Oncology Advanced Practice Nurse,* Pittsburgh, 2000, Oncology Nursing Press.
28. Moore G, Hayes C: *Maintenance of comfort: fatigue and pain: outcomes in radiation therapy,* Sudbury, MA, 2001, Jones and Bartlett.
29. Berendt MC: In Itano KN, Taoka N, editors: *Alterations in nutrition: core curriculum for oncology nursing,* ed 3, Philadelphia, 1998, WB Saunders.
30. Sugarbaker PH, Barofsky I, Rosenberg SA et al: Quality of life assessment of patients in extremity sarcoma clinical trials, *Surgery* 91(1):17-23, 1982.
31. Davis AM, Devlin M, Griffin AM et al: Functional outcome in amputation versus limb sparing of patients with lower extremity sarcoma: a matched case control study, *Arch Phys Med Rehabil* 80 (6):615-618, 1999.
32. Zunino JH, Johnson JO: Early results of lower limb surgery for osteogenic sarcoma of bone, *Orthopedics* 21(1):47-50, 1998.
33. Ham SJ, Schraffordt-Koops H, Veth RP et al: Limb salvage surgery for primary bone sarcoma of the lower extremities: Long-term consequences of endoprosthetic reconstruction, *Ann Surg Oncol* 5(5):423-436, 1998.
34. Enneking WF, Dunham W, Gebhardt MC et al: A system for the functional evaluation of reconstructive procedures after surgical treatment of tumors of the musculoskeletal system *Clin Orthop Rel Res* 286:241-246, 1993.
35. Robinson MH, Spruce L, Eeles R et al: Limb function following conservation treatment of adult soft tissue sarcoma, *Eur J Cancer* 27(12):1567-1574, 1991.
36. Karasek K, Constine LS, Rosier R: Sarcoma therapy: functional outcome and relationship to treatment parameters, *Int J Radiat Oncol Biol Phys* 24(4):651-656, 1992.
37. Cella DF, Tulsky DS, Gray G: The functional assessment of the cancer therapy scale: development and validation of the general measure, *J Clin Oncol* 11(3):570-579, 1993.
38. Aaronson NK, Ahmedzai S, Bergman B et al: The European Organization for Research and Treatment of Cancer QLQ-C30: a quality-of-life instrument for use in international clinical trials in oncology, *J Nat Cancer Inst* 85(5):365-376, 1993.
39. Davis AM, Wright JG, Williams JI et al: Development of a measure of physical function for patients with bone and soft tissue sarcoma, *Qual Life Res* 5(5):508-516, 1996.
40. Davis AM, Bell RS, Bradley EM et al: Evaluating functional outcome in patients with lower extremity sarcoma, *Clin Orthop Relat Res* Jan (358):90-100, 1999.

Chapter 18

Nonmalignant Tumors

Mary Ann Robbins

Nonmalignant tumors and benign diseases are the result of abnormal cell growth. They are not considered cancerous and do not metastasize to other sites, but can cause damage, discomfort, or harm to the area of growth. Order and Donaldson[1] compiled almost 100 indications for the use of radiation therapy for benign conditions, but only 10 of those would be treated by more than 90% of North American radiation oncologists, according to a 1990 survey (Table 18-1).

Biologic mechanisms of ionizing irradiation in the treatment of various benign disorders are not completely understood. To achieve an optimal effect, radiation therapy should be applied at the appropriate time over a suitable period of time and with sufficient dose. The dose can vary from disease to disease and also among individuals.[2]

This chapter reviews the use of radiation therapy for the most common nonmalignant/benign diseases. Other nonmalignant tumors are reviewed in other chapters; acoustic neuroma, for example, is discussed in the chapter on stereotactic radiosurgery (Chapter 24).

HETEROTOPIC BONE FORMATION

New bone formation occurs at sites of bone trauma as part of the normal healing process. When bone trauma occurs within the joint capsules, new bone formation can occur at that site. This heterotopic new bone formation can ossify normal mobile soft tissue structures, causing pain and/or restricting movement.[3] The formation of bone where it is neither needed nor wanted ranges from no significance to devastating clinical conditions that dramatically affects quality of life.[4]

The pathology of heterotopic bone formation is unknown. Patients at high risk for heterotopic bone formation include patients that have had a traumatic fracture/injury to the hip or elbow joints and those who are undergoing elective total hip replacement and who have a history of heterotopic bone formation, hypertrophic osteoarthritis, diffuse idiopathic skeletal hyperostosis, or ankylosing spondylitis.[3]

Heterotopic ossification is detectable on radiographs as late as 4 to 12 weeks after injury, when no effective therapy is available. Almost 30% of all patients develop symptoms, including pain, restricted motion, or fixation of the joint that may require a secondary surgical procedure.[5] Brooker's grading system has generally been accepted for classifying the extent of ossification (Table 18-2).

Radiation therapy has been used as an adjuvant treatment to reduce the risk of heterotopic bone formation. Nonsteroidal antiinflammatory drugs such as indomethacin have also been found to be effective in the prevention of heterotopic bone formation, but patient compliance and side effects are a drawback to this treatment.[6]

Radiation therapy can be given before surgery and up to 3 days after surgery, but most institutions try to administer the radiation treatment within 24 hours of surgery. Randomized trials have shown that a single fraction of 6 Gy to 8 Gy to be as effective as multifractions with a dose to 10 Gy to 20 Gy.[7] Treatment planning includes simulation, but because of patient mobility postoperatively and machine time, a clinical set-up on the treatment machine is most often done. In such cases, preports are taken to verify treatment field before administering the radiation treatment. The planning target volume includes the entire area encompassed by the relevant joint capsule. The treatment field is administered through an anteroposterior/posteroanterior (AP/PA) port prescribed to midline.[3]

Acute side effects of radiation therapy are minimal; however, aggressive pain management is needed for the treatment. Also these patients may be in intensive care units, which requires coordination with the intensive care staff for transportation. Long term, radiation therapy has been

Table 18-1 Benign Diseases and Radiation Therapy Doses

Diseases	Treatment
Acoustic neuroma	SRS at 12 Gy–13 Gy times 1 or SRT at 1.8 Gy per fraction for a total of 50 Gy–54 Gy
Arterial stenosis and restenosis	High dose rate: 2 Gy to the vessel wall
Arteriovenous malformations	SRS 14 Gy–18 Gy
Graves' ophthalmopathy	20 Gy in 10 × 2 Gy fractions
Gynecomastia	Total of 12 Gy; give 4 Gy × 3 (see Figure 20-7)
Heterotopic bone formation	Single fraction of 7 Gy–8 Gy
Hyperthyroidism	15–30 mCi of I-131
Keloids	8 Gy–15 Gy given in one to four divided doses
Pterygium	25 Gy–30 Gy given in one to three divided doses of Sr-90
Meningiomas	SRS 15 Gy–20 Gy or SRT 50 Gy–54 Gy

Data from Order SE, Donnaldson SS: *Radiation therapy of benign diseases*, ed 2, Berlin, 2003, Springer; and Perez CA, Brady LW: *Principles and practice of radiation oncology*, ed 3, Philadelphia, 1998, Lippincott-Raven.

SRS, Stereotactic radiosurgery; *SRT*, stereotactic radiotherapy; *mCi*, millicuries; *I-131*, iodine-131; *Sr-90*, strontium-90.

Table 18-2 Classifications of Heterotopic Ossifications About the Hip (on AP Radiographs)

Grade	Description
Grade 0	No bone islands visible
Grade 1	Islands of bone visible within soft tissue about the hip
Grade 2	Bone spurs from pelvis or proximal end of femur, leaving 1 cm or less between opposing surfaces
Grade 3	Like grade II, except that space between opposing surface is less than 1 cm
Grade 4	Apparent bony ankylosis

Modified by MacLennon et al. of the Brooker classification. Original source: Seegenschmiedt MH, Makoski HB, Micke O, German Cooperative Group on Radiotherapy for Benign Diseases: *Int J Radiat Oncol Biol Phys* 51(3): 756–765, 2001.

AP, Anteroposterior.

found to be safe, with little risk to the development of other cancers such as sarcomas, the inhibition of bone growth into the prostheses, or wound healing[7] (Figure 18-1).

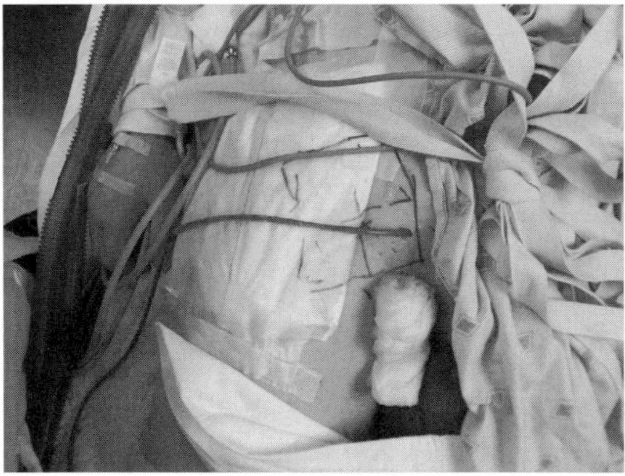

Figure 18-1 Heterotopic Hip Treatment Field.

KELOIDS

Keloids are caused by the overgrowth of collagen fibers and capillaries at the site of a surgical incision or trauma site to the skin such as piercing of the ears (Figure 18-2). Keloids differ from normal scars because they tend to increase in dimension over time causing deformities, numbness, tingling, itching, and pain. Surgical resections of the keloids alone have been shown to result in a recurrence in 50% to 80% of cases.[8] The growth of a keloid at the surgical incision site is often larger than the original keloid. Adjuvant therapies have been tried with minimal results. These therapies include constant pressure devices worn for 4 to 6 months, multiple intralesional injections of corticosteroids, and application of topical retinoic acid, methotrexate, or nitrogen mustard.[9] The most effective adjuvant treatment is postexcisional radiation therapy, which has been shown to reduce the recurrence rate to 12% to 28%.[9]

The radiation therapy dose ranges from 9 Gy to 15 Gy. The treatment field includes the surgical wound and a narrow band of skin on either side of the incision.[10] Electrons are the most commonly used energy. Some facilities administer the first dose before excision. Others begin treatment after the excision of the keloid, administering the radiation

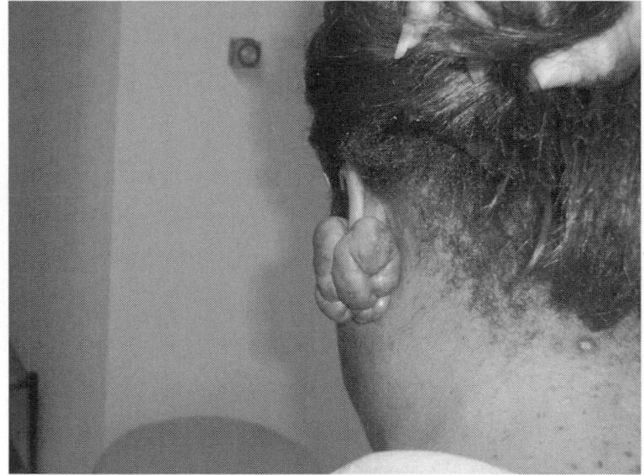

Figure 18-2 Keloid of the Ear From Piercing.

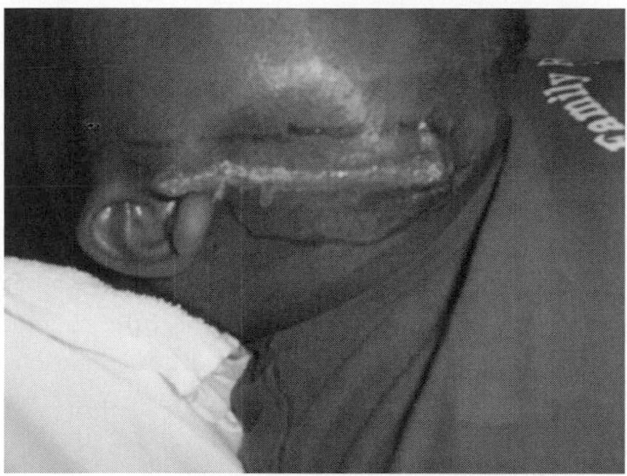

Figure 18-3 Treatment Set-up for Keloid of the Face.

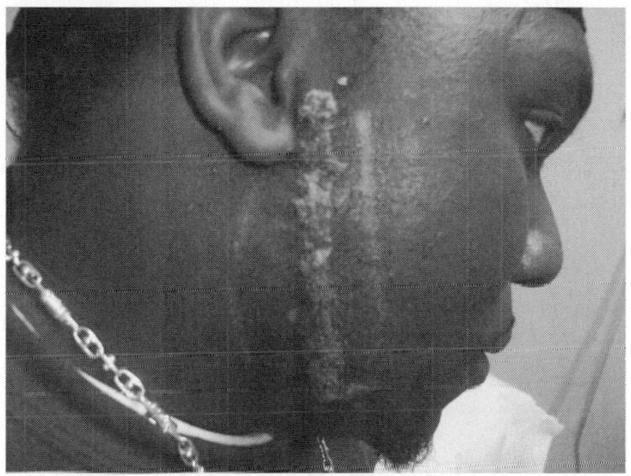

Figure 18-4 Keloid of the Face After Treatment.

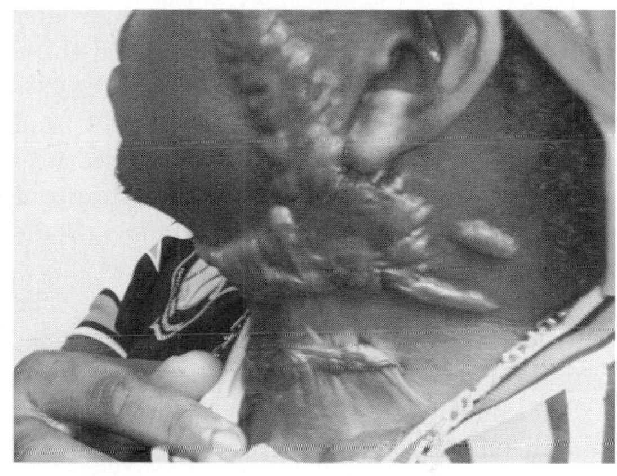

Figure 18-5 Keloid of the Face and Neck Before Surgery and Treatment.

therapy on three consecutive days, whereas others give a larger daily fraction 1 day a week for 3 weeks (Figures 18-3 through 18-6). Side effects from radiation treatment may include skin irritation or dryness, hair loss, and/or changes in pigmentation. Patients coming to the clinic from surgery should be assessed for pain and wound management.

High-dose-rate brachytherapy (^{192}Ir) has been used to treat keloids that have reoccurred after surgery and external beam radiation therapy. At the time of the keloid resection, hollow catheters are imbedded within the incision site and then secured with plastic or metal buttons. The patient is then transferred to the radiation therapy department for treatment planning and administration of the high-dose-rate radiation. The total treatment doseis 15 Gy given over 3 consecutive days (5 Gy/day).[8]

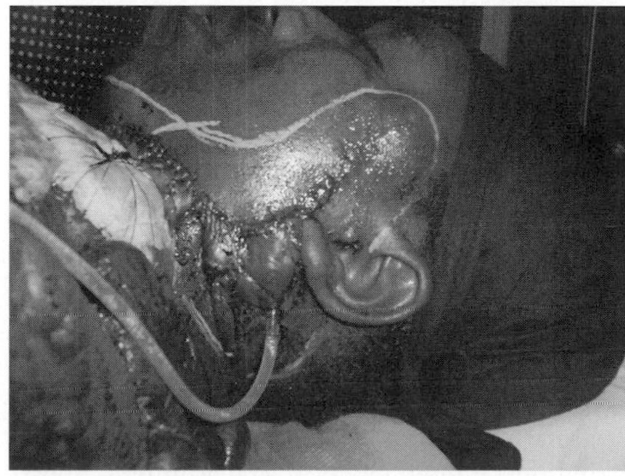

Figure 18-6 Keloid Treatment Set-up of Face and Neck After Surgery.

Pterygium

A pterygium is a chronic, fibrovascular, gray tissue that expands, invading and destroying the cornea of the eye. Most pterygiums originate in the conjunctival-cornea junction (94%), with altered limbal stem cells being the probable cells of origin.[11,12] The development of pterygiums generally occurs between ages 20 and 50.[12] Prevalence is increased in Mediterranean regions and in areas near the equator. Chronic exposure to dusty, dry, and hot conditions and ultraviolet rays are assumed to be the main factor for the development of pterygiums.[11] If untreated, the pterygium can cause irritation, photophobia, cosmetic problems, or visual loss from corneal astigmatism or growth over the pupil.[12]

Pterygiums are treated by surgical excision using the bare sclera technique, which is characterized by leaving a large portion of the sclera bare after removing the pterygium and a diamond-shape piece of conjunctiva. A relapse rate of 20% to 68% is seen with surgery alone.[12] Mitomycin C and thiotepa drops applied during and immediately after resection are used, but both have treatment complications such as edema and perforation of the cornea, acute mature cataracts, scleral calcifications, and increased pain or infections of the eye. The potential for severe side effects and complications limit the use of this adjuvant treatment.[11]

The combined treatment of surgery and radiation therapy shows a recurrence rate of 0% to 20%.[11] Strontium-90 is a beta source of radiation, usually measuring 12 to 15 mm in diameter, that is secured to the end of an applicator (Figure 18-7). The applicator is then placed on the excisional site. Treatment varies from a single dose of 25 Gy, 10 Gy in three doses, to 70 Gy over several weeks.[11] Treatment is typically initiated the day of surgery or as soon as possible.

Nurses play an active role in the treatment of pterygiums. Oxybuprocaine drops are placed in the eye to anesthetize the eye. An eye retractor is used to spread the eyelids open and a applicator is then placed on the excision. The duration of time the applicator is placed is determined by the age of the strontium source and the dose fraction being delivered. The applicator is cleaned according to institutional protocol.

Treatment sequelae are rare, but could include irritation, photophobia, scleral thinning, postoperative granulomas, cataracts, and infections[12] (Figure 18-8).

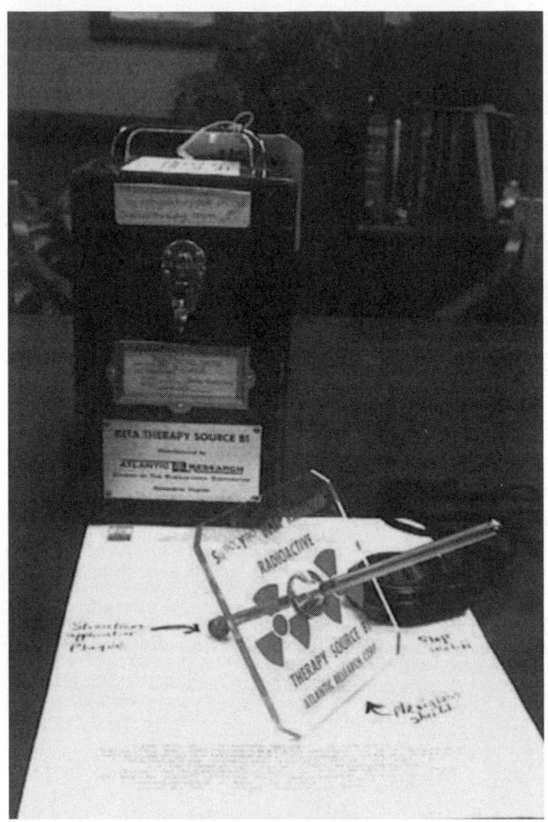

Figure 18-7 Strontium Applicator.
Courtesy of Florida Radiation Oncology Group.

GRAVES' OPHTHALMOPATHY

Graves' ophthalmopathy (GO) is the most common extrathyroidal expression of Graves' disease. GO is an autoimmune disease characterized by an inflammatory swelling of orbital fat and extraocular eye muscles.[13] The pathogenic mechanisms are not completely understood, but it is believed that GO is triggered by autoimmune reactions to antigens shared by the thyroid and the orbit. Clinical presentation includes eyelid swelling and retraction, proptosis, eye muscle impaired function, and optic neuropathy all caused by the increased volume of the orbital content (extraocular muscles, fibroadipose tissue).[14] In 90% of the cases, it is associated with hyperthyroidism. Most patients have mild and self-limiting symptoms, but 3% to 5% have severe GO expressions for which treatment is difficult.[15] Current treatments such as radiation or steroids are aimed at increasing orbital space by decompressing or diminishing the orbital tissue volume. Orbital surgery is aimed

Primary untreated pterygium left eye.

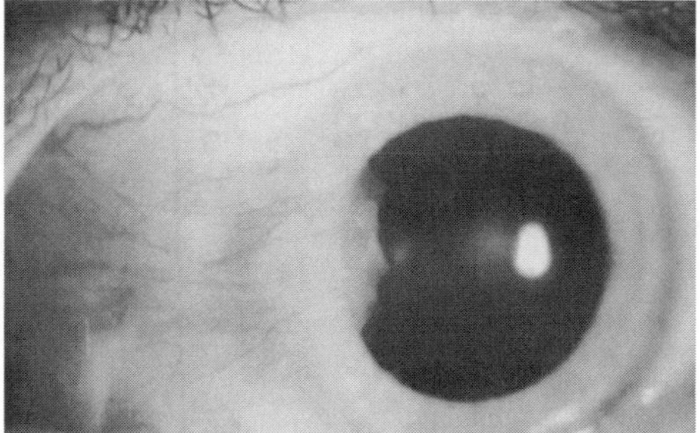

Same eye 6 weeks after combined treatment

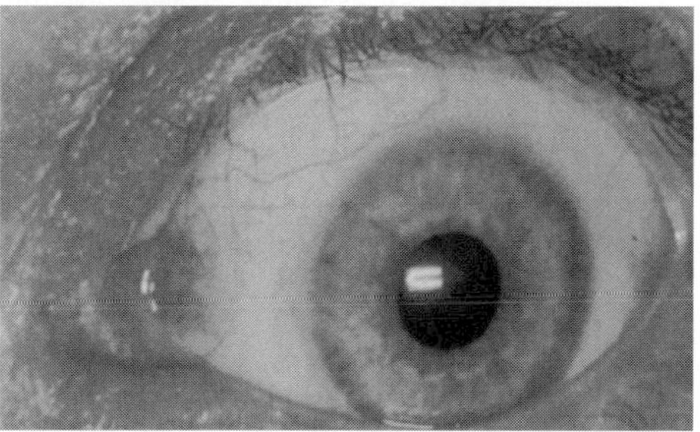

Same eye 2 years after combined treatment. Neither relapse nor complications.

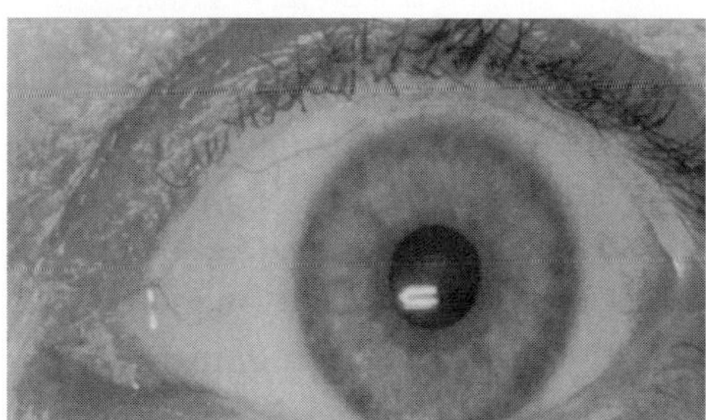

Primary untreated pterygium left eye.

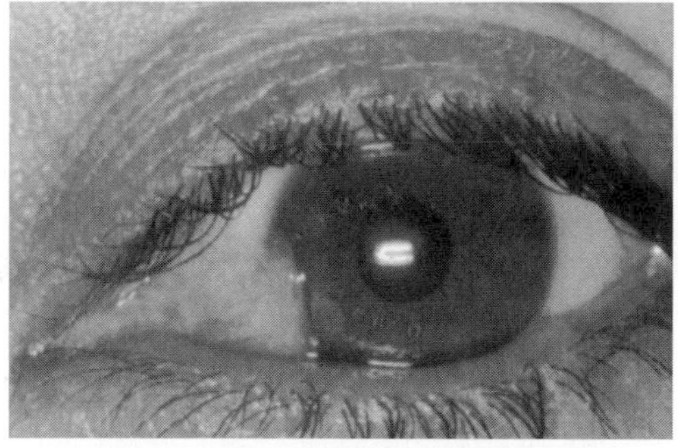

Same eye 6 weeks after excision only, post operative granuloma

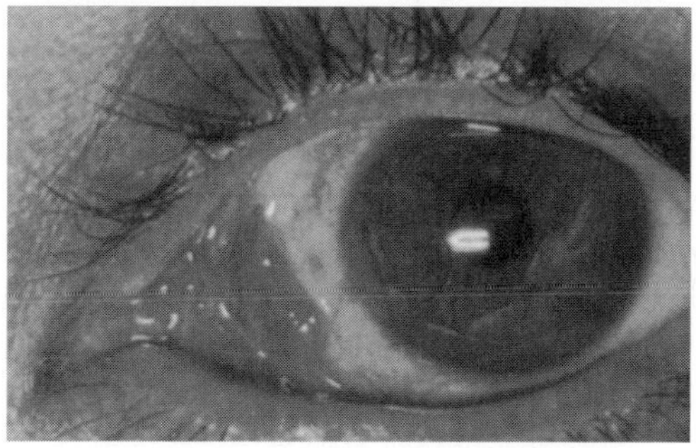

Same eye 2 years after excision only, pterygium relapse.

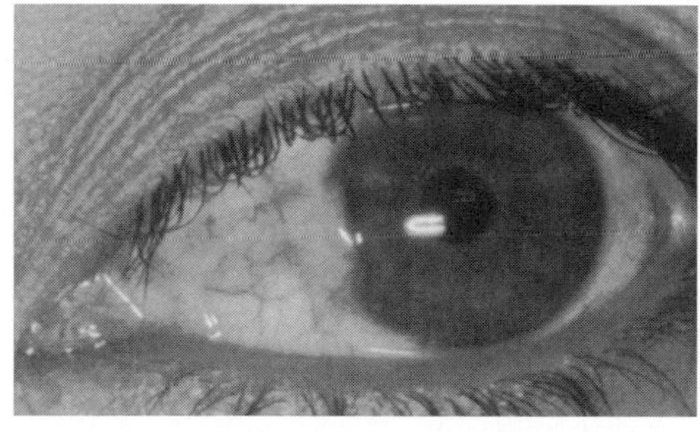

Figure 18-8 Pterygium With and Without Radiation.
From Jürgenliemk-Schulz I, Hartman L, et al: Int J Radiat Oncol Biol Phys 59(4):1138-1147, 2004.

at expanding the available space for the tissue. The combination of orbital radiation therapy and steroids appears to have more favorable results than either treatment alone. Smoking seems to reduce the effectiveness of medical treatment for GO. Treatment also has a better response if the disease is in the active phase.[14]

Oral corticosteroids, such as prednisone, have been shown to be an effective treatment for GO by acting as an antiinflammatory. Corticosteroids have been used before radiation as a first-line treatment for GO or after in cases of insufficient response to radiation therapy.[13]

Orbital radiation therapy is administered using lateral fields. The dose given is 20 Gy over 10 days (2 Gy/day).[16] Acute side effects from orbital radiation therapy include skin irritation and hair loss at the entry port, eye irritation, and some worsening of the soft tissue involved. It is important to educate the patient that these side effects could occur after treatment and will resolve shortly thereafter. The use of lubricating eyedrops may help with the eye irritation. Long-term sequalae include cataracts, retinopathy, or secondary tumors (although so far no cases of radiation-induced cancers have been reported).[14] Many of these sequalae are compounded by age and diabetes.

SUMMARY

Because the biologic mechanisms of radiation therapy used on benign diseases are still unknown; all means of protection must be applied. These protections include using the smallest but most effective dose and field size. Because many benign diseases receive one single fraction of radiation therapy, the treatment field must be verified and approved by the medical physicist and the physician before administrating the radiation therapy. Because radiation therapy is known to cause damage to normal tissue and second malignancies, the patient needs to be fully aware of possible short- and long-term side effects and be properly consented.[2]

REFERENCES

1. Order SE, Donnaldson SS: *Radiation therapy of benign diseases*, ed 2, Berlin, 2003, Springer.
2. Micke O, Seegenschmiedt MH: Consensus guidelines for radiation therapy of benign diseases: a multicenter approach in Germany, *Int J Radiat Oncol Biol Phys* 52(2):496-513, 2002.
3. Cornes PG, Shahidi M, Glees JP: Heterotopic bone formation: irradiation of high risk patients, *Br J Radiol* 75(893):448-452, 2002.
4. Kaplan FS, Glaser DL, Hebela N et al: Heterotopic ossification, *J Am Acad* Orthop *Surg* 12(2):116-125, 2004.
5. Seegenschmiedt MH, Makoski HB, Micke O, German Cooperative Group on Radiotherapy for Benign Diseases: Radiation prophylaxis for heterotopic ossification about the hip joint—a multicenter study, *Int J Radiat Oncol Biol Phys* 51(3):756-765, 2001.
6. Ashton A, Bruce W, Goldberg J et al: Prevention of heterotopic bone formation in high risk patients post-total hip arthroplasty, *J Orthop Surg* 8:53-57, 2000.
7. Healy W, Lo T, DeSimone A et al: Single-dose irradiation for the prevention of heterotopic ossification after total hip arthroplasty: a comparison of doses of five hundred and fifty and seven hundred centigray, *J Bone Joint Surg Am* 77A(4):590-595, 1995.
8. Garg M, Weiss P, Sharma A et al: Adjuvant high dose brachytherapy (Ir-192) in the management of keloids which have recurred after surgical excision and external radiation, *Radiother Oncol* 73(2):233-236, 2004.
9. Kovalic J, Perez C: Radiation therapy following keloidectomy: a 20-year experience, *Int J Radiat Oncol Biol Phys* 17(1):77-80, 1989.
10. Doornbos J, Stoffel T, Hass A et al: The role of kilovoltage irradiation in the treatment of keloids, *Int J Radiat Oncol Biol Phys* 18(4):833-839, 1990.
11. Pajic B, Pallas A, Aebersold D et al: Prospective study of exclusive, nonsurgical strontium-/yttrium-90 irradiation of pterygia, *Strahlenther Onkol* 8:510-516, 2004.
12. Jürgenliemk-Schulz I, Hartman L, Roesink JM et al: Prevention of pterygium recurrence by postoperative single-dose β-irradiation: a prospective randomized clinical double-blind trial, *Int J Radiat Oncol Biol Phys* 59(4):1138-1147, 2004.
13. Wakelkamp I, Tan H, Saeed P et al: Orbital irradiation for Graves' ophthalmopathy: is it safe? A long-term follow-up study, *Am Acad Ophthalmol* 111(8):1557-1562, 2004.
14. Bartalena L, Marcocci C, Gorman CA et al: Orbital radiotherapy for Graves' ophthalmopathy: useful or useless? Safe or dangerous? *J Endocrinol Invest* 26(1):5-16, 2003.
15. Heyd R, Seegenschmiedt M, Strassmann G et al: Radiotherapy for Grave's orbitopathy: results for a national survey, *Strahlenther Onkol* 6:372-376, 2003.
16. Perez CA, Brady LW: *Principles and practice of radiation oncology*, ed 3, Philadelphia, 1998, Lippincott-Raven.

Unit IV
Adjuvant Therapies

Chapter 19 Chemoradiotherapy

Wendy H. Vogel

Chemotherapy and/or radiation have been the standard treatment for many cancers, particularly following surgery, for the past 30 years. However, improvements in the survival of patients receiving these treatments was modest at best. Chemoradiotherapy is the concomitant administration of chemotherapy with radiation therapy and now has a recognized role as being either definitive therapy for unresectable disease or adjuvant therapy for high-risk surgical disease.[1,2] Positive effects are found in many cancers such as head and neck cancer, gastrointestinal cancers, advanced pelvic cancers, colorectal cancers, and lung cancers.[3-5] Chemoradiotherapy improves local-regional tumor control and enhances disease-free survival and overall survival when compared with the previously standard treatments for these diseases. However, this improvement comes with an increase in the toxicities normally seen with either modality of treatment.[6-8] These toxicities can result in significant morbidity and mortality.

As treatments for cancers become more aggressive and toxicities increase, the need for a team-based approach becomes more obvious. The use of chemoradiation validates the value of a multidisciplinary team that includes the surgical, medical, and radiation oncology nurses. It is equally important that each subspecialty nurse understands the treatment toxicities of each modality and the synergistic toxicity that can occur when combined modality treatment is prescribed and administered. Astute nursing care and collaboration between disciplines ensures the successful completion of the prescribed therapy, with the hope of improved patient outcomes. Although each subspecialty of nurses are experts in only their own field, they cannot ignore the toxicities caused by other modalities of treatment. Appropriate supportive care must be initiated at whatever stage of therapy the patient is in. Coordination between the subspecialties is crucial to the successful completion of the therapy. In the past, it was common for each discipline to blame the other's treatment for the toxicity or side effect that the patient was experiencing. Today, medical, surgical, and radiation oncology nurses all need to understand the synergistic effect of combined modality therapies and be accountable to provide coordinated patient care. No team member can assume that another team member initiated care for the patient's treatment side effects or disease symptomology. All team members must be familiar with the prevention and treatment of the toxicities associated with combined modalities. Each discipline should be involved in the education of the patient and family (or caregivers).

In addition to the coordination of toxicity management, treatment goals should be well defined and mutually agreed upon by each discipline involved in the multidisciplinary team. The goal of treatment could be cure, control, palliation or prophylaxis.[9] If the tumor is diagnosed at an early stage, cure could be possible. Curative therapy may be lengthy and aggressive. Certain cancers and cancers diagnosed in later stages are unable to be cured. For these, control of the disease is the goal. Control of the disease may range from months to years. Palliation is the goal when cure or control is not possible, and treatment may provide relief of symptoms. Prophylactic treatment goals are to eradicate any micrometastasis before it becomes clinically apparent or to treat a potential problem before it becomes clinically significant.[10] Multidisciplinary treatment conferences are ideal scenarios for discussing treatment goals and coordinating treatment and toxicity management.

Besides multidisciplinary treatment conferences, participation in round table discussion groups, grand rounds in the hospital setting, tumor board, and educational teleconferences affords opportunities to learn more about the other disciplines. Each multidisciplinary team member must share their expertise with the team to promote communication and coordination between the disciplines to obtain the most positive outcome for their mutual patient. Understanding the rationale for chemoradiotherapy will enhance each team member's functionality.

The rationale for chemoradiotherapy is based on the premise that chemotherapeutic drugs enhance the antitumor and cytotoxic effects of radiation. Each modality affects tumor cells differently.[10-12] Chemotherapy is effective in eradicating micrometastasis, and radiation is effective in achieving local, primary tumor control.[11] Chemotherapy enhances the initial radiation damage, inhibits cellular repair, affects cellular kinetics, and eliminates hypoxic cells.

To enhance the initial radiation cell kill, chemotherapy is used as a radiation sensitizer, making radiation more lethal. Chemotherapy affects cell growth and proliferation by producing damaging effects to DNA. This will accumulate the tumor cells in a radiosensitive phase or eliminate radioresistance.[11] If tumor growth does occur after radiation, it is slowed by the addition of chemotherapy. In many cases, because of DNA damage, chemotherapy will inhibit the cell's ability to repair itself after radiation damage. In addition, chemotherapy eliminates hypoxic cells and improves tumor oxygen supply by cytoreduction effects, thus maximizing radiation cell kill.[12] For full understanding of these concepts, it is necessary to understand the characteristics of cancer cells and how chemotherapy affects cancer cells and normal cells.

CHARACTERISTICS OF CANCER CELLS

Cancer is a malignant disease with a series of cellular and genetic aberrations that cause abnormal cell proliferation. Characteristics of cancer cells include unregulated growth and invasion of surrounding tissues and the ability to metastasize.[13] These differences of cancer cells occur because of multiple sequential alterations in a cell's genes. Different types of altered genes can interact to cause a cancer. The same gene may cause both inherited and noninherited versions of the same tumor.[14] One of the notable theories to explain these cellular alterations is the *three-stage theory,* also called the *multistage theory,* that originated during mouse skin chemical carcinogenesis studies.[15,16]

The three-stage theory explains the development of cancer. The first stage is *initiation.* An initiating agent (carcinogen) may be chemical, physical, or biologic.[17] Chemical carcinogens are the most common human carcinogens and are found in tobacco smoke, certain medications, and certain industrial products. Chemical carcinogens are classified as (1) *inorganic,* such as arsenic, nickel and chromium; (2) *organic,* including vinyl chloride and benzene; or (3) *hormones,* such as estrogenic compounds and androgenic steroids.

Physical carcinogens include radiation, fibers, or chronic irritation.[17] Radiation carcinogens include ultraviolet light and ionizing radiation. Skin cancers are associated with increased exposure to ultraviolet light. Exposure to asbestos fibers or silica fibers can lead to malignant changes. An example of chronic irritation is a mole subjected to daily irritation from a belt or collar.

Biologic carcinogens can include viruses, parasites, and bacteria. The Epstein-Barr virus has been associated with Burkitt's lymphoma and Hodgkin's lymphoma.[17] The papilloma virus has been implicated in cervical cancer. Parasites such as *Schistosoma haematobium* and bacteria such as *Helicobacter pylori* have been associated with cancer.

Some of the common carcinogens are found in Table 19-1. These carcinogens damage DNA by changing a specific gene. This gene then undergoes repair or becomes permanently changed. Changes do not cause cancer unless there is repeated exposure. When the gene does mutate, the change is irreversible, and it can produce a cancer cell line.[16] The cell then progresses to the second stage.

The second stage is *promotion.* Alteration of the genetic structure of a cell or the inhibition of apoptosis (cell death) may occur with exposure to a carcinogen. Carcinogens have time and dose limitations. Time between exposure to initiators and promoters and the development of cancer varies. This phase can be interrupted and reversed up to the point at which damage to the proliferation mechanisms of the cell occurs. Then it is irreversible, and the result is cancer cell transformation.[16] Some damage may be repaired by cancer-reversing or cancer-suppressing agents (vitamins, minerals, etc) or the host's own immune function. When transformation occurs, the cell moves to the third stage, progression.

In the *progression* stage, the cell has increasing genetic instability, that is, mutations. Mutations may provide tumor cells with a growth advantage.

Table 19-1 Common Carcinogens

Cancer-producing agent	Examples
Radiation (damages cellular DNA)	Ionizing and ultraviolet radiation
Organic chemicals	Benzene, asbestos, silica, ethanol, radon
Tobacco and tobacco smoke	Multiple carcinogens such as aromatic amines, nitrosamines, free radicals, N-nitrosamines, and many more
Hormones	Diethylstilbestrol
Charbroiled meat	Heterocyclic amines
Chemotherapeutic agents	Cyclophosphamide (Cytoxan), melphalan (Alkeran)
Mineral products	Chromium, nickel, arsenic
Industrial products	Benzene, tar volatiles, asphalt, coal tar and pitch, vinyl chloride, coal carbonization products, chloromethyl methyl ether
Environmental pollution	Combustion emissions
Bacteria	*Helicobacter pylori*
Parasites	*Schistosoma haematobium*
Viruses	Epstein-Barr virus and human papilloma virus

Data from Vulimiri S, Digiovanni J: Carcinogenesis. In Pollock R, Doroshow J, Khayat D, et al: *UICC manual of clinical oncology*, ed 8, Hoboken, NJ, 2004, John Wiley & Sons.

Cancer cells continue to divide without normal stop mechanisms and invade normal cells. During this stage, angiogenesis is stimulated. Angiogenesis is the ability to stimulate proliferation of new blood vessels from the host to feed itself. Because tumors larger than 0.5 mm require a vasculature to survive, the angiogenesis process allows tumors to thrive. Angiogenesis is modulated by VEGF (vascular endothelial growth factor).[13] The tumor continues to grow and to spread.

Metastasis is the spread of cancer from primary site to distant sites. Routes of metastases include direct invasion, seeding throughout a body cavity (peritoneal), and spread by way of the lymph system or by blood capillaries and veins. Metastasis is influenced by pattern of blood flow, cell receptors and genes that tell the cell to travel to specific sites, tumor cell production of adhesion molecules that prefer certain distant organs, chemical signals and growth factors (found in selected organs), or inhibitor substances produced by organs not typically sites for metastatic growth. Metastasis is the major cause of treatment failure and death.

The three-stage theory explains the development of a cancer and the process of its growth. Cancer is able to survive and grows within a host because cancer cells are different from normal cells. Cancer cells do not have the normal growth-control pathways and regulatory mechanisms.[18] Various characteristics of cancer cells are described in Box 19-1. Cancers cells may have various genetic changes as well. One type of genetic change is a germ-line mutation. This mutation affects the ova and sperm. This type of mutation confers the greatest risk for a cancer, and the mutation can be passed from generation to generation. The various types of genetic changes are listed in Box 19-2.

Box 19-1 Characteristics of Cancer Cells

- Pleomorphism (variable size and shapes)
- Hyperchromatism (nuclear chromatin more pronounced in staining)
- Polymorphism (nucleus enlarged and variable in shape)
- Cell membrane changes (production of surface enzymes that aid in invasion/metastasis)
- Loss of contact inhibition (caused by loss of glycoproteins)
- Defect in cell-to-cell recognition and adhesion
- Inability to control proliferation
- Increased mitotic index (percentage of cells that are in mitosis at any given time)
- Abnormal longevity
- Less dependent upon oxygen (caused by abnormal glycolysis)
- Abnormal cell differentiation

Data from Merkle C, Loescher L: Biology of cancer. In Yarbro C, Frogge M, Goodman M: *Cancer nursing principles and practice*, ed 6, Boston, 2005, Jones and Bartlett.

The growth of tumors depends on several factors.[19] One factor is the cell cycle time, which is the length of time for a cell that has just completed mitosis to grow, redivide, and again pass through mitosis. A second factor is the growth fraction of the tumor. This is the fraction, or percentage, of the cell population that is currently undergoing division. Another factor that affects tumor growth is the total number of cells in the population. As the number of cells increases, so does the number of resistant cells, which means decreased curability. Large tumors often have less of an adequate blood supply and oxygenation, which impairs drug delivery to the tumor cells and decreases the sensitivity of tumor cells to chemotherapy or radiation therapy. The last factor is the rate of intrinsic cell death. This is difficult to measure.

CHEMOTHERAPY

Chemotherapy is one of several treatment modalities used for cancer. Chemotherapy is a systemic therapy, rather than a local therapy such as radiation therapy. This means that the drug or drugs are distributed throughout the body by the blood stream. Significant advances have been made in the treatment of cancer with chemotherapy over the past 60 years. Today, several types of cancer can be cured with a combination of chemotherapy drugs. Adjunctive treatment with chemotherapeutic agents is intended to destroy any micrometastasis that could be left in the body after primary therapy. Chemotherapy may be employed to control the cancer and thus prolong life or to control cancer symptoms alone (palliation).

The use of chemotherapy requires a basic understanding of the cell cycle and tumor cell growth. Most chemotherapeutic agents affect tumor cell proliferation. Because most normal cells are also proliferating, damage to normal cells often occurs too, thus causing the side effects that are common to cytotoxic drugs.[9] These effects are more pronounced on cell populations that have a rapid rate of turnover, such as the bone marrow and the mucous membrane cells.

Five stages of the cell life cycle process occur in both normal and cancerous cells.[10] Table 19-2 lists each of the stages and describes the activity that occurs in each stage. Chemotherapeutic agents are generally classified by the phase of the cell cycle in which their activity occurs. Cell cycle–specific (or phase-specific) drugs work within one specific phase of the cell cycle. Cell cycle–nonspecific agents (phase-nonspecific) have activity within all phases of the cell cycle, including the resting phase, a period of reproductive quiescence. Differences in cell cycle–"specific" and "nonspecific" drugs are shown in Table 19-3. Table 19-4 lists the classifications of the chemotherapeutic agents. Although not every drug can be assigned to one classification exclusively, it is helpful to have a general understanding of the drug activity.

Box 19-2 Genetic Changes in Cancer Cells

- **Translocations:** exchange of material between chromosomes
- **Deletions:** loss of chromosome segments
- **Amplification:** increase in number of copies of DNA sequence
- **Aneuploidy:** abnormal number of chromosomes

Data from Loescher L, Whitesell L: The Biology of Cancer. In Tranin A, Masny A, Jenkins J: *Genetics in oncology practice: cancer risk assessment*, Pittsburgh, 2003, Oncology Nursing Society.

Table 19-2 The Life Cycle of Cells

Stage	Description	Activity
G0	Resting phase	Temporarily out of cycle, not actively proliferating
G1	Postmitotic phase	Begins active phase; proteins and RNA are synthesized
S	Synthesis phase	DNA is synthesized
G2	Premitotic phase	Further protein synthesis occurs; preparation for mitotic spindles
M	Mitosis phase	Cell division occurs; shortest phase
		At conclusion of M phase, two daughter cells have been formed that will either reenter the cycle or stay in G0 phase
		Insensitive to many chemotherapeutic agents

Data from Merkle C, Loescher L: Biology of cancer. In Yarbro C, Frogge M, Goodman M: *Cancer nursing principles and practice*, ed 6, Boston, 2005, Jones and Bartlett.

Table 19-3 Differences in Cell-cycle Specific and Cell-cycle Nonspecific Drugs

	Cell-cycle specific	Cell-cycle nonspecific
Method of administration	Divided, frequent doses or continuous infusions with short cycle times	Intermittent doses, allowing recovery from dose-limiting toxicities
Greatest cell kill	Limited as to number of cells killed with one drug exposure Proportional to length of drug exposure; higher dosing does not kill more cells For rapidly proliferating tumors	Proportional to amount of drug given-higher doses kill more cells For more slowly proliferating tumors

Data from Polovich M, White J, Kelleher L: *Chemotherapy and biotherapy guidelines and recommendations for practice, ed 2*, Pittsburgh, 2005, Oncology Nursing Press.

Table 19-4 Classifications and Examples of Chemotherapeutic Agents

Cell cycle	Classification	Examples
Cell-cycle specific	Antimetabolites	5-Fluorouracil (Adrucil) Methotrexate (Folex)
	Vinca alkaloids	Vinorelbine (Navelbine) Vincristine (Oncovin)
	Camptothecins	Irinotecan (Camptosar) Topotecan (Hycamtin)
	Epipodophyllotoxins	Etoposide (VePesid)
	Taxanes	Docetaxel (Taxotere) Paclitaxel (Taxol)
Cell-cycle nonspecific	Alkylating agents	Cyclophosphamide (Cytoxan) Cisplatin (Platinol AQ)
	Antitumor antibiotics	Doxorubicin (Adriamycin) Bleomycin (Blenoxane)
	Hormonal therapies	Tamoxifen (Nolvadex) Leuprolide (Lupron)
	Nitrosoureas	Carmustine (BiCNU) Streptozocin (Zanosar)

Data from Tortorice P: Chemotherapy: principles of therapy. In Yarbro C, Frogge M, Goodman M, editors: *Cancer nursing principles and practice*, ed 6, Boston, 2005, Jones and Bartlett, pp 315-350 and from Polovich M, White J, Kelleher L: *Chemotherapy and biotherapy guidelines and recommendations for practice, ed 2*, Pittsburgh, 2005, Oncology Nursing Press.

For many years, single-agent therapy (one chemotherapeutic agent given alone) was employed. Now, it is well established that the combination of various chemotherapeutic agents are often more effective.[10] Combination therapy often will combine a cell cycle–specific with a cell cycle–nonspecific agent, thus maximizing the cell kill by affecting cells that are dividing slowly or rapidly. Cell cycle–nonspecific agents often will assist in the recruitment of cells into a more actively dividing state, thus becoming more sensitive to the cell cycle–specific agents. Combination therapy also can prevent the development of resistance to treatment. The goal of combination therapy is that each agent will enhance the other's activity resulting in beneficial effects.

Dosing

Most adult chemotherapeutic agents are dosed by a calculation based on the patient's body surface area and are expressed in milligrams per square meter. The body surface area (BSA) is a calculation based on the patient's weight and height. The height and weight should be accurate and measured precisely, not recorded simply as stated by the patient.[9] BSA calculators are readily available in many forms:

textbooks, online, in handheld computer programs, and as a slide rule.

Although BSA dosing is used the majority of the time, some agents use the area-under-the-curve (AUC) dosing. AUC dosing is a reliable method for achieving the most accurate dose and balancing efficacy and toxicity for particular agents.[20] Patients with a more rapid clearance may need larger doses. The Calvert formula is the most often used formula for calculating the AUC dose. For example, AUC dosing is the standard of practice for determining doses of carboplatin. The AUC dose provides a measure of total systemic drug exposure and is expressed in concentration × units (mg/mL × min).[20] AUC dosing depends on drug administration and elimination. The target AUC is usually between 5 and 7 mg/mL/min for previously untreated patients. In previously treated patients or when combined with other modalities of treatment, such as radiation, the target AUC dose may be lowered.

Another method of dosing some chemotherapeutic agents is in milligram (mg) per kilogram (kg) of patient weight.[9] This method is more commonly used in children younger than 1 year of age or those who weigh less than 10 kg. Many biologic agents are dosed in this manner. When combined with radiation therapy, drugs dosed in this manner also will be given in lower doses.

The ideal dose and schedule of the drug is what provides the maximal benefit with the least toxicity.[19] The most limiting factor in the ability to cure patients is the drug toxicity at the doses required for total cell kill. At times, a patient may receive a lower than standard dose because of neutropenia from chemotherapy, other side effects of the chemotherapy (e.g., severe vomiting), or side effects of radiation therapy (e.g., severe esophagitis). Although dose reduction for concomitant therapy with radiation is necessary, reduced dosing for toxicities can result in lowered cure rates. A 20% dose reduction can result in about 50% less cure rate.[9] Inadequate dosing may occur more often in the elderly with doses given that are lower than standard dosing and not evidence based. Most standard chemotherapy schedules are based on how quickly the bone marrow recovers from exposure to cytotoxic agents.

Toxicities

Chemotherapeutic agents have a narrow therapeutic index, meaning there is little distance between the therapeutic dose and the toxic dose.[21] Because of this, the oncology nurse, whether in radiation oncology, surgical oncology, or medical oncology, must be knowledgeable about potential toxicities and their treatments. Side effects may appear within a few hours, a few days, a few weeks, or even months to years after chemotherapy administration.

One of the most common side effects or toxicities of chemotherapy is myelosuppression. Other toxicities associated with various chemotherapeutic agents include nausea and vomiting, diarrhea, constipation, mucositis, cystitis, sterility, myalgia, neuropathy, local reactions from extravasation (leaking of an irritant or vesicant chemotherapy drug into tissues surrounding the venipuncture site), cardiotoxicity, renal failure, allergic reactions, anaphylaxis, phlebitis, alopecia, and pulmonary fibrosis.[9] Each chemotherapeutic agent is associated with a unique side effect profile. Many of these toxicities also occur with radiation therapy but can be exacerbated by concomitant chemotherapy. The most common toxicities of chemotherapy and their causative agents are listed in Table 19-5. The most common side effects of various chemotherapeutic agents are listed in Table 19-6.

Myelosuppression

Most chemotherapeutic agents cause some degree of myelosuppression.[21] In chemotherapy-naïve patients (those who have never received prior chemotherapy), chemotherapy generally causes myelosuppression (lowered blood counts), specifically, leukopenia (lowered white blood cell counts [WBC]) and thrombocytopenia (lowered platelet counts) between days 7 and 10. The nadir blood count is the lowest point to which the blood counts drop. Depending on the agent(s) used, recovery usually begins by day 21, with complete recovery by day 28.[9] Patients treated previously may have a depleted stem cell pool in the bone marrow. This may shorten the time to the appearance of leukopenia and thrombocytopenia and prolong the recovery time. This is also true for patients with tumor cells in the bone marrow or for those who have received radiation therapy to wide radiation fields or in higher doses. It is important to note the duration of the nadir level of leukocytes and platelets, so that neutropenia or thrombocytopenia may be anticipated and treated promptly and appropriately.

Myelosuppression is the most common dose-limiting toxicity of chemotherapy[9] and is potentially lethal. To determine the risk of infection, the

Table 19-5 Cancer Therapy Toxicities and Common Causative Agents

Nephrotoxicity	Hepatotoxicity	Neurotoxicity	Pulmonary toxicity	Cardiotoxicity
Carmustine (BiCNU)	Cytarabine* (Cytosar-U)	Bortezomib (Velcade)	Bleomycin (Blenoxane)	Cyclophosphamide* (Cytoxan)
Cisplatin (Platinol AQ)	Methotrexate* (Folex)	Cisplatin (Platinol AQ)	Carmustine (BiCNU)	Daunorubicin (Daunomycin)
Cyclophosphamide (Cytoxan)		Docetaxel (Taxotere)	Cyclophosphamide* (Cytoxan)	Doxorubicin (Adriamycin)
Gemcitabine (Gemzar)		5-FU (Adrucil)	Cytarabine (Cytosar-U)	Epirubicin (Ellence)
Ifosfamide (Ifex)		Ifosfamide (Ifex)	Gemcitabine (Gemzar)	Paclitaxel* (Taxol)
Irinotecan (Camptosar)		Methotrexate* (Folex)	Mitomycin-C (Mutamycin)	
Lomustine (CCNU)		Oxaliplatin (Eloxatin)		
Methotrexate* (Folex)		Paclitaxel (Taxol)		
Mitomycin C (Mutamycin)		Vincristine (Oncovin)		
Streptozocin* (Zanosar)				

Data from Camp-Sorrell D: Chemotherapy toxicities and management. In Yarbro C, Frogge M, Goodman M: *Cancer nursing principles and practice*, ed 6, Boston: Jones and Bartlett and Chu E, Devita V: *Cancer chemotherapy drug manual, 2006*, Sudbury, MA, 2006, Jones and Bartlett.
*Causes this toxicity in higher doses.

Table 19-6 Side Effects of Cancer Therapy and Most Common Causative Agents

Nausea/vomiting	Alopecia	Rash	Diarrhea	Constipation
Carboplatin (Paraplatin)	Cyclophosphamide (Cytoxan)	Cytarabine (Cytosar-U)	Bortezomib (Velcade)	Vinblastine (Velban)
Cisplatin (Platinol AQ)	Dactinomycin (Cosmegen)	Daunorubicin (Cerubidine)	Capecitabine (Xeloda)	Vincristine (Oncovin)
Cyclophosphamide (Cytoxan)	Daunorubicin (Daunomycin)	Doxorubicin (Adriamycin)	Docetaxel (Taxotere)	Vinorelbine (Navelbine)
Dacarbazine (DTIC)	Doxorubicin (Adriamycin)	Epirubicin (Ellence)	Doxorubicin (Adriamycin)	
Doxorubicin (Adriamycin)	Etoposide (VePesid)	Methotrexate (Folex)	5-FU (Adrucil)	
Epirubicin (Ellence)	Idarubicin (Idamycin)	Procarbazine (Matulane)	gefitinib (Iressa)	
Ifosfamide (Ifex)	Ifosfamide (Ifex)	Topotecan (Hycamtin)	Irinotecan (Camptosar)	
Mechlorethamine (Mustargen)	Irinotecan (Camptosar)		Methotrexate (Folex)	
	Paclitaxel (Taxol)			
	Topotecan (Hycamtin)			
	Vincristine (Oncovin)			

Data from Chu E, DeVita V: *Cancer chemotherapy drug manual*, Sudbury, Mass, 2006, Jones and Bartlett.

absolute neutrophil count (ANC) should be calculated. To calculate this, the percentage of segmented neutrophils is added to the percentage of band neutrophils, then multiplied by the total percentage by the white blood cell (WBC) count (Box 19-3). In some cases, the total WBC count could be normal, and the ANC could be too low for the patient to be treated, so assessment of the WBC alone is insufficient. The highest risk for infection occurs when the ANC is lower than 500/dL. The highest risk of bleeding occurs when the platelet count is lower than 10,000/dL. If the nadir lasts only 4 to 7 days, patients usually tolerate leukopenia and thrombocytopenia well and recover without assistance. Signs and symptoms of leukopenia and thrombocytopenia are listed in Table 19-7.

Anemia also may occur in patients receiving chemotherapy, although less often than leukopenia or thrombocytopenia.[21] In general, chemotherapy is not withheld for anemia because this can be corrected with red blood cell transfusions. Signs and symptoms of anemia are listed in Table 19-7. Anemia may be a common cause of fatigue in cancer patients.

Until recently, the treatment for leukopenia, thrombocytopenia, and anemia was to hold the chemotherapy treatment or delay the treatment, or in the case of thrombocytopenia or anemia, to administer blood products when necessary. The introduction of growth factors for hematopoietic progenitor cells has changed this practice dramatically. Table 19-8 lists the various hematopoietic growth factors, indications, and potential side effects. The National Comprehensive Cancer Network[22] (NCCN) provided guidelines based on a consensus of experts in the oncology fields regarding their views of currently accepted approaches to treatment with myeloid growth factors. Patients who are at high risk for leukopenia can be prophylactically treated. Patients at lesser risk may have a growth factor added to their therapeutic regimen after a febrile neutropenic episode has occurred or chemotherapy treatment has been delayed because of neutropenia. It is important for both the medical and radiation oncology nurses to understand the appropriate indications for these medications and the possible side effects that can occur after administration.

For the treatment of anemia, the NCCN[22] also offers practices guidelines. Erythropoietin therapy should be considered for a hemoglobin (Hgb) of 10 to 11g/dL and titrated to maintain a hemoglobin of 12g/dL. The Federal Drug Administration (FDA) has approved the use of interleukin-11 (Il-11), the only FDA-approved agent for thrombocytopenia, but its use has been limited because of the toxicity profile of this drug and because thrombocytopenia is easily treated in the outpatient setting with platelet transfusions.[23]

Box 19-3 Calculating the ANC

Formula: % of segments + % of bands × WBC = ANC
Example:
WBC = 1500
Neutrophil percentage = 40%
Band percentage = 5%
(40% + 5%) × 1500 = 675
ANC = 675

ANC, Absolute neutrophil count; *WBC*, white blood cell count.

Nausea and Vomiting

Nausea and vomiting are two of the most feared toxicities of chemotherapy. Acute nausea and vomiting occurs with 1 to 2 hours after treatment administration and usually resolves within 24 hours.

Table 19-7 Signs and Symptoms of Myelosuppression

Leukopenia	Thrombocytopenia	Anemia
Normal signs of infection may be absent Fever may be only sign of infection	Easy bruising Bleeding from gums, nose, bowels, or urinary tract Petechiae	Pallor Hypotension Headaches Fatigue and weakness, not relieved by rest Irritability

Data from Camp-Sorrell D: Chemotherapy toxicities and management. In Yarbro C, Frogge M, Goodman M: *Cancer nursing principles and practice*, ed 6, Boston, 2005, Jones and Bartlett, pp 412-457.

Table 19-8 Hematopoietic Growth Factors in Oncology

Classification	Agents	Indication	Side effects
Granulocyte colony-stimulating factor (G-CSF)	Filgrastim (Neupogen) Pegfilgrastim (Neulasta)	Neutropenia	Musculoskeletal pain Injection site reaction Nausea Headache Hypotension Abdominal/flank pain Splenomegaly
Granulocyte-macrophage colony-stimulating factor (GM-CSF)	Sargramostim (Leukine)	Neutropenia	Fever Asthenia Chills Headache Nausea Diarrhea Myalgias and bone pain Rash, pruritis Edema, dyspnea Tachycardia Hypotension
Erythropoietin	Darbepoetin (Aranesp) Epoetin alfa (Procrit)	Anemia	Hypertension Pain at injection site May require iron supplementation for adequate erythropoiesis
Megakaryocyte and platelet growth factor (interleukin-11)	Oprelvekin (Neumega)	Thrombocytopenia	Edema Dyspnea Palpitations Dilutional anemia Pleural effusion Severe asthenia

Data from Fang E: Epocrates RX Pro®, Version 7.50, San Mateo, Calif, 2006, Epocrates, Inc.

Delayed nausea and vomiting persists or develops 24 hours after treatment administration. Anticipatory nausea and vomiting is a conditioned response that occurs before chemotherapy administration, usually occurring because of inadequately controlled emesis associated with a previous treatment.[21]

The management of nausea and vomiting has been greatly improved by the advent of the 5-HT_3 receptor antagonists. There are several 5-HT_3 receptor antagonists now on the market, and no one of the antagonists has proven to be superior to the others.[24] According to the NCCN guidelines,[24] chemotherapeutic agents can be classified according to their antiemetic potential, and prophylactic antiemesis treatment should be instituted accordingly. Combinations of antiemetic agents are often employed; for example, dexamethasone and a 5-HT_3 antagonist are often used together. Classes of drugs used in antiemetic therapy and examples of these are listed in Table 19-9. Oncology nurses need to be proactive in ensuring that patients are taught how to prophylactically medicate themselves to prevent nausea and vomiting. Inadequate nutritional intake can result from nausea and vomiting and is further addressed in Chapter 33.

Mucositis and Esophagitis

Many chemotherapeutic agents can cause mucositis to some degree. Mucositis is generally dose related, being more common in higher doses. Up to 40% of patients receiving standard doses of chemotherapy will experience mucositis.[25] Younger patients are more likely to have mucositis, but they recover more quickly. Chemoradiotherapy to the head or neck can exacerbate mucositis.[26]

There is no single, effective treatment for the prevention or management of mucositis.[25] Good oral hygiene using swabs instead of a toothbrush

Table 19-9 Antiemetic Drug Classes and Examples

Class	Example
5-HT_3 Receptor Antagonist	Dolasetron (Anzemet), granisetron (Kytril), ondansetron (Zofran), palonosetron (Aloxi)
Steroids	Dexamethasone (Decadron)
Neurokinin I Receptor Antagonist	Aprepitant (Emend)
Antihistamines	Diphenhydramine (Benadryl)
Phenothiazines	Prochlorperazine (Compazine), promethazine (Phenergan)
Cannabinoids	Dronabinol (Marinol)
Benzodiazepines	Lorazepam (Ativan)

Data from National Comprehensive Cancer Network (NCCN) *Practice Guidelines for Antiemesis*, v.1., 2006.

and nonalcohol-containing mouthwashes are useful. Avoidance of irritates such as hot or cold foods, spicy foods, alcoholic or carbonated beverages, smoking, and oral tobacco use should be advised.[21] If oral candidiasis is present, it should be properly treated with an antifungal agent. For severe mucositis, local anesthetics and narcotics may be required for adequate pain control.

Esophagitis also may occur with chemotherapy because the mucosal lining of the esophagus is the same as the mouth.[21] This symptom is intensified when chemotherapy is given concurrently with radiation therapy. This inflammatory response is similar to mucositis and ultimately affects nutrition. At times, chemotherapy and/or radiation therapy is withheld until esophagitis and mucositis resolves. When administered with head and neck radiation, esophagitis and mucositis may become so severe that a feeding tube may be necessary. Assessment before therapy, therefore, is essential. Esophagitis is further addressed in Chapter 8.

Neurotoxicity

Many patients undergoing chemotherapy experience some form of neurotoxicity, at least temporarily.[21] Severe neurotoxicity may cause chemotherapy to be withheld or delayed or the dose reduced. Neurotoxicity secondary to chemotherapy often manifests as peripheral neuropathy, constipation, peripheral sensory losses, muscle weakness, cerebellar ataxia, impotence, postural hypotension, and/or loss of deep tendon reflexes.[21] Neurotoxicity may be progressive and dose dependent. It is usually, but not always, reversible.

It is vital to have a baseline neurologic assessment in patients receiving neurotoxic chemotherapeutic agents. This assessment should include sensory and motor function, gait, range of motion, cranial nerves, and deep tendon reflexes.[21] Patients should be assessed before each chemotherapy administration for neurotoxicity. Amifostine (Ethyol) is a chemoprotectant agent approved for the prevention of mucositis and renal toxicity (see section on hemorrhagic cystitis and renal toxicity below), but is being used in clinical trials to minimize the neurotoxic effects of certain chemotherapeutic agents such as cisplatin.[27]

Pulmonary Toxicity

A rare side effect of a few chemotherapeutic agents is pulmonary toxicity. This toxicity is usually irreversible and progressive.[21] Bleomycin (Blenoxane) is known to cause pulmonary toxicity in approximately 5% to 10% of patients who reach a cumulative dose of 400 units when given without radiation therapy. When given with radiation therapy, the pulmonary toxicity will be enhanced.[9] The oncology nurse must be acutely alert to the possibility of pulmonary toxicity. Early discontinuation or dose reduction of the offending drug may prevent further damage to the lung.

Dermatologic Reactions

Various skin reactions can occur with chemotherapy and may intensify when given with radiation therapy. Some chemotherapeutic agents may cause hyperpigmentation of the skin and nails or dark streaking over veins.[21] Rashes also can occur with certain chemotherapeutic agents. Urticaria and pruritis may accompany hypersensitivity reactions and should be treated appropriately by stopping the infusion and using emergent medications as necessary. Photosensitivity can occur with many chemotherapeutic agents. Oncology nurses must educate patients on the dangers of sun exposure and the protective measures, such as the proper use of sunscreens.

Alopecia is one of the most noticeable dermatologic reactions of chemotherapy and one of the most psychosocially distressing. Not every chemotherapeutic agent will cause total alopecia, although most will cause at least some thinning.[21] Alopecia is dose dependent, and patients receiving low dose, continuous infusions often have less loss. Hair loss includes not only scalp hair but also eyebrows, eyelashes, and body hair. Hair loss usually begins within 2 to 3 weeks after the first chemotherapy administration. Alopecia caused by chemotherapy is temporary, and hair begins to regrow within 4 to 6 weeks after completion of chemotherapy. Regrowth may be different in color, texture, and type.[21] Patient education about hair loss is vital for adequate coping.

Cardiotoxicity

Cardiotoxicity can occur acutely in about 10% of patients who receive chemotherapy.[21] Acute cardiotoxicity is transient and does not cause long-term effects. However, late cardiotoxicity requiring cessation of therapy occurs in less than 5% of patients receiving chemotherapy. Cardiotoxicity can occur weeks to months after administration of a cardiotoxic agent and has a 60% mortality rate, being poorly responsive to cardiac medications.[21] Most chemotherapeutic agents with significant cardiotoxic effects have a lifetime maximum dose. An example of this is doxorubicin (Adriamycin), which has a lifetime maximum dose of 550 mg/m^2. The lifetime maximum dose decreases if mediastinal radiation was given in the past. Other drugs with a lifetime maximum cumulative dose include epirubicin (Ellence) and daunorubicin (Daunomycin).[27] Careful documentation of cumulative doses is essential.

Dexrazoxane (Zinecard) is approved by the FDA for metastatic breast cancer patients with a doxorubicin (Adriamycin) dose of more than 300 mg/m^2 (cumulative).[27] This may enable patients to receive greater cumulative doses of doxorubicin with decreased risk of cardiotoxicity. Cardiac function should be evaluated periodically, and if cardiotoxicity is noted, the cardiotoxic agent should be discontinued. Long-term follow-up for cardiac dysfunction is recommended.

Hepatotoxicity

When parenchymal cells of the liver are damaged by chemotherapeutic agents, hepatotoxicity can occur. This toxicity is usually reversible, unless extensive fibrosis or necrosis occurs.[21] Liver function tests should be monitored closely throughout chemotherapy treatments. Enzymatic changes are often the first clinical sign of hepatotoxicity.[21]

Hemorrhagic Cystitis and Nephrotoxicity

Hemorrhagic cystitis can result from chemotherapeutic agents such as cyclophosphamide (Cytoxan) and ifosfamide (Ifex). Signs of hemorrhagic cystitis could be as little as microscopic hematuria to frank bleeding.[21] Often chemotherapy-induced cystitis is transient, occurring soon after chemotherapy administration and lasting only a short while. However, if hemorrhagic cystitis occurs, the chemotherapeutic agent must be discontinued.

Many chemotherapeutic agents are metabolized and excreted by the kidneys, although some may be excreted as metabolites or unchanged drug.[21] If a patient has preexisting renal disease, the chemotherapy dose may need to be lowered. If a patient begins to exhibit signs of nephrotoxicity, the offending agent may need to be discontinued or the dose reduced.

Mesna (Mesnex) is a uroprotectant and is given before ifosfamide and then twice in 4 hour intervals.[27] The dose is calculated as 60% of the total ifosfamide dose (Ifex), divided into three doses.[22] Amifostine (Ethyol) is used to reduce renal toxicity caused by cisplatin. The dose is 910 mg/m^2 given over 15 minutes, after antiemetics, with a liter of fluids, and 30 minutes before the cisplatin dose is administered.[27] Transient systolic hypotension can occur during the administration; therefore, blood pressure should be monitored every 5 minutes throughout the infusion and 5 minutes after the infusion. It is important to note that the dose and administration schedule is different when this drug is given for reduction of xerostomia.[28]

Patients should be instructed on hyperhydration and frequent voiding.[21] Ideally, urotoxic agents should be given early in the day to allow adequate hydration and clearing of the agent from the bladder without the interruption of sleep as a result of frequent voiding. Diuresis, aggressive intravenous hydration, or urinary alkalinization may be necessary. The oncology nurse must carefully monitor renal function tests before administering nephrotoxic agents. The patient's renal function also should be assessed throughout the treatment and periodically thereafter.

PRETREATMENT EVALUATION AND EDUCATION

Before treating any patient with chemotherapy, it is important to perform a pretreatment evaluation to determine the patient's ability to tolerate the prescribed treatment.[21] A thorough baseline physical assessment is essential in order to determine the effects of the prescribed treatment. For most chemotherapeutic agents, it is of utmost importance to check the ANC and the platelet count before chemotherapy administration. Chemotherapy is usually withheld if the ANC is less than 1000 to 1500/mm^3 and/or the platelet count is less than 100,000/dL. Other areas to assess before chemotherapy treatment are listed in Box 19-4.

Some chemotherapeutic agents require premedications to ensure better tolerability of the drug. Some of these may be given orally the night before and the morning of chemotherapy, such as dexamethasone (Decadron) before docetaxel (Taxotere) or dexamethasone (Decadron), cimetidine (Tagamet), and diphenhydramine (Benadryl) before paclitaxel (Taxol).[28] These medications are used to reduce the incidence of infusion reactions and side effects such as lower extremity edema. The chemotherapeutic agent should not be given if the patient has not taken his premedications. Certain antiemetics, such as aprepitant (Emend), are given orally before chemotherapy. Aprepitant (Emend) is given orally 1 hour before chemotherapy and then daily for 2 days.[27] Side effects from premedications should be assessed. For instance, dexamethasone (Decadron) may cause insomnia in some patients.[27]

Box 19-4 Pretreatment Evaluation

- Overall physical condition
- Ability to perform self-care
- Baseline vital signs
- Prechemotherapy labs
  - ANC
  - Platelet count
  - Hemoglobin and hematocrit
- Labs specific to chemotherapy agent
  - BUN and creatinine when giving cisplatin
- Comorbid conditions
  - Renal dysfunction
  - Diabetes
  - Hypertension
- Present physical symptoms
  - Nausea and vomiting
  - Diarrhea
- Venous integrity (if chemotherapy is to be given intravenously)
- Psychologic readiness for treatment
- Ability to understand posttreatment instructions (such as treatment for nausea and vomiting)
- Ability to obtain needed prescriptive and/or over-the-counter medications for adequate symptom management posttreatment
- Concomitant medications for potential drug interactions
- Tolerance of last chemotherapy treatment

Data from Camp-Sorrell D: Chemotherapy toxicities and management. In Yarbro C, Frogge M, Goodman M: *Cancer nursing principles and practice*, ed 6, Boston, 2005, Jones and Bartlett, pp 412-457.
ANC, Absolute neutrophil count; *BUN*, blood urea nitrogen.

In addition to a pretreatment evaluation, the patient must be taught about their treatment before the administration.[21] Verbal and written information should be provided. The education should be documented in the patient's record. It is important for the nurse to explain how the treatment will be administered and how the treatment will affect the cancer. The patient can be taught to recognize and control potential treatment side effects. The patient should have a list of side effects that need to be reported to the healthcare professional immediately, instead of waiting until the next healthcare encounter. Lastly, the patient should be told when to return for blood counts and the next treatment. Coordination with radiation therapy department must occur as well if combined modality treatment is given.

Combining modalities has the potential of increasing toxicity, making symptom management more challenging, and requiring greater communication between radiation and medical oncology personnel. Being informed of all the planned components of treatment will help manage patients through therapy. One communication tool developed by Dr. Marilyn Haas, a nurse practitioner, and Jane Hudson, a medical oncology research nurse, entitled Patient Chemoradiation Therapy Communication Tool (CTCT), is a tool that is designed to inform the oncology team about the entire oncology treatment plan for individual patients (Figure 19-1) (Personal communication with Dr. Haas, 3/17/2006). The CTCT has information regarding diagnosis and staging, chemotherapy regimens, premedications planned for radiation and/or chemotherapy, initial symptom management medications, expected laboratory

Patient's Name : ______ Date of Birth: ______

Medical Oncology Dr./Medical Record #: ______ Radiation Oncology Dr./ Medical Record #: ______
Medical Oncology Fax #: ______ RT Fax #: ______
Chemo RN Contact: ______ RT RN Contact: ______

Diagnosis (Pathology/Location): ______ TNM/Staging: ______

Purpose of Combined Modality (Circle): Definitive Neoadjuvant Adjuvant Control Palliative

Pretreatment Data : Weight Loss Past 6 Months: Yes/ No Current Weight/Meter Squared: ______ Height (inches): ______
Type/Location IV Access: ______ Feeding Tube (Circle): PEG, J-PEG None Home Health Agency: ______
Allergies: ______ Labs: ______ Frequency ______ Drawn where? ______
Meds (all): ______

Present ECOG Scale: ______
0=Fully active, able to carry on all pre-disease performance
1=Restricted in physically strenuous activity but ambulatory
2=Ambulatory, capable of all selfcare but unable to carry out work
3=Capable of only limited selfcare,confined to bed/chair>50%
4=completely disabled, no selfcare, totally confined to bed/chair

Present Pain Level ______
Select Range 0= No pain to 10= Severe pain

Present Fatigue Level: ______
ONS Scale 1= No fatigue
2= Mild fatigue
3=Moderate fatigue
4=Extreme fatigue
5= Worst fatigue

Chemotherapy Orders:
Drug Names: ______
Routes (Circle): IV / PO
Dosing (Circle): Sequencing/ Daily/ Weekly / Continuous Infusion
Administration Day(s)/# cycles: ______
Planned Dates: ______
PreMeds (names): ______

Radiation Oncology Orders:
Prescription (cGy/fx): ______
Treatment Fields/Area: ______
Initiation & Anticipated Completion Dates: ______
PreMeds (names) ______

Mark Beside Any Anticipated Major Side Effects Chemoradiation: R= Radiation C= Chemotherapy

General		**Brain**	**Head/Neck**	**Respiratory**	**GI**	**GU**	**Other**
Alopecia	Myalgia	Headache	Dysphagia	Cough	Constipation	Cystitis	Financial Issues
Fatigue	Neuropathy		Esophagitis	Dypsnea	Diarrhea	Nocturia	Medicare D
Myelosuppression			Mucositis		Dyspepsia	Proctitis	Med. Assistance
Pain			Pharyngitis		Nausea		Risk for injury: ______
Radiodermatitis			Xerostomia		Vomiting		______
Weight Loss							Psychosocial Issues

Completing Form: Chemotherapy Nurse: ______ Radiation Therapy Nurse: ______

Figure 19-1 Combined Modality Communication Tool—Initial Treatment Plan.

requirements, total radiation doses (Gys), number of radiation treatments, daily radiation dose, and radiation treatment fields/site. Nurses who know the entire treatment plan via CTCT can provide a higher level of care, ultimately having an impact on patient outcomes.

BIOTHERAPY

Biotherapy is defined as the use of agents derived from biologic sources or agents that affect biologic responses.[29] As a cancer cell differentiates, it produces proteins called *antigens*. The host's immune system recognizes these as foreign and is then activated to destroy the foreign cell. Biotherapy manipulates the host immune system in some way to enhance cancer cell kill. Proposed mechanisms of action[9] include the following:

- Enhancing the host's own immune system
- Modifying the normal cells in the area of the tumor
- Increasing the vulnerability of cancer cells to the host's own immune system
- Preventing formation of cancer cells by altering the way normal cells transform into malignant cells
- Preventing metastasis of cancer cells
- Enhancing the repair of normal cells damaged by treatments
- Changing cancer cells in a way that makes them behave like normal cells

There are several different categories of biotherapy.[29] These are listed in Table 19-10, along with the therapeutic action and major side effects of each. Some biologicals are used for cure, either as a primary or adjuvant treatment. Biologicals can have at least six different effects; these include augmentation of immune system; modulation of the immune system; restoration of the immune system; differentiation or maturation of cells; interference with tumor-cell metastasis or transformation; or increase the ability of the host to tolerate side effects of cytotoxic treatment.[29]

Biologic agents of particular interest to radiation oncology are hematopoietic growth factors and the monoclonal antibodies. Hematopoietic growth factors are glycoproteins that activate the production of bone marrow cells. These growth factors are used both prophylactically and therapeutically by permitting the continuation of the chemotherapeutic maintenance dose in situations of otherwise dose-limiting cytopenias.[30] The major hematopoietic growth factors used in oncology, discussed earlier in this chapter, are listed in Table 19-8.

Monoclonal antibodies (MAB) are antibodies produced from a single clone of cells.[31] Producing MABs requires first immunizing an animal, usually a mouse. The mouse is injected with a specific antigen—a foreign substance that the animal's immune system can recognize and respond to by producing antibodies. After the mouse's immune system develops antibodies against the antigen, antibody-producing white blood cells (B-cells) are removed from the mouse's spleen. These antibody-secreting cells are then fused with myeloma cells, a rapidly multiplying white blood cell cancer, to make them immortal—that is, they will grow and divide indefinitely. This fusion of cells called a *hybridoma* secretes MABs. The main difficulty of MABs is that mouse antibodies are "seen" by the human immune system as foreign, and the human patient mounts an immune response against them, producing HAMA ("human anti-mouse antibodies"). These not only cause the therapeutic antibodies to be quickly eliminated from the host but also form immune complexes that cause damage to the kidneys.[31]

Side effects of MABs are generally infusion related and may include fever, chills, rigors, urticaria, flushing, and headache. Cytopenias can occur as well as nausea, rash, diarrhea, and anaphylaxis.[32] During intravenous administration of biotherapy, the patient should be monitored for infusion-related side effects.

COMBINED MODALITY THERAPY

Combined modality is chemotherapy (or biotherapy) administered before (neoadjuvant), after (adjuvant), or concurrently with surgery or radiation therapy.[9] Chemotherapy is used as a radiosensitizer in neoadjuvant, adjuvant, or concurrent treatment to enhance the effects of radiation therapy. One of the primary goals of using radiosensitizers is to prevent radiation resistance and to enhance local and regional control of the cancer by eliminating radiation-resistant cancer cells and increasing the oxygen supply to the tumor as it shrinks in response to the chemotherapy.[11] Box 19-5 lists the most common chemotherapy agents used as radiosensitizers. The use of radiosensitizers in combined modality treatment, however, will increase certain toxicities.

Table 19-10 Biotherapeutic Agents

Agent	MOA	Indications	Side effects
Interferons	Inhibit viral replication, antiproliferative effects on tumor cells, modulation of host immune response	Hairy cell leukemia, chronic hepatitis, CML, AIDS-related Kaposi's sarcoma	Flu-like symptoms: fever, chills, malaise, headache, anorexia, fatigue; depression, nausea, diarrhea, CNS changes, leukopenia, thrombocytopenia
Interleukins	Promotes proliferation, differentiation, and recruitment of T and B cell, NK cell, LAK cells; enhances tumor-killing capacity	Renal cell cancer, metastatic melanoma	Fever, chills, rigors, malaise, headache, myalgia, arthralgia, tachycardia, hypotension, capillary leak syndrome, dyspnea, nausea, diarrhea, dizziness, anemia, thrombocytopenia, leukopenia
Monoclonal antibodies	Dependent upon agent; bind to specific targeted surface antigen of tumor cell, thus inhibiting or initiating some action that causes tumor cell destruction	Alemtuzumab (Campath): B-cell CLL; bevacizumab (Avastin) and cetuximab (Erbitux): metastatic colorectal; denileukin (Ontak): T-cell lymphoma; gemtuzumab (Mylotarg): AML; ibritumomab (Zevalin), rituximab (Rituxan), and tositumomab (Bexxar): B-cell lymphoma;trastuzumab (Herceptin): breast cancer	Chills, fever, hypersensitivity reactions, headache, rash, infusion related reaction, neutropenia, anemia, thrombocytopenia, and other specific side effects related to specific agent
Hematopoietic growth factors	Promotes proliferation and differentiation of a particular stem cell line	Treatment or prevention of: neutropenia, thrombocytopenia, or anemia	Bone pain, flu-like symptoms, flushing, hypertension
Tyrosine kinase inhibitors	Inhibits the intracellular phosphorylation of tyrosine kinases associated with EGFR	Gefitinib (Iressa): CML Erlotinib (Tarceva): NSCLC	Rash, diarrhea, conjunctivitis, nausea, headache, edema, thrombocytopenia, neutropenia, other specific side effects of each agent

Data from Rieger P: *Biotherapy: a comprehensive overview*, ed 2, Sudbury, Mass, 2001, Jones and Bartlett.
MOA, Mechanism of action; *CML*, chronic myelogenous leukemia; *AIDS*, acquired immune deficiency syndrome; *CNS*, central nervous system; *NK*, natural killer; *LAK*, lymphokine-activated killer; *CLL*, chronic lymphocytic leukemia; *AML*, acute myelogenous leukemia; *EGFR*, epidermal growth factor receptors.

Although timing of each modality is important, the goals of chemotherapy differ from that of surgery or radiation alone. Radiation and surgery goals are to control and sterilized the tumor, whereas chemotherapy goals are to eradicate any distant micrometastases. When combining chemotherapy and radiation therapy (chemoradiotherapy), chemotherapy also serves as a powerful radiosensitizer, assisting in the reduction of locoregional disease.[4,33] Various approaches have been used including sequential chemotherapy followed by radiation, concurrent chemoradiotherapy, induction chemotherapy followed by concurrent chemoradiotherapy, and concurrent chemoradiotherapy followed by consolidation chemotherapy. Each approach has advantages and disadvantages.

Box 19-5 Commonly Used Radiosensitizing Agents

- Bleomycin (Blenoxane)
- Carboplatin (Paraplatin)
- Cisplatin (Platinol AQ)
- Dactinomycin (Actinomycin D)
- Docetaxel (Taxotere)
- Doxorubicin (Adriamycin)
- Etoposide (VePesid)
- Fluorouracil (Adrucil)
- Gemcitabine (Gemzar)
- Ifosfamide (Ifex)
- Methotrexate (Folex)
- Mitomycin-C (Mutamycin)
- Paclitaxel (Taxol)
- Vinblastine (Velban)
- Vinorelbine (Navelbine)

Data from Gosselin-Acomb T: Principles of radiation therapy. In Yarbro C, Frogge M, Goodman M, editors: *Cancer nursing principles and practice*, ed 6, Boston, 2005, Jones and Bartlett.

Sequential approaches can reduce distant failure rates whereas concurrent chemoradiotherapy can reduce local failure rates.[4,33]

Chemoradiotherapy combines the unique cytotoxic features of each modality to enhance cancer cell kill. However, chemoradiotherapy also will exacerbate many toxicities of both radiation and chemotherapy.[12] In general, the most common exacerbated toxicities occur in the gastrointestinal tract, skin, mucosa, and the bone marrow. The oncology nurse should understand the most common toxicities of the chemotherapy administered and be observant for overlapping toxicities expected from radiation therapy. Chemoradiotherapy also may increase late toxicity potential such as fibrosis of the lung or pneumonitis.

Because of its demonstrated effectiveness and despite the increase in toxicities, chemoradiotherapy is used in the treatment of many different cancers, including head and neck, gastric, rectal, anal, pancreatic, and others.[11,34] The next section describes the use of chemoradiotherapy in several of these cancers.

Head and Neck Carcinomas

Multimodality Treatment

According to the NCCN guidelines,[35] chemotherapy may be given in newly diagnosed, unresectable disease (M0) or T4b, any N or unresectable node-positive disease, or for recurrent disease. With an adequate performance status, concurrent chemotherapy that is platinum-based is recommended. For poorer performance status, induction chemotherapy, followed by radiation may be employed. Either cisplatin (Platinol AQ) or carboplatin (Paraplatin) may be used, because these agents have not been directly compared when combined with radiation therapy in any randomized trials. When given as induction therapy, three cycles of cisplatin (Platinol AQ) 100 mg/m^2 on day 1 and 5-fluorouracil (5-FU) (Adrucil) 1000mg/m^2 every 24 hours by continuous intravenous infusion for 120 hours is recommended.[35]

Cisplatin (Platinol AQ) is a heavy metal that acts like an alkylating agent. It inhibits DNA synthesis, preventing cell replication, and is considered cell-cycle phase nonspecific.[36] For radiosensitizing effect, it is usually administered 1 to 3 times per week at doses of 15 to 50 mg/m^2 for a total weekly dose of 50 mg/m^2 with concomitant radiation therapy. The nadir for cisplatin (Platinol AQ) is 2 to 3 weeks. Twenty to seventy-four percent is excreted in the urine within 24 hours, therefore, caution should be used if it is given to patients with renal dysfunction. Cisplatin (Platinol AQ) accumulates in the kidneys, causing necrosis of proximal and distal renal tubules. Damage to the renal tubules can prevent the reabsorption of magnesium, calcium, and potassium. Renal damage can be prevented by vigorously hydrating the patient before and after administration of this drug and by maintaining the urine output to at least 100 to 150 mL/hour.[36] Mannitol (Osmitrol) or furosemide (Lasix) diuresis may be necessary.

5-FU (Adrucil) is classified as a pyrimidine antimetabolite. It inhibits the formation of thymidine synthetase, an enzyme that is necessary for the synthesis of DNA. 5-FU (Adrucil) also incorporates into RNA, causing abnormal synthesis.[36] When given to those with head and neck cancers, this drug is usually dosed at 1000 mg/m^2 per day for 4 to 5 days as a continuous infusion.[36] Doses may need to be reduced in patients with liver, renal, or bone marrow dysfunction, or in those with malnutrition. The nadir for 5-FU (Adrucil) is 10 to 14 days after the drug dose.

Combinations of platinum-based agents with 5-FU (Adrucil) or taxanes may be used. However, combination therapy regimens are generally more toxic and have not been directly compared to single-agent regimens.[35] Platinum-based combination therapy has been shown to produce higher response rates, but no effect on overall survival has been demonstrated. The NCCN guidelines[35] recommend platinum-based chemotherapy combined with 5-FU (Adrucil) be given for the primary treatment of the nasopharynx. Combination therapy may be given in recurrent disease of the head and neck as well. Other combinations of chemotherapeutic agents with concomitant radiation are being evaluated in clinical trials. Table 19-11 shows the most common chemotherapeutic agents used in chemoradiotherapy in head and neck cancers and their side effects. Some combinations being studied in clinical trials include 5-FU (Adrucil) and mitomycin-C (Mutamycin);[37] gemcitabine (Gemzar) and vinorelbine (Navelbine);[38] gemcitabine (Gemzar), paclitaxel (Taxol) and 5-FU (Adrucil);[39] 5-FU (Adrucil), hydroxyurea (Hydrea) with either cisplatin (Platinol AQ) or paclitaxel (Taxol);[40] and induction chemotherapy with carboplatin (Paraplatin) and paclitaxel (Taxol) followed by concomitant TFHX paclitaxel (Taxol), infusional 5-FU (Adrucil), and hydroxyurea (Hydrea).[41]

The taxanes used in the treatment of head and neck cancers include paclitaxel (Taxol) and docetaxel (Taxotere).[35] They are considered mitotic inhibitors because they promote early microtubule assembly and prevent polymerization, resulting in cell death. The taxanes are considered phase specific agents, so frequent dosing is necessary.[42] They are mainly metabolized by the liver using the P-450 enzyme system. Because of the high risk of hypersensitivity reactions (around 10% of patients), premedications of dexamethasone (Decadron), cimetidine (Tagamet), and diphenhydramine (Benedryl) must be given with paclitaxel (Taxol) and dexamethasone (Decadron) with docetaxel (Taxotere). When given in combination with cisplatin (Platinol AQ) or carboplatin (Paraplatin), there is increased cytotoxic activity when paclitaxel (Taxol) is given first. When given as a radiosensitizer, weekly doses of 80 to 100 mg/m^2 are usually given as a 1-hour infusion. The nadir is 7 to 10 days after the drug administration of both drugs.[36]

Single chemotherapeutic agents that may be used to treat recurrent head and neck cancers include cisplatin (Platinol AQ), carboplatin (Paraplatin), paclitaxel (Taxol), docetaxel (Taxotere), 5-FU (Adrucil), methotrexate (generic only), ifosfamide (Ifex), bleomycin (Blenoxane), and gemcitabine (Gemzar).[35] Each agent has its own particular side effects, and many of these side effects are exacerbated by concomitant radiation therapy.

Future of Chemoradiotherapy in Head and Neck Carcinoma

Cetuximab (Erbitux), a human mouse chimeric monoclonal antibody is the first MAB to be used in the treatment of head and neck cancer. Cetuximab is approved for use in combination with radiation therapy for locally or regionally advanced squamous cell carcinoma of the head and neck or as a single agent in recurrent or metastatic disease in those who have previously failed platinum therapy.[43] Cetuximab has been shown to radiosensitize squamous cell carcinoma of the head and neck, by decreasing the cells' ability to recover from radiation by arresting the cells in the

Table 19-11 Agents Used in Chemoradiotherapy in Head and Neck Cancers

Agent	Nadir*	Side effects exacerbated by RT	Premeds
Cisplatin (Platinol AQ)	14–21 days	Mucositis, dysphagia, aspiration, poor nutrition, myelosuppression, ototoxicity	No
Carboplatin (Paraplatin)	18–28 days (thrombocytopenia)	Mucositis, dysphagia, aspiration, poor nutrition, myelosuppression	No
Docetaxel (Taxotere)	7–10 days	Myelosuppression, neurotoxicity, mucositis, dysphagia, poor nutrition	Yes
5-FU (Adrucil)	10–14 days	Mucositis, dysphagia, aspiration, poor nutrition	No
Paclitaxel (Taxol)	7–10 days	Myelosuppression, neurotoxicity, mucositis, dysphagia, poor nutrition,	Yes

Data from Carr E: Head and neck malignancies. In Yarbro C, Frogge M, Goodman M: *Cancer nursing principles and practice*, ed 6, Boston, 2005, Jones and Bartlett, pp 1294-1329.
*Refers to neutrophil count unless otherwise specified.
5-FU, 5-fluorouracil.

G1 phase of the cell cycle.[44] Many human cancers, including head and neck carcinoma, overexpress epidermal growth factor receptors (EGFR). Abnormal signaling of EGFR promotes deregulated cell proliferation and survival, promotes angiogenesis and metastases.

There are on-going trials that are examining the role of other biologic modifiers in the treatment of head and neck cancers. Gefitinib (Iressa) and erlotinib (Tarceva), tyrosine kinase–specific inhibitors, work in a similar manner as cetuximab and appear to have synergistic effects when combined with chemotherapeutic agents and/or radiation therapy.[44] Further research into this type of therapy will hopefully lead to increases in survival and better quality of life.

Gastric Carcinoma

Multimodality Treatment

Surgical resection alone of gastric carcinoma cures less than 40% of patients.[45] Single-modality treatment of gastric cancers with radiation therapy provides little palliation and no improvement in survival.[46,47] Chemotherapy as a single agent can provide palliation effects in gastric cancer. In general, as a single agent, only 5-FU (Adrucil), mitomycin (Mutamycin), etoposide (Etopophos), and cisplatin (Platinol AQ) are active in advanced gastric cancer. However, when radiation is given concurrently with 5-FU (Adrucil), survival benefits are seen. A small number of patients can be cured with combined modality treatment.[47] Common chemotherapeutic agents used in chemoradiotherapy in gastrointestinal and pancreatic cancers are listed in Table 19-12.

When combination chemotherapy is given in advanced gastric cancer, there is better quality of life and higher response rates over single agents,[46] and improvements in overall survival compared to best supportive care.[47] Response rates for combination chemotherapy fall in the 20% to 40% range and median survival is between 6 and 12 months.[46] FAM (5-FU [Adrucil], doxorubicin [Adriamycin], and mitomycin [Mutamycin]) was considered the standard of care in the 1980's for patients with advanced gastric cancer.[3,46]

Curatively resected patients (negative margins) and those with no metastatic disease are also candidates for adjunctive chemoradiation with a 5-FU–based regimen.[47,48] The INT0116 study completed in the United States strongly supported the use of adjuvant chemoradiotherapy.[45] This updated trial confirmed benefit and showed that chemoradiotherapy does not produce significant long-term toxicity.[45] Compared with surgery alone, adjuvant chemoradiotherapy increases overall survival by 9%. Relapse-free survival increases from 31% to 48%. At 5 years, overall survival is increased by 11.6%.[48] Other treatment options include chemotherapy that is 5-FU–based (Adrucil), cisplatin- (Platinol AQ)- or oxaliplatin (Eloxatin)-based agents, taxane-based agents, or irinotecan (Camptosar)-based.

Standard of care for medically fit patients with unresectable, locoregional disease is combination therapy with concurrent radiation and 5-FU–based chemotherapy.[47] For medically unfit patients, the above may be given or salvage chemotherapy may be given with 5-FU (Adrucil)-based agents, cisplatin- (Platinol AQ)- or oxaliplatin (Eloxain)-based agents,

Table 19-12 Agents Used in Chemoradiotherapy in GI and Pancreatic Cancers

Agent	Nadir*	Side effects exacerbated by RT	Premeds
Cisplatin (Platinol AQ)	14–21 days	Mucositis, dysphagia, aspiration, poor nutrition, myelosuppression, ototoxicity	No
5-FU (Adrucil)	10–14 days	Mucositis, dysphagia, aspiration, poor nutrition	No
Gemcitabine (Gemzar)	10–14 days	Diarrhea, nausea, vomiting, mucositis, myelosuppression, rash	No
Mitomycin-C (Mutamycin)	28–35 days	Myelosuppression, pulmonary fibrosis, nausea and vomiting	No

Data from Wilkes G: Colon, rectal, and anal cancers. In Yarbro C, Frogge M, Goodman M: *Cancer nursing principles and practice*, ed 6, Boston, 2005, Jones and Bartlett, pp 1155–1214, and Coleman J: Pancreatic cancer. In Yarbro C, Frogge M, Goodman M: *Cancer nursing principles and practice*, ed 6, Boston, 2005, Jones and Bartlett, pp 1523-1551.

* Refers to neutrophil count unless otherwise specified.

GI, Gastrointestinal; *RT*, radiation therapy; *5-FU*, 5-fluorouracil.

taxane-based agents, or irinotecan (Camptosar)-based agents.[47]

Future of Chemoradiotherapy in Gastric Carcinoma

New drugs and new combinations of chemotherapeutic agents are continually being assessed for the treatment of gastrointestinal cancers. Several oral chemotherapy agents are demonstrating promise. These include capecitabine (Xeloda) for rectal cancer treatment multimodality combinations[49] and capecitabine (Xeloda) and oxaliplatin (Eloxatin) in gastric cancers.[47] Because of the survival benefits seen with combined modality treatment, the newer radiosensitizing agents are being examined in more clinical trials.[47]

In gastric cancer, preoperative induction chemotherapy followed by chemoradiotherapy is showing great promise in durable survival times.[47] This area is continuing to be studied in clinical trials. Other areas of ongoing study in gastric carcinoma include neoadjuvant chemotherapy, neoadjuvant radiation, or immunotherapy either alone or in combination.[48] Biologic-based therapies also may prove beneficial as more is learned about the molecular basis of gastric cancer.[46]

Rectal Carcinoma

Multimodality Treatment

Radiation therapy was added to the adjunctive treatment of rectal cancer because of the large numbers of locoregional failure after curative surgery.[49] The efficacy of surgery alone (and survival) depends greatly on the degree of bowel wall invasion, lymph node involvement, and the margins of resection. Locoregional failure also can greatly affect quality of life. Because of its effectiveness in decreasing locoregional failure, chemoradiotherapy is now the standard of care for rectal cancer.[50,51] The timing of chemoradiotherapy in rectal carcinoma varies greatly between the United States and Europe.[49] Postoperative adjuvant chemoradiation is used in the United States and preoperative radiation therapy and chemoradiotherapy is preferred in Europe. Ongoing studies continue to evaluate the efficacy of preoperative chemoradiotherapy versus postoperative chemoradiotherapy with various chemotherapy combinations and the differences in toxicity and quality of life in rectal cancers.[50]

In rectal carcinoma, patients with pathologic lymph node–negative T3 or T4 lesions or any lymph node–positive cancer should receive postoperative adjuvant chemotherapy with 5-FU (Adrucil) (or 5-FU/leucovorin [Wellcovorin]), followed by concurrent 5-FU (Adrucil) and radiation therapy, then 5-FU (Adrucil) (or 5-FU/leucovorin [Wellcovorin]).[51] Patients with T3 or T4 disease should be considered for preoperative multimodality treatment to shrink the tumor burden and to preserve sphincter function.[51] Patients who receive preoperative radiation should receive postoperative adjuvant 5-FU (Adrucil) with or without leucovorin or infusional 5-FU (Adrucil), leucovorin (Wellcovorin), and oxaliplatin (Eloxatin).[51] If radical resection is not possible, adjuvant chemoradiotherapy is indicated after local excision to decrease local recurrence rates. Table 19-12 shows the most common chemotherapeutic agents used concurrently with radiation in gastrointestinal cancers. Patients with stage IV lesions may be candidates for palliative resection or radiation followed by systemic therapy. Recurrent disease is treated with single agents or combination therapy. Chemotherapeutic agents include 5-FU (Adrucil), irinotecan (Camptosar), bevacizumab (Avastin), cetuximab (Erbitux), and capecitabine (Xeloda).[51] First-line treatment combinations in metastatic disease have significantly prolonged survival in patients with metastatic colorectal cancer.[52] Survival rates in metastatic colorectal cancer are nearly double those of 5 years ago using combination therapy.

Anal Carcinoma

Multimodality Treatment

In the past, advanced anal cancer was routinely treated with abdominoperineal resection, but the 5-year survival was only 40% to 75% and patients were left with a permanent colostomy.[53] Chemoradiotherapy with 5-FU (Adrucil) and mitomycin (Mutamycin) is now the standard of care, replacing radical surgery, in the treatment of epidermoid and squamous cell carcinoma of the anal canal.[54,55] Chemoradiotherapy allows anal continence to be maintained. Abdominoperineal resection is reserved for recurrent or residual disease after primary chemoradiotherapy.[56] Anal cancer is one of the few cancers of the gastrointestinal tract that could possibly be cured without definitive surgery.[57]

Future of Chemoradiotherapy in Rectal and Anal Carcinoma

In rectal cancers, the roles of preoperative versus postoperative therapy continues to be examined.[58]

The optimal combination of chemoradiotherapy has not yet been determined in rectal or anal cancers.[58,59] In anal cancers, there are expectations of increasing incidence because of human papillomavirus (HPV) and human immunodeficiency virus (HIV) infection.[56] Clinical trials are also looking at the substitution of cisplatin (Platinol AQ) for mitomycin (Mutamycin).[57,60]

Pancreatic Carcinoma

Multimodality Treatment

Surgery is the only potentially curative measure for pancreatic cancer. However, patients with visceral, distant nodal, peritoneal, and pleural metastatic pancreatic cancer do not benefit from resection.[61] But even with the optimal resection, the median survival rate is 15 to 19 months and the 5-year survival rate is about 20%. Pancreatic cancer is prone to metastasize and to be locally resistant,[62] therefore, multimodality therapy is necessary.

Chemoradiotherapy is one of the standard treatment options, especially in locally advanced pancreatic cancer, and has been since the Gastrointestinal Tumor Study Group reported in 1985 that the median survival of patients who are treated with pancreaticoduodenectomy could be almost doubled by postoperative chemoradiotherapy.[63] The NCCN guidelines[61] recommend that postoperative radiation therapy should be given with concurrent 5-FU (Adrucil) regardless of the margin or nodal status. After chemoradiotherapy, additional chemotherapy with a 5-FU–based regimen or gemcitabine (Gemzar) is recommended. Gemcitabine (Gemzar) may be considered an alternative to 5-FU (Adrucil) –based chemoradiation for those with locally advanced, unresectable disease.[61] Some studies have reported that preoperative chemoradiotherapy is beneficial in some patients deemed inoperable in converting them to operable candidates,[61] but a randomized trial is needed to confirm these results.

In patients with advanced disease, chemotherapy is given for palliative effects.[61] For patients with locally advanced or metastatic disease, gemcitabine (Gemzar) as a single agent provides clinical benefit and slight survival advantage over treatment with 5-FU (Adrucil)[64] and thus is considered standard therapy for patients with metastatic disease.[61] When gemcitabine (Gemzar) is combined with other chemotherapeutic agents such as cisplatin (Platinol AQ), oxaliplatin (Eloxatin), and irinotecan (Eribitux) in patients with advanced pancreatic cancer, response rates are better and time to progression is longer, but no clear survival advantage has been shown.[61] Gemcitabine (Gemzar) may offer benefits in the second-line setting, as may capecitabine (Xeloda) or infusional 5-FU (Adrucil). Table 19-12 lists the most commonly used agents in chemoradiotherapy for gastrointestinal and pancreatic cancers. Besides these drugs, other chemotherapeutic agents have been found to act against these carcinomas, including paclitaxel (Taxol), docetaxel (Taxotere), irinotecan (Camptosar), oxaliplatin (Eloxatin), and bevacizumab (Avastin).[61] These may be used as single agents or in combinations. Cisplatin (Platinol AQ), 5-FU (Adrucil), and the taxanes were reviewed in the above head and neck section of this chapter, and drugs used in the treatment of gastrointestinal and pancreatic cancers are reviewed below.

Chemotherapeutic Agents Used in Gastrointestinal and Pancreatic Carcinomas

Mitomycin (Mutamycin) is often employed in the treatment of anal cancer[54] and is given with 5-FU (Adrucil). Mitomycin (Mutamycin) is an antitumor antibiotic that by alkylation and cross-linking interferes with the structure and function of DNA.[36] Major toxicities include myelosuppression that can be dose-limiting, cumulative and serious. The nadir is delayed at about 4 to 6 weeks, and recovery may be prolonged over many weeks. Nausea and vomiting is usually mild to moderate and dose dependent. Mucositis can occur, usually within the first week of treatment. Care should be taken with administration because of the potent vesicant properties of mitomycin (Mutamycin).[28] A vesicant drug can cause blistering, pain, erythema, and necrosis of the skin if the drug leaks out of the vein into the surrounding tissue (extravasation). Skin grafting may be needed in severe cases of extravasation. Interstitial pneumonitis is a rare event, but can occur with total cumulative doses of more than 60 mg.

Oxaliplatin (Eloxatin) is a drug similar to alkylating agents and is considered a platinum analog.[36] It inhibits DNA replication and transcription.[28] Oxaliplatin (Eloxatin) is cell-cycle nonspecific. Side effects include neurotoxicity, nausea and vomiting, diarrhea, and myelosuppression.[36] Paresthesias and cold-induced dysesthesias are common after the infusion of oxaliplatin and usually last less than

7 days. Chronic neuropathies can occur and may last for months. Mucositis is exacerbated when oxaliplatin is given in combination with 5-FU (Adrucil).[9] Oxaliplatin (Eloxatin) is given for colorectal cancers both adjuvantly and in treatment of recurrent or metastatic disease[36] in combination with 5-FU (Adrucil) and leucovorin (Wellcovorin).

Leucovorin (Wellcovorin) is not a chemotherapeutic agent in the sense that it is cytotoxic in its own right. This drug was originally developed as an antidote for antifolate therapy.[65] It is most commonly used to modulate the cytotoxicity of 5-FU (Adrucil). In the presence of increased folate pools, the active form of 5-FU (Adrucil) binds more tightly to the target enzyme. Side effects of leucovorin (Wellcovorin) are minimal and rarely could include nausea and vomiting and urticaria.[27]

Irinotecan (Camptosar) is a derivative of camptothecin, a topoisomerase I inhibitor. It is considered cell-cycle nonspecific. It causes protein-linked DNA single-strand breaks and blocks DNA and RNA synthesis in dividing cells, preventing cells from entering mitosis.[36] The most common side effects include diarrhea (both early and late), nausea and vomiting, myelosuppression, fever, and asthenia.[36] Early diarrhea is a syndrome that consists of diarrhea, diaphoresis, and abdominal cramping during the infusion or within the first 24 hours. Early diarrhea is best treated with atropine (0.25–1 mg) intravenously. Late diarrhea (24+ hours postadministration) can lead to severe dehydration if not managed carefully. Loperamide (Imodium) 4 mg should be taken immediately after the first loose stool and 2 mg every 2 hours around the clock until patient has been diarrhea free for 12 hours. Nighttime dosing can be extended to 4 mg every 4 hours.[36] The nadir occurs within 6 to 9 days. Anemia is common and thrombocytopenia is uncommon. Irinotecan (Camptosar) is given in treatment for colorectal cancer in combination with 5-FU (Adrucil) and leucovorin (Wellcovorin).[65]

Bevacizumab (Avastin) is a monoclonal antibody against VEGF.[27] It prevents the formation of new blood vessels for the developing malignancy. It is indicated for the first-line treatment of advanced colorectal cancers in combination with a 5-FU– (Adrucil) based regimen.[65] Common side effects include abdominal pain, asthenia, headache, hypertension, nausea, diarrhea, anorexia, stomatitis, constipation, epistaxis, dyspnea, and exfoliative dermatitis. In rare cases, hemorrhage and gastrointestinal perforation have been reported. Treatment with Bevacizumab should be delayed for at least 21 days before or from surgery.[65]

Gemcitabine (Gemzar) is considered an antimetabolite. It acts by inhibiting reductase and competes with deoxycytidine triphosphate for incorporation into DNA.[36] It is generally given over 30 minutes because prolongation of infusion time beyond 60 minutes can increase the toxicities. A major toxicity is myelosuppression that is dose related and common. The nadir occurs by day 14, and recovers by day 21. Nausea and vomiting is mild to moderate. Diarrhea and mucositis also can occur. A flu-like syndrome occurs in about 20% of patients. When combined with cisplatin (Platinol AQ), gemcitabine (Gemzar) enhances the cytotoxicity of cisplatin (Platinol AQ).[36] Gemcitabine (Gemzar) is also a potent radiosensitizer.

Non–Small Cell Lung Carcinoma

Multimodality Treatment

Several chemotherapy agents have proven active in non–small cell lung carcinoma (NSCLC). These include cisplatin (Platinol AQ), carboplatin (Paraplatin), docetaxel (Taxotere), gemcitabine (Gemzar), irinotecan (Camptosar), paclitaxel (Taxol), and vinorelbine (Navelbine). Aggregate data continue to show that in advanced NSCLC, both platinum-based chemotherapy and certain single agents improve survival over best supportive care.[33] Because of this, it is important to identify which patients might not benefit from chemotherapy. Performance status appears to be the best predictor of who will benefit from therapy. After this assessment, the decision becomes which type of therapeutic approach should be taken. In metastatic disease, the goal of therapy is to prolong life. However, increased survival must be balanced by quality of life. Platinum-based regimens consistently show higher response rates and slightly higher median response rates over single-agent regimens, although at the expense of increased toxicity.[33] Many practitioners routinely use a platinum agent and paclitaxel (Taxol) for first-line therapy in advanced NSCLC.[33]

Many randomized clinical trials and meta-analyses have examined the role of chemotherapy versus best supportive care in patients with advanced NSCLC. Overall, these support the role of chemotherapy in advanced NSCLC by suggesting that there is almost doubling of the 1-year survival rate in patients who receive chemotherapy.[33] Both combination and single-agent therapy showed survival benefit. Most platinum-based combination regimens had higher response rates over that of single-agent therapies. Most studies have shown that stage IV patients receiving platinum-based chemotherapy have a survival rate at 5 years of 4% to 5%[66] and a palliative benefit.[67] However, single-agent regimens often offer survival benefit with better quality of life, even in patients with a performance status of common toxicity grade 2, as well as the elderly patient.[33,67] Therefore therapy would be directed by the patient's overall health and ability to perform activities of daily living. Second-line and third-line therapy is often employed in the United States.[33] These continue to be addressed in clinical trials. Targeted therapy is also being extensively studied.

The National Comprehensive Cancer Network (NCCN) Practice Guidelines in Oncology[68] recommend that adjuvant chemotherapy may be employed in high-risk patients with stage IA (T1, N0) disease. High-risk patients are defined as those with poorly differentiated tumors, vascular invasion, wedge resections, or minimal margins. In stage IB (T2, N0) and IIA or B (T1–2, N1) disease, chemotherapy may be given alone if margins are negative or given adjuvantly if positive margins. Chemotherapy and radiation therapy may be used in stages IB and higher. Adjuvant chemotherapy usually consists of cisplatin (Platinol AQ) and vinorelbine (Navelbine) or paclitaxel (Taxol) and carboplatin (Paraplatin). In stages IIIA and IIIB, concurrent chemoradiotherapy may be used in certain patients.[68] In locally advanced NSCLC, concurrent chemoradiotherapy is superior to sequential chemoradiation. Table 19-13 represents the most commonly used chemotherapeutic agents used in lung cancers concomitantly with radiation.

In advanced or recurrent NSCLC, the NCCN guidelines[68] recommend that chemotherapy should be employed (with uniform consensus based on high or lower levels of evidence). A cisplatin-based therapy is superior to best supportive care with improvement in median survival of 6 to 12 weeks and a doubling of the 1-year survival rates.[68] Cisplatin (Platinol AQ) or carboplatin (Paraplatin) are effective in combination with paclitaxel (Taxol), docetaxel (Taxotere), gemcitabine (Gemzar), vinorelbine (Navelbine), irinotecan (Camptosar), etoposide (Etopophos), and vinblastine (Velban). In patients with performance status of common toxicity grade 2, single-agent therapy is a reasonable alternative. Chemotherapy is not indicated for patients with a performance status of common toxicity grade 3 or 4. In progressive disease, docetaxel (Taxotere), pemetrexed (Alimta), or erlotinib (Tarceva) are recommended as single agents for patients with a performance status of common toxicity grade 0 to 2. Pemetrexed (Alimta) has proven to be equivalent to docetaxel (Taxotere) with less toxicity. Third-line chemotherapy recommendations include erlotinib (Tarceva). Bevacizumab (Avastin) is also established in the treatment of NSCLC in combination with other agents.[68]

Table 19-13 Common Chemotherapeutic Agents Used With Radiation Therapy in Lung Cancers

Agent	Nadir*	Side effects exacerbated by RT	Premeds
Carboplatin (Paraplatin)	18–21 days (thrombocytopenia)	Mucositis, esophagitis, dysphagia, aspiration, poor nutrition, myelosuppression, fatigue	No
Cisplatin (Platinol)	14–21 days	Mucositis, esophagitis, dysphagia, aspiration, poor nutrition, myelosuppression, fatigue	No
Docetaxel (Taxotere)	7–10 days	Myelosuppression, neurotoxicity, mucositis, dysphagia, poor nutrition, fatigue	Yes
Gemcitabine (Gemzar)	10–14 days	Nausea, vomiting, mucositis, esophagitis, myelosuppression, rash, fatigue	No
Irinotecan (Camptosar)	7–10 days	Diarrhea, fatigue, nausea, vomiting, dyspnea, cough, esophagitis, poor nutrition, fatigue	No
Paclitaxel (Taxol)	7–10 days	Myelosuppression, neurotoxicity, mucositis, esophagitis, dysphagia, poor nutrition, fatigue	Yes
Vinorelbine (Navelbine)	Day 7	Myelosuppression, nausea, vomiting, diarrhea, mucositis, esophagitis, poor nutrition, fatigue	No

Data from Knop C: Lung cancer. In Yarbro C, Frogge M, Goodman M: *Cancer nursing principles and practice*, ed 6, Boston, 2005, Jones and Bartlett, pp 1379-1413.

*Refers to neutrophil count unless otherwise specified.

Benefit from chemotherapy appears to occur with the initial 3 to 4 cycles, and prolonged therapy is not indicated.[67] Second-line chemotherapy also appears to provide both survival and palliative benefits. In unresectable stage III NSCLC, the chemotherapy and radiation therapy improves long-term survival and may actually cure a few patients.[69]

Treatment of locally advanced, NSCLC (stages IIIA, IIIB without pleural effusions, and Pancoast tumors) continues to evolve.[8] Surgery or radiation therapy alone achieves long-term survival in less than 5% of these patients. Recent clinical trials have demonstrated that combined modality therapy (chemoradiation) in patients with good performance status and no significant comorbid conditions can provide better results.[8,33] Median survival times have increased from less than 10 months to more than 18 months[70] with chemoradiotherapy. A meta-analysis of the Cochrane Central Register of Controlled Trials, Medline, and Embase compared concurrent chemoradiotherapy with radiation therapy alone. This meta-analysis showed a 14% reduction in risk of death at 2 years with concurrent chemoradiotherapy compared with a 7% reduction with radiation therapy alone.[71] In general, when platinum-based chemotherapy is given before thoracic radiation or surgery, outcome is improved by decreasing distant metastases.[4] The ideal sequencing and combination of modalities remains unknown.

The fit, elderly patient also may benefit from the above recommended treatments. Even in patients with poor performance status, chemoradiation may be employed. However, comorbid conditions and functional impairment must be carefully assessed. In the palliative setting, carboplatin may be more appropriate for those patients with poorer performance status and perhaps the frail elderly too. Additional studies are needed to assess whether the treatment toxicities outweigh the benefits in survival.[33]

NSCLC has become a disease that requires a multidisciplinary treatment approach. The involvement of pulmonary physicians, thoracic surgeons, medical oncologists, and radiation oncologist before the initiation of any treatment is the ideal treatment planning method.[72]

Several agents have proven to be active in treatment of NSCLC, but are also used as radiosensitizers. These include cisplatin, carboplatin (Paraplatin), paclitaxel (Taxol), docetaxel (Taxotere), gemcitabine (Gemzar), vinorelbine (Navelbine), etoposide (VePesid, and irinotecan (Camptosar). Table 19-13 gives more information about these agents. These agents have been described earlier in the chapter with the exception of vinorelbine (Navelbine) and etoposide (VePesid).

Vinorelbine (Navelbine) is a semisynthetic vinca alkaloid derived from vinblastine. It inhibits mitosis at metaphase by interfering with microtubule assembly.[36] The usual dose is 30 mg/m^2 IV weekly. Common side effects include bone marrow suppression (with a nadir at 7 to 10 days), neuropathies, nausea, vomiting, mucositis, and hepatotoxicity. When given with cisplatin (Platinol AQ), increased neutropenia occurs.

Etoposide (VePesid) has often been combined with cisplatin (Platinol AQ) and radiation therapy because of its radiosensitizing properties and synergy with cisplatin.[73] The limiting toxicity of chemoradiotherapy with cisplatin (Platinol AQ) and etoposide (VePesid) is a significant increase in esophageal toxicity.[73] Etoposide (VePesid) is a plant alkaloid and inhibits DNA synthesis in the S and G2 phases so that cells do not enter mitosis. It is given orally or by the intravenous route. The oral route is twice that of the intravenous dose, rounded to the nearest 50 mg.[36] One major side effect of etoposide (Vepesid) is myelosuppression. The nadir occurs in 7 to 14 days, and neutropenia may be severe. The dose should be modified if there is any renal or hepatic dysfunction. Other side effects include hypersensitivity reactions, nausea, vomiting, anorexia, skin irritations, and neurotoxicity.[36] When concurrent therapy is used, radiation recall can occur.

Pemetrexed (Alimta) is a multitargeted antimetabolite and inhibits key steps critical to pyrimidine and purine synthesis, preventing DNA synthesis and cell division.[36] Premedication with a corticosteroid is required to help prevent skin rash, and daily folic acid supplementation is needed. Intramuscular injections of vitamin B_{12} before treatment and every three cycles throughout treatment also should be administered. Side effects include bone marrow suppression (neutropenia nadir day 8, recovery by day 15), nausea, constipation, diarrhea, anorexia, mucositis, and dyspnea.

There have been two molecularly targeted therapies approved for NSCLC. These are gefitinib (Iressa) and erlotinib (Tarceva). Gefitinib (Iressa) now has restricted access in the United States, with its use being limited to patients who are currently/previously benefitting from treatment or if enrolled in an institutional review board (IRB)-approved clinical trial.[27] Gefitinib (Iressa) is a small molecule that specifically inhibits the tyrosine kinase activity of the epidermal growth factor receptor (EGFR) type 1 by interfering with the adenosine triphosphate (ATP) binding site.[74] Gefitinib (Iressa) was previously approved for third-line treatment of NSCLC, but use is now restricted as noted above. The most common side effects of gefitinib (Iressa) are low-grade rash, diarrhea, nausea, and vomiting.[36] A rare, but serious, side effect is interstitial lung disease (ILD). It appears to be efficacious in nonsmokers, women, and patients with adenocarcinoma, and those with bronchioalveolar lung cancer.[74] Strong evidence suggests concurrent chemotherapy and gefitinib offers no benefit.[74] Preclinical evidence indicates that gefitinib (Iressa) is a radiosensitizer, but for now, there is no proven clinical benefit for concurrent treatment with radiation.[74] Gefitinib is an oral agent and should be administered about the same time every day.

Erlotinib (Tarceva) is another EGFR tyrosine kinase inhibitor and is also given orally, but should be given on an empty stomach.[27] Side effects are similar to gefitinib (Iressa) and include rash, diarrhea, conjunctivitis, eye dryness, mucositis, and anorexia. Rarely, erlotinib (Tarceva) also can cause ILD. Erlotinib (Tarceva) has proven statistically superior to best supportive care in respect to survival.[68]

Future of Chemoradiotherapy in NSCLC

Despite improvements in median survival in the recent years, a need for significant improvement in treatment still exists. The majority of patients with locally advanced NSCLC die within 5 years from locoregional or distant progression of disease.[75] New systemic agents are needed to reduce and to control distant metastasis, because this remains the major site of failure.[4] Preoperative chemoradiotherapy should be compared to preoperative chemotherapy.[72] The optimal approach for stages III and IV patients with poor performance status has not been defined.[67]

There are many on-going trials of biologic-based, targeted therapies for NSCLC. Multiple cellular targets have been identified including EGFR, the *ras* signaling pathway, tumor angiogenesis, and cyclooxygenase-2 (COX-2) expression.[76] These agents are being studied both as single agents and in combination with chemotherapy and/or radiation therapy.

An interesting area of study is the combination of COX-2 inhibitors and chemoradiation therapy. COX-2 upregulation occurs early in the development of NSCLC. COX-2 inhibitors are known to enhance chemosensitivity. This combination strategy could potentially target angiogenesis while maximizing quality of life.[76,77]

Small-Cell Lung Cancer

Multimodality Therapy

Chemotherapy has been employed in the treatment of small-cell lung cancer (SCLC) since the 1960s. Cyclophosphamide (Cytoxan), doxorubicin (Adriamycin), and vincristine (Oncovin) (CAV) was the standard treatment until the late 1970s when the etoposide (VePesid) and cisplatin combination proved effective in patients resistant to cyclophosphamide (Cytoxan). This combination therapy is now considered the standard of care because of its moderate side effects[78] for both limited and extensive stage disease. The NCCN guidelines[79] recommend concurrent chemotherapy with radiation in limited stage disease.

In extensive stage disease, irinotecan (Camptosar) and cisplatin (Platinol AQ) (IP) may given as an alternative. Studies of irinotecan (Camptosar) in preclinical models showed that this drug has a mechanism of action that is complimentary to cisplatin (Platinol AQ).[78] The Japan Clinical Oncology Group (JCOG) has extensively studied this combination.[80,81] JCOG 9511 compared irinotecan (Camptosar) and cisplatin (Platinol AQ) with etoposide (VePesid) and cisplatin (Platinol AQ) in patients with extensive stage small-cell lung cancer that had not been previously treated.[81] The response rate was significantly higher in the irinotecan (Camptosar) and cisplatin (Platinol AQ) arm versus the etoposide (VePesid) and cisplatin (Platinol AQ) arm (84% vs 68%; p = .02), and there was a statistically significant improvement in progression-free survival (6.9 vs 4.8 months; p = .003). Based on the results of JCOG 9511,[81] IP (irinotecan and cisplatin) appears to be another platinum-based model to consider for extensive stage disease. It is the new standard of treatment for patients with extensive stage disease in Japan.[78] In the United States, trials are underway to confirm these results.

Second-line chemotherapy for small-cell lung cancer includes ifosfamide, paclitaxel (Taxol), docetaxel (Taxotere), gemcitabine (Gemzar), irinotecan (Camptosar), topotecan (Hycamtin), CAV, etoposide (VePesid), and vinorelbine (Navelbine).[76] No standard therapy exists for recurrent SCLC after a complete response.[75] To date, no molecular-targeted agents have shown significant activity in small-cell lung cancer.

TREATMENT OF THE ELDERLY WITH CHEMORADIOTHERAPY

People who are age 85 and older are now the fastest growing segment of the U.S. population according to the U.S. Census Bureau. Over 50% of cancers occur in the 13% of the population that is aged 65 years or older.[81] Treatment of the elderly population with chemoradiotherapy deserves special consideration and astute physical assessment.[82,83]

Age is associated with certain physiologic conditions that could complicate the treatment plan for cancer. For instance, there is a decreased functional reserve in the elderly patient, meaning there would be a prolonged recovery time for treatment of the cancer or a comorbidity. Table 19-14 lists some physiologic changes related to aging and potential complications with chemoradiotherapy. One physiologic change is declining organ function. This may create problems in some elderly cancer patients. There is a decline in renal and pulmonary function in the elderly.[83] Decreases in gastric emptying and intestinal motility may result in drugs staying in the body for longer periods, increasing the likelihood of an adverse drug reaction or interaction with concomitant medication. Gastrointestinal absorption of dietary vitamin D, zinc, and calcium are decreased. Diets are often lacking in protein and are higher in fat and carbohydrates. Lower albumin levels in the elderly also increase the risk of drug toxicities. Changes in body water and body mass may alter drug distribution, affecting the drug's onset of action and elimination. The liver shrinks up to 25% as people age.[84] This means there is a loss of hepatocytes and the parenchyma is replaced by fibrosis and increased fat. The ability of the liver to metabolize certain drugs is decreased by the significant reduction of the presystemic (first-pass) metabolism.[85,86]

Because of physiologic changes, pretreatment assessment of the elderly patient should include a medication assessment that covers all over-the-counter (OTC) medications and alternative treatments. Patients who are 75 years or older are more likely to be taking more than four medications.[87] The elderly population takes 25% to 35% of all the prescription drugs ordered in the United States. The elderly patient is more likely to use OTC drugs and complementary and alternative therapies.[87] There is always a potential for drug-drug interactions, and this increases exponentially with each additional medication in the regimen.[87] Assessment of the elderly patient, beyond pharmaceutical assessment also should include general health status, performance status, nutritional

Table 19-14 Physiologic Changes in the Elderly and Potential Consequences With Chemoradiotherapy

Physiologic change	Potential consequence
Decreased functional reserve	Prolonged recovery time from chemoradiotherapy
Decreased range of motion	Falls, inability to perform activities of daily living
Skeletal instability	Falls, inability to perform activities of daily living, bone fractures
Decreased circulation to organs	Risk of organ failure
Decreased cough reflex	Aspiration, pneumonia
Decreased hepatic, cardiac, and renal function	Drug reactions or interactions with concomitant medications; increased drug toxicities
Less responsive immune system	Infection; prolonged recovery from infection and myelosuppression
Decreased cerebral blood flow	Decrease in cognitive functioning
Decrease in subcutaneous tissue, body fat, lean body mass	Malnutrition; impaired wound healing
Decrease in skin elasticity	Exacerbated skin reactions, impaired wound healing; infection

Data from Haas M: *Geriatric Nurs*, 25(5):355-360, 2004, and Repetto L: *J Supportive Oncol* 1(4, Suppl 2):18-24, 2003.

status, and fluid balance.[88] Comorbidities are a significant problem for the elderly as well. A large phase III trial in elderly NSCLC patients found that 11.2% of patients also suffered from diabetes.[89] The elderly have an average of three different diseases.

Recent trials that focused on the elderly patient proved that they receive the same beneficial results from chemotherapy as do younger patients.[67] For example, elderly patients with lung cancer have no difference in survival rates when compared with other populations, but the death rate resulting from toxicity is higher in this population.[75] Airoldi and colleagues[90] looked at adjuvant chemoradiotherapy in fit older patients with head and neck cancers. The results were better than those observed in a comparable group treated with radiation alone and were similar to a younger group with the same poor prognostic factors that were treated with adjuvant carboplatin plus radiation. Similar results have been noted in those with colorectal cancer.[83] Dose decreasing simply based on age is not evidence-based.[9] In short, effective treatments should not be withheld from the elderly population simply based on age, but rather on their functional ability.[91]

SUMMARY

Chemoradiotherapy has a valuable role in the treatment of several cancers, especially head and neck carcinomas, selected gastrointestinal carcinomas, and lung carcinomas. Chemotherapy is used as a radiation enhancer, and locoregional tumor control is enhanced and disease-free survival is improved in many cases. However, these improvements may come at the expense of additional toxicities, which can result in significant morbidity and mortality. Because of the aggressiveness and toxicities of chemoradiotherapy, a team-based approach between surgical, medical, and radiation oncology nurses is vital. Communication and collaboration will ensure the successful completion of the therapy with positive patient outcomes. Future directions in chemoradiotherapy will include combining chemotherapy, radiation, biologic therapy and gene therapy, producing a more targeted therapy that will maximize positive patient outcomes.

REFERENCES

1. Khuri F, Jain S: Novel agents and incremental advances in the treatment of head and neck cancer, *Semin Oncol* 31 (2 Suppl 4):3-10, 2004.
2. Haddad R, Wirth L, Posner M: Integration of chemotherapy in the curative treatment of locally advanced head and neck cancer, *Exp Rev Anticancer Ther* 3(3):331-338, 2003.
3. Macdonald J, Fleming T, Peterson R et al: Adjuvant chemotherapy with 5-FU, adriamycin, and mitomycin-C (FAM) versus surgery alone for patients with locally advanced gastric adenocarcinoma: a Southwest Oncology Group study, *Ann Surg Oncol* 2(6):488-494, 1995.
4. Gandara D, Green M, Lara P et al: *Treatment strategies for advanced non-small cell lung cancer* (website): www.medscape.com/viewprogram/2676. Accessed May 15, 2005.
5. Zackrisson B, Mercke C, Strander H et al: A systematic overview of radiation therapy effects in head and neck cancer, *Acta Oncol* 42(5-6):443-461, 2003.
6. Eisbruch A, Lyden T, Bradford C et al: Objective assessment of swallowing dysfunction and aspiration after radiation concurrent with chemotherapy for head-and-neck cancer, *Int J Radiat Oncol Biol Phys* 53(1):23-28, 2002.
7. Gopal R, Starkschall G, Tucker S et al: Effects of radiotherapy and chemotherapy on lung function in patients with non-small-cell lung cancer, *Int J Radiat Oncol Biol Phys* 56(1):114-120, 2003.
8. Edelman M, Suntharalingam M, Krasna M: The management of the patient undergoing combined modality therapy for locally advanced non-small cell lung cancer, *Curr Treat Opt Oncol* 4(1):45-53, 2003.
9. Polovich M, White J, Kelleher L: *Chemotherapy and biotherapy guidelines and recommendations for practice, ed 2*, Pittsburgh, 2005, Oncology Nursing Press.
10. Tortorice P: Chemotherapy: principles of therapy. In Yarbro C, Frogge M, Goodman M, editors: *Cancer nursing principles and practice*, ed 6, Boston, 2005, Jones and Bartlett Publishers, pp 315-350.
11. Nishimura Y: Rationale for chemoradiotherapy, *Int J Clin Oncol* 9(6):414-420, 2005.
12. Gosselin-Acomb T: Principles of radiation therapy. In Yarbro C, Frogge M, Goodman M, editors: *Cancer nursing principles and practice*, ed 6, Boston, 2005, Jones and Bartlett, pp 229-249.
13. Volker D: Biology of cancer and carcinogenesis. In Itano J, Taoka K: *Core curriculum for oncology nursing*, ed 4, St Louis, 2005, Mosby, pp 443-464.
14. Loescher L, Whitesell L: The Biology of Cancer. In Tranin A, Masny A, Jenkins J: *Genetics in oncology practice: cancer risk assessment*, Pittsburgh, 2003, Oncology Nursing Society, pp 23-56.
15. Trosko J, Chang C, Upham B et al: Ignored hallmarks of carcinogenesis: stem cells and cell-cell communication, *Ann NY Acad Sci* (Online) 1028:192-201, 2004.
16. Trosko J, Ruch R: Cell-cell communication in carcinogenesis, *Front Biosci* 3 (Feb 15):208-236, 1998.
17. Gil-Delgado M, Khayat D, Johnson S: Lymphomas. In Pollock R, Doroshow J, Khayat D: *UICC manual of clinical oncology*, ed 8, Hoboken, NJ, 2004, John Wiley & Sons, pp 641-659.
18. Merkle C, Loescher L: Biology of cancer. In Yarbro C, Frogge M, Goodman M, editors: *Cancer nursing principles and practice*, ed 6, Boston, 2006, Jones and Bartlett Publishers, pp 3-25.
19. DeVita V, Chu E: Principles of cancer chemotherapy. In Chu E, DeVita V: *Cancer chemotherapy drug manual, 2006*, Sudbury, MA, 2006, Jones and Bartlett, p 1-21.

20. Noronha V, Mota A, Fogarasi M et al: Guidelines for Chemotherapy and Dosing Modifications. In Chu E, DeVita V: *Cancer chemotherapy drug manual, 2006*, Sudbury, MA, 2006, Jones and Bartlett, pp 375-391.
21. Camp-Sorrell D: Chemotherapy toxicities and management. In Yarbro C, Frogge M, Goodman M: *Cancer nursing principles and practice*, ed 6, Boston, 2005, Jones and Bartlett, pp 412-457.
22. National Comprehensive Cancer Network: Myeloid growth factors, V1.2006. In *National Comprehensive Cancer Network clinical practice guidelines in oncology, 2005* (website): www.nccn.org. Accessed May 1, 2006.
23. Ozer H, Tfayli A: *Supportive care of cancer patients: hematopoietic growth factors* (website): www.medscape.com/viewprogram/2029-pnt. Accessed January 23, 2006.
24. National Comprehensive Cancer Network: Antiemesis, V1.2006. In *National Comprehensive Cancer Network clinical practice guidelines in oncology, 2006* (website): www.nccn.org. Accessed May 1, 2006.
25. Kostler W, Hejna M, Wenzel C et al: Oral mucositis complicating chemotherapy and/or radiotherapy: options for prevention and treatment, *CA J Clin* 51(5):290-315, 2001.
26. Maher K: Radiation therapy: toxicities and management. In Yarbro C, Frogge M, Goodman M, editors: *Cancer nursing principles and practice*, ed 6, Boston, 2005, Jones and Bartlett, pp 283-314.
27. Fang E: Epocrates RX Pro®, Version 7.50, San Mateo, Calif, 2006, Epocrates.
28. Chu E, Devita V: *Cancer chemotherapy drug manual, 2006*, Sudbury, MA, 2006, Jones and Bartlett.
29. Rieger P: *Biotherapy: a comprehensive overview*, ed 2, Sudbury, Mass, 2001, Jones and Bartlett Publishers, pp 3-37.
30. Wujcik D: Hematopoietic growth factors. In Rieger P: *Biotherapy: a comprehensive overview*, ed 2, Sudbury, Mass, 2001, Jones and Bartlett Publishers, pp 245-282.
31. DiJulio J: Monoclonal antibodies: overview and use in hematologic malignancies. In Rieger P: *Biotherapy: a comprehensive overview*, ed 2, Sudbury, Mass, 2001, Jones and Bartlett Publishers, pp 283-316.
32. Reiger P, Green M, Murray J: Monoclonal antibodies: application in solid tumors and other diseases. In Rieger P: *Biotherapy: a comprehensive overview*, ed 2, Sudbury, Mass, 2001, Jones and Bartlett Publishers, pp 317-355.
33. Gandara D, Edelman M, Lara P et al: Evolution of combined modality therapy for stage III non-small-cell lung cancer, *Oncology* 14(7 Suppl 5):35-41, 2003.
34. National Comprehensive Cancer Network: *National Comprehensive Cancer Network Clinical practice guidelines in oncology, 2006* (website): www.nccn.org. Accessed May 1, 2006.
35. National Comprehensive Cancer Network: Head and Neck Cancers, V1.2006. In *National Comprehensive Cancer Network clinical practice guidelines, 2006* (website): www.nccn.org. Accessed May 1, 2006.
36. Wilkes G, Barton-Burke M: *Oncology nursing drug handbook*, Boston, 2005, Jones and Bartlett.
37. Christiansen H, Hermann R, Hille A et al: Concomitant radiochemotherapy in primary inoperable advanced head and neck cancer with 5-fluorouracil and mitomycin-C, *Head Neck* 26(10):845-853, 2004.
38. Airoldi M, Cattel L, Cortesina G et al: Gemcitabine and vinorelbine in recurrent head and neck cancer: pharmacokinetic and clinical results, *Anticancer Res* 23(3C): 2845-2852, 2003.
39. Milano M, Harah D, Stenson K et al: Phase 1 study of concomitant chemoradiotherapy with paclitaxel, fluorouracil, gemcitabine and twice-daily radiation in patients with poor-prognosis cancer of the head and neck, *Clin Cancer Res* 10(15):4922-4932, 2004.
40. Argiris A, Haraf D, Kies M et al: Intensive concurrent chemoradiotherapy for head and neck cancer with 5-fluorouracil and hydroxyurea-based regimens: reversing a pattern of failure, *Oncologist* 8(4):350-360, 2003.
41. Haraf D, Rosen F, Stenson K et al: Induction chemotherapy followed by concomitant TFHX chemoradiotherapy with reduced dose radiation in advanced head and neck cancer, *Clin Cancer Res* 9(16 Pt 1):5936-5943, 2003.
42. Nabell L, Spencer S: Docetaxel with concurrent radiotherapy in head and neck cancer, *Semin Oncol* 30 (6 Suppl 18):89-93, 2003.
43. ImClone Systems Incorporated and Bristol-Myers Squibb Company. Erbitux® (Cetuximab) package insert. Princeton, NJ, 2006, Bristol-Myers Squibb.
44. Song J, Chen C, Raben D: Emerging role of EGFR-targeted therapies and radiation in head and neck cancer, *Oncology* 18(14):1757-1767, 2004.
45. Macdonald J: Roles of post-operative chemoradiation in resected gastric cancer, *J Surg Oncol* 90(3):166-170, 2005.
46. Meyerhardt J, Fuchs C: Chemotherapy options for gastric cancer, *Semin Radiat Oncol*, 12(2):176-186, 2002.
47. National Comprehensive Cancer Network: Gastric cancer, V1.2006. In *National Comprehensive Cancer Network clinical practice guidelines, 2006* (website): www.nccn.org. Accessed May 1, 2006.
48. Earle C, Maroun J, Zuraw L: Neoadjuvant or adjuvant therapy for respectable gastric cancer? A practice guideline, *Can J Surg* 45(6):438-446, 2002.
49. Glynne-Jones R, Debus J: Improving chemoradiotherapy in rectal cancer, *Oncologist* (6 Suppl 4):29-34, 2001.
50. Glimelius B: Chemoradiotherapy for rectal cancer—is there an optimal combination? *Ann Oncol* 12(8): 1039-1045, 2001.
51. National Comprehensive Cancer Network: Rectal cancer, V2.2006. In *National Comprehensive Cancer Network clinical practice guidelines, 2006* (website): www.nccn.org. Accessed May 1, 2006.
52. Hurwitz H: New combinations in metastatic colorectal cancer: what are our expectations? *Oncologist* 10(5):320-322, 2005.
53. National Comprehensive Cancer Network: Anal carcinoma, V2.2006. In *National comprehensive cancer network clinical practice guidelines, 2006* (website): www.nccn.org, Accessed May 1, 2006.
54. Flam M, John M, Pajak T et al: Role of mitomycin in combination with fluorouracil and radiotherapy and of salvage chemoradiation in the definitive nonsurgical treatment of epidermoid carcinoma of the anal canal: results of a phase III randomized intergroup study, *J Clin Oncol* 4(9):2527-2539, 1996.
55. Charnley N, Choudhury A, Chesser P et al: Effective treatment of anal cancer in the elderly with low-dose chemoradiotherapy, *Br J Cancer* 92(7):1221-1225, 2005.
56. Clark M, Hartley A, Geh J: Cancer of the anal canal, *Lancet Oncol* 5(3):149-157, 2004.

57. Gervaz P, Allal A, Roth A et al: Chemotherapeutic options in the management of anal cancer, *Exp Opin Pharmacother* 5(12):2479-2484, 2004.
58. Madoff R: Chemoradiotherapy for rectal cancer—when, why, and how? *N Engl J Med* 351(17):1790-1792, 2004.
59. Melcher A, Sebag-Montefiore D: Concurrent chemoradiotherapy for squamous cell carcinoma of the anus using a shrinking field radiotherapy technique without a boost, *Br J Cancer* 88(9):1352-1357, 2003.
60. Bendell J, Ryan D: Current perspectives on anal cancer, *Oncology* 17(4):492-497, 502-503, 2003.
61. National Comprehensive Cancer Network: Pancreatic adenocarcinoma, V2.2006. In *National comprehensive cancer network clinical practice guidelines, 2006* (website): www.nccn.org. Accessed May 1, 2006.
62. Oya N: Chemoradiotherapy for pancreatic cancer: current status and perspectives, *Int J Clin Oncol* 9(6):451-457, 2004.
63. Kalser M, Ellenberg S: Pancreatic cancer: adjuvant combined radiation and chemotherapy following curative resection, *Arch Surg* 120(8):899-903, 1985.
64. Berlin J, Catalano P, Thomas J: Phase III study of gemcitabine in combination with fluorouracil versus gemcitabine alone in patients with advanced pancreatic carcinoma, *J Clin Oncol* 20(15):3270-3275, 2002.
65. Wilkes G: Colon, rectal, and anal cancers. In Yarbro C, Frogge M, Goodman M, editors: *Cancer nursing principles and practice*, ed 6, Boston, 2005, Jones and Bartlett, pp 1155-1214.
66. Smith W, Khuri F: The care of the lung cancer patient in the 21st century: a new age, *Semin Oncol* 31(2 Suppl 4): 11-15, 2004.
67. Socinski M: The role of chemotherapy in the treatment of unresectable stage III and IV non–small cell lung cancer, *Respir Care Clin North Am* 9(2):207-236, 2003.
68. National Comprehensive Cancer Network: Non small cell lung cancer, V2.2006. In *National comprehensive cancer network clinical practice guidelines, 2006*, (website): www.nccn.org. Accessed May 1, 2006.
69. Socinski M, Zhang C, Herndon J et al: Combined modality trials of the Cancer and Leukemia Group B in stage III non-small cell lung cancer: analysis of factors influencing survival and toxicity, *Ann Oncol* 15(7):1033-1041, 2004.
70. Curran W: Evolving chemoradiation treatment strategies for locally advanced non-small cell lung cancer, *Oncology* 17(12 Suppl 13):7-14, 2003.
71. Rowell N, O'Rourke N: Concurrent chemoradiotherapy in non-small cell lung cancer, *Cochrane Database Syst Rev*, 4: CD002140, 2004.
72. Pisters K: Combined modality therapy of early stage non–small cell lung cancer, *Respir Care Clin North Am* 9(2): 191-205, 2003.
73. Reboul F: Radiotherapy and chemotherapy in locally advanced non-small cell lung cancer: preclinical and early clinical data, *Hematol Oncol Clin North Am* 18(1):41-53, 2004.
74. Birnbaum A, Ready N: Gefitinib therapy for non-small cell lung cancer, *Curr Treat Opt Oncol* 6(1):75-81, 2005.
75. Penland S, Socinski M: Management of unresectable stage III non-small cell lung cancer: the role of combined chemoradiation, *Semin Radiat Oncol* 14(4):326-334, 2004.
76. Vokes E, Choy H: Targeted therapies for stage III non-small cell lung cancer: integration in the combined modality setting, *Lung Cancer* 41(Suppl 1):S115-S121, 2003.
77. Saha D, Pyo H, Choy H: COX-2 inhibitor as a radiation enhancer: new strategies for the treatment of lung cancer, *Am J Clin Oncol* 26(4):S70-S74, 2003.
78. Horiike A, Saijo N: Small-cell lung cancer: current therapy and novel agents, *Oncology* 19(1):47-52, 2005.
79. National Comprehensive Cancer Network, Inc: Small cell lung cancer, V1.2006. In *National comprehensive cancer network clinical practice guidelines, 2006*, (website): www.nccn.org. Accessed May 1, 2006.
80. Kudoh S, Fujiwara Y, Takada Y et al: Phase II study of irinotecan combined with cisplatin patients with previously untreated small-cell lung cancer, *J Clin Oncol* 16(3): 1068-1074, 1998.
81. Noda K, Nishiwaki Y, Kawahara M et al: Irinotecan plus cisplatin compared with etoposide plus cisplatin for extensive small-cell lung cancer, *N Engl J Med* 346(2): 85-91, 2002.
82. National Comprehensive Cancer Network, Inc: Senior adult oncology, V1.2005. In *National Comprehensive Cancer Network clinical practice guidelines, 2005*, (website): www.nccn.org. Accessed December 28, 2005.
83. Lichtman S: Management of advanced colorectal cancer in older patients, *Oncology (Williston Park)* 19(5):597-602, 2005.
84. Vestal R: Aging and pharmacology, *Cancer* 80(7): 1302-1310, 1997.
85. Gridelli C, Aapro M: Factors influencing the choice of 5-HT3-receptor antagonist antiemetics: focus on elderly cancer patients, *Suppor Care Cancer* 12(7):487-496, 2004.
86. Repetto L: Greater risks of chemotherapy toxicity in elderly patients with cancer, *J Suppor Oncol* 1(4 Suppl 2):18-24, 2003.
87. Horiot J, Aapro M: Treatment-implications for radiation-induced nausea and vomiting in specific patient groups, *Eur J Cancer* 40(7):979-987, 2004.
88. Oncology Nursing Society: Demystifying CINV control in the complex aging patient: assessing the complexities of the aging oncology patient, *ONS News* 19(Suppl):5-8, 2004.
89. Gridelli C, Perrone F, Gallo C et al: Chemotherapy for elderly patients with advanced non small cell lung cancer: the Multicenter Italian Lung Cancer in the Elderly Study phase III randomized trial, *J Nat Cancer Inst* 95:362-372, 2003.
90. Airoldi M, Cortesina G, Giordano C et al: Postoperative adjuvant chemoradiotherapy in older patients with head and neck cancer, *Arch Otolaryngol Head Neck Surg* 130(2): 161-166, 2004.
91. Haas M: Utilizing geriatric skills in radiation oncology, *Geriatr Nurs* 25(5):355-360, 2004.

Chapter 20
Combined Chemoradiation Safety

Katen Moore and Martha Polovich

Preventing hazardous drug exposures in the radiation treatment facility is the focus of this chapter. Known health risks from occupational chemotherapy exposure are discussed, along with safe handling precautions aimed at reducing exposure in radiation therapy departments.

The extent of hazardous drug exposure for radiation oncology clinicians and others working in a radiation oncology facility is unknown. The frequency of chemotherapy infusions present in the radiation setting also has not been studied. Although the opportunity for hazardous drug exposure is lower for radiation oncology clinicians than for clinicians practicing in medical oncology or for oncology pharmacists, the potential for exposure does exist.

Perez and colleagues[1] have stated that 60% of all cancer patients will encounter radiation at some point in their cancer treatment, although this statistic has never been confirmed. Chemotherapy is also a common therapy, and it is possible for patients to receive both types of treatment. Radiation oncology clinicians may be directly exposed to chemotherapy through accidental spills when patients are treated with concurrent radiation and chemotherapy.

Clinicians specializing in the care of patients receiving radiation therapy should have a basic knowledge of how to protect themselves and others from accidental chemotherapy exposure. The fact that a patient is receiving chemotherapy may not be readily apparent to the radiation staff. With combined modality therapy, patients may receive chemotherapy immediately before their radiation treatments. Alternatively, patients may receive continuous infusion chemotherapy using a small pump with an unobtrusive intravenous line that is inadvertently hidden from view.

Institutions and/or radiation facilities may not have policies or procedures regarding chemotherapy handling and safety. Staff orientation may not include such information. Thus there is concern about the lack of knowledge regarding occupational risks of chemotherapy exposure among radiation oncology clinicians.

SYSTEMIC THERAPY FOR CANCER

Chemotherapy refers to the use of drugs for the systemic treatment of cancer. Chemotherapy has been used for cancer treatment since the 1940s, following the discovery of nitrogen mustard. In 1955, the federally funded National Chemotherapy Program provided financial support for the development of many new agents. The U.S. Food and Drug Administration (FDA) approved 85 drugs for the treatment of cancer between the years of 1949 and 1992, another 85 drugs were approved in the next 8 years (1993–2000), and an additional 34 drugs were approved during the 3-year period from 2001 to 2004.[2] Chemotherapy is now one of the most commonly administered treatments for certain solid tumors and for hematologic malignancies. Systemic chemotherapy can be administered intravenously, intramuscularly, subcutaneously, or orally.

Most chemotherapeutic agents exert their action by interfering with cell division and/or damaging deoxyribonucleic acid (DNA). They cause direct damage to DNA, disrupt DNA replication during its synthesis, or interfere with the repair of DNA. Any of these events may lead to cell death.[3] Harris[4] described the potential effects on cells exposed to cytotoxic agents: no effect, cell death, mutagenic changes, or possible cancer. The mechanisms of action that damage cancer cells may cause the same effects in normal cells. These result in the side effects that patients experience with chemotherapy, as well as the occurrence of secondary malignancies in a small percentage of patients.

Concurrent cancer therapies using intravenous chemotherapy and radiation may be used for head and neck, esophageal, lung, rectal, and bladder cancers. Continuous infusion chemotherapy regimens are the greatest source of potential chemotherapy exposure for radiation oncology clinicians.

Biologic therapy is another form of systemic therapy for cancer. The first such agents stimulated a generalized immune response, which sometimes resulted in regression of tumor growth.[5] New biologic agents are similar to proteins that occur naturally in the human body, or they target receptors that control cell growth. Their anticancer actions suppress tumor growth, inhibit tumor angiogenesis, or induce tumor cell death. Patients may receive a combination of chemotherapy, biotherapy, and radiation therapy.

HEALTH EFFECTS OF OCCUPATIONAL EXPOSURE

Occupational exposure to chemotherapy drugs may result in adverse health outcomes. These effects are based on the inherent toxicities of the agents (Box 20-1). Several published studies have demonstrated health risks for healthcare workers who were exposed to chemotherapy. The first was a small, controlled study by Falck and colleagues.[6] The authors reported finding mutagenic activity, as measured by the Ames test, in the urine of patients who received chemotherapy and also in the urine of the clinicians who administered it. The Ames test measures genetic mutations in bacteria following exposure to chemicals. Ninety percent of known carcinogens test positive on this test.[7] This study demonstrated that handling cytotoxic drugs during administration resulted in drug absorption by the clinicians and, consequently, also resulted in the potential for genetic changes.

Box 20-1 Criteria for Defining Hazardous Drugs

Drugs that meet one or more of the following criteria should be handled as hazardous:

- Carcinogenicity
- Teratogenicity or developmental toxicity
- Reproductive toxicity
- Organ toxicity at low doses
- Genotoxicity
- Structure or toxicity similar to drugs classified as hazardous using the above criteria

From National Institute for Occupational Safety and Health (NIOSH) (2004): *Preventing occupational exposure to antineoplastic and other hazardous drugs in health care settings* (website): www.cdc.gov/niosh/docs/2004-165. Accessed January 8, 2006.

Pharmacists and nurses have reported acute symptoms from chemotherapy exposure, such as skin irritation, sore throat, cough, dizziness, headache, allergic reaction, diarrhea, nausea, and vomiting as reported by Harrison.[8] Harrison also reviewed 14 studies of reproductive outcomes in healthcare workers exposed to hazardous drugs. Nine of the studies showed adverse outcomes. The reported problems included fetal loss, congenital malformations, and infertility. Other documented effects of occupational exposure include liver damage in nurses[9] and learning disabilities in the offspring of nurses who handled chemotherapy during pregnancy.[10] Polovich[7] provides a summary of frequently cited studies on the risks of occupational exposure to hazardous drugs.[7]

Many chemotherapy agents are carcinogenic[11] (Box 20-2). Exposure to known carcinogens should be avoided whenever possible, because no level of exposure is considered safe. By the 1970s it was well known that there is a risk of secondary leukemia and other malignancies in patients treated with chemotherapy for an unrelated primary cancer. This led some practitioners to suggest that a similar risk might exist for healthcare workers occupationally exposed to cytotoxic agents.[12,13]

Two European epidemiologic studies have demonstrated a small increased incidence of cancer in healthcare workers who handled chemotherapy. Skov and colleagues[14] used data from the Danish cancer registry from 1943 to 1987. The relative risk for leukemia among Danish nurses with a history of handling antineoplastic drugs was significantly increased (10.65), but was based on only two cases. Hansen and Olsen[15] found an increased risk for non-Hodgkin's lymphoma among long-term pharmacy handlers of chemotherapy. With a standardized incidence ratio [SIR] for cancer of 1.0, the pharmacists showed an SIR of 3.7, based on five cases.

Sessink and Bos[16] proposed a method to estimate the increased risk of cancer in pharmacists and nurses exposed to cyclophosphamide. By measuring the urinary excretion of cyclophosphamide, systemic absorption can be calculated. Using data from animal studies, the authors suggested that a healthcare worker's exposure of 3.6 to 18 mcg per day will result in an increased risk of cancer of 1.4

Box 20-2 Chemotherapy Agents With Carcinogenic Potential

KNOWN HUMAN CARCINOGENS (IARC GROUP 1)

Azathioprine
Cyclophosphamide
Melphalan
Chlorambucil
Busulfan
Thiotepa
Tamoxifen
MOPP (mechlorethamine, Oncovin, procarbazine, prednisone)

PROBABLE CARCINOGENS (IARC GROUP 2A)

Carmustine
Lomustine
Nitrogen mustard
Cisplatin
Doxorubicin
Procarbazine

POSSIBLE CARCINOGENS (IARC GROUP 2B)

Streptozocin
Dacarbazine
Daunorubicin
Bleomycin
Mitomycin
Mitoxantrone
Amsacrine

Data from International Agency for Research on Cancer (IARC) (2004): *Overall evaluations of carcinogenicity to humans* (website): www.cie.iarcfr/monoeval/crthall.html. Accessed May 21, 2005.

Box 20-3 Selected Biotherapy Agents Used in Cancer Treatment

ANGIOGENESIS INHIBITOR

Bevacizumab (Avastin)

CYTOKINES

Interleukin-2* (Aldesleukin)
Interferon* (Intron-a, Roferon-a)

GROWTH INHIBITORS

Erlotinib (Tarceva)
Gefitinib (Iressa)

HEMATOPOIETIC GROWTH FACTORS

Darbepoietin Alfa (Aranesp)
Epoetin Alfa (Procrit)
Filgrastim (Neupogen)
Pegfilgrastim (Neulasta)
Sargramostim (Leukine)

MONOCLONAL ANTIBODIES

Cetuximab (Erbitux)
Rituximab (Rituxan)
Trastuzumab (Herceptin)

RADIOLABELED MONOCLONAL ANTIBODIES:

Tositumomab and iodine 131* (Bexxar)
Ibritumomab tiuxetan and yttrium-90* (Zevalin)

*These drugs appear in Appendix A of the National Institute for Occupational Safety and Health (NIOSH) Alert. Safe handling precautions are recommended.[21]

to 10 additional cases per million workers per year. Absorption of 16 to 80 mcg per day, a level of exposure that has been measured in another study of nurses, is estimated to increase cancer risk by 7 to 50 excess cases per million.[17] Although the proposed increase in cancer cases is small, their estimate applies to the risk from a single cytotoxic agent and may apply to as many as 6 million healthcare workers.[18]

Little evidence about the risks of occupational exposure to biologic agents has been gathered (Box 20-3). Because most of these drugs do not affect DNA, they do not cause genetic changes.[5] The U.S. Department of Labor, Occupational Safety & Health Administration (OSHA) added the biologic agent interferon to its list of hazardous drugs in 1995 because of its reproductive toxicity.[19] Thus healthcare workers should avoid occupational exposure to interferon. Some biotherapy agents are irritating to the eyes, skin, digestive tract, and respiratory tract. For these reasons, it is generally accepted practice to avoid direct skin contact with biologic agents and to avoid generating aerosols.[5]

OSHA categorized chemotherapy drugs as hazardous substances and published guidelines for handling these agents. The American Society of Health System Pharmacists[20] (ASHP) asserted that drugs other than antineoplastic agents pose an occupational risk and proposed a class of agents called "hazardous drugs." OSHA drafted a list of 62 drugs for which special handling was recommended.[19] Recently, the National Institute for Occupational Safety and Health (NIOSH) published a list of 136 drugs considered hazardous, with a commitment to update the list annually.[21]

EXPOSURE PREVENTION

Although safe handling precautions have been available for many years, they have been aimed at those who prepare and administer chemotherapy. With the increased use of concurrent and synchronous chemotherapy and radiation, radiation therapy personnel should be aware of the possibility of occupational exposure and the precautions that can reduce their exposure.

The first recommendations for the safe handling of chemotherapy came from the ASHP in 1985, in their first *Technical Assistance Bulletin on Handling Cytotoxic Drugs*.[20] OSHA released guidelines in 1986, which drew heavily from the ASHP document. The Oncology Nursing Society (ONS) published safe handling recommendations in 1988. NIOSH summarized the most recent recommendations in *Preventing Occupational Exposures to Antineoplastic and Other Hazardous Drugs in Healthcare Settings*.[21]

All of the above-mentioned documents outline similar methods of reducing exposure to hazardous drugs. Specific equipment, work practices, and personal protective equipment (PPE)—garments that protect individuals from contact with hazardous chemicals—are described based on the drug-handling activity (Box 20-4). The interventions target the most likely routes of exposure: inhalation, dermal absorption, or ingestion. In a radiation treatment facility, exposure is possible by any or all of the three routes.

The greatest inhalation risk exists during drug preparation, which is not usually a concern for radiation oncology clinicians. For those clinicians who do mix chemotherapy, drug preparation should take place in a ventilated control, such as a biological safety cabinet (BSC). Generating aerosols is possible during spiking or unspiking of intravenous (IV) containers of chemotherapy or when expelling air from a drug-filled syringe. These activities should be avoided to prevent inhalation exposure.

Box 20-4 Personal Protective Equipment for Handling Hazardous Drugs

- Gloves made of latex, nitrile, or neoprene that are powder-free and have been tested with hazardous drugs
- Gowns that are disposable, have cuffs and back closure, and have been tested with hazardous drugs
- Eye and face protection, such as a face shield (when splashing is possible)
- Respirator/masks for aerosols and spill clean-up

Chemotherapy spills also result in the release of drug aerosols. A chemotherapy spill is possible for radiation oncology clinicians whenever a chemotherapy infusion is present. Respiratory protection, using a NIOSH-approved respirator appropriate to the agent, should be worn during clean up of a chemotherapy spill. Radiation oncology clinicians should be aware of the need for respiratory protection and have access to the appropriate equipment.

Dermal exposure is possible during drug handling activities that release hazardous drugs into the environment. Gowns and gloves should be worn to protect skin and clothing from contact with hazardous drugs. Dermal exposure is most likely to occur in a radiation facility during activities such handling an IV container or tubing during the positioning of a patient for treatment or examination.

In 1992, Sessink and colleagues[22] published the first of 14 studies that found hazardous drug residue on work surfaces in pharmacies and drug administration areas.[21] Results indicate that current methods of handling hazardous drugs do not prevent leakage of hazardous drugs. Leaking of drugs during handling causes surface contamination. Drug residue has been recovered from floors and work surfaces in drug preparation and administration areas, including over-bed tables, chair armrests, countertops, storage carts, tables, sinks, and the outside of infusion containers. Workers can be inadvertently exposed to chemotherapy by dermal absorption from touching contaminated surfaces with unprotected hands and from ingestion after hand-to-mouth contact. Surface contamination is a possible source of chemotherapy exposure for radiation oncology clinicians.

Chemotherapy drug residue is present in excreta (urine, stool) of patients who have recently received chemotherapy. Although the duration of detectable drug in urine varies from a few hours to several days, the most common recommendation is to follow safe handling precautions when handling the bodily wastes of patients for 48 hours after the completion of chemotherapy.[19,20] Universal precautions require the wearing of personal protective equipment by personnel when they are handling body fluids. Gloves (and gowns when there is a risk of contaminating the clothing) are recommended for all waste handling. OSHA[19] states that gloves made of latex or other materials tested with hazardous drugs are best for handling urine and stool contaminated with chemotherapy. Disposable diapers are preferred for incontinent patients.[23]

Any disposable item that is contaminated with chemotherapy must be handled with PPE and disposed of in a container designed to hold chemotherapy waste. Although no official color or warning label for this class of waste has been designated, the containers are traditionally yellow or white and yellow and are labeled with a warning such as "cytotoxic" or "chemotherapy waste." PPE used to handle drug-contaminated items also should be also be disposed of in a chemotherapy waste container. The containers should be closed and removed by trained personnel when full.[23] In settings where these containers are used infrequently, it is prudent practice to remove the containers on a timely schedule even if they are not full to avoid long-term storage of cytotoxic waste. All radiation facilities should have access to chemotherapy waste containers despite their infrequent use.

Linen that is soiled with chemotherapy contaminated bodily waste should be handled with gloves and a gown if there is a chance of soiling clothing. Dispose of chemotherapy contaminated linens in a leak-proof linen bag. Many facilities handle all linen as being contaminated; others may have designated linen bags for items soiled with chemotherapy. Disposable pads or other items soiled with body fluids from chemotherapy patients should be handled with gowns and/or gloves and discarded in containers used for potentially infectious materials.

A hazardous drug spill does not occur frequently, but can represent a serious exposure risk for many individuals. Prompt spill management is essential. This can be accomplished only with easy access to spill clean-up equipment and by having appropriately trained individuals available. Spill kits contain PPE, spill control "pillows" or absorbent towels, a scoop or utility gloves for picking up sharps, and plastic bags for disposable of the items used in the clean up.[23] These kits should be available wherever chemotherapy is administered and in the locations to which patients may be transported during a chemotherapy infusion. Unfortunately, there is no data on the frequency of chemotherapy spills in radiation facilities.

OPPORTUNITIES FOR EXPOSURE

Although the greater risk for hazardous drug exposure involves direct drug manipulations during the preparation and administration of these drugs, any contact with patients who are receiving chemotherapy represents an opportunity for exposure. Malfunctioning infusion devices, loose IV tubing connections, or kinking of IV tubing with pressure build-up can cause leaking or disconnection. Luer-lock connections help to prevent this from occurring. Patients' IV access devices can become dislodged. Clinicians also have reported accidental removal of administration sets from IV containers causing a spill of the entire contents of the bag or bottle.

Radiation clinicians should be knowledgeable about the care and assessment of central venous access devices (VADs). VADs include peripherally inserted central catheters (PICC lines), nontunneled central venous catheters, tunneled central venous catheters (including Hickman and Groshong catheters), and implanted venous ports that are accessed by Huber needles.[24] VADs can be kinked internally by anatomic structures such as bones causing "pinch-off syndrome," or by clots that can block or prevent proper flow of the infusion. Huber needles used to access ports can be pulled and dislodged when positioning a patient or assisting the patient onto the simulation or treatment table. A similar risk exists for all VADs; therefore, great care must be taken when working with patients with VADs. Clinicians also should monitor peripheral IV catheters that are placed in areas of flexion (such as the wrist or the antecubital area) or that have long tubing that may become caught on equipment or tangled.

Radiation clinicians should consider checking the integrity of a chemotherapy IV line when patients arrive for treatment. This assessment should include examining the infusion site, inspecting all tubing connections, and verifying the function of the infusion pump. The slow rates of some continuous infusions may not trigger pump alarms before a significant infiltration or spill. Pumps may not sound an alarm at all when the solution is infusing and the infusion line is separated from the access site.

Surface contamination has been found to exist where there has been no spill.[22] It is important that radiation oncology clinicians are aware of this "non-wet" type of accidental exposure risk. Radiation oncology clinicians and other radiation facility personnel can be exposed by skin absorption or hand to mucous membrane transfer after touching a chemotherapy-contaminated item. All current guidelines recommend that contaminated items should be handled with chemotherapy safe gloves. These may include infusion bags, tubing, pumps, and IV poles. Following any handling activity, the individual should remove the gloves carefully, turning them inside out, discard them in a chemotherapy waste designated container, and wash his or her hands.[21]

A number of studies have examined the compliance of chemotherapy clinicians with published safe handling recommendations.[25-28] All of the studies took place in settings with safe handling policies and procedures. Clinicians are generally expected to practice accordingly, and although most do, some others do not. There are no published studies examining the use of safe handling precautions in radiation oncology settings.

Many radiation facilities require that continuous chemotherapy is "capped" or stopped when a patient travels to the facility for treatment. Theoretically, this practice should reduce hazardous drug exposure for radiation oncology clinicians; however, there may be other implications to consider.

First, it is not known whether interrupting continuous infusion chemotherapy for radiation treatment has a negative effect on treatment or disease outcome.[29] Disconnecting chemotherapy infusions actually increases the risk of exposure to the individual doing so. IV tubing can leak, and clothes or linen may become contaminated during the capping or reconnecting procedure. Safe storage of the drug while the patient is undergoing radiation is an issue. Policies such as these also do not address outpatients who are receiving continuous chemotherapy using small infusion devices.

Body fluids such as blood, vomitus, stool, and urine represent an exposure risk when patients receive intermittent chemotherapy or continuous infusion chemotherapy that is interrupted for radiation. Several chemotherapy agents have been detected in patient excreta as long as 7 days after the drug's administration.[7] Radiation facility bathrooms are a potential source of chemotherapy exposure. It is not reasonable to clean bathrooms thoroughly after each use. Patients and personnel should not share a bathroom. Disposable towels should be used.

Chemotherapy infusing in the radiation facility presents a frank, or wet, accidental exposure risk. A small spill can be merely a damp intravenous access site (less than or equal to 5 mL or 1 teaspoon). Cleanup of any spill should be performed by personnel wearing a gown and gloves. A small spill requires first containment with an impermeable but absorbent towel. Discontinue the infusion if the spill is caused by an IV infiltration. A "large" spill—defined as any amount greater than the 5 mL or 1 teaspoon[7]—is visible on either clothing, furniture, or the floor. This type of spill requires the use of a spill kit. Large spills may require the assistance of the environmental management personnel. The responsibility of large chemotherapy spill cleanup should be addressed clearly in policy.

Patients receiving continuous infusion may arrive for treatment on foot, in a wheelchair, or on a stretcher. Patients can travel to the facility accompanied by transport personnel, by clinicians, or be unaccompanied, depending on the policy of the institution. Infusions may be administered by an infusions pump, in which case IV bags or bottles are hanging from an IV pole. IV poles can be unstable and are subject to tipping over. Patients may be tempted to use an IV pole for support while walking. Unsteady gait, awkward footing, wet floors, and uneven floor surfaces increase the risk of falling. Any of these factors can contribute to a chemotherapy spill and to patient injury.

Radiation therapists also should take care to protect the integrity of IV tubing and intravenous access sites when assisting or maneuvering a patient into position on the radiation treatment table. Infusion lines or tubing can tangle, kink, or disconnect. When central or peripheral lines become kinked or tangled, pressure buildup can increase the risk of a spill and extravasation of the fluid from the access site. A spill of this kind can expose the patient, the healthcare personnel, and the environment. If IV pump alarms are silenced or deactivated, it renders them useless in the event of a spill that is not immediately evident.

Immobilization devices restricting patient movement and blocks or cones that are inserted into the treatment machinery must be placed carefully by radiation therapists to avoid dislodging or displacing IV pumps or lines. IV poles or infusion pumps worn by patients must be safely placed or put out of the way of the radiation machinery to prevent damage and spills. It is very important to avoid contaminating the radiation treatment machines by improper chemotherapy handling or because of a spill.

IMPLICATIONS FOR PRACTICE

The radiation oncology clinician should obtain the patient's history, which includes all other providers. This information should include names of physicians and nurses, telephone numbers, and their role in the patient's treatment (e.g., medical oncologist or surgeon). The clinician should inquire about chemotherapy the patient is receiving before, during, or after radiation. This information should be documented in the patient's record. A radiation nursing documentation tool such as that developed by the Oncology Nursing Society is an excellent example of a radiation nursing–specific documentation tool.[30] This documents weekly changes, incorporating toxicity scales that show variations over time.

Radiation therapy facility personnel should receive training for chemotherapy safe handling and cleaning up spills. Safe handling competency should be validated before assuming radiation nursing duties and be reevaluated annually. Safety education must include the risks of exposure under the Hazard Communication Standard,[31] which states that all employees must be informed of the chemicals present in their workplace and the risks of those chemicals.

Safety standards should include policies and procedures regarding the safe handling of chemotherapy, patient transport with chemotherapy infusing, and appropriate personal protective equipment.

Policies should outline procedures for handling continuous chemotherapy infusions. Someone in the radiation facility should be assigned to monitor the patency and integrity of all IV infusions. The responsibility and the frequency of checking should be defined and addressed specifically. Policies should require that radiation departments have spill kits on site. The lack of these kits significantly increases the risk of direct chemotherapy exposure to personnel, patients, and others in the department. One solution might be that patients with continuous chemotherapy carry a spill kit with them during transport.

A chemotherapy safety policy should include procedures to follow when transporting patients to and from the radiation facility and to specifically delineate who can transport these patients and the competencies required to do so.

Appropriate PPE must be made available to radiation personnel when they are working with patients with continuous infusions. Policies should identify situations when PPE is required.

NEED FOR EVIDENCE AND RESEARCH

There are no published studies to date that have assessed the risk of chemotherapy exposure in a radiation department. Data on how many patients are transported to other departments with continuous infusions of chemotherapy is lacking in the literature. NIOSH recommends that employers "evaluate the workplace to identify and assess hazards before anyone begins work with hazardous drugs."[21] The evaluation should include the types of drugs being handled, the frequency, and the potential for exposures during work. The radiation therapy work environment has never been formally evaluated for this risk.

Environmental contamination studies in the radiation department might be helpful in determining the extent of surface contamination. Such studies perform wipe samples for evidence of hazardous drugs (e.g., treatment/simulation tables, exam rooms and tables, waiting rooms, phlebotomy areas, and restrooms). The results would help to evaluate the degree of chemotherapy exposure risk in radiation treatment facilities.

Medical surveillance of radiation personnel in direct contact with patients or patient waste (including physicians, clinicians, radiation therapists, aides, and environmental management) should be considered. Policies should address who will be monitored with annual medical surveillance, including health and reproductive history, blood work, and physical exam.[19,21] In some facilities where chemotherapy is administered, policies identify those with the highest exposure risk for medical monitoring. The frequency of potential exposure determines the degree of risk. Personnel with low exposure risk because of less direct patient contact, might not be followed as closely as personnel with high exposure risk. Acute exposure, such as after a chemotherapy spill, requires a health evaluation.

The materials used in the department's furniture should be able to be cleaned quickly and effectively. Upholstered furniture and carpets may not be appropriate in a medical setting. Seating arrangements in waiting areas are also important. Patients receiving continuous infusion chemotherapy might be segregated from other patients, although this has not been studied.

SUMMARY

All oncology clinicians need to advocate that chemotherapy safe handling recommendations be incorporated into practice regardless of the practice setting. Although guidelines are clearly defined for clinicians who prepare and administer chemotherapy, such clarity is lacking in radiation oncology. Radiation oncology clinicians should be proactive in developing policies regarding the safe handling of chemotherapy when administered in the radiation oncology facility. Evaluation of the radiation therapy environment, which identifies the opportunities for exposure, is a necessary first step.

Future research that quantifies the chemotherapy exposure risk in radiation oncology settings can lead to developing standards that will support safe practice. Guidelines are needed for the safety and well-being of all radiation therapy workers and patients.

REFERENCES

1. Perez CA, Brady LW, Halperin EC et al, editors: *Principles and practice of radiation oncology*, ed 4, Philadelphia, 2004, Lippincott Williams & Wilkins.
2. Food and Drug Administration: *Approval statistics: oncology tools* (website): www.accessdata.fda.gov/scripts/cder/onctools/statistics.cfm. Accessed May 14, 2005.
3. Devita VT, Hellman S, Rosenberg SA, editors: *Cancer: principles and practice of oncology*, ed 6, Philadelphia, 2004, Lippincott Williams & Wilkins.
4. Harris CC: The carcinogenicity of anticancer drugs: a hazard in man, *Cancer* 37(2 suppl):1014-1023, 1976.
5. Rieger PH, editor: *Biotherapy: a comprehensive overview*, ed 2, Boston, 2001, Jones and Bartlett.
6. Falck K, Grohn P, Sorsa M et al: Mutagenicity in urine of nurses handling cytostatic drugs, *Lancet* 1(8128):1250-1251, 1979.
7. Polovich M, editor: *Safe handling of hazardous drugs*, Pittsburgh, 2003, Oncology Nursing Society.
8. Harrison BR: Risks of handling cytotoxic drugs. In Perry MC, editor: *The chemotherapy source book*, Philadelphia, 2001, Lippincott Williams & Wilkins, pp 566-582.
9. Sotaniemi EA, Sutinen S, Arranto AJ et al: Liver damage in nurses handling cytostatic agents, *Acta Med Scand* 214(3):181-189, 1983.
10. Martin S: Chemotherapy handling and effects among nurses and their offspring (Abstract), *Oncol Nurs Forum* 32(2):425, 2005.
11. International Agency for Research on Cancer: *Overall evaluations of carcinogenicity to humans* (website): www-cie.iarc.fr/monoeval/crthall.html. Accessed May 21, 2005.
12. Donner AL: Possible risk of working with antineoplastic drugs in horizontal laminar flow hoods [letter], *Am J Hosp Pharm* 35(8):900, 1978.
13. Ng LM, Jaffe N: Possible hazards of handling antineoplastic drugs, *Pediatrics* 46(4):648-649, 1970.
14. Skov T, Lynge E, Maarup B et al: Risks for physicians handling antineoplastic drugs [letter], *Lancet* 336(8728): 1446, 1990.
15. Hansen J, Olsen JH: Cancer morbidity among Danish female pharmacy technicians, *Scand J Work Environ Health* 20(1):22-26, 1994.
16. Sessink PJ, Bos RP: Drugs hazardous to healthcare workers: evaluation of methods for monitoring occupational exposure to cytostatic drugs, *Drug Saf* 20(4):347-359, 1999.
17. Connor TH, Anderson RW, Sessink PJ et al: Surface contamination with antineoplastic agents in six cancer treatment centers in Canada and the United States, *Am J Health-Sys Pharm* 56(14):1427-1432, 1999.
18. Bureau of Labor Statistics: *Occupational employment statistics* (website): www.stats.bls.gov/oes/current/oes290000.htm. Accessed May 14, 2005.
19. Occupational Safety and Health Administration: *Controlling occupational exposure to hazardous drugs, OSHA Technical Manual, 1995* (website): www.osha.gov/dts/osta/otm/otm_vi/otm_vi_2.html. Accessed August 31, 2005.
20. American Society of Hospital Pharmacists: ASHP technical assistance bulletin on handling cytotoxic and hazardous drugs, *Am J Hosp Pharm* 47(11):1033-1049, 1990.
21. National Institute for Occupational Safety and Health: *Preventing occupational exposure to antineoplastic and other hazardous drugs in health care settings* (website): http://www.cdc.gov/niosh/docs/2004-165/. Accessed March 31, 2006.
22. Sessink PJ, Boer KA, Scheefhals AP et al: Occupational exposure to antineoplastic agents at several departments in a hospital: environmental contamination and excretion of cyclophosphamide and ifosfamide in urine of exposed workers, *Int Arch Occup Environ Health* 64(2):105-112, 1992.
23. Polovich M, White J, Kelleher LO, editors: *Chemotherapy and biotherapy guidelines and recommendations for practice*, ed 2, Pittsburgh, 2005, Oncology Nursing Press.
24. Camp-Sorrell D, editor: *Access device guidelines and recommendations for practice and education*, ed 2, Pittsburgh, 2004, Oncology Nursing Society.
25. Nieweg R, deBoer M, Dubbleman R et al: Safe handling of antineoplastic drugs: results of a survey, *Cancer Nurs* 17(6):501-511, 1994.
26. Martin S, Larson E: Chemotherapy-handling practices of outpatient and office-based oncology nurses, *Oncol Nurs Forum* 30(4):575-581, 2003.
27. Turk M, Davas A, Ciceklioglu M et al: Knowledge, attitude and safe behaviour of nurses handling cytotoxic anticancer

drugs in Ege University Hospital, *Asian Pac J Cancer Prev* 5(2):164-168, 2004.
28. Ritchie MA, McAdams C, Fritz N: Exposure risk in the handling and administration of chemotherapy agents: a review and synthesis of the literature, *Online J Knowl Synth Nurs* 7:4, 2000.
29. Schulmeister L: Transporting patients receiving continuous infusion chemotherapy, *Clin J Oncol Nurs* 8(4):419-420, 2004.
30. Caitlin-Huth C, Haas M, Pollock V et al: *Radiation therapy patient care record: a tool for documenting nursing care*, ed 2, Pittsburgh, 2002, Oncology Nursing Society.
31. Occupational Safety and Health Administration: *Hazard Communication Standard 1910.1200* (website): www.osha.gov/pls/oshaweb/owadisp.show_document?p_table=STANDARDS&p_id=10099. Accessed September 15, 2005.

Chapter 21

Interventional Radiology Procedures

Diana H. Wortham

Improvements in diagnostic and therapeutic capabilities have promoted the use of interventional radiology (IR) to offer a variety of services to clinicians and patients. IR plays a steadily increasing role in the supportive care of the cancer patient. This emerging arena is driven by three factors: (1) the need for effective treatments of therapeutically challenging diseases, (2) technical advancements, and (3) the expansive growth of knowledge and skills in this collaborative environment by practicing experts. To provide appropriate nursing care, nurses must understand disease processes, accurate patient selection and eligibility, and therapeutic appropriateness of various IR treatment options. The goal of this chapter is to heighten awareness and equip oncology nurses with knowledge to competently provide quality care for patients undergoing IR therapeutics.

STAFF AND WORK ENVIRONMENT

Interventional radiology and interventional neuroradiology are clinical subspecialties of radiology focused on minimally invasive image-guided therapy for numerous diseases. The terms *interventionalist, intervention,* or *interventional* are interchangeable terms commonly used to designate the radiology physician specialists, who provide specialized care and are uniquely trained to provide specific therapies. Of the 20,000 radiologists in the United States, only 4000 are interventionalists.[1]

In 2005, the American College of Radiology (ACR), the American Society of Interventional and Therapeutic Neuroradiology (ASITN), and the Society of Interventional Radiology (SIR) jointly developed the *"Practice Guidelines for Interventional Clinical Practice"* according to the process described in the ACR Practice Guidelines and Technical Standards books governed by the Guidelines and Standards Committee of the Interventional and Cardiovascular Radiology Commission in collaboration with ASITN and SIR based on ACR's March 2003 White Paper. Provisions of clinical practice were defined as "a longitudinal involvement of the interventionalist in patient care, beginning with the initial consultation often involving therapeutic interventions, and continuing through to eventual resolution of the clinical problems or establishment of an alternative care plan"[2] (Box 21-1).

The guidelines for Interventional Clinical Practice were written to educate numerous audiences including radiologists (interventionalists and non-interventionalist), physicians, hospital credentialing committees, administrators, payors, multidisciplinary team members, healthcare professionals, and lay consumers. This infrastructure and blueprint is essential to the development, standardization, and articulation of the defined roles, services, reimbursement strategies, treatment modalities, and delivery models of care in the area of interventional radiology[2] (Box 21-2).

Established in 1981, the American Radiological Nurses Association (ARNA) initiated a grassroots organization comprising 35 nurses from 15 states. By 1982, organizational bylaws were developed and adopted including the professional radiology nurse's role description followed by guidelines for Standards of Practice (1985) and lastly the attainment of national recognition by other specialty organizations and intersociety liaison positions including American Healthcare Radiology Administration (AHRA), Radiological Society of North America (RSNA), Society of Cardiovascular Interventional Radiology (SCVIR) and American Nurses Association (ANA) in 1991. In 1998, ARNA released the *Standards of Radiology Nursing Practice and Guidelines of Radiology Practice,* in which the philosophy, history, scope, generalist and advanced practice role descriptions, standards of care, and professional performance were ratified.[3,4] The goal of this professional organization is to promote and maintain quality patient

Box 21-1 Benchmarks of Interventional Clinical Practice

1. Accepts referrals for therapeutic interventions as the sole or primary consultant for the disease process
2. Routinely performs and bills for consultations for patients before and after planned or elective interventions
3. Routinely informs patients referred for diagnostic services about the spectrum of therapeutic options that might benefit them and provide interventional treatment if they desire
4. Routinely establishes treatment plans and implements them without requiring the participation of another specialist
5. Admits patients to the interventional service who require inpatient services after undergoing therapeutic interventions
6. Provides longitudinal patient care

Data from American College of Radiology, the American Society of Interventional and Therapeutic Neuroradiology, and the Society of Interventional Radiology: Practice guidelines for interventional clinical practice, *J Vasc Interven Radiol* 16:149-155, 2005.

care during diagnostic and therapeutic imaging procedures through education, standards of practice, professional growth, and collaboration with other multidisciplinary healthcare providers. ARNA in collaboration with the Association of Operating Room Nurses (AORN) addresses care provisions related to management of patients (including conscious sedation), specific invasive procedures, infection control, sterile environments and equipment, and radiation safety.[5] The certification examination for radiologic nursing (CRN) in imaging, interventional, and therapeutic environments was established in 1997 by the Radiologic Nursing Certification Board.[4] Table 21-1 lists selected resources affiliated with radiologic practice.

CLASSIFICATION AND CONSIDERATIONS OF VASCULAR AND NONVASCULAR APPROACHES FOR ABLATIVE MODALITIES

Goldberg and colleagues,[6] under the authority of the Society of Interventional Radiology Technology Assessment Committee and the International Working Group on Image-guided Tumor Ablation, ratified a standardization of terminology and reporting criteria related to image-guided tumor ablation. This framework provides the greatest accuracy in comparing emerging technologies, classification of therapies and procedure terms, methods for describing treatment-related risks, and patient outcomes that impact quality of care. The role of nonvascular and vascular ablative strategies is to decrease disease volume, prevent progression, and minimize the risk of new tumor growth in nonsurgical populations with selective advanced cancers. The focus of this discussion features an overview of the most commonly used interventional radiology procedures: nonvascular-based radiofrequency ablation (RFA) and percutaneous vertebroplasty (PV) and vascular-based superselective intraarterial chemotherapy (IA) *and* percutaneous transcatheter

Table 21-1 Selected Radiological Resources

Organization	Website	Journal
American College of Radiology	www.acr.org	Journal of American College of Radiology (JACR)
American Healthcare Radiology Administrators	www.ahraonline.org	Journal of the American Healthcare Radiology Administrators
American Radiological Nurses Association	www.arna.net	Journal of Radiology Nursing
American Roentgen Ray Society (ARRS)	www.arrs.org	American Journal of Roentgenology
American Society of Neuroradiology	www.asnr.org	American Journal of Neuroradiology
International Society of Radiology	www.isradiology.org	Online newsletter format
Radiology Central: General Radiology Information	www.radcentral.com	Multi-link source site
Radiological Society of North America	www.rsna.org	RadioGraphics Online
Society of Interventional Radiology (SIR)	www.sirweb.org	Journal of Vascular and Interventional Radiology
Society for Vascular Nursing	www.svnnet.org	Journal of Vascular Nursing

Box 21-2 Practice Guidelines for Interventional Clinical Practice

I. Clinical team
   a. Interventionalist
   b. Non-physician practitioner
   c. Nurses
   d. Radiological technologists
II. Administrative services
   a. Office manager
   b. Clerical support
   c. Scheduler
   d. Transcriptionist
   e. Coding and billing personnel
   f. Insurance precertification and compliance
   g. Data management and quality management databases
III. Outpatient clinic
   a. Space and equipment (office sharing or freestanding clinic)
   b. Personnel (see I and II)
   c. Time
      i. New consults—45–60 minutes
      ii. Follow up—20–30 minutes
      iii. Procedure volumes—
         1. =/< 999/year = 5 hours/week
         2. 1000–3000/year = 5–15 hours/week
         3. > 3000/year = 15 hours/week
   d. Communication of clinical care
IV. Inpatient requirements
   a. Admitting privileges
   b. Time allotment for inpatient clinical duties
   c. Scheduling of interventional procedures
V. Imaging requirements
   a. Fluoroscopy, vascular imaging, including vascular ultrasound (US) and angiography, CT, MRI, ± MR or CT angiography with future trend using PET, PET/CT
VI. Interventional suite requirements
   a. Setting
   b. Location
   c. Dedicated room with sterile equipment and conditions
   d. Radiographic equipment
   e. Patient preparation area and recovery room
   f. Medical/surgical supply inventory
   g. Nonradiographic equipment
   h. Staffing
   i. Physiologic monitoring equipment
VII. Quality improvement
   a. Clinical decision making of:
      i. Appropriateness of clinical diagnosis
      ii. Appropriateness of ordering laboratory and radiographic tests
      iii. Mechanisms of follow-up (FU) and patient failure to FU
   b. Monitoring thresholds and measures of clinical benefit of completed therapy
   c. Procedure complication and adverse event rates
VIII. Marketing and education

Data from American College of Radiology, the American Society of Interventional and Therapeutic Neuroradiology, and the Society of Interventional Radiology. Practice Guidelines for Interventional Clinical Practice. *J Vasc Interven Radiol, 16*, 149-155. (2005).
CT, Computed tomography; *MRI,* magnetic resonance imaging; *PET,* positron emission tomography.

embolization (PTE). This review addresses treatment descriptions, common indications and considerations from the interventionalist's cache to oncologic ablative options and their nursing care implications.

IMAGE GUIDANCE

Radiographically based image guidance refers to measures in which imaging techniques, such as fluoroscopy, ultrasound, angiography, computerized tomography (CT), or magnetic resonance imaging (MRI), are used and serve as the critical methodologic approach to ensuring IR procedural success. Imaging guidance is used in five distinct and separate ways: planning, targeting, monitoring, controlling, and assessing treatment response. Of these, fluoroscopy provides the interventionalist the interactive capabilities of multiplanar monitoring that permit simultaneous viewing of the ablative zone, enhanced applicator control and positioning and assist in the intentional avoidance of adjacent nontargeted structures. In conjunction with traditional radiographic planning techniques, advanced technology uses positron emission tomography (PET), PET/CT, CT, and MRI angiography. These tools assist the interventionalist to better identify and determine the patient's suitability before their respective procedure. Extrapolated data regarding tumor characteristics including size, shape, number, volume, and location with respect given to vital vascular and organ structures are essential to minimizing or eliminating injury and adverse events. Target imaging steers interventionalists intraprocedurally to map and isolate the precise tumor physicality. Using this "real-time" localization enables the use of "direct" treatment pathways such as intraarterial, transvertebral, or transcutaneous, compared to the general radiologist's traditional noninvasive oral or peripheral venous route. The route of instillation, substances injected, delivery vehicle (size and type of catheter, needle, probe), and rate of delivery (e.g., rapid or bolus injection or defined infusion time) are commonly detailed within these procedural descriptions. The delivery of all ablation methods is referred to as a "procedure" or "session," which defines the completed effort to ablate one or more tumors. In select circumstances, treatment encounters may involve either single or multiple visits to deliver the therapeutic goal. Based on procedure type, previous treatment, and disease progression localities may be reconsidered for retreatment in limited cases.

Nonvascular Ablative Modalities

The term *ablation therapy* is defined as the direct application of chemical or thermal therapies to specific focal tumor(s) in an attempt to achieve eradication or substantial tumor destruction that can lead to longer survival in select patient groups.[7]

There are two ablation methodologies currently used in practice: (1) *chemical ablation* and (2) *thermal ablation*. Classified universally by the chemical nomenclature of the agent(s), chemical ablation includes agents such as acetic acid or ethanol, which is referred to as percutaneous alcohol instillation (PAI) or percutaneous ethanol instillation (PEI) interchangeably. The purpose and action of chemical ablation is to introduce coagulation necrosis, which is the formative result of tissue destruction.[8] Conversely, thermal ablation involves energy sources to destroy tumors. Thermal conduction is achieved through various sources and applicator devices such as radiofrequency (RF) electrodes, microwave antennas, laser fibers, cryoablation cryoprobes, and ultrasound through either transcutaneous (extracorporeal) or percutaneous via needle-like applicators for intracavitary or intracardiac use.[6] Each technique has its strengths and weaknesses, discovered in part from successes and failures, which serve as provisions for identifying similar problems and technical shortfalls. Of the types of chemical and thermal ablation, radiofrequency ablation (RFA) is currently the front-runner among the many choices for local tissue ablation.[9]

Of these technologies, the basis of action can be divided into two major categories with regard to the physics and physiology of how the targeted cell is killed by either cooling or heating.[10] By in large, these methods are nonvascular in origin, based on their entry approach, delivery route, or site of tumor target destination. With all technical delivery, a concise documentation framework for standardized procedure reporting should include a critical comparison of the device; applicator with variations to number of probes, length, and dwell times; energy or chemical source; and if mechanically delivered, the settings and modifications of constant or pulsing energy algorithms. Additional technical variations in RF may describe *internal cooling* with saline or water within the electrodes or perfusion-cooled enhancement. This increasingly popular technical role transports perfusate directly into the tissues to avoid focal charring of the tumor, thereby diminishing the duration, quality, and optimal exposure of the thermal conduction. Conversely, during cryoablation, materials such as liquid or gaseous nitrogen or argon gas are chosen with the treatment specifications that describe the number of freeze-thaw cycles. If required by the size or location of the tumor, similar to RFA, as many as five probes can be inserted and cooled to -195° C simultaneously. The process of freezing is monitored by ultrasound, which displays a hypoechoic (dark) image when the tissue is frozen. Rapid freezing, slow thawing, and repetition of the freeze/thaw cycle are standard features of this technique. The pathophysiologic effects are related to direct cellular damage as a result of physicochemical effects, intracellular and extracellular ice crystal formation, and solute-solvent shifts that lead to cell dehydration and rupture.[11] Indirect cytotoxicity results from loss of structural integrity, as well as small-vessel obliteration with resulting hypoxia.[12]

Completing the list of therapies administered through a nonvascular route, *vertebroplasty (VP)* or *kyphoplasty* involves the percutaneously delivered genetic or cemented material injected under fluoroscopic guidance into a collapsed vertebra. Kyphoplasty also involves the introduction of inflatable bone tamps into the fractured vertebral body for elevation of the endplates before fixation of the fracture with bone cement. The purpose of both procedures is to minimize or alleviate osseous pain based on an admixture in which chemical reactions generate thermal reactions at extreme temperatures to impose cytotoxic effects in osseous tumors.

Vascular Ablative Modalities

In contrast, the purpose of vascular-based approaches are designed to "plug up" or chemically or mechanically infiltrate venous or arterial structures resulting in devascularization. This method of intentional reduction or cessation of blood flow to a targeted vascular bed or an entire organ is called *percutaneous transcatheter embolization.* Embolic agents are most commonly derived from particulate (e.g., gelatin, collagen, polypropylene, cellulose, and liquid embolic agents [e.g., glues, alcohol, polymers]); however, rarely used, mechanical barriers such as stainless steel coils, balloons, or glass beads yield selective treatment indications. When embedded into tissue, the result of this material causes both a temporary or permanent occlusion and accompanies a foreign body–associated inflammatory reaction.[13] These materials are instilled intravascularly by way of an interventionally placed microcatheter. Once localized in the desired target, these catheters can carry a selection of either beta-emitting sealed and unsealed radioactive sources or more commonly, chemotherapy based compounds in a technique called *transarterial chemotherapy embolization (TACE)* or concentrated, transient dosages of arterially delivered chemotherapeutic agents in a procedure called superselective *intraarterial chemotherapy (IA).*[14]

INTRODUCTION OF NONVASCULAR INTERVENTIONAL RADIOLOGY TECHNIQUES

Radiofrequency Thermal Ablation

Thousands of years ago, Hindu medics used heated metal bars to stop bleeding. Hippocrates said "what is not cured by the knife may be cured by fire." Electrocautery has been used for many decades in surgery to stop bleeding, coagulate blood vessels, and cut tissue. Therapeutic application of radiofrequency (RF) energy has been used in surgery since the late 1920s.[15] Historically, RF energy has been used for the treatment of cardiac arrhythmias, which lead into establishing indications for use in focal, nonmalignant conditions related to hyperactive neurologic foci in epilepsy, painful trigeminal neuralgia/nerve ganglion ablation, and osteoid osteoma.[16-19] Advancements in ablation research and technology yields RFA's continued time-tested, major role in the treatment of patients with unresectable tumors such as hepatocellular and metastatic liver lesions.[20,21] Promising new data and a growing body of knowledge are emerging in a variety of cancers that demonstrate treatment refractory activity in primary and metastatic lesions associated with osteolytic bone, cerebral metastases, renal cell, lung, breast, and the adrenals.[22-27]

Radiofrequency thermal ablation (RFA) is a minimally invasive, image-guided therapy that provides effective local treatment of a selection of isolated or localized neoplastic diseases. Used as a single strategy or adjunct to multimodality therapies such as conventional surgery, systemic chemotherapy, and radiation therapy, RFA also may be added to other treatments such as percutaneous ethanol injection (PEI), cryosurgical ablation, transarterial chemotherapy embolization (TACE), and for primary or metastatic liver lesions, with hepatic arterial infusion (HAI) chemotherapy. Recent developments in RFA technology make large-volume tissue ablation more effective and safer for local control of neoplastic disease when contrasted with initial clinical experiences. This precision enables clinicians, based on established criteria, to treat not only solitary but also multifocal lesions. Local tumor control is an attractive option for some patients who are not ideal surgical candidates, have failed conventional therapies, or have contraindications to surgery. Retreatment in the presence of tumor progression, regrowth, or incomplete treatment in some cases is attainable. Needle-based tissue ablation techniques provide a viable alternative to open surgery. Although no long-term, prospective, randomized clinical trials using RFA have been reported, the early results reveal optimism for safety, low complication rates, and efficacy and show it to be a beneficial alterative to managing anatomic or problematic tumors. Additionally, certain tumor responses may enhance surgical options by converting a patient who was once considered inoperable because of tumor burden or dissemination to a candidate for surgical resection.

Between 1999 and 2003, Tateishi and colleagues[28] studied over 1000 RFA sessions in 2140 hepatocellular carcinoma (HCC) tumors on 319 primary (naïve) treatment patients and 345 nonnaïve patients with recurrent disease whose treatment included percutaneous ethanol injection therapy (PEIT), microwave therapy, and transarterial embolization. Cumulative survival data beginning at year 1 demonstrated an overall slight advantage for naïve subjects (94.7%) compared to nonnaïve subjects (91.8%) with rising statistically significant morbidity occurring in both groups at the fifth year posttreatment of 54.3% versus 38.2%, respectively. Of the 40 major (4% per treatment) and 17 minor (1.7% per treatment) complications, only one surgical intervention was required for a duodenal perforation, and no treatment-related deaths were reported. This large-scale, longitudinal study suggests that RFA for primary or recurrent disease to be a safe and effective strategy for managing unresectable HCC.

The benefit of RFA relative to surgical resection for patients with potentially resectable HCC remains controversial. Few retrospective series report long-term outcomes from RFA, and there are no randomized trials that directly compare the two treatments. Most clinicians consider that surgery is preferable, if it is feasible. Nevertheless, with data on over 3000 patients treated with RFA, the safety and benefit has been supported, particularly in patients with unresectable HCC. With a successful ablation, overall 5-year survival rates of 40% to 50% can be achieved for small tumors (less than 5 cm), with complete local response averages of 70% to 75%, yet dropping to 25% in large tumors (greater than 5 cm). In patients with comorbidity associated cirrhosis, Child-Pugh class A fair better than those with advancing levels of liver dysfunction. Major side effects or complications of RFA in the liver are less than 2%, most of which do not require surgery. Although recurrence rates are determined predominantly by lesion size, with lesions less than 3 cm yielding a better local treatment rate, new intrahepatic or extrahepatic disease arises in 25% to 50% of patients.[9] The emergence of newer equipment, which can produce larger zones of ablation, the role of single-agent chemotherapy and the use of adjunctive therapies such as PEI, hepatic arterial chemoembolization, cryoablation, and microwave coagulation offer the potential of local tumor control and sometimes achieve long-term disease-free survival and are currently under investigation.[29,30]

Procedures and Technical Considerations

Radiofrequency energy is defined as 10 kHz to 2.59 GHz on the electromagnetic spectrum. During acceleration, energy creates elongated wavelengths by direct electrical or resultant thermal effects that can be exploited for therapeutic use. Before the RFA, needle-like electrodes are placed into the tumor under ultrasound, computed tomography (CT), or magnetic resonance (MR) image guidance. Similar to the operative suite, a grounding pad(s), also called a *reference electrode,* is placed on the patient's thigh or back muscles, thereby turning the patient into an electrical circuit. Connected to a radiofrequency (RF) generator that supplies the electrical current, the small needled RF electrode typically comprises an insulated metal shaft and an uninsulated, exposed conductive tip. This electrode is inserted through the skin into the tumor and becomes the direct electrical connection to the targeted tissue volume. The RF generator produces voltage between the RF and reference electrode to establish lines of electric field patterns (Figure 21-1, *C*). The intensity can be modified to gain adequate heat range. The mechanism of tissue heating with RFA is frictional (or resistive) energy loss associated with this ionic current causing molecules to become agitated to temperatures greater than 50° C; this leads to the breakdown of proteins and membranes resulting in cellular death.[31] Tissue heat deposition is more intense near the electrical probe where the current is greatest; however, device variables such as probe dimensions, tumoral configuration, and cylindrical transference of dose contribute to the quality and volume of tissue treated. An uncontrollable condition such as the dimpling of the treatment sphere caused by tissues being located next to blood vessels (higher blood flow increases the risk of lowered temperatures, hence altering the desired constant thermal state) contribute to poor conduction compared to tumors adjacent to healthy, soft tissue, which serve as a better conductor and have an optimizing treatment effect. Therefore, the parameter governing tumor destruction has been based on temperature distribution by inducing cellular death via coagulation.[32] The key to RFA is ensuring that adequate heat is delivered as characterized in the bio-heat equation of Pennes.[33] This

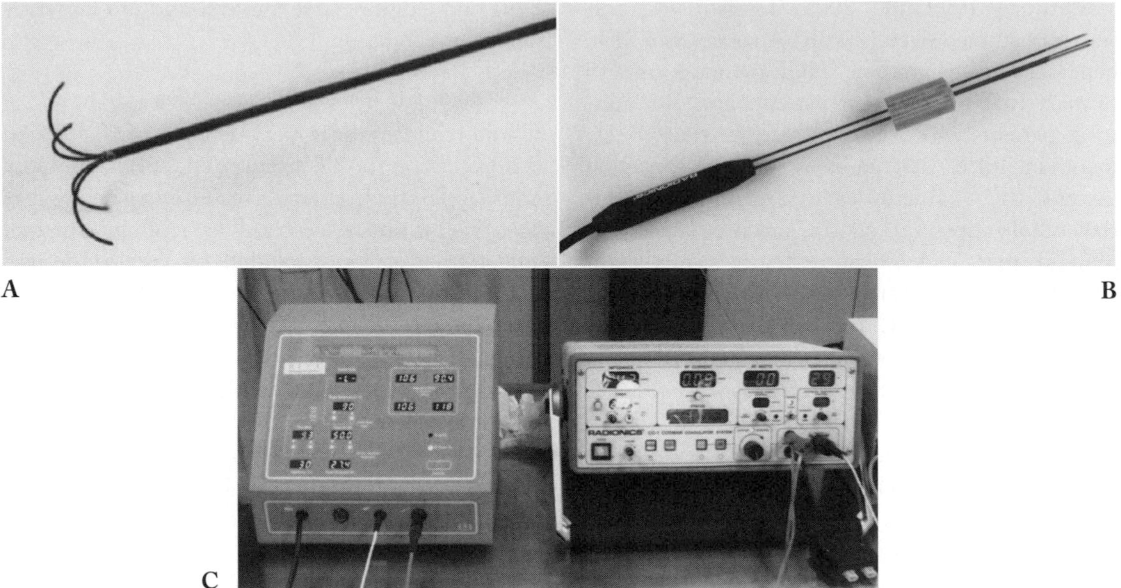

Figure 21-1 Radiofrequency Ablation. **A,** Tip of 15-gauge expandable needle shows four hook-shaped, expandable electrodes deployed. **B,** Cooled-tip triple-cluster needle with 2.5-cm exposed active parts shows probe-guiding device and stabilizer threaded onto needle. **C,** Two generators used for experiments. Generator for expandable needle is on left, and generator for cooled needle is on right.
From de Baere T, Denys A, Wood BJ, et al: AJR Am J Roentgenol 176(1):187-192, 2001.

relationship typifies the treatment's influence based on tissue/blood heat, density, conduction, and perfusion. The equation simplified is as follows:

Coagulation necrosis = Energy deposited × Local tissues interactions – Heat loss

Strategies designed to improve RFA efficacy are based on manipulating energy deposition, modulating tissue interactions, or decreasing blood flow.[34] Specific tumor types and anatomic locations are predeterminates for the treatment plan. For example, an encapsulated tumor's thermal conduction behaves similar to the likes of an "oven effect," which allows for greater heat deposition and tissue burn. Conversely, a "heat sink" effect occurs with extracapsular lesions or tumors adjacent to large vessels in which the body's blood inflow creates a counter-cooling effect. Impaired heating based on suboptimal temperatures increase the risk of tumor regrowth or incomplete therapy. Unlike classic hyperthermia requiring long courses of hours-long exposure, RFA consists of a single application, 10 to 30 minutes (depending on device type) with a desired temperature range from 50° to 100° C.[34] Impediments to attaining optimal temperatures negatively impact treatment outcome as evidenced by failure to induce coagulation at temperatures less than 50° C and tissue vaporization or "charring" resulting in local impedance causing a reduction or variable coagulation in temperatures greater than 105° C.[35] The aim of minimally invasive ablation is to destroy the targeted tumor and to reduce the incidence of margin recurrence while limiting injury of surrounding healthy tissue by minimizing the ablation margin to 5 to 10 mm of normal tissue.[36] Although complete tumor necrosis volume is not met, coagulation necrosis can be seen as early as 3 to 7 days after therapy, which is the result of the tissue's loss of enzymatic function, including cytosolic lactic dehydrogenase (LDH) activity and mitochondrial enzyme activity.[37]

Changing probe technology has significantly influenced the clinician's ability to diversify treatment considerations. Historically, the genesis of monopolar devices once limited amenable field sizes to 1.6 cm with probe lengths of 0.9 cm has given rise to evolving treatment dimensions. Standard technology includes probes equipped with up to twelve multitined, expandable electrodes dispersed approximately 2.5 cm apart, powered with 50-watt

RF generators producing a treatment radius measuring up to a 3.5-cm ablation diameter to emerging evaluation of 250-watt generators affording treatment geometries up to 5 cm to 6 cm in diameter.[38-39] The synergistic technique between internal probe cooling and pulsing has resulted in greater coagulation necrosis and tumor destruction than either method alone.[40] Recent advances in techniques have resulted in larger target volume of tissue ablation without compromising safety or promoting collateral damage, yielding to the feasibility of treating larger tumors. There are three 510-K FDA-approved systems used for radiofrequency ablation; however, the two main strategies that have been developed to enlarge radiofrequency-induced lesions are the expandable multiple-array needle electrodes (Figure 21-1, *A*) and the electrode cooling (Figure 21-1, *B*). The expandable multiple-array needle consists of an insulated needle containing hook-shaped inner electrodes that can be deployed like umbrella ribs once the outer needle has been inserted into the tissue targeted for destruction. In this manner, after a single-needle insertion, radiofrequency can be applied at multiple sites, which has an additive effect, thus increasing the area of radiofrequency destruction.[41] The cooled-tip needle is made of a cluster of three single electrodes welded into three separate dual-lumen insulated cannulas with exposed tips of 2.5 cm in length. The cannulas are perfused with chilled saline to reduce the heat accumulated at the tip of each electrode, thereby allowing a higher current intensity to be deposited in tissue, especially tissue that is remote from the electrode. Both methods rely on the fact that the sum of the simultaneous adjacent multiprong ablation is greater than if each prong had been inserted separately.[40] de Baere and colleagues[39] compared these two RF devices on an in vivo pig liver and explanted calf livers. The study concluded the cooled-tip needle induced significantly larger lesions than the expandable needle, but the lesions produced by the expandable needle are more reproducible, uniform, and spheric. The larger size of the lesions produced by the cooled-tip needle was hypothesized to be attributed to the higher maximum power used by the generator and the higher energy deposition, which results in the cooling of the needle electrode.

Percutaneous Vertebroplasty

Metastatic cancer to bone is a frequent outcome of common malignancies and is often associated with significant morbidity caused by osteolysis.[42] Osteolytic metastasis or pathologic vertebral bodies (e.g., multiple myeloma) is also selective in that a disproportionately small number of malignancies account for the majority of tumors such as breast, prostate, and lung cancers, which spread to bone. Compounding this prevalence are the many therapeutic regimens in cancer treatment that carry the risk of causing or favoring the development of osteoporosis. This skeletal loss, characterized by low bone mass and micro-architectural deterioration of the bone tissue, is the result of an increase in fragility and risk of fracture. Of the 700,000 new cases in the United States annually, which join the over 7.8 million cases with osteoporosis, constituting approximately $17 million in healthcare system costs, at the time of diagnosis, about two-thirds are asymptomatic or unassociated with injury.[43] Further underscoring the pervasiveness, the IMPACT trial, a multicenter, multinational prospective study evaluated the accuracy of radiographic diagnosis of vertebral fractures in postmenopausal women 65 to 80 years of age and newly diagnosed with osteoporosis. Of the 2451 participants, 34% demonstrated a false-negative rate illustrating the incidence of misdiagnosis based on radiographic misinterpretation or underreporting.[44] Vertebral compression fractures (VCF) are the most common type of osteoporotic fractures, occurring most commonly at either the T12–L1 or T7–T8. Melton and colleagues[45] published a population study reviewing 429 men who had orchiectomies from 1956 to 2000 and compared the fracture risk to the community and found a 3.5-fold increase in risk. Estimates of the overall lifetime risk of an osteoporotic fracture for women is 16%, which is 2 to 4 times that of men at a 5% incidence. Overall, VCF correlate with a poorer overall survival and are an associated risk of future fractures. Contributing effects of hypogonadal functioning from suboptimal levels of testosterone, androgen, and estrogen negatively affects bone development, reabsorption, and increase bone matrix production. With either etiology, hypogonadism or metastatic osteolytic lesions, VCF symptom sequelae is primarily pain and immobility. VCF management of either benign or metastatic origin has varied from conservative to aggressive management with opioid and nonopioid therapy, physiotherapy, orthotic braces, calcitonin, and hormonal replacement therapy to radiation therapy, surgical fixation, chemotherapy, and bisphosphonates, respectively. These fractures interfere greatly with activities of daily living, and all of them can have a substantial negative impact on quality of life.

Percutaneous vertebroplasty (PV) and most recently, a newer technique called *kyphoplasty* are designed to treat such painful, nonhealing compression fractures of the spine resulting from osteoporosis, tumors, or trauma. The use of these image-guided, minimally invasive, nonsurgical therapies has significantly increased over the past 5 years. The number of procedures performed between 2001 and 2003 for kyphoplasties was 16,000 and vertebroplasties increased 28% from 38,000 to 48,000.[46] Historically, PV and kyphoplasty have followed different paths of development and distribution. The review of literature on PV revealed more than 350 published articles, which is predominately based on its development by academic medicine with refinement disseminated through peer-reviewed literature during the past 15 years. Conversely, kyphoplasty was introduced in the mid-1990s and marketed through commercial investment. Of the 40 articles, more than 30 are review articles that reflect a discussion limited to the technique rather than outcomes from kyphoplasty. These VCF management procedures can increase the patient's functional abilities, allow a return to the previous level of activity, and prevent future vertebral collapse in the targeted treatment area. In spite of this, PV or kyphoplasty are contraindicated for healed VCF and do not serve as a preventative treatment to help patients avoid future fractures.

Procedures and Technical Considerations

Developed in the mid 1980s, PV uses a fluoroscopy-guided approach for the insertion of a 11- to 13-gauge needle through the pedicle into the collapsed vertebral body. Achieved while in the prone position, a variety of introductory routes for needle delivery are possible, including the most classical, transpedicular, followed by parapedicular, posterolateral, and anterolateral.[47] Through a technique called *intraosseous venography*, the interventionalist determines the safety and appropriate placement of the trocar within the targeted vertebral space. McGraw and colleagues[48] found value of venograms with respect to showing a high correlation between venographic findings and cement distribution. Conversely, critics report no advantage or change in safety while withholding venography in more than 1500 cases, but rather inexperience, improper needle placement, uncontrolled cement application, or improper patient selection as factors that heighten complications rate.[49] Therefore, some long-term proponents have belatedly stopped its routine use and have become reliant on equipment advancement such as dynamic biplane views or C-arm fluoroscopy.[50] Once the trocar is placed properly, acrylic or calcium phosphate bone cement with a radiopaque quality for visualization is then injected directly into the vertebral body. Local pain can be partially or totally relieved with the injection of 1% lidocaine into the marrow space.[51] Some patients experience considerable bone pain during the injection of the cement, therefore sedation with opioids and anxiolytics are associated with PV whereas general anesthesia is used with kyphoplasty. Although comfortable or slightly drowsy, the patient is educated to report local or radicular pain that extends into the extremities. Continuous fluoroscopic monitoring is mandatory to ensure proper instillation of the cement. A lapse or breach of the targeted structure signals perivertebral extravasation, warranting immediate cessation to abate the risk of neurologic complications. Any sign of an adverse event triggers immediate search of the explanatory cause using imaging modalities and potentially hospitalization. Acting as a chemical reagent with a toothpaste-like viscosity, the cement expands creating thermal heat and encases the internal structure, acting as a splint. In approximately 20 minutes, the cement solidifies within the fracture lines, forming a supportive structure by stabilizing the fracture, reducing or eliminating pain, and often preventing future collapse[52] (Figure 21-2, *A–F*).

An alternative procedure, kyphoplasty uses the insertion of a tiny balloon into the bone's interior to create a void or cavity within the VCF. Identical to the needle cannula placement during PV, the two technical differences in kyphoplasty include a small dermatotomy incision and the use of a slightly larger 8-gauge needle to achieve the pre-collapse or anatomic restoration. These requirements serve to accommodate the additional balloon that is passed through the cannula and inflated in the vertebral body to house the instilled cement. In the circumstance of VCF caused by metastatic disease, it is critical that all anteroposterior and bilateral vertebral walls are in intact without epidural intrusion. A breach of anatomic structural support, especially in the posterior wall,

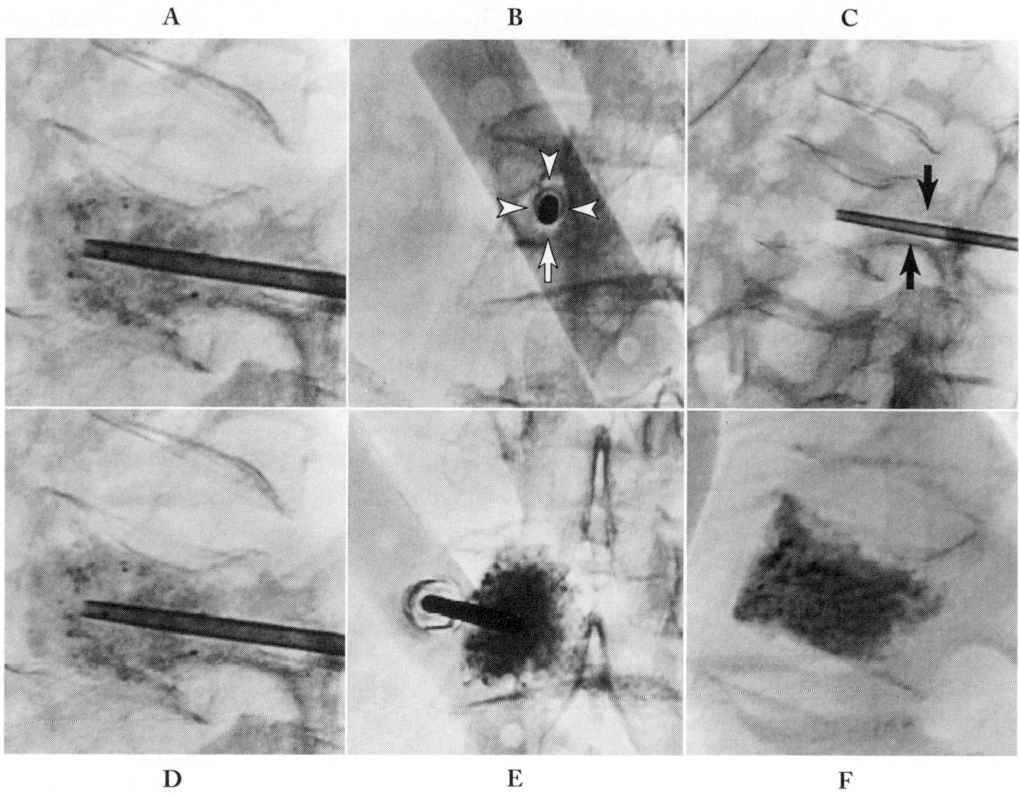

Figure 21-2 Vertebroplasty (VP). **A,** Percutaneous vertebroplasty. **B,** The pedicle to be punctured is marked and anesthetized. **C,** Biplane fluoroscopy is used to assess path of needle. **D,** Injection of PMMA is best seen on lateral fluoroscopy. **E,** PMMA usually respects the midline during instillation. **F,** Final image of vertebral stabilization
Courtesy of Asheville Radiology Associates.

may likely compromise the spinal canal causing paralysis. Palliative in nature, other therapies should be undertaken in the adjuvant management of malignant lesions. It is practical to sequence radiation therapy treatments after PV based on its often immediate analgesic effect when compared to the anticipated time-delayed pain reduction associated with external radiation. No modification of the radiation therapy protocols is necessary after cementation.[53]

In 2003, the Society of Interventional Radiology (SIR) Standards of Practice Committee convened a panel of experts who developed the quality improvement guidelines for PV.[54] Since that time, a gradually evolving body of knowledge related to definitions, indications, and outcome measures is emerging. Nevertheless, efficacy, outcome, and safety concerns regarding both treatment strategies remain unresolved. Yet, despite their inconclusive efficacy and safety profiles, PV and kyphoplasty are gaining rapid rising popularity and are expected to emerge as the greatest drivers of spinal surgery volume growth over the next several years, in part, because they offer the first advances in VCF treatment beyond bed rest and medication.[55] Limited, but promising, outcome data based on case reports suggest pain relief is achieved in 67% to 100% of patients with significant improvements in functioning and quality of life often occurring spontaneously or within 24 hours after intervention.[56-58] Mckiernan and colleagues[59] reported improvements in pain severity score and overall quality of life at 2 weeks, 2 months, and 6 months in all five domains of the Osteoporosis Quality of Life inventory ($p < 0.001$) in frail elderly subjects with a mean age of 73.4 years with a history of VCF on average of 2.5 months. The overall results of the procedure are individual based on subjective improvement in pain, reduction of analgesic therapy, enhanced ability for weight bearing, and restoration for range of motion and independence in performing activities of daily living. Partial or incomplete responses are measured as late as 7 days. Objective measures of improvement can be identified on plain films and contrast CT scans based on sagittal and coronal reconstructions of the intraosseous cement injection.

Long-term benefits have not yet been shown, but potentially include prevention of recurrent pain at the treated level(s) with both procedures and, with kyphoplasty, reversal of height loss and spinal deformity. Furthermore, the efficacy of these procedures has not been established in randomized, controlled trials. No studies have compared the two VCF treatments, and few studies compare either procedure to conventional treatment involving bed rest, bracing, and analgesics. One nonrandomized trial enrolled 79 consecutive patients with osteoporotic compression fractures and severe pain, of whom 55 chose vertebroplasty and 24 chose conservative therapy.[60] At 24 hours, pain scores had significantly decreased in the vertebroplasty group as compared with the conservative therapy group (55% versus 5% reduction in pain), and more patients were able to stop all analgesia (24% versus 0%). There were no significant differences in clinical outcomes at 6 weeks or at 6 to 12 months. Amidst safety concerns, these procedures are not without risk. To provide a broad view of the type and rate of complications in PV and kyphoplasty, the Food and Drug Administration's Manufacturer and User Facility Device Experience (MAUDE) database, details medical complications that occur with medical devices used in specific procedures.[61] A point of interest is that PV and kyphoplasty are classified and control guidance is addressed in this report as a medical device used in spinal vertebral body augmentation based on the bone cement polymethylmethacrylate (PMMA) classified under CFR 888.3027, class II (special controls).[62] In a document that outlined the scientific methodology for evaluating PMMA, on April 1, 2004, the FDA granted 510K approval for its use in VCF based on clinical trial considerations in the use of vertebral augmentation devices.[63] However, outside of a clinical trial, patients often were uninformed about the use of these non-FDA approved materials, assurance of safety, or description of delivery methods directed at PMMA variability such as cement admixture uniformity, consistent injection time, and the hydraulics associated with the administration.[64] Based on these early experiences and adverse events, the FDA issued in May 2004, a public health web notification based on complications related to the use of bone cement in the treatment of VCF.[65] Nussbaum and colleagues[66] reviewed the literature and manufacture's reports related to complications between 1999 and 2003 in PV and kyphoplasty procedures. Of the 53 patients, 33 underwent kyphoplasty with 5 lateral and 14 transpedicular approach vertebroplasties. Figure 21-3 demonstrates complication rates by procedure and/or needle approach. Kyphoplasty was associated with the largest number of acute procedural-related complications, yet both techniques have resulted in a variety of adverse events such as rare bleeding or anaphylaxis to increasing accounts of cement pulmonary embolism.[67,68] Spinal compressions occurred from either pedicle fracture or extravasations of cement requiring surgical decompression to prevent permanent paralysis.[69]

An overall comparison of PV's early complication occurrence rates reported a 1% to 3% incidence in the treatment of osteoporotic fractures and up to 10% for more serious metastatic lesions.[70] Possible long-term complications include local acceleration of bone reabsorption caused by the treatment itself or by foreign body reaction at the cement bone interface and increased risk of fracture in treated or adjacent vertebrae through changes in mechanical forces. A retrospective review of 177 patients treated with vertebroplasty found a high rate of new vertebral fractures.[71] Twenty-two patients developed 36 new vertebral body fractures. Of the 36 fractures, 67% involved vertebrae adjacent to a previously treated level, and 67% occurred within 30 days after the initial treatment.

Until there is conclusive evidence for efficacy and long-term safety, controlled clinical trials should be conducted in carefully selected patient populations using either procedure compared to a control group randomized to conservative management measures. Until this body of knowledge is generated, the current practice suggests that the best candidates appear to be older patients with focal, intense, deep pain, with evidence of a new or progressive vertebral fracture by plain radiography or MRI. Likewise, it is unknown whether the early management of new VCF is most beneficial in contrast to the period of time, costs, and sequelae in which conservative, noninvasive measures fail to yield benefit.

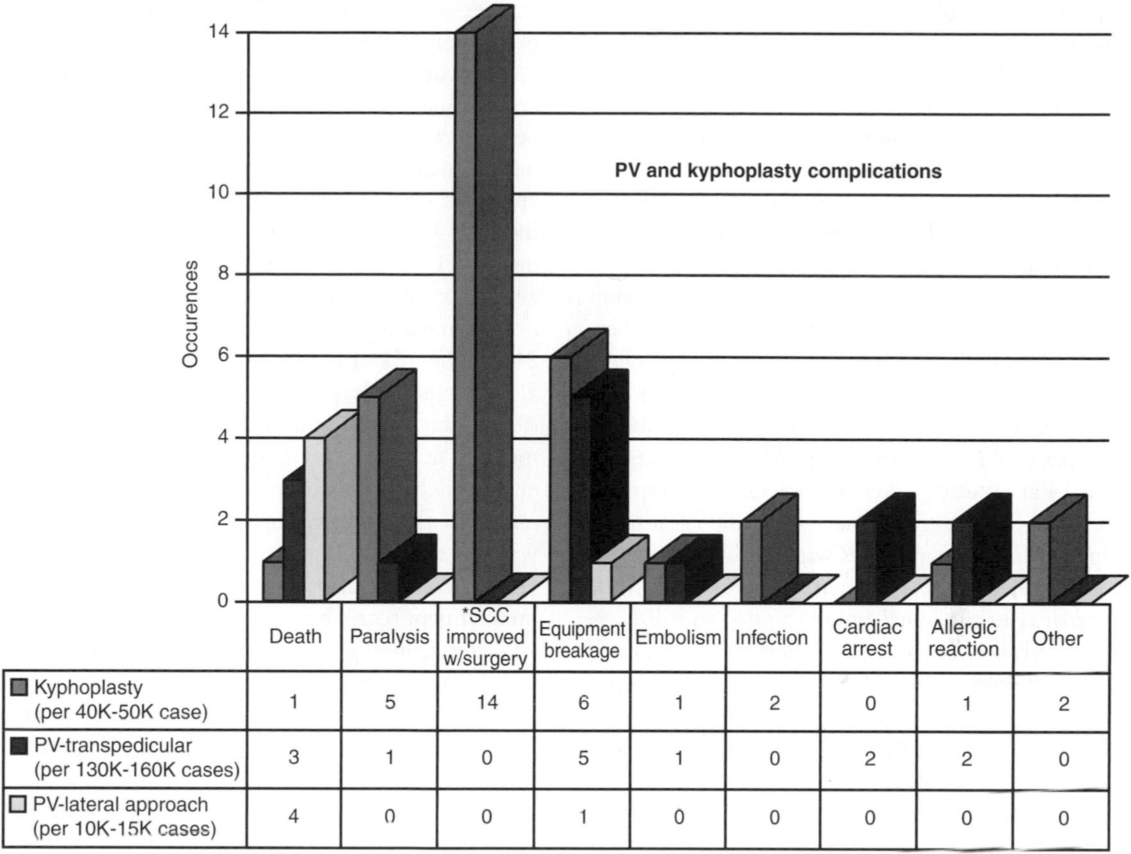

	Death	Paralysis	*SCC improved w/surgery	Equipment breakage	Embolism	Infection	Cardiac arrest	Allergic reaction	Other
Kyphoplasty (per 40K-50K case)	1	5	14	6	1	2	0	1	2
PV-transpedicular (per 130K-160K cases)	3	1	0	5	1	0	2	2	0
PV-lateral approach (per 10K-15K cases)	4	0	0	1	0	0	0	0	0

Figure 21-3 Percutaneous Vertebroplasty (PV) and Kyphoplasty Complication Rates by Event Type.
SCC, Spinal cord compression.
Data from Nussbaum DA, Gailloud P, Murphy K: A review of complications associated with vertebroplasty and kyphoplasty as reported to the Food and Drug Administration Medical Device related web site, J Vasc Interv Radiol 15(11):1185–1192, 2004.

INTRODUCTION OF VASCULAR INTERVENTIONAL RADIOLOGY TECHNIQUES

Superselective Intraarterial Chemotherapy

Head and neck cancers refractory to primary treatment present a therapeutic challenge at the time of recurrence. Various modalities including prolonged infusions followed by intraarterial (IA) chemotherapy were tested in the late 1970s; results were poor and excessive complications were noted. Recent developments challenging this notion suggest a need to reevaluate other promising strategies in the presence of these historically restricted options.[72] Under the direction of an interventional radiologist, newer and safer angiographic techniques now permit placement of microcatheters into the smallest arteries relative to a tumor's anatomic blood supply under direct vision using fluoroscopy.[73] Superselective intraarterial chemotherapy is usually limited to advanced/bulky or recurrent tumors of the oral cavity, oropharynx, hypopharynx, or larynx and which are functionally or anatomically unresectable and for which multimodality chemotherapy, radiation, ± surgery was initially used but failed to achieve durable response.[72] These advances make it possible to selectively and repeatedly infuse agents into the territory of a tumor bed's blood supply with minimal catheter-related complications.[74]

Procedures and Technical Considerations

Targeted superselective IA infusion permits the tumor bed to receive 5 times the drug level concentrations that otherwise are not tolerated because of organ toxicity. Robbins and colleagues[75] conducted a phase I study of 213 patients with advanced head and neck cancer to determine the maximum-tolerated dose (MTD) of cisplatin that could be administered intraarterially. The MTD was 150 mg/m^2/week for 4 weeks. When radiation therapy was administered concomitantly with targeted cisplatin chemotherapy, preliminary observations indicated an extremely high complete pathologic response rate, sustained disease control above the clavicles, and a relatively low rate of toxicity.[76] In an attempt to further answer the question of feasibility, tolerance, and efficacy, the Radiation Therapy Oncology Group (RTOG 96–15) opened a phase II study in which of the 61 eligible subjects, 87% were able to complete all proposed therapy (47 at inexperienced and 14 at experienced centers). Complete response (CR) was 85% at the primary site and 85% at nodal regions, and the overall CR was 80%. At the median follow up of 3.9 years (range, 0.9 to 6.1 years), the estimated locoregional tumor control and disease-free survival rates were 66% and 62% at 1 year and 57% and 46% at 2 years.[77] In 2004, Kovacs[78] replicated the RTOG study design; however, stages I to II treatment naïve patients were included. As a conclusion, it can be stated that IA high-dose chemotherapy with cisplatin and systemic neutralization in a neoadjuvant setting should be considered a feasible, safe, and effective treatment modality for resectable oral and oropharyngeal cancer. The overall clinical local response has been 69%. There was no interference with surgery, which was carried out 3 to 4 weeks later. Pathologic complete remission was assessed in 25%. The mean observation time was 3 years. A 3-year overall and disease-free survival was 82% and 69%, respectively, and at 5 years 77% and 59%, respectively.

The steps of technical administration require synchronization between the interventionalist, radiology technologists, and a chemotherapy certified nurse. Cisplatin (CDDP, cip-diaminedichloroplatinum) 150 mg/m^2 is arterially instilled rapidly by a pressure injector. Because of the chemotherapy concentration, which exceeds a systemically tolerable dose, a bolus dose of sodium thiosulfate at 9 g/m^2 IV is administered intravenous 30 seconds before the CDDP. A subsequent infusion of sodium thiosulfate at 12 g/m^2 IV over 6 hours acts as an antagonist to neutralize the CDDP before it recirculates through the venous system. After the CDDP passes through the tumor bed, the sodium thiosulfate's chelating effects abate potential organ and mucosal toxic effects. The optimal treatment cycle is 4 weekly based on acceptable arterial tolerance and patient response.[77]

Few studies have been conducted to evaluate the longitudinal impact of the patient's functional well-being. Ackerstaff[79] conducted the only study evaluating the quality of life of patients with advanced head and neck cancers who had undergone IA chemotherapy. Of the 26 patients available for QOL assessment at 1 year, the functional well-being and head and neck scales showed a statistically significant improvement over time ($P < .001$). After 12 months, 21 patients (81%) returned to an oral diet, whereas 5 patients still needed tube feeding. For 23 patients (88%), the quality and strength of the voice was more or less normal. Of the 18 patients who were employed before their treatment, 10 were able to return to their job within 12 months. Xerostomia was reported by 17 patients (65%). Further detailed analysis showed statistically significant differences in pretreatment scores between the 1-year QOL group and the failure group, when comparing physical well-being, functional well-being, and the head and neck scales ($P < .05$). Differences in these groups with respect to gender, age, tumor site, or stage could not be found.

Murray[80] studied the acute and chronic changes in swallowing and quality of life after intraarterial chemoradiation (CR) for organ preservation in patients with advanced head and neck cancer. The results indicate that QOL and swallowing function decrease acutely during chemoradiation ($p < .05$), but improvement begins shortly after the treatment-related decline. At 6 months after chemoradiation, mean QOL exceeded pretreatment level. The oropharynx patients have the poorest outcome when compared with laryngeal and hypopharyngeal patients. A stronger correlation exists between swallowing and QOL at 6 months after chemoradiation than during treatment ($R = .52$ versus $R = .30$). Quality of life and swallowing are compromised in advanced head and neck cancer patients before treatment. There was a further decrease in QOL and swallow function during chemoradiation. The results suggest that organ-preservation programs in head and neck cancer contribute to improved QOL and swallowing 6 months after treatment.

With respect to improving candidate eligibility, a study measuring a pretreatment probability model for predicting outcome after intraarterial chemoradiation for advanced head and neck carcinoma, van den Broek and colleagues[81] found that tumor volume was found to play a significant role in predicting local control and overall survival in patients with advanced-stage head and neck carcinoma who were treated with targeted chemoradiation.

The low toxicity of this local chemotherapy recommends usage especially in stage 1 to 2 patients. However, to thoroughly evaluate potential benefits, a prospective, controlled randomized trial is warranted to compare the role of superselective IA infusion to the present chemoradiation standard for the management of early head and neck cancer. Others argue that the best results of IA chemotherapy have not surpassed the best response rates from IV chemotherapy, and when combined with the increased risk of local toxicity, there is no advantage to this approach.[82]

Percutaneous Transcatheter Embolization

Percutaneous transcatheter embolization (PTE) is a safe and effective delivery method resulting in vascular channel occlusion or obliteration. Embolization, broadly defined, is the "plugging up" and is virtually transferable in every vascular territory to arrest hemorrhage, to occlude congenital and acquired vascular abnormalities, to palliate neoplasms, and to ablate tissue. Embolic vascular occlusion is accomplished by the intravascular deposit of chemical or radioactive particulate, liquid, mechanical agents, or autologous blood clot to produce intentional vessel occlusion. These obstructions may be performed at any level for large arteries or veins to the capillary beds and may be temporary or permanent in nature. The technique of transarterial chemotherapy embolization (TACE) or chemoembolization works in two ways: (1) by delivering high-concentration chemotherapy directly into the tumor to avoid systemic exposure of otherwise unsafe drug and (2) cutting off the tumor's blood supply, depriving oxygen and nutrients and trapping the drug at the tumor site to enhance and prolong cytotoxic exposure. With the advent of infinite access to lesions through microcatheter delivery systems, direct visualization enhancement with the use of low osmolarity contrast material, high-resolution digital imaging, and road mapping, percutaneous transcatheter embolization has transcended the historically limited inventory of disease-controlling and palliative measures now amenable by minimally invasive strategies.

Procedures and Technical Considerations

Numerous factors determine the technique and materials used for embolization procedures that influence the goals, response, and duration of benefit.

The Society of Interventional Radiologist's (SIR) *Quality Improvement Guidelines for Percutaneous Transcatheter Embolization* (2003) defined the important processes of care related to (1) patient selection, (2) procedure performance, and (3) patient monitoring in addition to prescribing definitions, indications, techniques, and outcome measures based on success and complication rates.[83] Successful embolization results in devascularization and intentional reduction or cessation of blood flow to a target vascular bed or an entire organ. The target area is defined as the focal lesion, vessel, vascular territory, or organ requiring an interruption of its nutrient blood supply by means of ischemia or obstruction within the immediate distributed target. Conversely, nontarget embolization is the unintentional deposition of embolic materials distant from the treatment site, which may be accompanied by increased complications and result in inferior management of the primary lesion. Strategic planning is required to ensure collateral circulation is preserved to organs or structures that are dependent and subordinate to the targeted treatment area, such as superior mesenteric artery branches supplying the vasa recta of the small and large bowel, which if interrupted may cause bowel infarction.[84]

Results and side effects are measured at the periprocedural, interim, and latent period longitudinally.

Success is measured by technical (immediate results evaluated by radiograph) and clinical outcomes (30 days immediately after the procedure determined by patient follow-up) and be complete (total resolve of presenting signs or symptoms) or partial (significant improvement, with a positive impact on the overall disease process; retreatment is often possible, yet often with a potential for diminished return) in nature. Palliative embolization is considered a success if there is reduction in symptom distress. Specific indications and relative criteria for patient referral should govern patients deemed potentially eligible for the procedures as well as calculated risk-benefit ratio necessary to safely and effectively execute the treatment plan. In oncology settings in which controlled trials, benchmarking, and case reports have illustrated therapeutic embolization, the primary indication is for the control of hemorrhage and the palliation of pain and other symptoms associated with malignant tumors. The incidences of complications are dependent on operator experience, vascular territory, the specific lesion addressed, and on the clinical condition of the patient. Oncology patients with hemodynamic instability, multiorgan failure, coagulopathy, and infection will have higher complication rates.[85] Complications are stratified on the basis of outcome and severity. Major complications result in unplanned admission or rise in level of care, prolonged hospitalization, permanent sequelae, or death. In experienced hands, the rate of severe complications is acceptable and ranges from 2% to 7%.[86] Known contraindications for this technique are portal vein thrombosis, encephalopathy, and biliary obstruction. Relative contraindications include serum bilirubin more than 2 mg/dL; LDH more than 425 U/L, AST more than 100U/L; tumor burden involving 50% of the liver, cardiac or renal insufficiency; ascites, recent cardiac bleed, or significant thrombocytopenia. Lladó and colleagues[87] described prognostic index and pretreatment independent predictors of worse survival were associated with the serum AFP concentration of more than 400U/L, tumor volume more than 50% of normal liver, and increasing Child-Pugh score. Posttreatment independent predictors of worse survival included the presence of portal vein thrombosis and diffuse heterogeneous uptake of lipiodol on CT.

Systemic toxicities in addition to the side effects from embolization include nausea, vomiting, low-grade fever (83%), right upper quadrant pain (100%), leukocytosis, and increased liver function tests that constitute *postembolization syndrome* (PES).[10] Leung and colleagues[88] performed 70 TACE procedures in 29 patients and found clinically relevant predictors of the severity of PES and length of postprocedural hospitalization. Embolization of the gallbladder and chemoembolic dose administered were found to be associated with an increased risk of PES, whereas previous embolization was associated with a reduced risk. However, in the absence of an evidence-based, predictive algorithm that can identify individuals at highest risk, the current review of literature places the incidence of PES between 15.1% and 100%. The etiology of pain is not well understood, but some theories postulated include distension of the liver capsule, acute ischemia of the liver parenchyma, and tumor necrosis. At the time of the instillation, patients may report an acute, sharp right upper quadrant pain, followed by a deeper visceral pain, most likely caused by the swelling of the liver and stretching of the capsule that contains the nerve fibers.[89] The most common strategy to pain management is the use of intravenous opioid; however, celiac plexus block intraarterial lidocaine studies yielded significant reductions in intra- and post-procedural pain, as did parenteral morphine compared to conventional intravenous opioid alone.[89,90] Depending on severity, this syndrome necessitates medication therapies to maximize relief of symptom distress consisting of patient-controlled analgesia (PCA) delivered opioids, antiemetics, and hydration. Prophylactic antibiotics may be used to offset fevers, which are common for up to 1 week posttreatment. This syndrome lasts for 2 to 3 days, with some symptoms lasting up to 10 days, with the resolution of symptoms coincident with liver function tests returning to close to baseline levels.

Hepatic Artery Embolization

The most common treatment indication is hepatic artery embolization (HAE), an alternative therapy for patients who have become refractory to other treatment modalities and are not candidates for hepatic resection from either primary hepatocellular cancer (HCC) or liver metastasis from colon, islet cell carcinomas, carcinoid tumors, or metastatic neuroendocrine tumors.[91-93] Surgical resection of HCC is the treatment choice and represents the only potentially curative option. However, only 10% to 15% of patients have disease that meets the criteria for surgical resection.[94] Llovet and colleagues[95] illustrate, as shown in Figure 21-4, a decision-making model for the management of HCC by stage and liver severity scores (Child-Pugh; Okuda) to derive a treatment base plan. The concept of HAE was developed in Japan in the early 1980s by Nakamura, who injected iodized oil (lipiodol) into HCC neovasculature.[96]

The liver is the second most common site of metastatic disease from extrahepatic primary tumors, following nodal spread, with approximately 30% of cancer patients having liver involvement at the time of death.[97] The liver is a unique organ in that it has a dual blood supply, receiving three-fourths from the portal vein and one fourth from the hepatic artery. The majority of the nutritive blood flow to the hepatocytes is via the portal vein, whereas the nutritive blood flow to hepatic tumor

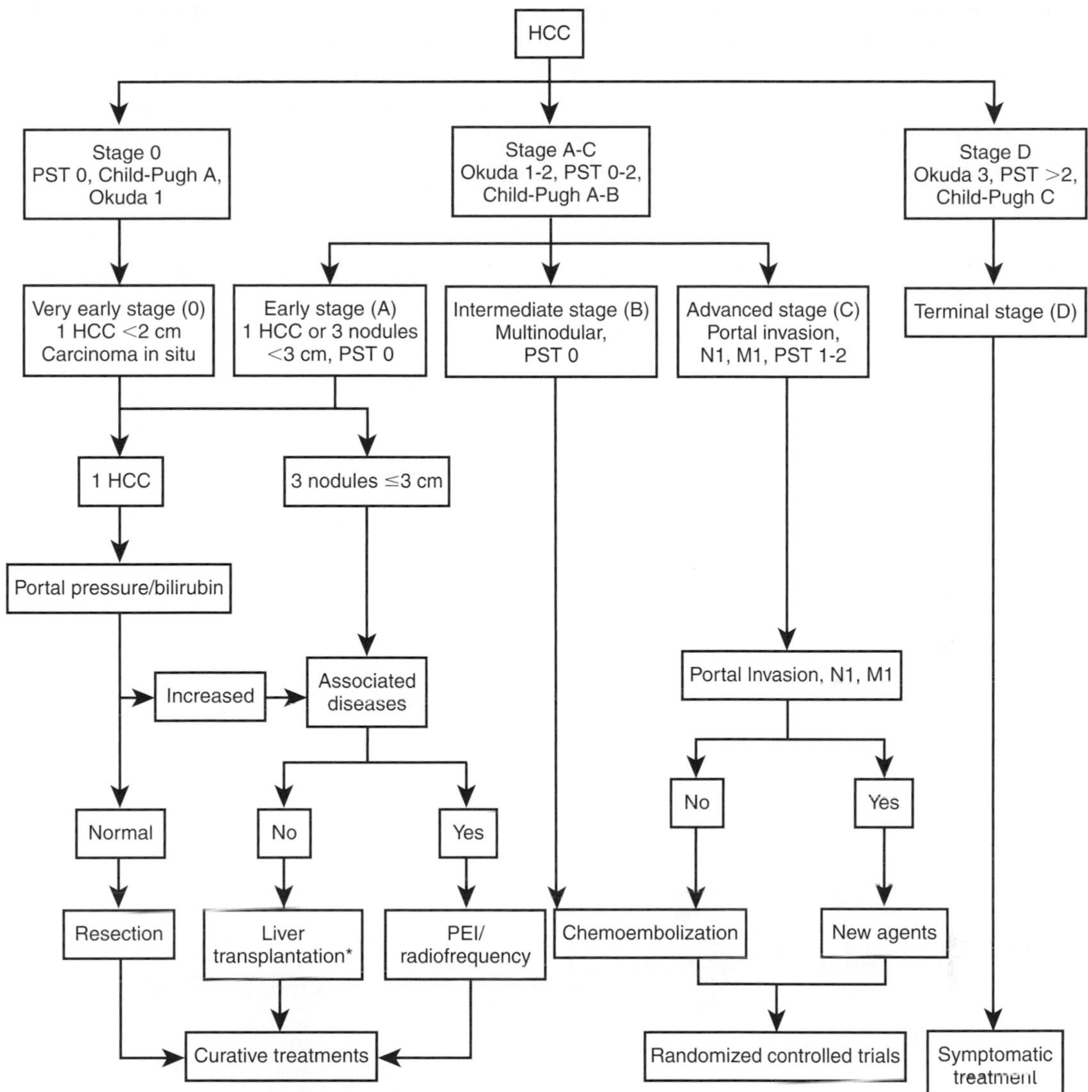

Figure 21-4 Barcelona-clinic Liver Cancer Staging Classification and Treatment Schedule. Illustrates a decision-making model for the management of HCC by stage and liver severity scores.
PST, Performance status test; *N*, nodules; *M*, metastases; *PEI*, percutaneous ethanol injection. *Cadaveric liver transplantation or living donor liver transplantation.
Reproduced with permission. Modified from Llovet JM, Burroughs A, Bruix J: Lancet 362(9399):1907-1917, 2003. Copyright © 2003 Elsevier.

cells is primarily via the hepatic artery.[98] Roughly 80% to 90% of any agent placed into the hepatic artery will lodge in the feeding arterioles to the tumor. This accounts for significant tumor necrosis. A range of materials may be used to embolize the affected arteries. Current techniques of HAE include embolization with particulate agents (polyvinyl alcohol, Gelfoam powder [UpJohn, Kalamazoo, Mich], microfibrillary collagen), synthetic microencapsulated chemotherapy drug(s), transcatheter oily chemoembolization with iodized oil mixed with a cytotoxic agent, and hepatic arterial chemoembolization with a single or combination of chemotherapeutic agents mixed with embolic particulates.[99] The strategic advantage of embolization is to allow greater concentrations of chemotherapeutic agents within a tumor. It has been reported that the concentration of chemotherapy within tumor tissue can be 10 to 100 times higher after chemoembolization than after systemic chemotherapy.[100] The collaborative decision between the oncologist and interventionalist as to which product or formula to use is individualized based on the treatment goals as to the effect, degree, and duration of the obstruction desired, technical strategies to select or protect adjacent vascular passages, and the intended confinement within the target. Based on this discernment, combinations of these embolic materials may be used in conjunction with certain single or combination chemotherapies such as doxorubicin, cisplatin, and mitomycin-C in a technique called *chemoembolization*[86,101] (Figure 21-5). Most chemotherapeutic agents (even a single agent) are often made by the oncologist in collaboration with the interventionalist at doses of 50 mg, 100 mg/m^2, and 20 mg/m^2, respectively. Most chemotherapeutic agents used have been those that either are activated by the liver or do not require systemic activation before they become tumoricidal. Once identified, a cocktail of chemotherapy drugs dissolved in contrast material and emulsified in a 1:1 ratio with Ethiodol are mixed to aid visualization of the selected embolic material to be instilled into the target. Several embolization materials commonly used include gelatin USP granules, polyvinyl alcohol particles, steel coils, detachable balloons, and glues with or without antineoplastic agents.

The present technical limitations leading to inferior treatment penetration include displacement of the embolic material including irregular separation of the admixture, intravascular loss of product outside the target through catheter misplacement, and particle aggregate and clumping.[102] The response

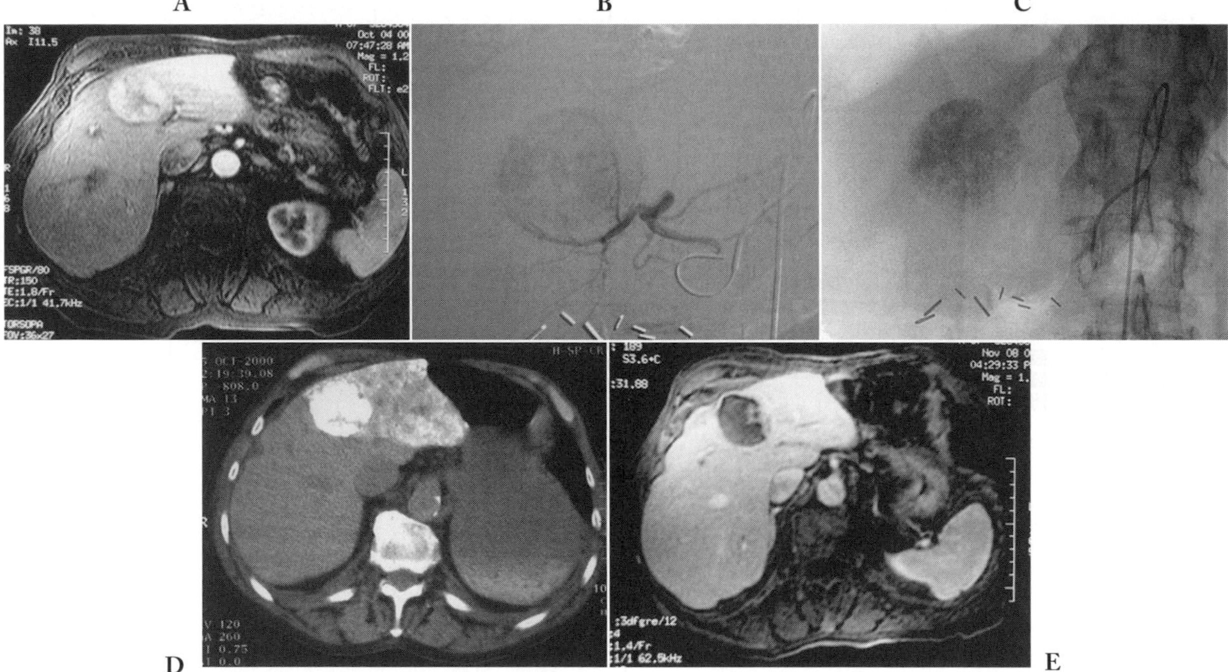

Figure 21-5 Chemoembolization. **A,** Gadolinium-enhanced magnetic resonance image (MRI) of the liver in a patient with a focal hepatoma located in segment 4. Note the fairly homogeneous enhancement pattern, which is suggestive of viable tumor. **B,** Selective left hepatic arteriogram obtained via a 3-F microcatheter that had been advanced farther distally coaxially through a 5-F catheter. In this case, given the single focus of tumor, superselective placement of the catheter was highly recommended. **C,** Postchemoembolization fluoroscopic image shows excellent distribution of the lipiodol within the tumor, which is consistent with technical success of the chemoembolization. **D,** Unenhanced CT scan of the abdomen helps confirm the findings in *C.* Again, this is consistent with the technical success of the chemoembolization procedure. **E,** Gadolinium-enhanced MR image of the liver obtained after chemoembolization. The tumor has been nearly completely destroyed, and no residual enhancement is visible.

From Ramsey DE, Kernagis LY, Soulen MC, et al: J Vasc Interv Radiol 13(9 Pt 2):S211–S221, 2002.

rates associated with embolization are measured by radiographic regression or a decrease in either hormonal secretion alpha fetoprotein (AFP) (carcinoid tumors), carcinoembryonic antigen (CEA). Hepatic arterial embolization and chemoembolization have demonstrated an objective tumor response ranging from 17% to 58% in selected cohorts of patients and have been shown to prolong survival only in nonrandomized studies with the transient duration of response ranging from 4 to 24 months in uncontrolled series.[92,99,103-105] In one of the largest series of 81 patients undergoing embolization or chemoembolization for carcinoid tumor, the median duration of response was 17 months, and the probability of progression-free survival at 1, 2, and 3 years was 75%, 35%, and 11%, respectively.[92] Follow-up hepatic and tumor marker values and cross-sectional imaging may be obtained 1 month after completion of therapy and every 3 months thereafter to monitor response. Additional chemoembolization procedures may be undertaken if there is evidence of tumor progression in terms of rising AFP levels or enlarging hepatic lesions.

Treatment-associated morbidity, which can include abdominal pain, nausea, elevated liver function tests, and infection, needs to be weighed against the potential benefits of this procedure. Brown and colleagues[106] compared two classifications systems that determine the severity of liver disease, the Child-Pugh and the Model for End-stage Liver Disease (MELD), to predict patient survival after TACE. Findings validated the scores correlated well between the two scales; however, Child-Pugh was a better predictor of overall survival ($r = -0.35$, $p = .04$) of the laboratory findings, albumin level was the most useful predictor of survival.

The future of HAE is evolving along with new techniques and combination interventional therapies. Microsphere technology advances provide an "all-in-one" delivery system of either chemotherapy or selective internal radioisotopes (yttrium-90; I-131 labeled lipiodol) combined with either a resorbable or nonresorbable embolization materials.[107] These microsphere brachytherapy yttrium-90 beta-emitting spheres (SIRsphere, Sirtex, Perth, Australia) have a half-life of 64.2 hours and a penetration depth in tissue of 4 to 8 mm. With the advent of new microdosimetry measures, most of the tumor can receive 1000 Gy, and the margin of the tumor can receive 100 Gy with a less than 30 Gy decline within 1 cm of the tumor margin.[108] In previously published work comparing the survival of patients with metastatic colorectal cancer with use of intraarterial 5-FU/leucovorin with or without a single administration of SIRsphere, a greater than double survival was found for the chemotherapy + SIRsphere group (27 versus 13 months).[109] Advances over the current sequential delivery of various agents translate to strengthening of carcinolytic effect, reduction in tumoral drug clearance, and prolonged tumor drug contact. In vivo and in vitro studies have shown that the microsphere's precise calibration and perfectly spherical shape ensures total occlusion with optimization of sterility, mechanical and thermal stability, and hydrophilic and cationic surface charges that initiate and improve cell adhesion with heighten particle penetration (75% to 100%) compared to nonparticle (66%).[110,111] In 2000 Dancey and colleagues[112] studied the use of intrahepatic arterial injection of yttrium-90 (90Y) microspheres in patients with HCC. Since then, emerging data has demonstrated treatment tolerability (radiation gastritis managed with antacids and H2 blockers), acceptable response rates (20%) with dose ranges on average of 104 Gy (range, 45 Gy to 145 Gy) higher than allowable through external beam. The median duration of response was 127 weeks, the median time to progression was 44 weeks, and the median survival was 54 weeks.[113] Ultimately, randomized controlled trials will be needed to compare the efficacy with historical nonsurgical therapies.[114]

CARE CONSIDERATIONS

The radiation oncology nurse needs to understand the procedural phases of delivering interventional therapies and the impact that they have on patients. Patient and family education includes a description of the underlying disease, thorough review of the risks, benefits, and alternatives to all treatment management strategies, ensuring steps to validate competency and obtain voluntary informed consent for pre-, intra-, and postprocedure care, a description of the IR equipment and environment, interactive reporting, and aggressive symptom management. The use of anatomic models and diagrams assists in simplifying the procedure description, reduces threatening terminology, and encourages one to ask questions and express concerns about the treatment. The following summation describes the procedural care strategies for vascular and nonvascular modalities.

Preprocedure Care

Multiple factors influence a treatment's efficacy, benefits, and risks. Risks are kept to a minimum when a comprehensive history and physical examination incorporate the use of the American Society of Anesthesiology (ASA) physical status classification preparation for sedation. Diagnostic radiographic images including CT, MRI, ultrasound, PET, and PET/CT also should be evaluated to determine the optimal treatment recommendation. Determining visceral organ targets, tumor measurement, location of intra- or extracapsular lesion(s) and proximity of vital organs and large vessels is done to predict the most safe and effective interventional approach. Conversely, prescreening of vertebral targets includes the presence of persistent pain correlated by CT or MRI radiographic confirmation of vertebra collapse, structural integrity of vertebra's posterior wall, and secondary origins of pain such as herniated disc have been eliminated.

In general, vascular and nonvascular modalities are performed on an outpatient basis under conscious sedation in a special procedure room in the radiology department. However, in complex cases often associated with larger lesions, general anesthesia and overnight observation is preferred, thereby enabling adequate supervision and nursing interventions for potential residual symptom distress.

Preprocedure blood tests including coagulation panels (PT [prothrombin time], a PTT [partial thromboplastin time], INR [international normalized ratio]), hematologic and organ functionality (CBC [complete blood count] with differential, BUN [blood urea nitrogen], creatinine, hepatic panel, and appropriate tumor markers) are analyzed for abnormalities. Medication therapies affecting coagulation, platelet aggregation inhibition, and agents used in the management of bleeding disorders or deficiencies require explicit instruction to modify or abstain dosages often 12 to 24 hours before procedure. If indicated, a pregnancy test for candidates of childbearing potential will in advance identify fetal presence and ultimately avoid unwarranted radiation exposure.

Information ascertained about current medications also should include drug allergies/intolerances, past experience with radiopaque contrast medium, and substance abuse history. Likewise, special considerations for diabetic patients require either holding or reducing oral hyperglycemic agents or insulin. Metformin use should be abated 48 hours before procedure because of the heightened risk of poor renal clearance associated with contrast dyes commonly used to assist in the target site localization process. Capillary blood glucose (CBG) levels are obtained before and every 4 hours throughout the procedure. Results ranging between 40 and 70 and more than 200 require intervention and prompt reporting to the physician.

An accurate account of the time and quality of oral intake leading into the event is critical to preventing avoidable physiologic complications. In both PTE and IA procedures, patients are generally admitted to the hospital the evening before for intravenous hydration at 150 mL/hr. Otherwise, unless contraindicated for fluid restricted patients, in both vascular- and nonvascular-based treatments withstanding PV, adjustments to assert oral hydration by 2 liters for 24 to 28 hours pre- and postprocedure is recommended to compensate for risks associated with rapid tumor necrosis. The day before, patients are usually restricted to clear liquids for 12 hours, followed by being NPO (nothing by mouth) past midnight. Conversely, in the case of emergent, nonelective cases, minimal fasting period of ingested materials is 2 to 4 hours for clear liquids or 6 hours for a light meal.[115] Invasive procedures, sedative and opioid agents, and supine positioning are known to heighten the emetogenic potential and are associated with an increased chance of inadvertent aspiration. Prokinetic medications, such as metoclopramide to increase gastric motility and emptying, histamine receptor antagonist to decrease gastric pH, and prophylactic antiemetics (5HT antagonist and dexamethasone) as single or combination agents are recommended to reduce the consequence of aspiration in patients prone to gastric reflux.

Infections remain one of the more common complications of invasive procedures. Despite minimally invasive procedures and aggressive technology, the risk for infection can never be eliminated based on the incidence of virulent strains, emerging antibiotic resistant clones, increasing immunocompromised populations, and more aggressive interventional procedures. The widespread use of prophylactic antibiotics in IR is believed to be beneficial and a practice standard, in spite of the lack of randomized controlled clinical trials demonstrating benefit of the use of antibiotics in this setting.[116] Patients also may be discharged on a short course of antibiotics to minimize risk postprocedure. Nevertheless, with most PTE and RFA used at discretion in IA cases, prophylactic antibiotics such as cefazolin 1 g then 500 mg Q8hr and metronidazole 500 mg Q12hr is prevalent in covering anaerobic and Gram + pathogens.[88]

Intraprocedure Care

Once positioned on the table in the IR suite, patients are advised to lay still, and passive immobilization devices are used to reduce injury associated with unanticipated or sudden patient movement. Under sterile conditions, a small skin incision is made to accommodate internalized devices such as microcatheters, probes, or needles that are being placed. The introduction of a single probe in RFA and a trocar needle in PV is placed directly over the targeted treatment site. However, in PTE and IA cases, an indirect entrance via the femoral artery houses the introduction of the microcatheter through which all agents are delivered. Through this catheter, angiography is performed by briskly delivering 1 to 2 mL of contrast material into the catheter to map the path through the artery leading to the targeted site. By fluoroscopic visualization, the anatomic destination is located by tracing these "puffs" of dye that guide catheter advancement to the final tumor destination.

Interventional procedures necessitate trained nursing personnel with expertise in the pharmacologic, physiologic, and clinical management of the patient receiving sedation and analgesia.[117] This prerequisite is essential in practice environments outside the operating room in which nonanesthesiologists are designated to conduct, monitor, and document level of consciousness, airway patency, oxygen therapy, continuous SpO_2 (functional oxygen saturation), end-tidal carbon dioxide ($ETCO_2$), vital signs, ECG (electrocardiogram), and administer pharmacologic agents that depress the central nervous system to promote conscious sedation.[118] The nurse monitoring the equipment communicates physiologic data throughout the procedure to other staff so early signs of potential complications can be minimized. Pre- and intraprocedural anxiolytics with midazolam and fentanyl are administered in titrated dosages for patient comfort in which the goal is to achieve moderate sedation while attempting to avoid deep sedation necessitating the introduction of mechanical airway protection. Prudent administration will reduce the chance of regular or premature use of reversal agents (opioid-naloxone; flumazenil-benzodiazepine antagonists), which can precipitate the patient's anxiety response. However, when spontaneous ventilatory efforts and airway or circulatory control are compromised, judicious use and appraisal of antagonists should be employed to ensure the duration of effect and reversal of the cardiorespiratory depression has been resolved. Although the "gold standard," pulse oximetry monitoring of oxygenation is not a substitute for monitoring ventilatory function. In a prospective trial comparing clinical detection of sedation levels using $ETCO_2$ monitoring devices in the presence of various anxiolytics, Miner and colleagues[119] compared pulse oximetry to $ETCO_2$ monitoring to determine levels of sedation and patient safety. Of those monitored, 80% had respiratory depression when combining opioids with anxiolytics, with the most sensitive indication associated with the $ETCO_2$ monitored group. Hence, deeply sedated patients can hypoventilate and become hypercapnic without being hypoxic if they are given supplemental oxygen.[120] End-tidal CO_2 monitoring allows noninvasive monitoring of respiratory rate and may detect respiratory depression sooner than pulse oximetry. In October 2005, the American Society of Anesthesiologists Task Force on Perioperative Management of Patients with Obstructive Sleep Apnea recommended that patients receiving moderate or deep sedation have continuous respiratory CO_2 monitoring.[121] Although specialized equipment is required, in-line $ETCO_2$ monitoring of exhaled CO_2 can be performed on a patient via devices that mutually deliver oxygen therapy and should be considered for all patients receiving moderate or deep sedation. Therefore, prudent application of agents should be employed based on patient characteristics; small, incremental dosages; allowance for time to effect; and the use of an evidenced-based scoring system that measures the depth of sedation, for example, the Ramsey scale. Known high-risk groups susceptible for heighten sedation effect include pediatric patients; the elderly; patients with pharmacologic naivety, airway restrictive conditions (COPD [chronic obstructive pulmonary disease], obstructive sleep apnea); obesity; or coronary artery disease; and those with renal and hepatic organ dysfunction. In a study of over 6500 diagnostic radiology tests that reported on safety, it was found that radiology nurses with specialized training demonstrated lower costs, shorter sedation periods, and few complications compared to general nursing personnel.[122] Findings further suggested that during inadequate sedation, prolonged procedure times were attributed to patient motion hampering imaging quality and increased need for midprocedural suspension because of the risk of movement-related injury leading to prolonged room use. Conversely, oversedation contributed to extended recovery time, delays in start times for subsequent cases, and increased complication rates.

The risk of bleeding may occur either at the site of insertion or within the depth of the treatment focus or as a complication from adjacent highly vascular anatomic structures. During intraarterial entrances, vascular damage, postprocedural insertion site bleeding and pseudoaneurysm formation are directly related to the puncture hole site most often with catheter sizes above 9 Fr.[13] During RFA, both the thermal treatment affects and cauterization of the probe's exit track ensure hemostasis at the procedure's closure accounting for the overall low rate of bleeding.[123] Intraarterial routed catheters may include the intraprocedural use of low-dose heparin for thrombosis prophylaxis. At the close of a vascular-based procedure but before the removal of the catheter sheath, prolonged activated partial thromboplastin time (aPTT) or activated clotting time (ACT) values ACT are performed to determine appropriate coagulation levels values based on physician or institutional protocol. Normalization of aPTT and ACT values is an indication that the sheath may be removed, and manual or a femoral compression device is then applied.

Postprocedure Care

Patients may continue to be at significant risk for developing complications after their procedures. Vital signs, procedural site inspection, and comprehensive pain assessment are performed per institutional protocol or a prudent schedule to include Q15 × 4, Q30 × 1 hour, and hourly × 4. Intravenous or oral opioid therapy is the gold standard for the visceral or somatic-oriented pain. Mild and transient osseous pain occurring during PV is often relieved with nonsteroidal antiinflammatory agents. For extreme pain severity associated with the targeted organ or radicular shoulder and flank pain unrelieved with intermittent opioids, hospitalization and patient-controlled analgesia (PCA) should be considered. Additional strategies to promote optimal pain relief include considering equianalgesic dosing or resuming maintenance regimens in patients with chronic pain. Conversely, monitoring of potential synergistic effects of procedural sedative agents should be considered in vulnerable populations such as medication naïve, elderly, or organ profusion compromised patients. Decreased procedural stimulation, delayed drug absorption, and slow elimination may contribute to residual respiratory sedation and cardiorespiratory depression during the recovery period. Hypotension or a change in level of consciousness should be aggressively investigated. For patients with pretreatment medication regimens, anticoagulation therapy can generally be safely resumed 12 to 24 hours postprocedure when it is established that the patient is having an uncomplicated recovery.

Adequate hydration following the procedure is important to limit the potential risk of a tumor-lysis-like syndrome or a postembolization-like syndrome, particularly noted in PTE, RFA, and IA cases. The exact rate of fluid administration is, of course, patient-specific and may depend on the size of the treatment volume and the underlying cardiovascular and renal medical issues. In general, oral fluids should be encouraged in the days after the procedure, in the absence of hypertension, congestive heart failure, renal failure, or other fluid management conditions.

Activity postprocedure consists of flat positioning and bed rest for 4 to 6 hours, with a gradual increase of the head of bed by 30 degrees followed by progressive, limited activity. PV patients are kept initially recumbent for 1 to 2 hours with bed rest recommended for the first 24 hours, although ambulation to the bathroom is permitted. Showering and activity can gradually resume after 24 hours. Driving should be avoided for the initial 2 to 5 days based on the speed for returning to general activity level. For procedures requiring hospitalization such as PTE and IA procedures, the length of hospitalization is anticipated to be 1 to 3 days. Residual side effects from PTE, including fatigue and lethargy, are expected and may last up to 6 weeks. Significant shifts in severity or duration beyond the symptoms described warrant patient contact with a physician.

SUMMARY

The role of interventional radiology is rapidly emerging as a viable treatment arena in which locoregional control of advanced cancers can be safely and effectively managed. It is imperative that the radiation oncology nurse be apprised of treatment options, clinical indications, and response rates to ensure the multimodality cancer patient receives the quality of care indicative of the latest therapeutic techniques. As research and the body of knowledge expands, the oncology nurse will be situated to facilitate patient and family education through comprehension and care management strategies to ensure the highest standards of oncology nursing practice.

REFERENCES

1. Murphy TP: American College of Radiology Practice Guideline for Interventional Clinical Practice: a commitment to patient care, *J Vasc Interv Radiol* 16(2 pt 1):157-159, 2005.
2. American College of Radiology, the American Society of Interventional and Therapeutic Neuroradiology, and the Society of Interventional Radiology: Practice guidelines for interventional clinical practice, *J Vasc Interv Radiol* 16(2 pt 1):149-155, 2005.
3. American Radiological Nurses Association: *Standards of radiology nursing practice*, Oak Brook, Ill, 1998, American Radiological Nurses Association.
4. American Radiological Nurses Association: *Guidelines of radiology practice: standards of radiology practice*, Oak Brook, Ill, 1998, American Radiological Nurses Association.
5. Weemering ML, editor: *Standards, recommended practices, and guidelines*, Denver, Colo, 2005, Association of Perioperative Nurses.
6. Goldberg SN, Grassi CJ, Cardella JF et al: Image-guided tumor ablation: standardization of terminology and reporting criteria. Society of Interventional Radiology Technology Assessment Committee and the International Working Group on Image-Guided Tumor Ablation, *Radiology* 235(3):728-739, 2005.
7. Dupuy DE, Goldberg SN: Image guided radiofrequency tumor ablation: challenges and opportunities, part II, *J Vasc Interv Radiol* 12(10):1135-1148, 2001.
8. Livraghi T, Giorgio A, Marin G et al: Hepatocellular carcinoma and cirrhosis in 746 patients: long-term results of percutaneous ethanol injection, *Radiology* 197(1):101-108, 1995.
9. Decadt B, Sriwardena AK: Radiofrequency ablation of liver tumours: systemic review, *Lancet Oncol* 5(9):550-560, 2004.
10. Coldwell DM, Sewell PE: The expanding role of interventional radiology in the supportive care of the oncology patient: from diagnosis to therapy, *Semin Oncol* 32(2):169-173, 2005.
11. Baust J, Gage AA, Ma H et al: Minimally invasive cryosurgery—technological advances, *Cryobiology* 34(4):373-384, 1997.
12. Seifert JK, Morris DL: Prognostic factors after cryotherapy for hepatic metastases from colorectal cancer, *Ann Surg* 228(2):201-208, 1998.
13. Conners JJ, Wojak JC, Qian Z: Tools of the trade. In Connors JJ, Wojak JC, editors: *Interventional neuroradiology: strategies and practical techniques*, Philadelphia, 1999, WB Saunders, pp 1-37.
14. Camma C, Scheis F, Orlando A et al: Transarterial chemoembolization for unresectable hepatocellular carcinoma: meta-analysis of randomized controlled trials, *Radiology* 224(1):47-54, 2002.
15. McLean A: The Bovie electrosurgical current generator, *Arch Surg* 18:1863-1873, 1929.
16. Huang SK, Graham AR, Hoyt RH et al: Transcatheter desiccation of the canine left ventricle using radiofrequency energy: a pilot study, *Am Heart J* 114(1 pt 1):42-48, 1987.
17. Patil AA, Andrews R, Torkelson R: Stereotactic volumetric radiofrequency lesioning of intracranial structures for control of intractable seizures, *Stereotactic Functional Neurosurg* 64(3):123-133, 1995.
18. Oturai AB, Jensen K, Eriksen J et al: Neurosurgery for trigeminal neuralgia: comparison of alcohol block, neurectomy, and radiofrequency coagulation, *Clin J Pain* 12(4):311-315, 1996.
19. Rosenthal DL, Hornicek FJ, Wolf MW et al: Percutaneous radiofrequency coagulation of osteoid osteoma compared with operative treatment, *J Bone Joint Surg Am* 80(6):815-821, 1998.
20. Seki T, Wakabayashi M, Nakagawa T et al: Ultrasonically guided percutaneous microwave coagulation therapy for small hepatocellular carcinoma, *Cancer* 74(3):817-825, 1994.
21. Solbiati L, Ierace T, Goldberg SN et al: Percutaneous US-guided radio-frequency tissue ablation of liver metastases: treatment and follow-up in 16 patients, *Radiology* 202(1):195-203, 1997.
22. Goetz MP, Callstron MR, Charboneau JW et al: Percutaneous image-guided radiofrequency ablation of painful metastases involving bone: a multicenter study, *J Clin Oncol* 22(2):300-306, 2004.
23. Anzai Y, Lufkin R, DeSalles A et al: Preliminary experience with MR-guided thermal ablation of brain tumors, *Am J Neuroradiol* 16(1):39-48, 1995.
24. Zagoria RJ: Imaging-guided radiofrequency ablation of renal masses, *Radiographics* 24(suppl 1):S59-S71, 2004.
25. Belfiore G, Moggio G, Tedeschi E et al: CT-guided radiofrequency ablation: a potential complementary therapy for patients with unresectable primary lung cancer—a preliminary report of 33 patients, *AJR Am J Roentgenol* 183(4):1003-1011, 2004.
26. Fornage BD, Sneige N, Ross MI et al: Small (=/< 2 cm) breast cancer treated with US-guided radiofrequency ablation: feasibility study, *Radiology* 231(1):215-224, 2004.
27. Brown DB: Concepts, considerations, and concerns on the cutting edge of radiofrequency ablation, *J Vasc Interv Radiol* 16(5):597-613, 2005.

28. Tateishi R, Shiina S, Teratani T et al: Percutaneous radiofrequency ablation for hepatocellular carcinoma: an analysis of 1000 cases, *Cancer* 103(6):1201-1209, 2005.
29. Goldberg SN, Kamel IR, Kruskal JB et al: Radiofrequency ablation of hepatic tumors: increased tumor destruction with adjuvant liposomal doxorubicin therapy, *AJR Am J Roentgenol* 179(1):93-101, 2002.
30. Barnett CC Jr, Curley SA: Ablative techniques for hepatocellular carcinoma, *Semin Oncol* 28(5):487-496, 2001.
31. Lorentzen T: A cooled needle electrode for radiofrequency tissue ablation: thermodynamic aspects of improved performance compared with conventional needle design, *Acad Radiol* 3(7):556-563, 1996.
32. Cosman ER, Nashold BS, Ovelman-Levitt J: Theoretical aspects of radiofrequency lesions in the dorsal root entry zone, *Neurosurgery* 15(6):945-950, 1984.
33. Pennes H: Analysis of tissue and arterial blood temperatures in the resting human forearm, *J Appl Physiol* 1:93-122, 1948.
34. Goldberg SN, Gazelle GS, Mueller PR: Thermal ablation therapy for focal malignancy: a unified approach to underlying principles, techniques, and diagnostic imaging guidance, *AJR Am J Roentgenol* 174(2):323-331, 2000.
35. Goldberg SN, Gazelle GS, Halpren EF et al: Radiofrequency tissues ablation: importance of local temperature along the electrode tip exposure in determining lesion shape and size, *Acad Radiol* 3(3):212-218, 1996.
36. Dodd GD III, Soulen MC, Kane RA et al: Minimally invasive treatment of malignant hepatic tumors: at the threshold of a major breakthrough, *Radiographics* 20(1):9-27, 2000.
37. Goldberg SN, Gazelle GS, Compton CC et al: Treatment of intrahepatic malignancy with radiofrequency ablation: radiologic-pathologic correlation, *Cancer* 88(11):2442-2463, 2000.
38. LeVeen R: Laser hyperthermia and radiofrequency ablation of hepatic lesions, *Semin Interv Radiol* 14:313-324, 1997.
39. de Baere T, Denys A, Wood BJ et al: Radiofrequency liver ablation: experimental comparative study of water-cooled versus expandable systems, *AJR Am J Roentgenol* 176(1):187-192, 2001.
40. Goldberg SN, Solbiait L, Hahn PF et al: Large-volume tissue ablation with radio frequency by using a clustered, internally cooled electrode technique: laboratory and clinician experience in liver metastases, *Radiology* 209(2):371-379, 1998.
41. Rossi S, Buscarini E, Gargagnait F: Percutaneous treatment of small hepatic tumors by an expandable RF needle electrode, *AJR Am J Roentgenol* 170(4):1015-1022, 1998.
42. Reddi AH, Roodman D, Freeman C et al: Mechanisms of tumor metastasis to the bone: challenges and opportunities, *J Bone Miner Res* 18(2):190-194, 2003.
43. National Osteoporosis Foundation: *Osteoporosis Clinical Practice Guideline: A physician's guide to prevention and treatment of osteoporosis*, Washington, DC, 2003.
44. Delmas PD, Van De Langerijt L, Watts NB et al: Underdiagnosis of vertebral fractures is a worldwide problem: the IMPACT Study, *J Bone Miner Res* 20(4):557-563, 2005.
45. Melton LJ, Alothman KI, Khosla S et al: Fracture risk following bilateral orchiectomy, *J Urol* 169(5):1747-1750, 2003.
46. Health Research Institute: US markets for adjunctive and non-fusion spine technologies, *Medtech Insights Report #103-1 US-0103*, 2003.
47. Mathis JM, Petri M, Naff N: Procedural techniques and materials: tumors and osteoporotic fractures. In Mathis JM, Deramond H, Belkoff SM, editors: *Percutaneous vertebroplasty*, New York, 2002, Springer-Verlag, pp 81-108.
48. McGraw JK, Heatwole EV, Strand BT et al: Predictive value of intraosseous venography before percutaneous vertebroplasty, *J Vasc Interv Radiol* 13(2 pt 1):149-153, 2002.
49. Wong W, Mathis J: Is intraosseous venography a significant safety measure in performance of vertebroplasty? *J Vasc Interv Radiol* 13(2 pt 1):137-138, 2002.
50. Gaughen JR, Jensen ME, Schweickert PA et al: Relevance of antecedent venography in percutaneous vertebroplasty for the treatment of osteoporotic compression fractures, *Am J Neuroradiol* 23(4):594-600, 2002.
51. Sesay M, Dousset V, Liguaro D et al: Intraosseous lidocaine provides effective analgesia for percutaneous vertebroplasty of osteoporotic fractures, *Can J Anesth* 49(2):137-143, 2002.
52. Mathis JM, Wong W: Percutaneous vertebroplasty: technical considerations, *J Vasc Interv Radiol* 14(8):953-960, 2003.
53. Murray JA, Bruels MC, Lindberg R: Irradiation of polymethylmethacrylate: in vitro gamma radiation effect, *J Bone Joint Surg Am* 56(2):311-312, 1974.
54. McGraw JK, Cardella J, Barr JD et al, Society of Interventional Radiology: Quality improvement guidelines for percutaneous vertebroplasty, *J Vasc Interv Radiol* 14(suppl):311-315, 2003.
55. Advisory Board. Technology Watch: Spinal surgery: vertebroplasty remains more profitable than kyphoplasty, but efficacy and safety questions linger (website): http://www.advisory.com/members/default.asp?contentID=51860&collectionID=1142&program=32&filename=51860.xml. Accessed June 13, 2005.
56. Watts NB, Harris ST, Genant HK: Treatment of painful osteoporotic vertebral fractures with percutaneous vertebroplasty or kyphoplasty, *Osteoporos Int* 12(6):429-437, 2001.
57. Zoarski GH, Snow P, Olan WJ et al: Percutaneous vertebroplasty for osteoporotic compression fractures: qualitative prospective evaluation of long-term outcomes, *J Vasc Interv Radiol* 13(2 pt 1):139-148, 2002.
58. Liberman IH, Dudeney S, Reinhardt MK et al: Initial outcome and efficacy of "kyphoplasty" in the treatment of painful osteoporotic vertebral compression fractures, *Spine* 26(14):1631-1637, 2001.
59. Mckiernan F, Faciszewski T, Jensen R: Quality of life following vertebroplasty, *J Bone Joint Surg Am* 86-A(12):2600-2606, 2004.
60. Diamond TH, Champion B, Clark WA: Management of acute osteoporotic vertebral fractures: a nonrandomized trials comparing percutaneous vertebroplasty with conservative therapy, *Am J Med* 114(4):257-265, 2003.

61. US Food and Drug Administration, Center for Devices and Radiology Health: *MAUDE Database, report number 2953769-2003-00007:* http://www.accessdata.fda.gov/scripts/cdrh/cfdocs/cfMAUDE/search.cfm. Accessed June 22, 2005.
62. US Food and Drug Administration, Center for Devices and Radiology Health, Orthopedic Devices Branch: *Class II special controls guidance document: polymethylmethacrylate (PMMA) bone cement: guidance for the industry and FDA July 17, 2002* (website): http://www.fda.gov/cdrh/ode/guidance/668.html. Accessed June 22, 2005.
63. US Food and Drug Administration, Center for Devices and Radiology Health: *Clinical trial considerations: vertebral augmentation devices to treat spinal insufficiency fractures October 24, 2004* (website): http://www.fda.gov/cdrh/ode/guidance/1543.pdf. Accessed June 22, 2005.
64. Mathis JM, Barr JD, Belkoff SM et al: Percutaneous vertebroplasty: a developing standard of care for vertebral compression fractures, *AJNR Am J Neuroradiol* 22(2):373-381, 2001.
65. US Food and Drug Administration, Center for Devices and Radiology Health, Orthopedic Devices Branch: *Complications related to the use of bone cement and bone void fillers in treating compression fractures of the spine, May 7, 2004* (website): FDAhttp://www.fda.gov/cdrh/safety/bonecement.pdf. Accessed June 22, 2005.
66. Nussbaum DA, Gailloud P, Murphy K: A review of complications associated with vertebroplasty and kyphoplasty as reported to the Food and Drug Administration Medical Device related web site, *J Vasc Interv Radiol* 15(11):1185-1192, 2004.
67. Bernhard J, Heini PF, Villiger PM: Asymptomatic diffuse pulmonary embolism caused by acrylic cement: an unusual complication of percutaneous vertebroplasty, *Ann Rheum Dis* 62(1):85-86, 2003.
68. Choe DH, Marom EM, Ahrar K et al: Pulmonary embolism of polymethylmethacrylate during percutaneous vertebroplasty and kyphoplasty, *AJR Am J Roentgenol* 183(4):1097-1102, 2004.
69. Shapiro S, Abel T, Purvines S: Surgical removal of epidural and intradural polymethylmethacrylate extravasation complicating percutaneous vertebroplasty for osteoporotic lumbar compression fracture (case report), *J Neurosurg* 98(1 suppl):90-92, 2003.
70. Depriester C, Deramond H, Toussaint P: Percutaneous vertebroplasty: indications, technique, and complications. In Connors JJ, Wojak JC, editors: *Interventional neuroradiology: strategies and practical techniques*, Philadelphia, 1999, WB Saunders pp 346-357.
71. Uppin AA, Hirsch JA, Centenera LV et al: Occurrence of new vertebral body fractures after percutaneous vertebroplasty in patients with osteoporosis, *Radiology* 226(1):119-124, 2003.
72. Rohde S, Kovács, AF, Turowski B et al: Intra-arterial high dose chemotherapy with cisplatin as part of a palliative treatment concept in oral cancer, *Am J Neuroradiol* 26(2):1804-1809, 2005.
73. Wolpert SM, Kwan ES, Heros D et al: Selective delivery of chemotherapeutic agents with a new catheter system, *Radiology* 166(2):547-549, 1988.
74. Robbins KT, Storniolo AM, Kerber C et al: Rapid superselective high dose cisplatin infusion for advanced head and neck malignancies, *Head Neck* 14(5):364-371, 1992.
75. Robbins KT, Storniolo AM, Kerber C et al: Phase I study of highly selective superdose cisplatin infusions for advanced head and neck cancer, *J Clin Oncol* 12(10):2113-2120, 1994.
76. Robbins KT, Kumar P, Regine WF et al: Efficacy of targeted supradose cisplatin and concurrent radiation therapy for advanced head and neck cancer: the Memphis experience, *Int J Radiat Oncol Biol Phys* 38(2):263-271, 1997.
77. Robbins KT, Kumar P, Harris J et al: Supradose intra-arterial cisplatin and concurrent radiation therapy for the treatment of stage IV head and neck squamous cell carcinoma is feasible and efficacious in a multi-institution setting: results of Radiation Therapy Oncology Group Trial 9615, *J Clin Oncol* 23(7):1447-1454, 2005.
78. Kovacs AF: Intra-arterial induction high-dose chemotherapy with cisplatin for oral and oropharyngeal cancer: long-term results, *Br J Cancer* 90(7):1323-1328, 2004.
79. Ackerstaff AH, Tan IB, Rasch CR et al: Quality-of-life assessment after supradose selective intra-arterial cisplatin and concomitant radiation (RADPLAT) for inoperable stage IV head and neck squamous cell carcinoma, *Arch Otolaryngol Head Neck Surg* 128(10):1185-1190, 2002.
80. Murray T, Madasu R, Martin A et al: Acute and chronic changes in swallowing and quality of life following intraarterial chemoradiation for organ preservation in patients with advanced head and neck cancer, *Head Neck* 20(1):31-37, 1998.
81. van den Broek GB, Rasch CRN, Pameijer FA et al: Pretreatment probability model for predicting outcome after intraarterial chemoradiation for advanced head and neck carcinoma, *Cancer* 101(8):1809-1817, 2004.
82. Marcial VA, Pajak TF, Mohiuddin M et al: Concomitant cisplatin chemotherapy and radiotherapy in advanced mucosal squamous cell carcinoma of the head and neck, *Cancer* 66(9):1861-1868, 1990.
83. Drooz AT, Lewis CA, Allen TE et al, Society of Interventional Radiology Standards of Practice Committee: Quality improvement guidelines for percutaneous transcatheter embolization, *J Vasc Interv Radiol* 14(suppl):237-242, 2003.
84. Novelline RA: Interventional radiology. In *Squire's fundamentals of radiology*, 6th Ed. Cambridge, Mass, 2004, Harvard University Press, pp 562-593.
85. Hemingway AP, Allison DJ: Complications of embolization: analysis of 410 procedures, *Radiology* 166(3):669-672, 1988.
86. Solomon B, Soulen MC, Baum RA et al: Chemoembolization of hepatocellular carcinoma with cisplatin, doxorubicin, mitomycin-C, ethiodol, and polyvinyl alcohol: prospective evaluation of response and survival in a U.S. population, *J Vasc Interv Radiol* 10(6):793-798, 1999.
87. Lladó L, Virgili J, Figueras J et al: A prognostic index of the survival of patients with unresectable hepatocellular carcinoma after transcatheter arterial chemoembolization, *Cancer* 88(1):50-57, 2000.

88. Leung DA, Goin JE, Sickles C et al: Determinants of postembolization syndrome after hepatic chemoembolization, *J Vasc Interv Radiol* 12(3):321-326, 2001.
89. Loper KA, Coldwell DM, Lecky J et al: Celiac plexus block for hepatic arterial embolization: a comparison with intravenous morphine, *Anesth Analg* 69(3): 398-399, 1989.
90. Molgaard CP, Teitelbaum GP, Pentecost MJ et al: Intraarterial administration of lidocaine for analgesia in hepatic chemoembolization, *J Vasc Interv Radiol* 1(1):81-85, 1990.
91. Ajani JA, Carrasco CH, Charnsangavej C et al: Islet cell tumors metastatic to the liver: effective palliation by sequential hepatic artery embolization, *Ann Intern Med* 108(3):340-344, 1988.
92. Gupta S, Yao JC, Ahrar K et al: Hepatic artery embolization and chemoembolization for treatment of patients with metastatic carcinoid tumors: the M.D. Anderson experience, *Cancer J* 9(4):261-267, 2003.
93. Gupta S, Johnson MM, Murthy R et al: Hepatic arterial embolization and chemoembolization for the treatment of patients with metastatic neuroendocrine tumors, *Cancer* 104(8):1590-1602, 2005.
94. Liu CL, Fan ST: Nonresectional therapies for hepatocellular carcinoma, *Am J Surg* 173(4):358-365, 1997.
95. Llovet J, Burroughs A, Bruix J: Hepatocellular carcinoma, *Lancet* 362(9399):1907-1917, 2003.
96. Nakamura H, Tashiro S, Hiraoka T et al: Studies on anticancer treatment with an oily anticancer drug injected into the ligated hepatic artery for liver cancer, *Cancer* 52(12):2193-2200, 1983.
97. Berger DH, Carrasco CH, Hohn DC et al: Hepatic artery chemoembolization or embolization for primary and metastatic liver tumors: post-treatment management and complications, *J Surg Oncol* 60(2):116-121, 1995.
98. Breedis C, Young G: The blood supply of neoplasm in the liver, *Am J Pathol* 30(5):969-977, 1954.
99. Tellez C, Benson AB 3rd, Lyster MT et al: Phase II trial of chemoembolization for the treatment of metastatic colorectal carcinoma to the liver and review of the literature, *Cancer* 82(7):1250-1259, 1998.
100. Konno T: Targeting cancer chemotherapeutic agents by use of lipiodol contrast medium, *Cancer* 66(9):1897-1903, 1990.
101. Kamada K, Nakanishi T, Kitamoto M et al: Long term prognosis of patients undergoing transcatheter arterial chemoembolization for unresectable hepatocellular carcinoma: comparison of cisplatin lipiodol suspension and doxorubicin hydrochloride emulsion, *J Vasc Interv Radiol* 12(7):847-854, 2001.
102. Laurent A, Beaujeux R, Wassel M et al: Trisacryl gelatin microspheres for therapeutic embolization, I. Development and in vitro evaluation, *AJNR Am J Neuroradiol* 17(3):533-540, 1996.
103. Eriksson BK, Larsson EG, Skogseid BM et al: Liver embolizations of patients with malignant neuroendocrine gastrointestinal tumors, *Cancer* 83(11):2293-2301, 1998.
104. Fong Y, Kemeny N, Lawrence TS: Cancer of the liver and biliary tree. In DeVita VT, Hellman S, Rosenberg SA, editors: *Cancer: principles & practice of oncology*, ed 6, Philadelphia, 2001, Lippincott Williams & Wilkins, pp 1162-1203.
105. Loewe C, Schindl M, Cejna M et al: Permanent transarterial embolization of neuroendocrine metastases of the liver using cyanoacrylate and lipiodol: assessment of mid- and long-term results, *AJR Am J Roentgenol* 180(5):1379-1384, 2003.
106. Brown DB, Fundakowski CE, Lisker-Melman M et al: Comparison of MELD and Child-Pugh scores to predict survival after chemoembolization for hepatocellular carcinoma, *J Vasc Interv Radiol* 15(11):1209-1218, 2004.
107. Vallée JN, Lo D, Guillevin R et al: In vitro study of the compatibility of tri-acryl gelatin microspheres with various chemotherapeutic agents, *J Vasc Interv Radiol* 14(5):621-628, 2003.
108. Kennedy DA, Coldwell DM, Nutting C: ^{90}Y Microspheres in the treatment of colorectal lever metastases: USA experience. International Congress on Anti-cancer Therapy Annual Meeting; Paris, France; February 2004.
109. Gray B, Van Hazel G, Hope M et al: Randomized trial of SIR-Spheres plus chemotherapy vs. chemotherapy alone for treating patients with liver metastases for primary large bowel, *Ann Oncol* 12(12):1711-1720, 2001.
110. Derdeyn CP, Graves VB, Salamant MS et al: Collagen-coated acrylic microspheres for embolotherapy: in vitro and in vivo characteristics, *Am J Neuroradiol* 18(4): 647-653, 1997.
111. Beaujeux R, Laurent A, Wassel M et al: Trisacryl gelatin microspheres for therapeutic embolization, II. Clinical evaluation in tumors and arteriovenous malformations, *Am J Neuroradiol* 17(3):541-548, 1996.
112. Dancey JE, Shepherd FA, Paul K et al: Treatment of nonresectable hepatocellular carcinoma with intrahepatic ^{90}Y microspheres, *J Nucl Med* 41(10):1673-1681, 2000.
113. Salem R, Thurston KG, Carr BI et al: Yttrium-90 Microspheres: radiation therapy for unresectable liver cancer, *J Vasc Interv Radiol* 13(9 pt 2):S223-S229, 2002.
114. Ramsey DE, Kernagis LY, Soulen MC et al: Chemoembolization of hepatocellular carcinoma, *J Vasc Interv Radiol* 13(9 pt 2):S211-S221, 2002.
115. American Society of Anesthesiologists, American Society of Anesthesiologists Task Force on Preoperative Fasting: Practice guidelines for preoperative fasting and the use of pharmacologic agents to reduce the risks of pulmonary aspiration, *Anesthesiology* 90(3):896-905, 1999.
116. Ryan JM, Ryan BM, Smith TP: Antibiotic prophylaxis in interventional radiology, *J Vasc Interv Radiol* 15(6):547-556, 2004.
117. Martin ML, Lennox PH: Sedation and analgesia in the interventional radiology department, *J Vasc Interv Radiol* 14(9 pt 1):1119-1128, 2003.
118. American Society of Anesthesiology: Practice guidelines for sedation and analgesia by non-anesthesiologists, *Anesthesiology* 96(4):1004-1017, 2002.
119. Miner JR, Heegaard W, Plummer D: End-tidal carbon dioxide monitoring during procedural sedation, *Acad Emerg Med* 9(4):275-280, 2002.

120. American Medical Association, Council on Scientific Affairs: The use of pulse oximetry during conscious sedation, *JAMA* 270(12):1463-1468, 1993.
121. American Society of Anesthesiologists, American Society of Anesthesiologist Task Force on Perioperative Management of Patients with Obstructive Sleep Apnea: Practice guidelines for the perioperative management of patients with obstructive sleep apnea. *Anesthesiology*, 104:1081-1093, 2006.
122. Bluemke DA, Breiter SN: Sedation procedures in MR imaging: safety, effectiveness, and nursing effect on examinations, *Radiology* 216(3):645-652, 2000.
123. Livraghi T, Solbiati L, Meloni FM et al: Treatment of focal tumors with percutaneous radio-frequency ablation: complications encountered in a multicenter study, *Radiology* 226(2):441-451, 2003.

Chapter 22

Radioprotectants

Carrie F. Daly and Annette Lea Jones

Radiation therapy, a local treatment that is often disease-site specific, often leads to significant damage to normal tissue exposed in the treatment field.[1] Acute adverse effects may lead to long-term complications. Xerostomia, mucositis, stomatitis, pneumonitis, pulmonary fibrosis, esophagitis, and rectal complications are some of the adverse effects that can occur. These can be serious complications in cancer patients. Multiple factors contribute to the incidence and severity of radiation-induced toxicities, including concurrent chemotherapy, total dose of radiation, dose fractionation schedule, volume of tissue irradiated, and the stage and extent of the disease.

Today, combined modality treatment is becoming the standard of care in treating a variety of cancers. An increasing body of evidence suggests that chemotherapy combined with radiation yields a survival advantage over radiation alone.[2-4] However, combining chemotherapy and radiation may cause further complications to occur, resulting in debilitating symptoms, hospitalization, treatment delays, and dose reductions.

A major dose-limiting effect of radiation therapy and/or chemotherapy is damage or toxicity to normal tissue, thereby compromising the efficacy of treatment. Protection of normal tissues against adverse effects from radiation therapy and/or chemotherapy may permit dose escalation, increased patient survival, and better quality of life for patients requiring cancer therapies.[5]

Selective cytoprotectants are used as supportive agents with chemotherapy. The cytoprotectants most commonly used are amifostine (Ethyol), mesna (Mesnex), and dexrazoxane (Zinecard). Cytoprotection is defined as the use of chemical modifiers designed to minimize normal tissue damage resulting from chemotherapy administration without compromising tumor control.[6,7] Amifostine is a cytoprotectant agent indicated for the reduction of cumulative renal toxicity associated with repeated administration of cisplatin in patients with advanced ovarian cancer or non-small-cell lung cancer (NSCLC).[8] Mesna is one of the oldest cytoprotectants used. It is a sulfhydryl compound that was developed as a prophylactic agent against ifosfamide- and cyclophosphamide-induced hemorrhagic cystitis. The major source of urothelial toxicity is believed to be a urinary excretion of acrolein, a metabolite of both ifosfamide and cyclophosphamide. Mesna was designed to function in the urinary tract to detoxify urotoxic metabolites. Dexrazoxane is a cytoprotectant that is a cyclic analog of EDTA (ethylenediamine tetraacetic acid) that prevents cytotoxicity by chelation of iron. Data from preclinical and clinical studies suggest that dexrazoxane protects against anthracycline-induced cardiomyopathy but not against other anthracycline-induced toxic effects. This agent may be for patients with metastatic breast cancer who received more than 300 mg/m^2 of doxorubicin in the metastatic setting and who may benefit from continued doxorubicin containing therapy.[9] Increased nausea and vomiting are evident with this therapy.

Other supportive agents used to decrease cancer treatment toxicities include leucovorin, granulocyte colony-stimulating factors (G-CSF), and granulocyte macrophage colony-stimulating factors (GM-CSF). Leucovorin is the active form of the B-complex vitamin folate. Leucovorin is used as an antidote to drugs that decrease levels of folic acid. In cancer-treatment regimens, leucovorin is used in patients receiving high-dose methotrexate and trimetrexate, the cytotoxic effects of which include myelosuppression and gastrointestinal toxicity. Leucovorin rescues normal cells threatened by such treatments by facilitating repletion of reduced levels of intracellular folate. G-CSF and GM-CSF are colony-stimulating factors, which are groups of glycoproteins that stimulate the growth and differentiation of myeloid cells from bone marrow and cytokines that stimulate or inhibit the chemotaxis and proliferation of white blood cells involved in immune response.

G-CSF has significantly reduced the incidence of febrile neutropenia following initial chemotherapy in patients with NSCLC. This therapy reduced the need for hospitalizations and antibiotics. GM-CSF has been shown to accelerate neutrophil recovery following autologous bone marrow transplantation.[10]

The goal of radiation therapy is to improve local control and decrease metastasis. A larger dose yields greater effects with greater toxicity; therefore, dose may be limited by toxicity. Amifostine is presently the only radioprotectant agent that the Food and Drug Administration (FDA) has approved to reduce the incidence of moderate to severe xerostomia in patients undergoing postoperative radiation therapy for head and neck cancer, where the radiation field includes a substatial portion of the parotid gland.[8] Figure 22-1 shows the molecular structure of amifostine. Based on extensive data, additions were made to the amifostine compendia usage and are included in the United States Pharmacopeia-Drug Information (USP-DI). The monographs provided data for the off-label uses of amifostine for mucosal protection in radiation therapy or radiation therapy combined with chemotherapy according to the USP-DI, June 2002 update.

In a review of the use of chemotherapy and radiation therapy protectants, the American Society of Clinical Oncology (ASCO) concluded that there was no evidence from the available clinical data to demonstrate that amifostine leads to tumor protection.[11] Numerous clinical trials have closely examined the safety and efficacy of amifostine in the prevention of mucositis from radiation and combined modality therapy in head and neck cancer, NSCLC, and pelvic cancer.[12-14] These areas are reviewed in this chapter.

Prevention of early and late toxicities is essential when providing radiation therapy and chemotherapy to cancer patients. Radioprotection/cytoprotection agents can selectively protect a broad assortment of normal tissues such as the oral mucosa, salivary glands, lungs, bone marrow, heart, intestines, and kidneys. These agents do not protect tumor cells, but reduce radiation-related and selected chemotherapy-related toxicities and improve long-term functioning and quality of life for the patient because they prevent treatment delays and thereby improve survival.[6]

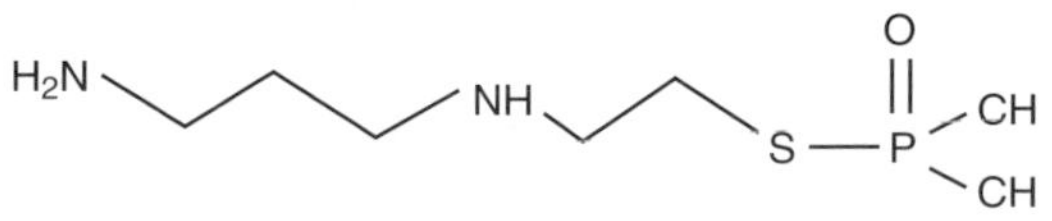

The goals of cytoprotection are to reduce early toxicities such as radiation and chemical mucositis; neurologic, renal, and skin toxicities; and immune suppression. Another goal in the use of cytoprotection is to reduce the late toxicities of radiation and chemotherapy, such as late xerostomia, esophageal or colon/intestinal stenosis, skin, muscle, breast, and lung fibrosis. Lastly, the use of cytoprotection can enhance the antineoplastic activity of radiation and chemotherapy with the increase in dose intensity chemotherapy and avoidance of unnecessary delays in radiation therapy treatments.

H_2N—NH—S—P(=O)(CH)(CH)

Figure 22-1 Molecular Representation of Amifostine.

UNDER INVESTIGATION

Numerous radioprotective or cytoprotective agents are being investigated. However, information concerning these agents is limited at this time. These investigational agents include gene therapy such as intratumor injection of manganese superoxide dismutase-plasmid/liposome (SOD2-PL); transforming growth factor-beta; glutamine; IL-15; melatonin; and omega-3 fatty acids.[15]

Of great interest is keratinocyte growth factor-2 (KGF-2) known as repifermin. This is a novel human protein discovery by Human Genome Sciences that stimulates the repair of injured mucosal tissues. Preclinical studies demonstrate that repifermin contributes to the healing of injured tissues containing keratinocytes, including internal wounds to the mucous membrane that lines the alimentary tract. Human Genome Sciences is developing repifermin as a potential treatment for cancer therapy–induced mucositis. Mucositis is an inflammation and ulceration of the lining of the mouth, throat, or gastrointestinal tract most commonly associated with chemotherapy or radiation therapy for cancer.[16] Currently, repifermin has completed a phase II clinical trial. It was administered intravenously both before the conditioning regimen and after autologous hematopoietic stem cell transplantation. Safety was the primary endpoint; secondary endpoints included incidence, severity, and duration of mucositis. Repifermin significantly reduced the incidence of grade 2 to 4 mucositis compared with the control patients.[17]

Amgen Incorporated also has completed a phase II clinical trial of KGF-1 (palifermin Kepivance), a protein that is related to repifermin, in cancer patients to reduce cancer-induced mucositis and has reported that KGF-1 significantly decreases the duration and incidence of oral mucositis.[18] Palifermin also demonstrated effectiveness in reducing the complications of oral mucositis with intensive chemotherapy and radiation therapy. The study measured severity and duration after intensive chemotherapy and radiation therapy for hematologic cancers. Results showed grade 3 to 4 mucositis was 63% in the palifermin group and 98% in the placebo group. The median duration of mucositis was 6 days in the palifermin group and 9 days in the placebo group. The study also demonstrated a significant reduction of grade 4 mucositis from the placebo group, 20% respectively versus 62%. Patient-reported soreness of the mouth was measured and the study revealed an area under the curve score of 29% versus 46.8%. The most common adverse events were rash, pruritus, erythema, mouth and tongue disorders, and taste alterations; they were mild to moderate in severity and were transient.[19] Based on research to date, it is believed that repifermin binds to receptors on cells in the mucous membrane at the site of an injury, causing cells to migrate to the injury, thus promoting wound healing by increased epithelial cell proliferation.[20] Cancer therapy–induced mucositis occurs with radiation or chemotherapy, which destroys rapidly dividing cancer cells and other rapidly proliferating cells that line the mouth, throat, and gastrointestinal tract.

With new radiation technology, including three-dimensional conformal radiation therapy (3D-CRT) and intensity-modulated radiation therapy (IMRT), higher doses of radiation can be used; therefore, protection against normal tissue toxicity becomes increasingly important. Additional clinical trials of radiation-protective agents will lead to more definitive conclusions regarding protection of radiation-induced mucositis in the head and neck, thorax, and pelvic region.

Amifostine is a supportive therapy, used as a cytoprotectant agent with both radiation and chemotherapy. Clinical trials have demonstrated favorable results in a number of trials involving a variety of cancers and treatment modalities. Results have suggested that amifostine protects against radiation-induced toxicity in patients receiving radiation alone and those receiving radiation and chemotherapy.[8,11,21] A reduction in the incidence of radiation-induced toxicities such as xerostomia and mucositis in head and neck cancer patients has been shown. Although not included in the product label, several studies have provided evidence that amifostine (at the higher IV dose of 300 to 340 mg/m^2) provides protection and may reduce the incidence of mucositis associated with radiation or radiochemotherapy.[22] Amifostine is an organic thiophosphate cytoprotective agent known chemically as ethanethiol, 2-[(3-aminopropyl) amino]-dihydrogen phosphate.[23] Amifostine was created by the U.S. Army in Nuclear Warfare Project (WR-2721). Amifostine is a pro-drug that is dephosphorylated by alkaline phosphate in tissues to a pharmacologically active free-thiol metabolite. The active free metabolite is believed to be responsible for the reduction of the toxic effects of radiation on normal tissue.[6] The free-thiol metabolite is much more readily absorbed by normal tissue than by tumor tissue. In fact, micro-environmental differences between normal tissue cells and tumor tissue cells result in free-thiol concentrations one-hundredfold greater in normal tissue. These higher concentrations of free-thiol protect normal tissue such as bone marrow, the kidneys, and the heart, but not tumor tissue.[3]

Head and Neck Cancer

It is estimated by the American Cancer Society that the number of new head and neck cancers will approach 51,000 in 2006. The estimated mortality from both new and current cases is estimated to reach 14,640 in 2006.[24] Squamous cell carcinoma (SCC) is the most common type of head and neck cancer (> 90%). The most common site is the oral cavity and the pharynx, estimated at 30,990 new cases in 2006. Men over age 50 are at the greatest risk, particularly men who use tobacco and/or consume excessive alcohol. Signs and symptoms of head and neck cancer include a sore in the mouth that does not heal, persistent red and white patches in the mouth, difficulty swallowing or chewing, and hoarseness.[24]

In an overview of clinical trials for head and neck cancer, it was found that there is a 40% survival rate for patients with resectable advanced SCC and a 20% survival rate for patients with unresectable SCC treated with radiation alone. The addition of chemotherapy to radiation therapy significantly increased survival rates in patients with advanced nasopharyngeal cancer from 10% to 40%. The 5-year survival rate in patients treated with chemotherapy plus radiation therapy compared to radiation alone increased to over 80%.[25] In a recent meta-analysis of 25 clinical trials that compared the addition of chemotherapy with local definitive treatment (surgery and/or radiation therapy), there was an 11% improved survival with the adjuvant chemotherapy group and a 22% improved survival with the concurrent chemotherapy group.[26]

With the addition of chemotherapy and radiation, there was an increase in toxicities including anorexia, weight loss, pain, xerostomia, mucositis/stomatitis, dysphagia, radiation necrosis, and candidiasis.[8] The addition of chemotherapy to radiation therapy in the treatment of head and neck cancers has been found to significantly increase treatment-associated toxicities, even though it increases long-term survival and improves other treatment goals. Other complications relative to the toxicities of radiation and chemotherapy include tooth decay, increased fatigue, treatment interruptions, dose limitations, hospitalization, and discontinuation of treatment—resulting in decreased survival, poor outcomes, and potential recurrences.

In a phase III randomized trial with amifostine as a radioprotector in SCC of the head and neck, amifostine reduced acute and chronic xerostomia while preserving antitumor efficacy and reducing the overall incidence of grade 2 or higher xerostomia (Table 22-1) from 78% to 51% ($P < 0.0001$).[8] The median time to onset of grade 2 or higher acute xerostomia was longer in the amifostine and radiation group at 45 days compared to the control group at 30 days ($P = 0.0001$). In addition, patients pretreated with amifostine were able to tolerate higher doses of radiation at 60 Gy compared to the radiation-alone group at 42 Gy ($P = 0.0001$) before experiencing a higher severity of symptoms. The radiation dose necessary to cause grade 2 or higher acute xerostomia was 40% higher in the amifostine and radiation group. In the Brizel follow-up study done in 2000, 18- and 24-month follow-up showed no statistically significant differences in locoregional control ($P = 0.610$; $P = 0.535$, respectively), progression-free survival ($p = 0.958$; $p = 0.982$, respectively) and overall survival rate ($P = 0.184$; $P = 0184$, respectively) between patients receiving amifostine and those in the control group, confirming that amifostine did not compromise antitumor efficacy of radiation therapy.[8]

An eight-item validated patient benefit questionnaire (PBQ) was done during and up to 11 months after completion of radiation therapy. Clinical benefit was measured by this questionnaire. Amifostine-treated patients consistently reported better PBQ scores beginning at week 4 of radiation ($p < 0.05$), which was indicative of improved oral

Table 22-1 Xerostomia: Radiation Therapy Oncology Group Grading Criteria

Grade 0	Grade 1	Grade 2	Grade 3	Grade 4
ACUTE XEROSTOMIA				
No changes over baseline	Mild mouth dryness: slightly thickened saliva may have slight metallic taste No change in baseline feeding behavior	Moderate to complete dryness: thick, sticky saliva; markedly altered taste	Not defined	Acute salivary gland necrosis
LATE XEROSTOMIA				
None	Slight dryness of mouth: good response with stimulation	Moderate dryness of mouth: poor response to stimulation	Complete dryness of the mouth: no response to stimulation	Fibrosis

Data from Cox JD, Stetz J, Pajak TF: *Int J Radiat Oncol Biol Phys* 31(5):1341-1346, 1995; Radiation Therapy Oncology Group (RTOG), American College of Radiology, Philadelphia, Penn, with support from the National Cancer Institute.

toxicity-related outcomes and improved clinical benefits.[5]

Antonadou and colleagues[27] administered amifostine (300 mg/m^2 by IV infusion) to head and neck cancer patients undergoing radiochemotherapy (2 Gy fractions 5 days weekly for a total of 60 Gy to 74 Gy and carboplatin 90 mg/m^2 once per week before radiation therapy). It was found that acute mucositis (Table 22-2) was almost nonexistent in the amifostine group (n = 22; 9% grade 2 mucositis at week 3 and 4.5% grade 4 mucositis at week 5) compared with the control group (n = 23; 100% grade 2 mucositis at week 3 and 54% grade 4 mucositis at week 5). Late-phase toxicity of xerostomia was similarly diminished in the amifostine group at the 3-month follow-up; only 27% of the amifostine group had a grade 2 xerostomia as compared to the control group at 74% grade 2 xerostomia.

LUNG CANCER

The American Cancer Society reports that lung cancer is the leading cause of cancer-related mortality in the United States, with an estimated 93,820 men and 73,230 women dying in 2006.[24] The overall 5-year survival rate for lung cancer for all stages of NSCLC is still only 15%. Signs and symptoms of lung cancer include persistent cough, bloody sputum, chest pain, chronic recurrent bronchitis, and pneumonia. Common presenting symptoms of acute pneumonitis are cough, dyspnea, congestion, fullness of the chest, mild to moderate fever, and possible shortness of breath (hypoxia). Lung cancer risk factors include cigarette smoking; exposure to radiation, organic chemicals, asbestos, and other agents; air pollution; and tuberculosis.[24]

Reducing Toxicities in Non–Small-Cell Lung Cancer

Radiation therapy to the lung and chest area for NSCLC has significant acute and chronic toxicities in many patients that may become dose limiting. Recent studies show that concurrent chemotherapy and radiation therapy has resulted in better tumor control. However, combining radiation and chemotherapy will result in increased toxicities. Toxicities from radiation include dysphagia, esophagitis, dyspnea, cough, pneumonitis, and fibrosis.[10,28,29] Twenty percent to 50% of patients with lung cancer suffer from severe esophagitis (grade 3 or higher). Pulmonary toxicity occurs in 10% to 20% of patients with lung cancer and can occur 1 to 4 months postradiation treatment or more than 1 year posttreatment; late effects of lung fibrosis can become life-threatening.[28,30] These toxicities can cause nutritional issues resulting in significant weight loss, pain requiring opioids, further respiratory complications or infections, hospitalizations, and an interruption in therapies (i.e., radiation and/or chemotherapy).

Multiple trials have shown a reduction in acute and late lung toxicity without affecting the antitumor efficacy of radiation treatments in advanced lung cancer. In one study, the incidence of esophagitis of grade 2 or higher during week 4 of treatment with daily fractionation of 2 Gy/5 days a week was 42% (31/73) in the radiation-alone

Table 22-2 Mucositis: Radiation Therapy Oncology Group Grading Criteria

Grade 0	Grade 1	Grade 2	Grade 3	Grade 4
ACUTE MUCOSITIS				
No change over baseline	Possible mild pain not requiring analgesia	Patchy mucositis that may produce inflammatory serosanguinous discharge; may include moderate pain requiring analgesia	Confluent fibrinous mucositis; may include severe pain requiring opioid analgesia	Ulceration, hemorrhage, or necrosis
LATE MUCOSITIS				
None	Slight atrophy and dryness	Moderate atrophy and telangiectasia; little mucus	Marked atrophy with complete dryness; severe telangiectasia	Ulceration

Data from Cox JD, Stetz J, Pajak TF: *Int J Radiat Oncol Biol Phys* 31(5):1341-1346, 1995; Radiation Therapy Oncology Group (RTOG), American College of Radiology, Philadelphia, Penn, with support from the National Cancer Institute.

group compared to 4% (3/73) in the group that also received amifostine ($p < 0.0001$). Amifostine was administered daily at 340 mg/m^2. Two months posttreatment, 43% (23/53) of patients in the radiation arm and 9% (4/44) in the amifostine-plus-radiation arm had changes representative of grade 2 or greater lung damage ($p < 0.0001$). Fibrosis was present in 53% (19/36) of patients receiving radiation alone versus 28% (9/36) of patients receiving radiation plus amifostine.[12]

In another study, 26 patients with lung cancer received thoracic radiation; 11 patients received concurrent hyperfractioned radiation with cisplatin and etoposide with amifostine. The cytoprotective benefit of amifostine in this study showed an increase in the threshold for the diffusing capacity of carbon monoxide (DLco). Amifostine was also found to reduce the decrease of lung function in DLco measurements from 42% to 24% in patients with NSCLC treated with chemoradiation. It is important to evaluate the relationship between local radiation dose and the loss of local diffusion capacity in the lung. The utilization of this information in combination with a dose-volume histogram, allows for the prediction of the expected loss of whole lung diffusion capacity associated with a treatment plan. Clinically this is important because the DLco should not decrease more than 50% if patients are to maintain a reasonable quality of life.[28]

DOSING AND ADMINISTRATION OF AMIFOSTINE

Data from preclinical studies support the hypothesis that cytoprotection in the clinical setting appears to be time- and dose-dependent.[31,32] It is recommended that amifostine be administered IV 20 to 30 minutes before daily radiation treatments.[8] Several large clinical trials have demonstrated significant cytoprotection with the use of amifostine as a single subcutaneous injection before each standard fraction of radiation treatment 5 days each week for 6 to 7 weeks.[8,12,14,33]

The recommended dose of amifostine to protect against xerostomia resulting from radiation therapy for head and neck cancer is 200 mg/m^2 once daily, administered as a 3-minute IV push 15 to 30 minutes before radiation.[23] However, recent studies of rapid IV push amifostine (less than 1 minute) have demonstrated that shorter infusion times reduced hypotension and nausea/vomiting and improved tolerability associated with the drug.[34] Although subcutaneous administration of amifostine is not currently FDA-approved, it seems to have some advantages over IV administration. Studies by Koukourakis[14] and Anne[21] showed the subcutaneous amifostine has comparable bioavailability and efficacy to IV amifostine with improved tolerability of common adverse effects such as nausea, vomiting, and hypotension. Hydration and appropriate oral antiemetics 90 to 120 minutes before injections are still necessary with subcutaneous amifostine. There may be a reduction in time required and staff needed to administer subcutaneous amifostine. Koukourakis and colleagues[14] recently tested the feasibility of amifostine administered by subcutaneous injection in 140 patients undergoing radiation therapy for head and neck, thoracic, and pelvic tumors. Patients were given a 500-mg dose of amifostine diluted in 2.5 mL of normal saline administered subcutaneously, 20 minutes before receiving daily radiation therapy. The results demonstrated that amifostine administered subcutaneously was well tolerated; the incidence of grade 1 nausea occurred in 29% of patients and hypotension in only 3%.

The rate of dissolution of amifostine is temperature- and volume-dependent. In mixing amifostine, reconstitution with normal saline may be easier at room temperature. After reconstitution, the vial should be inspected visually for particulate matter and discoloration before administration. It is recommended that a 500-mg vial is reconstituted with 2.9 mL of normal saline and given in two equally divided subcutaneous injections.[8,14,21,35-38] Proper technique for subcutaneous injection is recommended and site rotation is necessary.

ADVERSE EFFECTS OF AMIFOSTINE

The most common adverse effects associated with amifostine in oncology patients include nausea and vomiting, transient hypotension, local injection site reaction, and generalized rash. Other reported adverse effects include hypocalcemia, sneezing, sleepiness, dizziness, flushing, hiccups, and fevers/chills. Increased adverse effects are noted as the dose of amifostine is increased when used for chemoprotection IV at 740 mg/m^2 or 910 mg/m^2

compared to the radioprotection dose of 200 mg/m^2 or 500-mg flat dose given IV or subcutaneously.

Hypotension

The precise mechanism of action by which amifostine causes hypotension is unknown. Studies have suggested its aminothiol metabolites cause vasodilation via direct relaxation of vascular smooth muscle. Lowered blood pressure during amifostine administration is usually transient and easily reversible with placement of the patient in a flat or Trendelenburg position and administration of IV hydration bolus. It does not appear to cause long-term central nervous system, cardiovascular, or renal sequelae. Daily assessment includes baseline blood pressure and hydration status before administration. Patients who are hypotensive or dehydrated before injection may need amifostine to be held until hydration issues are resolved. If an antihypertensive is needed, it is recommended that it be taken at bedtime. Clinical studies to date have not evaluated the safety of amifostine in elderly patients or patients with cardiovascular, renal, or cerebrovascular disease.[35]

To minimize the risk of hypotension, the patient should be well hydrated before amifostine administration. The patient should drink one extra liter of fluid throughout the day, if not contraindicated, and at least 2 cups of fluid 30 minutes before administration. Amifostine should not be given if the patient is dehydrated. Signs and symptoms of dehydration include poor skin turgor, low blood pressure, increased heart rate, concentrated urine, sudden weight loss, and dry mucous membranes. Risk factors for dehydration include nausea/vomiting, diarrhea, excessive urine output, stomatitis/pharyngitis, loss of appetite, excessive sweating, poor oral intake, and diuretics. Adequate hydration before amifostine administration and a reclining position during IV administration will reduce the propensity for hypotension.

Nausea and Vomiting

Amifostine has the potential to be an emetogenic medication for cancer patients receiving radiation therapy and/or chemotherapy. Risk factors that increase the likelihood of nausea and vomiting include highly emetogenic chemotherapy; emesis with previous chemotherapy and/or amifostine; age (younger); poorly hydrated patients; women prone to nausea and vomiting during pregnancy, and patients with a history of motion sickness.[34] Lower-risk patients may include those receiving radiation therapy alone or with non-emetogenic chemotherapy, those with no nausea or emesis during previous chemotherapy and/or amifostine use, and those with increased alcohol intake or drug abuse.

Radiation-specific risk factors for nausea and vomiting include patients receiving a large single dose, large fields, concurrent chemotherapy, and radiation to the brain, upper abdominal area, or pelvis.[39] To minimize nausea and vomiting, antiemetic medication should be administered in a timely manner before, with, or after amifostine when needed. Giving oral antiemetics 90 to 120 minutes before amifostine administration reduces the potential for nausea and vomiting. Oral or IV 5-HT$_3$ receptor antagonists alone or with other antiemetics work well for patients receiving chemotherapy. Dexamethasone, lorazepam, or metoclopramide (Reglan) may be needed during radiation alone and during combined chemotherapy and radiation and for delayed nausea and vomiting.[40]

Cutaneous Reactions

Cutaneous reactions may occur with administration of amifostine. These reactions are categorized as a local injection site reaction or a patchy to generalized skin reaction. A general skin reaction is outside of the radiation treatment field or outside of the local injection site. A generalized skin reaction may appear as a macular-papular or urticarial rash, appearing initially on the chest or back and then spreading.

Rare generalized reactions are erythema multiforme, Stevens-Johnsons syndrome, toxic epidermal necrolysis, and exfoliated dermatitis. These reactions may be severe and require discontinuation of amifostine without re-challenging. For generalized skin reaction, treatment with corticosteroids and/or antihistamines will provide comfort. Aveeno bath, Aveeno soap, and use of calamine lotion also may provide comfort. At the discretion of the oncologist, a dermatology consult may be recommended in some cases of generalized reactions. Patients who develop early mucosal ulcerations or blistering reactions that are not considered to be radiation or chemotherapy-induced should have amifostine discontinued.[38]

Management of local injection site reactions depends on the severity of each reaction. Oral antihistamines daily before amifostine injections and local antihistamine cream or steroidal cream after injection may reduce the amount of local injection site reactions seen. For pain, ulceration, wet desquamation, or necrosis at the injection site, amifostine should be discontinued and the patient treated as medically indicated with the appropriate dressings and debridement measures.[41]

SUMMARY

It is important for oncology nurses to be familiar with the acute and late toxicities of cancer treatment and the impact that cytoprotectant agents can have on managing these toxicities. Nurses need to know their mechanism of action and how to safely administer them and manage their side effects. Proper patient management and assessment is critical and can significantly improve the tolerability of both the cytoprotectant and the cancer therapy. Numerous trials are studying multiple therapies and medications for the purpose of improving tolerance and reducing toxicities caused by radiation and chemotherapy. We need to continue to remember that the patient, not the cancer diagnosis, is the focus of our carc; if cytoprotectants can reduce treatment-related toxicities, decrease treatment breaks, and reduce long-term complications, then quality of life and survival may be positively impacted.

REFERENCES

1. Kostler W, Hejna M, Wenzel C et al: Oral mucositis complicating chemotherapy and/or radiotherapy: options for prevention and treatment, *CA Cancer J Clin* 51(5):290-315, 2001.
2. Wendt TG, Garbenbauer GG, Rodell CM et al: Simultaneous radio-chemotherapy versus radiotherapy alone in advanced head and neck cancer: a randomized multi-center study, *J Clin Oncol* 16(4):1318-1324, 1998.
3. Calais G, Alfonzsi M, Bardet E et al: Randomized trial of radiation therapy versus concomitant chemotherapy and radiation therapy for advanced-stage oropharynx carcinoma, *J Natl Cancer Inst* 91(24):2081-2086, 1999.
4. Brizel DM, Albers ME, Fisher SR et al: Hyper-fractionated irradiation with or without concurrent chemotherapy for locally advanced head and neck cancer, *N Engl J Med* 338(25):798-803, 1998.
5. Wasserman T, Mackowiak J, Brizel D et al: Effect of amifostine on patient assessed clinical benefit in irradiated head and neck cancer, *Int J Radiat Oncol Biol Phys* 48(4):1035-1038, 2000.
6. Capizzi RL, Scheffler BS, Oster W et al: Amifostine reduces cumulative cisplatin nephrotoxicity, *Eur J Cancer* 31a (suppl 5):577, 1995.
7. Kemp G, Rose P, Lurain J: Amifostine pretreatment for protection against cyclophosphamide-induced and cisplatin-induced toxicities: results of a randomized controlled trial in patients with advanced ovarian cancer, *J Clin Oncol* 14(7):2101-2112, 1996.
8. Brizel DM, Wasserman TH, Henke M et al: Phase III randomized trial of amifostine as a radioprotector in head and neck cancer, *J Clin Oncol* 18(19):3339-3345, 2000.
9. Product Insert: Dexrazoxane. Kalamazoo, Mich, Pharmacia & Upjohn Co.
10. Schuchter LM: Current role of protective agents in cancer treatment, *Oncology* (Huntingt) 11(4):505-512, 515-516, 1997.
11. Hensley ML, Schuchter LM, Lindley C et al: American society of clinical oncology clinical practice guidelines for the use of chemotherapy and radiotherapy protectants, *J Clin Oncol* 17(10):3333-3355, 1999.
12. Antonadou D, Coliarakis N, Synodinou M et al: Randomized phase III trial of radiation treatment +/- amifostine in patients with advanced-staged lung cancer, *Int J Radiat Oncol Biol Phys* 51(4):915-922, 2001.
13. Buntzel J, Kuttner K, Frohlich D et al: Selective cytoprotection with amifostine in concurrent radio-chemotherapy for head and neck cancer, *Ann Oncol* 9(5):505-509, 1998.
14. Koukourakis MI, Kyrias G, Kakolyris S et al: Subcutaneous administration of amifostine during fractionated radiation therapy: a randomized phase II study, *J Clin Oncol* 18(11): 2226-2233, 2000.
15. Jatoi A, Thomas CR: Esophageal cancer and the esophagus: *Semin Radiat Oncol*, 12 (suppl. 1), 62-67, 2002.
16. *Mucositis* [Data File] (website): http://www.hgsi.com/news/prcss/background_mucositis.html. Rockville, Md, May 2000, Backgrounder Human Genome Sciences.
17. Connolly K, Alderson R, Gohari-Fritsch S et al: Cancer Chemotherapy and Pharmacology Springer Berlin / Heidelberg Volume 50, Number 3 September, 2002 171-255 Rockville, Md, Human Genome Sciences Inc.
18. Product Insert: Kepivance™. Amgen Inc, Thousand Oaks, Calif.
19. Spielberger R, Stiff P, Bensinger W et al: Palifermin for oral mucositis after intensive therapy for hematologic cancer, *N Engl J Med* 351(25):2590-2598, 2004.
20. Connolly K, Alderson R, Gohari-Fritsch S et al: Cancer Chemotherapy and Pharmacology Springer Berlin / Heidelberg Volume 50, Number 3 September, 2002 171-255 Rockville, Md, Human Genome Sciences Inc. Connolly K, Alderson R, Gohari-Fritsch S et al: Rockville, Md, Human Genome Sciences Inc.
21. Anne P, Curran W, Machtay M et al: A phase II trial of subcutaneous amifostine and radiation therapy in patients with head and neck cancer (WR-B060), *Int J Radiat Oncol Biol Phys* 51(3[suppl]):84, 2001.
22. *Amifostine, finalized drug information,* Rockville Md, 2002, United States Pharmacopeia.
23. *Ethyol PI* (Product Information) (website): http://www.medimmune.cim/products/htmlpis/ethyolpi.html. Accessed May 19, 2005.
24. American Cancer Society: *Cancer facts and figures,* Atlanta, 2006, American Cancer Society.
25. Dimery IW, Hong WK: Overview of combined modality therapies for head and neck cancer, *J Natl Cancer Inst* 85(2):95-111, 1993.

26. El-Sayed S, Nelson N: Adjuvant and adjunctive chemotherapy in the management of squamous cell carcinoma of the head and neck region: a meta-analysis of prospective and randomized trials, *J Clin Oncol* 14(3):838-847, 1996.
27. Antonadou D, Synodinou M, Boufi M et al: Amifostine reduces acute toxicity during radiochemotherapy in patients with localized advanced stage non small cell lung cancer. ASCO 2000 Convention. Ref Type: Abstract.
28. Gopal R, Tucker SL, Komaki R et al: The relationship between local dose and loss of function for irradiated lung, *Int J Radiat Oncol Biol Phys* 56(1):106-112, 2003.
29. Komaki R, Lee JS, Milas L et al: Effects of amifostine on acute toxicity from concurrent chemotherapy and radiotherapy for inoperable non–small-cell lung cancer: report of a randomized comparative trial, *Int J Radiat Oncol Biol Phys* 58(5):1369-1377, 2004.
30. Werner-Wasik M, Axelrod RS, Friedland DP et al: Phase II: trial of twice weekly amifostine in patients with non-small cell lung cancer treated with chemo-radiotherapy, *Semin Radiat Oncol* 12(1 suppl 1):34-39, 2002.
31. Bachy CM, Fazenbaker CA, Kifle G et al: Daily dosing with amifostine is necessary for full protection against oral mucositis caused by fractionated radiation in rats: Protection and pharmacokinetics. ASCO 2003 Abstract (2081).
32. Fazenbaker CA, Bachy CM, Kifle G et al: Dose and schedule dependency of amifostine protection against hyperfractionated radiotherapy in a rat model. *Proc Am Soc Clin Oncol* 22:518, 2003 (abstr 2083).
33. Antonadou D, Pepelassi M, Synodinou M et al: Prophylactic use of amifostine to prevent radio-chemotherapy-induced mucositis and xerostomia in head and neck cancer, *Int J Radiat Oncol Biol Phys* 52(3):739-747, 2002.
34. Boccia R: Improved tolerability of amifostine with rapid infusion and optimal patient preparation, *Semin Oncol* 29(6 suppl 19):9-13, 2002.
35. Ethyol® (amifostine) for injection prescribing information, In Ethyol PI (Product Information).(5/19/05). Retrieved from http://www.medimmune.cim/products/htmlpis/ethyolpi.html: 2000, MedImmune Oncology.
36. Cassatt DR: Extended window of mucosal radioprotection with intravenous or subcutaneous amifostine in rats. *Proc Am Soc Clin Oncol, 20:* 279a, 2001.
37. Werner-Wassik M, Axelrod RS, Friedland D et al: Preliminary report on reduction of esophagitis by amifostine in patients with non-small cell lung cancer treated with chemo-radiotherapy, *Clin Lung Cancer* 2(4):284-289, 2001.
38. Daly C, Ameen D, Holloway N: Subcutaneous Administration of Amifostine during Radiotherapy: A Clinical Perspective. ASCO 2003 Convention. 2003. (Abstract 315)
39. The Italian Group for Antiemetic Research in Radiotherapy: Radiation-induced emesis: a prospective observational multicenter Italian trial, *Int J Radiat Oncol Biol Phys* 44(3):619-625, 1999.
40. Gralla RJ, Osoba D, Kris M et al: Recommendations for the use of antiemetics: evidence-based, clinical practice guidelines, *J Clin Oncol* 17(9):2971-2994, 1999.
41. Boccia R, Anne PR: Assessment and management of cutaneous reactions with amifostine administration: findings of the Ethyol (amifostine) Cutaneous Treatment Advisory Panel (Ectap), *Int J Radiat Oncol Biol Phys* 60(1):302-309, 2004.

Chapter 23

Radiopharmaceuticals

Susan Vogt Temple

Radiopharmaceuticals are actually radioactive medications. They are chemical or biochemical entities that either contain radioactive agents or have radioactive agents attached to them. Radiopharmaceuticals may be administered to patients orally, intravenously, interstitially, intradermally, inhaled, or instilled into an organ or cavity for either diagnostic or therapeutic purposes.[1] The majority of radiopharmaceuticals on the market today are used for diagnostic purposes; however, the use of radiolabeled antibodies and small molecules as a form of targeted radiation therapy is expected to increase as understanding of appropriate targets in molecular oncology increases.[1-3] Radiation oncology clinicians should be familiar with both the diagnostic testing required to stage/restage patients and the various therapeutic options available to treat them. Thus they will be in a unique position to effectively counsel patients when radiopharmaceuticals will be given as part of the initial staging and diagnostic work-up, the restaging evaluation, or as a therapeutic intervention.

Diagnostic radiopharmaceuticals are designed and prepared to specifically target radioactivity to an organ or system. This targeting allows for imaging and assessment of particular organs and systems for morphologic evaluation or physiologic function.[1,2] Imaging procedures using diagnostic radiopharmaceuticals are generally performed in the nuclear medicine department. Table 23-1 lists examples of the radionuclide, radiopharmaceutical, nuclear medicine procedure and the form of administration used in the diagnosis, staging, and follow-up of malignancies.

Images obtained from the administration of radiopharmaceuticals are static or dynamic depending on the type of information required. Organ morphology including size, shape, position, and presence of space-occupying lesions can be observed on static images. Dynamic studies provide information on function by way of measuring rate of accumulation and clearance of the radiopharmaceutical.[1]

Therapeutic applications of radiopharmaceuticals use particulate radiation (generally, beta particles) for cytotoxicity. The therapeutic dose of a radiopharmaceutical may be designed to cure or control disease in radiosensitive tumors; for example, radioisotopes have been attached to monoclonal antibodies and used in the treatment of patients with non-Hodgkin's lymphoma.[1] Other agents—radioactive pharmaceuticals such as ^{89}Sr-strontium chloride and ^{153}Sm-samarium lexidronam—have been developed to ameliorate pain associated with osseous lesions.[2]

The classic therapeutic use of a radiopharmaceutical in oncology is the use of ^{131}I-sodium iodide for thyroid carcinoma. ^{131}I-sodium iodide emits both beta and gamma radiation and can be used diagnostically and therapeutically, however, the dose required for thyroid ablation (therapeutic application) is significantly higher than the dose required for diagnosing and evaluating thyroid function (diagnostic application).[1]

Concepts of time, distance, appropriate shielding, and radiation exposure are fundamental to radiation oncology nursing practice. These concepts are integrated into the care of the patient receiving diagnostic and therapeutic doses of a radiopharmaceutical; the amount of radioactivity, type of emissions, half-life, elimination, and exposure concerns must be considered in the plan of care and patient/family education.[4,5] This chapter focuses on therapeutic applications of select radiopharmaceuticals.

RADIOIODINE THERAPY FOR THYROID CANCER

Radioactive iodine (RAI) has been used in the treatment of metastatic thyroid cancer for over 50 years and is considered a mainstay of therapy

Table 23-1 Examples of the Radioisotopes and Radiopharmaceuticals Used in Nuclear Medicine Procedures for Oncology Diagnosis and/or Staging Purposes

Radionuclide	Radiopharmaceutical	Test performed	Use	Route
Fluorine (^{18}F-)	^{18}F-Fluorodeoxyglucose (FDG) injection	FDG-positron emission tomography (PET)	Measure glucose use differential—biochemical and metabolic activity of tissue	IV
Technetium (^{99m} TC-)	^{99m} TC-sodium pertechnetate injection	Radionuclide ventriculogram (MUGA)	Measure ventricular ejection fraction	IV
Technetium (^{99m} TC-)	^{99m} TC-medronate injection	Bone scan	Bone imaging for altered osteogenesis	IV
Carbon (^{11}C-)	^{11}C-methionine injection	MET-PET	Imaging of neoplastic brain lesions	IV
Indium (^{111}In-)	^{111}In-pentetreotide injection	OctreoScan	Localization of neuroendocrine tumors with somatostatin receptors	IV
Indium (^{111}In-)	^{111}In-Capromab Pendetide injection	ProstaScint	Localization of prostate cancer	IV

Data from Kowalsky RL, Falen SW: *Radiopharmaceuticals in nuclear pharmacy and nuclear medicine*, ed 2, Washington, DC, 2004, American Pharmacists Association.
MUGA, Multiple gated acquisition (blood pool scan).

for thyroid cancer today.[6] Papillary and follicular thyroid carcinomas may be treated with oral ^{131}I-sodium iodide to ablate any functional, metastatic, or residual remnant of thyroid tissue.[7,8] Additionally, larger doses of ^{131}I are administered with RAI therapy for recurrent or metastatic disease. Iodine uptake is heterogeneous in both normal and malignant thyroid tissue.[8] The metabolism of radioiodine is altered in papillary and follicular thyroid carcinoma because iodine uptake is decreased and the half-life of iodine is shorter.[7-9]

Radioiodine Remnant Ablation

Radioiodine remnant ablation (RRA) is used to destroy residual macroscopic normal thyroid tissue after surgical thyroidectomy.[7,8] Radioactive iodine is usually administered 4 to 6 weeks after surgery; proposed advantages of RRA include the following[7]:

- Microscopic foci of disease present within normal thyroid tissue are eradicated
- Persistent or recurrent disease may be detected early because all remaining normal tissue has been eradicated
- Follow-up serum thyroglobulin (Tg) measurements are more sensitive

An RRA follow-up whole-body scan is performed to screen for any nonphysiologic uptake outside the thyroid area. The first scan is generally obtained 2 to 3 months after radioiodine therapy; subsequent scans are obtained periodically in high-risk patients or when clinical findings suggest possible tumor recurrence.[7-9]

The dose of RAI for RRA has ranged from 25 to 29.9 mCi in low dose regimens and up to 75 to 150 mCi in standard dosages. There is no current consensus for the appropriate dose of RAI for remnant ablation.[7]

Radioactive Iodine Therapy

The most common metastatic sites for thyroid cancer are the lungs, spine, and bone.[7-9] Small nodal metastatic follicular cell lesions are treated with 100 to 175 mCi of RAI; locally recurrent, invasive lesions are usually treated with 150 to 200 mCi. Patients with distant metastatic sites may be treated with dosages up to 200 mCi.[7-9] Older patients with progressive disease that demonstrates minimal radioiodine uptake may be given dosages as high as 300 mCi.

Metastatic sites may have limited avidity for iodine (used in follow-up whole-body scans to ascertain areas of recurrence/metastases).[7] Caution should be used in evaluating iodine whole-body scans for response to high-dose iodine therapy because metastatic lesions with low affinity for iodine may not be seen on imaging. Additionally, subsequent high-dose ^{131}I therapy should be abandoned if the patient does not show a clinical response to RAI. Lesions that are resistant to high-dose RAI often evidence high avidity for ^{18}F-FDG/PET (18-fluorine-fluorodeoxyglucose/positron emission tomography).[7-8]

Oral ^{131}I is available as a liquid solution or capsules for administration; intravenous administration is reserved for those patients unable to swallow the liquid or capsules. The capsule formulation is better tolerated; the product is quickly and completely absorbed in the upper intestine.[8] Patients should be instructed to force fluids; copious amounts of fluid will modulate the dose of radiation to the gastric walls before dissolution of the capsule.[8]

The most clinically relevant side effects of RAI therapy for thyroid carcinoma are limited in duration and severity. Side effects of therapy include nausea and gastric pain lasting a few days, salivary gland inflammation, loss of taste, ocular dryness, nasolacrimal drainage system obstruction, fatigue, headache, marrow suppression, and rare reports of pulmonary fibrosis.[7-9]

Administration of ^{131}I is contraindicated in pregnant and lactating women. Additionally, conception should be delayed for 1 year after RAI because the risk of miscarriages and fetal anomalies is higher in the first year after treatment with ^{131}I. Based on current data, there is no evidence to suggest women of childbearing potential exposed to RAI should avoid subsequent pregnancy.[8,10] Repeated administration of ^{131}I may lead to decreased sperm production, increased levels of follicle-stimulating hormone (FSH), and decreased levels of inhibin B in men.[8,10] Data regarding secondary malignancies and exposure to RAI are inconclusive.[8,9]

Written and oral instructions should be given to the patient before treatment.[8] Nursing care should focus on ameliorating the patient's perception of isolation while the patient is hospitalized; measures to avoid contamination of the hospital room, bathroom, and facility should be implemented. Detailed recommendations and procedures to be followed are site specific and should be obtained from the facility radiation safety officer.[8,9]

RADIOIMMUNOTHERAPY

Systemic administration of radiolabeled antibodies or small molecules enables precise targeting of radioactivity via an antigen or receptor site.[2] Antibodies, small molecules, peptide receptors, or other target carriers are radiolabeled and infused or instilled as part of a therapeutic regimen. At the present time, the commercial use of therapeutic radioimmunotherapy is limited to patients with CD20+ relapsed or refractory low-grade, follicular, or transformed B-cell non-Hodgkin's lymphoma. However, clinical trials have reported on the use of radiolabeled antibodies or other small molecules either as single agents or in combination with chemotherapy in the management of patients with numerous malignancies including metastatic colorectal cancer, ovarian cancer, malignant gliomas, prostate cancer, hepatocellular carcinoma, advanced non–small cell lung cancer, gastroenteropancreatic malignancies, and breast cancer.[11-21]

Radioimmunotherapy for Non-Hodgkin's Lymphoma

Malignancies with accessible tumor-specific antigens or receptors are candidate diseases for rationally designed antibody/ligand therapy. Indeed, monoclonal antibody therapy is considered one of the first successful target-specific therapies for cancer.[22] Monoclonal antibodies are "Y" shaped structures that bind to cell surface antigens with high affinity.[11,22] The *variable* region of the antibody (the upper portion of the Y) can be engineered to bind to a known antigen or receptor; thus the shape of this portion of the antibody will vary according to target morphology.[11,12] Monoclonal antibodies can be unlabeled—sometimes referred to as "cold" or "naked"—or labeled with cytotoxic agents including radioisotopes ("hot").

Desired characteristics of target antigens or receptor sites include the following[23]:

- Target is only present on tumor cells (tumor specific)—so only tumor cells would be accessible to antibody-antigen/receptor site binding and therefore exposed to the treatment
- Target is present or expressed on all malignant progeny—so all tumor cells are exposed to treatment
- Target is stable on the surface of the cell membrane (not found or shed in the circulation, modulated or internalized)

One such antigen, the CD20 antigen, does not shed or modulate (internalized into the cell upon antibody-antigen binding) and is, therefore, an excellent target.[23-25] The CD20 antigen is found on most mature and malignant B cells; unfortunately it is not a target limited to malignant cells. Ninety percent of B-cell lymphomas are CD20+.[22] The CD20 antigen does not shed off the surface of the cell membrane, modulate its structure, or internalize within the cell upon binding, and is present in high density on the surface of most B-cell malignancies.[23-25]

The antineoplastic effects of antibody-antigen binding or receptor/ligand binding are believed to include: 1) complement dependent cellular cytotoxicity (CDCC), 2) antibody dependent cellular cytotoxicity (ADCC), and/or 3) inducement of the affected cell into the apoptotic pathway.[22-26]

In 1997, rituximab (Rituxan; Genentech Inc, South San Francisco, Calif., and Biogen Idec Inc, Cambridge, Mass), an unlabeled antibody directed against the CD20 antigen, was the first monoclonal antibody approved by the U.S. Food and Drug Administration (FDA) for the treatment of low-grade non-Hodgkin's lymphoma.[22,25] Patients with low grade or indolent forms of non-Hodgkin's lymphoma commonly present with advanced stage disease, eventually become refractory to chemotherapy/biotherapy, and succumb to drug-resistant disease. A significant number of these patients will have disease that transforms to a more aggressive form of lymphoma; most are generally considered incurable at presentation.[25,27] Thus there is a need for new therapeutic agents, including biologicals such as rituximab, with novel mechanisms of action.[25,27]

As a single agent, rituximab had limited activity in clinical trials. Results of the pivotal multicenter phase II trial in 166 patients with relapsed low-grade lymphoma showed an overall response rate of 48% with a 6% complete response rate and a 42% partial response rate in patients with recurrent follicular and low-grade lymphoma. The median number of prior therapies was 3; the median duration of response was slightly less than 1 year at 11.2 months.[28]

Studies investigating the combination of rituximab with chemotherapy, duration of therapy with rituximab (including number/sequence of cycles, maintenance therapy), line of therapy, and incorporation of rituximab in combination with other biologic agents are ongoing.[25,28-32] The combination of rituximab and CHOP (cyclophosphamide, hydroxydaunomycin, vincristine [Oncovin], prednisone) chemotherapy in patients with CD20+ aggressive non-Hodgkin's lymphoma improved the complete response rate (76%) compared to chemotherapy alone (63%, $p = 0.005$).[33]

Radioimmunotherapy, or the combination of directed radiation therapy via a radioisotope bound to a target-specific monoclonal antibody or receptor, may overcome inherent or acquired resistance to chemotherapy and/or monoclonal antibody therapy, including rituximab-resistant disease.[24,26] Lymphomas are considered one of the most radiosensitive cancers.[34] Localized disease is curable with external beam radiation therapy; yet only a small portion of these patients are diagnosed when treatment with external beam for curative intent is an option.[34] Therefore, systemic delivery of specifically targeted cytotoxic particles of radioactivity is an attractive alternative.[35]

The resultant targeting of the radiolabeled monoclonal antibody (radioimmunoconjugate) to the CD20 antigen on lymphoma cells may surmount some of the impediments found in unlabeled antibody therapy.[23,24,26] Tumor cell heterogeneity in antigen expression and/or the lack of CD20 antigen accessible sites because of poor tumor vascularity potentially limit the effectiveness of unlabeled antibodies.[23,24,26,35] Antibody/antigen binding initiates CDCC, ADCC, and apoptotic pathways.[26,35,36]

In radioimmunotherapy, the presence and length of the radionucleotide emissions may mitigate some of these obstacles (heterogeneity in antigen expression, lack of accessible sites for antigen/antibody binding) through the *"crossfire" effect*. The crossfire effect refers to collateral damage to adjacent tumor cells caused by the cytotoxicity of beta particles emitted by the radionucleotide attached to the antibody bound to those neighboring tumor cells that express the antigenic target.[23,26,35-37]

Two similar yet different radiolabeled monoclonal antibody regimens have been approved by the FDA for the treatment of patients with indolent forms of non-Hodgkin's lymphoma that have relapsed following primary therapy. Both regimens include an infusion of unlabeled monoclonal antibodies before the infusion of both the tracer and therapeutic doses of the radiolabeled antibodies, have the CD20 antigen as the target receptor, and have demonstrable activity and durable responses in patients with indolent forms of lymphoma such as follicular lymphomas and the follicular lymphomas that have transformed.[22,24,26,35,36] The initial infusion of unlabeled antibodies—given before each of the radiolabeled infusions—optimizes the biodistribution of the radiolabeled antibodies by binding to CD20-accessible sites in the spleen and circulation.[35,36] Additionally, patients who relapse after radioimmunotherapy can often receive additional courses of chemotherapy or immunotherapy without undue concern regarding toxicity. Table 23-2 provides a comparison of the major properties associated with the two radioisotopes used in the therapeutic portion of the Bexxar (^{131}I) and Zevalin (^{90}Y) radioimmunotherapy regimens. Table 23-3 lists the infused components of both radioimmunotherapies.

Potential patients should be evaluated for appropriateness of radioimmunotherapy before scheduling the infusions. Data to be obtained and reviewed includes tumor histopathology reports (type of lymphoma and if CD20 ±, results of a recent bone marrow biopsy and aspirate including marrow cellularity and percent involvement by lymphoma), lab work including a creatinine and blood urea nitrogen (BUN), and a complete blood count with differential and platelets, patient history and physical, treatment history including chemotherapy flow sheets, performance status, and computed tomography/positron emission topography (CT/PET) results. Previous exposure to both chimeric and murine antibody therapy should be noted. The choice of radioimmunotherapeutic agent (Bexxar or Zevalin) is based, in part, on a variety of patient variables including current and possible living arrangements, the patient's ability to understand and comply with modified living arrangements to delimit radiation exposure to others (pregnant women and children, co-workers, caregivers, members of the general public), urinary continence, and patient tolerance/intolerance or exposure to previous monoclonal antibody therapy.[35,36] Patients with significant symptomatology also may need to be evaluated for electron beam radiation therapy (EBRT).

Bexxar Therapeutic Regimen

Bexxar is indicated for the treatment of patients with CD20 antigen–expressing relapsed or refractory, low-grade, follicular, or transformed non-Hodgkin's lymphoma, including patients with rituximab-refractory non-Hodgkin's lymphoma. Bexxar is not indicated for the initial treatment of patients with CD20-positive non-Hodgkin's lymphoma. The

Table 23-2 Characteristics of ^{90}Y and ^{131}I

Radionuclide for therapeutic application	Physical half-life	Decay type	Particulate energy	Primary gamma energy	Particle length in tissue	Biologic clearance	Nontumor potential for uptake
Yttrium (^{90}Y)	2.7 days	β	2.3 MeV	None	5.3 mm	Slower	Bone
Iodine (^{131}I)	8.01 days	β, γ	0.606 MeV	0.364	0.8 mm	Rapid	Thyroid

Data from Bush S: *Semin Oncol Nurs* 18(Suppl 1):16-21, 2002; Hendrix C: *Semin Oncol Nurs* 20(Suppl 1):14-19, 2004.

Table 23-3 Infused Components of the Zevalin and Bexxar Regimens

	Zevalin	Bexxar
Predose unlabeled monoclonal antibody	Rituximab 250 mg/m^2	Tositumomab 450 mg
Imaging radioimmunoconjugate	^{111}In-ibritumomab tiuxetan 5 mCi	^{131}I-tositumomab 5 mCi
Therapeutic radioimmunoconjugate	^{90}Y-ibritumomab tiuxetan 0.4 mCi for platelet count >150,000 or 0.3 mCi for platelet count 100,000 to 149,000	^{131}I-tositumomab 75cGy for platelet count > 150,000 or 65cGy for platelet count 100,000 to 149,999

Data from Bush S: *Semin Oncol Nurs* 18(Suppl 1):16-21, 2002; Hendrix C: *Semin Oncol Nurs* 20(Suppl 1):14-19, 2004; Wahl R: *J Nucl Med* 46(Suppl 1):128S-140S, 2005.
^{111}In, Indium-111; *^{90}Y,* yttrium-90.

Bexxar therapeutic regimen consists of two steps—a dosimetric phase and a therapeutic phase. In the dosimetric phase, the patient is infused with 450 mg of tositumomab (unlabeled antibody) followed by a dosimetric dose (5 mCi) of radiolabeled iodine-131 (^{131}I) tositumomab. The therapeutic portion consists of an infusion of 450 mg of tositumomab followed by a patient-specific dose of radiolabeled ^{131}I-tositumomab calculated to deliver a particular total-body radiation absorbed dose.[35,36] The entire treatment can be administered in nuclear medicine or in radiation oncology on an outpatient basis and is completed in 14 days or less.[35,36]

^{131}I is a gamma and beta emitter and was chosen as the radiolabel for the monoclonal antibody for the following reasons[35]:

- Gamma emissions would allow noninvasive imaging to determine biodistribution, whole-body clearance, and dosimetry
- Properties of free ^{131}I in regards to chemistry, path length of emissions, biodistribution, and toxicity profile are known
- Free ^{131}I is primarily cleared via the renal system in patients on thyroid-protecting agents; does not bind to bone cortex
- Half-life of ^{131}I is well matched to the antibody in regards to localization, retention, and clearance

The total-body clearance of radioactivity administered as ^{131}I-tositumomab is monoexponential. This relatively linear clearance allows for a patient-specific dose that is calculated from data (gamma camera counts) obtained at three time points (dosimetry).[35] Patients are dosed to achieve a 65cGy (platelet count of 100,000-149,999/mm^3) or 75cGy total-body absorbed dose for patients with a platelet count greater than 150,000/mm^3. The significance of a patient-specific calculation cannot be underestimated because the interpatient variability in doses of ^{131}I-tositumomab required to obtain a 65cGy or 75cGy total-body absorbed dose can be significant; patients with large spleens, bulky tumors, or significant marrow involvement require greater mCi activity to be administered to achieve the desired total-body dose (cGy), whereas patients with a normal-sized spleen, limited or no marrow involvement, and a small tumor burden will require less mCi activity to achieve that same target total-body absorbed dose (cGy).[35]

Before the initial infusion of Bexxar, patients are prescribed a thyroid-protecting agent and begin thyroid blockade at least 24 hours before the dosimetric infusion. This thyroid blockade, delimiting uptake of the radioactive iodine into the thyroid, should be continued throughout the regimen and continue for 14 days after the therapeutic infusion (between 23 and 30 days inclusive depending on the patient infusion schedule).[35,36]

The dosimetric step, the first part of the therapeutic regimen, includes a 60-minute infusion of 450 mg of unlabeled tositumomab followed by a 20-minute infusion of radiolabeled tositumomab (5 mCi ^{131}I-tositumomab/35 mg unlabeled tositumomab). The patient should be premedicated with diphenhydramine and acetaminophen before the unlabeled antibody infusion; vital signs (temperature, pulse, respiration, and blood pressure) are obtained immediately before, during, and after the infusion according to institution protocol. Imaging with the gamma camera follows the infusion of the radiolabeled component; anterior and posterior gamma camera counts are obtained as well. Images and gamma camera counts are obtained at three different time points (on day 0 immediately after the radiolabeled infusion; on day 2, 3, *or* 4; and again on day 6 *or* 7); the counts are used to determine the clearance/residence time of the ^{131}I-tositumomab. Images are evaluated for biodistribution.[35,36]

The therapeutic portion of the regimen consists of two infusions—a 60-minute infusion of 450 mg of unlabeled tositumomab followed by a 20-minute infusion of radiolabeled ^{131}I-tositumomab/35 mg unlabeled tositumomab. The mCi dose of the ^{131}I component to be delivered is, as described earlier, variable and individualized to the patient; the dose is calculated to achieve a 65cGy or 75cGy total-body absorbed dose. Patients with a platelet count of 100,000/mm^3 to 149,999/mm^3 should receive a target dose of 65cGy; patients with platelet counts greater than 150,000/mm^3 should have a dose targeted for 75cGy. Patients with less than 100,000/mm^3 platelets should not be treated with Bexxar. Patients are premedicated as during the first infusion; vital signs are obtained immediately before, during, and following the tositumomab infusions and according to institutional guidelines.[35,36]

A syringe pump capable of holding a 60-mL syringe and delivering the total volume of 30 mL over 20 minutes is used for the infusion of the radioactive component. Lead shields for shielding the syringe pumps can be bought; some institutions use a lead "cave" or "fort" for shielding during the infusion.

Figure 23-1 depicts the Bexxar therapeutic regimen.

Patients are evaluated for releasability immediately after the therapeutic infusion. Calculations using both the residence time and the measured exposure rates (at 1 meter from the patient after the infusion) are used to determine timeframes for minimizing exposure to others. Recently revised guidelines from the Nuclear Regulatory Commission (NRC) enable most patients treated with Bexxar to be released after the therapeutic infusion; data from the University of Nebraska revealed that the average exposure to caregivers was less than 150 milliroentgens (mR) when following posttreatment release instructions—certainly less than the limit of 500 mR recommended by the NRC.[35] Patients are given specific written instructions detailing measures to limit exposure to others. Corresponding timeframes for following the instructions are also reviewed with the patient and caregiver(s) before discharge.[35,36]

Overview of Efficacy and Safety Studies With ^{131}I-tositumomab

Early studies with ^{131}I-tositumomab were performed at the University of Michigan; the *phase I study* included a protein-mass dose escalation and a radiation-absorbed dose escalation. The optimal dose for the unlabeled antibody infusion was determined to be 450mg; the total-body absorbed radiation dose was escalated in 10cGy increments with the maximally tolerated dose determined to 75cGy in patients with platelet counts greater than 150,000/mm^3, 65cGy in patients with platelets counts greater than 100,000/mm^3 and less than 150,000/mm^3, and 45cGy in patients who had undergone prior bone marrow transplantation. Fifty-nine patients were entered into the study and 53 patients were treated. Most patients had been heavily pretreated with a mean of 3.9 prior therapies including chemotherapy, radiation therapy, and biologic therapy. Almost half of the patients had no response to their last chemotherapy and most had a number of poor prognostic indicators. According to investigators, 71% of patients responded; 34% of patients achieved complete responses. For responders, the median progression-free survival for all patients was 12 months and 20.3 months for those patients with a complete response. Toxicities included reversible grade 3–4 hematologic toxicity, hypothyroidism (approximately 10%), seroconversion to positive human antimouse antibody (17%), and myelodysplastic syndrome (in approximately 10%).[35,38]

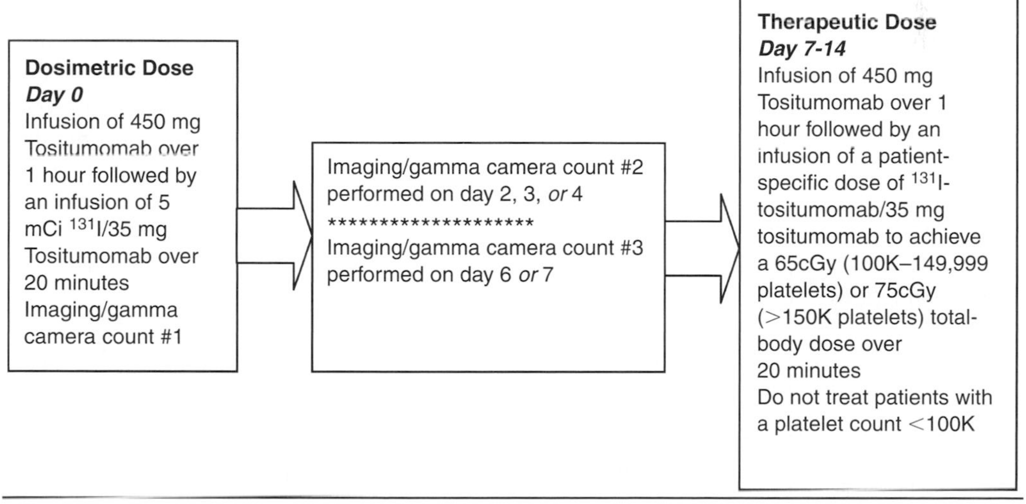

Figure 23-1 Bexxar Therapeutic Regimen.

The efficacy and safety of ^{131}I-tositumomab in patients with B-cell lymphoma that progressed after rituximab was further evaluated in a phase II multicenter study of 40 patients. Twenty-four subjects were considered non-responders to rituximab; over half of the patients were deemed resistant to chemotherapy. According to Horning and colleagues[39] the median number of prior therapies in this patient group was four. The confirmed overall response rate was 65% with a complete response rate of 38%. The median progression-free survival was 24.5 months for responders and has not been reached for complete responders. Approximately 50% of patients experienced transient grade 3–4 myelosuppression. The median time to a complete response was 13 weeks.

Davies and colleagues[40] conducted an open-label phase II study of ^{131}I-tositumomab in patients with indolent or transformed B-cell lymphoma at first or second recurrence; 76% of patients responded with 49% of patients achieving a complete response and 27% achieving a partial remission. The overall median duration of response was 1.3 years; the median duration of response has not been reached in patients with a complete response. Eleven of 31 responders (confirmed and unconfirmed) remain in a complete remission for a minimum of 2.6 years with a median of 4.1 years. Toxicity was considered mild and easily manageable; grade 3 or 4 anemia, neutropenia, and thrombocytopenia was seen in 5%, 45%, and 32% or patients, respectively.

Finally, Kaminski and colleagues[41] evaluated ^{131}I-tositumomab therapy as initial treatment for follicular lymphoma. The study included 76 patients; results indicated that 95% of the patients had a response with 75% of patients achieving a complete response. The median progression-free survival was 6.1 years. Approximately 77% of patients with a complete response remain disease-free for over 5 years. Toxicity included mild to moderate hematologic toxicity with a median neutrophil nadir of 1300/mm^3 and a median platelet nadir of 83,000/mm^3. No cases of myelodysplastic syndrome (MDS) or acute myelogenous leukemia (AML) have been reported in this group of patients.

Zevalin Therapeutic Regimen

Zevalin is indicated for the treatment of patients with relapsed or refractory low-grade, follicular, or transformed B-cell non-Hodgkin's lymphoma, including patients with rituximab refractory follicular non-Hodgkin's lymphoma.[42] The Zevalin therapeutic regimen also consists of two steps and can be completed in 7 to 9 days (Figure 23-2). Step one, the dosimetric step, includes an infusion of 250 mg/m^2 of rituximab followed within 4 hours by a 5 mCi imaging dose of indium-111 (^{111}In)-ibritumomab tiuxetan. The ^{111}In-ibritumomab tiuxetan is given IV push over 10 minutes. Whole body images via a gamma camera are obtained at one time point—between 48 to 72 hours to determine biodistribution; a second scan is optional and may be performed 90 to 120 hours after the dosimetric infusion if the results of the first scan are ambiguous.[42] The regimen is completed on day 7, 8, *or* 9 with another infusion of 250 mg/m^2 of rituximab followed by the therapeutic injection

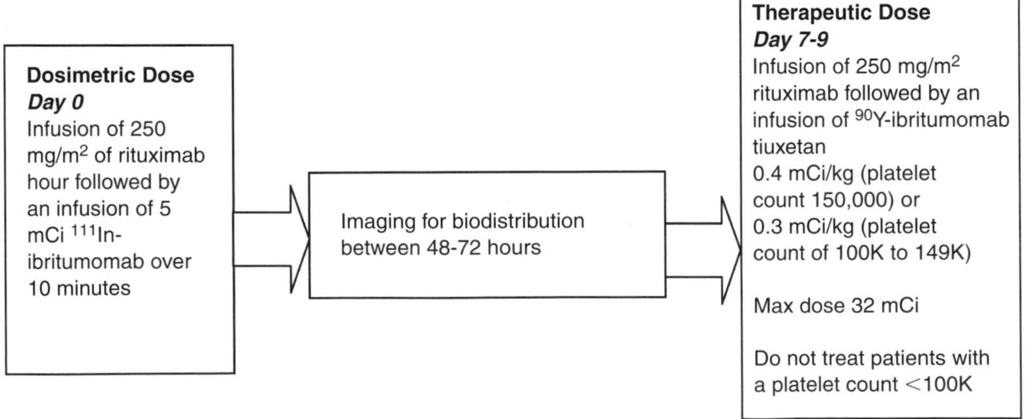

Figure 23-2 Zevalin Therapeutic Regimen.

of yttrium-90 (^{90}Y)-ibritumomab tiuxetan over 10 minutes.

The rituximab is administered in the oncology infusion center; the radiolabeled component is administered in nuclear medicine and/or radiation oncology.[43] Infusion reactions, which may be severe, are most often associated with the rituximab infusion and are primarily seen with the first infusion.[42,43]

^{90}Y-ibritumomab tiuxetan is dosed by weight; patients with a platelet count of more than 150,000/mm^3 should receive 0.4 mCi/kg and patients with a platelet count between 100,000/mm^3 and 149,999/mm^3 should be dose reduced to 0.3 mCi/kg. Patients with less than 100,000/m^3 of platelets should not receive ^{90}Y-ibritumomab tiuxetan. The maximum allowable dose of ^{90}Y-ibritumomab tiuxetan is 32.0 mCi.[42-45]

Ibritumomab is the murine monoclonal antibody "parent" of rituximab, a chimeric monoclonal antibody. Ibritumomab is linked to ^{111}In, a gamma emitter, for imaging purposes, and to ^{90}Y, a pure beta emitter, for therapeutic purposes. Dissociation of the radionucleotide in vitro is less than 1% per day; there is little interpatient variability in urinary clearance. Urinary clearance of ^{90}Y-ibritumomab tiuxetan is the primary route of excretion; only 7.3% ± 3.2% of the administered dose is found in the urine in the first week after therapy. Hematologic toxicity correlates with the administered dose and does not correlate with the radiation absorbed dose to either total body or red marrow.[42-45]

^{90}Y is a pure beta emitter and cannot be used for imaging for biodistribution, which is why ^{111}In is used as a surrogate radiolabel in evaluating biodistribution. Acrylic vial and syringe shields are required with the ^{90}Y-ibritumomab tiuxetan; lead shielding should not be used with ^{90}Y-ibritumomab tiuxetan because interaction of the beta emissions with high atomic weight materials will produce bremsstrahlung.[43-45]

^{90}Y-ibritumomab tiuxetan is administered on an outpatient basis; the radiolabeled antibody is injected over 10 minutes at both time points. Patients can be discharged immediately after treatment with ^{90}Y-ibritumomab tiuxetan with few restrictions or modified living arrangements. Patients should be instructed regarding appropriate handling of urine spills, importance of handwashing after urination, and use of condoms for sexual relations.[43-45]

Overview of Efficacy and Safety Studies With ^{90}Y-ibritumomab tiuxetan

Long-term follow-up data of the *phase I and II* study were reported in 2004.[46] Fifty of fifty one patients received study drug; all subjects had received prior chemotherapy and had received a median of two prior regimens. Eighteen percent of participants were resistant to their last chemotherapy. The overall response rate in this study was 73%, and 51% of patients obtained a complete response (confirmed and unconfirmed complete responses). The median time to progression for responders was 12.6 months; the median duration of response was 11.7 months. Patients treated with 0.4 mCi of ^{90}Y-ibritumomab tiuxetan achieving a complete response had a median time to progression of 45 months. The primary systemic side effect seen was reversible hematologic toxicity. There has been no increase in MDS or AML incidence seen in this study group.[46,47]

Witzig and colleagues[48] compared single-agent standard dose rituximab (375 mg/m^2 q week × 4 weeks, n = 70 patients) with ^{90}Y-ibritumomab tiuxetan (0.4 mCi/kg, n = 73 patients) in a phase III randomized study. ^{90}Y-ibritumomab tiuxetan had overall response rates (80% versus 56%) and complete response rates (30% versus 16%) significantly higher than those of rituximab in patients with relapsed or refractory low-grade, follicular, or transformed B-cell non-Hodgkin's lymphoma. The difference in response duration, however, was not statistically significant; the study was not powered adequately to detect differences in time to event variables/response duration.[47,48] The median time to progression for patients (all inclusive) treated with the radiolabeled antibody was 10.6 months and 10.2 months for patients treated with the unlabeled antibody.[47,48]

Earlier use of radioimmunotherapy (^{131}I-tositumomab and ^{90}Y-ibritumomab tiuxetan) is associated with higher overall and complete response rates and is associated with longer, more durable responses. Integrated data analyses of both Bexxar and Zevalin supports the earlier use of radioimmunotherapy as a therapeutic modality. First relapse patients achieve a higher overall response rate than patients with two or more prior therapies. Additionally, both the median time to progression and response durations are longer in patients treated at first or second relapse than in patients treated at fourth or fifth relapse.[49]

There is no data from a direct comparative trial of the two radioimmunotherapies—^{131}I-tositumomab and ^{90}Y-ibritumomab tiuxetan—available at present. Given that there is no data, it is and would be inappropriate to compare data across trials. Significant similarities and differences in the regimens exist that may make one product more appropriate than the other in individual patient situations. Both products have similar toxicity profiles with a prolonged hematologic nadir; both require interim blood counts (CBC) for monitoring and intervention (typically begin drawing the CBC 3 weeks after the therapy and continuing weekly for 10 to 12 weeks through the nadir). Patients treated with ^{131}I-tositumomab should have a thyroid-stimulating hormone (TSH) level drawn before therapy and repeated yearly because the incidence of hypothyroidism after Bexxar therapy is approximately 10%.[26,36,37,43,44] Bexxar is dosed by clearance (gamma camera counts) and Zevalin is dosed by patient weight.

Future Implications

Early data supports the use of radiolabeled antibody therapy as part of the initial therapy of indolent non-Hodgkin's lymphoma. The Southwest Oncology Group is currently conducting a trial of Rituxan/CHOP chemotherapy versus CHOP chemotherapy followed by ^{131}I-tositumomab; data from the phase II study revealed an overall response rate of 90% including 67% complete remissions (confirmed and unconfirmed) and 23% partial remissions. Therapy with ^{131}I-tositumomab improved the overall response rate to chemotherapy significantly. Furthermore, toxicities recorded after the radiolabeled antibody therapy were generally more mild than those seen after CHOP chemotherapy.[50]

MANAGEMENT OF PAIN ASSOCIATED WITH OSSEOUS LESIONS

Bone (osseous) metastases are a significant complication of a number of solid tumors including breast, prostate, lung, renal, and thyroid cancers. Pain associated with these metastases can certainly diminish the patient's quality of life and decrease their performance status. Clinical complications of osseous lesions can include hypercalcemia of malignancy (HCM) and fractures. Over 50% of patients with breast and prostate cancer who develop boney metastases suffer significant pain associated with the osseous lesions. Therapeutic options include chemotherapy, hormonal therapy, nonsteroidal antiinflammatory drugs, narcotic analgesics, steroids, radiofrequency ablation, external beam radiation, bisphosphonates, and systemically administered radiotherapeutic agents including phosphorus-32, strontium-89, and samarium-153.[51-57] At the present time, treatment is palliative and a combination of systemic and localized therapies may be required for optimum patient management.

Several radiopharmaceuticals have been developed to treat osseous lesions; most are administered systemically (intravenously) and target lesions by accretion to reactive sites. The two most common bone-seeking radiopharmaceuticals used in the management of painful osseous lesions in the United States include strontium chloride (^{89}SrCl, Metastron) and samarium (^{153}Sm) lexidronam (Quadramet) (Table 23-4).[52,53]

Single injections of the systemic radioisotope target all boney lesions, whether symptomatic or not, and are not limited to osteoblastic bone metastases. Lesions that are osteolytic and osteoblastic are targeted. Pain relief can be achieved within a week, depending on the radiopharmaceutical used, and can last for months after a single injection. Over half of the patients treated with targeted radioisotope therapy report a decreased need for analgesics, an increase in quality of life, and improved mobility. Thus the goals of systemic radioisotope therapy include amelioration of pain or substantial pain relief, improved quality of life, decreasing dependence on alternative forms of pain relief, and improved outcomes/survival.[51-54]

Patients referred for bone pain palliation therapy should have blood counts drawn within 1 week of therapy; due consideration should be given to the length of the nadir and impact of resultant myelosuppression on the overall clinical course. A bone scan is used to ascertain that metastatic disease is indeed the etiology of the pain. Acute or chronic renal failure, significant renal insufficiency, hypersensitivity to any of the components of therapy, the need for emergent EBRT, platelet count of less than 60,000/mm^3 or a neutrophil count of less than 1500/mm^3 are general contraindications.[51-53]

Metastron (^{89}SrCl)

Strontium-89 (^{89}Sr) has been used in the management of painful boney metastases for over 30 years. Similar to calcium, ^{89}Sr is biodistributed to areas

Table 23-4 Characteristics of Radiopharmaceuticals Used in Pain Palliation of Osseous Metastases

Isotope	Radiopharmaceutical	Half-life (d)	β-energy (MeV) max/mean	γ-energy (MeV) [%]	Soft-tissue range (mm) max/minimum
Strontium (^{89}Sr)	$^{89}SrCl$	50.5	1.46/0.58	0.91/(0.01)	2.4
Samarium (^{153}Sm)	^{153}Sm-EDTMP	1.93	0.81/0.23	0.103 (29)	0.6
Rhenium (^{186}Re)	^{186}Re-HEDP	3.7	1.07/0.349	0.137 (9)	2.4
Rhenium (^{188}Re)	$^{188}ReHEDP$	0.7	2.12	–	3
Tin (^{117m}Sn)	^{117}mSn-DTPA	14	None—emits conversion electrons	0.158 (86)	0.3/0.2

Data from Serafini A, Houston SJ, Resche I, et al: *J Clin Oncol* 16:1574-1581, 1998; Pandit-Taskar N, Batraki M, Divgi CR: *J Nucl Med* 45:1358-1365, 2004; Serafini A: *J Nucl Med* 42:895-906, 2001; Pagliaro LC, Delpassand ES, Williams D, et al: *Cancer* 97: 2988-2994, 2003; Scuito R, Festa A, Pasqualoni R, et al: *Br Cancer Res Treat* 66:101-109, 2001; Li S, Liu J, Zhang H, et al: *Clin Nucl Med* 26:919-922, 2001; Palmedo H, Manka-Waluch A, Albers P, et al: *J Clin Oncol* 21:2869-2875, 2003.

Cl, Chloride; *EDTMP,* ethylenediaminetetramethylene phosphonic acid; *HEDP,* hydroxyethylidenediphosphonate; *DTPA,* diethylenetriaminepentaacetic acid.

of the skeleton that normally metabolize calcium to create new bone. Approximately 30% of ^{89}Sr is excreted in the urine and gastrointestinal tract; the rest is retained in the skeleton. The degree of retention is variable; more of the radioisotope is retained in the bone when more of the skeleton is involved. The biologic half-life is profoundly affected by the presence of osseous lesions; the biologic half-life is approximately 2 weeks in normal bone, whereas the biologic half-life may be closer to 50 days in reactive bone around metastases.[51-53] Approximately 20% may be retained for over 90 days.[52] Transient flare reactions may occur in 2 to 3 days after treatment, is self-limiting, and usually implies a therapeutic benefit. A fixed dose of 148 MBq (4 MCi) is used most commonly.[51-53] Patients may be retreated after 3 months, with cumulative marrow toxicity being the primary deterrent.[52,53]

Numerous studies with ^{89}Sr have been reported using varied protocols and dosing schedules. Randomized phase III studies evaluated efficacy and safety of Metastron to local or hemibody EBRT; most studies involved subjects with prostate cancer.[53]

Quadramet

The most commonly used bone-seeking radiopharmaceutical for pain palliation in the United States today is samarium (^{153}Sm) lexidronam injection, or Quadramet. Quadramet concentrates in the skeleton in proportion to osteoblastic activity. Less than 1% remains in the circulation at 5 hours after injection; with approximately 65% remaining in the skeleton. Urinary clearance is virtually complete at 6 hours. The dose of Quadramet is 37 MBq/kg or 1 mCi/kg. The dose-limiting toxicity is myelosuppression with a platelet nadir between days 16 and 45 (median is 28 days); the neutrophil nadir occurs at 3 to 4 weeks, with hematologic recovery at 2 months for the majority of patients. Hematologic toxicity is more common in patients with extensive boney metastases, and pretreatment platelet count, hormonal therapy, tumor pathology, and percentage of Quadramet uptake impact the degree of myelotoxicity more than the dose of Quadramet.[51-53]

A transient flare reaction may occur within 72 hours of the injection in 10% of patients, is self-limiting, and is usually responsive to analgesics. A dose of Quadramet can provide pain relief for up to 4 months, with onset of relief occurring as early as 1 week after injection and maximum relief occurring approximately 1 month after administration.[52,53]

Pivotal prospective controlled studies have been performed in Asia, Europe, and North America. Serafini and colleagues[51,53] randomized 118 patients to placebo or one of two doses of ^{153}Sm-lexidronam. Pain scores were unchanged in the placebo group, whereas pain scores revealed relief primarily in patients receiving a 37 MBq/kg (1.0 mCi/kg) dose of the radiopharmaceutical. Pain relief was experienced early on and was durable; findings were supportive of the short half-life and high dose rate of ^{153}Sm. Additionally studies by Sartor [54], Resche and colleagues [55], and Bushnell and colleagues[56] support the earlier findings reported by Serafini.[51,53]

Other Agents

Rhenium-labeled radiopharmaceuticals also have been used as alternative agents for bone pain palliation. According to Sciuto and colleagues[58] approximately 92% of patients with breast cancer achieved overall pain relief with ^{186}Re-HEDP (hydroxyethylidenediphosphonate); pain relief of 50% to 100% has been reported in various other cancers including androgen-independent prostate cancer.[58-60] Thrombocytopenia is the dose limiting toxicity; marrow recovery generally occurs within 4–6 weeks for most patients. Flare reactions have been reported which last up to 4 days.[52,58-60] This agent is not available in the United States.[52]

^{117m}Sn-DTPA (diethylenetriamine pentaacetic acid)/^{117m}Sn-pentetate is an experimental radiopharmaceutical with a low incidence of myelosuppression. Pain palliation response rates are reported to be around 75% and may be seen within 1 week of injection.[52,61]

SUMMARY

The use of radiopharmaceuticals in oncology nursing practice is expanding beyond traditional diagnostic applications. Historically, ^{131}I has been used in the management of patients with certain forms of thyroid carcinoma. Radioimmunotherapy—an infused form of radiation therapy—is an emerging option for patients with relapsed or refractory CD20+ low-grade, follicular, or transformed lymphoma. Data regarding response rates, the potential for complete responses, and duration of response are particularly encouraging.

The infusion components for radioimmunotherapy are completed in two visits within a 2-week window; nadirs occur approximately 30 to 45 days after the therapeutic dose. Most patients will recover their counts within 3 months.

Patients should be evaluated for appropriateness of radioimmunotherapy before treatment. There are significant similarities and differences in the two radioimmunotherapies approved for clinical use in the United States, and the choice of agent depends, in part, on individual patient variables. Additionally, patients should be educated about principles of radioimmunotherapy, outpatient release instructions, potential adverse events, and other practical considerations.

Finally, radiopharmaceuticals are also used in the management of pain associated with metastatic disease. Patients with metastatic prostate cancer and metastatic breast cancer make up the majority of patients enrolled in clinical trials evaluating ^{89}SrCl (Metastron) and ^{153}Sm-lexidronam (Quadramet). Systemically administered bone-seeking radiopharmaceuticals have been associated with improved patient performance status, pain control, and quality of life. Additional radiopharmaceuticals are under investigation and show promise; they are relatively simple to administer, are well tolerated by the patient when used appropriately, and can be used in combination with other treatment modalities.

REFERENCES

1. Kowalsky RL, Falen SW: *Radiopharmaceuticals in nuclear pharmacy and nuclear medicine,* ed 2, Washington, DC, 2004, American Pharmacists Association.
2. Goldman B: Next generation of targeted radiotherapy drugs emerging from the clinical pipeline, *J Natl Cancer Inst* 96(12):903-904, 2004.
3. Weber W: Use of PET for monitoring cancer therapy and for predicting outcome, *J Nucl Med* 46(6):983-995, 2005.
4. Gosselin-Acomb TK: Principles of radiation therapy. In Yarbro C, Frogge M, Goodman M, editors: *Cancer nursing principles and practice,* ed 6, Sudbury, Mass, 2005, Jones and Bartlett, pp 229-249.
5. Behrend SW: Radiation treatment planning. In Yarbro C, Frogge M, Goodman M, editors: *Cancer nursing principles and practice,* ed 6, Sudbury, Mass, 2005, Jones and Bartlett, pp 250-282.
6. Seidlin S, Oshry E, Yallow AA: Spontaneous and experimentally induced uptake of radioactive iodine in metastases from thyroid carcinoma, *J Clin Endocrinol Metab* 8(8):423-425, 1948.
7. American Association of Clinical Endocrinologists/ American Association of Endocrine Surgeons: Medical/ surgical guidelines for clinical practice: management of thyroid cancer, *Endocr Pract* 7(3):203-220, 2001.
8. Robbins RJ, Schlumberger MJ: The evolving role of ^{131}I for the treatment of differentiated thyroid carcinoma, *J Nucl Med* 46 (Suppl):28S-33S, 2005.
9. Grigsby P: Thyroid. In Perez CA, Brady LW, Halperin EC et al, editors: *Principles and practice of radiation oncology,* ed 4, Philadelphia, 2004, Lippincott-Raven, pp 1179-1200.
10. Fraker DG, Skarulis M, Livolsk V: Thyroid cancers. In DeVita V, Hellman S, Rosenberg S, editors: *Cancer: principles and practice of oncology,* ed 6, Philadelphia, 2001, Lippincott Williams & Wilkins, pp 1740-1763.
11. Forero A, Meredith RF, Khazaeli MB et al: A novel monoclonal antibody design for radioimmunotherapy, *Cancer Biother Radiopharmaceut* 18(5):751-759, 2003.
12. Meredith RF, Alvarez RD, Partridge EE et al: Intraperitoneal radioimmunochemotherapy of ovarian cancer: a phase I study, *Cancer Biother Radiopharmaceut* 16(4):305-315, 2001.
13. Akabani G, Reardon DA, Coleman RE et al: Dosimetry and radiographic analysis of ^{131}I-labeled anti-tenascin 81C6 murine monoclonal antibody in newly diagnosed

patients with malignant gliomas: a phase II study, *J Nucl Med* 46(6):1042-1051, 2005.

14. Bander NH, Trabulsi EJ, Kostakoglu L et al: Targeting metastatic prostate cancer with radiolabeled monoclonal antibody J591 to the extracellular domain of prostate specific membrane antigen, *J Urol* 170(5):1717-1721, 2003.
15. Milowsky MI, Nanus DM, Kostakoglu L et al: Phase I trial of 90Y-labeled anti-prostate specific membrane antigen monoclonal antibody J591 for androgen-independent prostate cancer, *J Clin Oncol* 22(13):2522-2531, 2004.
16. Bander NH, Milowsky MI, Nanus DM et al: Phase I trial of ^{177}lutetium-labeled J591, a monoclonal antibody to prostate-specific membrane antigen, in patients with androgen-independent prostate cancer, *J Clin Oncol* 23(21): 4591-4601, 2005.
17. Chen S, Beilei L, Hong Xie et al: Phase I clinical trial of targeted therapy using ^{131}I hepama-1 mab in patients with hepatocellular carcinoma, *Cancer Biother Radiopharmaceut* 19(5):589-600, 2004.
18. Buck RH, Robert F, Meredith RF et al: Phase I study of 90Y-CC49 monoclonal antibody therapy in patients with advanced non-small cell lung cancer, *Proc Am Assoc Cancer Res* 41(3):634, 2000 (abstract).
19. Robert F, Busby EM, LoBuglio AF: Chemotherapy tolerance after radioimmunotherapy with ^{90}Y-CC49 monoclonal antibody in patients with advanced non-small cell lung cancer: clinical effects and hematologic toxicity, *Cancer Biother Radiopharmaceut* 18(3):317-325, 2003.
20. Kwekkeboom DJ, Mueller-Brand J, Paganelli G et al: Overview of results of peptide receptor radionuclide therapy with 3 radiolabeled somatostatin analogues, *J Nucl Med* 46(suppl 1):62S-66S, 2005.
21. DeNardo S: Radioimmunodetection and therapy of breast cancer, *Semin Nucl Med* 35(2):143 151, 2005.
22. Forero A, LoBuglio A: History of antibody therapy for non-Hodgkin's lymphoma, *Semin Oncol* 30(6 suppl 17): 1-5, 2003.
23. Maloney DG: Concepts in radiotherapy and immunotherapy: anti-CD20 mechanisms of action and targets, *Semin Oncol* 32(1 suppl 1):S19-S26, 2005.
24. Horning SJ: Future directions in radioimmunotherapy for B-cell lymphoma, *Semin Oncol* 30(6 suppl 17):29-34, 2003.
25. Foon KA, Safa MM: Biologic therapy of lymphoma. In Mauch PM, Armitage JO, Coiffier B, et al, editors: *Non-Hodgkin's lymphoma,* Philadelphia, 2004, Lippincott Williams & Wilkins.
26. Riley MB, Byar K: The rationale for and background of radioimmunotherapy: an emerging therapy for B-cell non-Hodgkin's lymphoma, *Semin Oncol Nurs* 20(1 suppl 1):1-7, 2004.
27. DeNardo G: Concepts in radioimmunotherapy and immunotherapy: radioimmunotherapy from a Lym-1 perspective, *Semin Oncol* 32(1 suppl 1):S27-S35, 2005.
28. McLaughlin P, Grillo-López AJ, Link BK et al: Rituximab chimeric anti-CD20 monoclonal antibody therapy for relapsed indolent lymphoma: half of patients respond to a four-dose treatment program, *J Clin Oncol* 16(8):2825-2833, 1998.
29. Davis TA, White CA, Grillo-Lopez AJ et al: Single-agent monoclonal antibody efficacy in bulky non-Hodgkin's lymphoma: results of a phase II trial of rituximab, *J Clin Oncol* 17(6):1851-1857, 1999.
30. Feuring-Buske M, Kneba M, Unterhalt M et al: IDEC-C2B8 (rituximab) anti-CD20 antibody treatment in relapsed advanced-stage follicular lymphomas: results of a phase II study of the German Low-Grade Lymphoma Study Group, *Ann Hematol* 79(9):493-500, 2000.
31. Hainsworth JD, Burris HA III, Morrissey LH et al: Rituximab monoclonal antibody as initial systemic therapy for patients with low grade non-Hodgkin's lymphoma, *Blood* 95(10):3052-3056, 2000.
32. Hainsworth JD, Litchy S, Burris HA III et al: Rituximab as first-line and maintenance therapy for patients with indolent non-Hodgkin's lymphoma, *J Clin Oncol* 20(20):4261-4267, 2002.
33. Coiffer B, Lepage E, Briere J et al: CHOP chemotherapy plus rituximab compared with CHOP alone in elderly persons with diffuse large B-cell lymphoma, *N Engl J Med* 346(4):235-242, 2002.
34. Mauch PM, Ng AK, Wu EJ et al: Principles of radiation therapy. In Mauch PM, Armitage JO, Coiffier B, et al, editors: *Non-Hodgkin's lymphoma,* Philadelphia, 2004, Lippincott Williams & Wilkins.
35. Wahl R: Tositumomab and 131I therapy in non-Hodgkin's lymphoma, *J Nucl Med* 46 (suppl 1):128S-140S, 2005.
36. Bush S: Monoclonal antibodies conjugated with radioisotopes for the treatment of non-Hodgkin's lymphoma, *Semin Oncol Nurs* 18(16 suppl 1):16-21, 2002.
37. Hendrix C: Radiation safety with yttrium 90 ibritumomab tiuxetan (Zevalin™) radioimmunotherapy, *Semin Oncol Nurs* 20(1 suppl 1):14-19, 2004.
38. Kaminski M, Estes J, Zasadny KR et al: Radioimmunotherapy with iodine 131I tositumomab for relapsed or refractory B-cell non-Hodgkin's lymphoma: updated results and long-term follow-up of the University of Michigan experience, *Blood* 96(4):1259-1266, 2000.
39. Horning S, Younes A, Jain V et al: Efficacy and safety of tositumomab and iodine-131 tositumomab (Bexxar) in B-cell lymphoma progressive after rituximab, *J Clin Oncol* 23(4):712-719, 2005.
40. Davies AJ, Rohatiner AZS, Howell S et al: Tositumomab and iodine-131 tositumomab for recurrent indolent and transformed B-cell non-Hodgkin's lymphoma, *J Clin Oncol* 22(8):1469-1479, 2004.
41. Kaminski MS, Tuck M, Estes J et al: ^{131}I-tositumomab therapy as initial treatment for follicular lymphoma, *N Engl J Med* 352(5):441-449, 2005.
42. Zevalin™ (ibritumomab tiuxetan) prescribing information, Cambridge, Mass, 2006, Biogen Idec Inc.
43. Riley MB, Gordon LI: Efficacy and safety of radioimmunotherapy with yttrium 90 ibritumomab tiuxetan (Zevalin), *Semin Oncol Nurs* 20(1 suppl 1):8-13, 2004.
44. Hendrix C: Radiation safety with yttrium 90 ibritumomab tiuxetan (Zevalin) radioimmunotherapy, *Semin Oncol Nurs* 20(1 suppl 1):14-19, 2004.
45. Gordon LI: Practical considerations and radiation safety in radioimmunotherapy with yttrium 90 ibritumomab tiuxetan (Zevalin), *Semin Oncol* 30(6 suppl 17):23-28, 2003.
46. Gordon LI, Molina A, Witzig T: Durable responses after ibritumomab tiuxetan radioimmunotherapy for CD20^{+} B-cell lymphoma: long term follow-up of a phase 1/2 study, *Blood* 103(12):4429-4431, 2004.

47. Witzig T: Efficacy and safety of 90Y ibritumomab tiuxetan (Zevalin) radioimmunotherapy for non-Hodgkin's lymphoma, *Semin Oncol* 30(6 suppl 17):11-16, 2003.
48. Witzig TE, Gordon LI, Cabanillas F et al: Randomized controlled trial of yttrium 90-labeled ibritumomab tiuxetan radioimmunotherapy versus rituximab immunotherapy for patients with relapsed or refractory low-grade, follicular, or transformed B-cell non-Hodgkin's lymphoma, *J Clin Oncol* 20(10):2453-2463, 2002.
49. Emmanouilides C, Silverman D, Witzig TE: Treatment with yttrium 90 ibritumomab tiuxetan (Zevalin) radioimmunotherapy at first relapse in patients with B-cell non-Hodgkin's lymphoma is associated with higher response rates and longer durations of response than as a more delayed treatment option: results from a retrospective analysis, *Int J Radiat Oncol Biol Phys* 60(suppl 1):S541, 2004.
50. Press OW, Unger JM, Braziel RM et al: A phase 2 trial of CHOP chemotherapy followed by tositumomab/iodine I-131 tositumomab for previously untreated follicular non-Hodgkin's lymphoma: Southwest Oncology Group Protocol S9911, *Blood* 102(5):1606-1612, 2003.
51. Serafini A, Houston SJ, Resche I et al: Palliation of pain associated with metastatic bone cancer using samarium-153 lexidronam: a double-blind placebo controlled clinical trial, *J Clin Oncol* 16(4):1574-1581, 1998.
52. Pandit-Taskar N, Batraki M, Divgi CR: Radiopharmaceutical therapy for palliation of bone pain from osseous metastases, *J Nucl Med* 45(8):1358-1365, 2004.
53. Serafini A: Therapy of metastatic bone pain, *J Nucl Med* 42(6):895-906, 2001.
54. Sartor O: Overview of samarium sm 153 lexidronam in the treatment of painful metastatic bone disease, *Rev Urol* 6 (Suppl 10):S3-S12, 2004.
55. Resche I, Chatal JF, Pecking A et al: A dose-controlled study of Sm-153 EDTMP in the treatment of patients with painful bone metastases. *Eur J Cancer* 33(10): 583-1591, 1997.
56. Bushnell D, Quick D, Reid R et al: Multiple administration of Sm-153 lexidronam in the treatment of painful bone metastases, *J Nuc Med* 37 (Suppl 1) p 31, 1996.
57. Pagliaro LC, Delpassand ES, Williams D et al: A phase I/II study of strontium-89 combined with gemcitabine in the treatment of patients with androgen independent prostate carcinoma and bone metastases, *Cancer* 97(12): 2988-2994, 2003.
58. Sciuto R, Festa A, Pasqualoni R et al: Metastatic bone pain palliation with 89-SR and 186-Re-HEDP in breast cancer patients, *Breast Cancer Res Treat* 66(2):101-109, 2001.
59. Li S, Liu J, Zhang H et al: Rhenium-188 HEDP to treat painful bone metastases, *Clin Nucl Med* 26(11):919-922, 2001.
60. Palmedo H, Manka-Waluch A, Albers P et al: Repeated bone-targeted therapy for hormone-refractory prostate carcinoma: randomized phase II trial with the new, high-energy radiopharmaceutical rhenium-188 hydroxyethylidenediphosphonate, *J Clin Oncol* 21(15):2869-2875, 2003.
61. Srivastava SC, Atkins HL, Krishamurthy GT et al: Treatment of metastatic bone pain with tin-117m stannic diethylenetriaminepentaacetic acid: a phase I/II clinical study, *Clin Cancer Res* 4(1):61-68, 1998.

Unit V

Special Treatment Modalities

Chapter 24
Stereotactic Irradiation

Susan D. Bruce and Annette Martin Quinn

The principles of radiosurgery (RS) evolved in 1951 from the work of Lars Leskell, a Swedish neurosurgeon. This was during a time when mortality from neurosurgery alone was approximately 40%.[1] Radiosurgery became an established treatment modality for certain benign intracranial disorders about 30 years ago. Leskell and colleagues are credited with the development of the first stereotactic radiosurgical tool, known as the Gamma Knife (Elekta Oncology Systems Inc., Norcross, Ga.). The application of the Gamma Knife radiosurgery during the 1970s was used to destroy vascular malformations in the brain, benign brain tumors, and small brain tumors. The 1980s saw major growth in the development of stereotactic radiosurgery (SRS) techniques at many sites around the world. In 1980, SRS was performed at two centers in the United States (Boston and Berkeley). Now over several hundred centers offer radiosurgery.

Stereotactic techniques have evolved beyond the scope of neurosurgical sequelae. As a result of success with radiosurgery, researchers began looking at using stereotactic irradiation to treat tumors elsewhere in the body. Researchers at the Karolinska Hospital in Stockholm, Sweden, are credited with the development of stereotactic body radiation therapy (SBRT). Work with SBRT has been ongoing since 1992. The first treatment in the United States was performed in 1997 at Indiana University. During the last decade, SBRT has been investigated as a focal noninvasive fractionated radiation modality for a limited number of localized malignant lesions in the liver, pancreas, and lung.[2] SBRT adds to the current arsenal of treatment modalities and provides a noninvasive treatment alternative when curative treatment modalities cannot be applied. SBRT is now being implemented in some centers in the United States.

STEREOTACTIC RADIOSURGERY SYSTEMS FOR INTRACRANIAL LESIONS

Four primary radiosurgery systems are currently being used to deliver SRS. Each system has some inherent differences in the way planning is done or radiation is delivered. Each has its own advantages and disadvantages. Clinical results suggest similar local control rates irrespective of the stereotactic irradiation methods used.[3] Although there are subtle differences in the dose distribution between Gamma Knife and linac-based systems, they have not translated into differences in clinical outcomes. This conclusion is based on phase III studies of the Radiation Oncology Therapy Group (RTOG), which demonstrated no differences in outcomes or toxicities between the two techniques in the treatment of brain metastases and malignant gliomas.[4] In general, the treatment modality selected is influenced by the shape, size, and location of the target. These systems include the Gamma Knife, the linac (linear accelerator)-based system, CyberKnife (Accuray, Inc., Sunnyvale, Calif.) and the cyclotron.

The Gamma Knife is a dedicated radiosurgery unit and is used only for that purpose. The use of Gamma Knife is limited to SRS because fractionated stereotactic irradiation usually is not delivered with this modality. The cost of the Gamma Knife system ranges from approximately $3.5 million to $4.2 million inclusive of new facility construction.[5] It uses cobalt sources that must be replaced frequently because of decay and have a half-life of 5.26 years.[3] Gamma Knife works by delivering 201 beams of gamma radiation focused precisely on the lesion with 0.1 mm accuracy. The "blades" of the Gamma Knife are the beams of gamma radiation programmed to target the lesion at the point where they intersect.[6] Gamma Knife uses sophisticated three-dimensional software, which allows the

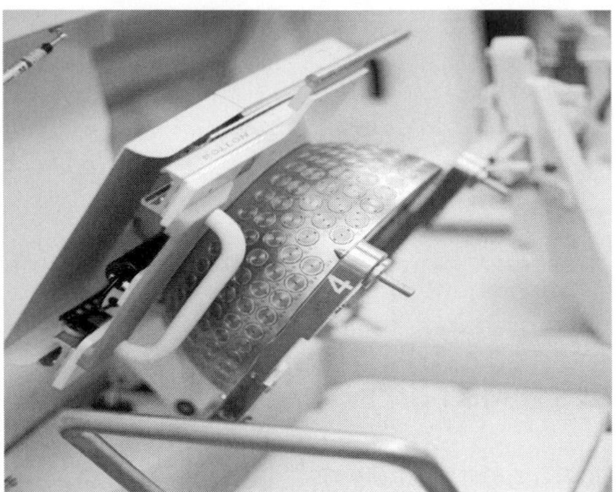

Figure 24-1 Gamma Knife Collimator Helmet.
Courtesy of Elekta Oncology Systems, Inc., Norcross, GA.

radiation to be focused only on the abnormal tissue, thereby sparing surrounding normal brain tissue. After treatment, the abnormal tissue slowly decreases in size and dissolves.

The process of delivering Gamma Knife radiosurgery is similar to that of linac-based radiosurgery, which is outlined in more detail later in this chapter. The primary difference is the use of the Gamma Knife helmet (Figure 24-1). This radiosurgery system attaches the head frame to a 500-pound collimator helmet. The collimator helmet is supported by the treatment couch, and as it moves automatically into the Gamma Knife machine, the helmet clicks into place to prevent head movement during treatment. There are 201 holes in the collimator helmet, and it is through these holes that the radiation is focused on the target. The Gamma Knife emits 201 beams of cobalt radioactive sources. Each beam alone is too weak to damage the normal tissues. As the beams intersect on their way to the target, they become powerful enough to destroy the tumor with a high degree of precision and accuracy. The Gamma Knife has the ability to tailor the shape of the radiation administered to irregularly shaped lesions. These finely focused beams of gamma radiation minimize the radiation effect on the surrounding normal tissues. Tumors up to 3.5 cm in size can be treated using this modality. The name may imply a surgical incision, but it is actually a noninvasive tool that replaces the scalpel and can be used to destroy deep-seated brain tumors that were once inoperable. Pin care, treatment toxicity, follow-up, and nursing implications are similar to those for the linac-based radiosurgery.

Linear accelerators, commonly referred to as *linac-based* radiosurgery, are machines that can be used to deliver conventional radiation, but can be modified to deliver a single-dose high-energy, computer-shaped treatment to the tumor. Linear accelerators can be modified to perform SRS at a cost of $50,000 to $300,000 depending on whether external treatment planning devices need to be purchased.[5] The cost of linear accelerators compared to other systems makes radiosurgery more widely available. The linac-based system consists of using four or five noncoplanar arcs of circular (or dynamically shaped) beams converging on the machine isocenter, which is stereotactically placed at the center of the imaged target volume.[7]

CyberKnife is a type of linac-based system that uses image-guided robotic stereotactic irradiation techniques. The CyberKnife device combines a linear accelerator tube and target assembly with a computer-controlled robotic arm that can orient the linac to more than 100 specific locations.[3] The CyberKnife maneuvers better than a conventional linac. Unlike other systems, it uses a real-time stereotactic imaging device, relies on a very large number of digitally reconstructed radiographs (DRRs), and compares these with real-time x-ray planar images acquired to resolve the current patient position.[3] This system uses the skeletal structure of the skull or spine as a reference frame, so it eliminates the need for a stereotactic head ring. A conventional thermoplastic mask is used for patient immobilization. Another advantage of the CyberKnife is that larger lesions (up to 6 cm) can be treated.[5]

The last radiosurgery system is the cyclotron, or proton beam treatment. It is a nuclear reactor capable of smashing atoms to release proton, neutron, and helium ions that can be harnessed for radiosurgery purposes. When using these charged particles, a few fixed beams and one isocenter are usually adequate in generating plans that are of high-dose conformality and homogeneity. This allows a significantly decreased integral dose to the adjacent normal tissues compared with the Gamma Knife or linac-based system, which usually use a large number of convergent beams with larger portions of normal tissue receiving a low dose.[8] The side effects from this type of therapy are similar to those experienced with standard external beam radiation therapy (EBRT). Nursing implications (education, side effect management, and follow-up) are also similar to external beam radiation therapy. The use of charged particle beams is not widely available because of the cost of installation. Currently only two proton beam facilities are in the United States, the Harvard Cyclotron Laboratory in Massachusetts and Loma Linda Medical Center in California.

In patients with metastatic cancer, metastases to the brain is a common complication of systemic cancer. Brain metastases occur in up to 40% of all patients with systemic cancer and 30% to 40% present with a single metastasis.[9] The brain is recognized as one of the most debilitating sites of metastatic disease as a result of the profound impairment of functional mobility, neurocognition, and emotional well-being. The incidence of brain metastases is increasing because people with cancer are experiencing increased survival. Further, the ability to detect small tumors with magnetic resonance imaging (MRI) has improved, and newer treatments responsible for better control of systemic cancer are in place.

The optimum therapy for treating brain metastases has yet to be determined. Historically the treatment options for patients with brain metastases included medical management with the use of corticosteroids, surgical resection, and whole brain fractionated radiation therapy. Whole brain radiation therapy (WBRT) was the mainstay of treatment. Surgical resection was typically reserved for solitary, accessible, and symptomatic brain metastases. Up to 50% of individuals with brain tumors will not be surgical candidates because the lesion may be surgically inaccessible or widespread disease may be present.[10]

During the past 15 years, significant advances have been made in the diagnosis and treatment of brain metastases. Stereotactic irradiation, more commonly known as *stereotactic radiosurgery (SRS)*, has emerged as an effective treatment modality for achieving local tumor control in brain metastases. SRS is a highly focused and precise form of radiation that is delivered to a well-defined area of the brain. This treatment modality uses a focused radiation beam in a single treatment to produce maximal damage to the tumor while sparing adjacent normal tissue from receiving high doses of radiation and associated toxicity. The entrance and exit doses are distributed in such a way that tissue outside the target area is minimally affected.[11]

Initial Evaluation of Intracranial Lesions

Preparation of the patient, as well as the patient and family education, is an essential component of care for the patient undergoing SRS and is the primary responsibility of the radiation oncology clinician. Upon the initial consultation with the radiosurgery team, the clinician begins the assessment of the patient. The goal is to identify any physical or psychological needs of the patient. The clinician begins with a complete review of the patient's medical history, being careful to note any drug allergies, use of anticoagulants, steroids, or antiepileptic medications, and the current medications the patient is taking. Assessment of psychosocial needs involves evaluating the patient's level of anxiety and need for antianxiety premedications before the procedure. It is important that the clinician identify the patient's primary caregiver so as to include them when teaching is initiated.

Patients and their families are often given printed material or brochures and given detailed verbal instructions on the radiosurgery procedure and care involved. Videotapes or CD-ROM programs detailing this same content can be used to augment the printed and verbal instruction. This is particularly beneficial to patients who learn best by visualizing what is going to occur. In lieu of a videotape, photos showing the headframe, the treatment machine, and treatment area can be just as useful to illustrate the concept of treatment. A tour of the treatment area, when possible, is a good way to alleviate any anxiety the patient or family may experience.

Following the initial consultation with the radiosurgery team, the radiation oncology clinician will schedule appropriate lab work and additional radiologic imaging exams required. Lab work includes checking a serum creatinine to determine normal kidney function, because the patient will have a planning computed tomography (CT) scan the day of the radiosurgery procedure and receive intravenous contrast. Serum creatinine parameters vary among radiosurgery facilities. It is essential for any patient on anticoagulants to have a recent coagulation panel drawn to check the International Normalizing Ratio (INR). Patients also require instructions on when to discontinue anticoagulant therapy prior to the radiosurgery procedure. Patients on antiepileptics should have serum drug levels obtained to ensure therapeutic levels are maintained.

Usually by the time of consultation with the radiosurgery team, the patient will have had a diagnostic magnetic resonance imaging (MRI) scan. A planning MRI is obtained about 1 to 2 weeks before the radiosurgery procedure. This MRI uses fine-cut 3-mm slices and gives precise imaging of the lesion(s) and surrounding critical structures. The smaller slices are used to achieve greater image resolution for target definition. CT images, that include target volumes, are outlined slice by slice and correlated with MRI through fusion techniques.[7]

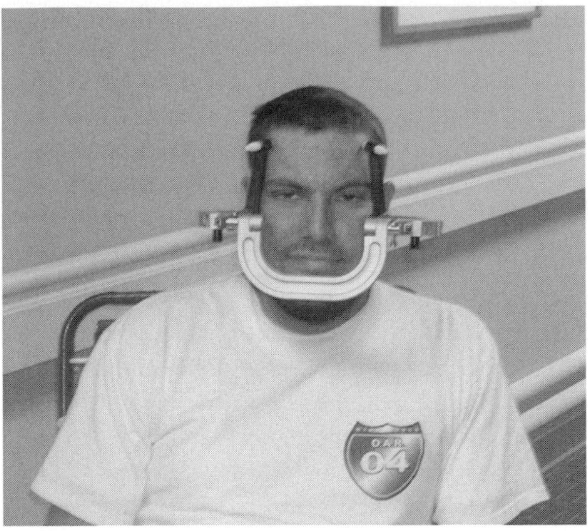

Figure 24-2 Patient With Brown-Roberts-Well (BRW) Head Frame.
Courtesy of Department of Radiation Oncology, Duke University Hospital, Durham, NC.

SRS Treatment Day

The patient and accompanying family members are asked to arrive at the treatment facility in the early morning. The patient's radiology studies are reviewed before the placement of the stereotactic head frame. An assessment of the patient is performed to ensure that no changes in the patient's condition have occurred. An intravenous heparin lock is placed in preparation for the patient receiving intravenous contrast during the planning CT scan. An oral or intravenous anxiolytic may be administered before the placement of the head frame or if requested by the patient.

Head Frame Placement

The patient's forehead and the scalp are cleansed with an antiseptic solution. The Brown-Roberts-Well (BRW) head frame (Figure 24-2), with four attached posts, is placed by the neurosurgeon at the desired position. The head frame provides accurate landmarks for localization of intracranial targets using an *x*, *y*, and *z* coordinate system. The system defines the shape and extent of the target lesion. The location of the head frame position depends on the location of the lesion(s) as determined by the radiation oncologist and neurosurgeon.[12] The radiation clinician helps support the head frame while a local anesthetic is injected into the four identified sites. The two sites in the front are located anteriorly above the supraorbital ridge and the two in the back are located posteriorly above the occipital protuberance.[3] It is important to warn the patient that he or she may experience a burning sensation from the local anesthetic that usually lasts for several minutes. To minimize the initial burning sensation of the local anesthetic, a buffering solution, such as sodium bicarbonate may be mixed with the local anesthetic. The head frame is then secured tightly using pins that penetrate about 2 mm into the outer table of the skull. While the pins are being tightened in place, the patient may experience a brief pressure sensation or discomfort. If the patient experiences sharp pain, additional local anesthetic can be administered. Stabilization of the patient's head is critical for SRS. The head frame allows therapy to be administered within millimeter accuracy and is used for localization of the target as well as immobilization of the patient during treatment.

Computerized Tomography Scan

After placement of the head frame, the patient will undergo a planning CT scan. This CT scan will be fused with the planning MRI to help establish the radiosurgery treatment plan. The patient will be in a supine position, and the posterior portion of the head frame is secured to the CT table to immobilize the head. A device known as a *depth helmet* (Figure 24-3) is attached, and markings are made with a felt-tip pen through the helmet openings onto the scalp. Measurements are taken of the distance from the helmet to the cranium and will be repeated before treatment to ensure that the head frame has not shifted.[12] Once measurements are taken, a CT localizer frame (Figure 24-4) is

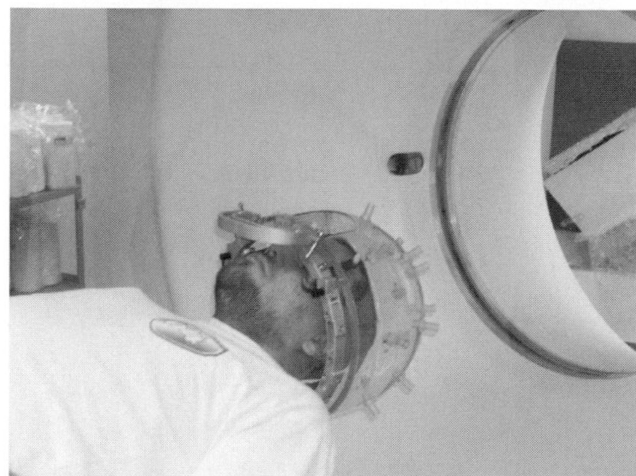

Figure 24-3 Depth Helmet.
Courtesy of Department of Radiation Oncology, Duke University Hospital, Durham, NC.

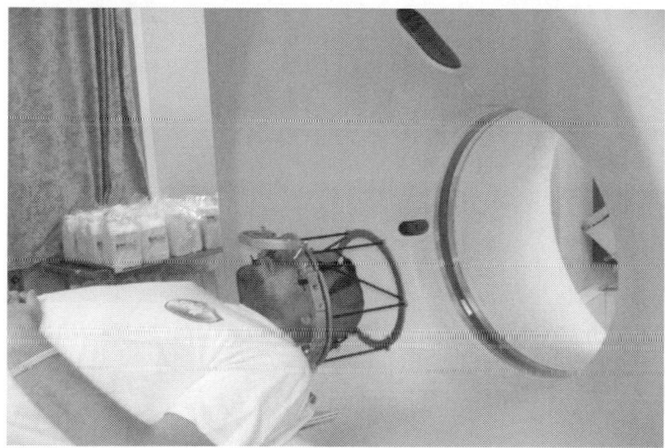

Figure 24-4 Localizer Frame.
Courtesy of Department of Radiation Oncology, Duke University Hospital, Durham, NC.

attached and used during the CT scan. These images are taken in 3-mm slices just as is done with the planning MRI. The localizer rods are visible on each image of the CT scan and are used as reference points to determine stereotactic coordinates when planning treatment.[12] The radiation oncology physicist uses information obtained from imaging studies to assist in the development of a personalized three-dimensional computerized treatment plan.

Once the CT scan is completed, the patient begins a period of waiting while the treatment plan is being developed. During this time the clinician is frequently assessing the patient for pain or discomfort throughout the day. Patients may need periodic medication with acetaminophen or anxiolytics. Depending on the location of the tumor, some patients may experience mild nausea and require antiemetics. Most patients are given a dose of dexamethasone before treatment to minimize cerebral edema that may occur as a result of the treatment. Patients are usually provided with a wheelchair for the day and asked not to be up ambulating while the head frame is in place. The patient could be at risk for falling, because there may be some compromise in peripheral vision while the head frame is on. A family member is encouraged to stay with the patient the entire day.

Linear Accelerator Treatment Planning

The time required to develop the treatment plan varies and depends on the number of lesions being treated and complexity of the plan. All radiologic images are transferred electronically to a designated treatment planning computer where they are digitally fused. Collaborative planning occurs between the radiation oncologist, neurosurgeon, and the medical physicist to delineate the target and surrounding critical structures. The goal is to select the optimal plan that will allow the target volume of the tumor to be treated while minimizing dose to normal brain tissue. An isocenter is selected as the central point to the target.[12] Multiple isocenters may be selected for a large target with an irregular shape or near a critical structure, such as the optic chiasm, optic nerves, or brainstem.[13] A three-dimensional model of the target lesion(s) and surrounding critical structures is created (Figures 24-5 and 24-6).

Dose Selection

Dose selection is of extreme importance in SRS because dose is strongly correlated with local control and complications.[3] Complications with stereotactic radiation therapy (SRT) are unusual because this technique uses conventional dose and fractionation schedules. Currently, dose selection is determined while taking into consideration the following criteria: (1) lesion size, (2) lesion location, (3) type of lesion, (4) presence of neighboring critical structures, and (5) preexisting neurologic symptoms, comorbid conditions, and previous surgical resections.

The relationship between size and dose is one of the most important determinants of complications.[3] The larger the lesion, the prescribed dose must be reduced to avoid brain injury to the

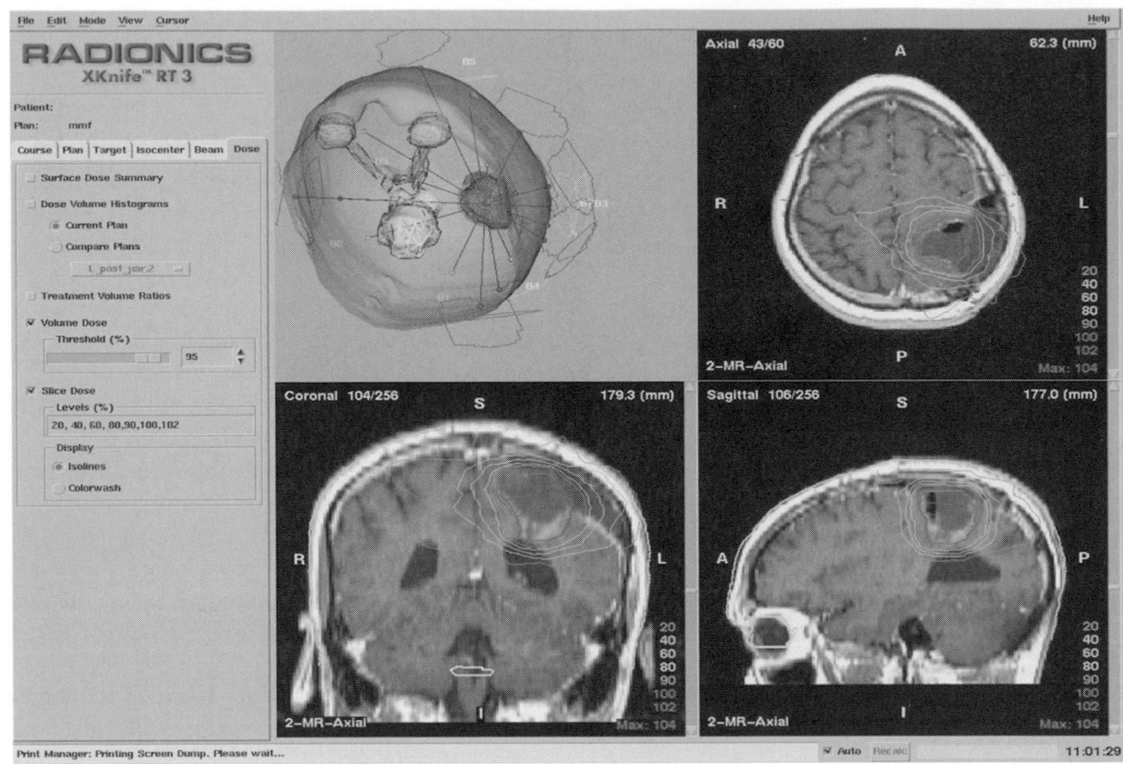

Figure 24-5 Computer-generated Plan.
Courtesy of Department of Radiation Oncology, Duke University Hospital, Durham, NC.

normal brain tissues adjacent to the target volume. Therefore, lesions that exceed 4 cm in greatest diameter are generally not treated with SRS because required reductions of dose would render SRS biologically ineffective in the treatment of the target.[3] The volume of the brain receiving a single dose of 12 Gy has been shown to correlate with complications.[14]

The doses used in radiosurgery are partially determined by the location of the lesion and are adjusted based on location. Radiation-induced injury is more likely to occur in critical areas of the brain, such as the brainstem, thalamus, and areas of the cerebral cortex responsible for speech and motor function. Lesions in the frontal lobe generally are treated with higher doses than lesions of corresponding size in the motor strip.[3]

The type of lesion is taken into consideration when determining the dose used and the aggressiveness of treatment. Caution must be taken to limit high-dose sensitive regions to the greatest extent possible because a patient's increased life expectancy increases the risk of developing long-term complications.[3] Patients whose life expectancy is less than 1 year may receive palliative doses to avoid causing acute toxicities.

In cases where the lesion abuts a critical structure, such as the optic chiasm/nerve or the brainstem, great care is necessary in minimizing the dose to these areas. The distance between the tumor margin and the chiasm/optic structures should be at least 4 mm.[3] The dose delivered to the optic chiasm/nerves and the surface of the brainstem should be limited to less than 8 Gy and 12 Gy, respectively.[15]

Patients with preexisting neurologic deficits are at higher risk of developing complications, and should be treated with lower radiation doses if radiosurgery is used.[3] The risk for complications is higher for patients that have undergone previous surgical resection(s) or have diabetes mellitus because of decreased tolerance of adjacent normal critical structures, most likely resulting from vascular compromise.[16]

The Radiation Therapy Oncology Group (RTOG) has established guidelines for doses used in the treatment of recurrent gliomas and brain

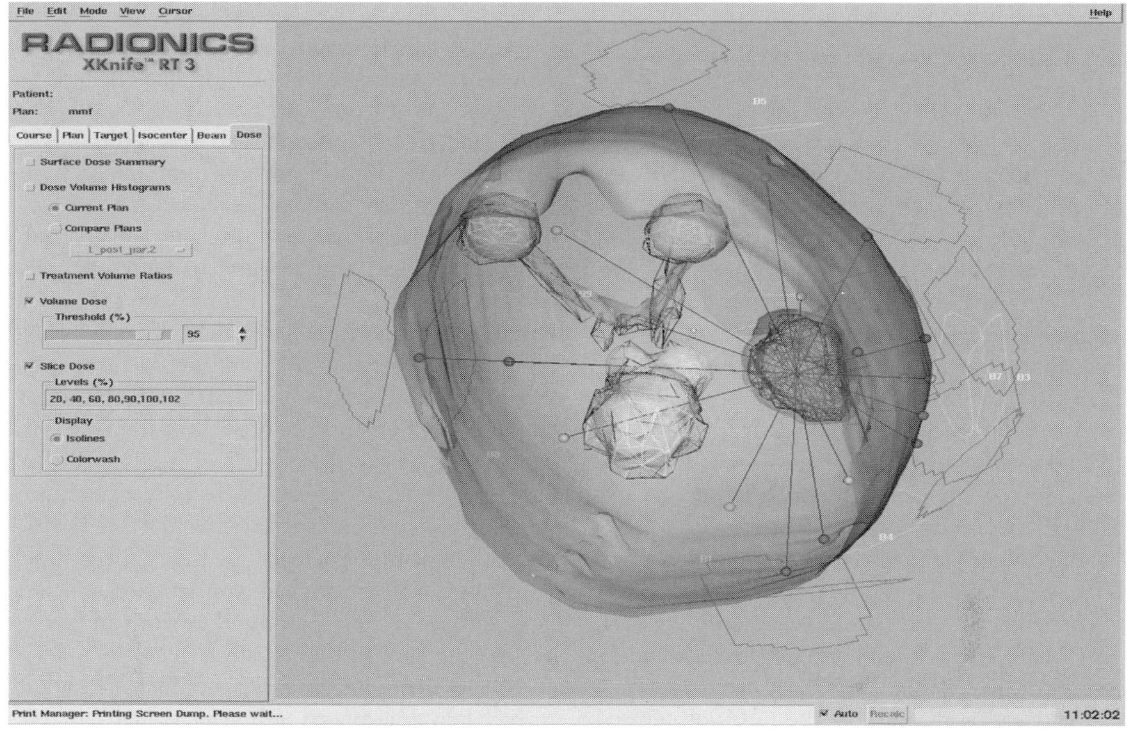

Figure 24-6 Multidimensional Representation of Patient's Anatomy.
Representation includes target area.
Courtesy of Department of Radiation Oncology, Duke University Hospital, Durham, NC.

metastases; for single fraction SRS, the maximum tolerated doses are 24 Gy, 18 Gy, and 15 Gy for tumors less than or equal to 20 mm, 21 to 30 mm, and 31 to 40 mm in maximum diameter, respectively.[17]

Stereotactic Radiosurgery Treatment Delivery

Upon completion of quality assurance indicators, the linear accelerator is ready for the treatment of the patient. The final preparations of the treatment machine are made with the installation of a multileaf collimator unit (MLC). The collimator unit is attached to the linear accelerator and contains dozens of tiny leaves (which are similar to blocks made of metal) that move in and out to conform the shape of the radiation beam to the shape of the target.[12] In some cases, the MLC is self-contained within the linear accelerator, and attaching a separate unit is not necessary. The patient is assisted onto the treatment table (couch) and is placed in a supine position (Figure 24-7). The stereotactic head frame is secured to the couch mount for stability of the head position during treatment. Measurements with the depth helmet are performed by the radiation oncologist to ensure that there has been no shifting of the head frame. The radiation therapist checks the laser lights to verify patient

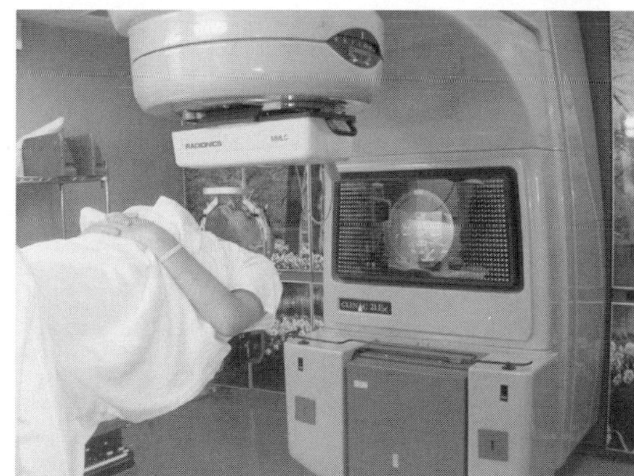

Figure 24-7 Patient on Treatment Couch (table).
Courtesy of Department of Radiation Oncology, Duke University Hospital, Durham, NC.

position. These laser lights are used to align the treatment isocenter to the linac isocenter.

The patient remains in a supine position on the couch (table) as the gantry rotates around the couch for delivery of each beam (Figure 24-8) while the multileaf collimation unit shapes the beams of radiation. A few minutes are required between rotations while the apparatus is set to the target from a new angle. During each rotation all personnel leave the room. Each isocenter requires approximately 30 to 45 minutes to fully treat. Overall treatment time depends on the total number of isocenters treated. During treatment, the patient is constantly monitored by the radiation therapist via video monitor outside of the treatment room. The patient can be heard at all times through the use of an intercom system.

Once treatment has been completed, the patient is assisted off the couch and taken to a room where the stereotactic head frame is removed. Opposing pins are unscrewed simultaneously to facilitate the frame's release. Patients are instructed they may feel a sense of pressure as the pins are released.

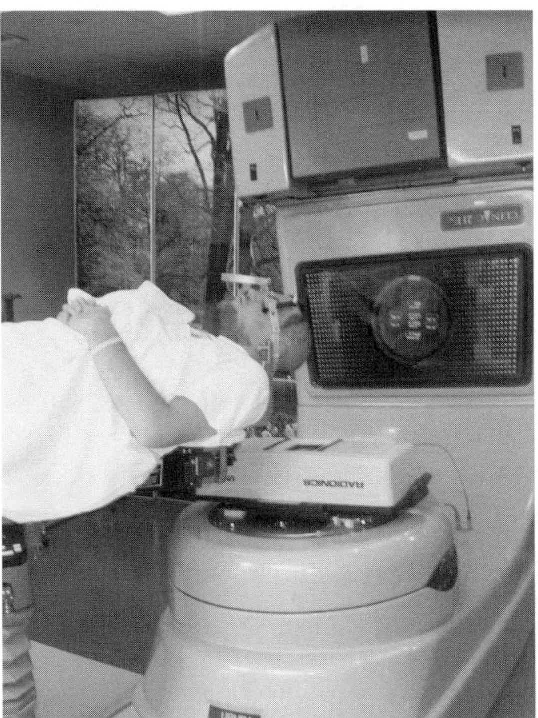

Figure 24-8 Gantry Rotation.
Courtesy of Department of Radiation Oncology, Duke University Hospital, Durham, NC.

Minimal bleeding may occur when the pins are removed, which usually subsides by applying pressure to the sites. Once bleeding has resolved, an antibiotic ointment is applied to all the pin sites and bandaids are applied to the frontal pin sites. In rare cases in which bleeding cannot be controlled with pressure, sutures may be required.

The clinician reviews discharge instructions with the patient and family. It is helpful to have written instructions to send home with the patient for future reference. The patient should be told that he may experience a mild headache or pressure sensation that is usually relieved with acetaminophen. Patients are often sent home on oral steroids to be taken for a brief period to alleviate any swelling that may result from treatment. Steroid administration instructions and a taper schedule should be provided to the patient upon discharge. Other discharge instructions include care of the pin sites, postprocedure signs and symptoms to report to the radiation oncologist, and a contact telephone number. Patient follow-up, which may be arranged at this time, usually involves an MRI scan. The timing of the MRI is usually 3 to 6 months after radiosurgery so as to monitor for edema, radiation sequelae, and response to treatment. The positron emission tomography (PET) scan has emerged as a way to differentiate tumor from necrosis in previously irradiated patients.[5] In many radiation oncology centers, the radiation oncology clinician contacts the patient the day after treatment to assess for complications related to the radiosurgery procedure, answer questions, and reinforce discharge teaching and follow-up appointments.

Treatment Toxicity

The risk of complications after single fraction SRS is low (3%–15%) in most reported series.[18] Toxicities of radiosurgery often are related to tumor and brain tissue response to high doses of radiation.[19] Radiobiologic effects on proliferating tumor cells and normal parenchymal cells within the target account for the desired clinical outcome and the toxicities of stereotactic radiosurgery.[12] The proliferating tissues exhibit an early response whereas normal tissues exhibit a late response.

Neurologic toxicity from SRS may be classified as acute, subacute, or chronic.[12,13] Acute side effects are caused by cerebral edema or bleeding and generally occur 24 to 48 hours after treatment.

During this time, the patient may present with headache, vertigo, fatigue, nausea and vomiting, swelling or bruising around the eyes, or seizures.

Patients with a history of seizures may, for the first 24 hours, be at a greater risk for seizure activity even if they are on antiepileptic medications.

Subacute toxicities are those that occur in the first 6 months after SRS. Destruction of proliferating tissue and death of tumor cells may cause persistent cerebral edema in surrounding tissues, presenting as a worsening or recurrence of the initial neurologic symptoms.[12]

Chronic toxicities are those that occur 6 months or longer after treatment with SRS. These may include persistent headaches, asymptomatic or symptomatic cerebral edema, cerebral radionecrosis, cranial nerve deficits (cranial nerves III–VII), hemorrhage, cyst formation, changes in cognitive function, hormonal deficiency, and scattered or incomplete alopecia.[20] The risk of chronic toxicities increases in patients who have a large tumor volume, multiple isocenters, high radiosurgical dose, prior or concurrent whole brain irradiation, treatment with certain chemotherapy agents, and other underlying medical problems.[21] Stereotactic radiosurgery can induce focal radionecrosis (tissue damage to the white matter of the brain), which is a complication that produces symptoms of mass effect that may require surgical resection to remove the necrotic debris. It is estimated to occur in less than 5% of patients with brain metastases and may present as a worsening of neurologic symptoms.[10] Management with corticosteroids may help control edema around the radionecrotic area. Surgery may be indicated to remove the necrotic debris so as to alleviate symptoms.

Clinical Outcomes

Identification of patients whose tumor size and location are amenable to SRS is crucial to obtaining good clinical outcomes. Radiosurgery has had the best outcomes in patients who meet the following criteria: absence of extracranial disease, Karnofsky performance scale (KPS) score greater than 70%, single intracranial metastases, age less than 45, response to steroid treatment, and site of primary tumor.[18] Other variables reported by Boyd and Mehta[13] that favor good prognosis include stable systemic disease, radiosensitive tumors, tumor size less than or equal to 3 cm, tumor volume of 2 mL or less, and age 60 years or younger. The most important prognostic factor is the KPS at the time the brain metastases is diagnosed.[22]

Despite treatment, brain metastasis is associated with a poor prognosis. Untreated patients have a median survival time of approximately 4 weeks and nearly all untreated patients die as a result of the brain tumor exerting increasing intracranial pressure, ultimately leading to terminal cerebral herniation.[23] Data from large retrospective studies[24-26] have shown that WBRT increases the median survival time to 3 to 6 months and that more than half of patients treated with WBRT die from progression of systemic cancer and not as a direct result of brain metastases. The best results from surgery are seen in those patients with a single surgically accessible lesion and either no remaining systemic disease or with controlled systemic cancer limited to the primary site only.[23]

The role of radiosurgery has been the subject of three randomized trials to date. As a result of using nonstandard endpoints or methodologic problems, data from two of the studies is uninterruptible or conclusions cannot be drawn.[23] The RTOG 90-05 was the first successful radiosurgical trial that determined the maximum tolerated radiosurgical dose in the treatment of recurrent previously irradiated primary brain tumors and brain metastases. This phase I study used a dose escalation schema with 10 to 15 patients per arm based on the tumor size and dose. Metastases up to 2 cm were treated with 24 Gy; 2 cm to 3 cm with 18 Gy; and larger than 3 cm, but less than 40 cm, with 15 Gy.[17]

The largest phase III study to date is the RTOG 9508 multi-institutional prospective randomized comparison of WBRT with or without SRS that included patients with one to three brain metastases. The patients were randomized to receive WBRT (37.5 Gy over 3 weeks) or WBRT (37.5 Gy over 3 weeks) followed by SRS boost. SRS doses were based on the earlier dose-escalation RTOG radiosurgery trial (90-05). Although it failed to show a benefit of radiosurgery in the treatment of multiple brain metastases, when radiosurgery was given in the initial management of newly diagnosed tumors, patients with a single brain metastasis did benefit. The results of this study showed that there is a survival advantage in the WBRT plus SRS group in patients with a single brain metastasis (median survival time 6.5 months versus 4.9 months, $p = 0.0393$).[9] Patients in the SRS group were also more likely to have a stable or improved KPS score at 6 months follow-up than were patients allocated WBRT alone (43% versus 27%, respectively, $p = 0.03$).[9] This study favors WBRT plus SRS to be the standard treatment for patients with a single unresectable brain metastasis and should be considered for patients with two to three brain metastases. Also noted were significantly greater complete response and local control rates in the SRS boost group. The rates of local control and overall survival with radiosurgery and WBRT are comparable to that in patients treated with conventional surgery plus WBRT.[23] The results of RTOG 9508 have caused a major reevaluation of the use of radiosurgery in the treatment of brain metastases.[23] The Eastern Cooperative Oncology Group (ECOG) and the American College of Surgeons Oncology Group (ACOSOG) are currently doing trials to compare SRS alone with SRS plus WBRT for patients with one to three brain metastases.

Advantages of Stereotactic Radiosurgery

Stereotactic radiosurgery has many advantages. It has been used as sole therapy, as a boost to WBRT, or for recurrent lesions in patients with brain metastases. Radiosurgery is a noninvasive single-day procedure and is performed in the outpatient setting. Only patients with extenuating circumstances, such as bleeding or uncontrolled seizure activity, may require overnight hospitalization. SRS has a favorable toxicity profile and minimal side effects that generally are self-limiting and respond to conventional management strategies. Treatment with radiosurgery has the added advantage of not delaying other treatment modalities.

Brain metastases are particularly amenable to treatment with radiosurgery. Metastatic tumors do not tend to infiltrate the brain and have well-defined borders, making it easier to target the tumor with a highly focused dose of radiation. Up to 50% of individuals with brain tumors will not be surgical candidates because the lesion may be surgically inaccessible or widespread systemic disease may be present.[10] Radiosurgery is a treatment option for patients who are not surgical candidates because of other comorbid conditions. It is a good treatment option for elderly patients who are at risk for surgical morbidity.

Radiosurgery has shown superior cost outcomes on all measures compared to surgery.[27] Rutigliano and colleagues (1995)[28] also found radiosurgery had lower average complications per case, lower total cost per procedure, and lower uncomplicated procedure cost and had better incremental cost effectiveness than resection.[18]

STEREOTACTIC RADIATION THERAPY

Stereotactic radiation therapy (SRT) delivers the same precise form of radiation as SRS, but it is given in smaller doses (daily fractionation) over an extended period of time. SRT combines the precision of stereotactic positioning with the radiobiologic biologic advantage of fractionation.[3] It has been referred to as "frameless radiosurgery." SRT uses a custom-made, frameless immobilization device, as opposed to the rigid head frame secured to the skull. The frame is relocatable and noninvasive. The Gill-Thomas-Cosman (GTC) head ring is used and consists of a BRW-compatible base ring, occipital mold support, and an individually customized dental appliance that attaches either directly to the anterior portion of the base ring or to a metal extender plate.[3] Head straps are used to achieve frame positioning and immobilization. At the time of the original frame fitting and prior to daily treatment, a depth confirmation helmet is affixed to the base ring and a set of helmet-to-scalp measurements is made.

The delivery of SRT is usually given in 1.8 Gy to 2.0 Gy per day for a full course of 5 to 6 weeks.[3] Standard fractionation avoids the toxicities associated with large single doses, and tumors located near critical structures may be more successfully treated with the precision of the stereotactic technique.[10] SRT is used primarily for the treatment of acoustic neuromas, low-grade astrocytomas, optic pathway gliomas, meningiomas, craniopharyngiomas, and pituitary adenomas. SRT is now commonly used to treat malignant brain tumors, especially those in proximity to critical structures, such as the brainstem and optic pathways.[7] Treatment takes approximately 45 to 60 minutes each day.

STEREOTACTIC RADIOSURGERY FOR EXTRACRANIAL LESIONS

For over 3 decades, physicians have been using stereotactic radiosurgery to treat tumors in the brain and head or neck region. As previously described, these highly focused radiation beams are delivered from several different angles. With older systems, such as the Gamma Knife, a metal frame is secured into the patient's skull in order to immobilize the patient during treatment. This minimizes the chance that a patient's movement will cause damage of surrounding healthy tissue. Frame-based SRS for the treatment of malignant and benign intracranial lesions has become widely accepted and has shown excellent long-term outcomes and minimal toxicity.[29-31] Unfortunately, such frame-based technology has limited the use of radiosurgery to treatment of intracranial lesions.

There are now several modalities for extracranial SRS using frameless fixation for target immobilization.[32-35] The CyberKnife (Figure 24-9) is one such technology that has gained considerable recognition in the field of extracranial radiosurgery. Developed at Stanford University, the CyberKnife was cleared for commercial applications by the Food and Drug Administration (FDA) in August 2001 and is currently the only FDA-approved system for such treatment. Consisting of an advanced, lightweight linear accelerator used to produce a high energy (6 MV) "killing beam" of radiation; a robotic arm that possesses six degrees of freedom and can point the linear accelerator from a wide variety of angles; and several x-ray cameras combined with powerful software to track patient position. These cameras obtain frequent pictures of the patient during treatment and use this information to target the radiation beam emitted by the linear accelerator.

The robot portion is instrumental in precisely aiming the radiation. The robotic arm can position the linear accelerator to more than 100 specific locations, with each location having 12 possible approach angles. This translates into 1200 possible beam angles. The system monitors internal reference points in the anatomy (skeletal landmarks or small implanted markers) to correct for patient movement in real time during actual treatment. When a patient moves during treatment, the cameras detect the change in position and the robot compensates by retargeting the linear accelerator before administering the radiation beam. This process of continually checking and correcting ensures accurate radiation targeting throughout treatment. The use of a head frame is now replaced with an image-guided localization system. Because of this technology, the CyberKnife can be used for radiosurgical applications outside the brain. Current research has focused on its use in treating malignant tumors of the head and neck, spine, lung, abdomen, and pelvis.[3,36-39] Benign extracranial lesions, including recurrent lesions previously resected or irradiated, are also an area of interest for clinical research using CyberKnife technology.[40]

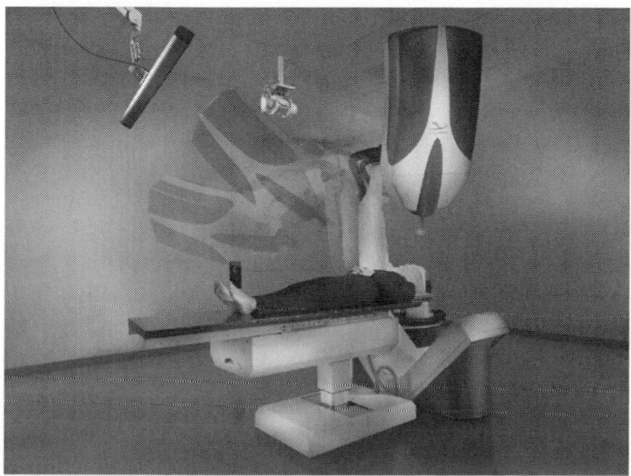

Figure 24-9 CyberKnife Treatment Machine. *Courtesy of Accuray Inc., Sunnyvale, Calif.*

Patient Selection and Treatment Process

Because the CyberKnife can be used to treat both malignant and benign lesions outside the brain where radiation therapy is currently indicated or has previously been administered, patient selection becomes a crucial step decided on carefully by the radiation oncologist and surgeon. Through a multidisciplinary approach consisting of review of patient records, imaging studies, and patient performance status, the radiation oncologist together with the surgeon determine whether radiosurgery is the most desirable form of treatment. Lesions that have already received the maximum dose of conventional external beam irradiation and have a maximum volume of under 250 mL are most desirable. Lesions with a volume greater than 250 mL will decrease the conformity of the dose. It is also important to mention that the diameter of the collimator allows for treatment of lesions as small as 5 to 6 mm.

Treatment for extracranial lesions also may require placement of fiducials near the tumor. Fiducials are small metal markers that track the tumor's position during treatment. These markers, which are approximately 3 mm to 4 mm in length, are visible to normal diagnostic x rays and are tracked by the CyberKnife to determine the

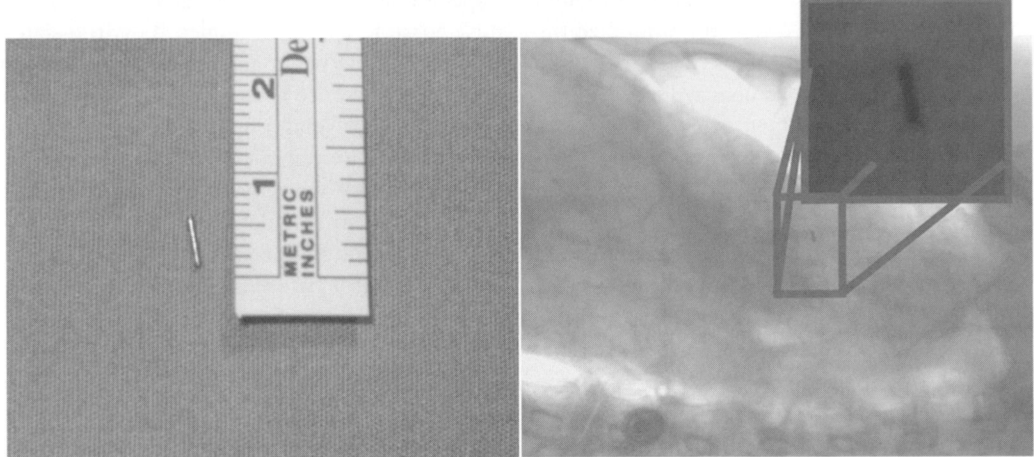

Figure 24-10 Gold Fiducial Markers Used for CyberKnife Tracking.
Courtesy of University of Pittsburgh Cancer Centers, Pittsburgh, Penn.

precise position of the tumor throughout radiosurgery (Figure 24-10). The markers are placed through a needle under CT guidance by an interventional radiologist or surgeon in an outpatient procedure and can take anywhere from 15 minutes to 1 hour to perform depending on location of lesion. A single fiducial marker can be tracked, but the more fiducials that are placed, the more accurate the tracking becomes. Thus typically 3 to 5 markers are placed around a tumor target. Currently, spine-tracking software, to eliminate the need for fiducials in the delivery of radiosurgery treatments to the spine, is being investigated.

Once the fiducials have been implanted, the treatment process consists of three basic steps:

1. Treatment set-up
2. Treatment planning
3. Treatment delivery

Unlike frame-based procedures, in which the entire process must be performed in a single day, a patient treated with the CyberKnife does not need to wait in the hospital while the treatment plan is being developed. As a result, a patient can go home after setup and return on a separate day for treatment delivery.

Treatment Setup

With the assistance of image guidance, the CyberKnife tracks the target throughout the treatment process. The system repeatedly confirms target location in relationship to skeletal structure by processing radiographic images and correlating them to previously obtained CT scans. The imaging cameras detect any patient movement, and the CyberKnife system's linac is accurately repositioned with respect to the target.

Although the technology can compensate for minimal movements, more exaggerated patient movements are limited by fitting the patient with an immobilization device. A custom-fit, flexible mesh mask (for head/neck treatments) or body cradle is formed and is used to help minimize movement during the treatment and ensures patient comfort. Creating the mask or body cradle is a simple, painless process and is often performed by a radiation therapist. Proper immobilization is a vital step in the treatment process because patient positioning is critical with any type of radiosurgery. Within days after the fiducials are implanted and before the treatment planning CT scan is acquired, the immobilization device is constructed.

After proper immobilization has been obtained, the patient then undergoes a CT scan to create the computerized images of the tumor for planning. The CT scan is centered on the implanted fiducials, and consists of a minimum of 180 slices in 1.25-mm thickness and must include the entire circumference of the patient. At this point, the patient is sent home and the treatment planning process begins.

The Planning Process

The CyberKnife system provides a wide range of treatment options, including the ability to use either forward or inverse treatment planning, allowing the physician to customize each patient's treatment plan. With forward treatment planning, the physician determines what dose to deliver from a particular targeting position. The planning software then calculates the total dose within the lesion for the physician.

When inverse treatment planning is used, the physician specifies the total dose to be delivered to the tumor and sets boundaries to protect the critical structures. The software then determines the targeting positions and dose to be delivered from a particular targeting position. Although CyberKnife is capable of both options; inverse treatment planning is preferable for the majority of CyberKnife extracranial cases.

Without the use of a rigid stereotactic frame, fractionation is feasible with this system. Head and neck tumors are typically given 36 Gy over 5 fractions and a preliminary report of a phase I trial examining SRS for stage I lung tumors suggests that 60 Gy in 3 fractions is feasible and well tolerated.[41] Spinal lesions are typically given 16 Gy to 20 Gy in one fraction.

Treatment Delivery

At some point after planning, typically 1 to 5 days, the patient returns for treatment administration. The patient is fitted with the custom plastic mask (for head and neck tumors) or body cradle (extracranial tumors) and lies on the treatment table. Before beginning the actual radiation treatment, the imaging system acquires digital x rays of the patient position. This information is used to move the linear accelerator to the appropriate position. Subsequently, the robot moves and retargets the linear accelerator at a large number of positions around the patient. At each position or "node," a small radiation beam is delivered. This process is repeated at 50 to 300 different positions around the patient to complete the treatment. At various intervals, the linear accelerator stops and additional pictures are obtained of the patient, thereby allowing the CyberKnife to track and compensate for small amounts of patient movement. These intervals can be as frequent as every node.

The entire process is painless and typically takes between 30 to 120 minutes to deliver all radiation beams depending on tumor location. Most typically a patient can go home immediately upon completion and return to normal activities. If the treatment prescription is for fractionated radiosurgery, the patient will return on a separate visit and repeat the above process for treatment delivery.

Delivering dynamic radiosurgery to targets that move with respiration, such as lung, liver, kidney, and pancreatic tumors, has always been a challenge and typically is accomplished through a breath-holding technique. Currently, Synchrony (Accuray Inc., Sunnyvale, Calif.) software has eliminated that problem and has allowed for the delivery of dynamic radiosurgery to tumors that are affected by the respiratory cycle. With the use of a complex system of cameras, motion-tracking software, fiber-optic sensing technology, infrared emitters, and a special formfitting, highly elastic patient garment, Synchrony corrects for any movement of the lesion incurred by breathing. In conjunction with CyberKnife, the system identifies, updates, and then correlates external body surface movement with movement of the internal tumor fiducials. Throughout the procedure, Synchrony technology monitors the target and readjusts its calibrations to assure that it is locked on the tumor, thus allowing the physicians to know exactly where the tumor is in real time, and giving them the ability to deliver the maximum dose of radiation without harm to normal surrounding tissue.

CLINICAL OUTCOMES

The CyberKnife was first developed for the treatment of intracranial lesions, and treatment outcomes have closely mirrored the results of conventional frame-based radiosurgery.[43] With the ability to treat lesions outside of the skull using fiducial tracking, a growing interest in treating lesions of the spine, lung, head and neck, and abdomen and pelvis has emerged. The indications for CyberKnife radiosurgery have evolved over time and will continue to evolve as clinical experience increases. At the University of Pittsburgh, CyberKnife has shown both feasibility and clinical efficacy of spinal radiosurgery for both benign and malignant lesions. Their outcomes 1 month after CyberKnife radiosurgery reflected a decrease in pain, no new neurologic deficits, decrease in tumor volume within the spinal canal, significant decompression of the spinal cord, and no evidence of further vertebral body collapse.[37] Stanford University has completed significant work in the area of lung tumors and has found that single-fraction stereotactic radiosurgery is safe and feasible for the treatment of selected lung tumors. Their outcomes from treatment of 23 patients reported no grade 3 to 5 radiation-related complications. Of the 23 patients treated in this phase I trial, radiographic response was scored as complete in 2 patients, partial in 15, stable in 4, and progressive in 2. Follow-up ranged from 1 to 26 months.[38] Currently, work in the area of lung tumors focuses on optimal radiation dose and fractionation.

In contrast to the chest, head and neck lesions are more amenable to treatment with stereotactic radiosurgery because of ease of immobilization and the lack of requirement for surgically implanted fiducials. A recent study reported a remarkably high response rate (70%) in 13 squamous cell carcinoma patients of the head and neck treated with image-guided radiosurgery.[40] At the University of Pittsburgh a current study examining the therapeutic efficacy of stereotactic radiosurgery for recurrent squamous cell carcinoma of the head and neck is underway. Because the optimum dose and fractionation schedule of stereotactic radiosurgery for patients presenting with this histology has not yet been determined, this study also will include a dose escalation portion to be examined as a secondary analyses.

IMPLICATIONS FOR NURSING PRACTICE

Although over several hundred centers offer radiosurgery, specific training or orientation that focuses on the nursing role related to radiosurgery rarely exists. As a result, clinicians often educate themselves independently and define their role specific to their practice setting.

Radiosurgery patients are treated to sub-millimeter accuracy for an extended period of time with extremely limited movement throughout the treatment process. Treatment, depending on the site, could take up to 2 hours. It is the role of the clinician to provide extensive patient education and clinical expertise so as to make the patient as comfortable as possible for the duration of treatment. Pain management becomes crucial, as does relief of anxiety that may be related to the procedure.

Clinicians caring for patients undergoing radiosurgery must understand the potential side effects related to the treatment. Side effects, as with any type of radiation therapy, are limited to the area being treated; thus it becomes prudent that the clinician in the radiosurgery suite review with patients the side effects they may experience and pre-medicate the patient appropriately with antiemetics, anxiolytic, or pain medicine as appropriate. For example, patients receiving CyberKnife to the lower thoracic and lumbar spine should receive pre-medication for nausea and education that nausea, vomiting, diarrhea, or abdominal cramping are potential side effects to treatment of this area.

Patients are instructed that they may experience temporary changes in any area that received the radiation. These changes may include redness, dryness, flaking, and/or itching of the treated area. Skin changes normally occur 1 to 2 days after treatment and may last 1 to 2 weeks following. For interventions related to skin care, please refer to Chapter 30. Permanent skin changes include increased sensitivity to summer and winter temperatures. Although skin reaction with radiosurgery techniques is far less advanced than with external beam radiation therapy, patients are still instructed to apply sunscreen with a sun protection factor of 30 or higher when the treated area is exposed to sunlight.

Patient preparation and education of the patient and family is an essential component of care for the patient undergoing radiosurgery. The radiation oncology clinician is actively involved in all aspects of care for the patient receiving stereotactic radiosurgery. The multidisciplinary collaborative role of the clinician is critical to the success of any radiosurgery treatment program. As radiosurgery continues to evolve as a treatment modality, it is essential for radiation oncology clinicians to acquaint themselves with the basic principles and responsibilities associated with radiosurgery technology.

QUALITY ASSURANCE

Quality assurance (QA) is an integral part of any radiosurgical program. The QA system serves to verify that the treatment apparatus is operating within the proper parameters and that the patient is being treated according to the treatment prescription. A quality assurance program needs to be comprehensive and should involve both the clinical and physical aspects of radiosurgery, regardless of which technology is used. The stereotactic radiosurgery quality assurance program involves medical physics and dosimetry for successful implementation.

The clinical component of QA involves verification of the procedure and treatment parameters based on each individual patient. The objective should be to ensure procedural accuracy during each step of the planning and treatment process so as to minimize the chance of a treatment error.[7] The physical component of quality assurance involves routine checks and safeguards performed on the actual equipment used to administer treatment. The quality assurance process is designed to inspect hardware and software performance so as to ensure compliance with the original accuracy and safety specifications.

SUMMARY

The advantages of radiosurgery include a favorable toxicity profile and minimal side effects, which are generally self-limiting and respond to conventional management strategies. Radiosurgery is an appealing treatment option for patients because of its noninvasive nature and low associated morbidity. Radiosurgery continues to offer options to patients who may not be surgical candidates or have other comorbidities that make surgery a high risk. Treatment with radiosurgery can have a significant impact on the quality of life for the patient and in many cases may extend the life of the patient. Patient outcomes are comparable to, if not better than, other treatment modalities.

REFERENCES

1. Alexander E III, Loeffler J, Lunsford L, editors: *Stereotactic radiosurgery,* New York, 1993, McGraw Hill.
2. Fuss M, Thomas C: Stereotactic body radiation therapy: an ablative treatment option for primary and secondary liver tumors, *Ann Surg Oncol* 11(2):130-138, 2004.
3. Chan A, Cardinale R, Loeffler J: Stereotactic irradiation. In Perez CA, Brady LW, Halperin EC et al, editors: *Principles and practice of radiation oncology*, ed 4, Philadelphia, 2004, Lippincott Williams & Wilkins, p 410.
4. Perez CA, Brady LW, Halperin EC et al, editors: *Principles and practice of radiation oncology,* ed 4, Philadelphia, 2004, Lippincott Williams & Wilkins.
5. Behrend S: Radiation treatment planning. In Yarbro C, Frogge M, Goodman M, editors: *Cancer nursing: principles and practice*, ed 6, Boston, 2005, Jones and Bartlett, pp 250-282.
6. *Gamma Knife surgery* (website): www.irsa.org/gamma_knife.html. Accessed December 28, 2004.
7. Khan F: Stereotactic radiosurgery. In Khan F, editor: *The physics of radiation therapy*, ed 3, Philadelphia, 2003, Lippincott Williams & Wilkins, pp 507-520.
8. Harsh G, Loeffler J, Thornton A et al: Stereotactic proton radiosurgery, *Neurosurg Clin N Am* 10(2):243-256, 1999.
9. Andrews D, Scott C, Sperduto P et al: Whole brain radiation therapy with or without stereotactic radiosurgery for patients with one to three brain metastases: phase III results of the RTOG 9508 randomized trial, *Lancet* 363(9422):1665-1672, 2004.
10. Belford K: CNS cancers. In Yarbro C, Frogge M, Goodman M, editors: *Cancer nursing: principles and practice*, ed 6, Boston, 2005, Jones and Bartlett, pp 1089-1136.
11. Gnanadurai A, Purushotamam L, Rajshekhar V et al: Stereotactic radiosurgery for brain lesions: an observation and follow-up, *J Neurosci Nurs* 36(4):225-227, 2004.
12. Law E, Mangarin E, Kelvin J: Nursing management of patients receiving stereotactic radiosurgery, *Clin J Oncol Nurs* 7(4):387-392, 2003.
13. Boyd T, Mehta M: Stereotactic radiosurgery for brain metastases, *Oncology* (Huntingt) 13(10):1397-1408, 1999.
14. Flickinger J, Kondziolka D, Lunsford L et al: Development of a model to predict permanent symptomatic postradiosurgery injury for arteriovenous malformation patients, *Int J Radiat Oncol Biol Phys* 46(5):1143-1148, 2000.
15. Foote K, Friedman W, Buatti J et al: Analysis of risk factors associated with radiosurgery for vestibular schwannoma, *J Neurosurg* 95(3):440-449, 2001.
16. Debus J, Hug E, Liebsch N et al: Brainstem tolerance to conformal radiotherapy of skull base tumors, *Int J Radiat Oncol Biol Phys* 39(5):967-975, 1997.
17. Shaw E, Scott C, Souhami L et al: Single dose radiosurgical treatment of recurrent previously irradiated primary brain tumors and brain metastases: final report of RTOG protocol 90-05, *Int J Radiat Oncol Biol Phys* 47(2):291-298, 2000.
18. Armstrong T, Gilbert M: Metastatic brain tumors: diagnosis, treatment, and nursing interventions, *Clin J Oncol Nurs* 4(5):217-225, 2000.
19. Gelbaum D, Lee H, Bilsky M et al: Radiographic findings and morbidity in patients with stereotactic radiosurgery, *Int J Radiat Oncol Biol Phys* 42(2):391-395, 1998.
20. Moore-Higgs G: Stereotactic radiosurgery/radiotherapy. In Watkins Bruner D, Haas M, Gosselin-Acomb TK, editors: *Manual for radiation oncology nursing practice and education*, Pittsburgh, 2005, Oncology Nursing Society.
21. Shaw E, Coffey R, Dinopoli R: Neurotoxicity of radiosurgery, *Semin Radiat Oncol* 5(3):235-245, 1995.
22. Patchell R: Treatment of brain metastases. In Perry M, editor: *American Society of Clinical Oncology 2002 educational handbook,* Alexandria, Va, 2002, American Society of Clinical Oncology, pp 383-391.
23. Patchell R: The management of brain metastases, *Cancer Treat Rev* 29(6):533-540, 2003.
24. Posner J: Management of brain metastases, *Rev Neurol (Paris)* 148(6-7):477-487, 1992.
25. Cairncross J, Posner J: The management of brain metastases. In Welker MD, editor: *Oncology of the nervous system,* Boston, 1983, Martinus Nijhoff, pp 341-377.
26. Berk L: An overview of radiotherapy trials for the treatment of brain metastases, *Oncology Williston Park* 9(11): 1205-1219, 1995.

27. Mehta M, Noyes W, Craig B et al: A cost effectiveness and cost utility analysis of radiosurgery versus resection for single brain metastasis, *Int J Radiat Oncol Biol Phys* 39(2): 445-454, 1997.
28. Rutigliano M, Lunsford L, Kondziolka D et al: The cost effectiveness of stereotactic radiosurgery versus surgical resection in the treatment of solitary metastatic brain tumors, *Neurosurgery* 37(3):445-453, 1995.
29. Kondziolka D, Nathoo N, Flickinger JC et al: Long-term results after radiosurgery for benign intracranial tumors, *Neurosurgery* 53(4):815-821, 2003.
30. Flickinger JC, Lunsford LD, Coffey RJ et al: Radiosurgery for acoustic neuromas, *Cancer* 67(2):345-353, 1991.
31. Flickinger JC, Pollack BE, Kondziolka D et al: A dose-response analysis: arteriovenous malformation obliteration after radiosurgery, *Int J Radiat Oncol Biol Phys* 36(4): 873-879, 1996.
32. Blomgren H, Lax I, Naslund I et al: Stereotactic high dose fraction radiation of extracranial tumors using an accelerator: clinical experience of the first thirty-one patients, *Acta Oncol* 34(6):861-870, 1995.
33. Adler JR Jr, Chang SD, Murphy MJ et al: The CyberKnife: a frameless robotic system for radiosurgery, *Stereotact Funct Neurosurg*, 69(1-4 pt 2):124-128, 1997.
34. Shiu AS, Chang EL, Ye JS et al: Near simultaneous computed tomography image-guided stereotactic spinal radiotherapy: an emerging paradigm for achieving true stereotaxy, *Int J Radiat Oncol Biol Phys* 57(3):605-613, 2003.
35. Takeuchi H, Yoshida M, Kubota T et al: Frameless stereotactic radiosurgery with mobile CT, mask immobilization and micro-multileaf collimators, *Minim Invas Neurosurg* 46(2):82-85, 2003.
36. Adler JR Jr, Murphy MJ, Chang SD et al: Image-guided robotic radiosurgery, *Neurosurgery* 44(6):1299-1306; discussion 1306-1307, 1999.
37. Gerszten PC, Ozhasoglu C, Burton SA et al: CyberKnife frameless stereotactic radiosurgery for spinal lesions: clinical experiences in 125 cases, *Neurosurgery* 55(1):89-98; discussion 98-99, 2004.
38. Whyte RI, Crownover R, Murphy MJ et al: Stereotactic radiosurgery for lung tumors: preliminary report of phase I trial, *Ann Thorac Surg* 75(4):1097-1101, 2003.
39. Koong AC, Le QT, Ho A et al: Phase I study of stereotactic radiosurgery in patients with locally advanced pancreatic cancer, *Int J Radiat Oncol Biol Phys* 58(4):1017-1021, 2004.
40. Bhatnager AJ, Gerszten PC, Ozhasaglu C et al: CyberKnife frameless radiosurgery for the treatment of extracranial benign tumors, *Technol Cancer Res Treat* 4(5):571-576, 2005.
41. Timmerman R, Papiez L, McGarry R et al: Extracranial stereotactic radioablation: results of a phase 1 study in medically inoperable stage I non-small cell lung cancer, *Chest* 124(5):1946-1955, 2003.
42. Ryu SI, Chang SD, Kim DH et al: Image-guided hypofractionated stereotactic radiosurgery to spinal lesions, *Neurosurgery* 49(4):838-846, 2001.
43. Ryu S, Khan M, Yin FF et al: Image-guided radiosurgery of head and neck cancers, *Otolaryngol Head Neck Surg* 130(6):690-697, 2004.

Chapter 25
Accelerated Partial Breast Irradiation

Anita Axiak and Christine Flynn

For most women with early-stage breast cancer, breast-conserving therapy (BCT) is now a widely accepted treatment option.[1] The components of breast-conserving therapy include surgical resection of the tumor with negative margins, lymph node dissection, and radiation therapy. An important benefit of BCT is the overall cosmetic result and the associated decrease in psychologic trauma to the patient. According to Recht,[1] randomized trials and retrospective studies of relatively unselected individuals have generally shown unacceptably high local failure rates after breast-conserving surgery without radiation therapy.

However, there is no significant difference in overall long-term survival between mastectomy and breast-conserving therapy plus radiation for women with early-stage breast cancer.[2] This has been demonstrated in several phase III trials.[3] Standard whole breast radiation therapy after lumpectomy includes prophylactic irradiation of clinically uninvolved breast tissue and therefore is associated with significant acute and chronic toxicities. Additionally, a time commitment of 6 to 7 weeks is required to complete a standard course of external beam radiation to the whole breast. Furthermore, it has been well established that most recurrences of disease occur in or near the tumor bed.

The potential to reduce toxicities, time obligations, and the overall cost of treatment, while at least maintaining current control rates, prompted the development of alternative methods of accelerated partial breast irradiation (APBI) or limited field radiation (LFR). LFR delivers radiation to the region of the tumor bed only. With these types of breast radiation, therapy is delivered only to the site (lumpectomy cavity) with a small margin of surrounding normal tissue, thus sparing the remaining breast. APBI allows that smaller treatment volumes may enable practitioners to administer larger fractions of radiation over a shorter time interval without an increase in toxicity. Clearly, this would offer an attractive option to a selective group of women with early-stage disease.

Accelerated partial breast irradiation includes the following types of radiation:

- *External beam quadrant breast irradiation.* This type of treatment delivers radiation to only a portion of the breast rather than the whole breast.
- *Interstitial brachytherapy.* This method allows radioactive sources to be delivered directly into the lumpectomy cavity and surrounding tissues usually in the form of a hollow catheter/needle.
- *Needle implant* (interstitial brachytherapy). Hollow needles/catheters are systematically placed throughout the lumpectomy cavity to deliver the radiation treatment.
- *Balloon implant/MammoSite* (a type of intracavitary brachytherapy). A balloon with a thin catheter is strategically placed in the lumpectomy cavity to administer radiation therapy.
- *Intraoperative radiation therapy (IORT).* This treatment refers to the delivery of a single dose of radiation during the lumpectomy surgery.

The prescribed dose of radiation varies depending on the type of treatment administered. Table 25-1 shows the recommended doses of radiation in terms of the type of APBI used.[4-7] The selection criteria for ABPI has been defined by two professional societies (American Brachytherapy Society and American Society of Breast Surgeons) and are listed in Table 25-2. These groups offer guidelines only. The radiation oncologist and surgeon must ultimately use their best clinical judgment in patient selection. Candidates for treatment should *not:*

- Have a serious medical illness or condition that may affect the use of the MammoSite applicator
- Be pregnant or breastfeeding
- Have collagen-vascular disease

- Have an extensive intraductal component (Harvard definition, more than 25% ductal carcinoma in situ [DCIS])
- Have an infiltrating lobular histology
- Have pure DCIS

HISTORY

According to Recht,[1] accelerated partial breast irradiation began in the early 1980s in England with the first of the formal studies. In the 1990s, Europe, Canada, and the United States recorded preliminary data for APBI using interstitial brachytherapy.[1] From 1992 through 1993, Kuske and colleagues[8] explored patients receiving low-dose-rate (LDR) interstitial implants and high-dose-rate (HDR) implants. Later, through retrospective review, these same patients were compared with 94 other patients eligible for brachytherapy but received external beam radiation with no significant differences in end results.[4] The group at William Beaumont Hospital recently reported the largest patient population (199) and longest follow-up (5 years) of these patients treated with LDR/HDR brachytherapy as compared with whole breast irradiation.[3] No statistically significant differences in measurable outcomes were reported. Perera and colleagues[9] from the London Regional Cancer Center in Canada achieved less successful 5-year follow-up results. The local recurrence rate of 39 patients treated with HDR brachytherapy from 1992 to 1996 was 16%. Differences in outcomes from this study to more successful ones could possibly be attributed to less rigorous patient selection criteria and the very limited implantation volume. Several early European groups' results were also less successful than those reported by researchers in the United States.[10] Again, the authors concluded that these failures could be attributed to inadequate patient selection criteria and/or suboptimal treatment technique.[10] The failures of these early trials prompted a number of European researchers to create trial protocols that required strict patient selection criteria and systematic quality assurance protocols. Outcomes from these later studies are similar to those of whole breast irradiation.[10] In 2002, so as to address issues of complex and time-consuming treatment planning associated with multicatheter brachytherapy, the MammoSite balloon brachytherapy catheter (Cytyc Corporation, Marlborough, Mass.) was approved by the Food and Drug Administration.[6] Original approval of the MammoSite catheter was as an addition to whole breast irradiation, and its use as sole therapy was considered "off-label." Currently, MammoSite brachytherapy is offered as one of three forms of accelerated partial breast irradiation (external beam and multicatheter brachytherapy comprising the other two) versus conventional whole breast radiation in the NSAPB B39/RTOG 0413 randomized phase III multicenter trial.

Intraoperative radiation therapy, another form of partial breast irradiation, recently has been used with promising results,[7] but is not included in the current NSABP/RTOG trial. With this modality, a single dose of radiation is delivered to the tumor bed immediately after surgical removal of the cancerous

Table 25-1 Recommended Doses For APBI[4-7]

Treatment modality	Total dose
EBRT quadrant	38.5 Gy
Interstitial LDR	50 Gy
Interstitial HDR	32 Gy–34 Gy
Intracavitary/MammoSite	34 Gy
Intraoperative	21 Gy

EBRT, External beam radiation therapy; *LDR*, low dose rate; *HDR*, high dose rate.

Table 25-2 Selection Criteria Recommendations for APBI

	American Brachytherapy Society	American Society of Breast Surgeons
Age	> 45	> 50
Diagnosis	Unifocal, invasive ductal carcinoma	Invasive ductal carcinoma or ductal carcinoma in situ
Tumor size	< 3 cm	< 2 cm
Surgical margins	Negative microscopic surgical margins of excision	Negative microscopic surgical margins of at least 2 mm in all directions
Node status	NO	NO

APBI, Accelerated partial breast irradiation.

mass. Work conducted at the European Institute of Milan on 558 patients between May 2000 and December 2003 indicates that the cumulative risk of in-breast recurrence was very low, but also cautions that specific criteria for patient selection need to be refined, and continued long-term follow-up is needed to evaluate outcomes.[7]

Only very limited data is available on external beam partial breast irradiation. Before the advent of computed tomography (CT)-based simulation for treatment planning, accurately locating the excisional cavity of the tumor proved to be very difficult.[11] Presently, the few published studies existing include a randomized trial in England comparing partial breast and whole breast irradiation and pilot studies from groups at the University of Southern California, New York University, and William Beaumont Hospital. Additionally, a multi-institutional pilot trial conducted by the Radiation Oncology Group (RTOG 0319) to explore feasibility of partial breast radiation in the supine position quickly completed target accrual and is presently ongoing.

EXTERNAL-BEAM QUADRANT BREAST RADIATION

In early 2003, Baglan and colleagues[12] reported results from a pilot study of nine patients with early-stage breast cancer using accelerated partial breast irradiation in the supine position. The purpose of their investigations was to develop and test the clinical practicability of an innovative approach of three-dimensional conformal external beam radiation therapy (3D-CRT). When planning for such an innovative treatment approach, highly sophisticated software and imaging studies are used to simulate beam alignment in regard to patient anatomy (Figure 25-1). The investigators' predicted advantages over brachytherapy included elimination of additional surgery to implant needles/catheters or the MammoSite applicator and improved radiation dose homogeneity within the target volume. This would potentially improve cosmetic outcomes and decrease the risk of symptomatic fat necrosis, a side effect associated with brachytherapy. Additionally, the risks of infection and hemorrhage that accompany any invasive procedure would likely be eliminated. Moreover, most radiation therapy facilities already have the tools and equipment to deliver 3D-CRT, and no special training for staff is needed.

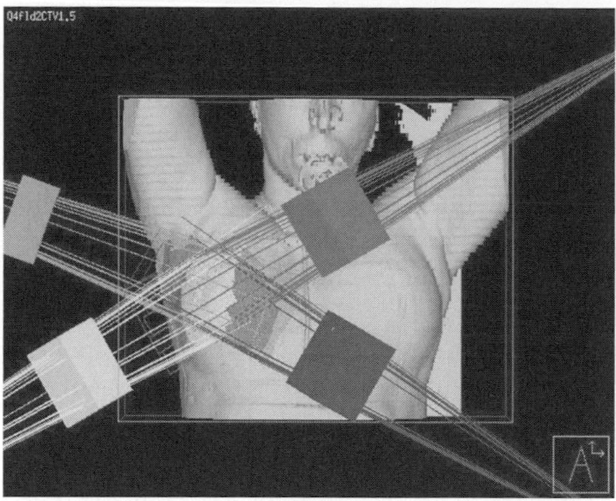

Figure 25-1 Virtual Beam Alignment for External Quadrant Irradiation.

To be eligible, patients' age was 40 or older, tumor size 3 cm or less with invasive ductal histology, surgery consisted of lumpectomy with negative surgical margins by 2 mm or more with a minimum of 6 axillary lymph nodes all reported as negative for disease. Additional criteria included the lack of an extensive intraductal component (EIC), absence of skin involvement, and absence of Paget's disease of the nipple. These factors seem to be consistent with a low risk of possible significant residual carcinoma adjoining the excisional cavity and the presence of occult multicentric disease. All clients also had radiopaque surgical clips outlining the tumor cavity placed at the time of lumpectomy. The first five women enrolled were treated with a total of 34 Gy, given twice daily, at least 6 hours apart and divided into 10 fractions over 5 consecutive days, identical to previously used brachytherapy dosing and fractionation. Because these patients encountered very little acute toxicity, the next four women were treated with 3.85 Gy per fraction for a cumulative dose of 38.5 Gy. The results were promising. Overall, patient tolerance was excellent, and acute toxicity was minimal with no observed skin changes during treatment. At first follow-up 4 to 6 weeks after completion of treatment, some women reported mild fatigue, mild breast tenderness at lumpectomy site, mild hyperpigmentation or mild to moderate erythema, and small areas of dry desquamation limited to the treated quadrant. Median follow-up at conclusion of the pilot trial was 8 months, so long-term tumor control, cosmetic end results, and late toxicities could not be assessed.

Based on this early data, Vicini and colleagues[13] continued the research with a phase I-II study of 31 patients with similar eligibility criteria. Twenty-nine of 31 patients had surgical clips placed to define the lumpectomy cavity, the clinical target volume (CTV) extended 10 to 15 mm beyond the cavity margin, and the planned target volume (PTV) included the CTV plus an additional 1 cm margin to include variations of breathing motion and daily treatment setup. During treatment, the only side effect noted was grade I erythema. Toxicities reported at the first follow-up 4 to 8 weeks after treatment completion were grade I and grade II erythema. Cosmetic results were rated as good or excellent in all patients evaluated at different time intervals, some up to longer than 2 years after radiation was completed. Based on the success of this study, the RTOG 0319 multicenter phase I-II trial to evaluate 3D-CRT confined to the region of the lumpectomy cavity for stage I and II breast cancer was initiated. Client eligibility requirements included negative excisional margins by at least 2 mm, tumor size 3 cm or smaller, 3 or fewer positive lymph nodes, and absence of lobular histology or an extensive intraductal component. A total dose of 38.5 Gy was given in twice-daily fractions at least 6 hours apart for 5 consecutive days. Results are not available at this time. Other institutions such as Evanston Northwestern Health Care in Illinois and Dana Farber/Harvard Cancer Center in Massachusetts used somewhat different doses and fractionation schedules (43.2 Gy in 16 twice daily fractions with intensity-modulated radiation therapy [IMRT] and 32 Gy in 8 fractions twice a day with conformal photon or mixed photon-electron plans), respectively. Very early results confirm feasibility of such treatment with little acute toxicity.

Common problems of such treatment noted by researchers include accurate identification of the excised cavity and time elapsed between surgery and treatment planning. Surgical clips placed at the time of lumpectomy permanently mark the extent of the cavity, but migration of clips has been reported and thus incorrect outlining and treatment planning are possible. The partial mastectomy cavity is normally identified without difficulty within a few weeks of surgery. This is due to the seroma that fills the surgical bed and is easily seen on CT as a fluidlike density at the time of treatment planning, unless the interval between surgery and simulation is too long. On the other hand, if treatment planning is done too soon after surgery, the size and configuration of the lumpectomy bed or the breast may change by the time treatment is initiated. These changes include decrease in edema of the breast and absorption of fluid or air accumulation within the cavity. Other concerns include adequacy of doses high enough to achieve tumor control and effects on normal tissues (late toxicities) resulting from increased doses and hyperfractionation.

Risks and Side Effects

Likely side effects that occur in about 10% of patients receiving external beam radiation to the breast include the following[14]:

- Erythema during treatment and for several weeks after treatment
- Hyperpigmentation of skin that may last months and could be permanent
- Slightly smaller size of breast or change in appearance of breast
- Fatigue and weakness during treatment and for several weeks after treatment
- Tightness or tenderness of muscles in chest wall under the treated breast
- Edema of breast

Side effects that about 3% to 9% of patients receiving external beam radiation to the breast experience are as follows[14]:

- Desquamation of the skin in the treated area
- Pain/discomfort at the site of treatment with radiation

Rare but serious side effects that may occur in a very small percentage (less than 3%) of patients receiving external beam breast radiation include the following[14]:

- Cough
- Difficulty breathing
- Pericardial irritation
- Cardiac muscle inflammation
- Rib fracture

Nurses caring for patients receiving this novel form of breast irradiation must be aware of protocol requirements, which include additional consent forms, testing such as CT scans, bone scans, and x rays, blood tests and more frequent follow-up visits. Clients and their family members will present with multiple questions, and nurses must be sensitive to their concerns and provide additional emotional support that is necessary because of the uncertainty of outcomes when participating in a clinical trial.

Nursing interventions to assist patients during their treatment course need to include education regarding skin care and wearing a soft cotton bra without underwire (i.e., sports bra) to avoid unnecessary skin irritation. Specific nursing interventions regarding skin care can be found in Chapter 30. Additionally, the client needs to be aware of signs and symptoms of infection of the breast (redness, swelling, tenderness, fever, chills), how to manage fatigue (frequent rest periods, increasing or reducing activity, maintaining proper nutrition), and management of discomfort or pain of the affected breast. Nurses must stress to their patients the importance of reporting any adverse effects so that they can be properly documented and the necessary interventions can be taken to reduce these toxicities.

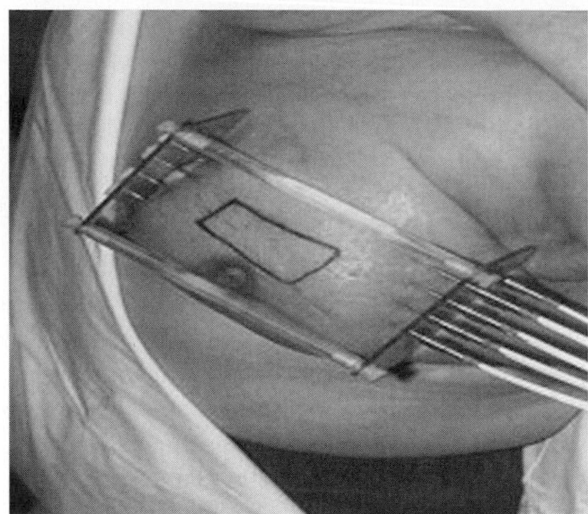

Figure 25-2 High-Dose-Rate Interstitial Needle Breast Implant.

INTERNAL INTERSTITIAL BRACHYTHERAPY

Needle Breast Implant

Needle breast implants are brachytherapy treatments that consist of surgical placement of either LDR or HDR implants. The LDR interstitial needle breast implant is done as an inpatient procedure and typically requires a 2- to 4-day stay in the hospital. The HDR interstitial needle breast implant is an outpatient procedure and allows the patient to go home with the implant in place and then return twice a day for treatment. The course of treatment for HDR implants is completed over a 4- to 5-day period. Interstitial brachytherapy to the breast may be considered primary (alone) therapy or boost (in addition to external beam) therapy to the tumor area. This technique allows for a series of needles to be systematically placed throughout the lumpectomy area via ultrasound guidance (Figure 25-2). Nursing and follow-up care are similar for both implants.

Low-Dose-Rate Implant

LDR implants receive a curative dose of 50 Gy. The difference between the HDR and LDR needle implants is that the total dose for the LDR is delivered continuously over 96 hours on an inpatient basis, therefore requiring inpatient hospitalization. This continuous dose is administered via ribbons of radioactive seeds. The radioactive source for these implants is iodine-125 (^{125}I). These seeds are threaded (loaded) into the hollow needles/catheters. The patient is radioactive and per Nuclear Regulatory Commission regulations remains in a private room.[15] The patient may have visitors but there are some radiation safety restrictions implemented. Persons under the age of 18 and pregnant women are not allowed in the room.[15] A sign is placed on the door explaining the precautions. After the total dose is achieved, the needles/catheters are removed. The area is dressed and the patient is discharged. The patient is not radioactive. Follow-up care and side effects are managed the same as for the HDR breast patients. At William Beaumont Hospital, through in-house protocols, accelerated partial breast irradiation via LDR or HDR was examined and later established its relative safety.[8,16-18] These two treatment modalities were found to be tolerable, feasible, and acceptable.[3] At many institutions, LDR breast implants have been replaced by HDR implants. By using HDR as the sole radiation treatment modality, significant benefits over the LDR treatments were realized, such as termination of radiation exposure to staff, elimination of inpatient costs, and significant dosimetric advantages (improvement in radiation delivery). However, the data from the LDR in-house protocol was available first and formed the foundation for the HDR implant.

High-Dose-Rate Implant

The goal of HDR brachytherapy when used as the sole method of radiation therapy for patients with early-stage breast cancer is to deliver a curative dose of radiation to the targeted area via the implant. This technique also allows for a reduction in dose to surrounding tissues and structures. The rationale behind APBI is that the most likely site of recurrence is the biopsy cavity.[3] Therefore, another benefit of this method of treatment is that a decreased volume of breast tissue is treated, thereby lending to a shorter course of treatment and requiring much less time to complete. In some cases, when the HDR implant cannot be used as the primary treatment, it can be used as a boost along with external beam irradiation. According to Vicini and colleagues[19] there were no statistically significant differences in the median time to local recurrence of disease between the APBI group and the whole breast RT group.

Women who undergo a lumpectomy for stage I and II carcinoma of the breast are considered for inclusion in this type of radiation treatment. Patients with tumors pathologically greater than 3 cm in maximum dimension are not eligible. Other selection criteria for the implant include no evidence of an extensive intraductal component (EIC) in the primary tumor and negative lumpectomy margins (2 mm or more) by microscopic exam.[18,20]

The HDR needle implantation can be performed either at the time of reexcision/axillary dissection (open cavity) or up to 1 week after the surgery has been completed (closed cavity). The total radiation dose delivered is 32 Gy. The radioactive source expended is iridium-192. This dose is delivered by administering eight fractions (4 Gy) twice a day over 4 days.[18] Each treatment must be at least 6 hours apart and is performed on an outpatient basis. Therefore, the patient may go home between treatments.

The patient is sent to an operating room in the hospital to have the needles placed into the breast tissue and lumpectomy cavity. A plastic template is placed on each side of the breast to help guide the needles and secure the implant. After the needles are in place, the ends of the needles are fastened with plastic stops at one end and plastic caps on the other end. Once the needle placement is complete, the patient is taken to the postanesthesia care unit to recover. The next appointment is for the simulation or treatment planning session. At that time, x rays are taken of the implant to verify placement of the needles. From these films, the specific radiation treatment is planned. Once the radiation oncologist and medical physicist verify dose calculations, the needles are connected to the high dose rate treatment machine (Figure 25-3).

The radiation is administered with the assistance of a device called a *high-dose-rate remote after-loading machine* that enables each radiation treatment to be given in approximately 10 to 20 minutes. The needles are uncapped and connected to the after-loader

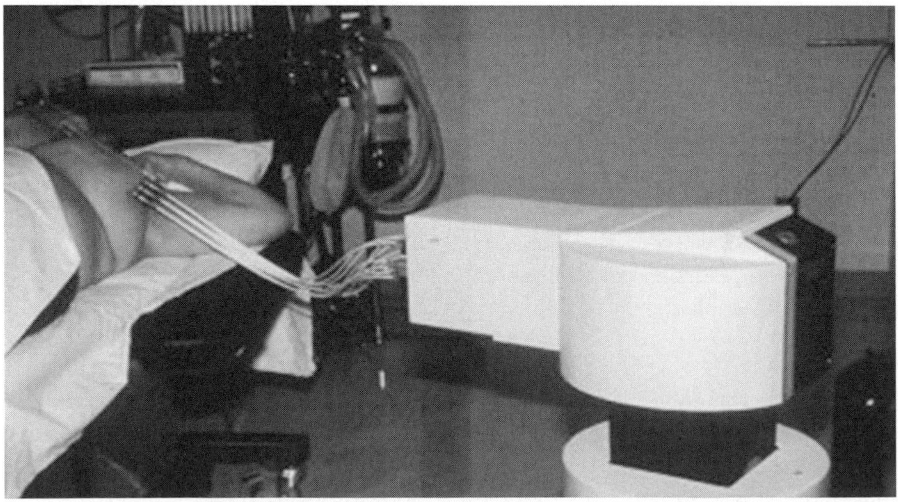

Figure 25-3 The High-Dose-Rate Unit. This unit houses the radioactive source (iridium-192).

via transfer tubes. The radioactive source travels through each needle in the breast for a prescribed amount of time. The medical physicist, using a sophisticated computerized calculation system, determines the amount of time the source dwells in each needle. Once the appropriate dose is delivered, the radioactive seed retracts back into the after-loader and the transfer tubes are disconnected from the patient. The patient is radioactive only while the source is dwelling in the breast tissue.

Again, regulations from the Nuclear Regulatory Commission mandate that the patient be left alone in the treatment room for the duration of the treatment.[15] A monitor and intercom outside the treatment room allow for the staff to see and communicate with the patient during the treatment.

Nursing measures call for ongoing monitoring of the implant site for toxicity assessment. This is done by inspecting the treatment area for infection, measuring the effectiveness of the analgesic prescribed and cleansing the needle sites daily as well as changing and securing the dressing after each treatment.

Risks and Side Effects

All patients receiving multicatheter/needle breast brachytherapy[14] (LDR and HDR) treatments are at risk for side effects. Most of these side effects resolve shortly after the completion of the radiation treatments. Likely effects include the following:

- Mild redness of the skin over the treatment area
- Mild scar tissue
- Flaking or peeling of dry skin over the treatment area
- Slightly smaller breast size or change in the general appearance of the breast
- Swelling of the breast
- Bruising
- Mild breast pain

Less likely effects, which occur in 3% to 9% of patients receiving multicatheter brachytherapy, include the following:

- Infection
- Telangiectasia
- Increased firmness of the breast tissue
- Slight change in color of the skin over the treatment area
- Thickening of the skin over the treatment area (fibrosis)
- Damaged fat cells in the breast that cause a red, swollen, or tender area in the breast

Rare but serious effects, which occur in less than 3% of patients receiving this treatment, include the following:

- Severe scar tissue
- Severe infection
- Breast pain lasting more than 1 year

As a result of the placement of the implant, side effects such as breast pain/discomfort and drainage (from needle insertion site) are treated with pain and antibiotic medications immediately after surgery until radiation treatment is completed.

The nurse should encourage the use of pain medications for patients experiencing discomfort during treatment. It is recommended that moisturizing lotion be applied to the treatment area after needle/catheter entrance and exit sites have healed. In order to facilitate compliance with the overall treatment plan, the nurse must properly educate the patient and caregiver. This begins with the nurse coordinating appointments and providing proper direction for the patient. Instructions regarding the procedure, preparations, and possible side effects must be reviewed via telephone, face-to-face conversation, or written instructions. After implantation, safety measures must be reviewed. Restrictions such as no driving (if using narcotics), riding in the front seat (if there is a passenger airbag), or showering (for protection of the implant) must be enforced. Instructions regarding the importance of stabilizing the implant via a binding surgical bra are conveyed. The patient is also instructed to leave the surgical bra on at all times to sup-port the implant device and immobilize the breast. The patient is instructed to not clean or change the dressing. This is the nurse's responsibility after daily treatment. The nurse explains to patients the necessity for taking prophylactic antibiotics as prescribed and instructs them to watch for signs and symptoms of infection before, during, and after completion of treatment. A follow-up appointment with the radiation oncologist is scheduled for 2 to 6 weeks from completion of treatment. A clinical examination is performed every 3 months by the surgeon or radiation oncologist (physicians may rotate). Every 3 to 6 months an evaluation of cosmetic result should be performed by the radiation oncologist.[18] Typically, a bilateral mammogram 6 months after radiation therapy will be ordered and then every 12 months thereafter.

INTRACAVITY BRACHYTHERAPY

MammoSite

Intracavity brachytherapy, as a form of APBI, can be administered using the MammoSite radiation therapy system (RTS). This multilumen silicone catheter with an inflatable balloon assembly at the distal end is designed to position a radioactive source inside the cavity created by the lumpectomy (Figure 25-4). Early experience with the MammoSite RTS has been positive. Eligibility for an initial trial to test the safety and performance of the device included age more than 45 years, tumor less than 2 cm, invasive ductal histology, negative nodal status, negative margin status, applicator placement within 10 weeks of final lumpectomy procedure, and a cavity after lumpectomy with one dimension at least 3.0 cm. In all cases, 34 Gy was delivered at a point 1 cm from the surface of the balloon in 3.4 Gy fractions (twice daily) over 5 to 7 elapsed days. Interfraction separation was a minimum of 6 hours. Initial reports of 43 patients treated in this manner showed no adverse events. Patients received 100% of the prescribed dose and most experienced mild to moderate, dry or moist desquamation. At 1 month, 88% of patients were evaluated as having good to excellent cosmetic results.[22] Long-term data has yet to be published from this initial clinical experience.

Use of the MammoSite RTS, a 5-day internal treatment program, would replace the standard 6- to 7-week regimen of external beam radiation therapy (EBRT). The MammoSite RTS program functions by dispensing radiation from inside the lumpectomy cavity directly to the area surrounding the cavity where the cancer is most likely to recur.[21,23] The applicator is inflated and expands to fill the cavity. The central source allows for a symmetrical delivery of radiation from inside the cavity (Figure 25-5). The goal of HDR brachytherapy is to cure early-stage breast cancer and reduce the length of treatment by up to 5 weeks. Again, this type of radiation treatment decreases the exposure of normal tissue to damaging radiation, thus improving the quality of life of the patient and minimizing the potential damage of the radiation therapy.[21,24] The rationale for MammoSite RTS therapy is that it offers significant benefits over other methods of brachytherapy. With interstitial breast brachytherapy, approximately 16 to 18 needles are implanted with both an entrance and an exit site wound. However, MammoSite RTS, with just one exit site, decreases the risk of infection and lends to a more comfortable implant, which is easier for the patient to tolerate.

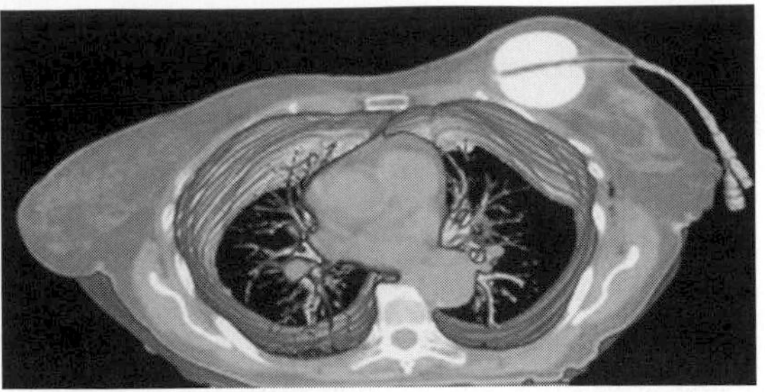

Figure 25-5 Implanted MammoSite Balloon. Computed tomography (CT) scan of an implanted MammoSite balloon with excellent tissue/balloon conformance.

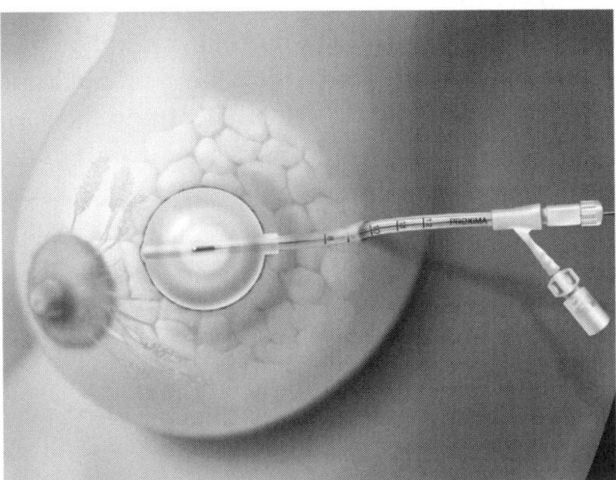

Figure 25-4 MammoSite® Radiation Therapy System. *Courtesy of Cytic™ Corporation and affiliates.*

Often, the goal of radiation therapy is to cure cancer. In most cases, the MammoSite radiation therapy system will be used to destroy cancer cells that may be left behind after breast-conserving therapy and may reduce the risk that the cancer will recur.[21,24] The MammoSite RTS may be used as the primary treatment to deliver the radiation dose to the lumpectomy cavity or be used as the localized boost dose of radiation that goes along with external beam treatments.

According to Keisch,[21] standard brachytherapy treatment planning should be performed employing commercially available software and equipment. The treatment should be conducted using HDR brachytherapy protocols. The radiation source, iridium-192, can be delivered via MammoSite's center nylon tube. The most common treatment scheme with this system is 3.4 Gy in 10 fractions given twice daily, over 5 treatment days, to a volume covering the lumpectomy cavity with a margin of 1 cm to 2 cm (see Figure 25-4).

The method of placement for the MammoSite system is influenced by two components such as timing and placement technique. The balloon may be placed at the time of the lumpectomy or reexcision (open cavity) or after lumpectomy (closed cavity). The open cavity procedure is performed at the time of the lumpectomy. Under general anesthesia, a trocar is used to create an 8-mm pathway into this lumpectomy cavity. The uninflated MammoSite balloon is advanced into the cavity through the trocar pathway and inflated.[23] Inflation of the balloon allows the MammoSite to position the tissue to receive the radiation therapy. However, the balloon is deflated before closing the cavity to avoid puncture during suturing. It is then re-inflated with saline and contrast after the cavity is closed. If placement of the balloon does not occur during the lumpectomy or reexcision, it may be inserted into a closed cavity as a separate procedure. If the timing of the implant is after lumpectomy, it can be achieved with either the scar entry technique (SET) method or the ultrasound lateral technique. With the SET technique, the cavity size is confirmed via ultrasound, and a narrow section of the lumpectomy scar is opened. Fluid is drained from the cavity and the MammoSite catheter is inserted and inflated with saline and contrast.[23] The ultrasound lateral placement technique is done by creating a skin nick and then inserting the trocar to create a MammoSite pathway.[23] Again, fluid is drained from the cavity and the MammoSite catheter is inflated with saline and contrast. Placement, conformance, and skin depth are verified under ultrasound. The balloon is accessed via a portion of the catheter that remains outside the breast. This is how the saline and contrast are instilled into the balloon. The balloon is inflated with enough saline so that it should conform to the lumpectomy cavity, enabling breast tissue to be in contact with its entire surface (see Figures 25-5 and 25-6). Different balloon sizes and shapes are available that make it possible to achieve this goal. The 4-cm to 5-cm MammoSite applicator can be inflated from 35 mL up to 70 mL. The 5-cm to 6-cm balloon, also a

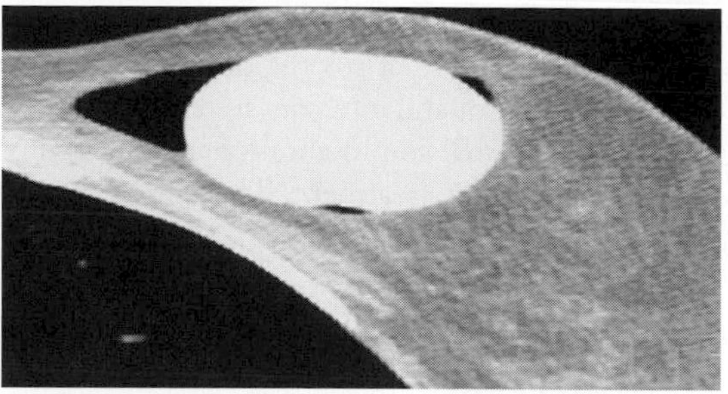

Figure 25-6 Implanted MammoSite Balloon. Computed tomography (CT) scan of an implanted MammoSite balloon with poor tissue/balloon conformance.

variable volume sphere, may be inflated with from 70 to 125 mL. The elliptical balloon is designed for irregularly shaped or unusually located lumpectomy cavities and has a single volume limitation.[23] Before the first treatment, regardless of which technique was performed, CT imaging is used. The information obtained at this time is tissue conformance the width of the MammoSite, distance to the skin surface, and balloon symmetry. Before each fraction is delivered, a repeat x ray/simulation film is done to compare with the previous CT scan and assess inflation status of the balloon.

The catheter exit site is dressed with a bandage and secured in place with tape and a surgical bra until treatment. The balloon is the device that will provide the means to position the radioactive source. After pathology is verified, treatment planning is completed and the applicator placement is verified by imaging, the first dose may be delivered. This is achieved by connecting the transfer tube to the Luer-Lock end of the external portion of the MammoSite RTS catheter. The opposite end of the transfer tube is locked into the computer-controlled machine (after-loader), which houses the radioactive source. A single radioactive source travels through the transfer tube to the MammoSite RTS catheter and delivers the radioactive source into the balloon. The radioactive source remains in the balloon for approximately 10 minutes to deliver treatment. After the completion of treatment, the source retracts into the safe in the after-loader. Depending on the number of fractions and the prescribed dose, the radioactive source will deliver the radiation therapy to the breast tissue over a course of 1 to 8 days (weekend interruptions are acceptable). The regulations from the Nuclear Regulatory

Commission mandate the patient be left alone in the brachytherapy suite for the duration of treatment.[21] A monitor and intercom system outside the suite enables verbal communication and a visual of the patient during treatment. The patient is not radioactive after treatment.

Risks and Side Effects

The MammoSite balloon method of APBI has risks and side effects.[14] Side effects that occur in 10% or more of patients receiving radiation therapy with the MammoSite balloon method include the following:

- Mild redness of the skin over the area of the balloon
- Mild scar tissue
- Flaking or peeling of dry skin over the area of the balloon
- Slightly smaller breast size or change in the way the breast looks
- Swelling of the breast
- Bruising
- Mild breast pain

Less likely effects, which occur in 3% to 9% of patients receiving the MammoSite balloon method, include the following:

- Infection
- Telangiectasia on the skin surface over the area of the balloon
- Increased firmness of the breast tissue
- Slight change in color of the skin over the area of the balloon
- Fibrosis
- Damaged fat cells in the breast that cause a red, swollen, or tender area in the breast

Rare but serious effects, which occur in less than 3% of patients receiving this type of treatment, include the following:

- Severe scar tissue
- Severe infection
- Breast pain lasting longer than 1 year

While the patient is under treatment, the nurse carefully monitors for infection and assesses the patient's pain level twice daily (documented on flowsheet). The patients are advised to keep the area dry (no showering), use a bra for support, and not remove any caps from the end of the catheter. Before the delivery of treatment, the area is undressed and cleaned with a mixture of sterile water and hydrogen peroxide, and a topical antibiotic ointment is applied to the incision. After treatment, the nurse redresses the area and secures the dressing with tape and the bra until the next treatment. The MammoSite balloon is explanted after the last fraction of radiation is delivered. The balloon is deflated by aspirating the saline/contrast from the access port of the MammoSite catheter via a 60-mL Luer-Lock syringe. This is done under sterile conditions. The nurse documents removal, reviews discharge instructions, and schedules the follow-up appointment. Discharge instructions include reporting of fever higher than 100°, redness or red streaks on the treated breast, swelling or warmth to the touch, large amounts or foul smelling drainage (a small amount of clear or reddish drainage is expected).

Since the approval by the Federal Food and Drug Administration, the MammoSite has been used to treat more than 12,000 women. Along with convenience (decrease in overall treatment time and a more tolerable implant) the MammoSite applicator addresses the disadvantages of brachytherapy by allowing easier implantation with a stronger reproducibility of radiation to the targeted breast tissue.

INTRAOPERATIVE RADIATION THERAPY

IORT as a form of accelerated partial breast irradiation can be applied in a single fraction during surgery, after the excision of the tumor.[7] Advantages to this form of radiation therapy over conventional external beam radiation include the direct visualization of the area/volume to be treated and therefore the potential protection of healthy tissues. Treatment volume can be reduced and the possibility of tumor control with any absorbed dose of radiation is lessened with an increase in the initial number of malignant cells. This is due to repopulation from neoplastic cells that are potentially present in residual disease and can occur during time elapsed between surgery and start of external radiation therapy. Additionally, "accelerated repopulation," the growth of neoplastic cells at an exponential rate, occurs after surgery. Therefore, IORT given directly after surgery (as a boost or as the only treatment) is theoretically eliminating this problem.

Few patients have been treated with IORT as a boost. In a recent trial in Austria, 188 clients with invasive breast cancer were treated with a conventional boost (12 Gy in 6 fractions) and 190 patients received a boost of intraoperative electrons (9 Gy in a single fraction). All patients additionally received external whole breast irradiation (51 Gy–56.1 Gy in 1.7 Gy fractions). Median follow-up periods were 55.3 and 25.8 months, respectively. Local recurrence rates were 4.3% in the conventional external radiation boost group and 0% in the IORT boost group, which seems to present an effective option to the traditional external boost.

IORT as the exclusive form of radiation therapy after lumpectomy was explored in Milan first as a dose escalation study from July 1999 to May 2000. Fifty-eight patients received increasing doses from 10 Gy to 21 Gy intraoperatively with or without external radiation.[7] The investigators observed no major side effects, and patients were followed every 2 to 3 months at a minimum of 4 years. Final conclusions determined a single dose of 21 Gy to be equivalent to a full course of external radiation therapy and to be well tolerated by patients.

In subsequent phase II and III trials from May 2000 to July 2003, the same investigators enrolled 558 patients who received 21 Gy as a single intraoperative dose. The average patient age was 61 years old. Breast tumors were unifocal, no larger than 2.5 cm, with ductal (78%) and lobular or mixed histology (11%). Follow-up examinations were done at 1 month, then at 3, 6, and 12 months and every 6 months afterwards, with data reported up to June of 2004. Analyzed data concluded that the risk of recurrence in the breast is very low. Three patients experienced local recurrence, three different patients developed carcinoma in another quadrant of the same breast, five women developed contralateral breast carcinoma, and an additional three patients were diagnosed with other primary tumors. A total of 13 patients developed distant metastases without local recurrence. The investigators determined the toxicity of IORT to be very low. Less than 3% of women developed fibrosis, which regressed within 36 months of treatment. Fat necrosis was noted in 2.5% of women, but resolved spontaneously except for one patient who required curettage of the tissue.

Delivery of IORT is accomplished through the production of electrons by a linear accelerator.[7] The most often used method is to transfer the patient from the operating room to a shielded radiation area after excision of the tumor, deliver radiation therapy to the open wound, and then return the patient to the operating room for closure of the cavity. A more recent development of miniature mobile accelerators actually allows for radiation therapy to be delivered in the operating room, thus avoiding transport of the anesthetized patient, coordination of facilities, and time constraints. These accelerators have the ability to deliver electrons at adjustable energies from 3 to 12 MeV and can be used in any operating room without structural modifications. Only limited shielding (15 cm wide) around the operating room table is necessary. The mobile accelerator is easily positioned alongside the operating room table and has the ability to conduct precisely controlled small movements to align and dock with the applicator that is placed in the breast. Applicators come in various shapes, diameters (4 cm–10 cm), and positions relative to the tumor bed (perpendicular or oblique at angles from 15 to 45 degrees).

Electron intraoperative treatment (ELIOT) requires the coordination of a multidisciplinary team of physicians, anesthesiologists, medical physicists/dosimetrists, radiation therapists, and nurses. Patients undergo lumpectomy with sentinel lymph node biopsy. An aluminum-lead shield disk is placed between the remaining parenchyma and the pectoralis fascia to protect the thoracic wall, the heart, and the lung. The breast tissue is temporarily sutured to expose the clinical target volume, which includes the entire surgical scar plus a safety margin of 1.5 cm to 3 cm. A metallic ring with hooks is applied to hold the skin open and the applicator is placed (Figure 25-7). Wet sterile gauze is positioned between the applicator and adjacent tissues to absorb any low energy electrons that scatter around the edge of the applicator.[7] Next, the head of the linear accelerator is connected to the applicator, and radiation therapy is delivered at the calculated dose with the appropriate energy

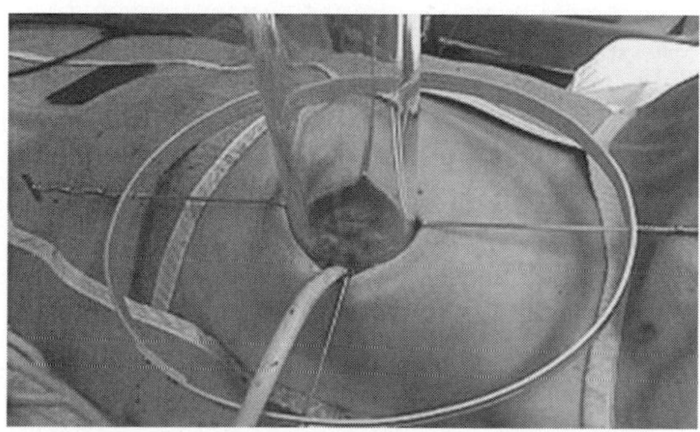

Figure 25-7 Placement of Applicator for Delivery of Intraoperative Radiation Therapy (IORT).

electron beam. Treatment time is less than 2 minutes, and the entire process lasts about 15 to 20 minutes. All materials are removed and the surgeon completes cosmetic reconstruction of the breast. The patient is then taken to the recovery room before being discharged to home.

Nursing care and instructions should include educating the patient about the signs and symptoms of infection (erythema, swelling, yellowish or greenish colored discharge from the incisional site, increased tenderness or discomfort, fever or chills). Additionally the patient will need a prescription for pain medication for postoperative discomfort to be taken as needed. Follow-up appointments with the surgeon and radiation oncologist should be scheduled. Patients need to be informed of when and where to call if any adverse reactions occur, such as fevers, chills, increased pain, or redness of breast tissue before the scheduled return visit. As with any surgical procedure, the patient may experience alterations in the perception of body image along with signs and symptoms of anxiety and depression. Nurses must remember to provide emotional support and be prepared to answer questions related to the diagnosis of cancer, the treatment, and its side effects and possible changes in personal relationships or family dynamics. If indicated, a social service consultation should be initiated.

SUMMARY

In summary, BCT is a curative treatment for early-stage breast cancer with improved cosmetic results. Accelerated partial breast irradiation delivers the radiation component of BCT in a shorter, more convenient amount of time than standard whole breast irradiation. Regardless of how it is delivered, via external beam quadrant treatment, brachytherapy, or intraoperatively, this technique allows for a decreased volume of breast tissue to be treated and a reduction of radiation to surrounding tissues and structures.

REFERENCES

1. Recht A: Introductory seminars in radiation oncology, *Semin Radiat Oncol* 15(2):67-132, 2005.
2. Hannoun-Levi JM, Mazeron JJ, Marsiglia H et al: Partial breast irradiation: revolution or evolution, *Cancer Treat Rev* 30(7):599-607, 2004.
3. Vicini FA, Kestin L, Chen P et al: Limited-field radiation therapy in the management of early stage breast cancer, *J Natl Cancer Inst* 95(16):1205-1210, 2003.
4. Chen PY, Vicini FA, Benitez P et al: Long-term cosmetic results and toxicity after accelerated partial-breast irradiation, *Cancer* 106(5):991-999, 2006.
5. Weed DW, Edmundson GK: Accelerated partial breast irradiation: a dosimetric comparison of three different techniques, *Brachytherapy* 4(2):121-129, 2005.
6. Shah NM, Wazer DE: The MammoSite balloon brachytherapy catheter for accelerated partial breast irradiation, *Semin Radiat Oncol* 15(2):100-107, 2005.
7. Orecchia R, Veronesi U: Interoperative, *Semin Radiat Oncol* 15(2):76-83, 2005.
8. King TA, Bolton JS, Kuske RR et al: Long-term results of wide-field brachytherapy as the sole method of radiation therapy after segmental mastectomy for T(is, 1,2) breast cancer, *Am J Surg* 180(4):299-304, 2000.
9. Perrera F, Engel J, Holliday R et al: Local resection and brachytherapy confined to the lumpectomy site for early breast cancer: a pilot study, *J Surg Oncol* 65(4):263-268, 1997.
10. Polgar C, Strnad V, Major T: Brachytherapy for partial breast irradiation: the European experience, *Semin Radiat Oncol* 15(2):116-122, 2005.
11. Formenti SC: External beam partial breast irradiation, *Semin Radiat Oncol* 15(2):92-99, 2005.
12. Baglan K, Sharpe MB, Laffaray D et al: Accelerated partial breast irradiation using 3D conformal radiation therapy (3DCRT), *Int J Radiat Oncol Biol Phys* 55(2): 302-311, 2003.
13. Vicini FA, Remonchamp V, Wallace M: Ongoing clinical experiences utilizing 3D conformal external beam radiotherapy to deliver partial breast irradiation in patients with early-stage breast cancer treated with breast conserving therapy, *Int J Radiat Oncol Biol Phys* 57(5):1247-1253, 2003.
14. Wolmark N, Curran WJ, Vicini FA et al: A randomized phase III study of conventional whole breast irradiation (WBI) versus partial breast irradiation (PBI) for women with stage 0, I, or II breast cancer, *NSABP B-39/RTOG 0413* [protocol]. Pittsburgh, NSABP, 2004.
15. Title 10 Code of Federal Regulation Part 35.615. *Safety precautions for remote afterloader teletherapy unit and gamma stereotactic radiosurgery units.*
16. Vicini FA, Chen PY, Fraile M et al: Low-dose rate brachytherapy as the sole radiation modality in the management of patients with early-stage breast cancer treated with breast conserving therapy: preliminary results of a pilot trial, *Int J Radiat Oncol Biol Phys* 38(2):301-310, 1997.
17. Vicini FA, Kini VR, Chen PY et al: Irradiation of the tumor bed alone after lumpectomy in selected patients with early-stage breast therapy, *J Surg Oncol* 70(1):33-40, 1999.
18. Baglan KL, Martinez, AA, Frazier RC et al: The use of high-dose rate brachytherapy alone after lumpectomy in patients with early-stage breast cancer treated with breast-conserving therapy, *Int J Radiat Oncol Biol Phys* 50(4): 1003-1011, 2001.
19. Vicini FA, Arthur DW: Breast brachytherapy: North American experience, *Semin Radiat Oncol* 15(2):108-115, 2005.

20. Benitez PR, Chen PY, Vicini FA et al: Partial breast irradiation in breast conserving therapy by way of interstitial brachytherapy, *Am J Surg* 188(4):355-364, 2004.
21. Keisch ME: Accelerated partial breast irradiation: the case for current use, *Breast Cancer Res* 7(3):106-109, 2005.
22. Keisch M, Vicini F, Kuske RR et al: Initial clinical experience with the MammoSite breast brachytherapy applicator in women with early-stage breast cancer treated with breast-conserving therapy, *Int J Radiat Oncol Biol Phys* 55(2):289-293, 2003.
23. Keisch ME: MammoSite, *Expert Rev Med Devices* 2(4): 387-394, 2005.
24. A multi-center, open-label clinical study to evaluate the performance and safety of the Proxima MammoSite Radiation Therapy System, *MammoSite* [protocol], Alpharetta, Ga, Proxima Therapeutics, August 2, 2000, Rev D.

Chapter 26

Total Body Irradiation and Total Lymphoid Irradiation

Joni Dunn and Catherine M. Comeau Lew

Total body irradiation (TBI) is a technique of delivering a uniform radiation dose to the entire body unlike total skin irradiation that treats only the skin. This method has the ability to provide shielding to particular organs of the body as needed.[1] TBI treatments have been in existence for over 25 years and have been used to treat various cancers since the turn of the twentieth century. Initially it was used for palliation in patients with advanced lymphoma. This use of TBI therapy greatly decreased with the development of more effective chemotherapy in the 1960s. TBI for palliative care is rarely used today. TBI's clinical use increased again after E.D. Thomas and associates' pioneered work in 1976. Such work demonstrated that curative treatment of refractory cancers could be obtained by the administration of sublethal TBI in conjunction with myeloablative chemotherapy followed by bone marrow rescue.[1,2]

TBI use has grown from a conditioning treatment used in a small number of bone marrow transplant (BMT) protocols to being used today with a multiple of hematopoietic stem cells transplants (HSCT). Sources of today's transplants are not only from donor bone marrow cells used with BMTs but also include donor peripheral stem cells and umbilical cord stem cells.[3]

TOTAL BODY IRRADIATION OVERVIEW

The role TBI plays in HSCT preparatory conditioning varies with the transplant protocol and can be either conventional or low-intensity TBI. In conventional allogeneic HSCT, TBI's role includes the destruction of residual malignant cells, or in the case of genetic disorders, (i.e., Fanconi's anemia) destruction of bone marrow cell populations.[4] The other purposes of TBI with allogeneic HSCTs include ablating the marrow to allow room for engraftment of the transplanted cells and suppressing the host immune system to allow engraftment of the donor cells. The bone marrow is specifically targeted to achieve immunosuppression. Bone marrow primitive precursor cells are extremely radiosensitive, and bone marrow cells progressively drop in number after the destruction of these precursor cells by TBI. One of the most important functions of TBI and its primary goal is the achievement of immunosuppression, which allows engraftment of donor cells. TBI's cytotoxic effects are a secondary goal.[2,4] Engraftment is typically defined as reaching an absolute neutrophil count (ANC) greater than 500/millimeters $(mm)^3$ for 2 to 3 consecutive days after receiving the HSCT.[4] Platelet engraftment is commonly defined as a platelet count of greater than 20,000/mm^3 without platelet transfusion in the previous 7 days.[5] Graft versus tumor response theory proposes that the engrafted allogeneic transplant has its own cytotoxic effect on the patient's remaining malignant cells, which reduces the need for cytotoxic therapy. This theory has been supported by evidence of lower relapse rates that have been seen in allogeneic HSCT patients as compared to those seen in autologous HSCT patients. Lower allogeneic relapse rates have been documented in all HSCT-treated malignancies.[6-8] TBI use with autologous HSCT is much more infrequent than its allogeneic HSCT counterpart. TBI's role in autologous HSCT is primarily cytoreduction (tumor kill) with a secondary goal of providing marrow space for engraftment of transplanted cells.[2,4,9] Resistance to engraftment appears to be mediated by the patient's lymphocyte precursors that survive myeloablative conditioning.[5] The high doses of TBI required to achieve immunosuppression and total tumor kill with HSCTs would result in unacceptably high toxicity.[4] However, both goals can be achieved when chemotherapy conditioning regimens are used in conjunction with lower TBI doses.[4,10]

Indications for Treatment

TBI is used with both adult and pediatric autologous and allogeneic HSCTs. TBI usage in pediatric diseases is presented later in this chapter. Adult hematologic malignancies such as acute lymphocytic leukemia (ALL), acute myelogenous leukemia (AML), chronic lymphocytic leukemia (CLL), and chronic myelogenous leukemia (CML) are commonly treated with HSCT with TBI conditioning.[4] TBI is used as part of treatment protocols for breast cancer, multiple myeloma, non-Hodgkin's lymphoma (NHL), aplastic anemia and congenital abnormalities.[4,10,11] See Table 26-1 for diseases treated with TBI as an HSCT conditioning regimen.

In treatment for AML, HSCT is usually done in first remission and usually with an allogeneic HSCT. Whereas in ALL, HSCT treatment is typically used for refractory ALL or Philadelphia chromosome positive ALL in which there is a high risk for relapse. Meta-analysis indicates that HSCT is now the best form of post-remission treatment for ALL.[5] CML patients have better survival rates if they are transplanted early in their disease (i.e., in the chronic phase). Refractory, relapsed, or high-risk NHLs have been treated with autologous HSCT with TBI conditioning. Of note, lymphoma patients with presenting high lactate dehydrogenase (LDH) levels, bulky mediastinal, and abdominal disease are considered to have high-risk disease. Hodgkin's patients who are refractory or relapsed may be eligible for TBI conditioning if they had no previous or just minimal radiation treatment (RT). Autologous HSCT with TBI in conjunction with chemotherapy has been used in treatment for multiple myeloma.[4] Ideally aplastic anemia HSCT patients are treated with total lymphoid irradiation. However, if these patients have been sensitized by receiving several blood transfusions, they may require TBI conditioning.[4,5]

Dosing/Scheduling

TBI in daily doses of 1.5 Gy to 7.5 Gy causes a rapid depletion of vital stem cells within 1 week of treatment. Bone marrow regeneration is very gradual, with total recovery taking 1 to 5 years after TBI completion.[2] When 25% to 50% of bone marrow is exposed to RT, permanent ablation occurs at single doses of 20 Gy or a fractionated total dose of 30 Gy.[12] Death usually occurs after myeloablative TBI without HSCT because of granulocytopenia and thrombocytopenia that leads to infection and hemorrhage. HSCT is possible because the microvasculature of the marrow continues to support implantation and growth of transplant stem cells

Table 26-1 TBI Uses in Adult Diseases[2,4,5,6,7,8,10,11,16,17,21,30,43]

Type	Manifestation	Disease
Malignant	Hematologic	Acute lymphoblastic leukemia*
		Acute myeloid leukemia*
		Chronic myeloid leukemia
		Hairy-cell leukemia
	Myeloproliferative	Non-Hodgkin's lymphoma*
		Refractory Hodgkin's disease (minimal prior irradiation)
		Myelodysplasia
		Multiple myeloma
	Solid tumors	Small cell carcinoma of lung
		Testicular carcinoma
Nonmalignant	Immune disorders	Aplastic anemia
	Genetic disorders	Osteopetrosis
		Wiskott-Aldrich syndrome
		Thrombocytopenia-absent radii syndrome
		Fanconi's anemia with leukemic conversion

*Most common diseases.
TBI, Total body irradiation.

even after doses of 7.5 Gy to 10.5 Gy TBI have been administered.[4]

A single TBI dose of 1 Gy to 2 Gy without HSCT has been used for inducing remissions and providing palliation care for advanced stages of CML and NHLs.[5] Typically regimens consisted of radiation doses of 0.1 Gy to 0.15 Gy per day, 2 to 3 times a week to a total dose of 1.5 Gy to 2 Gy. In such regimens it is recommended that a treatment break of 4 to 8 weeks after each 0.5 Gy of TBI be taken to avoid severe thrombocytopenia.[4,5,13] It is not well understood how a low dose of 0.5 Gy to 1.5 Gy can have anti-tumor effects. Some investigators attribute this to an initial low dose hypersensitivity of the cancer cells.[14]

The initial TBI method used in conjunction with BMT was a single dose of 8 Gy to 10 Gy.[2] Animal studies in dogs showed that a dose of greater than 9.2 Gy was needed in allogeneic HSCTs to prevent graft rejection when TBI was the only conditioning treatment.[2] Fractionated TBI significantly reduces immunosuppression, and theory proposes that an increase in TBI total dose (TD) with the fractionated method would be needed to maintain the equivalent cell kill achieved with single high-dose treatments. Studies in the late 1980s and 1990s showed that reduced toxicities were obtained with fractionated treatments without detrimental effect from the use of the higher TD given. Higher TDs have been found to decrease relapse rates.[2,4] However, the increase in TD with dose rates of 0.8 Gy/minute has failed to improve overall survival because of increased treatment-related toxicities such as graft-versus-host disease (GVHD).[2] Studies have shown that increasing the number of fractions to reach the TD contributes to a decreased incidence of interstitial pneumonitis (IP) and possibly a decrease in the incidence of parotitis.[4] The smaller fraction size appears to be associated with a significantly shorter cell repair time than larger size fractions.[2]

Animal studies have shown that TBI hyperfractionation method decreases TBI immunosuppressive effect and could possibly lead to decreased engraftments. Single doses of 7.5 Gy to 10 Gy have been shown to be more effective in preventing rejection than comparable total fractioned TBI doses.[4] International bone marrow transplant registry (IBMTR) reported in 1992 that single TBI doses greater or equal to 11 Gy and dose rates greater or equal to 1.4 Gy/minute were associated with significantly fewer rejections.[4] However, in a CML 5-year follow-up study, survival rates were found to be better with fractionated versus single dose TBI. AML HSCT studies have attributed low relapse rates reported to hyperfractionated TBI with total dose of 13.2 Gy to 14.4 Gy, testicular boosting, and sequencing TBI after cyclophosphamide conditioning.[4] Another study by Redei and colleagues 5 of 19 patients receiving partially mismatched related HSCTs with TBI hyperfractionated conditioning using fractions of 2 Gy to TD of 12 Gy followed by thiotepa, fludarabine, and antithymocyte antisera resulted in donor engraftment in 17 patients and platelet engraftment in 15 patients. Two of the 19 patients died because of sepsis on day 6 and 8 post transplant. The authors concluded that TBI hyperfractionation had been well tolerated and had provided sufficient immunosuppression to allow rapid engraftments.[5] At Mount Sinai Medical Center the use of 1.5 Gy fractions 2 times per day in nonmyeloablative HSCT protocols achieved the same immunosuppression as 1.25 Gy 3 times a day with no untoward side effects.[4] At this time, there is no gold standard for optimal administration of TBI delivery method. Method of delivery varies between treatment centers and the disease being treated. Today many HSCT centers use the fractionated TBI method.[4,6,9,10,13,15]

Most TBI conditioning protocols use more than 9 Gy TD to prevent graft rejection.[2] However, some studies have found that immunosuppression can be accomplished with fractionated doses 1.5 Gy to total dose of 3 Gy.[4] Fractionated TBI TD ranges from 5 Gy to 16 Gy with fraction sizes varying from 1.2 Gy to 4 Gy. A common fractionated dosing schedule consists of 1.5 Gy or less with dose rates of 0.5 Gy to 1.8 Gy/minute. The fraction size most commonly used is between 1.5 Gy to 2 Gy. Accelerated hyperfractionated doses are also being used. In this method 2 fractions a day are administered with optimally 6 hours between fractions.[2,4,14]

Because there is no standard treatment method for the delivery of TBI, differences in dose distribution delivered at different treatment facilities can be significant. Treatment variations make it difficult to assess clinical effectiveness between multiple treatment centers. Subsequently, a method has been developed that allows for better comparison of clinical outcomes between treatment sites.

Such a method uses a single point prescription, that is, midpoint at the level of the umbilicus, and specifies limits for the highest and lowest dose levels for any point in the body and sets dose limits for specific tissues such as the lungs. A typical prescription might read: dose to midpoint at the level of the umbilicus as 8 Gy. All points in the body should fall within the limits of 8.4 Gy and 7.2 Gy or +5% and -10%. A total dose to greater than 50% of one lung must not exceed 8 Gy.[2]

Dose Rates

Dose rate, fraction size, time interval between fractions, and TD are factors that influence the biologic effects of TBI. Animal studies have shown that the immunosuppression effect in relationship to graft rejection is influenced by dose rate and dose fractionation. A lower TD of 4.5 Gy given at high dose rate of 0.7 Gy/minute can prevent graft rejection.[2] Data on the need to modify TBI dose rates is conflicting. A TD of 4.5 Gy given in fractions using the same dose rate or given as a single dose at a low dose rate of .07 Gy/minute is much less effective in accomplishing engraftment. Yet, one study found no dose rate effects on acute side effects when given with either single-dose or hyperfractionated TBI treatments.[4]

Low dose rates have been well documented in humans and animals for their effectiveness in reducing the incidence of pulmonary complications. It has been reported that a low dose rate of 0.5 Gy/minute is needed to decrease the risk of IP. At this rate, however, to deliver a single dose of 10 Gy, it would take 3 hours.[2] A lower TBI dose rate via the single-dose method could be equivalent to the fractionated method in decreasing toxicity. But at such a rate, it would require as much as 24 hours to complete the treatment.[4]

Typical dose rates reported in the literature range from .05 Gy to .18 Gy per minute when used with 1.5 Gy or less fractionated doses.[4,14]

Administration

Both cobalt and linear accelerator machines are used to deliver TBI.[9] Linear accelerators have a propensity for breakdown. Therefore it is useful to have a back-up treatment machine available to be able to keep the tight treatment time constraints of HSCTS protocols.[2] Three methods of TBI patient treatment positioning have been described in the literature. One has the patient standing upright. A bicycle-like seat is use to give the patient some support while in this standing position. The second position has the patient sitting on a couch or cart with the knees drawn up. The third position has the patient lying on a table.[1,2,4] Close monitoring of patients is especially needed for the standing position because this position requires more physical endurance. Patients treated in the standing position may need treatment interruptions because of their fatigue, dizziness, or nausea and vomiting.[4] On the other hand, a disadvantage of the sitting position is the difficulty involved with applying lung shields. Lung shielding in the sitting position can be accomplished without the use of metal shields by having patients cross their arms over their chests.[2]

Anteroposterior (AP) and Posterioanterior (PA) or parallel-opposed lateral techniques TBI delivery methods can be used. A major disadvantage of the AP/PA method is the need to use lung shields or other means to reduce lung dose. There are advantages and disadvantages to either the AP/PA or lateral treatment positions.

Shields

In the past, TBI studies have shown that 50% of patients receiving single high-dose TBI developed IP and half of those patients died. Past studies also have shown that the maximum tolerated TBI dose to the lungs without shielding is 16 Gy. This lung threshold dose, however, is not fixed and depends on the method of radiation administration.[2] Lungs are air-containing organs rather than solid tissue, which results in the lungs receiving a 10% to 20% higher dose than the prescribed single-point TBI dose. Lung shielding is used by some treatment centers to decrease TBI toxicity to the lung, but its use is not universal.[6] Some centers use attenuator thickness of 1 to 3 mm to ensure the lungs receive the same dose as other tissue.[4,16] Doses to the lung with shielding are usually around 10 Gy for an overall TBI prescription dose of 13.5 Gy.[2] However, there is a fear that shielding the lungs will lead to an increase in the relapse rate. This fear is based on the fact that the lungs contain a large pool of blood that may harbor circulating leukemic or lymphoma cells.[2] Lung shields usage increases the complexity of TBI delivery. Lung shields ideally will achieve the same lung dose as prescribed to the designated single point in the treatment prescription. Some treatment centers use lung shields for one treatment and none for the remaining treatments to achieve a total uniform dose. Other treatment centers may use thinner shields with every treatment fraction. The ribs under the lung shields may need to be treated with electron boost to bring them to single-point prescription dose. As previously discussed, lung shielding in the sitting position can be accomplished without the use of metal shields by having the patient cross their arms over their chests.[16] However, there are mixed opinions concerning the use of patients' arms to shield the lungs as this method is more difficult to replicate with each fraction.[4]

Shielding also may be used for other areas of the body that may be of concern. If a patient has history of elevated blood urea nitrogen (BUN) and creatinine levels or is receiving cytarabine and cyclophosphamide conditioning, renal shields may be employed. Reports using liver shielding to decrease the incidence of veno-occlusive disease (VOD) have been seen in the literature. No long-term results have been reported on the effect on relapse/survival rates related to the use of liver shields. Some authors have reported on the use of eye shields. One retrospective study of children with hematologic diseases found the use of eye shields accomplished a total TBI dose reduction of 55% to 58% to the children eyes and an increase in the latency time of cataract development without resulting in an increased incidence of central nervous system (CNS) relapses.[17]

Bolus

It is assumed that leukemic cells may be anywhere throughout the body, including the skin. Linear accelerators delivering TBI have a dose buildup region upon entering tissue that could potentially result in under-dosing the skin.[4] Therefore, with linear accelerators, the delivery of the prescribed TBI dose to the skin surface requires the use of a bolus or a scatter screen between the radiation source and the patient to provide dose homogeneity. The use of blankets between the radiation source and the patient also can provide an equivalent 8-mm tissue bolus. Numerous treatment centers use a plastic screen in front of the patient to scatter photons into electrons to achieve prescription dose to the skin surface. Some institutions use compensators at the neck, feet, and other areas to improve dose distribution homogeneity.[4]

Boosting

Theoretically, boosting the ribs that have been shielded by lung shields ensures homogeneity dose distribution to shielded ribs. However, there has been at least one study reporting no difference in relapse rates when not using electron rib boosting, and many treatment centers no longer administer rib boosts.[4] Testicular boosting with TBI is a method used by some treatment centers. A high testicular relapse rate among leukemic patients was seen in the 1980s, which resulted in some centers using a 0.4 Gy testicular boost for leukemic patients. Memorial Sloan-Kettering Cancer Center (MSKCC) reported that since incorporating testicular boosts, no further testicular relapses have occurred in more than 300 treated leukemic patients. CML patients, especially when patients' spleens are enlarged, are at increased risk for harboring leukemic cells in their spleens. Because of this increased risk, splenic boosting is sometimes administered before TBI. Although CML studies have shown a trend toward improved survival when boosting the spleen, no conclusive studies on its survival effect have been reported. Boosting of residual disease or areas of initial disease involvement such as the mediastinum is often prescribed with TBI treatments of patients with lymphoma.[4]

Sequencing With Other Modalities

There are theoretical advantages of TBI conditioning over chemotherapy conditioning regimens. Namely, there are no malignant cell sanctuary sites from TBI as there are with chemotherapy conditioning, and treatments are not dependent on blood flow to provide homogenous dose delivery. Tumor cells have fewer resistance mechanisms to TBI as compared with chemotherapy and TBI shielding, and boosting techniques can be used to alter dose delivery to sensitive tissues or increase dose to areas at risk for recurrence.[2,4,10] TBI is combined with chemotherapy to allow reduction of TBI's TD and toxicities whereas still achieving tumor kill and the immunosuppression, which aids engraftment. The chemotherapy conditioning regimens used in conjunction with TBI varies by treatment protocol. The most commonly used HSCT chemotherapy conditionings used in conjunction with high-dose TBI are cyclophosphamide, fludarabine, and etoposide.[2,13,16] Various protocols also use melphalan with etoposide or thiotepa with fludarabine.[5,18] Low-dose TBI

(2 Gy) is commonly used with fludarabine in combination with busulfan, thiotepa, or melphalan.[7] Cyclophosphamide is frequently used in chemotherapy conditioning in combination with TBI because of its greater immunosuppression effect as compared to etoposide and cytarabine. In a 30-year follow-up study of HSCTs with AML patients, no overall survival differences were seen between the conditioning regimens using TBI and cyclophosphamide and those using TBI and melphalan.[19]

Animal studies have found more lung toxicity occurs when TBI follows chemotherapy conditionings, and some authors report less nausea and vomiting with TBI if given before chemotherapy conditioning, especially when TBI is given in a standing position.[4] Therefore, in many protocols, TBI is prescribed to be administered before the chemotherapy conditioning. Chemotherapy agents have their own dose-limiting toxicities as seen in Table 26-2.

Many HSCT protocols also use one or a combination of the following drugs to help attenuate immunosuppression: antithymocyte antisera, cyclosporine, methotrexate and tacrolimus.[2,5,7] New clinical trials are using iodine-labeled anti-CD33 antibody M195, CD 34 enriched hematopoietic progenitor cells, and anti-CD45 antibody and rhenium-labeled anti-CD66 antibody in combination with chemoradiation conditionings as a means to increase radiation dose without increasing toxicities.[5,19] Alemtuzumab usage is being explored in Britain, with some studies showing low treatment-related mortality.[7]

Reduced Intensity Conditioning

Many investigators are studying variations in HSCT conditioning treatment modalities in an attempt to decrease the concomitant related toxicities.[20] A relatively new area of investigation is using nonmyeloablative reduced-intensity conditioning (RIC) protocols for allogeneic HSCT. In these protocols, TBI has been administered in lower doses solely to suppress the immune system to aid engraftment and not to destroy residual malignant cells.[2,7,10,21,22] Investigators have recognized the importance of graft versus tumor effect for tumor kill in allogeneic transplants, which, in theory, may allow the use of nonmyeloablative conditionings without effecting survival rates. Some investigators are using nonmyeloablative TBI doses as low as 1 Gy to 2 Gy along with immunotherapy such as donor lymphocyte infusions to achieve chimerism. Chimerism is a bone marrow state in which host and donor cells exist compatibly without signs of GVHD.[7,22] Similar investigations are showing a renewed interest in using single 4.5 Gy to 5 Gy fractionations at a high dose rate of 0.7 Gy/minute.[2] Some investigators in out-patient HSCT centers are using 5 Gy single-fraction TBI in conjunction with chemotherapy conditioning for autologous HSCT treatment for multiple myeloma or low-grade lymphoproliferative disorders.[23] Investigators at Washington University in St. Louis have used a single dose of 5.5 Gy with a dose rate of 0.3 Gy/minute for allogeneic HSCTs. Their results have shown durable engraftment with low treatment toxicities and mortality rates.[24] Their study found no difference in incidence of GVHD and, on the other hand, found significantly fewer grade II to IV GVHD as compared to myeloablative regimens. However, a nonmyeloablative study involving AML patients reported a high rate of relapse. It is notable that the lower TBI total dose used in these investigations achieved a lower incidence of IP.[19]

The clinical challenge in RIC is to reduce morbidity without compromising tumor kill. Some novel approaches involve the use of radioimmunotherapy using the monoclonal antibody tositumomab.[8] TBI single-dose immunosuppression conditioning of 1 Gy to 2 Gy is presently being used in conjunction with immunotherapy (donor lymphocyte infusions) to help secure engraftment.[4] Many RIC variations are seen in the literature. TBI has been found to be more effective for immunosuppression than the highest tolerated doses of busulfan/cyclophosphamide conditioning in randomized trails.[1] Fludarabine is the most commonly used single-agent conditioning drug.[14] An alternative single-agent drug is busulfan. Busulfan/

Table 26-2 Dose-Limiting Toxicities of Commonly Used Chemotherapeutic Agents

Chemotherapy agent	Dose-limiting toxicity
Cyclophosphamide	Interstitial pneumonitis
Melphalan	Stomatitis and veno-occlusive disease
Cytarabine	Skin erythema and central nervous system (CNS) symptoms
Etoposide	Stomatitis and hepatic toxicities

cyclophosphamide is another common chemotherapy regimen used for conditioning allogeneic HSCTs.[19] However, significant toxicities, which include a 19% incidence of VOD compared with 1% with TBI conditioning exists. Of note there has been less IP incidence in patients with history of prior chest radiation treatments, 5% compared with TBI-related incidence of 32%.[4]

Leukemias

Animal studies have shown that host resistance to engraftment could be eliminated by giving large doses of T cell–depleted donor stem cells. A human study using large doses of T cell–depleted donor cells without any conditioning treatments reported full donor engraftment in the treatment of high-risk ALL patients.[5]

A prospective nonrandomized study of 18 patients with hematologic malignancies (CML, AML) compared the use of RIC with fludarabine/busulfan/antithymocyte globulin (ATG) and fludarabine/cyclophosphamide/ATG with myeloablative conditioning using TBI/cyclophosphamide. It is well known that intestinal integrity is impaired by myeloablative protocols.[21] Therefore, it was not surprising that patients in this study who received myeloablative therapy had significantly increased intestinal permeability and gastrointestinal toxicity. However, no significant differences were found in the incidence, time of presentation, or severity of acute GVHD.

TBI/cyclophosphamide versus busulfan/cyclophosphamide conditioning in clinical trials with CML patients have found no statistically significant differences in the incidence of morbidity or mortality.[25]

A review of the AML studies containing at least 20 patients over the last 30 years found that the two most common myeloablative regimens, busulfan/cyclophosphamide and TBI/cyclophosphamide, had no significant difference in engraftment rates or survival rates. A significant decrease in relapse rate was seen with the TBI regimen, whereas significant increase in the incidence of VOD was found with the chemotherapy regimens. No difference was seen in the incidence of acute or chronic GVHD. A consistent finding was the increase in VOD, hemorrhagic cystitis, and seizures seen with busulfan/cyclophosphamide regimens. An increase in CNS relapse was seen with the chemotherapy only regimens, which suggests that TBI is more effective in treating occult CNS disease. Conflicting reports were found on the incidence of IP with TBI regimens. However, TBI fractionation and the use of lung shields have been found to reduce the incidence of IP. Each of the regimens had disadvantages. The authors concluded that neither regimen is suitable for all patients. For example, busulfan/cyclophosphamide is not suitable for patients with elevated liver function tests, nor is TBI regimen the first choice for patients with prior lung radiation therapy.[19]

Lymphomas

Superiority of any specific regimen with or without TBI in the treatment of stage III and IV Hodgkin's disease has not been demonstrated.[10] A retrospective study of 92 Hodgkin's patients receiving either TBI/cyclophosphamide/etoposide or busulfan/melphan/thiotepa conditioning found the median time to engraftment to be similar. No statistically significant differences were found in regards to morbidity or mortality.[10]

The role of preparative regimens for autologous HSCT for patients with NHL was retrospectively studied in Spain. Three hundred forty-eight patients were treated with different chemotherapy conditioning regimens including busulfan, etoposide, cyclophosphamide, vincristine, and doxorubicin. Forty-seven patients received a TBI/cyclophosphamide regimen. Faster engraftment was found with the chemotherapy only regimens and a higher early mortality was found with the TBI regimen. A multivariate analysis revealed that patients conditioned with chemotherapy only regimen had improved overall survival, disease-free, and relapse-free survival when compared with the TBI/cyclophosphamide treated patients.[9]

A 2001 nonrandomized study of 85 NHL patients compared the use of TBI/cyclophosphamide/etoposide preparatory regimen to busulfan/melphalan/thiotepa regimen in patients receiving autologous HSCT. Regimen-related morbidity for the TBI arm was 8% compared with 11% in the chemotherapy only arm. More IP was found with the TBI arm, but more VOD was seen in the chemotherapy only arm. A statistically higher percentage of patients in the TBI arm had received immunotherapy. No significant difference was found in the treatment-related mortality between the two arms. Follow-up was 5 years for the TBI arm and 3.5 years for the chemotherapy only arm.[9]

Investigators of HSCT for follicular lymphoma have recommended that RIC be used for follicular lymphoma only when myeloablative conditioning is contraindicated. It was felt that although myeloablative regimens are associated with increased treatment-related mortality, it provides lower relapse rates.[8]

The third European Bone Marrow Transplant Group Workshop group, which met in February 2003, reached a consensus on the use of RIC with HSCT. It was concluded that RIC with HSCT was feasible for all diseases and allowed allogeneic HSCT to be offered as treatment for older patients. It was felt RIC achieved consistent engraftment and enduring donor chimerism in the majority of patients treated with or without low-dose radiation. In addition, it was felt that the phase of the disease had an impact on the outcome, that is, poorer outcomes with higher disease phases. Acute and chronic GVHD and post-transplant infections remained a significant RIC problem. The panel concluded that the optimal RIC had yet to be determined.[7]

TOTAL BODY IRRADIATION IN CHILDREN

TBI is a fundamental component of many pediatric HSCT protocol regimens. It may be combined with high-dose chemotherapy to provide myeloablation (total hematopoietic and immunosuppression) before bone marrow transplantation or peripheral stem cell transplantation.[26]

HSCT in the pediatric population is a consideration for children in whom no other alternative option would provide long-term disease-free survival. HCST is used in patients with acute lymphoblastic leukemia (high-risk ALL, Philadelphia chromosome positive), acute myelogenous leukemia, chronic myelogenous leukemia, myelodysplastic or myeloproliferative syndromes, leukemia patients in second remission with appropriate HLA-matched sibling donor, refractory or relapsed Hodgkin's disease, NHL, neuroblastoma, and some solid tumors. It has been shown to improve the overall survival rate in children with hematological disorders such as Fanconi's anemia, aplastic anemia, immunodeficiency diseases, and diseases of inborn errors of metabolism.[3,27]

As part of the preparative regimen for HSCT, the timing, selection of total dose to be delivered, fractionation schedule, and selected organ shielding are protocol driven and are determined by the specific disease being treated. The underlying principle goals of TBI, as covered earlier in this chapter, are the same in both pediatric and adult protocols. The indications for TBI in pediatric malignancies or immunologic/metabolic disorders are presented as an overview. Table 26-3 lists specific pediatric diseases for which TBI is used as part of their preparative regimens.

The long-term side effects of total body irradiation can be quite profound, particularly in very young children. These may include growth impairment, endocrine imbalance, cataracts, gonadal failure, risk of second malignancy, and neurocognitive impairment.

Several other factors are taken into consideration before HSCT is considered: the ability to successfully achieve long-term disease survival for the particular disease; the potential chemotherapeutic toxicities and additive effect using TBI in preparative regimens; the ability to achieve successful T-cell depletion to minimize GVHD; age of the child; and history of previous radiation therapy.

The decision to undergo transplantation is profound and can bring with it a mixture of emotions and stressors. Several strategies may be incorporated into the orientation of the radiation therapy department, which might help in alleviating some of the apprehension. A pre-bone marrow transplant orientation might include a tour of the

Table 26-3 TBI Uses for Diseases in Children

Malignant diseases	Nonmalignant diseases
Acute lymphoblastic leukemia*	Fanconi's anemia
Acute myelogenous leukemia	Aplastic anemia
Hodgkin's disease†	Wiskott-Aldrich syndrome
Lymphoma‡	Immunodeficiency diseases
Ewing's sarcoma§	Metabolic diseases
Neuroblastoma¶	Hurler's syndrome
Myelodysplastic syndrome	

*High-risk disease/features (Ph+ chromosome, translocation (9:22), t(4,11) ploidy.)
†Refractory or relapsed disease.
‡Relapsed disease.
§Advanced metastatic disease.
¶Double autologous transplant.
TBI, Total body irradiation.

treatment room and an opportunity to meet the staff who will be caring for the patient; medical play with the child life specialist; and interviewing the parents to find out about the child's ability to cooperate with medical procedures based on his or her previous experiences. Many children feel more relaxed if they can bring a special comfort object with them, or would prefer to watch a favorite video; listen to music, or have someone read them a story during the procedure to help distract them. When interacting with children, it is important to approach them from a developmental perspective and to appreciate their unique personalities and ability to deal with stress. When presenting instructions to children, one should provide simple but clear directions, and give specific behavioral expectations so that the child will know what is expected. Young children (usually under 4 years of age) and those who are developmentally delayed, or experiencing psychological, distress/anxiety may require anesthesia or sedation in order to help them achieve the degree of compliance and immobilization necessary to receive TBI. If the child is cooperative but a little apprehensive, distraction techniques, (e.g., videos to watch, music, reading a book) can be used to gain cooperation during the treatment session. If needed, a small dose of an anti-anxiety medication such as Ativan may help to alleviate stress.

Open communication between the transplant team and the radiation therapy staff is critical for ensuring optimum care for the child and family. This is particularly true for children undergoing anesthesia sedation, which requires the coordination of anesthesia, nursing, and radiation therapists. For children about to receive anesthesia, it is important to communicate changes in the child's status, which can directly impact on the child's tolerance of anesthesia. Such changes include problems with fluid and electrolyte balance, suspected infection, diarrhea, vomiting, fever, and need for transfusion support. The pediatric transplant team members have specific protocols and guidelines for management of symptoms and clinical problems. The treatment of children can present a variety of challenges to the radiation team. It is important to consider the child's age and developmental stage when planning and delivering care. Please see the Pediatric Considerations box for a list of considerations when caring for children in the radiation oncology setting.

Acute Lymphoblastic Leukemia

Children with standard risk acute lymphoblastic leukemia (ALL) achieve overall disease-free survival rates of 80% to 90% with current treatment protocols. Indications for bone marrow transplant in ALL would be early relapse (within 3 years of initial remission), poor initial response to induction therapy, and high-risk disease, which includes Philadelphia chromosome (+) and BCR-ABL or MLL-AF4 fusion genes.[28] The overall survival rate of children transplanted in first relapse is greater the 65%.[28]

Pediatric Considerations

- Does child require anesthesia for treatment?
  - Conscious sedation policy
  - Staff adequately trained
  - Adequate staffing available
- Role of child life therapist
  - Family-focused care
  - Parent and sibling guilt/grieving
  - Sibling alienation
  - Access to care
  - Medical bills
- Role of dietitian
  - Nutritional screening
  - Considerations related to age, growth and development, disease process
- Care coordination across the continuum
  - Ongoing quality-of-life assessment
  - Transition from pediatric to young adult to adult practitioners
- Age-specific milestones
  - Growth and development
  - Attainment of independence
  - Social skills
  - Peer acceptance
  - Self-image
- End-of-life issues
  - Hospice
  - Patient/family anger or grief
- Ethical and legal considerations
- Late effects from treatment
  - Fertility
  - Cognitive changes
  - Genetic testing for other primary malignancy
  - Secondary malignancies
- Long-term survivorship implications
  - Access to care
  - Ongoing surveillance
  - Disability?
  - Discrimination?

Davies and colleagues[29] provided a large retrospective comparison of preparative regimens in transplants for children with ALL from HLA-matched sibling donors, using data from the International Bone Marrow Transplant Registry. They compared the use of cyclophosphamide plus TBI (CY/TBI) versus busulfan plus cyclophosphamide (Bu/CY) for pre-transplant conditioning in children younger than age 20. Children receiving CY/TBI had reduced rates of relapse (55% versus 40%), reduced treatment-related mortality, reduced rates of overall treatment failure, and reduced overall mortality.[29]

Children who present with sites of extramedullary disease relapse, such as the CNS or testes, may require additional radiation immediately before the start of the conditioning regimen for transplantation. The dose of cranial irradiation may be 9 Gy to 10.8 Gy given at 1.8 Gy once daily a few days before TBI. The use of testicular boost before transplantation is somewhat controversial, and is not used in all institutions. Shank and colleagues[28] at Memorial Sloan-Kettering Cancer Center advocate the addition of testicular boost to eliminate testicular relapse. For this reason, many current protocols recommend 2 Gy given on 2 consecutive days, or a boost of 4 Gy in one fraction to the testes, using en face electrons.[28]

Acute Myeloblastic Leukemia

The overall disease-free survival of children with AML is less than 50%.[28] The most important prognostic indicators for AML are the disease's cytogenetic features. AML subtypes associated with good outcome after chemotherapy are FAB M2 with translocation + (8;21), FAB M3 with translocation + (15;17), and FAB M4 with inversion. Poor response to chemotherapy and poor disease-free survival has been noted in patients with the cytogenetic features of monosomy 5 and monosomy 7.[30]

HSCT remains the most important treatment modality for patients beyond complete remission.[13] A large retrospective review performed from 1991 to 1997, by the International Bone Marrow Tumor Registry, noted that 50% of patients who were in complete second remission and younger than 20 years survived 3 years after allogeneic transplantation.[30] In the prospective studies comparing consolidation chemotherapy and HSCT, improved disease control has been noted after allogeneic and autologous transplantation in Children Cancer Group and Pediatric Oncology Group Regimens.[28] It has been observed that those predictive factors that determine which relapsed AML patients are the best candidates for disease-free survival after HSCT include length of first complete remission, achievement of second remission, and absence of extramedullary disease.[30] Patients with favorable cytogenetics have improved outcome.

Conditioning regimens for allogeneic and autologous transplants in AML vary from cyclophosphamide/etoposide/TBI to busulfan and cyclophosphamide. The overall comparisons between multicenter clinical trials suggests greater leukemic control with the addition of TBI in children and adults; although overall survival rates are comparable, based on somewhat higher regimen-related mortality in the TBI-based transplants.[28] In autologous transplantation, leukemic contamination of the harvested bone marrow has been demonstrated to contribute to relapse after HSCT. A variety of methods have been employed to treat the bone marrow with chemotherapy or antibodies against myeloid cells.[30] In some situations this can contribute to the delayed engraftments and increased transplant morbidity.

Myeloproliferative and Myelodysplastic Disorders

Myelodysplastic syndrome (MDS) and myeloproliferative syndrome (MPS) represent a heterogeneous group of clinical stem cell disorders that are characterized by ineffective hematopoietic cells; impaired maturation of hematopoietic cells; progressive cytopenias in MPS disorders. In MPS there is an increased risk of developing acute myeloid leukemia.[26] These disorders are very rare in children. The MPS disease most commonly seen in children is chronic myelogenous leukemia. There are several congenital anomalies such as Down syndrome, neurofibromatosis type 1; and bone marrow failure syndromes including Kostmann's congenital neutropenia, Schwachmann syndrome, Blackfan-Diamond syndrome, thrombocytopenia, trisomy D, Klinefelter's syndrome, familial thrombocytopenia, and Fanconi's anemia, which have been shown to predispose children to an increased probability of developing MDS and subsequent AML.[26] In addition, exposure to alkylating agents (such as cyclophosphamide, nitrogen mustard) and topoisomerase 11 agonists and antagonist (etoposide) and ionizing radiation also have been identified as potential causative agents of MDS and AML.[26]

The treatment of choice for MDS is stem cell transplantation, from an HLA-matched donor.[26] Most of the series evaluating various chemotherapy regimens, and the success of allogeneic transplantation, involve both children and adults. The most common regimens use TBI with cyclophosphamide or busulfan with cyclophosphamide, using HLA-matched related donors or matched unrelated donors.[26]

The Seattle group at the Fred Hutchinson Cancer Research Center had the largest reported series of children and adults with MDS (1981-1996).[26] Their findings were similar to those previously reported for transplantation using unrelated donors, HLA-matched donors, and HLA-mismatched donors. The 3-year cumulative incidence of relapse was 17%, in patients with advanced disease, poor risk cytogenetics, and children treated in the earlier cohorts of HSCT. The disease-free survival was found to be 41%, in younger patients, less advanced morphology, and having favorable risk cytogenetics.[26]

Hodgkin's Disease

The choice of therapy for patients with refractory or relapsed Hodgkin's disease depends on several factors, including the initial treatment provided and the characteristics of the disease at time of relapse.[31] It is estimated that between 50% and 80% of patients who relapsed after radiation-alone therapy can be salvaged with chemotherapy or combined modality treatment.[31]

For children who have relapsed after initial treatment with radiation therapy alone, salvage chemotherapy regimens provide an effective means of achieving an overall disease-free survival of 55% to 80%. The addition of radiation to the site of relapsed disease, if feasible, along with chemotherapy may help improve outcome.[31]

In the setting of relapsed disease after chemotherapy, conventional salvage chemotherapy regimens are of limited success, increasing disease-free survival rates in only 10% to 50% of cases.[31] In some situations radiation alone, administered as a standard dose total lymphoid irradiation, may be curative.[31] However, total lymphoid irradiation is associated with many toxicities and may be difficult to administer in patients who have had problems with poor marrow reserve after aggressive high-dose chemotherapy.

Radiation therapy's role in the setting of high-dose chemotherapy and stem cell rescue is to provide treatment to relapsed disease sites. It may be administered in combination with chemotherapy conditioning regimens as total body irradiation, involved field irradiation, or as total lymphoid irradiation (TLI).[31]

Total body irradiation or total lymphoid irradiation usually includes cyclophosphamide with or without etoposide in the preparative regimen for stem cell rescue. The typical dose of TBI is 12 Gy to 14 Gy delivered over 4 to 5 days in twice daily fractions ranging from 1.5 Gy to 2.5 Gy. TLI is usually 18 Gy delivered in 0.9 Gy fractions twice daily over 2 weeks.[31]

TBI and TLI are not administered in those patients who have received previous mediastinal radiation because of the potential lethal toxicities of pneumonitis and pulmonary alveolar hemorrhage.[31]

Involved field radiation therapy (treatment of the site of primary disease presentation and adjacent lymph nodes) has been shown to play a positive role in treatment regimens using high-dose chemotherapy and stem cell rescue. The doses of radiation used in involved field radiation therapy are 20 Gy to 36 Gy in 1.5 Gy to 2.0 Gy fractions. The radiation volume may vary based on the pattern of disease presentation and the persistence of disease either after salvage chemotherapy or after the preparative regimen for transplantation.[31] In a series reported by the researchers at Stanford, patients with stage I to III disease at relapse who received high-dose therapy involved field irradiation, and autologous bone marrow transplant for relapsed or refractory Hodgkin's disease had a 3-year freedom from relapse of 100% and overall survival of 85%.[31]

Other novel approaches for relapsed Hodgkin's disease are currently under investigation. These include immunotoxin therapy; the use of low-dose TBI or fludarabine to provide nontoxic immunosuppression. This is done in an attempt to establish a graft versus lymphoma effect and to set the groundwork for adaptive immunotherapy.[31,32]

Lymphomas

Radiation plays a limited role in the treatment of childhood NHL due to the success of chemotherapy in treating the disease. Radiation is indicated in the following situations: for disease outside the CNS in pedi-atric NHL; as emergency treatment for medias-tinal disease or spinal cord compression; as treatment for patients who fail to achieve complete remission after induction chemotherapy, palliation of pain, or mass effect; and for consolidation of regions of local disease before or after bone marrow transplantation in patients' recurrent disease.[33]

Pediatric patients with lymphoma who fail to go into remission, or who relapse, are rarely cured using conventional chemotherapy doses.[26] Autologous HSCT has been used to provide an opportunity for dose escalation in chemotherapeutic regimens. The conditioning regimens may include one of the following combinations with or without the addition of total body irradiation: CBV (cyclophosphamide, carmustine, and etoposide) BEAM (carmustine [BCNU], etoposide, cytarabine [Ara C], and melphalan) and BEAC (carmustine [BCNU], etoposide, cytarabine [Ara C], and cyclophosphamide).[26]

If TBI is a component of the preparatory regimen for transplant, it is usually given in a fractionated course to total dose of 1.2 Gy to 1.4 Gy. Boosts to sites of local disease before or after transplant are limited to 20 Gy because of normal tissue tolerances.[33]

Solid Tumors

The overall survival rate for high-risk patients who fail conventional therapy remains poor. HSCT is being offered in an attempt to improve outcome and disease-free survival in these diseases. Clinical trials are currently investigating the role of autologous stem cell transplantation (ASCT) in patients with recurrent medulloblastoma, primary brain tumors, pontine brain tumors, neuroblastoma after induction without progressive disease, Ewing's sarcoma in first or second remission, rhabdomyosarcoma after induction without progression, and Wilms tumor with poor prognostic features or recurrent disease.[30] Radiation therapy as part of the conditioning regimen for ASCT plays a limited role in most of the above mentioned diseases, because many of the children may have already received radiation to their sites of initial disease presentation and the additional toxicity would not be justified.

Neuroblastoma

Children with neuroblastoma can be reliably assigned to risk groups (low-risk, intermediate-risk, and high-risk disease) by assessment of certain clinical, biologic, and genetic features. These prognostic features include age at diagnosis, international neuroblastoma staging system category (INSSC), certain biologic characteristics such as tumor histopathology, tumor cell DNA Index, and MYCN amplification status.[34] In addition, specific biologic markers, including ferritin, NSE, membrane proteins, and ganglioside, LDH, catecholamines, chromogranin A, and certain cytogenetic features, such as hyperdiploidy karyotype and chromosomal deletions, helped to provide important insights into tumor behavior and serve as predictors of response to therapy.[34,35]

Treatment of Low-Risk Neuroblastoma Disease

Low-risk disease patients are those with INSS stage 1 or 2 disease and infants with stage 4S disease with tumors that display hyperdiploidy, favorable histopathology, and single-copy MYCN. Most children in this group are under 1 year of age at presentation. Treatment for this group is limited to surgery, unless the child has symptomatic cord compression or respiratory compromise necessitating chemotherapy and, in very rare instances, low-dose radiation. Extensive neurosurgical procedures and spinal irradiation are best avoided in very young children because of the potential for long-term morbidity.[35] Children who present with INSS stage 3 disease and have MCYN amplification, and children with stage 4 disease with no amplification MCYN and favorable histopathology are considered to be at intermediate risk. Children in this group receive radiation therapy to sites of residual disease after chemotherapy with the intent of prolonging survival and controlling local tumor.[34]

Radiation plays a limited role in children with INSS stage 3 disease with favorable biology and in children less than 1 year of age with INSS stage 4 disease. Chemotherapy (cyclophosphamide, doxorubicin, carboplatin, and etoposide) followed by surgical resection of the primary tumor is the preferred mode of treatment.[33] Radiation therapy is employed for disease that persists or remains aggressive despite chemotherapy and as an adjunct after surgical resection.[34]

Treatment of Intermediate-Risk Neuroblastoma Disease

Children who present with INSS stage 3 disease and have MCYN amplification and children with stage 4 disease with no amplification MCYN and favorable histopathology are considered to be at intermediate risk. Radiation plays a limited role in children with intermediate risk. Chemotherapy (cyclophosphamide, doxorubicin, carboplatin, and etoposide) followed by surgical resection of the primary tumor is the preferred mode of treatment and has an overall clinical response rate of 60% to 90%. Radiation therapy is employed for disease that persists or remains aggressive despite chemotherapy and as an adjunct after surgical resection.[34]

Treatment of High-Risk Neuroblastoma Disease

Almost half of children with neuroblastoma present with advanced disease: INSS stage 4 in children more than 1 year of age; stage 3 disease with MYCN amplification; stage 3 disease in children more than 1 year of age with unfavorable histopathology; INSS stage 2 patients with amplified MYCN and unfavorable histopathology, and INSS stage 4S patients with MYCN amplification.[35] The 5-year survival in this group of children is less than 30%.[34]

Efforts to improve outcome for high-risk children have included aggressive induction chemotherapy, myeloablative consolidation therapy with stem-cell rescue, and targeted therapy for minimal residual disease.[36,37] The Children's Cancer Group (CCG 3891 Trial) reported a 3-year disease-free survival of 43% in newly diagnosed high-risk patients treated with myeloablative chemotherapy and TBI with purged bone marrow followed by oral cis-retinoic acid.[4] In addition, those patients who had gross residual disease after induction chemotherapy and surgery received external-beam radiation therapy.[37] Disease recurrence at the site of primary disease continues to be a problem after bone marrow transplantation for neuroblastoma. Newer clinical trials are directed towards intensification of treatment, using peripheral blood stem cells (PBSCs) to shorten time to engraftment and using non–cross-resistant agents and CD34-selected PBSCs for rescue. Double autologous stem cell transplants are spaced 4 to 6 weeks apart using both chemotherapy and TBI.[36] In high-risk patients, radiation therapy is given to sites of residual disease after high-dose chemotherapy to improve local control, and to sites of surgical resection to prevent disease recurrence, because relapses usually occur at original sites of presentation. TBI is employed in many treatment protocols that use autologous stem cell transplantation.

NURSING IMPLICATIONS FOR THE ACUTE SIDE EFFECTS OF TOTAL BODY IRRADIATION

Please see Section VI of this text, Special Supportive Nursing Care, for detailed radiation-induced symptom management. Table 26-4 shows TBI dose-limiting toxicities by organ site. Side effects from HSCT with TBI and chemotherapy conditioning have been well documented. Yet the exact contributing effect from TBI versus chemotherapy conditionings is difficult to determine. Specific toxicities have been seen with certain combinations of TBI and chemotherapy conditioning regimens. For example, IP and hemorrhagic cystitis have been documented with TBI and cyclophosphamide regimens, whereas a high risk of renal toxicity exists with the use of TBI and cytarabine.

Table 26-4 Organ Site TBI Toxicities

Gray total dose	Organ site	Toxicity
20-30	Liver	Veno-occlusive disease
20	Renal	Hemolytic uremic syndrome
15	Gastrointestinal	Enteritis
10 Single 15 Fractionated	Pulmonary	Interstitial pneumonitis
3-4	Hematopoietic	Hematopoietic syndrome
30	Central nervous system	Maximum dose tolerated
20	Mediastinum	Maximum dose tolerated

Data from Gutierrez-Delgado F, Holmberg L, Hooper H et al: Autologous stem cell transplantation for Hodgkin's disease; busulfan, melphalan, and thiotepa compared to radiation based regimen, *Bone Marrow Transplant* 32(3):279–285. 2003
TBI, Total body irradiation.

Both cyclophosphamide and cytarabine can cause IP. Therefore it is difficult to sort out their contributing factor to IP when they are used in conjunction with TBI.

Time definitions found in the literature for acute versus late effects of HSCTs and its conditioning regimens differ. For discussion purposes within the context of this chapter, acute effects are those that usually occur within the first 6 months after a patient's transplant. Whereas, late side effects are those that are usually seen 6 months or longer after transplant care. The most prominent acute effects after HSCT with TBI/chemotherapy conditioning include nausea and vomiting, parotitis, mucositis, enteritis, bone marrow suppression, VOD, IP, and acute GVHD. Other untoward effects can include fever, erythema/hyperpigmentation, alopecia, xerostomia, fatigue, ocular and renal toxicities, headaches, and other CNS symptoms. Recently tumor lysis syndrome was reported in a patient with refractory T-cell ALL who had received only 2 fractions (TD 4 Gy) of his TBI conditioning.[38] See Table 26-5 for a complete listing of HSCT acute side effects, incidence, onset, and duration. Please note that the table incorporates reports of side effects both from TBI and chemotherapy conditionings because both are usually used together as preparatory regimens for HSCT.

As can be seen from Table 26-5, only some of the HSCTs conditioning–related side effects occur during patients' TBI treatment days. Radiation nurses need to frequently assess TBI patients and offer symptomatic care as needs arise. The most common symptoms that arise during TBI treatment days are fever, nausea and vomiting, fatigue, parotitis, skin reactions, xerostomia, mucositis, and

Table 26-5 TBI/Chemotherapy Conditioning Side Effects/Presentation Ranges[2,4,7,14,17,19,22,24]

Side effect	Incidence	Onset from first TBI treatment	Duration
Fever	—	Hours	1 day
Nausea and vomiting	100%	Hours	3–4 days
Fatigue	100%	1–4 days	Variable, may last for months
Parotitis	50%	12 hours–1 day	1–3 days
Skin reactions	—	Hours–10 days	3–21 days
Xerostomia	100%	2–10 days	Variable
Mucositis	90%–100%	3–10 days	21–8 days
Enteritis [diarrhea]	33%–50%	3–14 days	3–5 days
Veno-occlusive disease	10%–60%	6–30 days	Variable
Reversible alopecia	100%	7–14 days	90–180 days
Central nervous system			
Neurologic sequelae	60%–70%	7 days	Variable
Leukoencephalopathy	50%	Variable	Variable
Decreased lacrimation	—	10 days	—
Ocular dryness			
Immune/bone marrow suppression			
Neutropenia	100%	7–10 days	14–28 days
Thrombocytopenia	100%	14–21 days	Variable
Anemia	100%	60–90 days	Variable
Acute graft-versus-host disease			
HLA identical match	30%–50%	7–90 days	Variable
Reduced intensity conditioning	39%	7–90 days	Variable
HLA unrelated mismatch	75%	7–90 days	Variable
Interstitial pneumonitis—idiopathic	0%–16% [auto's] 0%–32% [allo's]	30–more than 100 days	Variable
Renal	14%	30 days	Variable

TBI, Total body irradiation.

enteritis. Many of the major HSCTs conditioning–related side effects occur days to months after patients have completed their TBI treatments. It is important that radiation oncology nurses be knowledgeable about both acute and later side effects in order to provide TBI/HSCT patient education and answer patients' treatment-related questions.

Nausea and Vomiting

Nausea and vomiting can be extremely hard to manage with TBI patients even after only one TBI treatment. The severity of nausea and vomiting has been reported to be less with fractionated TBI doses and lower dose rates.[2,4] Studies have shown ondansetron (Zofran) versus placebo is effective in minimizing TBI-related nausea and vomiting when administered 1.5 hours before treatment.[4,11,39] Standard anti-emetics in addition to ondansetron are also used, namely Compazine, Ativan, and Decadron. The University of Colorado Hospital has added a scopolamine patch to TBI patients' anti-emetic regimens and has found its use to be especially helpful in reducing nausea in TBI patients being treated in the upright position. A recent study of 167 patients found that nausea and vomiting could be well managed in an outpatient HSCTs program with fractionated TBI conditioning. All patients were started on IV fluids before TBI and continued during TBI. Anti-emetics using ondansetron 8 milligrams (mg) every 12 hours, Decadron 8 mg twice daily, and Compazine as needed were started before TBI treatments and repeated before afternoon TBI treatments.[23]

Fatigue

All HSCTs patients develop fatigue, which is attributed to the conditioning regimens. Routine light exercise has been found to help minimize fatigue. Physical therapy programs and energy conservation techniques have been included in HSCT programs to help minimize this symptom.[40]

Parotitis

This is a common and quite painful side effect unique to TBI-treated patients. It manifests as post-auricular pain and swelling that affects the jaw.[2] It has been reported to occur less often with the use of the hyperfractionated TBI method.[4] Treatment includes the use of steroids and pain medications. Luckily this painful side effect usually resolves spontaneously after a few days.[1,2]

Skin Reactions

Generalized erythema and tanning skin pigmentation changes do occur after TBI treatments.[4] Standard skin moisturizers used to treat radiodermatitis are employed to minimize this condition. (See Chapter 30 for management of radiodermatitis.)

Xerostomia

TBI is considered to be the most likely causative agent in the occurrence of HSCTs-related xerostomia.[4] As with head and neck cancer patients, prophylactic dental care and fluoride treatments are needed for all TBI patients before treatment.[4] Pilocarpine to manage the oral dryness is not reported in recent TBI literature. This might be due to the transient nature of xerostomia in the TBI setting. It is important that nurses review with patients at their initial radiation therapy consultation the need for prophylactic dental care and fluoride treatments, as well as good oral hygiene care before, during, and after treatment. Frequent mouth rinses with water or saline are helpful for managing the discomfort caused by xerostomia.

Mucositis

Mucositis is seen in both autologous and allogeneic HSCT patients receiving TBI.[10] Ninety to 100% of HSCT patients develop grade III to IV mucositis. TBI contribution as a causal factor is hard to define because all myeloablative conditionings cause varying degrees of mucositis.[20,21] The hyperfractionated method of TBI delivery has been purported to help reduce the severity of HSCT-related mucositis. Risk factors for the development of severe mucositis include prolonged neutropenia, the development of GVHD, and unrelated donor HSCTs.[21] Bearman criteria is a specific mucositis grading scale developed for HSCT patients. It provides a scale from 1 to 3 for all major organs including oral mucositis. A newer scoring system found in the TBI literature is the oral mucosal assessment score that was validated in a large study.[21]

Results in the literature regarding the effectiveness of using acyclovir to reduce the severity of mucositis in TBI patients is mixed.[4,11] To date, there is no known effective mucositis prophylaxis,[11] nor is there a best-known treatment. Symptomatic resolution has been associated with patients' rising ANC.[2]

One study of 97 patients receiving 12 Gy TBI conditioning examined the use of Caphosol mouth rinse (calcium and phosphorous mixture) in managing HSCT TBI/chemotherapy mucositis. In this study, patients were randomized to either receiving fluoride gel treatments before TBI and HSCT followed by the use of Caphosol mouth rinses 4 times a day or the control arm in which patients had no fluoride treatments and used a placebo mouthwash 4 times a day. The authors reported a statistically significant decrease in the severity of mucositis and the number of days of patient pain complaints, reduction in intensity of pain scores, a decrease in the number of milligrams of morphine used by patients, and a reduction in the number of days that patients used morphine. The authors concluded that Caphosol administration had a significant effect in ameliorating oral mucositis associated with TBI and chemotherapy conditioning.[41] It should be noted that patients in the placebo arm were not provided fluoride treatments. Therefore the benefits found in this study may have been due to the use of fluoride rather than Caphosol. More studies on the effectiveness of Caphosol are needed. Many transplant centers use chlorhexidine mouthwash as a standard of care for HSCT treatment induced mucositis. Yet, a study on the use of chlorhexidine study that included 100 patients found no advantage to the use of this mouthwash versus the use of a placebo mouthwash.[21]

Several drugs are currently being tested in the search for mucosal protection. These studies include the use of epithelial growth factors, amifostine, keratinocyte growth factor, transforming growth factor beta, and interleukin-11.[5,10,20] These agents show promise and further trials are needed. Other prophylaxis trials include investigations of oral glutamine, decrease in TBI total dose and decreased methotrexate dosages. Methotrexate, a GVHD prophylaxis agent has been thought to contribute to the occurrence and severity of mucositis seen in HSCT patients.

Current clinical guidelines point to the need of systematic oral care protocols, patient education, and the use of pain medications.[14] Treatment may at times include parenteral nutrition. Nursing care includes patient teaching at the time of initial consultation about the need for pretreatment oral and dental evaluation and frequent oral hygiene before, during, and after treatment. Some treatment centers prescribe pretreatment fluoride teeth treatments for all their HSCT patients. Pain management is an essential part of patients' nursing care, which necessitates frequent evaluation of patients' pain and around-the-clock pain control medication.

Enteritis (Unrelated to GVHD)

It is well documented that gastrointestinal integrity is compromised by myeloablative conditioning, which can lead to the entry of bacteria and endotoxins into patient's circulation. Enteritis can be potentially life threatening if infection develops. Diarrhea is the clinical manifestation of enteritis. A known risk factor for the development of enteritis is prolonged neutropenia, which can occur after the HSCT conditioning regimens.

Sucralfate has been used with some effectiveness in reducing the incidence of TBI-related diarrhea. A 1999 placebo-controlled, randomized study of 105 HSCT patients having TBI conditioning found significant decrease in diarrhea seen with both TBI and the non-TBI patients on the sucralfate arm of the study.[42] Patients took either a placebo or sucralfate 2 grams every 3 hours during the day and once at night if awakening with a maximum of 7 doses per 24 hours starting 1 day before any conditioning. Patients continued to take the sucralfate/placebo until their ANCs were equal or greater than 500 mm ($.5 \times 10^6$) or the end of symptomatic oral mucositis. More studies examining the use of sucralfate in this patient population are needed. The same agents being studied to control oral mucositis are also under investigation for their potential benefit in controlling HSCT TBI/chemotherapy conditioning–related diarrhea.

Nursing care of patients with enteritis includes close monitoring of patients' vital signs, intake and output, weights, and peri-rectal skin integrity. Fluid replacement is given as needed. All fevers are worked up for source of infection including blood and stool cultures. Sitz baths are used for both cleaning and comfort purposes as needed. Antidiarrheals including the octreotide acetate are administered for severe diarrhea.[1] (See Chapter 34 for more symptom management information.)

Veno-Occlusive Disease

VOD is a condition in which endothelial damage has caused hepatic luminal narrowing or occlusion in the hepatic venules or small sublobular veins resulting in liver damage.[2,43,44] HSCT's VOD morbidity is 21% to 50%,[44,45] and it is fatal in 33% to

50% of patients affected.[1,44] It is a common toxicity associated with myeloablative HSCT conditionings, and its incidence also has been reported as being less with nonmyeloablative immunosuppressive protocols.[44] Animal studies suggest that the toxic metabolites of cyclophosphamide play a major role leading to the development of VOD. The incidence of VOD is significantly increased with the use of busulfan and cyclophosphamide conditioning. TBI has been reported to be an independent factor linked to the development of VOD.[2] Some clinical trials have reported reduction in the incidence of VOD with the use of fractionated versus single-dose TBI.[2]

Risk factors for the development of VOD include age greater than 15 and a history of hepatitis, high-dose chemotherapy before conditioning treatment, mismatched donors, an elevated transaminase level before conditioning, and the concurrent use of acyclovir and amphotericin treatments.[18,44,45] High transforming growth factor-beta (TGF-β levels before or after chemotherapy conditioning regimens have been shown to be a predictor for patients at risk for developing VOD.[46] The use of progestin to minimize menstrual bleeding has been theorized as a VOD risk factor. A multivariate analysis showed that norethindrone levels, a progestin, to be an independent predictor of VOD.[44]

Other investigators have found that the diffusing capacity of carbon monoxide corrected for hemoglobin (DLCO) levels less than 70% was predictive of an increased VOD risk and that a decreased DLCO level was reflective of prior systemic endothelial damage.[44]

Some investigators found that an increased need for platelet transfusions in any one week was predictive for the development of VOD. Typically VOD presents with symptoms of fluid retention and hepatomegaly followed by increasing jaundice. Bilirubin levels then rise and a slight rise is seen in alkaline phosphatase levels. The severity of VOD is also strongly associated with the amount of pathologic changes seen in zone 3 of the liver.[44] This zone is located around central veins, where oxygenation is poor.[47] Coagulation abnormalities occur as well as an increase in liver function tests.[2] Right upper quadrant pain and liver tenderness develop, as does weight gain caused by fluid retention and ascites. A rapid increase in bilirubin levels in conjunction with an increase in patients' weight has been correlated with increased disease severity. Ascites develops in 20% of patients with mild VOD and in 48% of patients with severe VOD. Encephalopathy occurs in approximately half of patients affected.[2,44]

Some centers have investigated the use of low molecular weight heparin 100 units per kilogram (kilo) per day with prostaglandin E IV infusions of .075 mg to 0.5 mg/kilo per hour.[2] The use of prophylactic heparin has been studied and found to help reduce only the incidence of moderate VOD but not severe VOD. These studies, however, only involved patients who were at a low risk for developing VOD. Therefore, the benefits of prophylactic heparin remain questionable.[44]

In studies using antithrombin III (ATIII) compared to historical controls not treated with ATIII showed a decrease in VOD symptoms including a decreased mortality rate, platelet consumption, painful hepatomegaly, and fluid retention. The use of pentoxifylline has been found to be ineffective in treating VOD. However, one small study reported 61% response rate with the use of methylprednisolone 500 mg/meters squared (m^2) every 6 hours for 6 doses.[44]

Some authors have reported using liver shielding during TBI in an attempt to prevent VOD yet there are very few reports on this practice in the literature.[2]

Ursodiol, a bile steroid, as been shown to decrease VOD incidence but has not had an effect on survival rates. Just how it works is unclear. It may work by preventing endothelial cell and hepatocyte injury. Future studies are needed in the protection of the liver endothelium and subsequently in the reduction of liver fibrosis.

One theory proposes that hepatocyte integrity might be protected by supporting glutathione levels, thereby preventing or reversing VOD.[44] Some studies have reported some success in the use of n-acetylcysteine, a precursor of glutathione synthesis, to reverse VOD in patients, but more studies are needed. Other studies have investigated the use of glutamine to replenish intracellular glutathione, but again, more studies are needed because the results of these studies have not been conclusive.[44] VOD is the most common non-relapse life-threatening complication of HSCTs, and there is no known 100% prevention.[45]

Surveillance nursing care includes twice daily patient weights, daily measurement of patients' abdominal girth, close monitoring of fluid intake and output, and daily monitoring of blood counts and blood chemistries. Nursing care includes close monitoring of blood chemistry levels in relation to the patient's weight and fluid balance. VOD treatment includes fluid management with diuretics and fluid restrictions.[1,45] Blood transfusions are administered to keep patients' hematocrit levels equal or greater than 35% with the goal of maintaining intravascular volumes and renal perfusion.[45]

Alopecia, Central Nervous System, and Acute Ocular Toxicities

Reversible alopecia occurs in most all HSCT patients.[14] Neurologic compromise has often occurred with HSCT patients and can consist of short-term memory loss, decreased attention spans, and impaired verbal skills.[45] Such compromises have been linked to the conditioning treatments and CNS infections.[45] Acute leukoencephalopathy has been reported in relationship to chemotherapy conditioning. Acute leukoencephalopathy risk factors include prior high-dose chemotherapy; intrathecal methotrexate, and prior cranial irradiation.[1,45] Acute global headaches can affect one-third of all patients. Narcotic pain medication may be needed for some patients to gain headache relief.[1] Decreased lacrimation and ocular dryness related to TBI has been seen in some patients starting about 10 days after completion of TBI.[14] Treatment consists of the administration of moisturizing eye drops such as methylcellulose.

Immunosuppression

Immunosuppression in allogeneic HSCTs is necessary to prevent rejection of donor cells and thereby ensure engraftment. Immunosuppression is accomplished by the singular use or the combination of TBI and chemotherapy conditionings and the use of other immunosuppressive agents such as methotrexate, cyclosporine, and tacrolimus. T-cell antibodies such as thymocyte globulin or monoclonal antibodies, namely, alemtuzumab also has been used to gain immunosuppression.[7,45] Immunosuppression comes hand in hand with bone marrow suppression, resulting in neutropenia, thrombocytopenia, and anemia. Thrombocytes are extremely sensitive to ionizing radiation, and thrombocytopenia is usually seen after TBI TD exceeds 1 Gy to 1.5 Gy.[2]

Daily and often twice daily CBC and platelet level monitoring is needed in caring for HSCT patients. Supportive treatment for neutropenia includes precautions to minimize the high risk of infection associated with neutropenia. These precautions include HEPA-filtered controlled environment and reverse isolation precautions for hospitalized patients.[1] Outpatients should be instructed to monitor their temperatures at least twice daily, report any fevers greater than 100.5° F. Patients should be taught to avoid indoor crowds and friends or family members who have cold or flu symptoms. Colony-stimulating factors are given to patients' whose neutropenia persists after engraftment is achieved. Some non-Hodgkin HSCT protocols routinely start patients on colony-stimulating factors on day 1 of patients' transplants.[2,9,10]

Cultures for bacteria, fungus, and viral illness are done upon fever presentation. Antibiotics/antifungal/antiviral agents are given based on the fever's causative factor. Nursing surveillance consists of frequent vital signs and daily oral and total skin integrity assessment. Early detection and treatment of oral and skin lesions is needed to minimize the patients' risks for developing infections. Thrombocytopenia risk requires frequent patient skin evaluations for the occurrence of petechiae associated with low platelet counts or compromised platelet function. Supportive blood and platelet transfusion are frequently needed until hemoglobin levels and platelet function and levels return to normal. This may not take place for months after engraftment.

Acute Graft-Versus-Host Disease

GVHD is solely an allogeneic HSCT complication.[48] Specific conditions must exist for GVHD to occur. First the donor cells must contain competent T-lymphocytes. Secondly, a histoincompatibility must exist between the patient's cells and the donor cells. Lastly, the patient must have the inability to reject the donor lymphocytes.[45]

This complication is due to donor cells interpreting patient's cells as foreign to themselves and then attempting to reject the patient's cells.[2,45] This is the opposite process seen in solid organ transplants where the patients' cells attempt to reject the donor cells. GVHD is one HSCT side effect with acute (70–90 days) and chronic (> 100 days) presentation timeframes that are consistently reported in the literature.[2] GVHD is thought to be mediated by inflammatory cytokines that are simulated by endotoxins.[21] Animal studies have found that its development is related to conditioning treatments. These studies have found intestinal damage and increased levels of endotoxins in animals are related to dose escalations of conditioning treatments.[20] TBI's contribution to this complication is unclear. It may contribute to GVHD due to its untoward effect on the endothelial mucosa.

Although the occurrence of GVHD is associated with lower relapse rates and better failure-free survival, it remains a major complication even with reduced-intensity conditioning protocols in which it has a 20% mortality rate.[7,20,22] GVHD risk factors include greater than 8 years of age, mismatched donor transplants, and negative cytomegalovirus (CMV) titers in either patient or donor.[45]

GVHD symptoms usually begin with a maculopapular rash just about the time that white cell engraftment is seen. It occurs on the nape of the neck, ears, shoulders, palms, and soles but may progress to the entire body and blisters may develop. The liver is almost always affected by GVHD at the time the skin rash appears. Blood test abnormalities include increased bilirubin, alkaline phosphatase, and transaminase levels. Jaundice closely follows. GVHD gastrointestinal tract symptoms include nausea/vomiting, anorexia, abdominal cramping, and diarrhea (greater than 2 liters/day). A severe ileus can develop.[45] Allogeneic HSCT patients' deaths during the first 100 days of transplant are most commonly caused by the combination of GVHD and infection leading to multi-organ failure.[4]

Immunosuppressive agents have been used to reduce GVHD incidence and its severity. The most common prophylaxis agents include methotrexate, cyclosporine, tacrolimus, and T-cell antibodies such as thymocyte globulin or monoclonal antibodies, namely, alemtuzumab.[7,45] Some studies in Britain are showing lower GVHD incidence with the use of alemtuzumab but with an associated high reactivation of CMV, although with a low CMV infection rate. Studies using T-lymphocyte donor depletions have shown a decrease in GVHD incidence, but this decrease has been associated with an increase in graft failure and relapse rates.[7,19] Donor lymphocyte infusions after transplant have been found to have little value in the treatment of severe GVHD cases or in GVHD in patients with mismatched HSCTs. However, they have been found to help moderate GVHD cases.[30] Despite the use of a wide variety of GVHD prophylactic agents, there is no known totally effective prophylaxis.

Animal studies have shown that GVHD decreases when intestinal integrity is protected by the use of keratinocyte growth factor before lethal chemotherapy is administered. Protection appears to result from the trophic effects on the intestinal epithelium and the improved intestinal crypt stem cell survival. Other animal studies have found a decrease in GVHD incidence with prophylactic use of interleukin-11, which has been found to decrease serum endotoxin levels.[20] Ongoing investigations are studying means to reduce this prominent allogeneic HSCT complication.

Nursing care entails early detection of symptoms by monitoring daily blood work, and a daily total body assessment of patients and symptomatic nursing care. Corticosteroids, intestinal rest, parental nutrition, fluid and electrolyte management, skin care, pain medications, anti-emetics, and antidiarrheals, including the use of octreotide acetate, are some of the major care needs of these patients.[1]

Pulmonary and Interstitial Pneumonitis Complications

Restrictive lung disease is often observed 3 to 6 weeks after allogeneic stem cell transplantation in patients conditioned with one or both TBI and chemotherapy conditioning regimens.[49] IP typically occurs within 90 days of transplantation and accounts for more than 40% of transplant-related mortality in children.[50] IP is a complication of both autologous 0% to 16% and allogeneic 32% to 60% HSCTs.[2,10,14]

Pathologic changes that occur with IP include alveolar capillary injury leading to leakage of plasma into the pulmonary interstitium. Chest x-ray findings show interstitial infiltrates.[18,45] Types of IP include, idiopathic, bacterial, viral (CMV), fungal (Aspergillus Candida, Cryptococcus), and opportunistic (*Pneumocystis jiroveci,* which has been historically identified as *Pneumocystis carinii*).[2]

CMV-related IP has an incidence of 42% compared with 26% TBI (fractionated, low dose rate) related idiopathic IP.[2] TBI, especially high-dose TBI, is considered the causative agent in idiopathic IP and is one of the most significant of the TBI dose-limiting toxicities.[1,2,18,45] The lung appears to have a threshold tolerance to radiation dose below which none or very low incidence of IP has been found to occur. The theory to explain this phenomenon is that lung cells have the capacity to repair themselves from sub-lethal injury. Radiation treatment–related IP occurs at a TBI dose of approximately 7.5 Gy to 8 Gy.[2]

Risk factors for the development of IP include previous thoracic radiation treatment, history of pulmonary disease, decreased pulmonary functions tests, history of smoking, concurrent infections, and the presence of GVHD.[4,18]

Prophylaxis treatment for TBI-related IP has included lung shielding as described earlier in this chapter.[10] Investigators are studying variations in TBI total dose, dose rates, and fractionation to reduce its incidence.[18] Sulfamethoxazole-trimethoprim is given to HSCT patients as a prophylaxis for *Pneumocystis jiroveci.*[2] Acyclovir is used as a prophylactic agent for CMV-positive patients. Some authors report the prophylactic use of systemic antibiotics starting when patient's ANC is less than 500 mm (0.5 × 10^9) and discontinuing them at the time patient has engraftment, namely an ANC of 500 mm (0.5 × 10^9) for 3 days.[9]

Pulmonary fibrosis may be manifested by cough, reduced exercise tolerance, orthopnea, cyanosis, rales, or cor pulmonale. Dyspnea with a rapid onset is the main presenting symptom seen with IP. Other IP symptoms include dry cough, hypoxia, and fever.[18,45] Treatment is based on causative factors, antibiotics for bacterial infections, antifungal (amphotericin) for fungal infections, sulfamethoxazole-trimethoprim for *Pneumocystis jiroveci,* and supportive care for CMV- or TBI-related IP. There is no known specific treatment other than supportive care for CMV- or TBI-related IP.[51]

Surveillance monitoring includes blood and sputum cultures upon symptom presentation. Supportive care can include the use of steroids, anti-tussive agents, antipyretics, fluid management, and oxygen. Nursing care includes close monitoring of temperatures for presentation of fevers and frequent assessment of patient's respiratory status including monitoring oxygen saturations and the promotion of rest and undisturbed sleep for patients.

Renal Toxicity

Renal toxicity can be an acute side effect of HSCT conditioning that may become a chronic condition. Fractionated radiation doses of 10 Gy to 20 Gy may cause decrease in glomerular filtration rate that results in significant reduction in renal plasma flow for up to 12 months after treatment despite clinically normal blood urea levels.[2] Radiation-related renal damage can be progressive as a result of the gradual degeneration of renal arterioles or capillaries.[14] TBI usage and the presence of GVHD has been associated with renal dysfunction.

Prevention measures may include renal shielding for TBI patients with a history of elevated BUN and creatinine levels or patients receiving combined cytarabine/cyclophosphamide and TBI conditioning.[2]

Renal toxicity symptoms include anemia, increased BUN, creatinine, and LOH levels, hypertension, decreased urine output, and edema.[4] Nursing care entails close monitoring of patients' renal function tests and fluid intake and output and changes in patients' fluid management as needed.

Nursing Implications for the Late Effects of Total Body Irradiation and Subsequent Hematopoietic Stem Cell Transplant

HSCT is a life-saving measure for many patients. However, with survivorship comes the risk of late complications, which can significantly impair the quality of life. The late effects of HSCT are diverse and may involve any body system or tissue. Many factors contribute to late morbidity: prolonged immunosuppression; infections; chronic GVHD; the use of irradiation in post-transplant conditioning regimens; prior treatment (surgery, radiation, chemotherapy); underlying disease status at the time of transplant; organ tolerance; and the age of the patient.[52] The type of transplant being performed influences the intensity of the conditioning chemoradiation regimens. This may involve giving additional radiation just before autologous stem cell transplantation, which is done frequently for neuroblastoma and relapsed leukemia. In the case of allogeneic HSCT, the incidence of chronic GVHD is being sustained by use of matched, unrelated donors, stem cell transplantation in older patients, and the increased use of donor lymphocyte infusions to treat relapsed disease or achieve full donor chimerism after nonmyeloablative transplantation.[49]

The late effects of autologous and allogeneic HSCT in children are primarily the result of conditioning chemotherapy and radiation therapy. The additive effect of combining these two modalities can contribute to lower organ/tissue tolerance. In addition, GVHD and the consequences of underlying disease and its prior treatment can further compound toxicities. There is an increasing incidence of second malignancies after HSCT, which may occur many years after transplantation. This emphasizes the need for long-term follow-up, patient/family education, and early detection and intervention. Table 26-6 summarizes late effects for children. Table 26-7 provides recommendations for long-term follow-up of adult transplant patients.

Pulmonary Toxicity

Pulmonary toxicity is a common complication of pre-transplantation regimens, which occurs by way of injury of the type II pneumocytes, endotracheal cells, fibroblasts, and macrophages. In transplanted patients, pulmonary toxicity may manifest as interstitial pneumonitis, idiopathic pneumonia syndrome, bronchiolitis obliterans, pulmonary hemorrhage, and pulmonary edema. Children who have received prior lung irradiation have been shown to have a decrease in lung capacity and failure of alveolar development. Several chemotherapy agents have been linked with pulmonary toxicity. These include nitrosoureas, cyclophosphamide, melphalan, busulfan, chlorambucil, and methotrexate.[50] Many of these agents are used as part of the preparative regimens for HSCT. Carmustine is used in patients receiving stem cell transplantation for brain tumors, busulfan and cyclophosphamide for leukemias, and melphalan for lymphomas. Prior treatment of underlying disease can also compound the risk of pulmonary complications in Hodgkin's disease (Adriamycin, bleomycin, vinblastine, and dacarbazine [ABVD] chemotherapy plus lung irradiation) and Wilms tumor (Adriamycin, vincristine, doxorubicin, and cyclophosphamide [Adria-VAC] chemotherapy plus lung irradiation). Chronic pulmonary toxicity can be either constrictive or obstructive in nature. Significant late toxicity involving airway and lung parenchyma affects 15% to 40% of patients after stem cell transplantation. The predisposing factors contributing to this include sensitivity to cytotoxic agents, irradiation, infection, and immune-mediated sensitivity associated with GVHD.[49]

Chronic obstructive lung disease can be detected in 20% of long-term survivors. It has been associated with chronic GVHD, TBI, hypo-gammaglobulinemia, methotrexate, and infection.[49] Late-onset pulmonary symptoms include bronchiolitis obliterans (BO), bronchiolitis obliterans with organizing pneumonia (BOOP), and diffuse alveolar pneumonia.[52] Patients with BOOP typically present with flu-like illness, cough, and dyspnea. This complication usually is managed by administration of immune globulin, antibiotics, and corticosteroids, if needed. BO usually presents in 2%-14% of allogeneic HSCT patients, with expiratory wheezing, cough and dyspnea, and it has a mortality rate of 50%-75% when it occurs with GVHD.[49,50]

The frequency and severity of pulmonary impairment after HSCT can vary with time. Several longitudinal studies have reported restrictive defects, such as reduced lung volume and/or diffusion capacity, in the first few months after transplantation, with only partial improvement by 1 year in 40% to 100% of long-term survivors.[52]

Baseline and serial post-transplant pulmonary function tests are recommended. Prophylaxis against *Pneumocystis jiroveci* with trimethoprim/sulfamethoxazole, atovaquone, or dapsone usually is administered for the first year after HSCT or during immunosuppressive therapy. Serial monitoring for CMV antigen and serial measurements of immunoglobulin G (IgG) and IgG subclasses should be conducted, and prophylaxis with immunoglobulin should be given, if needed. Immunization with diphtheria, tetanus, Haemophilus influenza type B, hepatitis A and B, pneumococcal, influenza, meningococcal, and inactivated poliovirus vaccines should begin at 12 months after transplantation. The Centers for Disease Control and Prevention (CDC) provide a comprehensive source of information on prophylaxis and immunizations for HSCT patients.[53]

Cardiac Toxicity

Children who receive hematopoietic stem cell transplantation are vulnerable to cardiac toxicity, because they often receive anthracyclines as a part of their initial cancer therapy or will receive conditioning regimens that require high-dose cyclophosphamide. Cardiac complications after HSCT include arrhythmias, pericarditis, cardiomyopathy, pericardial effusions, and valvular disease. The doses of anthracycline associated with cardiomyopathy are those greater than 300 mg/m^2 or 200 mg/m^2 with radiation therapy to the mediastinum of 25 Gy. Signs and symptoms of cardiac complications include cough, dyspnea on exertion, hypertension, rales, cardiomegaly, hepatomegaly, syncope, palpitations, and arrhythmias.[54]

Baseline screening before transplantation should include an electrocardiogram, echocardiography,

(Text continued on p. 476)

Table 26-6 Late Effects of Bone Marrow Transplantation in Children

Organ/system/Toxicity primary causative treatment(s)*	Other potential risk factors	Clinical features and consequences	Frequency†	Impact of allogeneic BMT‡	Comments
NEUROLOGICAL TOXICITY					
Before or during BMT: • Chemotherapy (CT)—methotrexate (systemic or intrathecal) • Cranial radiation therapy (RT)§	• Prolonged immunosuppression increases risk of CNS infection, especially with opportunistic organisms	• Leukoencephalopathy—variable symptoms/signs • Vascular episodes—cerebrovascular accidents, vasculitis, 'migraine-like' episodes • Infections—meningitis or focal disease; wide variety of causative organisms • CNS tumors—gliomas, lymphomas, meningiomas (attributed to RT); see 'Secondary malignancy'	• Leucoencephalopathy—7% in patients receiving both CNS-directed treatment pre-BMT (RT and/or intrathecal CT) *and* intrathecal methotrexate post-BMT[72] • CNS infections—7% (adults)[73] • CNS tumors—risk increases with time post-BMT, overall incidence 46 times expected[66]	• Link suggested[70, 71] between cGvHD and: • Vasculitic syndromes • Polymyositis • Myasthenia gravis • Peripheral neuropathy	• Note probable additive effect of multiple episodes of CNS-directed treatment, including CT plus RT, or two episodes of RT
NEUROPSYCHOLOGICAL TOXICITY					
Before or during BMT: • Chemotherapy—methotrexate (systemic or intrathecal), busulphan • Cranial RT§	• Higher cumulative RT doses, especially prior cranial RT followed by TBI • Young age at treatment (especially less than 3 years) • Female gender • Longer duration of follow-up	• Wide range and severity of neuropyschological functional impairment—memory, attention, intelligence, visual-spatial, verbal skills, fine motor skills, educational achievement • Cognitive function may deteriorate gradually over 10 years or more • Impaired psychosocial function	Patients receiving 2 RT treatments (i.e., cranial RT + TBI, or 2 episodes of cranial RT): • Impaired memory—46%[74] • Impaired verbal comprehension—50%[74] • Need for formalized extra educational support—36%[74] Patients receiving ≤ 1 RT treatment: • No measurable cognitive deficit in CT alone or CT + TBI groups, but sporadic cases of substantial toxicity[75]	cGvHD may have further profound effects on psychosocial adaptation post-allogeneic BMT	Note additive effects of multiple treatment episodes (as for neurological toxicity), aggravated by shorter intervals between episodes

(continued)

Table 26-6 Late Effects of Bone Marrow Transplantation in Children—cont'd

Organ/system/toxicity primary causative treatment(s)*	Other potential risk factors	Clinical features and consequences	Frequency†	Impact of allogeneic BMT‡	Comments
			• Variable IQ changes from pre- to 1 year post-BMT—no change[75] 20% fell ≥ 10 points[76] 44% fell ≥ 2 SEs[77] • Fall ≥ 2 SEs in adaptive behavior scale—39%[78]		
DENTAL/ORAL TOXICITY Before or during BMT: • Chemotherapy • RT to field including jaws§	• Young age at treatment • Prior RT	Dental: • Root—hypoplasia • Teeth—microdontia, enamel hypoplasia, dental aplasia • Impaired craniofacial skeletal growth (primarily due to RT) Oral: • Xerostomia due to reduced saliva formation • Oral/salivary gland tumors—see 'Secondary malignancy'	• Root hypoplasia—94%[79] • Microdontia—75%[79] • Enamel hypoplasia—44%[79] • Dental aplasia—56%[79] • Impaired craniofacial skeletal growth—100%[82] • Xerostomia, reduced salivary flow rate—43%[80] NB All above figures relate to TBI, and are higher than after chemotherapy only[79,81,82] • Oral/salivary gland tumor—overall incidence 500–>2500 times expected[66]	1. Xerostomia linked with RT to field including salivary glands (usually TBI) and/or cGvHD[80, 81] 2. Secondary malignancy related to RT (usually TBI) and/or cGvHD[83]	Unclear (due to conflicting evidence) whether risk of caries is increased
VISUAL/OCULAR TOXICITY Before BMT: • Previous RT to field including eyes§ During BMT:	• High dose/dose rate and/or unfractionated TBI (cataracts) • Prolonged use of steroids (cataracts)	Anterior segment: • Posterior subcapsular cataract	• Cataract—5.5% (no RT),[84] up to 34% (fractionated TBI),[85] up to 100% (unfractionated TBI)[84]	1. Keratoconjunctivitis sicca associated with cGvHD, but can occur in unaffected patients[85]	Latent period before cataract formation (classically 3–4 years) may be longer

RT to field including eyes§ • Chemotherapy • Corticosteroids		• Keratoconjunctivitis sicca, with reduced tear secretion, leading to corneal/conjunctival ulceration/scarring Posterior segment: • Chorioretinitis (viral e.g., CMV, VZV; toxoplasmosis)	• Keratoconjunctivitis sicca—6%[85] • Chorioretinitis—rare (<1%) after 1 year post-BMT[86]	2. Uncertain If cGvHD, or its treatment with corticosteroids, is an independent risk factor for cataract development	after fractionated TBI, not yet clear whether this will increase ultimate incidence
AUDITORY TOXICITY Before or during BMT: • Platinum agents • Aminoglycosides • RT to field including ears§	• Younger age at treatment increases risk of impaired speech development	• Sensorineural hearing impairment • Impaired speech development	• Variable, but high in vulnerable patient groups, e.g., hearing loss at speech frequencies in young children treated with platinum agents or aminoglycosides before and during BMT—22%–82%[87, 88]		
CARDIOTOXICITY Before or during BMT: • Chemotherapy—principally anthracyclines, but also high-dose cyclophosphamide and other alkylating agents • RT to a field including heart§	• Pre-BMT iron overload in thalassemia • Sepsis	• ECG abnormalities including arrythmias • Myocardial toxicity ranging—from subclinical damage (e.g., echocardiographic) to clinical cardiac failure • Pericardial disease, including effusions • Valvular disease	• ECG abnormalities—16%[89] • Subclinical left ventricular impairment—25%[90] • Abnormal exercise testing—74%[89] • Cardiomyopathy—7%[92] • Cardiac failure—3%[78] • Incidence of very late toxicity not yet known	Pericardial effusions related to cGvHD in some patients[91]	Not yet proven that BMT causes additional cardiac impairment in children who have already received cardiotoxic treatment

(continued)

Table 26-6 Late Effects of Bone Marrow Transplantation in Children—cont'd

Organ/system/toxicity primary causative treatment(s)*	Other potential risk factors	Clinical features and consequences	Frequency†	Impact of allogeneic BMT‡	Comments
NEPHROTOXICITY Before or during BMT: • Chemotherapy—especially platinum agents, ifosfamide • RT to fields including kidneys§ Before, during or after BMT: • Nephrotoxic antiinfective agents	• Sequelae of acute renal failure during BMT • Hepatic veno-occlusive disease • Young age	• Glomerular hyperfiltration • Radiation nephritis—chronic renal (glomerular) impairment, hypertension, anemia, hematuria • + hemolysis (in acute form) • Proximal tubular impairment • Isolated hypertension	• Subclinical glomerular impairment—28%[93,94] • Subclinical tubular impairment—45%[95] • Subacute radiation nephritis—46%[96] • Hypertension—16%[94] • Chronic renal, failure—up to 28%[94,99] depending on criteria • End-stage renal failure—rare	1. cGvHD may present rarely with proteinuria, or even nephrotic syndrome[97,98] 2. Additive effect of nephrotoxic immunosuppressive agents, especially cyclosporin A and tacrolimus[94]	Acute presentation of renal toxicity (up to 1 year post-BMT), presumably due to radiation nephritis, may resemble hemolytic uremic syndrome (HUS)
ENDOCRINE TOXICITY Before and during BMT: • RT to field including affected gland§ • Chemotherapy (including busulphan and cyclophosphamide, BuCy)	• Unfractionated TBI	Pituitary: • Growth hormone—see Growth impairment • No conclusive evidence of TSH, ACTH, LH/FSH, prolactin deficiency post-BMT Thyroid: • Hypothyroidism (often compensated), may be transient • Hyperthyroidism reported after neck RT, not yet described after TBI • Thyroid tumors—see 'Secondary malignancy' Adrenal: • No conclusive evidence of cortisol deficiency post-BMT	• Hypothyroidism—compensated more common than overt; fractionated TBI—25%, mostly compensated, may be transient; unfractionated TBI—58%, overt in 15%,[191] clinical symptoms—1.1% (adults)[102] • Thyroid tumors (adenomas, carcinomas)—overall incidence 125 times expected[66] • Metabolic syndrome—39%; type 2 diabetes—17% (single report)[103] • Type 1 and 2 diabetes mellitus—8% (single report)[104]	Autoimmune disturbances, including thyroid disease but also diabetes, described particularly in patients with cGvHD[101]	1. Longer-term studies required, especially after fractionated TBI 2. Uncertain whether occurrence of metabolic syndrome post-BMT is related to GH deficiency

		Pancreas: • Metabolic syndrome—hyperinsulinemia, impaired glucose tolerance, hypertriglyceridemia, ± hypertension ± obesity • Type 1 diabetes mellitus • Type 2 diabetes mellitus			
GROWTH IMPAIRMENT Before and during BMT: • RT—TBI, total lymphoid irradiation (TLI), cranial, craniospinal • Chemotherapy before, during, and after BMT: • Corticosteroids	• Younger age (<6 years) at BMT • Underlying diagnosis, e.g. thalassemia (iron overload) • Chronic illness • High total RT dose (especially >1 RT episode); unfractionated TBI • Growth hormone deficiency • Poor nutrition • Constitutional bone marrow failure syndromes (e.g., Fanconi anemia)	• Short stature due to growth impairment • Skeletal disproportion • Reduced bone mineral density in adulthood due to GH deficiency • Adult GH deficiency syndrome	• Short stature (final height below—2 standard deviation scores)—21% of mixed pediatric population (80% of whom received RT during prior or conditioning treatment)[105] • Mean final height loss (SDS) of -1.17 in males, -0.56 in females; greatest loss (-2.07) after prior cranial RT and unfractionated TBI[105] • Mean final height loss (SDS) greater with younger age at TBI, -3.49 if <6 years at BMT, -1.92 if 6–12 years, -0.37 if 12–15 years[107] • Final height loss after TBI (14 patients)—males 8.6 cm, females 7.9 cm; but not significantly different from target height.[108]	1. Association with cGvHD and prolonged use of steroids 2. In general, patients with major postallogeneic BMT complications suffer greater degrees of impaired growth[106]	Not possible to predict precisely the impact of GH treatment on final height in children with TBI-associated GH deficiency; prospective randomized controlled trials, with follow-up to final height, are not yet available

(continued)

Table 26-6 Late Effects of Bone Marrow Transplantation in Children—cont'd

Organ/system/toxicity primary causative treatment(s)*	Other potential risk factors	Clinical features and consequences	Frequency†	Impact of allogeneic BMT‡	Comments
REPRODUCTIVE TOXICITY Before and during BMT: • RT to field including gonads (and uterus in females)§ • Chemotherapy especially alkylating agents, e.g., high-dose cyclophosphamide (HD Cy), BuCy, melphalan (males)	• Older age at BMT • Gender • High total RT dose; unfractionated TBI • Total dose of alkylating agents (i.e., including prior treatment)	• Delayed/arrested puberty • Impaired fertility • Requirement for hormone replacement treatment in adult life in those patients with Leydig cell or ovarian failure Males: • Leydig cell dysfunction—low testosterone, raised gonadotrophins • Germ cell failure—azoospermia/ oligospermia Females: • Ovarian failure—amenorrhea, low estradiol, raised gonadotrophins • Pregnancy may occur, but uterine damage may lead to miscarriage, or premature delivery and low birthweight, especially if prepubertal at BMT • Even if ovarian recovery occurs, early menopause may follow	Males: • Delayed puberty after fractionated TBI, requiring HRT—7%[109] • Overt Leydig cell failure, requiring HRT—7%,[109] increasing with age (Dr A. Leiper, unpublished observations) • Germ cell failure—recovery reported, even after TBI, but conception rare, 24% after HD Cy, 7% after BuCy, 1% after TBI[110] Females: • Delayed menarche after fractionated TBI, requiring HRT—44%[109] • Overt ovarian failure, requiring HRT—recovery may occur after HD Cy (54%), but only rarely after TBI (10%), very rarely after BuCy (1%)[110] • Pregnancy—24% after HD Cy, 1% after TBI, 0% after BuCy[110]		1. Longer follow-up needed to assess full impact of reproductive toxicity 2. Fertility preservation techniques under active investigation

MUSCULOSKELETAL TOXICITY					
Before or during BMT: • Chemotherapy, especially methotrexate (reduced bone mineral density, BMD) • Cranial RT, leading to endocrinopathy (reduced BMD) During BMT: • RT to field including affected bone (AVN and OC)[§] Before, during, or after BMT: • Corticosteroids (AVN, reduced BMD)	• Older age (> 16 years), rare < 10 years age (AVN) • Male gender (AVN) • GH deficiency, hypogonadism (reduced BMD)	Muscular: See 'Neurological toxicity' Skeletal: • Avasular necrosis (AVN)—hip most commonly affected, often bilaterally • Osteochondroma (OC)—often multiple, malignant change rare • Reduced BMD • Others—including slipped epiphysis, scoliosis	• Avascular necrosis—0.6% at 5 years in patients < 16 years age at BMT[111] • Osteochondroma—26%[112] • Reduced BMD—varies considerably with methodology, especially choice of controls; whole body bone mass only minimally reduced compared to similar childhood ALL survivors treated without BMT,[113] but BMD reduced more in 10 children (using age but not height-matched controls) than in 13 adults[114]	Association with GvHD and hence steroid usage (AVN, BMD in adult studies)	Important need for long-term prospective studies of BMD with appropriate age-/height-matched controls
SECONDARY MALIGNANCY					
Before or during BMT: • Chemotherapy, especially alkylating agents, topoisomerase II inhibitors (especially epipodophyllotoxins) • RT	• Young age • Cranial RT, especially in younger children • High RT dose	• Solid tumors—late onset, median 4–8 years post-BMT; brain and thyroid tumors especially common in young (<5 years age) recipients of cranial RT	• Solid tumors—risk increases with time, cumulative 4% at 10 years, 11% at 15 years post-BMT; greater increased relative risk compared to normal population (60 times expected at > 10 years)[66]	1. Note influence of cGvHD (especially in skin and oral tumors), immunosuppressive treatment and prior diagnosis of Fanconi anemia in allogeneic BMT	1. Prognosis of secondary malignancy post-BMT is variable, but often poor 2. Lympho-proliferative disease may be treated by donor-derived cytotoxic T lymphocytes

(continued)

Table 26-6 Late Effects of Bone Marrow Transplantation in Children—cont'd

Organ/system/toxicity primary causative treatment(s)*	Other potential risk factors	Clinical features and consequences	Frequency†	Impact of allogeneic BMT‡	Comments
		• Acute myeloid leukemia/ myelodysplasia—early onset, median 2½ years post-BMT, often associated with cytogenetic abnormalities, especially deletions or monosomy of chromosomes 5 or 7	• AML/MDS—predominantly occur after autologous BMT; very rare in children (age >35 years at BMT is a recognized risk factor)[115]	2. Posttransplant lymphoproliferative disease, often EBV-related, usually donor-derived, occurs in severely immunosuppressed (often mismatched) allogeneic BMT patients—usually early-onset (<1 year post-BMT)[116]	

From Skinner R, Leiper A: Late effects of bone marrow transplantation in children. In Wallace H, Green D, editors: Late effects of childhood cancer, London, 2004, Arnold, pp 307–312.

*†Note that the etiology of late adverse effects is often multifactorial.

††The figures given for the frequency of the particular toxicities listed in this table are approximate and representative, and may vary considerably with study methodology (cross-sectional, prospective cohort, etc.) and the patient group (diagnosis, age at and type of BMT, presence of risk factors, etc.). Many studies include both allogeneic and autologous BMT recipients, and some include adult patients.

‡†This column highlights additional toxicity due to specific complications of allogeneic BMT (discussed in more detail in 'Selected late adverse effects of BMT in children—complex presentations and multifactorial etiology' in this chapter).

§†Including TBI.

ACTH, Adrenocorticotrophin; *ALL*, acute lymphocytic leukemia; *AML*, acute myeloid leukemia; *AVN*, avascular necrosis: *BMD*, bone mineral density; *BMT*, bone marrow transplantation; *BuCy*, busulphan and cyclophosphamide; *cGvHD*, chronicgraft-versus-host disease; *CMV*, cytomegalovirus; *CNS*, central nervous system; *CT*, chemotherapy; *EBV*, Epstein-Barr virus; *ECG*, electrocardiogram; *GH*, growth hormone; *HDCy*, high-dose cyclophosphamide; *HRT*, hormone replacement therapy; *LH/FSH*, luteinizing hormone/follicle-stimulating hormone; *MDS*, myelodysplasia; *OC*, osteochondroma; *RT*, radiation therapy; *SDS*, standard deviation scores; *TBI*, total body irradiation; *TSH*, thyroid-stimulating hormone; *VZV*, *Varicella zoster* virus.

Table 26-7 Recommendations for Long Term Follow-up after Transplantation

Complication	Group of hematopoietic-cell recipients at highest risk	Duration of increased risk after transplantation	Transplantation-related cause	Treatment or prophylaxis	Suggested monitoring interval and tests
ORAL CAVITY					
Lichen planus	Recipients of allogeneic transplants	3 mo to 2 yr	Chronic GVHD	Immunosuppressants, topical lubricants (cevimeline or oral pilocarpine), oral fluoride rinse	Every 1 to 3 mo
Symptoms of sicca syndrome	Recipients of allogeneic transplants	Lifelong	Chronic GVHD radiation therapy		Every 1 to 3 mo for GVHD
EYES					
Symptoms of sicca syndrome	Recipients of allogeneic transplants	Lifelong	Chronic GVHD radiation therapy	Immunosuppressants, topical lubricants (cevimeline or oral pilocarpine), surgery to alleviate lacrimal-duct obstruction	Eye examinations at least every 6 mo if there is corneal damage
Cataracts	Recipients of allogeneic transplants	≥ 6 mo	Radiation therapy and corticosteroids	Surgery when necessary	Every 12 mo
HEART					
Atherosclerotic cardiovascular disease	Recipients of allogeneic transplants	Years	Diabetes mellitus, hyperlipidemia, or hypertension related to drugs; premature ovarian failure; possibly radiation therapy	Standard therapy	Screening for cardiac risk factors, exercise testing
LUNGS					
Bronchiolitis obliterans	Recipients of allogeneic transplants	6 mo to 2 yr	Chronic GVHD	Immunosuppressants, possibly bronchodilators	Pulmonary-function tests
Bronchitis and bronchiectasis	Recipients of allogeneic transplants	6 mo to 2 yr	Defects in immunity and possibly ciliary function	Prophylactic antibiotics and immune globulin replacement for recurrent infections and bronchiectasis	No specific monitoring of pulmonary function usually required in an asymptomatic patient, shortness of breath and cough should trigger an infectious-disease workup, increasing symptoms or the absence of improvement should prompt chest radiographs and pulmonary-function tests

(continued)

Table 26-7 Recommendations for Long Term Follow-up after Transplantation—cont'd

Complication	Group of hematopoietic-cell recipients at highest risk	Duration of increased risk after transplantation	Transplantation-related cause	Treatment or prophylaxis	Suggested monitoring interval and tests
LIVER					
Chronic GVHD	Recipients of allogeneic transplants	First month	GVHD	Immunosuppression	Liver-function tests every 12 mo
Viral infection	Recipients of allogeneic transplants	6 mo to 2 yr	Hepatitis B and C virus	Antiviral therapy	Liver biopsy if warranted
Iron overload	Recipients of allogeneic transplants	Varies	Multiple causes	Phlebotomy or deferoxamine infusions	Viral testing as indicated, baseline ferritin measurement
KIDNEY					
Hypertension	Recipients of allogeneic transplants	First month	Drugs (e.g., corticosteroids, cyclosporine), hemolytic-uremic syndrome	Antihyperintensive agents, alterations in immunosuppressant regimen in patients with hemolytic-uremic syndrome, plasmapheresis	
Azotemia	Recipients of allogeneic transplants	0 to 6 mo	Drugs, hemolytic-uremic syndrome	Cautious use of nephrotoxins, supportive measures designed to prevent the progression of renal failure, antihypertensive agents	Annual monitoring of creatinine is probably sufficient, unless an abnormality is identified
ENDOCRINE					
Thyroid	Recipients of either allogeneic or autologous transplants	6 mo to many years	Radiation therapy	Levothyroxine replacement for hypothyroidism, aspiration or surgical excision of nodules	Measurement of thyrotropin and thyroid examination every 12 mo
Ovary	Recipients of either allogeneic or autologous transplants	First month	Radiation therapy	Hormone-replacement therapy or alternative treatment for symptoms associated with low estrogen levels	Mammogram and breast and pelvic examinations every 12 mo, bone-density study
Testes	Recipients of either allogeneic or autologous transplants	First month	Radiation therapy	Usually none Androgen patch if testosterone level is low	None
Osteopenia and osteoporosis	Recipients of either allogeneic or autologous transplants	Mo to yr	Corticosteroids, gonadal failure, chemotherapy and radiation therapy	Supplemental calcium and vitamin D, exercise, bisphosphonates or other antiresorptive agents	Initial bone-density study, repeated as indicated clinically

Secondary cancers	Recipients of allogeneic transplants	≥ 3 mo	Radiation, immunosuppressant agents	Disease-specific therapy	Physical examination, including skin and thyroid examinations, every 12 mo; mammogram and Papanicolaou smear at standard intervals; screening for colorectal cancer, possibly measurement of prostate-specific antigen
Skin cancer	Recipients of allogeneic transplants	Variable	Radiation therapy, chronic GVHD	Lifelong avoidance of exposure to ultraviolet light, local excision	6 to 12 mo

From Antin J: Long-term care after hematopoietic cell transplantation in adults, N Engl J Med 347:40–41, 2002.
*†GVHD denotes graft-versus-host disease.

radionuclide angiography, and chest x ray. These are repeated every 1 to 5 years, depending on risk factors. Management of symptoms may include diuretics, digoxin, anti-arrhythmics, cardiac transplantation, and education about risk reduction through exercise, decreased alcohol consumption, and avoidance of smoking and drug use. Patients and their families also should be alerted to the added cardiac risks associated with pregnancy and anesthesia.[54]

Neuropsychologic Complications

Long-term survivors of stem cell transplantation are at risk for cognitive deficits arising from their exposure to potentially neurotoxic agents (such as cyclosporine), GVHD and its treatment, high-dose ablative chemotherapies (such as busulfan/methotrexate), and TBI.[55] CNS events occurring during the early post-transplant period, such as cerebral hemorrhage, infection, viral encephalitis, and metabolic encephalopathy, are associated with a high risk of mortality and can impose significant long-term impairments.[55] Surveys of CNS complications after HSCT generally include mixed adult/pediatric populations and report varying complication rates ranging from 10% to 70%.[55]

Age is an important determinant of neurocognitive outcome. In their review of neurocognitive outcomes in HSCT, Dreyer and colleagues[55] concluded that, "HSCT, even with TBI, poses a low to minimum risk for late cognitive and academic deficits in patients who are at least 6 years of age at the time of transplant. The risk for cognitive impairment, sensorimotor delays, and decline in academic skills is increased in children <6 years of age, particularly in those <3 years of age, regardless of whether or not TBI is used as part of the conditioning regimen."[55]

When assessing neurocognitive and neuropsychologic changes after transplantation, one must consider what prior therapies the patient may have received. Children with high-risk ALL, ALL with CNS relapse, or brain tumors may already have received substantial doses of CNS irradiation and chemotherapy. Risk factors associated with neurocognitive impairments in survivors of childhood leukemia include age, gender (female greater than male), lower socioeconomic status, baseline intelligence, prior therapy for cancer, and duration of therapy.[56] Young age, female gender, low socioeconomic status, and higher doses of chemotherapy (especially methotrexate) are associated with intelligence quotient (IQ) decline in children treated for ALL.[56]

Combined chemotherapy and radiation therapy have been associated with decline in intellectual and academic function; particularly in the areas of information processing, working memory, and IQ.[56] Patients who have received triple intrathecal chemotherapy without cranial irradiation for CNS prophylaxis have a slightly higher risk of cognitive impairment than those who have received single-agent methotrexate.[55]

Leukoencephalopathy, demyelination, cerebral vasculopathy, and radionecrosis are some of the less common neurotoxicities exhibited by long-term survivors who have received combined-modality therapy for intracranial tumors and radiation doses to the cranium of 50 Gy to 60 Gy.[55]

Interventions for minimizing the toxicities of CNS therapies and providing structured cognitive rehabilitation are being explored. Specific radiotherapeutic interventions include eliminating cranial irradiation in very young children, or delaying it until children are older, dose reduction, volume reduction, and conformal treatments (such as stereotactic radiation therapy [SRT], stereotactic radiosurgery [SRS], three-dimensional conformal plannings). Participation in cognitive rehabilitation programs, such as the program sponsored by the National Cancer Institute for brain tumor and ALL survivors, may help to validate methods for teaching patients new cognitive skills and learning techniques by permitting formal assessment of a large cohort of patients.[55]

Neuropsychologic testing before, immediately after, and for several years beyond treatment is imperative for early detection of learning problems. This information should be shared with parents, teachers, pediatricians, and social workers to facilitate the child's transition to school, society, and long-term survivorship.

Oral Complications

Conditioning regimens for HSCT, particularly those employing high-dose chemotherapy and TBI, have been associated with severe damage to the enamel organ and developing teeth.[49,57] Dental defects caused by radiation may include tooth dwarfism, dental underdevelopment (blunting, shortening), premature apical closure, delayed or arrested root development, and failure of eruption.[57,58] Children less than 5 years of age who receive radiation to the head and neck at or above 24 Gy (neuroblastoma, Hodgkin's disease mantle field radiation, TLI) are at greatest risk for serious dental complications. Underdevelopment of the mandible and anomalies of the temporomandibular joint may occur after TBI in children.[49] Recent data in older children suggests that chemotherapy plus radiation in doses of 10 Gy to 18 Gy can produce apical root distortion.[58]

Chemotherapy is a contributor to dental complications because of its adverse effects on developing dentition, tooth enamel, and salivary function. Changes in the enamel may increase susceptibility of teeth to bacterial colonization, demineralization, and caries. Chemotherapy and radiation–induced changes in the oral environment can lead to periodontal disease, caries, and increased plaque accumulation. Changes in salivary function can be compromised for long periods of time, predisposing to dental caries. Studies in patients who have received TBI in doses of 10 Gy demonstrate decreased saliva production, which begins to decline 5 to 10 days into preconditioning with TBI, falls to approximately 50% of normal, and remains at 25% of normal for 2 to 3 months after transplantation.[58] General return to normal salivary function may take up to 4 years in TBI/chemotherapy patients and up to 1 year in patients who receive chemotherapy alone. Bleomycin, busulfan, and doxorubicin all have been identified as contributors to xerostomia.[58]

Allogeneic transplantation patients with chronic GVHD receiving cyclosporine A have been observed to have nongingival soft tissue growths. Children and adults with chronic GVHD also may exhibit oral changes, such as erythema, atrophy, mucoceles, ulceration, and mucosal lichenoid changes.[58] Consultation with a dental specialist before transplantation and at yearly intervals after transplantation would be beneficial to the management of post-transplant oral complications and would facilitate early intervention for dental problems in children. Specific efforts should be focused on strengthening the tooth enamel, use of fluoride, active oral hygiene, minimizing the effects of xerostomia, and treating oral mucosal infections.

Ocular Complications

Patients undergoing HSCT can suffer severe and potentially vision-threatening complications from the combined effects of chemotherapeutic agents, radiation, and GVHD.[59] In a large retrospective study of pediatric HSCT recipients, Suh and colleagues[60] noted that "certain diagnoses carried a higher risk for ocular complications; these include patients with ALL, acute myelocytic leukemia, myelodysplastic syndrome, thrombocytopenia, and Wiskott-Aldrich syndrome. Patients with allogeneic HSCT were 2 to 3 times more likely to develop ocular complications than autologous transplant patients.[60]

It is estimated that ocular complications occur in 60% of patients with GVHD.[59] The onset of acute GVHD occurs within the first 3 months after transplantation, and its sequelae can be long-lasting. Ocular effects of GVHD are keratoconjunctivitis sicca and dry eye syndrome (DES). DES may develop from inflammation of the lacrimal glands or lacrimal stasis, and occlusion in 59% to 75% of patients with GVHD.[59] Acute and chronic GVHD also may result in pseudomembranous conjunctivitis, keratitis, and infection, infectious ulceration of the cornea, eyelid changes, and destruction of the lacrimal and meibomian glands.[59]

Late-onset keratoconjunctivitis sicca syndrome can approach a 20% incidence 15 years after stem cell transplantation, and it occurs in almost 40% of patients with chronic GVHD. Identified risk factors for late-onset keratoconjunctivitis include GVHD, age more than 20 years, female gender, and use of methotrexate for GVHD prophylaxis.[49] Treatment for this may include topical lubricants, judicious use of topical steroids, and retinoic acid. Cataracts are the most common ocular complication of HSCT, with a reported incidence of 8.5% to 80%.[59,60] Associated risk factors for the development of cataracts include corticosteroids, GVHD, TBI, cranial irradiation, and chemotherapeutic agents such as busulfan.[60]

Patients treated with TBI are at greater risk for development of cataracts. The risk percentage varies from 10% to 60% at 10 years, depending on the total dose given and the fractionation scheme.[54] A decrease in the incidence of cataracts is noted in those patients who receive a lower dose rate (0.04 Gy/minute, or less) and six or more fractions of radiation.[54] One of the largest reported studies of the development of cataracts after TBI was in a group of 1064 survivors of leukemia treated with HSCT from the European Group for Blood and Marrow Transplantation. The study noted an overall 10-year cataract incidence of 50%. The rate was 60% in patients treated with single-fraction TBI, 43% in those treated with six fractions or less, and only 7% in patients treated with more than six fractions of TBI.[54] The independent risk factors for the development of cataracts were older age (>23 years), higher dose rate (>0.04 Gy/minute), allogeneic HSCT, and use of corticosteroids.[49,54,59]

Complications in the posterior segment of the eye occur in approximately 13% of patients.[59] These include ischemic retinopathy (cotton wool spots), focal intraretinal hemorrhage, telangiectatic vessels, and in very rare instances, retinal detachment.[59]

Prolonged immune deficiency and ocular complications of GVHD can predispose patients to ocular infections and potential visual deficits. Ocular infections commonly seen in bone marrow transplant HSCT patients include pseudomonal corneal ulcers, herpes simplex keratitis, herpes zoster retinitis, CMV chorioretinitis, Toxoplasma chorioretinitis, and fungal endophthalmitis.[59] Pre-transplant consultation with ophthalmology specialists and long-term follow-up of these patients is indicated to help prevent or reduce the severity of ocular complications.

Endocrine Complications

Changes in endocrine function after allogeneic HSCTs may be attributed to chemotherapy—specifically busulfan, cyclophosphamide, BCNU—and to irradiation to the fields that contain the affected glands, especially the pituitary, thyroid, and gonads. Thyroid dysfunction is one of the most common late complications after allogeneic HSCT. It can be classified into three distinct categories: subclinical compensated hypothyroidism, overt hypothyroidism, and autoimmune hypothyroidism.[49] Subclinical hypothyroidism occurs in 7% to 15.5% of patients during the year after HSCT and is detected by high serum thyroid stimulating hormone (TSH) and normal free T4 levels.[49] Early intervention with l-thyroxine is not usually indicated, because many episodes of subclinical hypothyroidism resolve spontaneously, and there is some speculation that l-thyroxine may stimulate osteoporosis in young women who have developed gonadal failure secondary to HSCT.[49]

Overt hypothyroidism after allogeneic HSCT is caused by direct damage of the thyroid gland and is usually detected during the fourth year after transplantation.[49] The incidence of overt hypothyroidism seems to vary according to the pre-transplant conditioning regimen. It can be 20% to 25% in children treated with fractionated TBI to doses less than 15 Gy.[52] Socie and colleagues[49] reported an incidence of overt hypothyroidism of up to 90% in patients receiving single-fraction TBI to a dose of 10 Gy and a reduction in incidence to 15% of patients after fractionated TBI.[49]

Thyroid hormone replacement is indicated in all patients with elevated serum TSH levels and low free T4 levels. Serum thyroid hormone and TSH levels should be monitored at baseline, 4 to 6 weeks after initiation of replacement therapy, and every 6 months thereafter.[49]

Autoimmune hypothyroidism has been reported in approximately 5% of patients after irradiation for Hodgkin's disease, prior head and neck irradiation, and after preparation for HSCTs.[49] Follow-up recommendations for patients experiencing treatment-related thyroid dysfunction include long-term monitoring of serum thyroid function studies, avoidance of concurrent use of radiation and iodine–containing materials, and periodic physical examinations to screen for the presence of thyroid gland abnormalities.

Growth Impairment

Normal linear growth in children may be affected by several factors, including genetic, nutritional, hormonal, and physiologic interference imposed by intensive cancer therapies. Children undergoing HSCT form a heterogeneous group because they undergo treatment at different stages of development and receive varying treatment modalities (chemotherapy and radiation therapy) before HSCT.

The risk of growth hormone deficiency is increased in children who receive TBI, particularly single-fraction, and in those who are treated with pre-transplant cranial irradiation, are female, and receive therapy for post-transplant GVHD with long-term steroids.[49,54] Socie and colleagues[49] in a recent review of late effects after HSCT made several important observations about growth impairment. Children who received transplants at ages less than 10 years and those who received cranial radiation therapy have more pronounced growth hormone deficiency than others. Children who receive pre-transplant conditioning with chemotherapy alone (either cyclophosphamide or busulfan/cyclophosphamide) usually grow normally. The average loss of height in the high-risk group was approximately 6 cm.[49]

Decreases in growth noted in children receiving radiation to the thoracic/abdominal field are attributable to direct effects on the gonads, the thyroid gland, and bone epiphyses.[49]

Many transplant recipients experience reduced bone mineral density and are at future risk for developing osteoporosis. After hematopoietic stem cell transplantation in adults, osteopenia occurs in 50% to 60% of patients, and osteoporosis develops in as many as 20%.[53] Factors contributing to bone loss include pre-transplantation chemotherapy, gonadal suppression from chemotherapy, use of corticosteroids, and reduced physical activity.[53] Avascular necrosis, primarily affecting the hips, occurs as a late effect in approximately 5% of patients.[53]

Gonadal Dysfunction

Radiation and chemotherapy may produce temporary and permanent effects on reproductive capacity, endocrine integrity, sexual development, and sexual function in patients undergoing transplantation.

Radiation to the ovary may reduce the numbers of small follicles, impair follicular maturation, and produce cortical fibrosis, cortical atrophy, generalized hypoplasia, and hyalinization of the capsule.[54] Alkylating agents affect the ovaries by causing a depletion of oocytes and disruption of follicular function. Arrested follicular maturation and decreased estrogen may be the consequence of these effects.[54] Disruption of ovarian function also may have negative effects on vaginal integrity and development, breast development, bone mineralization, the integrity of the cardiovascular system, and libido.

The dose of radiation that will produce ovarian failure depends on age and the radiation fractionation scheme. Friedman and Constine[54] have noted that the ovaries of younger girls are somewhat more resistant to the effects of radiation therapy than those of adolescents. Temporary sterility can occur after single-fraction treatments of 1.7-6.4 Gy, and permanent sterility after 3.2 Gy to 10 Gy. Whole-abdomen doses of 20 Gy to 30 Gy are associated with primary and secondary ovarian failure.[54] Dose fractionation may reduce the impact of radiation treatment on ovarian function. Pre-pubertal girls treated with fractionated TBI to a total of 12 Gy are 5 times more likely to have spontaneous recovery to normal ovarian function than girls receiving single-dose TBI.[49] Ovarian tolerance of radiation decreases with the onset of puberty.

TBI can have additive effects on reproductive function when it is administered (14.4 Gy) after prior irradiation of the whole abdomen (20 Gy to 30 Gy). Radiation may impair uterine development, if it is administered during pre-pubescence. Changes to the developing uterus may include reduction in length, compromised vasculature, disruption in blood flow, and premature menopause.[61]

Alkylating agents, such as cyclophosphamide and busulfan, have long been known to impair gonadal function.[61] Other chemotherapeutic agents associated with gonadal toxicity include ifosfamide, nitrosoureas, chlorambucil, melphalan, vinblastine, cytarabine, cisplatin, and procarbazine.[61] Many of these agents are used in combination to treat adult and childhood malignancies, so their additive effects of gonadal function are also appreciated.

Patients should be monitored for signs and symptoms of delayed, arrested, or absent pubertal development. In adolescents and sexually mature women, menstrual cycles should be observed for changes, and classic symptoms of estrogen insufficiency, such as hot flashes, vaginal dryness, dyspareunia, altered libido, and infertility, should be noted. Long-term management should include routine Tanner staging and monitoring of luteinizing hormone (LH), follicle stimulating hormone (FSH) and estradiol levels. Monitoring should begin at 12 years of age and continue as needed to facilitate hormone replacement through puberty into adulthood. Hormone replacement is indicated in adult women to promote cardiovascular and skeletal health. Referrals to reproductive endocrinologists and gynecologists specializing in oncology patients may help to address some of the unique challenges that these women experience.

In males, cytotoxic chemotherapy and radiation therapy can produce damage to the testes and cause hormone insufficiency and sterility. The pre-pubertal testis is susceptible to the effects of radiation, which can produce Leydig cell dysfunction, vascular changes, and decreases in testosterone production. Chemotherapy, especially alkylating agents, such as busulfan, cyclophosphamide, the combination of these two, and melphalan, are associated with reproductive toxicity and may produce oligospermia, azoospermia, and testosterone deficiency.[62]

The severity of radiation-induced testicular damage depends on total dose, fractionation, and field. Testicular irradiation in doses of greater than 20 Gy have been associated with Leydig cell dysfunction in prepubertal boys, whereas in sexually mature men, Leydig cell function is preserved up to 30 Gy.[62] Most men have normal testosterone and luteinizing hormone levels but are azoospermic.[53]

Loss of Leydig cell function in pre-pubertal male children necessitates androgen supplementation to help induce and support pubertal growth. In adults, testosterone replacement is indicated for men who exhibit symptoms of testosterone deficiency, for example, reduced energy level, impaired libido, anxiety/depression, and alterations in body composition and bone mineral density.[62]

Long-term follow-up and evaluation of male patients should include screening for signs and symptoms of testicular atrophy, delayed, arrested, or absent pubertal development, and Tanner staging. Measurements of serum LH, FSH, and testosterone levels are indicated for failure of pubertal development, as baselines for sexually active males, and to monitor for infertility. Sperm analysis should be obtained to check for potency and recovery.[52] Patients should be instructed in testicular examination and provided with referrals to reproductive endocrinologists and fertility specialists, as needed.

Impaired Fertility

Fertility after HSCT and the overall incidence of pregnancy are low, except for patients who have been treated for aplastic anemia.[49] Most patients who have received TBI conditioning as part of their pre-transplant regimen experience gonadal failure. In women, recovery of gonadal function occurs in 10% to 14% of cases, and the incidence of pregnancy is less than 3%.[49] In men, recovery of gonadal function is less than 20%.[49] Although infertility is a likelihood, it is not an absolute. Patients should receive counseling in safe sexual practices and contraception, because pregnancy during the first year after transplantation carries a high risk for complications.

Pre-transplant counseling should include a discussion about the risk of gonadal dysfunction, the potential for infertility, and the significance of this situation to the patient. Considerations for adolescents and young adults of reproductive age who might wish to have children in the future might include egg harvesting, sperm banking, and assisted contraception.[49]

Chronic Graft-Versus-Host Disease

Chronic graft-versus-host disease (cGVHD) and/or its treatment and the use of radiation in pre-transplantation conditioning regimens have both been identified as major risk factors for the development of nonmalignant complications after HSCT.[49]

The incidence of cGVHD is variable and depends on the source of hematopoietic cells. In fully histocompatible transplants, the incidence is 30%, and when cells from matched unrelated donors or mismatched hematopoietic cells from unrelated donors are used, the incidence is 60% to 70%.[53]

Graft versus host disease that occurs more than 100 days after HSCT transplantation is typically classified cGVHD.[53] Factors that have been associated with risk for development of cGVHD include donor and recipient age, prior acute GVHD, use of alloimmune female donors, the type of GVHD prophylaxis employed, and history of herpesvirus infection.[49]

Clinical manifestations of cGVHD are lichenoid changes in the skin and mucous membranes, vitiligo, periorbital hyperpigmentation, odynophagia, nail dysplasia, keratoconjunctivitis, sicca, xerostomia, alopecia, scleroderma, cholestasis, and increased susceptibility to infection. Gynecologic manifestations in women may include dyspareunia and vaginal strictures.[53]

Immune reconstitution after HSCT depends on several variables. Recovery of cellular immunity after allogeneic transplantation is influenced by patient age, disease factors, conditioning regimen, and type of transplant being performed.[49] Chronic GVHD can be a major obstacle to recovery, because of the need to treat it with prolonged courses of immunosuppressive medications and corticosteroids. Chronic GVHD is a major factor affecting immune reconstitution of B cells, CD4, and CD8 T cells.[49] Delays in cellular and humoral immune recovery are associated with a high risk for severe infections.[49,53]

There is an increased susceptibility to infections caused by encapsulated bacteria (*Streptococcus pneumoniae, Haemophilus influenzae* type B, and *Neisseria meningitides*), particularly in patients with cGVHD or past history of cGVHD.[49] The highest period for reactivation of CMV is 1 to 24 months after transplantation. Reactivation of varicella zoster virus typically occurs in 20% to 50% of patients within several months of transplantation, usually after acyclovir prophylaxis has been discontinued.[49] The risk for development of infections caused by *Pneumocystis jiroveci* and *Toxoplasma gondii* remains highest during the first year after transplantation or while patients are receiving immunosuppressive therapy for cGVHD.[49,53] Patients should receive prophylaxis to protect against these infections.

Specific recommendations and protocols for reimmunizing patients and family members may be found in guidelines published by the Centers for Disease Control and Prevention (CDC website for prophylaxis guidelines, www.cdc.gov/nip/publications/hsct-recs.pdf).

Secondary Malignancies

Patients undergoing HSCT are at increased risk for developing second malignancies. Bhatia and colleagues[63] analyzed 2129 patients who underwent HSCT for various hematologic malignancies at the City of Hope Medical Center from 1976 to 1998. They reported that 29 patients developed solid malignancies after HSCT, which represents a twofold increase in risk compared to the healthy population. The risk for developing liver cancer, cancer of the oral cavity, cervical cancer, and skin cancer was 6.1% at 10 years.[63]

In a 10-year follow-up study conducted from 1982 to 1997 on 605 patients who underwent autologous HSCT for B cell NHL with a conditioning regimen of cyclophosphamide and TBI followed by prolonged administration of anti-B cell monoclonal antibodies, a 21% higher than normal incidence of second malignancies was noted.[64] The incidence of solid tumors (thyroid, skin, oropharynx, brain, and soft tissue) was 10%, and the incidence of myelodysplastic syndrome (MDS) and/or acute myelogenous leukemia (AML) was 11%.[64] Risk factors for developing MDS/AML included prior radiation therapy, conditioning with TBI, older age, low stem cell dose, use of peripheral stem cells, and intensity of prior chemotherapy.[65]

Socie and colleagues[66] evaluated the risk of second malignancies after HSCT for childhood leukemia and found that risk increased over time to 11% at 15 years and was highest for children younger than 10 years at the time of transplantation. Multivariate analysis revealed increased risk associated with high-dose TBI and younger age at transplantation. Patients who received pretransplant conditioning with high-dose TBI of 10 Gy single-dose or a 13 Gy fractionated dose) had an increased risk for development of secondary cancers. Children who developed cGVHD had a lower risk of developing solid cancers. Solid tumors observed in this cohort of patients arose in brain, thyroid, tongue, and salivary gland.[66]

These studies demonstrate that there is a risk for second malignancies after HSCT and that the risk is sustained over many years. As length of follow-up increases, an increasing number of radiation- and chemotherapy-associated tumors may emerge. This underscores the importance of long-term follow-up of HSCT patients and educating healthcare providers and patients about the risks of second malignancies. Early detection and screening should be initiated soon after transplantation, and patients should be instructed in self-examination techniques and informed about lifestyle measures that minimize risk.

OVERVIEW OF TOTAL LYMPHOID IRRADIATION

TLI was developed by Kaplan and his colleagues in the late 1970s for the treatment of patients with stage III Hodgkin's disease. High-dose TLI (44 Gy) was well tolerated during the acute and late phases of treatment and provided the first curative treatment for stage III Hodgkin's disease. This early success led to extension of the use of TLI to stage I and stage II Hodgkin's disease and temporary acceptance as a standard for curative treatment of early-stage disease. Subsequently, it was established that subtotal lymphoid irradiation could be used to manage stage I or stage II Hodgkin's disease in patients with disease limited to locations above the diaphragm.[67] TLI also has been supplanted by high-dose combination chemotherapy regimens, such as MOPP (mechlorethamine, vincristine, procarbazine, and prednisone), or combined-modality regimens for treatment of Hodgkin's patients with stage III disease. TLI also was tried in treatment regimens for various forms of NHL, but for a variety of reasons, this modality met with little success and is rarely employed in contemporary regimens for NHL.[67,68]

Technique

TLI requires sequential irradiation of the mantle and inverted-Y fields. The mantle field contains all of the significant lymph node regions above the diaphragm and includes the cervical, supraclavicular, axillary, infraclavicular, mediastinal, and pulmonary hilar lymph node groups. The inverted-Y field encompasses lymph node groups below the diaphragm and includes the para-aortic, splenic hilar, common, internal and external iliac, the inguinal and femoral lymph node groups, plus the spleen itself. Megavoltage irradiation equipment is required to permit treatment of these large areas while sparing the overlying skin from radiation injury.

Immunologic Effects

TLI produces long-lasting effects on the composition of cells in lymph node and splenic tissue. Histologic preparations show depletion of lymphocytes, apparent hypertrophy of sinusoids, and infiltration by fat cells. Concomitantly, there is a marked depression of peripheral lymphocyte counts, which can last 2 years or more, and longer term depression of circulating T cells, with reversal of the normal T:B cell ratio. T cells undergo differential decreases in the numbers of helper ($CD4^+$) T cells and suppressor ($CD8^+$) T cells, and there is an increase in circulating T cells with absent surface markers, such as CD3. There also is a long-term increase in the number of natural killer cells ($CD16^+$). Corresponding functional abnormalities include reduced responsiveness in vitro to standard mitogens and reduced reactivity to allogeneic and autologous cells in mixed lymphocyte reaction (MLR) assays. Long-lasting clinical abnormalities include reduced delayed hypersensitivity responses to standard skin test antigens, an increased incidence of herpes zoster infections, and increased risk for life-threatening bacterial infections. Irradiation of the spleen may confer increased risk of overwhelming sepsis caused by encapsulated bacterial pathogens, such as Streptococcus pneumoniae and Neisseria meningitidis.[67]

The above immunologic effects constitute the principal theoretical and clinically observed risks of TLI and have served as a major barrier to widespread use of this modality.[67,68]

Studies in Animals

TLI has been studied in rodent models that produce immunosuppression that is roughly equivalent to that observed in humans treated with this technique. In this model, primary antibody responses to antigenic stimuli are seriously impaired, although secondary antibody responses in animals, which had received primary immunization before administration of TLI, are not affected. This implies that TLI does not abolish immunologic memory. Responsiveness to T cell–independent antigens recovers promptly after TLI, whereas there is a protracted delay in recovery of responsiveness to T cell–dependent antigens. In vitro production of lymphokines in response to standard stimuli also is impaired for prolonged periods after TLI.

TLI increases the survival of allogeneic skin grafts and bone marrow grafts, and it reduces the incidence and severity of GVHD. Survival of transplanted allogeneic solid organs is enhanced, when TLI-treated animals also are infused with bone marrow cells from the donor animal at the time of transplantation. TLI also confers improved tolerance of xenogeneic proteins, such as monoclonal antibodies.[67]

TLI in Autoimmune Diseases

Most clinical trials involving humans are flawed by limitations and variables in study design and technique. Radiation techniques (shielding, total dose, fractionation scheme) and concomitant or post-irradiation immunosuppressive regimens differ widely from study to study. Sample sizes usually are small, and use of historical controls is the rule. The timing of radiation before organ transplantation often is a variable, even within studies, that is greatly affected by the availability of suitable donor organs.[67]

The use of TLI has been reported for a small number of renal transplant recipients. The studies are largely reliant on historical controls. The underlying causes of the end-stage renal disease have varied, as have the post-transplant pharmacologic immunosuppressive regimens.[67]

Uncontrolled studies of TLI in cardiac transplant recipients with myocardial biopsies indicating rejection have met with some apparent success in limiting subsequent rejection episodes in a small number of patients.[67]

TLI plus cyclophosphamide has been studied with bone marrow transplantation principally in patients being treated for aplastic anemia and/or thalassemia major. TLI also has been used to boost the effects of TBI and chemotherapy for patients receiving T cell–depleted allogeneic HSCT.[67]

In rheumatoid arthritis, TLI has produced long-term improvement in disease activity, but no concomitant improvement in serologic markers, such as rheumatoid factor, production of which may be T cell–independent. Use of higher doses of radiation in these studies was associated with increased morbidity in the form of infections, cardiopulmonary toxicity, and xerostomia with significant weight loss.[67]

TLI has been studied in a small number of patients with lupus nephritis that has been refractory to standard immunosuppressive therapy. Reductions in urine albumin excretion, with concomitant rises in serum albumin concentrations, and reductions in mean daily doses of prednisone have been achieved. The durability of these benefits is unclear.[67]

TLI was employed in a prospective study of patients with multiple sclerosis, which used sham-treated controls. Patients in the treatment group experienced delays in functional decline, which appeared to correlate with decreases in the $CD4^+/CD8^+$ ratio.

SUMMARY AND FUTURE DIRECTIONS

Hematopoietic stem cell transplantation can be a life-sustaining treatment for many children and adults with diseases that previously were considered fatal. As more individuals survive the early complications of HSCT, they join an ever-growing cohort of patients at risk for late adverse effects. There are many potential factors that contribute to the development of late adverse effects after HSCT. These include the age of the patient, the use of high-dose chemotherapy and radiation therapy, the increasing use of matched unrelated donors, and GVHD.[52] Long-term survivors should remain in close follow-up and be referred to the appropriate specialists as needed.

New treatment approaches eliminating the use of TBI in conditioning regimens for chronic myelogenous leukemia, aggressive or relapsed lymphoma, aplastic anemia, and breast cancer are being explored. The long-term efficacy of these measures remains to be defined. The use of targeted radiolabeled monoclonal antibodies also is being investigated in patients undergoing autologous HSCT for acute leukemia and myelodysplastic syndromes. The outcomes of these phase I trials may provide insights into the use of preparative regimens that are more specific to the sites of disease and eliminate toxicity to normal tissues.

Further refinements in treatment regimens are needed to reduce the frequency and severity of toxicities associated with HSCT. The avoidance of TBI, especially in young children, is a desirable goal. Until this is feasible, the use of low-dose fractionated TBI can help reduce organ toxicity. The use of selective shielding (i.e., lungs), fractionation, and delivery of radiation doses over several days are the first steps toward reducing toxicity and improving the tolerability of HSCT. As can be seen from the RIC clinical trials, the verdict is still out on a single best conditioning regime for HSCT in all situations. We therefore predict that TBI in some form will continue to be used as a preparatory HSCT regime for several years to come. Radiation oncology nurses will need to be knowledgeable about the different TBI treatment methods, doses, and the related patient care needs. The ultimate goal is the advancement of primary cancer treatment that would eliminate the need for HSCT and its associated toxicities.

TLI now is used sparingly and has limited application in oncology. Even in Hodgkin's disease, for which it initially was developed, TLI has been largely supplanted by other treatment modalities. Some investigators still argue for use of TLI for stage III follicular NHL. TLI offers no survival advantage over other treatment modalities for any form of early NHL, and recurrences in NHL often assume a more aggressive cell type than the primary tumor.[68] The major inadequacy of TLI is long-term immunosuppression, which imposes limitations on the use of high-dose chemotherapy for recurrent disease. Future use of TLI in oncology, for autoimmune disorders, and in transplantation medicine awaits improvements in delivery techniques and better understanding of dosage, timing, and concomitant use of chemotherapy and immunosuppressive agents.[68,69]

REFERENCES

1. Salar A, Sierra J, Gandarellas M et al: Autologous stem cell transplantation for clinically aggressive non-Hodgkin's lymphoma: the role of preparative regimens, *Bone Marrow Transplant* 27(4):405-412, 2001.

2. Hsiu-San L, Drzymala E: Magna-field irradiation. In Perez CA, Brady LW, Halperin EC, Schmidt-Ullrich RK, editors: *Principles and practice of radiation oncology,* ed 4, Philadelphia, 2004, Lippincott Williams & Wilkins, pp 400-409.
3. Pierce M: Total body irradiation. In Bruner D, Haas M, Gosselin-Acomb TK, editors: *Manual for radiation oncology nursing practice and education,* ed 3, Pittsburgh, 2005, Oncology Nursing Society, pp 185-197.
4. Shank B: Total body irradiation. In Liebel S, Phillips T, editors: *Textbook of radiation oncology,* ed 2, Philadelphia, 2004, WB Saunders, pp 323-347.
5. Redei I, Langston A, Lonial S et al: Rapid hematopoietic engraftment following fractionated TBI conditioning and transplantation with CD 34 enriched hematopoietic progenitor cells from partially mismatched related donors, *Bone Marrow Transplant* 30(6):335-340, 2002
6. Lerner R, Burns L: Transformed lymphoma: an Achilles' heel of non-Hodgkin's lymphoma, *Bone Marrow Transplant* 31(7):531-537, 2003.
7. Bacigalupo A: Third EBMT/Amgen Workshop on reduced-intensity conditioning allogeneic haemopoietic stem cell transplants (RIC-HSCT) and panel consensus, *Bone Marrow Transplant* 33(7):691-696, 2004.
8. Tse W, Lazarus H, van Besien K: Stem cell transplantation in follicular lymphoma: progress at last? *Bone Marrow Transplant* 34(11):929-938, 2004.
9. Gutierrez-Delgado F, Maloney D, Press O et al: Autologous stem cell transplantation for non Hodgkin's lymphoma: comparison for radiation based and chemotherapy only preparatory regimens, *Bone Marrow Transplant* 28(5): 455-461, 2001.
10. Gutierrez-Delgado F, Holmberg L, Hooper H et al: Autologous stem cell transplantation for Hodgkin's disease: busulfan, melphalan, and thiotepa compared to radiation based regimen, *Bone Marrow Transplant* 32(3):279-285, 2003.
11. Rutledge D: Oncology nurses look to the latest evidence to treat mucositis, *ONS News* 20(2):1, 4-6, 2005.
12. Thomas E: Bone marrow transplantation; a review, *Semin Hematol* 36(4 suppl 7):95-103, 1999.
13. Specht L: History of radiation therapy of lymphomas and description of early trials. In Mauch P, Armitage J, Coiffier B, editors: *Non-Hodgkin's lymphomas,* Philadelphia, 2004, Lippincott Williams & Wilkins, p 36 and p 1191.
14. Constine L, Williams J, Morris M: Late effects of cancer treatment on normal tissues. In Perez CA, Brady LW, Halperin EC, Schmidt-Ullrich RK, editors: *Principles and practice of radiation oncology,* ed 4, Philadelphia, 2004, Lippincott Williams & Wilkins, pp 357-390.
15. van Bekkum D: Conditioning regimens for the treatment of experimental arthritis with autologous bone marrow transplantation, *Bone Marrow Transplant* 25(4):357-364, 2000.
16. Beriwal S, Brady L, Vonderheid C: Cutaneous T-cell lymphoma. In Perez CA, Brady LW, Halperin EC, Schmidt-Ullrich RK, editors: *Principles and practice of radiation oncology,* ed 4, Philadelphia, 2004, Lippincott Williams & Wilkins.
17. van Kempen-Harteveld, van Weel-Sipman M, Emmens C et al: Eye shielding during total body irradiation for bone marrow transplantation in children transplanted for a hematological disorder: risks and benefits, *Bone Marrow Transplant* 31(12):1151-1156, 2003.
18. Chen C, Abraham R, Tsang R et al: Radiation-associated pneumonitis following autologous stem cell transplantation predictive factors; disease characteristics and treatment outcome, *Bone Marrow Transplant* 27(2):177-182, 2001.
19. Gupta V, Lazarus H, Keating A: Myeloablative conditioning regimens for AML allografts: 30 years later, *Bone Marrow Transplant* 32(10):969-987, 2003.
20. Johansson J, Brune M, Ekman T: Reduced intensity conditioning: the gut mucosa barrier is preserved during allogeneic, haemopoietic stem cell transplantation with reduced intensity conditioning, *Bone Marrow Transplant* 28(8):737-742, 2001.
21. Filicko J, Lazarus H, Flomenberg N: Mucosal injury in patients undergoing hematopoietic progenitor cell transplantation: new approaches to prophylaxis and treatment, *Bone Marrow Transplant* 31(1):1-10, 2003.
22. Clarkson B, Strife A, Wisniewski D: Chronic myelogenous leukemia as a paradigm of early cancer and possible curative strategies, *Leukemia* 17(7):1211-1262, 2003.
23. Bredison C, Perry G, Martins C et al: Outpatient total body irradiation as a component of a comprehensive outpatient transplant program, *Bone Marrow Transplant* 29(8):667-671, 2002.
24. Adams MJ, Hardenbergh PH, Constine LS et al: Radiation-associated cardiovascular disease, *Crit Rev Oncol Hematol* 45(1):55-75, 2003.
25. Bunin N, Aplene R, Kamani N et al: Randomized trial of busulfan vs. total body irradiation containing conditioning regimens for children with acute lymphoblastic leukemia: a Pediatric Blood and Marrow Transplant Consortium study, *Bone Marrow Transplantat* 32(6):543-548, 2003.
26. Smith F, Woods W: Myeloproliferative and myelodysplastic disorders. In Pizzo PA, Poplack DG, editors: *Principles and practice of pediatric oncology,* ed 4, Philadelphia, 2002, Lippincott Williams & Wilkins, pp 614-628.
27. Tarbell NJ, Chin LM, Mauch PM: Total body irradiation for bone marrow transplantation. In Mauch P, Loeffler J, editors: *Radiation oncology: technology and biology,* Philadelphia, 1994, WB Saunders.
28. Kun LE: Leukemias in children. In Halperin EC, Constine LS, Tarbell NJ et al, editors: *Pediatric radiation oncology,* ed 4, Philadelphia, 2005, Lippincott Williams & Wilkins, pp 15-39.
29. Davies SM, Ramsay NK, Klein JP et al: Comparison of preparative regimens in transplants for children with acute lymphoblastic leukemia, *J Clin Oncol* 18(2): 340-347, 2000.
30. Guinan E, Krance R, Lehmann L: Stem cell transplantation in pediatric oncology. In Pizzo PA, Poplack DG, editors: *Principles and practice of pediatric oncology,* ed 4, Philadelphia, 2002, Lippincott Williams & Wilkins, pp 428-478.
31. Hudson MM, Constine LS: Hodgkin's disease. In Halperin EC, Constine LS, Tarbell NJ et al, editors: *Pediatric radiation oncology,* ed 4, Philadelphia, 2005, Lippincott Williams & Wilkins, pp 223-259.
32. Hudson MM, Donaldson S: Hodgkin's disease. In Pizzo PA, Poplack DG, editors: *Principles and practice of pediatric*

oncology, ed 4, Philadelphia, 2002, Lippincott Williams & Wilkins, pp 644-657.

33. Halperin EC, Constine LS, Tarbell NJ et al: Non-Hodgkin's lymphoma. In Halperin EC, Constine LS, Tarbell NJ et al, editors: *Pediatric radiation oncology,* ed 3, Philadelphia, 1999, Lippincott Williams & Wilkins, pp 233-244.
34. Matthay K, Haas-Kogan D, Constine L: Neuroblastoma. In Halperin EC, Constine LS, Tarbell NJ et al, editors: *Pediatric radiation oncology,* ed 4, Philadelphia, 2004, Lippincott Williams & Wilkins, pp 191-222.
35. Brodeur G, Maris J: Neuroblastoma. In Pizzo PA, Poplack DG, editors: *Principles and practice of pediatric oncology,* ed 4, Philadelphia, 2002, Lippincott Williams & Wilkins, pp 895-923.
36. Guinan E, Krance R, Lehmann L: Stem cell transplantation in pediatric oncology. In Pizzo PA, Poplack DG, editors: *Principles and practice of pediatric oncology,* ed 4, Philadelphia, 2002, Lippincott Williams & Wilkins, pp 429-478.
37. Matthay KK, Villablanca JG, Seegor RC et al: Treatment of high-risk neuroblastoma with intensive chemotherapy, radiotherapy, autologous bone marrow transplantation, and 13-cis-retinoic acid. Children's Cancer Group. *N Engl J Med* 341(16):1165-1173, 1999.
38. Linck D, Basara N, Tran V et al: Per-acute onset of severe tumor lysis syndrome immediately after 4 GY fractionated TBI as part of reduced intensity preparative regimen in a patient with T-ALL with high tumor burden, *Bone Marrow Transplant* 31(10):935-937, 2003.
39. Spitzer T, Friedman C, Bushnell W et al: Double-blind, randomized, parallel-group study on the efficacy and safety of oral granistron and oral ondansetron in the prophylaxis of nausea and vomiting in patients receiving hyper fractionated total body irradiation, *Bone Marrow Transplant* 26(2):203-210, 2000.
40. Magnan M, Mood D: The effects of health state, hemoglobin, global symptom distress, mood disturbance, and treatment site on fatigue onset, duration, and distress in patients receiving radiation therapy, *Oncol Nurs Forum* 30(2):E38-E39, 2003.
41. Papas A, Clark R, Martuscelli G et al: Post transplant complications: a prospective randomized trial for the prevention of mucositis in patients undergoing hematopoietic stem cell transplantation, *Bone Marrow Transplant* 31(8):705-712, 2003.
42. Castagna L, Benhamou E, Pedraza E et al: Prevention of mucositis in bone marrow transplantation: a double blind randomized controlled trial of sucralfate, *Ann Oncol* 12(7):953-955, 2001.
43. Woywodt A, Haubitz M, Buchholz S: Counting the cost: markers of endothelial damage in hematopoietic stem cell transplantation, *Bone Marrow Transplant* 34(12): 1015-1023, 2004.
44. Bearman S: Avoiding hepatic veno-occlusive disease: what do we know and where are we going, *Bone Marrow Transplant* 27(11):1113-1120, 2001.
45. Buchsel P: Bone marrow transplantation. In Miaskowski C, Buchsel P, editors: *Oncology nursing,* St. Louis, 1999, Mosby pp 143-303.
46. Ancher M, Peters W, Reisenbichler H et al: Transforming growth factor β as a predictor of liver, lung fibrosis after autologous bone marrow transplantation for advanced breast cancer, *N Engl J Med* 328(22):1592-1598, 1993.
47. The Internet Pathology Laboratory for Medical Education *medlib.med.utah.edu/WebPath/webpath.html.* Accessed July 16, 2005.
48. Bacigalupo A, Palandie F: Management of acute graft versus host disease, *Hematol J* 5(3):189-196, 2004.
49. Socie G, Salooja N, Cohen A et al: Nonmalignant late effects after allogeneic stem cell transplantation, *Blood* 101(9):3373-3385, 2003.
50. Marina N, Sharis C, Tarbell N: Respiratory complications. In Wallace H, Green D, editors: *Late effects of childhood cancer,* London, 2004, Arnold, pp 114-124.
51. *Mosby's medical, nursing and allied health dictionary,* ed 6, St. Louis, 2002, Mosby, p 473.
52. Skinner RT, Leiper A: Bone marrow transplantation. In Wallace H, Green D, editors: *Late effects of childhood cancer,* London, 2004, Arnold, pp 304-320.
53. Antin J: Long-term care after hematopoietic-cell transplantation in adults, *N Engl J Med* 347(1):36-41, 2002.
54. Friedman D, Constine L: Late effects of cancer treatment. In Halperin ER, Constine LS, Tarbell NJ et al, editors: *Pediatric radiation oncology,* ed 4, Philadelphia, 2004, Lippincott Williams & Wilkins, pp 523-611.
55. Dreyer Z, Blatt J, Bleyer A: Late effects of childhood cancer and its treatment. In Pizzo PA, Poplack DG, editors: *Principles and practice of pediatric oncology,* ed 4, Philadelphia, 2002, Lippincott Williams & Wilkins, pp 1431-1461.
56. Mulhern R, Phipps S, White H: Neuropsychological outcomes. In Wallace H, Green D, editors: *Late effects of childhood cancer,* London, 2004, Arnold, pp 18-37.
57. Holtta P, Alabuusua S, Saarinen-Pihkala U et al: Long term adverse effects on dentition in children with poor-risk neuroblastoma treated with high-dose chemotherapy and autologous stem cell transplantation with or without total body irradiation, *Bone Marrow Transplant* 29(2): 121-127, 2002.
58. Sonis A: Craniofacial development, teeth, and salivary glands. In Wallace H, Green D, editors: *Late effects of childhood cancer,* London, 2004, Arnold, pp 176-185.
59. Ober M, Beaverson K, Abramson D: Ocular complications. In Wallace H, Green D, editors: *Late effects of childhood cancer,* London, 2004, Arnold, pp 37-48.
60. Suh D, Ruttman M, Bradley J et al: Ocular findings after bone marrow transplantation in pediatric populations, *Ophthalmology* 106:1564-1570, 1999.
61. Critchley H, Thomson A, Wallace W: Ovarian and uterine function and reproductive potential. In Wallace H, Green D, editors: *Late effects of childhood cancer,* London, 2004, Arnold, pp 225-238.
62. Thomson A, Wallace W, Sklar C: Testicular function. In Wallace H, Green D, editors: *Late effects of childhood cancer,* London, 2004, Arnold, pp 239-256.
63. Bhatia S, Louie A, Bhatia R et al: Solid tumors after bone marrow transplantation, *J Clin Oncol* 19(2):464-471, 2001.
64. Brown J, Yeckes H, Friedberg J et al: Increasing incidence of late second malignancies after conditioning with cyclophosphamide and total-body irradiation and autologous

bone marrow transplantation for non-Hodgkin's lymphoma, *J Clin Oncol* 23(10):2208-2214, 2005.
65. Krishnan A, Bhatia S, Slovak D et al: Predictors of therapy-related leukemia and myelodysplasia following autologous transplantation for lymphoma: an assessment of risk factors, *Blood* 95(5):1588-1593, 2000.
66. Socie G, Curtis R, Deeg H et al: New malignant diseases after allogeneic marrow transplantation for acute childhood leukemia, *J Clin Oncol* 18(2):348-357, 2000.
67. Hoppe RT: Total lymphoid irradiation. In Mauch P, Loeffler J, editors: *Radiation oncology technology and biology*, Philadelphia, 1994, WB Saunders, pp 416-436.
68. Mauch PM, Ng AK, Wu ET et al: Principles of radiation therapy. In Mauch P, Armitage J, Coiffier B et al, editors: *Non-Hodgkin's lymphomas*, Philadelphia, 2004, Lippincott Williams & Wilkins, pp 173-199.
69. Serber W, Brady W, Zhang M et al: Radiation treatment of benign disease. In Perez CA, Brady LW, Halperin EC et al, editors: *Principles and practices of radiation oncology*, ed 4, Philadelphia, 2004, Lippincott Williams & Wilkins pp 2332-2351.
70. Padovan CS, Bise K, Hahn J et al: Angiitis of the central nervous system after allogeneic bone marrow transplantation? *Stroke* 30:1651-1656, 1999.
71. Patchell RA: Neurological complications of organ transplantation, *Ann Neurol* 36:688-703, 1994.
72. Thompson CB, Sanders JE, Flournoy N et al: The risks of central nervous system relapse and leukoencephalopathy in patients receiving marrow transplants for acute leukemia, *Blood* 67:195-199, 1986.
73. Padovan CS, Yousny TA, Schleuning M et al: Neurological and neuroradiological findings in long-term survivors of allogeneic bone marrow transplantation, *Ann Neurol* 43:627-633, 1998.
74. Christie D, Battin M, Leiper AD et al: Neuropsychological and neurological outcome after relapse of lymphoblastic leukaemia, *Arch Dis Child* 70:275-280, 1994.
75. Kupst MJ, Penati B, Oebban B et al: Cognitive and psychosocial functioning of pediatric hematopoietic stem cell transplant patients: a prospective longitudinal study, *Bone Marrow Transplant* 30:609-617, 2002.
76. Phipps S, Dunavant M, Srivastava DK et al: Cognitive and academic functioning in survivors of pediatric bone marrow transplantation, *J Clin Oncol* 18:1004-1011, 2000.
77. Kramer JH, Crittenden MR, DeSantes K et al: Cognitive and adaptive behavior 1 and 3 years following bone marrow transplantation, *Bone Marrow Transplant* 19:607-613, 1997.
78. Leiper AD: Non-endocrine late complications of bone marrow transplantation in childhood: part I, *Br J Haematol* 118:3-22, 2002.
79. Nasman M, Forsberg CM, Dahllof G: Long-term dental development in children after treatment for malignant disease, *Eur J Orthod* 19:151-159, 1997.
80. Dahllof G, Bagesund M, Ringden O: Impact of conditioning regimens on salivary function, caries-associated microorganisms and dental caries in children after bone marrow transplantation: a 4-year longitudinal study, *Bone Marrow Transplant* 20:479-483, 1997.
81. Woo S-B, Lee SJ, Schubert MM: Graft-vs.-host disease, *Crit Rev Oral Biol Med* 8:201-216, 1997.
82. Oahllof G, Forsberg CM, Ringden O et al: Facial growth and morphology in long-term survivors after bone marrow transplantation, *Eur J Orthod* 11:332-340, 1989.
83. Curtis RE, Rowlings PA, Deeg HJ et al: Solid cancers after bone marrow transplantation, *N Engl J Med* 336: 897-904, 1997.
84. Calissendorff BM, Bolme P: Cataract development and outcome of surgery in bone marrow transplanted children, *Br J Ophthalmol* 77:36-38, 1993.
85. De-Marco R, Dassio DA, Vittone P: A retrospective study of ocular side effects in children undergoing bone marrow transplantation, *Eur J Ophthalmol* 6:436-439, 1996.
86. Coskuncan NM, Jabs DA, Dunn JP et al: The eye in bone marrow transplantation. VI. retinal complications, *Arch Ophthalmol* 112:372-379, 1994.
87. Parsons SK, Neault MW, Lehmann LE et al: Severe ototoxicity following carboplatin-containing conditioning regimen for autologous marrow transplantation for neuroblastoma, *Bone Marrow Transplant* 22:669-674, 1998.
88. Liesner RJ, Leiper AD, Hann IM et al: Late effects of intensive treatment for acute myeloid leukemia and myelodysplasia in childhood, *J Clin Oncol* 12:916-924, 1994.
89. Eames GM, Crosson J, Steinberger J et al: Cardiovascular function in children following bone marrow transplant: a cross-sectional study, *Bone Marrow Transplant* 19:61-66, 1997.
90. Pihkala J, Saarinen UM, Lundstrom U et al: Effects of bone marrow transplantation on myocardial function in children, *Bone Morrow Transplant* 13:149-155, 1994.
91. Nysom K, Holm K, Hesse B et al: Lung function after allogeneic bone marrow transplantation for leukaemia or lymphoma, *Arch Dis Child* 74;432-436, 1996.
92. Leung W, Hudson MM, Strickland DK et al: Late effects of treatment in survivors of childhood acute myeloid leukemia, *J Clin Oncol* 18:3273-3279, 2000.
93. Kist-van Holthe JE, van Zwet JML, Brand R et al: Bone marrow transplantation in children: consequences for renal function shortly after *and* 1 year post-BMT, *Bone Marrow Transplant* 22:559-564, 1998.
94. Van Why SK, Friedman AL, Wei LJ et al: Renal insufficiency after bone marrow transplantation in children, *Bone Marrow Transplant* 7:383-388, 1991.
95. Patzer L, Ringelmann F, Kentouche K et al: Renal function in long-term survivors of stem cell transplantation in childhood. A prospective trial, *Bone Marrow Transplant* 27:319-327, 2001.
96. Tarbell NJ, Guinan EC, Niemeyer C et al: Late onset of renal dysfunction in survivors of bone marrow transplantation, *Int J Radiat Oncol Biol Phys* 15:99-104, 1988.
97. Oliveira JSR, Bahai D, Franco M et al: Nephrotic syndrome as a clinical manifestation of graft-versus-host disease (GVHO) in a marrow transplant recipient after cyclosporine withdrawal, *Bone Marrow Transplant* 23: 99-101, 1999.
98. Gomez-Garcia P, Herrera-Arroyo C Torres-Gomez A et al: Renal involvement in chronic graft-versus-host disease: a report of two cases, *Bone Marrow Transplant* 3: 357-362, 1988.
99. Frisk P, Bratteby LE, Carlson K et al: Renal function after autologous bone marrow transplantation in children:

a long-term prospective study, *Bone Marrow Transplant* 29:129-136, 2002.
100. Sherer Y, Shoenfeld Y: Autoimmune diseases and autoimmunity post-bone marrow transplantation, *Bone Marrow Transplant* 22:873-881, 1998.
101. Thomas BC, Stanhope R, Plowman PN et al: Endocrine function following single fraction and fractionated total body irradiation for bone marrow transplantation in childhood, *Acta Endocrinol* 128:508-512, 1993.
102. Al-Fiar FZ, Colwill R, Upton JH et al: Abnormal thyroid stimulating hormone (TSH) levels in adults following allogeneic bone marrow transplants, *Bone Marrow Transplant* 19:1019-1022, 1997.
103. Taskinen M, Saarinen-Pihkala UM, Hovi L et al: Impaired glucose tolerance and dyslipidaemia as late effects after bone-marrow transplantation in childhood, *Lancet* 356:993-997, 2000.
104. Traggiai C, Stanhope R, Nussey S et al: Diabetes mellitus after bone marrow transplantation in childhood, *Med Pediatr Oncol* 40:128-129, 2003.
105. Cohen A, Rovelli A, Bakker B et al: Final height of patients who underwent bone marrow transplantation for hematological disorders during childhood: a study by the Working Party for Late Effects—EBMT, *Blood* 93: 4109-4115, 1999.
106. Adan L, de Lanversin M-L, Thalassinos C et al: Growth after bone marrow transplantation in young children conditioned with chemotherapy alone, *Bone Marrow Transplant* 19:253-256, 1997.
107. Sanders JE: Growth and development after hematopoietic cell transplantation. In Thomas ED, Blume KG, Forman SJ, editors: *Hematopoietic cell transplantation,* ed 2, Malden, 1999, Blackwell Science, pp 764-775.
108. Holm K, Nysom K, Rasmussen MH et al: Growth, growth hormone, and final height after BMT. Possible recovery of irradiation-induced growth hormone insufficiency, *Bone Marrow Transplant* 18:163-170, 1996.
109. Sarafoglou K, Boulad F, Gillio A et al: Gonadal function after bone marrow transplantation for acute leukemia during childhood, *J Pediatr* 130:210-216, 1997.
110. Sanders JE, Hawley J, Levy W et al: Pregnancies following high-dose cyclophosphamide with or without high-dose busulfan or total-body irradiation and bone marrow transplantation, *Blood* 87:3045-3052, 1996.
111. Socie G, Cahn JY, Carmela J et al: Avascular necrosis of bone after allogeneic bone marrow transplantation: analysis of risk factors for 4388 patients by the Societe Francaise de Greffe de Moelle (SFGM), *Br J Haematol* 97:865-870, 1997.
112. Harper GD, Dicks-Mireaux C, Leiper AD: Total body irradiation-induced osteochondromata, *J Pediatr Orthop* 18:356-358, 1998.
113. Nysom K, Holm K, Michaelsen KF et al: Bone mass after allogeneic BMT for childhood leukaemia or lymphoma, *Bone Marrow Transplant* 25:191-196, 2000.
114. Bhatia S, Ramsay NK, Weisdorf D et al: Bone mineral density in patients undergoing bone marrow transplantation for myeloid malignancies, *Bone Marrow Transplant* 22:87-90, 1998.
115. Bhatia S, Ramsay NKC, Steinbuch M et al: Malignant neoplasms following bone marrow transplantation, *Blood* 87:3633-3639, 1996.
116. Deeg HJ, Socie G: Malignancies after hematopoietic stem cell transplantation: many questions, some answers, *Blood* 91:1833-1844, 1998.

Chapter 27 Hyperthermia

Tracy K. Gosselin-Acomb

Hyperthermia (HT) is the use of heat to kill cancer cells. Records dating back to Homer's era (800 B.C.) describe the healing qualities of hot steam baths in the treatment of many illnesses.[1] Hyperthermia has been used since the late 1800s, and one of the first written reports on the effects of hyperthermia was by Busch, reporting the disappearance of tumors after episodes of high fever.[2,3] Other authors reported similar occurrences of tumor regression following periods of fever. Warren[4] described the effects of heating patients after irradiation and produced hyperthermia by using a heating cabinet that contained carbon filament bulbs. Immediate improvement in the patient's condition and tumor shrinkage was observed. Hornback[1] noted that although there was continued interest in hyperthermia during the first half of the twentieth century, the development of radiation therapy was underway, and many scientists were more enthusiastic about improving x rays than continuing hyperthermia studies.

The 1970s and 1980s brought about new interest in the field of HT. Significant improvements were made in equipment, techniques, and thermometry (measurement of temperatures). A worldwide interest in hyperthermia was initiated by the first International Congress on Hyperthermia Oncology in 1975.[5] Grant funding increased and commercial development was instrumental in the progression of HT to an accepted treatment modality.

In the late 1980s and early 1990s funding for HT research decreased. The Food and Drug Administration (FDA) increased regulations on manufacturers of hyperthermia equipment and insurance reimbursements also decreased. The Radiation Therapy Oncology Group (RTOG) conducted a study (1981–2004) comparing radiation therapy (RT) to RT combined with HT. The complete response (CR) rate in the combined arm was 32% and in the RT arm alone 28%.[6] Poor quality control and overall outcome of this trial dealt clinical hyperthermia a possibly lethal blow in this country.[7] Recently, renewed interest in HT has been seen as a result of the results of positive clinical trials in a variety of disease sites (Table 27-1).

Hyperthermia is rarely used alone in the treatment of cancer. It may be administered in the neoadjuvant or adjuvant setting or in combination with chemotherapy (CT) and/or RT. Studies have evaluated its role with other treatments for cure, control, and palliation of disease. The combination of RT and HT produce greater cell kill than either treatment alone. Hyperthermia enhances the effect of radiation through an additive and synergistic effect, with the most therapeutic benefit attained when the irradiation is followed by hyperthermia.[8] When HT is given, the goal is to heat the targeted area to 40° C to 44° C. A variety of biologic events occur as a result of HT that impact tumors.[6,9,10]

1. Heat is directly cytotoxic and kills cells in a predictable and repeatable way. It has been shown that temperatures of 42° C produce cell killing.
2. Radioresistant S-phase cells are sensitive to the effects of HT.
3. Cells that are nutrient deficient or have a low pH are more sensitive to heat. Tumors tend to be hypoxic because of poor vascularity and thus are radioresistant. By combining the two modalities, RT will destroy the vascular (nutrient and oxygen) enriched peripheral cells, whereas the HT will be effective on the hypoxic components.
4. Heated cells develop a thermotolerance (resistance to further heating). This has been shown to be a significant effect. Cell thermotolerance does decrease; however, it has been shown to last as long as 80 to 100 hours and is associated with cell cycling time and

Table 27-1 Hyperthermia Clinical Trials

Author/study	Disease site	Treatment	Results
Anscher N = 15	Locally advanced, unresectable, or recurrent adenocarcinoma of the rectum	CI of 5-FU 250 mg/m²/day, 7 days a week during RT RT 1.8 Gy/day to 45 Gy total, M-F Regional whole pelvis HT on days 3, 8, 15, 22, and 29 Surgery 3–6 weeks after above treatment	All patients completed chemoradiotherapy Eleven of 15 patients completed all HT treatments Eleven patients had resectable disease One had pathologic CR
Blackwell N = 21	Locally advanced breast carcinoma	Dose-escalation schema of 4 cycles every 3 weeks of liposomal doxorubicin and paclitaxel followed by 1 hour of HT	Clinical CR 33% Partial clinical response 56% Clinically stable disease 11%
Jones N = 12*	Locally advanced cervical carcinoma	Weekly cisplatin 40 mg/m² RT 1.8 Gy/day to 45 Gy–50.4 Gy, M-F LDR tandem and ovoid to a cumulative dose of 80 Gy, followed by a EBRT sidewall boost Regional whole pelvis HT weekly for 5 treatments	Ten patients had a clinical CR Two experienced recurrence outside the pelvis Initial CR rate 92% and local CR 83%
Jones N = 122†	Superficial tumors of the breast/chest wall, head and neck, melanoma, and other sites	RT 1.8 Gy–2.0 Gy/day, to 30 Gy–66 Gy for previously treated patients and 60 Gy –70 Gy for previously unirradiated patients, M-F and no HT or RT 1.8 Gy–2.0 Gy/day, to 30 Gy–66 Gy for previously treated patients and 60 Gy–70 Gy for previously unirradiated patients, M-F and HT twice a week for a maximum of 10 treatments	CR in the HT arm 66% vs. 42% in the non-HT arm OS not significantly different between the groups
Sneed N =112	Glioblastoma multiforme	RT Brachytherapy boost or RT Brachytherapy boost with HT	Median time to progression 33 weeks non-HT arm and 49 weeks HT arm Two-year survival of 15% non-HT vs. 31% HT
van der Zee N = 115	Locally advanced cervical carcinoma	RT or RT and HT	CR rates improved from 57% to 83% with HT Survival at 3 years was 52% (RT and HT) and 27% (RT alone)

Data from Anscher MS, Lee C, Hurwitz H, et al: *Int J Radiat Oncol Biol Phys* 47(3):719-724, 2000; Blackwell KL, Vujaskovic Z, Rosen E, et al: *Proc Am Soc Clin Oncol* 21:200a, 2002 (abstract); Jones EL, Samulski TV, Dewhirst MW, et al: *Cancer* 98(2):277-282, 2003; Jones EJ, Oleson JR, Prosnitz LP, et al: *J Clin Oncol* 23(13):3079-3085, 2005; Sneed PK, Stauffer PR, McDermott MW, et al: *Int J Radiat Oncol Biol Phys* 40(2):287-295, 1998; van der Zee J, Gonzalez D, van Rhoon GC, et al: *Lancet* 355(9210):1119-1125, 2000.

*Ten patients treated at initial diagnosis.

†Thirteen patients were deemed to be unheatable, 109 randomly assigned.

CI, Continuous infusion; *5-FU*, 5-fluorouracil; *RT*, radiation therapy; *M-F*, Monday to Friday; *HT*, hyperthermia; *CR*, complete response; *LDR*, low dose rate; *EBRT*, external beam radiation therapy; *OS*, overall survival.

lowered pH. The interaction between RT and HT is described by the "thermal enhancement ratio" (TER), which is analogous to a dose-modifying factor for any adjuvant to radiation. This may allow less RT to be used.
5. Heat inhibits the repair of RT damage and increases the therapeutic ratio.
6. Heat increases vascularity and permeability of certain CT agents, thus improving the effect.

Mechanisms of action appear complimentary to radiation effects with regard to inhibition of potential lethal damage, sublethal damage repair, cell cycle sensitivity, and effects of hypoxia and nutrient deprivation.[9] By having a direct effect on the vasculature and blood flow of the tumor, CT may enter the tumor more readily. Higher perfusion can increase drug delivery and reoxygenation (increasing the efficacy of RT).[11] However, more recent studies claim not the hypoxia per se but the low pH associated with hypoxia is responsible for the increased thermosensitivity of cells.[2]

HT is typically used with CT and/or RT and may be used before surgery with CT/RT to downstage the disease and decrease the extent of surgery required. It has been shown that the addition of HT to mitomycin-C, nitrosureas, cisplatin, doxorubicin, and mitoxantrone can counteract drug resistance.[5] Liposomal doxorubicin also may be used to minimize the systemic effects. CT is typically given before or during the HT session for optimum benefit. The most important mechanisms for an interactive effect are an increased intracellular drug uptake, enhanced DNA damage, and higher intratumor drug concentrations, resulting from increased blood flow.[5] Clinical trials may employ a tri-modality approach with CT, HT, and RT.

TREATMENT

HT can be used to treat a wide variety of diseases in combination with CT and/or RT or may be used alone in certain clinical conditions (Box 27-1). Patients requiring HT typically enroll in a clinical trial. Type of disease, location, and size of the tumor are critical factors that need to be considered. Depending upon these variables, patients may receive local, regional, or whole-body hyperthermia. The heating is accomplished by exposing the area to conductive heat sources or nonionizing radiation sources such as electromagnetic and ultrasound heating devices. Local hyperthermia pertains to heating only a tumor-bearing area. In most cases, these are superficial skin or subcutaneous masses that can be easily defined and evaluated. The primary target is the tumor mass only, with very little margin of normal tissue included in the heating field. Intracranial malignancies also may be treated with local HT. Regional HT refers to treating a tumor site and surrounding normal tissue. These are usually situations in which the tumor volume is diffuse and difficult to define, necessitating treatment of a whole region rather than a localized area. Whole-body HT is a method that elevates the temperature of the whole body (core temperature) and is used for disseminated disease.

Box 27-1 Cancers Treated With Hyperthermia

Breast
Cervical
Glioblastoma multiforme
Head and neck
Malignant melanoma
Rectal
Sarcomas

HT is commonly given one to two times a week after an RT and/or CT treatment. Certain protocols may have the patient receiving infusional CT and HT at the same time. These patients are typically on a 21- or 28-day cycle. Some patients with inflammatory breast cancer may receive HT every day while undergoing RT, because of the size of the treatment field. Other protocols may have the patient receive HT with CT and/or RT preoperatively. Then after surgery the HT and CT may continue for a few more cycles.

Patients receiving HT should undergo a thorough evaluation before treatment. Treatment is not feasible in patients with metallic implants such as orthopedic rods and plates, as well as patients with surgical clips, shrapnel, and other foreign bodies. Because of the electromagnetic nature of the HT treatment device, excessive heat may result in pain and tissue damage. Patients with significant cardiovascular disease or other medical conditions that would put them at risk for physiologic stress should not be treated with HT; this also applies to those who are pregnant, have severe neuropathy, or who have grafts and skin flaps.[12] Pacemakers also present a contraindication to HT.

General Procedures

Before the initiation of treatment, patients may receive anxiolytics or pain medications to assist with comfort during treatment. Depending on the tumor location and size, a sterile, blind-ended interstitial catheter will be placed in the tumor after local anesthetic of lidocaine and sodium bicarbonate is administered. Imaging of the catheter(s) after placement, verifies the temperature measurement or heating source locations. It is extremely important to have this information during the treatment execution and when achieved temperatures are being analyzed.[13] Imaging is usually done on a CT scanner in the radiation oncology department.

The patient is then assisted onto a stretcher and escorted to the treatment room where a fiberoptic thermometer(s) will be placed in the catheter(s) for temperature monitoring. The thermometer may then be attached to a mechanical device that will move it within the tumor for automated temperature mapping within the tumor. Additional thermometry devices may be placed on the skin and scar areas to monitor normal tissue temperatures. The actual treatment time itself is 60 to 90 minutes. The treatment room may have shielding to minimize exposure to staff from electromagnetic radiation during the heating process.

Once the patient has achieved optimum heating time, the treatment is then stopped. The thermometry is removed, and depending on the patient, the catheter may or may not be removed. The catheter site is then cleaned and an antibiotic ointment and dry sterile dressing are applied. For patients who have catheters left in, they may be sutured into place so they do not fall out. The treated area is inspected for any sign of thermal changes (erythema, blisters, extremely warm to touch). Patients are instructed to contact their physician or nurse if they experience an elevation of temperature, pain, sign of infection, or catheter displacement. The patient should be assisted to a sitting position because some patients may experience hypotension. The patient should not drive home if anxiolytics or pain medicine were administered. Discharge instructions should include contact information, side effects that may arise, catheter site care, and the need to increase fluids during the next 24 hours.

The importance of continuous monitoring and documentation during each treatment is critical. Blood pressure, pulse, applicator position, patient comfort, and acute symptoms must be assessed and monitored throughout the treatment. The use of distraction techniques such as music, guided imagery, puzzle books, and conversation with the patient may assist in distracting him or her during treatment time.

Local

Local hyperthermia is used to treat superficial tumors of the skin or those tumors that can be directly palpated below the skin. Local HT can be delivered by external, intraluminal, or interstitial methods.[5] Patients receiving local HT may not require anxiolytics or pain medicine if a catheter is not placed within the tumor. A variety of different treatment devices can be used for superficial treatment including waveguide applicators, spiral applicators, and current sheet applicators (Figure 27-1).

Regional

Regional hyperthermia is used to treat deep-seated tumors in the abdomen and pelvis. It also may be used to treat extremity sarcomas. Catheters may be placed in the vagina, rectum, and/or the tumor, depending on the location. Additional thermometry may be placed in a Foley catheter and/or on the skin. Regional deep hyperthermia is often associated with physiologic stress similar to that seen in an exercise workout.[9] Several challenges are associated with heating deep-seated tumors including (1) heating of tumors when the body thickness is more than 25 cm and in the peripheral region of the tumor, (2) use of an external heating technique, (3) blood flow within the tumor and inhomogeneity of tissues make it difficult to keep the minimum tumor temperature of 41° C or more; and (4) because 1 kW of power is necessary to raise the tumor temperature to 42° C or more in the visceral organs such as the liver, the gallbladder, and the pancreas, consequently the whole body temperature may rise to as high as 39.5° C.[14]

When regional HT is applied to limbs, without a cytotoxic agent, the temperature can be increased to ≈43° C for a duration of 2 hours, but must be lower in combination with cytostatic drugs to

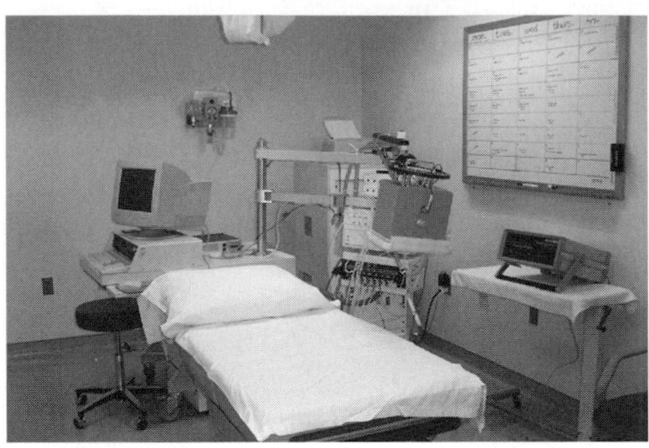

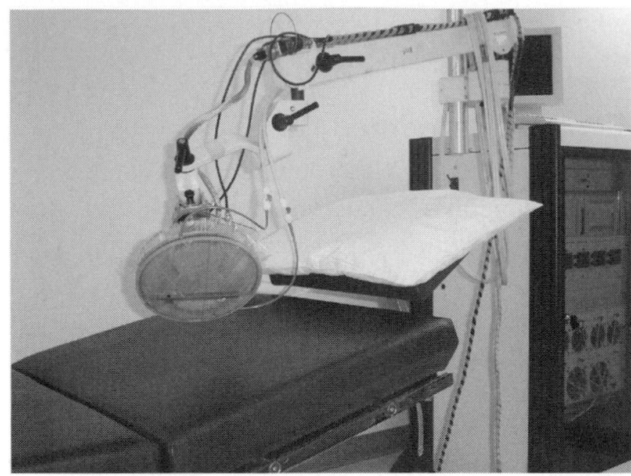

Figure 27-1 Superficial Treatment Devices.
Courtesy of the Department of Radiation Oncology, Duke University Hospital.

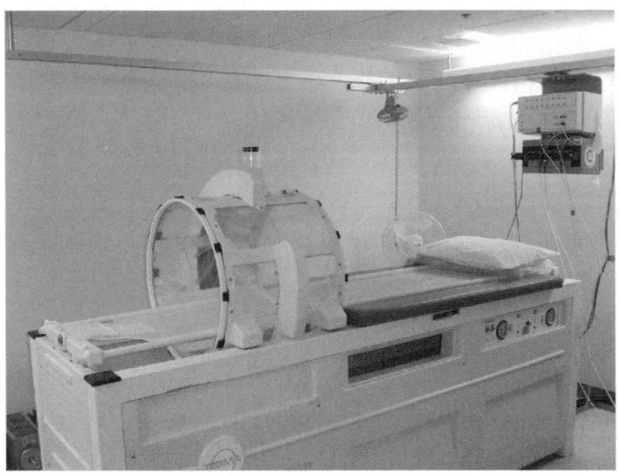

Figure 27-2 Deep-Seated Treatment Device.
Courtesy of the Department of Radiation Oncology, Duke University Hospital.

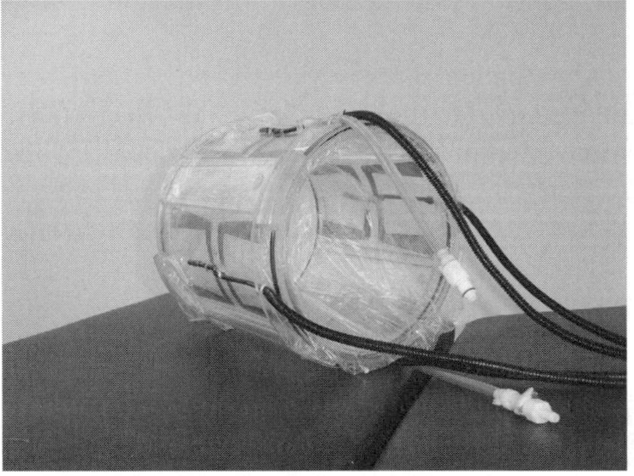

Figure 27-3 Extremity Treatment Device.
Courtesy of the Department of Radiation Oncology, Duke University Hospital.

avoid unacceptable toxicity.[5] The treatment device for deep-seated (Figure 27-2) and extremity treatment (Figure 27-3) are similar, with the exception of the extremity device being built to smaller scale. Magnetic resonance tomography may be used so the treatment team can see how the area is perfusing and heating during treatment. At Duke University Medical Center, researchers developed a hybrid system of treatment integrating a hyperthermia unit with a 1.5 T (Tesla) tunnel magnet to monitor heat and perfusion of patients.

Whole-Body

Whole-body HT (WBH) represents the only HT technique that enables systemic heat treatment in patients with disseminated malignancies and is therefore usually combined with systemic chemotherapy.[15] The aim of extreme WBH is to raise the temperature of the entire body to 41.5° C to 42° C over 90 to 150 minutes using a safe power input and to maintain this temperature for at least 60 minutes.[15] WBH is not as common as superficial and regional HT in the United States. Its efficacy has yet to be proven in the scope of a randomized clinical trial.[15]

Patients undergoing WBH require intensive monitoring during and after the treatment. The Interdisciplinary Working Group for Hyperthermia have specific eligibility criteria (Box 27-2) and treatment recommendations for patients who undergo WBH.[15] Patients should receive venous access placement and prehydration before treatment. Deep sedation or general anesthesia is given so the patient can tolerate treatment. The patient's entire body, excluding the head, are placed within the treatment device (Figure 27-4).

The most important side effects of WBH are skin burns, peripheral neuropathy, psychogenic disorders, and arrhythmias.[15] The rate of severe side effects was approximately 3% (neutropenic sepsis and multiorgan dysfunction) in 450 patients who received 1500 treatments in clinical trials.[15]

Heating Techniques

Heating of tumors is achieved through ultrasound, interstitial, and electromagnetic techniques. Treatment devices that employ a water bolus are heated by electromagnetic or ultrasound sources that include microwaves and radiofrequency. Although these modalities deposit energy in tissue by different physical mechanisms, they have general similarities. They are sensitive to the heterogeneity of tissue properties, geometry of blood flow, and the practical problems of coupling the energy source with tissue.[9] The temperature increase is induced by applying a power-density specific absorption rate (SAR; measured W/kg).[16] Temperature distributions achieved to date have limited absolute values and homogeneity (minimal temperatures typically lie between 39.5° C and 40.5° C), mainly because of physical and physiologic characteristics such as electrical tissue boundaries, local perfusion variations, and perfusion regulations.[11] Spatial and temporal variations for perfusion, changing of the tumor size, gas in the intestines, or the difference between the absorbed power displayed on the monitor of the heating equipment and the actual power absorbed in the patient's body are some of the heating challenges encountered in regional HT.[14]

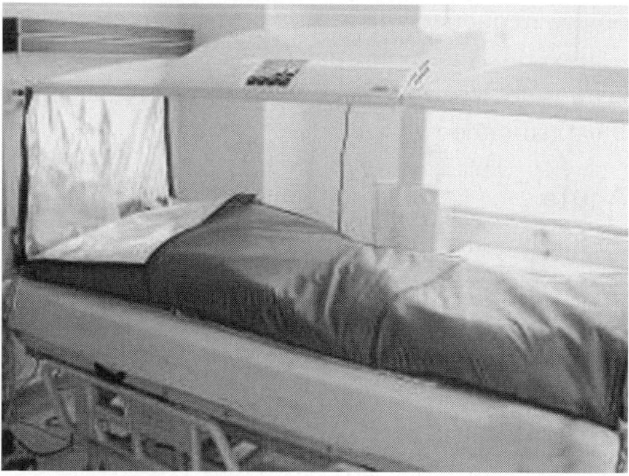

Figure 27-4 Whole-Body Treatment Device. *Courtesy of the Center for Thermal-Therapy Cancer Treatment in the Clinical Research Unit of Memorial Herman Hospital and the University of Texas Medical School-Houston.*

Box 27-2 General Eligibility Criteria for Whole-Body Hyperthermia

- ECOG (WHO)—Performance status index: 0, 1, 2
- Life expectancy of more than 12 weeks
- Creatinine clearance greater than 60 mL/min-1, if potentially nephritic substances (e.g., carboplatin, ifosfamide) are to be applied
- Left ventricular ejection fraction more than 60%, no evidence of relevant arrhythmias or other dysrhythmias, normal findings in resting and exercise ECG respiration stress echocardiography
- No current treatment with β-receptor antagonist
- No hyperthyroidism
- Pulmonary vital capacity more than 50%, FEV more than 50%, CO-diffusion capacity more than 50%
- No evidence of brain metastases
- No fracture-prone osteolysis
- Measurable disease
- Possibility of a regular, long-term follow-up

Data from Hildebrandt B, Hegewisch-Becker S, Kerner T, et al: *Int J Hyperthermia* 21(2):169-183, 2005.
ECOG, Eastern Cooperative Oncology Group; *WHO*, World Health Organization; *ECG*, electrocardiogram; *FEV*, forced expiratory volume.

Quality Assurance

A comprehensive quality assurance program is essential to ensure proper delivery of heat treatment to a specific area at a specific temperature for a specific amount of time. Strict guidelines are necessary to accomplish this repeatedly. Nurses, physicians, physicists, and therapists must collaborate to establish safe treatment practices.

NURSING IMPLICATIONS

The toxicity from HT varies based on type of disease, treatment site, and the heating mechanism used. These variables can be impacted by performance status and other treatment modalities that are being used. In regional and whole-body HT, larger volumes of tissue and deeper planes are heated. The areas, depth of heating, blood flow, power, frequency, and temperature are components that could cause potential side effects. Overall, the acute and late toxicities of HT are tolerable for most patients.

Acute

The acute side effects of HT arise during treatment or posttreatment. The most common side effect is superficial or subcutaneous tissue burn of first or second degree, which occurs in approximately 5% of all hyperthermia treatment sessions.[9] The skin should be assessed before and after each treatment for any skin reactions. Reactions can range from brisk erythema to blisters to moist desquamation. Pain may be associated with the skin reaction, infection, or irritation to the catheter site. Patients who have skin grafts need to be monitored closely. If pain or pressure arises during treatment, it is important that the patient report this so the power can be redirected if necessary so a "hot spot" is not created and thereby the potential for a skin reaction increases. Patients who have undergone surgery or have existing peripheral neuropathy may not feel the pain or pressure associated with treatment.

Subcutaneous fat or muscle tissue burns do not usually cause much discomfort: the patient feels a subcutaneous lump, which is tender for a few days to a maximum of a few weeks and then disappears spontaneously. Subcutaneous fat burns were seen in 3% to 12% of patients with deep hyperthermia.[5] Experimental studies have shown that most normal tissues are not damaged when the temperature over 1 hour of treatment does not exceed 44° C.[16] Patients who have undergone surgery in the past may have decreased sensitivity to feeling the pressure. During any application of hyperthermia, it is important to avoid pressure sites, because hypoxic normal tissues will be more sensitive to hyperthermia.[5]

During the treatment, patients are at risk for becoming dehydrated. This may be related to the CT, RT, HT, or a combination of factors. Patients may experience diaphoresis, flushing, and increased thirst. Patients can have ice chips during the treatment and are encouraged to increase their fluid intake after treatment. Nausea and vomiting associated with large amounts of heat given in a short period of time is usually short-term and resolves after the power is turned off and the treatment has stopped.[11] Patients receiving regional HT to the abdominal/pelvic area are more at risk for nausea because of the placement of the treatment device and the pressure that they may feel.

Patients are at risk for bleeding and/or infection related to the catheter placement and should be educated. Pressure should be applied to the site if it should start to bleed. If the catheter site requires a dressing, the patient should be taught how to assess the site and how to perform the dressing change. The incidence of myelosuppression can increase if combined modality therapy is used. Blood counts should be monitored for anemia, neutropenia, and thrombocytopenia.

Fatigue is a common side effect of many cancer therapies. Patients receiving combined modality therapy may experience fatigue for a variety of reasons. Patients receiving regional or WBH may experience more fatigue than those who receive superficial HT. Patients are encouraged to rest after the treatment and usually are able to return to their normal activities within 1 to 2 days.

Late

The two most common late effects of HT are fat necrosis and thermal injury. Fat necrosis can take several months to heal and currently there are no treatment options for it. Third-degree burns from HT often may require a skin graft. Fertility may be impacted depending on the treatment site, especially if HT is combined with another treatment modality. Other organ sites are also sensitive to the effects of HT and therefore ongoing monitoring and continued follow-up of patients is critical to identifying side effects and developing interventions as needed.

Patient Education

Patient education is an essential component of the care provided to patients who are going to receive HT. HT is very different than other cancer treatments, and it is important that the patient fully understand the treatment plan and see the treatment device before the initiation of therapy to decrease any anxiety that they may have in relation to the treatment. The side effects, self-care interventions, and follow-up plan should also be discussed with the patient.

SUMMARY

Hyperthermia is a specialized treatment that is not provided at all facilities because of resource needs and expertise in the field. Patients often have to travel to academic medical centers. Ongoing clinical trials employing different treatment regimens, better heating techniques, and quality thermal dosimetry continue to enhance the efficacy of HT. For chest wall recurrence of the breast, head and neck cancer, esophageal cancer, and melanoma, HT has shown to significantly increase the complete response rate.[17] Research in the area of liposomal agents in combination with HT, gene therapy, and isolated perfusion techniques continues to show promise. The ongoing development of three-dimensional techniques with magnetic resonance imaging (MRI) for monitoring and controlling of heat delivery will assist in facilitating this treatment. The need for quality of life and symptom management studies in this area is critical to understanding the patient experience.

REFERENCES

1. Hornback N: Hyperthermia and cancer: human clinical trial experience. 1. Boca Raton, 1984, CRC Press.
2. Gurkan Zorlu C, Eylem Seker Ari P: Hyperthermia in gynecologic cancers, *Eur J Gynaec Oncol* 24(3-4):282-286, 2003.
3. Busch W: Uber den Einfluss Welchen Heftigere Erysipein Zuweillen Auf Organisierte Neubildunge Ausuben, *Verhandlung-gen des Naturhistorischen Vereines der Preussischen Rheinlande und Westphalens* 23:28, 1866.
4. Warren SL: Preliminary study of the effect of artificial fever upon hopeless cases, *AJR Am J Roentgenol* 33:75, 1935.
5. van der Zee J: Heating the patient: a promising approach? *Ann Oncol* 13(8):1173-1184, 2002.
6. Perez CA, Pajak T, Emami B et al: Randomized phase III study comparing irradiation and hyperthermia with irradiation alone in superficial measurable tumors: final report by the Radiation Therapy Oncology Group, *Am J Clin Oncol* 14(2):133-141, 1991.
7. Storm FK: What happened to hyperthermia and what is its current status in cancer treatment? *J Surg Oncol* 53(3): 141-143, 1993.
8. Martin CW, Whitehead T: Radiation modifiers chemical and thermal. In Watkins-Bruner D, Moore-Higgs G, Haas M, editors: *Outcomes in radiation therapy*, ed 1, Boston, 2001, Jones and Bartlett, pp 102-116.
9. Jones EL, Samulski TV, Vujaskovic Z et al: Hyperthermia. In Perez CA, Brady LW, Halperin EC, Schmidt-Ullrich RK, editors: *Principles and practice of radiation oncology*, ed 4, Philadelphia, 2004, Lippincott Williams & Wilkins, pp 699-735.
10. Hall EJ, Roizin-Towle L: Biological effects of heat, *Cancer Res* 44(10 suppl):4708s-4713s, 1984.
11. Wust P, Hildebrandt B, Sreenivasa G et al: Hyperthermia in combined treatment of cancer, *Lancet* 3(8):487-497, 2002.
12. Gosselin-Acomb TK: Hyperthermia. In Bruner DW, Haas M, Gosselin-Acomb TK, editors: *Manual for radiation oncology nursing practice and education*, ed 3, Pittsburgh, 2005, Oncology Nursing Society, pp 205-207.
13. Hynynen K, Lulu BA: Hyperthermia in cancer treatment, *Invest Radiol* 25(7):824-834, 1990.
14. Kato H, Koyama T, Nikawa Y: Research and development of hyperthermia machines for present and future clinical needs, *Int J Hyperthermia* 14(1):1-11, 1998.
15. Hildebrandt B, Hegewisch-Becker S, Kerner T et al: Current status of radiant whole-body hyperthermia at tem peratures >41.5°C and practical guidelines for the treatment of adults. The German Interdisciplinary Working Group on Hyperthermia, *Int J Hyperthermia* 21(2):169-183, 2005.
16. Fajardo LF: Pathological effects of hyperthermia in normal tissues, *Cancer Res* 44(10 suppl):4826s-4835s, 1984.
17. Jones EJ, Oleson JR, Prosnitz LP, et al: Randomized trial of hyperthermia and radiation for superficial tumors, *J Clin Oncol* 23(13):3079-3085, 2005.

Chapter 28

GliaSite Radiation Therapy System

Eileen Maloney Wilensky, Marilyn L. Haas, and William P. Hogle

The American Cancer Society estimates that 18,820 cases of brain and central nervous system (CNS) tumors will be diagnosed in 2006, almost evenly distributed between men (10,730) and women (8090).[1] Malignant glioma accounts for 40% of CNS tumors diagnosed annually.[2] These brain tumors, although uncommon, are aggressively devastating because of the infiltration of the tumor cells into the surrounding healthy brain tissue, thus causing high fatality rates. Surgical resection of malignant brain tumors may leave behind cancerous cells surrounding the excised brain tumor, thus limiting the effectiveness of surgical resection. Therefore, treatment failure is associated more with local recurrence, often within 2 cm of the primary site.[3-5]

Radiation therapy is the most effective mode of treatment for malignant glioma after resection.[6] Radiation delivery methods include external beam with a stereotactic frame, interstitial seeds (which has a high incidence of radionecrosis), or intracavitary using the GliaSite Radiation Therapy System (Cytyc Corp., Marlborough, Mass.). The GliaSite radiation therapy system (RTS) is a brachytherapy device designed to improve tumor control and minimize damage to healthy tissue by delivering a conformal dose of radiation to the tumor cavity.[7] This brachytherapy, or intracavitary RTS, can deliver a large, spherically uniform dose of radiation to the tissue around the resection cavity while sparing surrounding normal brain tissue. This mode of therapy targets tumor cells while salvaging normal tissue, which can lead to preservation of cognition and function, thereby improving quality of life. Even at the time of first recurrence, a boost of radiation using the GliaSite RTS can be given locally to the resection cavity even though previous external beam irradiation treatment was administered.[8]

It is known that treatment of intracranial gliomas with interstitial iodine has yielded positive dose response effects and improved quality of life in most patients.[2,6,9,10] The GliaSite RTS attempts to extend survival time while minimizing side effects through the use of a unique treatment delivery system. Initial studies examining experimental validation of dose calculation algorithms and biodistribution and dosimetry of Iotrex radiation therapy solution (a liquid ^{125}I [iodine-125] radiation source) were favorable.[5,11] Stubbs and colleagues[11] examined rodents to determine radioactive clearance in urine and organ tissues after injection of Iotrex solution. Radioactivity was rapidly cleared from the brain (98% at 2 hours) and total body (urinary clearance 93% at 2 hours). It was determined that if the maximum clinical load of Iotrex were to be released intracerebrally, the radiation dose to all organs would be below the thresholds for deterministic effects.

In 2003, Tatter and colleagues[12] examined the safety and feasibility of GliaSite RTS in humans. Twenty-one patients with recurrent high-grade astrocytomas were successfully implanted, treated, and explanted using this treatment modality. At least 40 Gy to 60 Gy was delivered to all tissues within the target volume. Median survival for these patients was 12.7 months (see Figure 28-1) and no symptomatic radiation necrosis was reported at 21.8 patient-years of follow-up. It was reported that one patient had a pseudomeningocele, one patient had a wound infection, and three patients had meningitis (one bacterial, one chemical, and one septic).

More recently, Gabayan and colleagues[13] reported on a retrospective multi-institutional analysis of GliaSite RTS for treatment of recurrent malignant gliomas. Ninety-five patients with recurrent grade 3 or 4 gliomas who had previously undergone resection and external beam radiation were selected and agreed to receive GliaSite RTS. After recurrence, the device was placed and treatment consisting of a median dose of 60 Gy to an average depth of 1 cm with a median dose rate of

52.3 Gy/hr was administered. Median survival for all patients was 36.3 weeks with an estimated 1-year survival of 31.1%. The median survival was 35.9 weeks for patients with glioblastoma multiforme (GBM) and 43.6 weeks for those with non-GBM malignant gliomas. There were three cases of pathologically documented radiation necrosis.

Despite limited published studies examining the clinical effectiveness of GliaSite RTS, some data exists to suggest modest survival benefit in patients with recurrent malignant gliomas.

The Food and Drug Administration (FDA) approved the GliaSite RTS for commercial distribution on April 25, 2001.[14] The device consists of a proximal double-lumen subcutaneous injection port attached to a shaft catheter that leads to a distal inflatable balloon (Figure 28-2). The radiation oncologist instills Iotrex inside the balloon using a shielded syringe and needle several days or weeks after the device is implanted. After completion of RTS, the Iotrex is retrieved and the GliaSite RTS catheter is removed from the brain.

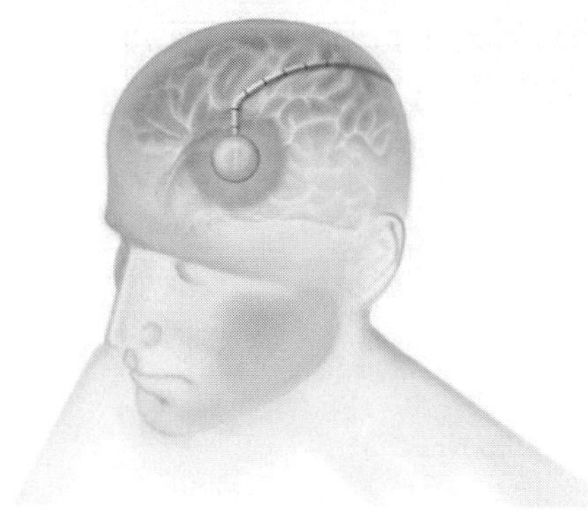

Figure 28-2 GliaSite® Radiation Therapy System With Catheter in Place. The prescribed dose can be delivered to within 1 cm of the tumor resection site (the highest area of recurrence).
Courtesy of Cytyc™ Corporation and affiliates.

PATIENT SELECTION

The GliaSite RTS is a modality used to treat patients with cancerous cranial lesions. These patients may have newly diagnosed or recurrent malignant brain tumors, as well as metastatic tumors.[14,15] Treatment for malignant cranial tumors depends on a number of factors, including tumor type, location, and size. Because this procedure requires surgery, the patient's general health and age are also determining factors.

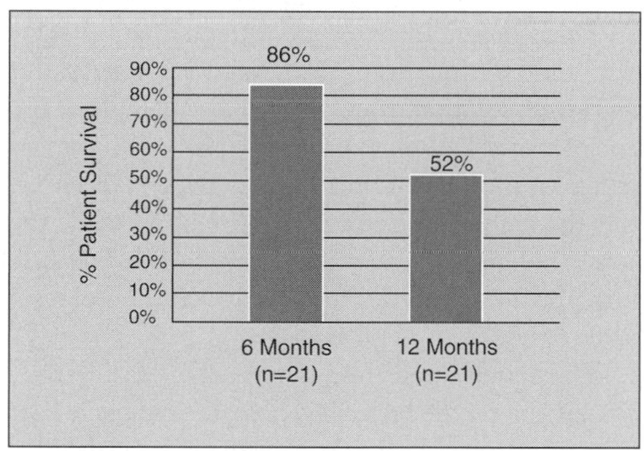

Figure 28-1 Survival Time of Patients Treated With GliaSite RTS® from Time of Treatment for Recurrent Primary Tumor.
Data extrapolated from Tatter SB, Shaw EG, Rosenblum ML, et al: An inflatable balloon catheter and liquid ^{125}I radiation source (GliaSite Radiation Therapy System) for treatment of recurrent malignant glioma: multicenter safety and feasibility trial, J Neurosurg 99(2):297–303, 2003 by Proxima Therapeutics, currently Cytyc Corporation. Originally retrieved from www.gliasite.com/glia_abogliarts.asp. Courtesy of Cytyc™ Corporation and affiliates.

TREATMENT

Surgical Phase: Catheter Placement

Placement of the GliaSite balloon is done by the neurosurgeon at the completion of tumor resection. Balloon size is determined by the neurosurgeon based on the cavity volume. A cross-section diameter is measured and the appropriate device is selected for placement. The GliaSite RTS catheters are available in diameters of 2, 3, and 4 cm. The system's integrity is confirmed by the surgical nurse before its use. The initial balloon test is completed by placing the maximum volume of sterile saline within the balloon while assessing the balloon, catheter shaft, and access port for fluid leakage. Once no leaks are found, the saline is removed from the balloon and a 75% sterile normal saline to 25% nonionic contrast agent mixture is prepared. The neurosurgeon then determines the final fluid volume, inflating the balloon with the saline and contrast solution to the desired circumference in the surgical cavity. The amount of fluid infused into or withdrawn from the balloon is recorded on a fluid status chart. Operating room guidelines are

Box 28-1 GliaSite Radiation Therapy System

GliaSite BALLOON FILL VOLUMES

Product code	Description	Min. fill volume	Max. fill volume
1020	2-cm catheter	4 mL	5 mL
1030	3-cm catheter	5 mL	15 mL
1040	4-cm catheter	15 mL	35 mL

SUPPLIES NEEDED

1 each, 10-mL and 20-mL syringes
Nonionic contrast solution
Sterile injectable saline (approximately 50 mL)

- Use only noncoring needles provided in the GliaSite catheter tray when accessing the GliaSite injection port
- Use nonionic contrast solution (Isoview, Omnipaque, etc.); ratio of contrast to saline should be no more than 25%/75%
- Screws for securing port

PREIMPLANTATION TEST*

- Select appropriate GliaSite ballon for cavity
- Fill balloon with saline to MAX fill volume indicated for size (see above)
- Check balloon to make sure it is free of leaks and is a round shape
- Deflate balloon and prepare for implantation
- Record on the *Fluid Status Chart* and place in the Progress Note Section of the patient's chart; note the final fill volume of saline and contrast placed in the balloon

*If balloon leaks or is not round in shape do not use. Select back up balloon and return failed balloon to Cytyc for replacement.

helpful to ensure that appropriate documentation and product testing occurs. Additionally, these guidelines ensure availability of needed supplies (Box 28-1).

Once the GliaSite balloon is in place, the dura and the bone flap are closed to ensure an adequate pathway for future removal of the GliaSite RTS catheter. Any rough edges around the exit burr hole are filed or shaved to prevent damage to the GliaSite RTS catheter. The catheter shaft is threaded through the burr hole. The bone flap is secured after dural closure, and a site is selected for placement of the access port. It is very important to secure the infusion/access port, avoiding kinks in the catheter shaft and positioning the port away from the suture line. Placement of the GliaSite RTS catheter is confirmed with magnetic resonance imaging (MRI) or x ray.[15] A copy of the final MRI and the fluid status chart should be sent to the radiation oncology department for treatment planning and to determine the amount of Iotrex to be ordered for that patient.

Brachytherapy Phase: Iotrex Infusion

The radiation oncologist schedules the patient for infusion of Iotrex radiation therapy solution, typically starting 3 days to 3 weeks after surgery and completed within 29 days after catheter implantation.[3] Twenty-four hours before and continuing throughout brachytherapy, the patient receives Lugol's solution, or saturated solution of potassium iodide (SSKI), to block the thyroid as prescribed by the radiation oncologist. SSKI solution is used as an oxidizing agent for removal of mercurial fixation artifacts. This protects the thyroid from the Iotrex radiation therapy solution while it is dwelling within the GliaSite balloon in the rare event that the balloon leaks the Iotrex solution. The SSKI also is administered to decrease the potential for accumulation of ^{125}I in the patient's thyroid. Iotrex can be harmful to the thyroid gland and can cause cancer of the thyroid if no prophylactic measures are taken.[16] Patients are to begin taking the solution 24 hours before injection of Iotrex radiation solution and continue until 24 hours after retrieval of the Iotrex solution from the GliaSite balloon at the end of therapy. A typical dose of SSKI is 0.3 g mixed in a glass of water or juice. The nursing staff monitors the daily administration of the SSKI while the Iotrex radiation therapy dwells in the GliaSite balloon and 24 hours after the Iotrex radiation solution is retrieved.[16]

The Iotrex dwell time is typically 3 to 7 days.[17] Depending on the prescribed dose, the patient is kept in a private room for the duration of radiation delivery. During that time, the patient is under strict radiation precautions, with signs warning of radiation exposure in place. Standard institutional procedures for therapeutic use of radiopharmaceuticals is followed for use with this treatment modality. Since radioactive ^{125}I solution is a low-energy x ray and gamma (γ) emitter, no external shielding is necessary.[16,18]

Some centers performing GliaSite treatments allow higher functioning patients to remain at home during the Iotrex dwell time. If this is permitted, patients must be given strict guidelines to ensure their safety and the safety of others in the home. The following should be included in the guidelines for outpatient treatment:

- Avoid traveling except to attend physician appointments.
- Remain home from work.
- Sleep alone.
- Maintain a distance of at least 3 feet from others.
- Avoid prolonged contact with children and pregnant women.
- Terminate breastfeeding (if applicable).

Patients also should be told whom to contact in the event of an emergency or if they have further questions. Additionally, they should be informed of the return-to-clinic date and time.

Source preparation and calibration is done under the direct supervision of the medical physicist. A running inventory of the liquid source should be maintained for each case. The syringe dose is to be delivered to an authorized user in the patient's room with the assistance of the medical physicist and/or radiation safety personnel. Room preparation, room surveys, in-service for the nursing staff, radiation waste disposal, and release of the patient is done by the radiation safety staff in a manner consistent with U.S. Nuclear Regulatory Commission (NRC) Regulatory Guide 10.8, rev. 2, 1987. For personnel handling Iotrex and for other support staff in the same room where Iotrex is being manipulated, a thyroid bioassay between 6 and 72 hours after the procedure is recommended.[16,19]

Iotrex Afterloading

There are three main steps to Iotrex afterloading: (1) injection site access, (2) fluid removal, and (3) securing the Iotrex.[19] Iotrex fluid insertion is done with the GliaSite RTS access tray supplemented with sterile gloves, additional syringes, and sterile normal saline for injection.

The radiation oncologist performs a standard aseptic site preparation. The scalp is palpated to locate the infusion port and is marked with a surgical marking pen at the location of needle entry into the infusion port. Next, the fenestrated drape is unfolded and draped over the patient's head, with the drape hole centered over the infusion site. A transparent dressing is placed over the infusion site to cover the skin and edges of drape hole. The pouch containing the infusion set with the noncoring needle should be opened and primed with saline solution. The clamp on the infusion set should be closed and then a noncoring needle inserted into the infusion port. Secure the noncoring needle with the steri-strips provided in the tray.

The next step is to remove the fluid with the 20-mL syringe. The noncoring needle of the syringe is inserted into the infusion set injection site, and the clamp is fully opened. Once the fluid has drained, the clamp should be closed before withdrawing the needle from the infusion site. The catheter and balloon should be flushed with saline solution after fluid removals using a 5-mL syringe. The syringe should be discarded in accordance with hospital procedure.

The last step is to prepare for instillation of the Iotrex solution. Two fluid-filled syringes, one containing the prescribed Iotrex solution and the other containing normal saline solution, are to be prepared in advance. The needle of the syringe containing the Iotrex solution is inserted into the infusion set injection site. After it is confirmed that the needle is completely inserted into the injection site, the clamp is opened and the Iotrex is slowly infused. The used needle and syringe containing the Iotrex should be measured for residual activity. The needle of the syringe containing the saline solution is inserted into the infusion set injection site and infused. Once all fluid has been delivered, the needle and syringe are removed from the infusion set injection site and discarded as radioactive waste. All of the dressings and drapes should be handled as radioactive waste. The volume of Iotrex and saline solution infused is to be recorded on the patient's fluid status chart.

Radiation safety staff perform a radiation survey on the patient, the patient's personal belongings, and hospital room contents and surfaces. Any contaminated materials are removed and quarantined or destroyed according to hospital policy and procedures. Surfaces contaminated with radioactivity must be appropriately cleansed and cleared by the radiation safety officer before the room can be approved for future patient use.

GliaSite Catheter Removal

The patient is prepared for surgical removal of the device once the bedside retrieval and radiation safety clearance is obtained. The FDA approved the GliaSite RTS for 29 days or less from time of implant.[4,14] This ruling was based on the fact that testing was done to support maximum duration of implantation of 29 days. Generally, catheter removal can be performed under conscious sedation instead of general anesthesia, thus eliminating the recovery time of general anesthesia and anesthesia side effects.

The explanted GliaSite catheter is radioactive and is disposed of by a radiation safety officer in accordance with NRC requirement. Radiation safety staff should be present during the explant procedure for disposal of catheter and for patient room survey. A radiation survey is done on the patient before release from the hospital.[16]

RISKS OF INTRACAVITARY PROCEDURE

Risks and discomforts are involved in this special procedure. First, placing the GliaSite RTS in the tumor space may cause bleeding during or after surgery. If bleeding occurs, it may result in temporary or permanent loss of some brain functions, and/or a second operation may be required to remove a blood clot. Second, besides the possible bleeding problems, the device itself may press on normal brain tissue, causing a decrease in some normal brain function. If this occurs, any solution, including the radioactive solution, will have to be emptied before the intended dwell time. A third risk involves overfilling the balloon, because this could result in temporary or permanent loss of some brain functions. If overfilling occurs and the patient becomes symptomatic, the infusion port can be accessed to remove some of the fluid, thus relieving the resulting intracranial pressure. Additionally, the device may become infected, causing abscess or chemical meningitis. It is also possible that the catheter shaft and infusion port may cause tension to the scalp, resulting in a break in skin integrity. Astute evaluation of the incision and port/catheter site is essential in the postoperative phase of treatment. A final risk includes the inability to complete a watertight dural closure after device placement. In patients whose tumor resection includes ventricular wall compromise, the device placement may maintain an opening for central spinal fluid outflow, leading to pseudomeningocele or externalized hydrocephalus.[1,20]

Besides the technical risks of placement and maintenance, radiation therapy to the brain may cause swelling of the normal brain tissues. If brain swelling occurs during the radiation treatment, the radioactive fluid may have to be taken out and the treatment canceled. Radiation also may result in necrosis of normal brain tissue. Radiation-induced necrosis is a late effect of treatment and may result in tissue edema resulting in headache, nausea, or vomiting. Brain swelling and radiation necrosis also may cause temporary or permanent loss of some brain functions.[20] In many cases, brain swelling can be controlled with corticosteroids and other medications. Surgery may again be necessary to remove swollen or necrotic tissue. Surgery, however, does not always reverse radiation necrosis. Such necrosis can progress like a tumor and result in death. Patients who receive radiation therapy for brain tumors have a slightly greater risk for developing a second primary brain tumor or another metastatic brain tumor in a different part of the brain.

Standard protection of the thyroid during brachytherapy is achieved with the medication SSKI. Again, SSKI is prescribed 24 hours before treatment and continues until 24 hours after treatment. Possible side effects of potassium iodide include rashes, swelling of the salivary glands, "iodism" (metallic taste, burning mouth and throat, sore teeth and gums, signs of a head cold, and sometimes stomach upset and diarrhea), and allergic reactions (fever and joint pains, swelling of parts of the face and body and, at times, severe shortness of breath requiring immediate medical attention). Rarely, overactivity or underactivity of the thyroid gland or enlargement of the thyroid gland (goiter) may occur. A very small amount of the brachytherapy solution will diffuse out of the balloon and into the brain and eventually into the urine, saliva, sweat, and stool. In other research studies, liquid radioactive materials were injected directly into brain tumors without a balloon, and these patients had no unusual problems. If the balloon integrity is compromised, the radiation safety officer and radiation oncologist are consulted to prescribe additional radiation safety precautions and additional doses of SSKI.

NURSING CONSIDERATIONS

Patients with the implanted GliaSite balloon should be admitted to a private room on the general ward with trained nursing staff. The final dwell (treatment) time is determined by the medical physicist and radiation oncologist, based on the net activity injected and the prescribed dose.[18] The patient is instructed to remain in the room. Visitors are allowed during designated times and at a designated area to be determined by the radiation safety officer in a manner consistent with state and NRC requirements.

To ensure balloon catheter integrity, the radiation safety officer and/or medical physicist should survey the patient's head and bladder daily. This is checked from 30 cm away from the head to confirm that the balloon has not failed. If measurements are above baseline value, physics, radiation safety, and neurosurgery need to be notified immediately. All measurements are maintained in the patient record.

During a course of treatment, small quantities of ^{125}I diffuse through the GliaSite catheter and are excreted in the urine.[12] Therefore, all clothing, bandages, and linens that come into contact with body fluids are to be kept for survey by radiation safety staff. All contaminated articles should be disposed of as radioactive waste. The radiation safety officer should be available at all times for any questions relating to patient care.[16] For example, if the toilet requires cleaning before the patient completes the radiation dwell time, the safety officer should be notified of any urine spills. However, nursing can use universal precautions while emptying urinary drainage bags and flushing twice. Not all items that come in contact with the patient will be radioactive. For example, nursing can remove dietary trays from the room without scanning and return them to the dietary cart. However, pregnant staff should not care for a patient who is receiving treatment with the GliaSite RTS. If the patient must leave the room, as for diagnostic testing, the patient should wear a lead-lined cap at all times, and unnecessary waiting times in other departments should be avoided. Ideally, portable scans should be used if possible.

In the event of a patient emergency, notify the radiation oncologist, radiation safety officer, and neurosurgeon immediately. Prepare liquid radioactive ^{125}I access tray. Retrieve the Iotrex from the patient. Recover all radioactive material and all contaminated items. Immediately call the operating room and schedule the patient for removal of the implanted balloon catheter.

SUMMARY

The GliaSite RTS is designed for local treatment of newly diagnosed, metastatic, and recurrent brain tumors by delivering radiation from within the tumor resection cavity. This type of brachytherapy is designed to deliver site-specific internal radiation therapy while minimizing radiation exposure to healthy brain tissues. GliaSite delivers radiation with Iotrex, a proprietary ^{125}I radiation source that is placed inside a balloon catheter. Targeted tissues receive high doses of radiation, while exposure to healthy tissue is minimized, and the treatment time lasts only 3 to 7 days.[3-5] The GliaSite RTS is another treatment option for patients that minimizes radiation exposure to healthy brain tissue and limits the side effects associated with external beam radiation. Some patients have gained additional survival time with this treatment modality (median 387 days from time of treatment for recurrent primary tumor).[9,10]

REFERENCES

1. Jemal A, Siegel R, Ward E et al: Cancer statistics, *CA Cancer J Clin* 56(2):106-130, 2006.
2. Mehta MP, Sneed PK: *Interstitial radiation therapy for brain tumors: principles and practice of brachytherapy*, Armonk, NY, 1997, Futura, pp 247-261.
3. Dempsey JF, Williams JA, Stubbs JB et al: Dosimetric properties of a novel brachytherapy balloon applicator for the treatment of malignant brain tumor resection cavity, *Int J Radiat Oncol Biol Phys* 42(2):421-429, 1998.
4. Stubbs JB, Frankel RH, Schultz K et al: Preclinical evaluation of a novel device for delivering brachytherapy to the margins of resected brain tumor cavities, *J Neurosurg* 96(2):335-343, 2002.
5. Monroe JI, Dempsey JF, Dorton JA et al: Experimental validation of dose calculation algorithms for the GliaSite RTS, a novel I-125 liquid-filled balloon brachytherapy applicator, *Med Phys* 28(1):73-85, 2001.
6. Wen PY, Alexander E 3rd, Black PM et al: Long term results of stereotactic brachytherapy used in the initial treatment of patients with glioblastomas, *Cancer* 73(12):3029-3036, 1994.
7. Shaw E, Mikkelson T, Kleinberg L et al: *The GliaSite Radiation Therapy System (RS): a novel approach to brain brachytherapy for recurrent malignant glioma.* Presented at the Annual Meeting of the American Society of Therapeutic Radiology and Oncology, 2001.
8. Chan TA, Weingart JD, Parisi M et al: Treatment of recurrent glioblastoma multiforme with GliaSite brachytherapy, *Int J Radiat Oncol Biol Phys* 62(4):1133-1139, 2005.
9. Leibel SA, Gutin PH, Wara WM et al: Survival and quality of life after interstitial implantation of removable high-activity iodine-125 for the treatment of patients with recurrent malignant gliomas, *Int J Radiat Oncol Biol Phys* 17(6):1129-1139, 1989.
10. McDermott MW, Gutin PH, Larson DA et al: Interstitial brachytherapy, *Neurosurg Clin N Am* 1(4): 801-824, 1990.
11. Stubbs JB, Strickland AD, Frank RK et al: Biodistribution and dosimetry of an aqueous solution containing sodium

3-(125I) iodo-4-hydroxybenzenesulfonate (Iotrex) for brachytherapy of resected malignant brain tumors, *Cancer Biother Radiopharm* 15(6):645-656, 2000.
12. Tatter SB, Shaw EG, Rosenblum ML et al: An inflatable balloon catheter and liquid ^{125}I radiation source (GliaSite Radiation Therapy System) for treatment of recurrent malignant glioma: multicenter safety and feasibility trial, *J Neurosurg* 99(2):297-303, 2003.
13. Gabayan AJ, Grenn SB, Sanan A et al: GliaSite brachytherapy for treatment of recurrent malignant gliomas: a retrospective multi-institutional analysis, *Neurosurgery* 58(4): 701-709, 2006.
14. *Brain Cancer Therapy with GliaSite* (website): http://www.gliasite.com/index_glia.asp. Accessed June 22, 2006.
15. Matheus MG, Castillo M, Ewend M et al: CT and MR imaging after placement of the GliaSite radiation therapy system to treat brain tumor: initial experience, *AJNR Am J Neuroradiol* 25(7):1211-1217, 2004.
16. deGuzman AF, Kearns WT, Shaw E et al: Radiation safety issues with high activities of liquid I-125: techniques and experience, *J Appl Clin Med Phys* 4(2):143-148, 2003.
17. Mayr MT, Crocker IR, Butker EK et al: Results of interstitial brachytherapy for malignant brain tumors, *Int J Oncol* 21(4):817-823, 2002.
18. Patel S, Breneman JC, Warnick RE et al: Permanent iodine-125 interstitial implants for the treatment of recurrent glioblastoma multiforme, *Neurosurgery* 46(5):1123-1130, 2000.
19. *GliaSite® Instruction Manual*, Atlanta, 2001, Proxima Therapeutics (now Cytyc Pharmaceuticals).
20. Marquardt G, Setzer M, Lang J et al: Delayed hydrocephalus after resection of supratentorial malignant gliomas, *Acta Neurochir* (Wien) 144(3):227-231, 2002.

Chapter 29

Total Skin Electron Beam Therapy

Tracy K. Gosselin-Acomb

Total skin electron beam therapy (TSEBT) is also known as total skin irradiation (TSI). This modality was first described in 1953 and historically is considered the single most effective method in treating cutaneous T-cell lymphoma (CTCL).[1] TSEBT is most commonly used to treat patients with CTCL. CTCL results from the development of abnormal T-lymphocytes, and therefore is a cancer of the lymphocytes (lymphoma).[2] This disease is typically confined to the skin and in advanced cases may involve other organs. Mycosis fungoides (MF) is the preferred name for CTCL. MF is a mature T-cell lymphoma that infiltrates the epidermis and dermis of the skin with small- to medium-sized T cells. These cells then contribute to the development of the patches/plaque that most patients develop. Sézary syndrome is a variant of MF, but the clinical behavior is much more aggressive and it is characterized by erythroderma, lymphadenopathy, and malignant T cells in the blood.[3]

Patients who require TSEBT typically have skin lesions that cover a large percentage of their body. These patients, unlike those receiving focal radiation, receive radiation to their entire skin/integumentary system. These lesions may appear as patches, plaque, erythroderma and/or as a tumor and may cause the patient discomfort depending on the severity. Patients typically presenting with this disease complain of dry, red, scaly, itchy skin that typically starts on the trunk and spreads to the limbs over the course of several years. This often can make the diagnosis difficult as a result of the lesions being confused with other dermatologic conditions. Patients who require TSEBT may have failed other therapies including topical chemotherapy, phototherapy, or photochemotherapy using an oral photosensitizing drug followed by ultraviolet light exposure (psoralen ultraviolet A-range [PUVA]), and systemic chemotherapy.

TSEBT may be used as neoadjuvant or adjuvant therapy with systemic or topical chemotherapy agents/targeted therapies (Box 29-1) or as part of a conditioning regimen. Patients with extracutaneous disease may receive systemic therapy for disease management. Photon irradiation may play a role as well.

Outcomes for patients receiving TSEBT vary based on staging. The majority of patients respond to the treatment, but overall survival is influenced by severity of the disease. Better control is seen in patients with early-stage disease who do not have generalized plaques and/or tumors. At Stanford University Hospital, response rates for plaque, generalized plaque, tumor, and erythroderma were found to be 98%, 71%, 35%, and 64%, respectively. Relapse occurred in 50% of patients with limited plaque and 80% in patients with generalized plaque.[4] In 48 patients with advanced disease who received a combination of TSEBT and photon irradiation, 5-year survival rates were 37% in patients with T3 disease and 44% in patients with T4 disease,[5] but such patients are rarely free of disease.

In a retrospective study of 148 patients who received TSEBT with or without adjuvant topical nitrogen mustard or nitrogen mustard alone, patients with T2 and T3 disease yielded a significantly higher complete response than topical nitrogen mustard alone (76% versus 39%, $p = 0.03$ for T2, and 44% versus 8%, $p < 0.05$ for T3).[6] TSEBT also may be administered before the use of adjuvant oral PUVA light. Studies have shown that this adjuvant treatment improves disease-free survival, but not overall survival, and may be an effective salvage therapy in patients who have already received TSEBT.[7]

TREATMENT

The treatment objectives for TSEBT are listed in Box 29-2.[8] TSEBT is typically administered 4 to 5 consecutive days a week over the course of 6 to 10 weeks. This time course varies based on individual patient needs and that of the treatment center.

Box 29-1 Common Agents Used to Treat Cutaneous T-Cell Lymphoma*

- Alemtuzumab (Campath, Genzyme Corp., Cambridge, Mass.)
- Bexarotene (Targretin, Ligand Pharmaceuticals, Inc., San Diego, Calif.)
- Denileukin diftitox (Ontak, Ligand Pharmaceuticals, Inc., San Diego, Calif.)
- Interferon (Intron A, Schering Corporation, Kenilworth, NJ)
- Mechlorethamine hydrochloride—topical (Mustargen, Merck & Co., Whitehouse Station, NJ)
- Methotrexate (generic, multiple manufacturers)
- Pentostatin (Nipent, SuperGen, Dublin, Ohio)
- Variety of alkylating agents in advanced disease

*NOTE: This is not meant to be an all-inclusive list, but a sample of the biologic and chemotherapeutic agents used.

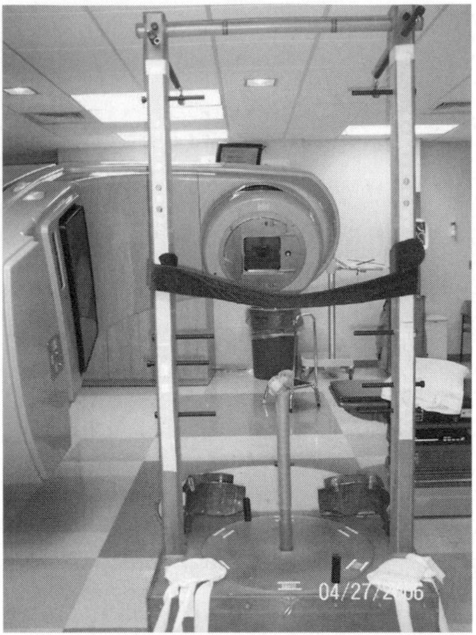

Figure 29-1 Treatment Stand.
Courtesy of Department of Radiation Oncology, Duke University Hospital.

Box 29-2 Objectives of Any Method of Total Skin Electron Radiation

- To align the distribution of dose to the target volume
- To be practical, comfortable, and efficient for the patient
- To provide sufficient dose within the target volume
- To reliably attain cutaneous remission
- To minimize toxicity
- To produce beneficial long-term clinical results
- To accommodate repeated administration as required

Data from Jones GW, Hoppe RT, Glatstein E: *Hematol Oncol Clin North Am* 9(5):1057-1076, 1995.

Treatment is typically delivered via a linear accelerator with 6 MeV electron beam, but may be as low as 3 MeV for optimum dose distribution. The optimal source-to-patient distance is between 3 to 8 meters, and when the distance is less than 3 meters, it is difficult to obtain dose homogeneity and limit photon contamination.[9] The treatment time is approximately 30 to 45 minutes per day.

A six-field treatment approach is commonly used to cover the entire body surface for dose heterogeneity. Self-shielded areas such as the soles of the feet, inframammary folds, perineum, and panniculus of obese patients may be boosted with additional electrons or photons. Patients are typically positioned on a treatment stand (Figure 29-1). This treatment stand assists the patient in maintaining one of the six positions required for treatment, with small straps used for additional support. The positions include straight anterior, left anterior oblique, right anterior oblique, straight posterior, left posterior oblique, and right posterior oblique. Patients receive treatment to three alternating fields per day.

During treatment patients may have their eyes, hands, and feet shielded. Eye shields are commonly used to protect the eye; these may be internal or external (Figure 29-2) and may change during treatment so that the eyelid may receive appropriate treatment if needed. The hands and feet are typically treated separately with bolus material because of their anatomic shape. Boost treatments also may be administered prior to the initiation of TSEBT to areas of the body that are symptomatic with ulcers.

The total dose of radiation prescribed is usually between 30 Gy and 36 Gy for the skin and varies from 18 Gy to 20 Gy for the hands and feet. The dose of radiation being delivered can be measured using a thermoluminescent dosimeter (TLD) or film dosimeter (Figure 29-3). This is often done during the first few weeks of therapy to ensure treatment accuracy and dose delivery.

Precautions need to be taken in positioning patients on the stand. The stand often requires the

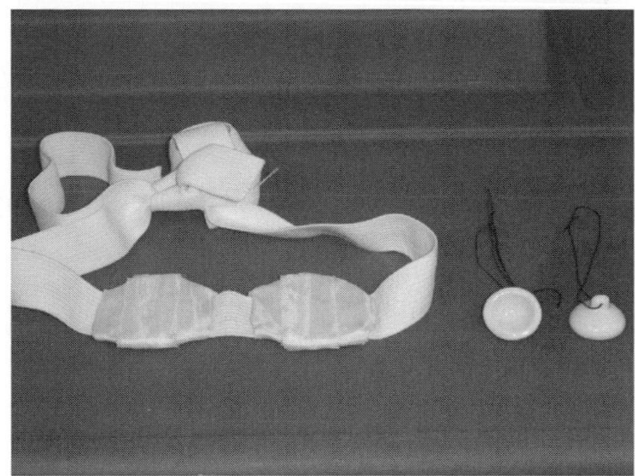

Figure 29-2 External and Internal Eye Shields.
Courtesy of Department of Radiation Oncology, Duke University Hospital.

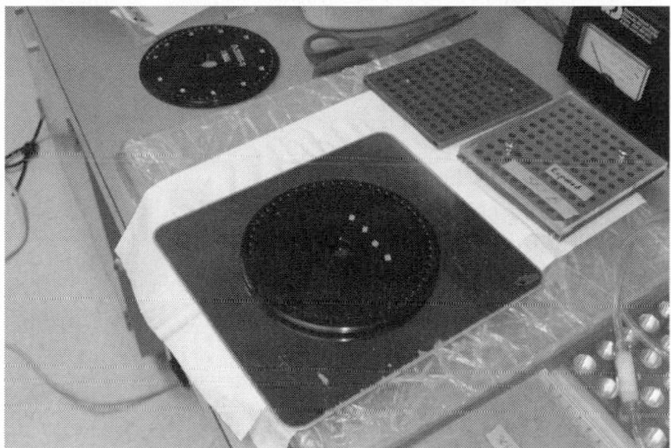

Figure 29-3 Thermoluminescent or Film Dosimeter.
Courtesy of Department of Radiation Oncology, Duke University Hospital.

patient to step up and this could potentially put some patients at risk for a fall when they are getting on or off the stand. Patients undergoing this treatment are not considered to be radioactive.

NURSING IMPLICATIONS

Treatment of MF with TSEBT affects all domains of quality of life (QOL). The acute side effects can often be profound and have a significant impact on the patient's QOL. The physical domain of QOL has the most prominent changes; patients experience itching and skin changes, along with generalized fatigue. These side effects impact the functional domain, and the patient may experience difficulty with activities of daily living and sleeping. The patient may not work during this time because of the severity of the skin reaction. Patients with MF may experience social issues before the use of TSEBT because of the nature and appearance of their disease. These patients may be embarrassed or ashamed of their body image and socially isolate themselves because of how they look. Lastly, from an emotional perspective, these patients may experience anxiety and/or have difficulty coping with the side effects if they do not have a support system in place. A referral to behavioral medicine or a cancer patient support program may be of benefit.

Patients undergoing TSEBT experience a variety of side effects. Prompt assessment, education, and intervention by the healthcare team (Table 29-1) can assist patients in performing self-care and can provide a time for patients to discuss other concerns they may have. Acute side effects arise while the patient is undergoing treatment, and late effects typically arise months to years after treatment.

The most common acute side effects include alopecia, fatigue, nail loss or stasis, and skin changes. It is expected that the patient will undergo a variety of acute skin changes including pruritus, erythema, dry desquamation, and moist desquamation. The skin reaction is self-limiting and appropriate supportive care is critical. Late skin changes may include atrophy, pigmentation changes, telangiectasia, and xerosis. Although rare, higher doses may cause permanent alopecia, frank poikiloderma (mottled skin appearance), skin fragility, and subcutaneous fibrosis.[10]

Patients undergoing TSEBT should be evaluated at least weekly by the physician and radiation oncology nurse while undergoing treatment. This may then be done more frequently as the patient's skin becomes more compromised and the risk of infection increases. The progressive changes of the skin from erythema to dry and then moist desquamation often can be problematic in this population because it may cause difficulties with activities of daily living. The patient should continue to bathe and to keep the skin clean and well moisturized. Antibiotic ointment may be used on fissures and other areas of skin breakdown. The severity of the skin reaction may be similar to a moderate to severe sunburn and may place the patient at risk for sepsis and require specialized nursing care when the patient experiences total body moist desquamation. Patients may be admitted to the hospital for pain control, intravenous fluids, and monitoring.

Table 29-1 Nursing Care of the Patient Receiving TSEBT

Symptom	Nursing interventions
Fatigue	Encourage patient to drink plenty of fluids and eat a well-balanced diet Recommend naps and energy-conserving techniques Encourage delegation of tasks
Itching	Consult with healthcare team about over-the-counter and prescription medications Encourage skin care recommendations noted below
Pain	Consult with healthcare team about over-the-counter and prescription medications Determine whether pain increases with ADLs Verify whether patient has allergies Review use of prescribed pain medications—short-acting and/or long-acting—and side effects
Psychosocial	Consider social work referral and behavioral medicine consultation Consider referrals to: American Cancer Society, "Look Good Feel Better" Program Leukemia and Lymphoma Society Mycosis Fungoides Foundation Local cancer patient support group
Skin care	Encourage patient to wear loose cotton clothing, nothing constricting or tight Bathe daily and apply moisturizer immediately afterwards Moisturize skin daily and as needed (Aquaphor, Beiersdorf AG, Hamburg, Germany) (Eucerin, Beiersdorf AG, Hamburg, Germany) Monitor skin for signs of infection Consult wound care nurse regarding skin products for patients with blisters and moist desquamation Consider use of special care bed for patients with full body desquamation Consider hydrocolloid dressings, Kerlex and Coban for areas of desquamation with edema Consult with healthcare team about the use of antibiotic ointment on fissures and other impaired skin areas Educate immobile patients about positioning SPF sunblock of 30 with UVA/UVB is recommended if the patient is going to be outside any time during the scheduled treatment regimen and after treatment is completed

Some patients may use oral medications to manage the itching whereas others may use topical medications. Oral agents typically cause central nervous system (CNS) depression and may make the patient groggy or tired. Patients typically are not bothered by the itchiness as much because of the CNS depression. Other measures used to palliate the itchiness include topical anti-itch medications, lidocaine jelly, and ice patches. Evidence-based strategies in this population are lacking.

All patients will experience some degree of transient edema of the hands and ankles at doses of 25 Gy. Blisters also may arise requiring shielding of the affected area, or the patient may be placed on a treatment break. Half of the patients experience minor edema of the hands and feet, but this may sometimes be more severe and protracted for several months when patients remain physically active during a course of TSEB or if they have an underlying condition such as diabetes mellitus.[9] Patients should be taught proper body positioning techniques as well as active and passive exercises if they become immobilized. Consultation with a wound care nurse regarding symptom management strategies and skin care products is often beneficial. Patients with lower extremity edema may benefit from daily wrapping of the legs with hydrocolloid dressings, Kerlex and Coban to minimize edema and to improve pain control. Male patients also may experience gynecomastia. Special care should be given to elderly patients who may already have thin or frail skin. These patients may be more susceptible to moist desquamation and therefore at higher risk for complications.

Late effects of the treatment typically manifest in the skin. Changes may include atrophy, fibrosis, frank poikiloderma, permanent alopecia, and telangiectasia. Patients who experience permanent alopecia may choose to wear a hat, wig, or scarf. Xerosis or difficulty sweating after TSEBT varies in each patient. The sweat glands, which are located close to the skin surface, are affected by the TSEBT and may not function as well as they did before TSEBT. Patients should be encouraged to drink plenty of fluids during warm weather and while exercising.

Patient education and understanding of TSEBT are essential elements of the treatment process. When a patient agrees to undergo TSEBT, a consent form should be signed that outlines the treatment and potential side effects. Patients and their families need to understand that the treatment is 4 to 5 days a week and often can take up to 45 minutes. With this being a total skin treatment, the patient needs to change into a cloth or paper gown and potentially have parts of their body exposed for treatment. For many patients, this can be awkward. However, a discussion at the time of consultation about treatment and treatment set-up can help alleviate these fears.

Male patients may be at risk for infertility; appropriate counseling and sperm banking should be performed if the patient wishes to have children at a later time. However, a number of young men have fathered children within a few months or several years after TSEBT.[9] The location of the testes make them sensitive to the radiation whereas a woman's ovaries are located deeper within the body cavity. Contraception should be used during and 6 months after treatment in case the disease does not go into remission or recurs.

Patients may initially continue to work during treatment, but once skin reaction arises, they may choose to stop. Many patients with MF who require TSEBT may not go out in public often because of the nature of the disease and, once the treatment is initiated, may become even more reclusive. Patients who live alone or who are in need of resources should be referred to a social worker.

Once treatment is completed and patients are in the follow-up phase, they may be seen by care providers more frequently at first depending on the severity of any skin reaction. A dermatologist and radiation oncologist will continue to follow patients to monitor treatment results and any new lesions that may arise. Patients should be reminded to consistently use sunscreen and to avoid direct sun exposure as much as possible. A more detailed discussion regarding sunscreen can be found in Chapter 15.

SUMMARY

Patients undergoing TSEBT for MF face a variety of physical and psychosocial issues related to the disease and treatment. Most patients receive some benefit from the treatment, but many go on to adjuvant treatment. Patients receiving TSEBT typically are treated at larger institutions that have experience with TSEBT and the care of such patients. The impact of treatment on disease-free survival and overall survival continues to be studied in clinical trials, as does the use of TSEBT with other treatment modalities. Studies need to continue to look at the impact of treatment on QOL and the impact that nursing interventions may have on side-effect management.

REFERENCES

1. Becker M, Hoppe R, Know S: Multiple courses of high-dose total skin electron beam therapy in the management of mycosis fungoides, *Int J Radiat Oncol Biol Phys* 32(5):1445-1449, 1995.
2. Reavely MM, Wilson LD: Total skin electron beam therapy and cutaneous T-cell lymphoma: a clinical guide for patients and staff, *Dermatol Nurs* 16(1):36, 39, 57, 2004.
3. Manson SD, Porter C: Lymphomas. In Yarbro CH, Frogge MH, Goodman M, editors: *Cancer nursing, principles and practice*, ed 6, Sudbury, Mass, 2005, Jones and Bartlett, pp 1414-1459.
4. Hoppe R: The management of mycosis fungoides at Stanford: standard and innovative treatment programs, *Leukemia* 5(suppl 1):46-48, 1991.
5. Maingon P, Truc G, Dalac S et al: Radiotherapy of advanced mycosis fungoides: indications and results of total skin electron beam and photon beam irradiation, *Radiother Oncol* 54(1):73-78, 2000.
6. Chinn DM, Chow S, Kim YH et al: Total skin electron beam therapy with or without adjuvant topical nitrogen mustard or nitrogen mustard alone as initial treatment of T2 and T3 mycosis fungoides, *Int J Radiat Oncol Biol Phys* 43(5):951-958, 1999.
7. Quirós PA, Jones GW, Kacinski BM et al: Total skin electron beam therapy followed by adjuvant psoralen/ultraviolet-A light in the management of patients with T1 and T2 cutaneous T-cell lymphoma (mycosis fungoides), *Int J Radiat Oncol Biol Phys* 38(5):1027-1035, 1997.
8. Jones GW, Hoppe RT, Glatstein E: Electron beam treatment for cutaneous T-cell lymphoma. *Hematol Oncol Clin North Am* 9(5):1057-1076, 1995.
9. Jones GW, Kacinski BM, Wilson LD et al: Total skin electron radiation in the management of mycosis fungoides: consensus of the European Organization for Research and Treatment of Cancer (EORTC) Cutaneous Lymphoma Project Group, *J Am Acad Dermatol* 47(3):364-370, 2002.
10. Gosselin-Acomb TK: Total skin irradiation. In Bruner DW, Haas M, Gosselin-Acomb TK, editors: *Manual for radiation oncology nursing practice and education*, ed 3, Pittsburgh, 2005, Oncology Nursing Society, pp 204-205.

Unit VI

Special Supportive Nursing Care

Chapter 30

Radiodermatitis

Shelia G. Sparks

During the cancer experience, approximately 60% of all patients receive radiation therapy at some point during their illness.[1] Although the aim of radiation therapy is to give maximum treatment with a minimum of side effects, it is still expected that approximately 87% to 90% of people will develop skin reactions to some extent during or shortly after treatment.[2-4] Skin reactions are the most frequently experienced side effect of radiation therapy, with the reactions ranging from minimal (e.g., mild erythema and dry desquamation) to severe (e.g., moist desquamation or necrosis). These various skin reactions can occur because of treatment-related and patient-related risk factors. Reactions are usually acute in nature and resolve within a short time after treatment. However, they can last indefinitely as in the case of chronic or late reactions. Skin reactions are often associated with significant pain and distress and may impact the patient's quality of life, ability to perform activities of daily living, and self-esteem as a result.[5]

The management of skin reactions demands a multidisciplinary approach in which nursing plays an important part.[6] Nursing care aims at creating an ideal environment to promote healing and to reduce possible pain and infection.[6] This chapter reviews the pathophysiology of normal skin, describes the stages of radiation-induced skin reactions, and discusses commonly used skin care practices.

ANATOMY AND PHYSIOLOGY OF NORMAL SKIN

The skin is the largest organ of the body and serves as the first line of defense against infection and trauma. It consists of three layers—the epidermis, dermis, and subcutaneous tissues (Figure 30-1).

Epidermis

The epidermis (30–300 μm thick) is the outer layer of the skin that is derived from a basal layer of actively proliferating cells, which is covered by several layers of nondividing differentiating cells to the surface. This is where the most superficial keratinized cells are desquamated.[7] It takes about 12 to 48 days from the time a newly formed cell leaves the basal layer to the time it is desquamated from the surface. The target cells for radiation damage are the dividing stem cells in the basal layer.[7] No blood vessels or nerves are located in the epidermis.[8] The primary function of the epidermis is to act as a barrier to prevent water loss.[9,10]

Dermis

The dermis is a dense connective tissue (1–3 mm thick) within which scattered fibroblasts produce most of the dermal proteins.[7] The dermis contains the hair follicles, lymphatics, sebaceous (oil secreting) glands, blood vessels, sweat glands, and nerves. The dermis and the subcutaneous tissue provide support, elasticity, and nourishment for the epidermis.[11] Regulation of body temperature and assistance in wound healing are major functions of the dermis. The vasculature of the dermis plays a major role in the radiation response. The target cells there are the fibroblasts and the vascular endothelial cells.[7]

Subcutaneous Tissue

The subcutaneous tissue, primarily a fat storage area, provides support for the blood vessels and nerves passing to the dermis.[12] Other functions of the subcutaneous tissue include protecting deeper structures from trauma, assisting in body temperature control, and serving as an energy reservoir.[11]

RADIATION-INDUCED SKIN CHANGES

Radiation therapy is a local treatment modality, and only tissues within the designated treatment field are affected. Because treatment beams must pass through the skin to reach their target tissue,

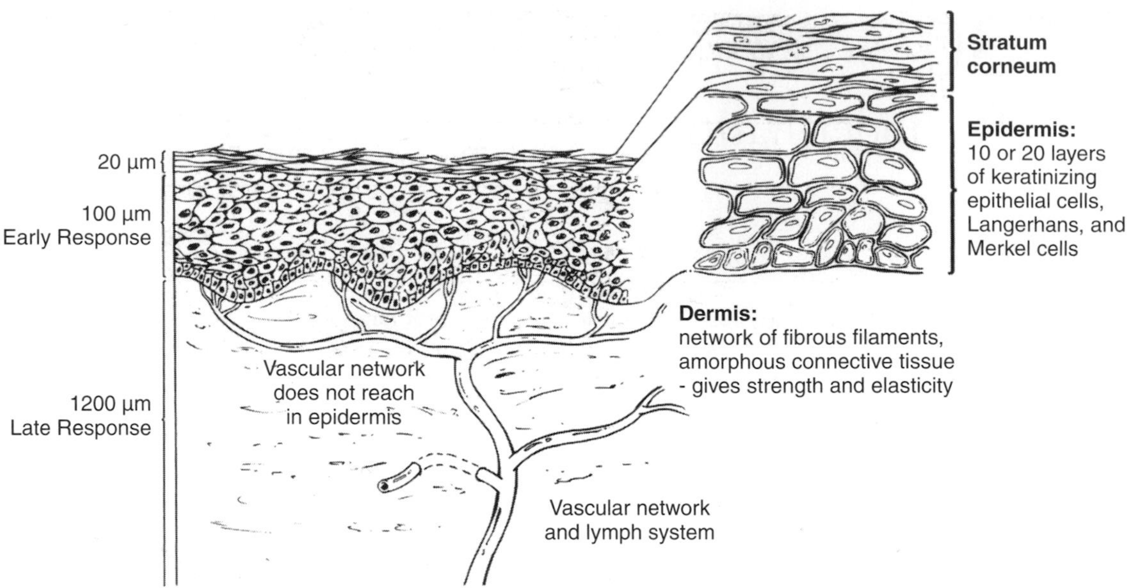

Figure 30-1 Skin Anatomy From the Perspective of the Radiation Biologist. The epidermis has a thickness of about 100 μm, although it varies with body site (30–300 μm). It consists of 10 to 20 layers of keratinizing epithelial cells. This is a self-renewing tissue. The stem-cell compartment forms part of the basal layer and has an unlimited capacity for proliferation. Cells produced in the basal layer migrate to the surface, differentiating as they do so, but retaining some proliferative potential. Cells in the surface layer are fully differentiated and keratinized and gradually are sloughed off and lost. The transit time for an epidermal cell to pass from the basal layer to the surface is 12 to 48 days depending on skin thickness. The dermis is about 1200 μm thick (1000–3000 μm) and consists of a dense network of fibrous filaments and connective tissue. The vascular network, capillaries, and lymph system are in the dermis. The vascular network does not extend into the epidermis. Two distinct waves of reactions are observed in the skin following irradiation. An early, or acute, reaction is observed about 10 days after a single dose and results from damage to the epidermis. Late reactions occur months later, mediated through damage to the dermis, principally to the vasculature. In clinical radiation therapy, late damage is now the dose-limiting reaction, because the buildup associated with megavoltage beams spares the epidermis. *From Hall EJ, Giaccia AJ: Radiobiology for the radiologist, ed 6, (Figure 19-2) (p 336), Philadelphia, 2006, Lippincott Williams & Wilkins.*

some degree of damage is an accepted side effect [13] Acute radiation damage is most prominent in tissues with rapidly proliferating cells, such as in epithelial surfaces of the skin or alimentary tract. Symptoms develop when functional cells are lost as part of normal tissue turnover and are not replaced because of damage to the stem-cell compartment.

In the early years of radiation therapy, skin changes, specifically stages of erythema (degrees of redness), were the measurement used to estimate the amount of therapeutic radiation administered. By the 1940s skin changes were replaced as the measurement of therapeutic radiation by a physical unit of measure, the roentgen (rad),[14] later replaced by the *gray* (Gy) as the radiation unit of measure. Until the 1960s, orthovoltage treatment machines were used to deliver radiation treatment. The majority of radiation energy was deposited on or below the skin surface, resulting in a severe skin reaction. The current use of megavoltage equipment (i.e., linear accelerators) has resulted in less severe skin reactions because of the skin-sparing technology and improved treatment techniques.[15]

Acute Skin Reactions

The skin is extremely sensitive to radiation because of rapid cellular mitosis with basal cell destruction.[16] Table 30-1 provides a summary of effects of radiation on the skin. Acute skin reactions occur during treatment and for a few weeks after radiation therapy are completed. Acute skin reactions are reversible and include erythema,

Table 30-1 Effects of Radiation on the Skin

Skin effect	Time factor	Description	Healing time
Erythema, pigmentation, epilation	Hours to 3 weeks	Increased blood volume beneath epidermis (erythema) Cell destruction due to activation of proteolytic enzymes (pigmentation and epilation)	May be up to several months posttreatment
Dry desquamation (basal cell damage)	3–6 weeks	Atypical keratinization due to reduction on linolenic cells in basal layer resulting in reduced reproduction	6–8 weeks after treatment
Moist desquamation (mostly skin folds)	4–6 weeks	Loss of epidermis due to sterilization of linolenic cells leaving nerves exposed	3–6 weeks after treatment
Secondary ulceration	6 weeks	Secondary damage to epidermis due to dehydration and infection from protracted moist desquamation	Permanent damage
Dermal necrosis	10 weeks	Due to vascular insufficiency	Permanent damage
Dermal atrophy	>26 weeks	Due to contraction of radiated area	Permanent damage
Telangiectasia	52 weeks	Atypical dilation of superficial dermal capillaries	Permanent damage
Invasive fibrosis	No time frame	Healing associated with acute ulceration leading to scar formation	Permanent damage
Acute ulceration	<10 days	Early loss of epidermis due to cellular death in interphase—unusual reaction	Scarring permanent
Acute epidermal necrosis	<10 days	Unusual response to low energy high-dose beta-radiation causing death of keratinocytes	Permanent damage

Reproduced with permission: Maddocks-Jennings W, Wilkinson JM, Shillington D: Novel approaches to radiotherapy-induced skin reactions: a literature review, *Complemnt Therap Clin Pract* 11(4):224-231, 2005. Table 1 on page 225.
Data from Nenot JC: *Int J Radiat Biol* 57(4):783-795, 1990; Hopewell JW: *Int J Radiat Bio,* 57(4):751-753, 1990; Barkam AM: *Prof Nurse* 8(11):732-736, 1993.

hyperpigmentation, dry desquamation, moist desquamation, and epilation (hair loss) within the treatment field.[16,17]

The severity of skin reactions depends on a number of variables. The variables include the type of treatment modality (electrons or lower-energy photons produce higher skin doses); larger total dose, larger fractional dose, location of the treatment field (e.g., sites where two skin surfaces are in contact including the breast and buttocks) and the use of a bolus material to increase the dose deposited in the skin, the size of treatment field, and any previous radiation exposure.[17-19] Certain chemotherapeutic agents such as fluorouracil, methotrexate, and adriamycin used in the combined/concurrent modality setting potentiate radiation effects, thus increasing the severity of skin reactions and also causing them to occur at a lower dose and possibly prolong the reaction.[14,20]

Patient-related variables impacting skin reaction include age (older patients are at increased risk), compromised nutritional status, low performance status, anatomic location of treatment area (skinfolds, body contour), individual radiosensitivity, compromised skin integrity (e.g., scars, surgery, lesions), sites of inflammation, compromised lymph drainage (e.g., the breast), chronic sun exposure, and comorbidities, especially those involving impaired vascularity such as hypertension and/or diabetes, preexisting collagen vascular disease, and smoking.[10,11,14,17-21]

Erythema

Erythema is characterized as reddened skin that may be edematous and feel hot.[6] The redness usually begins 2 to 3 weeks after treatment is initiated. Occasionally, a transient mild erythema may develop after the first treatment as a result of capillary dilation and increased vascular permeability.[8,22] The redness is caused by the histamine-like substance released by damaged cells located at the basal level.[16] This skin reaction may result in patient complaints of itching, tingling, and a feeling of warmth, tenderness, discomfort or pain, and swelling of the treated area.[23] The erythematous reaction usually resolves within 2 to 3 weeks after completion of treatment.

Hyperpigmentation

Hyperpigmentation is a darkening of the skin within the treatment field that begins approximately 2 to 3 weeks after treatment is initiated. It is a result of increased production of melanocytes attempting to protect the basal layer from further radiation-induced damage.[14,22] Varying degrees of hyperpigmentation are a result of complexion type. Patients with a darker complexion produce more melanin and may have more hyperpigmentation than a person with a lighter complexion. In some patients, the hyperpigmentation eventually resolves, whereas in others it can be permanent.

Dry Desquamation

Dry desquamation begins approximately 2 to 3 weeks into therapy and results from depletion of the basal cell population. It is characterized as reddened skin that is dry, flaky, or peeling. It is the result of damage to the sebaceous and sweat glands. The area of dry desquamation may itch and burn. Most of the symptoms resolve within 1 to 2 weeks after completing therapy.[14,16] Temporary epilation of the treatment area occurs during this same timeframe.

Moist Desquamation

Moist desquamation is painful peeling skin with exposure of the dermis and exudate production and ulceration.[6] The basal cell layer is completely destroyed, with blister or vesicle formation, nerve exposure with pain, and serous drainage.[19] It is observed in 10% of patients in selected groups.[6] Since the introduction of megavoltage linear accelerators in radiation therapy, skin reactions rarely deteriorate to the ulcerative stage.[3] Moist desquamation results when the basal cells are unable to produce sufficient amounts of new cells to maintain cellular equilibrium as the epidermal cells are destroyed, thus exposing the dermal layer.[22] At lower doses, islets of skin may regrow from surviving stem cells; at higher doses, at which no stem cells within the treated area survive, moist desquamation is complete and healing must occur by migration of cells from outside the treated area.[7] This reaction begins after approximately 4 weeks of treatment.[16] In some instances, a treatment break may be necessary.

Areas at risk for moist desquamation include those where two skin surfaces contact one another, (inframammary fold) and areas of friction such as the axilla, buttocks, perineum, genitals, and head and neck area.[24] Re-epithelialization occurs in approximately 2 to 4 weeks in the area of moist desquamation.[14,19,25] The newly formed epidermis will be thinner and more prone to injury than before treatment. Complete re-epithelialization and healing of acute skin reaction occurs within 1 to 2 months.[12]

It is not unusual for a patient to have all the previously described stages of reactions—erythema, dry desquamation, and moist desquamation—at the same time. The presence of a fever, foul odor, purulent drainage and/or pain and swelling extending outside of the radiation area are signs of infection.[19] As combined treatment modalities and more intensive radiation regimens are employed, more frequent and intense skin reactions will result for the patient.

Radiation Recall

Radiation recall is an inflammatory skin reaction at a previously irradiated field subsequent to the administration of a variety of pharmacologic agents.[26] Although the skin is the major site of radiation recall toxicity, instances involving other organs have been reported in the literature. It was first described with the antineoplastic agent dactinomycin, but can be observed with other pharmacologic agents. In a recent literature review, Azria and colleagues[26] identified reports of radiation recall in patients receiving anthracyclines, alkylating agents, antimetabolites, nucleoside analogs, taxanes, antituberculosis drugs, antibiotics, tamoxifen citrate (Nolvadex), simvastatin, and exposure to ultraviolet light. Taxanes and anthracyclines are responsible for the majority of cases, 20% and nearly 30%, repectively.[26]

Radiation recall is a poorly understood phenomenon; the precise mechanism is unknown. The dermatologic reaction may include maculopapular eruptions with erythema, vesicle formation, and desquamation of the affected skin areas.[26] The reactions can range in intensity from a mild rash to severe skin necrosis. The manifestations can occur when the precipitating agent is administered within days or even years after radiation in at the sharply defined area corresponding to the treatment field, which shows no or minimal residual reaction because of the previous radiation.[26] It appears to be most severe when the period of time between the radiation therapy and the administration of the chemotherapy is short.

The treatment of radiation recall reactions depends on the organ system involved. However, universally, corticosteroids (topical, oral, or intravenously), or the use of nonsteroidal antiinflammatory agents in conjunctions with the withdrawal of the offending agent, produce prompt and often dramatic improvement.[26]

Chronic or Late Skin Reactions

Chronic or late skin reactions typically occur months, years, and even decades after treatment. Patients who received treatment to a large area with high radiation doses over a shorter time are more likely to experience chronic reactions. Late reactions in the skin include alopecia, pigmentation changes, telangiectasia, atrophy, retraction, fibrosis, slow healing of trauma, necrosis, and carcinogenesis of the treatment area.[27,28] Although acute effects occur mostly in rapidly proliferating cells of the epidermis, the fibrosis, retraction, edema, lymphedema, and atrophy that develop later largely reflect damage to the vascular and connective tissues. The microscopic picture is of atrophy, atypical cells, vascular lesions, and fibrin exudates leading to collagen deposition.[29] The skin becomes more susceptible to infection, trauma, and irritation) and is less likely to heal.[18] In the event there is skin breakdown in the previously treated area that will not heal, a recurrence of the cancer should be ruled out before developing a wound care plan.[30]

Hypopigmentation

Hypopigmentation is a lightening of skin color that may occur after an injury to the skin from a previous surgical procedure or from trauma. It also may be related to conditions such as albinism or vitiligo. Some patients who receive radiation therapy may also experience patches of hypopigmentation within their treatment fields as a result of destruction of melanocytes by the radiation. This is often seen as a late effect with high-dose fields (i.e., mastectomy scar boost).[27] Complete radiation-induced depigmentation of the skin in patients with a history of vitiligo is a potential side effect of radiation therapy, and patients should be educated in advance of their risk of this permanent reaction.

Telangiectasia

Telangiectasia appears as small reddish/purple spider veins in the skin within the treatment field. These changes develop because of radiation damage to the small vessels near the skin surface causing them to stretch.[15] The development of telangiectasia appears to be associated with the occurrence of moist desquamation, loss of the endothelial cell's epidermal protection, and exposure to infectious, inflammatory, chemical, and/or mechanical irritants.[9]

Fibrosis

Fibrosis occurs because of the scarring of the subcutaneous tissue from the radiation and is more commonly seen after radiation therapy for breast cancer, head and neck cancer, and extremity sarcomas resulting in skin tightness, pain, neuropathy, loss of joint range of motion, and lymphedema.[31] It is often accompanied by local and/or regional lymphedema contributing to soft tissue induration. The underlying mechanisms of radiation-induced fibrosis originally were thought to be a result of impaired circulation causing tissue hypoxia and nutritional deficits.[31] More recent theories include the roles of cytokines and growth factors as additional underlying factors contributing to fibrosis formation.[31]

Other factors contributing to an increased risk of developing radiation-induced fibrosis include combined treatment modality, large area of treatment, high total radiation dose, high radiation dose per fraction of treatment, infection or operative complication, and inhomogeneity of treatment delivery.[9] The concurrent use of Nolvadex and radiation therapy has shown an increased incidence of subcutaneous fibrosis in breast cancer patients.[32]

For many years, fibrosis was considered irreversible and an unfortunate by expected side effect of therapy. Recent clinical studies have provided evidence that in some situations reversal of fibrosis is possible. Strategies that have been used in the treatment of fibrosis include pharmacologic, hyperbaric oxygen therapy, physiotherapy, and microcurrent (electric) therapy, although more studies are needed in this area.[9] Some of the most promising data comes from several studies evaluating the using of pentoxifylline and tocopherol (vitamin E).[20,33,34] However, a number of issues still need to be addressed including the appropriate time to initiate the therapy, appropriate dose, and appropriate length of treatment.

Secondary Malignancies

As patients become long-term cancer survivors, the risk of the development of secondary cancers increases. Most solid tumors do not develop for 10 years or longer after radiation.[20] Radiation-induced sarcomas of the bone and soft tissue are the most often seen secondary cancers.[20] Angiosarcoma is one type of secondary malignancy found in the skin, often in women treated with whole breast radiation therapy. It presents as a reddish or purple spot(s) on the skin within the treatment field. It is often misdiagnosed as either a rash or bruise until the disease is more extensive. Careful evaluation by a radiation oncologist and biopsy of the nodule is necessary for diagnosis. Patients should be educated to report changes in the skin immediately.

Another phenomenon that also has been recently addressed in the literature is postradiation vascular proliferations with reportedly benign clinical behavior.[35] These changes are described with a variety of designations including atypical vascular lesions, acquired lymphangiectasis, and lymphangioma. They are rare but well-documented complications of radiation that appear to be increasing in frequency, particularly in women treated with breast-conserving therapy.[35] They present clinically as being usually less than 5-mm papules, commonly showing red to brown discoloration and are often multifocal.[5] Currently more research is needed to determine the appropriate management for such lesions, particularly in light of their similar appearance to angiosarcoma and the possibility that they may be a precursor for this disease.

It is imperative for patients to understand the concept of lifelong radiation-induced skin changes requiring special care and attention to the skin. Patients often share the misconception that the longer the timeframe since completion of radiation therapy, the less likely it is side effects or problems will arise in the skin.

In the event of injury/trauma to an irradiated area resulting in ulceration and/or necrosis, surgical intervention and/or hyperbaric oxygen therapy may be necessary to enhance the healing process. Surgery should be performed by a physician familiar with radiation-induced tissue changes and considered only after other local measures have been tried unsuccessfully. Occasionally, these areas never heal completely.

SKIN CARE DURING RADIATION THERAPY

As previously described, skin reactions are one of the most commonly occurring side effect experienced during radiation therapy. Although the reactions are not as severe as in the past, proper care of the skin during treatment and lifelong thereafter is imperative. The goals of the care of radiation skin reactions include (1) to minimize radiation skin reactions; (2) to maintain and restore skin integrity when possible; (3) to control symptoms, promote comfort, and enhance quality of life.[19]

Nursing Assessment

A baseline nursing assessment should be performed before initiation of treatment. Expected radiation skin reaction is multifactorial and complex.[19] Therefore the assessment should include a careful evaluation of the condition of skin, particularly in the treatment field, and identification of potential risk factors for enhanced skin reactions (e.g., open or delayed wound healing, stoma(s), drain site(s), skin breakdown (*Candida,* bacterial or viral infection), allergic reactions, and the use of photosensitive medications). All identified risk factors should be factored into the planning phase of the consultation.

During the treatment phase, a weekly skin assessment should be performed to evaluate and document skin reactions. It may be necessary to evaluate the skin more frequently in patients with identified risk factors or in those who experience the beginning of skin breakdown. This will ensure that symptom management is adequate (e.g., pain management) and that the patient and/or family understand the daily skin care routine. Also, this is a good time to evaluate for evidence of infection. To enhance consistency of information, the National Cancer Institute's Common Toxicity Criteria, version 3.0,[36] grading system (found in the Oncology Nursing Society [ONS] Radiation Oncology Documentation Tool[37]) should be used for acute and late skin reactions documentation purposes.

Basic Skin Care Instructions

Internationally, wide variations are found in the care of irradiated skin, many based on anecdotal experience or institutional preference. It can vary considerably between institutions and often also between individual practitioners within an institution. Inconsistencies between practitioners can lead to patients receiving conflicting, or even erroneous, information.[38]

Areas of care in which opinions differ are whether to allow washing and use of soap, creams, or deodorants in the management of dry and moist desquamation; the use of steroid creams, saline soaks, gel or occlusive dressings; or use of topical antibiotics.[38] Only a limited amount of research has attempted to address these issues. In a systematic review of the literature, Bolderston and colleagues[38] found no systematic reviews, meta-analyses, or evidence-based guidelines and only two practice guidelines (based on expert opinion and consensus)—one by the British Columbia Cancer Agency[19] and one by the Oncology Nursing Society.[16] In a recent study evaluating the consensus of skin care advice given by nurses during radiation therapy, D'Haese and colleagues[6] found the highest consensus was seen in advice given to patients who developed dry and moist desquamation. Less agreement was found in the case of erythema, and even less consensus was found in preventative advice. These researchers found that some skin care techniques that were frequently used by nurses could not be supported by the literature, reinforcing the belief that the domain of nursing care is strongly influenced by traditional practice. Throughout nursing documents there does appear to be consensus in some general skin care recommendations. These include the following[13]:

- Keep the treatment field clean and dry.
- Use a mild soap of pH 7.5 or less.
- Wash skin gently with no rubbing or scrubbing of the skin.
- Use no irritants (e.g., perfumes, deodorants).
- Use no starch-based products (risk of infection) in areas of moist desquamation.
- Wear and use natural fibers (i.e., cotton clothing) next to the skin.
- Avoid extremes of temperature.

Patient education should be the starting point of the skin care routine and be initiated before the first day of therapy and reinforced on a regular basis (Box 30-1). Patient information should include a review of expected skin reactions, the anticipated timeframe for the stages of reaction, and the skin

Box 30-1 Methods to Reduce the Risk of Radiation-Induced Skin Reactions

- Identify factors that may increase the skin reaction, and take measures to reduce the impact of each factor.
- Delay beginning treatment until surgical wound has healed.
  - Confirm drug/dose of adjuvant chemotherapy to avoid treatment with drugs that may cause a radiation recall effect.
  - Obtain nutritional evaluation by dietician.
  - Obtain evaluation by internist to maximize stability of comorbid conditions.
- Educate patient and family to enhance compliance with the following skin care protocol.
  - Explain expected skin reaction and pattern of alopecia.
  - If departmental protocol includes use of a product to reduce symptoms of skin reaction, discuss appropriate cleansing and use of product. Provide schedule of appropriate times to perform skin care that do not conflict with treatment time.
- Teach patients to minimize skin trauma by reducing friction to the skin.
  - Patients should avoid tight clothing, clothing that increases skin moisture (nylon)
  - Avoid sun exposure and temperature extremes
  - Use an electric razor to shave in treatment fields
- Evaluate skin on a regular basis, and manage skin reactions proactively.
  - If skin integrity is compromised by tumor in the treatment field, a plan should be developed to prevent infection, absorb exudate, and decrease odor, as well as to minimize further trauma and irritation to the area.
  - Dressings that will compromise intact skin should be avoided.
  - Maintain adequate nutritional and fluid intake.
  - Identify signs and symptoms of skin reaction and infection to report.

Modified from Moore-Higgs GJ, Amdur RA: Sustained integrity of protective mechanisms (skin, oral, immune system). In Watkins-Bruner D, Moore-Higgs G, Haas M, editors: *Outcomes in radiation therapy: multidisciplinary management*, Sudbury, Mass, 2001, Jones & Bartlett.

care routine pertinent to the stage of reaction. Marks designating the treatment area may be placed on the patient's skin with semipermanent products such as carfusion dye and paint pens or tattoos that will remain permanently. The semipermanent marks fade during treatment and are reapplied by the radiation therapist as needed. At the conclusion of therapy, the semipermanent marks may be removed or simply worn off.

Management of Acute Skin Reactions

Unfortunately, the expense and difficulties encountered in performing clinical trials have led to a relatively slow growth of new treatment options for radiation wound management. Research efforts attempting to examine wound pathophysiology are hampered by the lack of an adequate chronic wound healing model, and the complexity of the wound healing cascade has limited attempts at pharmacologic modification. As such, currently available wound healing therapies are only partially effective. Many new therapies are emerging that target various aspects of wound repair, and the promise of new therapeutic interventions is on the horizon.

Skin Cleansing

The traditional recommendation was to avoid wetting the skin or washing the skin within the treatment field with any type of soap or cleansing agent. This was based on the idea that the soap may further dry the skin and increase the symptoms of pruritis and erythema. This restrictive approach can interfere with normal hygiene and can be very distressing to the patient. When asked to suspend normal hygiene practices, the patient may feel socially unacceptable at a time when the maintenance of existing social support is very important.[39] Three randomized control trials have compared washing the skin to not washing during radiation therapy.[40-42] None of these studies found washing to contribute to increasing the skin reactions and may actually reduce the severity in some patients. Based on this information, the British Columbia Cancer Agency[19] and the Supportive Care Guidelines Group[38] recommend washing with lukewarm water alone or gentle washing with mild unscented soap (e.g., Dove, Ivory, Neutrogena, Basis or baby soap). The scalp may be washed with lukewarm water and a mild, nonmedicated soap such as baby shampoo.

A sitz bath for treatment of perineal and rectal areas may be used from the beginning of treatment.[19] Luke-warm normal saline or water (40° to 43° C; 104° to 109° F) should be used for 10 to 15 minutes and repeated up to 4 times a day and/or after each bowel movement. Normal saline solution can be made by boiling 1 liter of water and adding 1.5 to 2 teaspoons of salt. It should be allowed to cool overnight before using.

Skin Care Products

A number of products have been used to prevent and treat acute skin reactions including hydrous lanolin, Aquaphor, Eucerin, aloe gel, A&D ointment, silver sulfadiazine, topical steroids, and moisturizing lotion. Few randomized trials have been performed to evaluate the efficacy of these different products in either the prevention or treatment of acute skin reactions. There is insufficient evidence to support or refute most specific topical agents, oral agents (e.g., enzymes, sucralfate) or intravenous agents (e.g., amifostine) for the prevention of or management of acute radiation skin reactions.[38] However, the following is a review of some of the data available on these products[30]:

Aloe vera gel: *Aloe barbadensis* Miller is a fleshy-leafed member of the Liliaceae family.[13] The mucilaginous gel of the leaf contains at least 27 different constituents and is incorporated into many skin and sun care products. It is theorized that aloe vera has a modulating effect on the skin by preventing ultraviolet sunrays from sensitizing the skin, especially in the first 24 hours after exposure and may also penetrate deeply into the skin, enhancing the passage of nutrients. It is also thought to have antibiotic, anticoagulant, and antiviral properties. Pilot data and clinical experience show that aloe vera gel may help prevent radiation therapy–induced dermatitis. In two phase III randomized trials conducted on women receiving breast or chest wall irradiation, no difference in skin dermatitis scores was found among the group using a placebo gel, the no-treatment group, and the group using aloe gel.[43] In fact, aloe gel has been found to delay the healing of wounds left open to heal by secondary intention.[44] The gel may provide some relief of symptoms associated with radiation-induced dermatitis, but will not prevent it, and should be used with caution in areas of moist desquamation because it may delay healing.

Topical steroids: Topical steroids have been used extensively in radiation therapy to manage the pruritus and burning sensation associated with radiodermatitis. However, little research has been conducted on its effectiveness, either as a prevention or treatment of symptoms. It is unknown whether the effect is primarily through miniaturization of the affected skin or as an antiinflammatory agent. Potera and colleagues[45] evaluated the effectiveness of 0.2% hydrocortisone valerate versus placebo in reducing acute radiation dermatitis. No statistically significant difference was found between the 0.2% hydrocortisone valerate and the placebo in the acute skin response, the symptoms of radiation dermatitis, or late skin effects (3 months). In another study, 1% hydrocortisone cream was compared with 0.05% clobetasone butyrate cream.[46] The cream was applied starting at 20 Gy. The majority of patients using either cream derived benefit in its soothing effect. However, a significant difference was seen in the intensity of skin reactions. Patients using clobetasone butyrate developed more severe reactions. Topical steroid creams may soothe the symptoms associated with acute skin reactions, but should not be used to prevent these reactions. They should not be used if infection is suspected or present in the skin.

Hydrocolloid dressings: These dressings provide moderate absorption and hydrate the wound by interacting with the wound fluid to form a gel-like substance resulting in increased epithelial proliferation and reduction in exposure to external pathogens. Margolin and colleagues[47] found that these dressings provide pain relief and timely healing (average 13 days). They should not be used if infection is present. Caution should be taken when removing the dressing because these dressings may damage friable skin. They also should not be used if daily radiation treatment is ongoing because they need to be removed before treatment so as not to create a bolus effect with the radiation dose.

Bepanthen cream: Patients who used this cream were compared to a group of patients who received no topical ointment in a prospective study of 86 patients.[48] The study did not find any benefit for ameliorating radiation-induced skin reactions.

Sucralfate cream: Delaney and colleagues[49] evaluated the use of sucralfate cream in the management of moist desquamation during radiation therapy. Patients were randomized to receive sorbolene alone or 10% sucralfate in sorbolene cream. Despite a small accrual of patients, the two groups did not differ significantly in time to healing or pain relief. Further studies are needed to completely evaluate this approach.

Silver sulfadiazine cream: Silver sulfadiazine cream has been used extensively in the treatment of burns to cover and prevent infection. This cream can be used to manage moist desquamation. However, the downside is that the cream is difficult to remove from the wound, which impacts the clinician's ability to assess the wound and also can increase the discomfort the patient experiences with dressing changes. However, it is inexpensive and readily available in most pharmacies. It should be applied generously and can be mixed with a hydrocolloidal gel to make it easier to apply and remove. A nonstick dry dressing can be applied over the area. A burn net can be used to hold the dressing in place.

However, disadvantages of silver sulfadiazine include the need for dressing changes at least once daily, pain, and the potential for inducing an allergic reaction and argyria. Argyria is the general term used to denote a clinical condition in which excessive administration and deposition of silver causes a permanent irreversible gray-blue discoloration of the skin or mucous membranes. Recent advances in topical wound care products have led to the development of moisture-retention dressings that have the advantages of improved exudate management, less frequent dressing changes, an improved barrier to microorganisms, reduced exposure to airborne microorganisms at dressing change, less disruption of newly healed tissue than gauze, less wound pain, and greater patient comfort. Some of these dressings incorporate silver sulfadiazine and ionic silver. To date, no data is available on the use of such dressings in the radiation therapy setting, but it may prove to be beneficial in the future.

Hyaluronic acid cream: This cream was evaluated in a randomized, double-blind, placebo-controlled study.[50] Acute radiation-induced dermatitis was significantly higher in the placebo group than in the group using hyaluronic acid cream. In addition, the cream appeared to delay slightly the onset of reactions (from week 1 to week 2) in this group.

Amifostine: Amifostine has been used to reduce the risk of mucositis associated with radiation therapy. One nonrandomized trial evaluated its role in 30 patients receiving radiation and chemotherapy.[51] They found a significantly lower maximal erythema score in the amifostine group. Further evaluation is needed with randomized trials to determine the benefit in different patient populations.

Specific Symptom Management

Pruritis

Pruritis is often associated with the early signs of dry desquamation and is a commonly reported symptom in the first 2 or 3 weeks. It can impact the patient's ability to concentrate and to sleep. Excessive scratching can increase the risk of a superficial infection. Warm air temperatures and perspiration can make the symptoms worse. The patient should be advised to cleanse the skin with tepid water. Dry cornstarch may be used as long as there is no evidence of moist breakdown because this may contribute to a fungal or skin infection. Some patients have used an oatmeal colloidal soap to cleanse the skin followed by oatmeal colloidal lotion to provide some temporary relief. The British Columbia Cancer Agency[19] and the Supportive Care Guidelines Group[38] suggest that a non-scented, lanolin-free hydrophilic cream is helpful to patients and should be applied after treatment and before bedtime. This type of cream attracts and traps moisture at the skin surface to increase the skin's moisture. Well-hydrated skin promotes healing and comfort and reduces the potential for trauma.[19,39,40] Examples of hydrophilic cream include Lubriderm, Glaxal Base, Eucerin, Keri Lotion, Dermal Therapy, and Aquaphor.[19]

Normal saline compresses also may help alleviate burning, itching, or shearing.[19] Aloe vera may be used to soothe and cool the skin. In severe cases, a mild steroid cream (e.g., 1%) maybe applied to provide a local antiinflammatory effect. However, this product should be discontinued if moist desquamation occurs. Products with alcohol, perfumes, or additives and products containing alpha hydroxy acids (AHA) should be avoided because they may increase the skin reaction. Petroleum-based products also should be avoided because they are poorly absorbed, provide minimal hydration, and are difficult to remove.

Dry Desquamation and Alopecia

Dry desquamation and alopecia can be managed using the same approach as that used for pruritis. The primary aims are to alleviate patient discomfort because there is no skin breakdown and potential for infection.[38]

Moist Desquamation

Treatment for moist desquamation has changed as a result of the extensive research into the mechanisms of wound healing. The skin becomes open and susceptible to infection, and antibacterial or antifungal medication with or without soaks and dressings are often prescribed. However, when there is no proven infection, the routine use of antiseptics, antibiotics and disinfectants is questionable.[38] Current wound healing policy is to support the wound with moisture and a protective dressing rather than allow the wound to air dry.

In radiation-induced moist desquamation, a number of different types of wound dressings have been tried with mixed success. Individual departments should have several different dressings that are recommend based on availability and expense. Other key factors that should be considered before selecting a wound care plan for an individual patient are the size and site of the wound, presence of infection, the radiation treatment plan, and the ability of the patient and/or family to comply with wound care plan.

The area should be gently cleansed with lukewarm water or normal saline and a mild soap. This is particularly useful if there are small friable areas that are bleeding; silver nitrate sticks or a sucralfate paste (1-g sucralfate tablet crushed into in 2 to 3 mL of hydrogel) may reduce sites of oozing blood.[52] A moisture-retentive protective barrier ointment or hydrogel should be applied.[19] Examples of these products include ProShield, DuoDerm Gel, and IntraSite Gel. For patients who are going to continue with treatment, products that act as a bolus should be avoided. For patients who are not going to continue with treatment or who are taking a treatment break, a product that provides moisture with or without an antibacterial or antifungal effect should be selected (e.g., silver sulfadiazine), which is effective against gram-positive and gram-negative organisms and *Candida albicans*.

A protective nonstick absorbent dressing should be applied to cover the entire wound area to avoid placing additional stress on surrounding skin that has been exposed to radiation. Hydrocolloid, occlusive, and moisture-vapor-permeable dressings may be used. However, the dressing must be removed before daily treatment and therefore may cause more desquamation and pain. If dressings stick to the wound, they can be soaked with normal saline or tepid water.

If there is evidence of a bacterial infection, a wound culture may be beneficial. Oral antibiotics should be initiated immediately, and the patient should be carefully monitored for response. Fungal infections can be managed with antifungal medications as needed. Moist desquamation is painful, and the patient should be provided with adequate analgesics that will reduce both physiologic and psychologic distress and enhance participation in twice daily wound care.

If tumor is present in the wound, a chronic wound-care program should be initiated that includes cleansing the wound, debridement, controlling bleeding, controlling odor, protecting the wound from further damage, and controlling pain. Metronidazole 0.8% gel, charcoal dressings, a suspension of aluminum hydroxide/magnesium hydroxide, or yogurt may be applied to the wound to reduce the odor.[52]

Management of Late Skin Reactions

Late skin reactions progress slowly and subclinically from 6 months to many years later. Each patient needs an individualized plan to improve skin texture and elasticity and to reduce risks for injury or trauma. If skin breakdown or necrosis occurs, a local recurrence of the cancer should be ruled out before referral to a chronic wound care specialist. In an attempt to prevent some of these affects, patients may want to follow these simple instructions.

Skin texture and elasticity improvement may be accomplished with the application of a moisturizing lotion to the treatment field at least once a day. The patient should be advised to avoid exposure to the sun or generously apply an appropriate sunscreen and repeat during sun exposure (minimum of 15 SPF).[19] Physical therapy with gentle massage or myofascial release may help increase elasticity and reduce fibrosis and scar formation.

Reduction of trauma risk may be accomplished by avoiding activities that increase the risk of a skin break or bruising. The patient should be taught to avoid scratching and avoid the use of adhesive tape and other activities that increase skin friction or damage in the treatment fields. The patient should continue to avoid temperature extremes including hot water bottles, heating pads, ice packs, and use of sunlamps and tanning beds. Activities that increase the risk of lymphedema also should be avoided whenever possible. The patient should report any skin changes or injury immediately.

SUMMARY

Radiation-induced skin changes can impair a patient's quality of life. Patient education related to expected skin reactions, institute-specific methods of skin care, and astute nursing assessments with prompt interventions specific to the level of skin reaction may prevent the patient unnecessary discomfort. More research must be conducted to establish evidence-based skin care regimens in radiation therapy. Until this occurs the regimens remain preferences of each institution.

REFERENCES

1. Naylor W, Mallett J: Management of acute radiotherapy induced skin reactions: a literature review, *Eur J Oncol Nurs* 5(4):221-233, 2001.
2. Fisher J, Scott C, Stevens R et al: Randomised phase III study comparing best supportive care to Biafine as a prophylactic agent for radiation-induced skin toxicity for women undergoing breast irradiation: Radiation Therapy Oncology Group, *Int J Radiat Oncol Biol Phys* 48(5):1307-1310, 2000.
3. Porock D, Kristjanson L: Skin reactions during radiotherapy for breast cancer: the use and impact of topical agents and dressings, *Eur J Cancer Care (Engl)* 8(3):143-153, 1999.
4. Porock D, Nikoletti S, Kristjanson L: Management of radiation reactions: literature review and clinical applications, *Plastic Surg Nurs* 19(4):186-193, 1999.
5. Noble-Adams R: Radiation-induced reactions, Pt 3: evaluating the RISRAS, *Br J Nurs* 8(19):1305-1312, 1999.
6. D'Haese S, Bate R, Claes S et al: Management of skin reactions during radiotherapy: a study of nursing practice, *Eur J Cancer Care* 14(1):28-42, 2005.
7. Hall EJ, Giaccia AJ: *Radiobiology for the radiologist,* ed 6, Philadelphia, 2006, Lippincott Williams & Wilkins.
8. Sitton E: Managing side effects of skin changes and fatigue. In Dow KH, Bucholtz JD, Iwanmoto RR, editors: *Nursing care in radiation oncology*, Philadelphia, 1999, WB Saunders, pp 79-100.
9. O'Sullivan B, Levin W: Late radiation-related fibrosis: pathogenesis, manifestations, and current management, *Semin Radiat Oncol* 13(3):274-289, 2003.
10. Pearce JD: Alterations in mobility, skin integrity, and neurologic status. In Itano JK, Taoka KN, editors: *Core curriculum for oncology nursing,* ed 4, St Louis, 2005, Mosby, pp 245-258.
11. Casey L: Skin and hair changes. In Varricchio CG, editor: *A cancer source book for nurses,* ed 8, Sudbury, Mass, 2004, Jones and Bartlett, pp 435-446.
12. Shimm DS, Cassady JR: The skin. In Cox JD, editor: *Moss' radiation oncology: rationale, technique and results,* ed 7, St Louis, 1994, Mosby, pp 99-120.
13. Maddocks-Jennings W, Wilkinson JM, Shillington D: Novel approaches to radiotherapy-induced skin reactions: a literature review, *Complement Ther Clin Pract* 11(4): 224-231, 2005.
14. Maher KE: Principles of radiation therapy. In Nevidjon BM, Sowers KW, editors: *A nurse's guide to cancer care,* Philadelphia, 2000, Lippincott, pp 215-240.
15. Campbell MK, Pruitt JJ: Radiation therapy: protecting your patient's skin, *RN* 59(1):46-47, 1996.
16. Haas ML: Skin reactions. In Bruner DW, Haas ML, Gosselin-Acomb TK, editors: *Manual for radiation oncology nursing practice and education,* ed 3, Pittsburgh, 2005, ONS Press, pp 323-351.

17. Maher KE: Radiation therapy: toxicities and management. In Yarbro CH, Goodman M, Frogge MH et al, editors: *Cancer nursing: principles and practice*, ed 5, Sudbury, Mass, 2000, Jones and Bartlett, pp 323-351.
18. Hom DB, Adams G, Koreis M et al: Choosing the optimal wound dressing for irradiated soft tissue wounds, *Otolaryngol Head Neck Surg* 121(5):591-598, 1999.
19. *Care of radiation skin reactions*, Vancouver, BC, 2006, British Columbia Cancer Agency.
20. Maher KE: Radiation therapy: toxicities and management. In Yarbro CH, Frogge MH, Goodman M, editors: *Cancer nursing: principles and practice,* ed 6, Sudbury, Mass, 2005, Jones and Bartlett, pp 283-314.
21. Delanian S, Porcher R, Rudant J et al: Kinetics of response to long-term treatment combining pentoxifylline and tocopherol in patients with superficial radiation-induced fibrosis, *J Clin Oncol* 23(24):8570-8579, 2005.
22. Wickline MM: Prevention and treatment of acute radiation dermatitis: a literature review, *Oncol Nurs Forum* 31(2): 237-247, 2004.
23. Noble-Adams R: Radiation-induced reactions 1: an examination of the phenomenon, *Br J Nurs* 8(17):1208-1211, 1999.
24. Warmkessel JH: Beaming in on radiation therapy, *Nursing* 28(11):65-67, 1998.
25. Campbell J: Skin care for patients undergoing radiotherapy. In Feber T, editor: *Head and neck oncology nursing*, Philadelphia, 2000, Whurr Publishers, pp 219-228.
26. Azria D, Magne N, Abderrahim Z et al: Radiation recall: a well recognized but neglected phenomenon, *Cancer Treat Rev* 31(7):555-570, 2005.
27. Constine LS, Williams JP, Moris M et al: Late effects of cancer treatment on normal tissues. In Perez CA, Brady LW, editors: *Principles and practice of radiation oncology*, ed 4, Philadelphia, 2003, Lippincott Williams & Wilkins, pp 357-390.
28. Witt ME: Nursing implications of radiation therapy. In Itano JK, Taoka KN, editors: *Core curriculum for oncology nursing,* ed 4, St Louis, 2005, WB Saunders, pp 748-762.
29. Fajardo LF: Morphology of radiation effects on normal tissues. In Perez CA, Brady LW, editors: *Principles and practice of radiation oncology,* ed 2, Philadelphia, 1997, JB Lippincott, pp 143-154.
30. Moore-Higgs GJ, Amdur RA: Sustained integrity of protective mechanisms (skin, oral, immune system). In Watkins-Bruner D, Moore-Higgs G, Haas M, editors: *Outcomes in radiation therapy: multidisciplinary management*, Sudbury, Mass, 2001, Jones and Bartlett, pp 493-518.
31. Chiao TB, Lee AJ: Role of pentoxifylline and vitamin E in attenuation of radiation induced fibrosis, *Ann Pharmacother* 39(3):516-521, 2005.
32. Azria D, Gourgou S, Sozzi WJ et al: Concomitant use of tamoxifen with radiotherapy enhances subcutaneous breast fibrosis in hypersensitive patients, *Br J Cancer* 91(7): 1251-1260, 2004.
33. Delanian S, Balla-Mekias S, Lefaix J-L: Striking regression of chronic radiotherapy damage in a clinical trial of combined pentoxifylline and tocopherol, *J Clin Oncol* 17(10): 3283-3290, 1999.
34. Okunieff P, Augustine E, Hicks JE et al: Pentoxifylline in the treatment of radiation induced fibrosis, *J Clin Oncol* 22(11):2207-2213, 2004.
35. Brenn T, Fletcher CD: Postradiation vascular proliferations: an increasing problem, *Histopathology* 48(1):106-114, 2006.
36. *Cancer therapy evaluation program, common terminology: criteria for adverse events (CTCAE), Version 3.0,* Washington, DC, 2003, National Cancer Institute.
37. Radiation Therapy Special Interest Group Documentation Project Core Committee: *Radiation therapy patient care record: a tool for documenting nursing care*, Pittsburgh, 2002, Oncology Nursing Press.
38. Bolderston A, Lloyd NS, Wong RK et al, the Supportive Care Guidelines Group of Cancer Care Ontario Program in Evidence-Based Care: The prevention and management of acute skin reactions related to radiation therapy: a systematic review and practice guideline, *Support Care Cancer* 14(8):802-817, 2006.
39. Campbell IR, Illingworth MH: Can patients wash during radiotherapy to the breast or chest wall? A randomized controlled trial, *Clin Oncol* 4(2):78-82, 1992.
40. Campbell L: Developing a skin-care protocol in radiotherapy, *Prof Nurse* 12(2):105-108, 1996.
41. Roy I, Fortin A, Larochelle M: The impact of skin washing with water and soap during breast irradiation: a randomized study, *Radiother Oncol* 58(3):333-339, 2001.
42. Wesbury C, Hines F, Hawkes E et al: Advice on hair and scalp care during cranial radiotherapy: a prospective randomized trial, *Radiother Oncol* 54(2):109-116, 2000.
43. Williams MS, Burk M, Loprinzi CL: Phase III double-blind evaluation of an aloe vera gel as a prophylactic agent for radiation-induced skin toxicity, *Int J Radiat Oncol Biol Phys* 36(2):345-349, 1996.
44. Schmidt JM, Greenspoon JS: Aloe vera dermal wound gel is associated with a delay in wound healing, *Obstet Gynecol* 78(1):115-117, 1991.
45. Potera ME, Lookingbill DP, Stryker JA: Prophylaxis of radiation dermatitis with a topical cortisone cream, *Radiology* 143(3):775-777, 1982.
46. Glees JP, Mameghan-Zadeh H, Sparkes CG: Effectiveness of topical steroids in the control of radiation dermatitis: a randomized trial using 1% hydrocortisone cream and 0.05% clobetasone butyrate (Eumovate), *Clin Radiol* 30(4): 397-403, 1979.
47. Margolin S, Breneman J, Denman D et al: Management of radiation-induced moist skin desquamation using hydrocolloid dressing, *Cancer Nurs* 13(2):71-80, 1990.
48. Lokkevik E, Skovlund E, Reitan JB et al: Skin treatment with Bepanthen cream versus no cream during radiotherapy—a randomized controlled trial, *Acta Oncol* 35(8):1021-1026, 1996.
49. Delaney G, Fisher R, Hook C et al: Sucralfate cream in the management of moist desquamation during radiotherapy, *Australas Radiol* 41(3):270-275, 1997.
50. Liguori V, Guillemin C, Pesce GF et al: Double-blind, randomized clinical study comparing hyaluronic acid cream to placebo in patients treated with radiotherapy, *Radiother Oncol* 42(2):155-161, 1997.
51. Koukourakis MI, Kyrias G, Kakolyris S et al: Subcutaneous amifostine during fractionated radiotherapy: a randomized phase II study, *J Clin Oncol* 18(1):2226-2233, 2000.
52. Waller A, Caroline NL: *Handbook of palliative care in cancer*, Boston, 1996, Butterworth-Heinemann.

Chapter 31
Pain

Karen Snow Kaiser and Micke A. Brown

Pain—has an Element of Blank—
It cannot recollect
When it begun—or if there were
A time when it was not[1]
Emily Dickinson

Pain in radiation oncology patients is not uncommon. These patients suffer from pain related to two major causes—from the cancer itself and from associated treatment or other etiologies. Regardless of the cause, pain is significantly undertreated and is feared by most patients. The American Pain Foundation estimates over 75 million Americans experience pain each year, with approximately 25 million experiencing acute pain and the remaining living with chronic or persistent pain.[2] The number of people suffering with chronic pain outnumbers those with breast cancer, AIDS, and nearly all other serious or terminal diseases.[3] Magnify these numbers to include the many others who live in pain on planet earth and it becomes obvious why pain is a healthcare crisis. With such a high prevalence, it would not be unusual for a patient receiving radiation therapy to experience pain. Because pain has deleterious effects, prompt assessment and management of pain is imperative no matter the cause.

As nurses, whose primary ethical tenet is to decrease the suffering of others, uncontrolled pain is an unacceptable societal norm that must be addressed. By understanding the pathophysiology of pain, using the essential components of a comprehensive pain assessment, linking physiology and assessment findings to the appropriate treatment options, and being an advocate for the patient, the nurse can have a major impact on the reduction of pain. This chapter provides information on pathophysiology of pain, pain assessment, treatment options, and patient advocacy to assist you with the management of pain in the radiation oncology patient.

PAIN IN THE RADIATION ONCOLOGY SETTING

Although pain is one of the most common clinical problems in healthcare today, little literature is focused on pain in the radiation oncology setting. Understanding the scope of the pain problem as it relates to cancer can provide some insight into the scope of the problem as it relates to radiation oncology because the patients evaluated and treated in radiation oncology most often are cancer patients in one or another of the many disease stages. In the United States, approximately 1.4 million new cancer cases are diagnosed every year[4] and more than 500,000 people die each year from the disease.[5] Added to these numbers are the millions of cancer survivors. Cancer pain epidemiologic studies suggest wide variations in the number of patients that experience pain from cancer, with overall estimates of pain ranging from 14% to 100%.[6] Upwards to 75% are reported to experience pain at the time of diagnosis, upwards to 57% experience pain during treatment for the disease, and anywhere from 23% to 100% report pain in advanced stages of the disease.[7] With these rates, it is worrisome that numerous cancer pain studies consistently show that such pain is undertreated. For example, one study reports 50% of those with advanced disease who are undergoing active treatment receive adequate pain management.[8]

Cancer pain can occur at any stage of the disease, including during survivorship, and may be the result of:

1. Tumor progression or related pathology (e.g., nerve damage)
2. Invasive diagnostic or therapeutic procedures and operations
3. Chemotherapy and radiation related toxicities
4. Infections
5. Muscle fatigue and atrophy from decreased physical activity

6. Emergence of other pain disorders caused by immune system changes (e.g., herpes zoster, polyarthritis)[9]

Some pain syndromes are common in cancer patients. It is important to recognize these syndromes so patients can receive prompt attention and treatment. These syndromes may be unrecognized or dismissed by the patient, the cancer survivor, or healthcare providers.[10] After surgery, common cancer pain syndromes caused by peripheral nerve injury include postmastectomy pain, postthoracotomy pain, postnephrectomy pain, postradical neck dissection pain, and phantom limb pain. Antineoplastic agents such as platinum-based drugs, vinca alkaloids, and taxanes also can cause peripheral neuropathy.

Radiation therapy may cause mild to severe pain from many sources. Some examples include local or distant skin irritation/desquamation caused by the radiation alone or from associated side effects such as diarrhea; disruption of mucous membrane integrity anywhere throughout the gastrointestinal (GI) tract; and swelling from tumor destruction (such as headache or nerve impingement). Radiation therapy sequelae also may be a source of pain. According to Campa and Payne,[11] radiation treatments can cause pain due to fibrosis, soft tissue ischemia, necrosis, inflammation, and peripheral nerve tumors in deep or superficial nerves that develop in a genetically predisposed person. Specifically, fibrosis may compress nearby neural tissue resulting in plexopathies (e.g., radiation-induced brachial plexopathy), acute and chronic skin changes can occur, a peripheral nerve plexus or an element of the spinal cord can be injured directly by radiation, or patients may develop osteoradionecrosis, myelopathy, or fibrosarcoma.

Pain can exist at the time of evaluation for radiation therapy, can be caused by the radiation treatment itself, can be aggravated by positioning, or can occur as an aftermath of radiation therapy. Whether radiation therapy is recommended for prevention, cure, or palliation, or whether the patient is being seen during active treatment or for follow-up, identifying the presence of pain, analyzing for possible causes, and intervening for effective management are critical elements of quality nursing care. Awareness of how and why pain may emerge is the first step in early intervention and promotes more effective management of pain.

Why is treatment of pain so important? The undertreatment of cancer pain leads to a diminished quality of life. Persistent pain causes alterations in function, a depressed mood, inability to sleep, changes in appetite, and often social isolation.[12-15] The burden of pain in cancer patients goes beyond the experience of pain itself, touching many aspects of a person's and their loved ones' lives.[16-18,19]

Uncontrolled acute pain can lead to increased morbidity and mortality.[20,21] Acute pain initiates the metabolic stress response,[22] placing additional stress on already compromised physiologic systems in those fighting a serious illness such as cancer. Immune competence may be altered resulting in an increased risk of infection,[21] which may subsequently delay cancer treatment. More importantly, poor pain control promotes tumor growth in metastatic prone tumors after surgery by suppressing natural killer (NK) cell activity, which recognizes and kills neoplastic cells.[23] Because immunocompetence varies over time, the effect of chronic pain on NK cells is unknown. However, a large prospective longitudinal epidemiologic human study suggests a relationship between chronic pain and cancer.[24] In this study, individuals suffering from widespread or regional pain had higher death rates after controlling for preexisting disease and other confounding factors, with most deaths attributed to cancer. It is possible that this phenomenon was at least partially related to immunocompetence.

Pain also can hinder mobility, contributing to thromboembolic complications[25] in a population that is already at high risk for thrombolytic events. Thrombolytic events are associated with an increase in intensive care unit (ICU) admissions[26] and may lead to death. Uncontrolled pain may be the causative factor for prolonged hospital stays[27] and hospital readmissions.[28] Pain also has been shown to predict postprocedural confusion in the elderly.[29-31] In contrast and contrary to popular belief, analgesic use does not predict confusion.[29]

Since cancer pain is common, acute or persistent pain is harmful, and inadequate management is unethical and substandard, why does it continue to be poorly treated? Studies have shown that physicians underprescribe, patients request less medication than they need, and nurses administer suboptimal doses of analgesics[32-37] even though the end results of ineffective pain management may be more deleterious than analgesic treatment. Misconceptions about pain physiology[25,38] may contribute to undermedication.[39] Inadequate assessment[40] and lack of integration of evidence-based pain management principles into clinical practice[41,42] are other common reasons for inadequately controlled pain.

The causes of undertreatment must be addressed in order to improve outcomes. The first step in improving pain management is through awareness and education. The next step is adopting new knowledge in clinical practice. This chapter reviews pain types and pain physiology and discusses how various pain interventions work. Then it explores pain assessment, pain management strategies, and general principles of pain care using best practice information for the care of the radiation therapy patient with pain. Because patients undergoing radiation therapy often have complex medical treatment plans, a variety of pain disorders that may be related to the disease or its management, as well as a dynamic clinical picture, this chapter provides general information to enable the radiation therapy nurse to make informed choices in the management of the radiation therapy patient with pain.

DEFINITION AND CLASSIFICATION

Pain *(poena)* translated from Latin means "a punishment or penalty;" the word itself reflects biases that may be found in modern society and health care. Definitions that are recognized in the specialty of pain management are as follows:

- "An unpleasant sensory and emotional experience associated with actual or potential tissue damage or described in terms of such damage"[43,44]
- "Whatever the experiencing person says it is, existing whenever the experiencing person say it does"[45]

Pain is a subjective experience that can occur in the absence of observable tissue damage[46] and can be classified as acute or chronic. Acute pain is often ascribed as our biologic red flag. It is a protective mechanism that signals during times of injury from disease, accident, or an invasive procedure.[27] Acute pain is often sudden in onset, short in duration (usually less than 6 months)[47] and may signal the stress response, which is self-limiting. It is expected that as the body heals, acute pain wanes. Acute pain tends to be the most intense during the first 48 to 72 hours after an invasive procedure or injury. It can vary in its presentation. Acute pain can be constant, intermittent, fluctuate in intensity and be caused by precipitating factors such as movement or occur spontaneously. Though beneficial in the short-term, prolonged or uncontrolled moderate to severe pain can be harmful.

Studies provide evidence that uncontrolled acute pain may set the stage for the development of chronic pain caused by nervous system changes in response to a constant bombardment of pain signals. Even brief episodes of acute pain can lead to chronic pain[27,48,49] by changing the neural wiring and increasing sensitization to stimuli.[27] Although acute pain may serve as a protective function, chronic pain appears to have no physiologic function.[39] "Chronic pain... is a destructive disease with physical, psychological, and behavioral consequences."[50]

In comparison to acute pain, chronic pain lasts beyond the original physical injury or acute disease. It is usually present for 6 months or more; however, it varies in its onset, duration, and character. The physical cause or associated pathology may be unknown[51] or due to a chronic pathologic process that leads to continuous pain or pain that recurs at intervals over time.[52] According to Brookhoff,[50] chronic pain is different than a prolonged version of acute pain. The repeating pain signals cause physiochemical changes in neural pathways resulting in hypersensitivity to pain signals and resistance to antinociceptive input. These signals leave a permanent imprint on the nervous system after acute injury has resolved.

Chronic pain also may be referred to as persistent pain and may be subdivided into malignant and nonmalignant pain. Malignant and nonmalignant pain may be present simultaneously. Acute and chronic pain also may coexist, arising from the same (e.g., chronic bone pain from a bony metastasis with acute bone pain due to stabilization) or different locations/causative factors (e.g., chronic osteoarthritis knee pain along with acute pain from a pathologic hip fracture). Patients with chronic pain also may have episodic breakthrough pain, transitory episodes of pain superimposed upon persistent pain that is generally well controlled.[53] Chronic pain may be nociceptive, neuropathic, or a mixture of the two. Nociceptive and neuropathic pain is described below.

Besides classifying pain based on time, it also may be classified based on the underlying mechanism causing the pain, which may be more helpful in the clinical setting because it aids in the selection of effective treatments. In this classification schema, pain may be nociceptive or neuropathic. Nociceptive pain is divided into somatic or visceral pain. Somatic pain arises from soft tissue, bone, and joints that contain nociceptors,[51] receptors that are sensitive to noxious stimuli and cause tissue damage.[43] It can be superficial (cutaneous), such as from a radiation burn, or deep, such as from a bony metastasis. In contrast, neuropathic pain is caused by injury to peripheral or central nerves, with resultant abnormal spontaneous nerve firings that may be accompanied by allodynia (exaggerated response to nonpainful stimuli), dysesthesias (unpleasant sensations such as tingling, skin crawling, or pins and needles), or paresthesia,[54] which are abnormal sensations that are not unpleasant.[43] Similar to its symptomatology, the underlying pathology of neuropathic pain is heterogeneous.[55] Various inflammatory or infectious processes are thought to be responsible for approximately half the cases of neuropathic pain.[56] According to Watkins and Maier,[56] these processes increase nerve excitability, alter the blood-nerve barrier, damage myelin, and activate the spinal cord glia—modulators of spinal pain transmission. Nociceptive and neuropathic pain may coexist, such as when a cancerous vertebral tumor impinges upon a nerve root.

Although classification of pain is helpful in determining management (e.g., use of short-acting drugs for acute pain and long-acting drugs for chronic pain or use of special classes of drugs for neuropathic pain), information about pain pathophysiology and where and how drugs work to control pain is also needed. The following section reviews this information.

PHYSIOLOGY OF PAIN AND HOW PAIN THERAPIES WORK

The theories about pain processing have evolved significantly since Descartes described pain in 1644. Though simplistic in its hypothesis, it has served as the framework for current understanding. Descartes explained pain as a reaction caused by an injury sending a message to the brain, where a signal (bell ring) activated a response. Current knowledge is multifarious but begins with the concept of injury. Nociception, "the process by which information about tissue damage is conveyed to the CNS"[57] is complex. Four basic physiologic processes occur during nociception—transduction, transmission, perception, and modulation. Each of these processes is briefly described below, and examples are provided to demonstrate how pain interventions work. Some pain management strategies affect more than one process because of the method of administration or multiple mechanisms of action. In general, the pain treatment's primary mechanism of action is described. The discussion primarily focuses on the physiologic processing of nociceptive pain because the physiology of neuropathic pain is not as well understood. However, neuronal plasticity, the active neurobiologic process by which the nervous system changes and modulates responses to any stimulus, is responsible for reversible exaggerated pain sensitivity or hypersensitivity and permanent changes in the pain processing system that causes chronic inflammatory or neuropathic pain.[58] Optimal treatment selection depends on these normal and abnormal physiologic processes, so sensitization that causes chronic inflammatory and neuropathic pain is integrated into the following discussion.

Transduction

"Transduction is the conversion of energy from a noxious thermal, mechanical, or chemical stimulus into electrical energy (nerve impulses) by sensory receptors called *nociceptors*."[57] Nociceptors are free nerve endings at the distal end of primary afferent (first order) neurons. Two major types of primary afferents that carry pain messages are A-delta and C-fibers. In general, A-delta fibers respond to high intensity mechanical stimuli, whereas C-fibers respond primarily to firm pressure, irritants, and heat.[39,59] Tissue damage from chemicals, heat, or pressure causes cell membranes to break down and causes release of chemical mediators such as prostaglandins, bradykinin, serotonin, substance P, histamine, and other substances, which activate nociceptors (generate impulses) and sensitize nociceptors (increasing excitability and discharge frequency).[57] When this occurs, the body mounts a localized inflammatory response, which includes redness, warmth, swelling, and increased pain. As the chemically mediated response changes into an action potential or electrical charge, transduction occurs.[60] During transduction, the cell depolarizes because there is an influx of sodium into the cell and a efflux of potassium out of the cell until the threshold is reached, at which point the transmission phase begins.[39]

Before discussing the transmission phase it is important to further discuss the inflammatory response and its relationship to pain and pain management interventions that may affect transduction. The inflammatory response triggers the release of additional chemical mediators that decrease the threshold for primary afferent nerve fiber activation, shortens the latency period (resting phase or lag time between nerve firings), and increases the response to stimuli.[39] As a result, the noxious stimulus that previously would not trigger a nociceptor does, causing pain. This phenomenon is called *peripheral sensitization*.[61] Nociceptors involved in the inflammatory response also release neuropeptides, causing autosensitization of the nerve and sensitizing other primary afferent fibers nearby,[39] in effect recruiting previously unsensitized nociceptors causing secondary hyperalgesia and extending the area of pain and inflammation beyond the original injury. This can cause additional peripheral sensitization. So, once pain begins, it can become self-sustaining. Whereas peripheral sensitization is protective during healing, the increased transduction associated with peripheral sensation can cause allodynia and hyperalgesia, and if chronic, neuropathic pain may develop.[62,63]

A variety of pain interventions affect transduction. *Nonsteroidal antiinflammatory drugs (NSAIDs)* exert their primary effect by inhibiting cyclooxygenase (COX-1 and COX-2), which catalyzes arachidonic acid transformation into prostaglandins and causes pain and inflammation. Thus nonspecific COX inhibitors (NSAIDs) such as ibuprofen and specific COX-2 inhibitors such as celecoxib modulate the inflammatory process. *Capsaicin,* a topical cream made from hot pepper extract, exerts its primary effect in the transduction phase and has an impact on the inflammation process as well. It causes intense irritation and rapidly depletes substance P here and elsewhere throughout the nociceptive system, reducing pain after an initial short period of intense pain.

Local anesthetics and *anticonvulsants* stabilize cell membranes. When administered systemically, topically (e.g., local anesthetic creams and gels), or intradermally, local anesthetics work by blocking ion channels,[39] preventing depolarization and the process of transduction. This is how intradermal injections of local anesthetic given before shallow procedures, such as placing an intravascular port, prevent pain. Anticonvulsants and local anesthetics may be used in neuropathic pain conditions to reinstitute normal, or more near normal, membrane stability throughout the nervous system, slowing the generation of pain signals in patients experiencing neuropathic pain. Unfortunately, it takes a few weeks to months to achieve maximum pain relief and usually requires titration to determine the optimal dose.

The salient point related to the transduction phase is to minimize the vicious cycle of peripheral sensitization. This suggests use of preemptive analgesia, the administration of analgesia before the advent of pain. Unfortunately, the results from systematic reviews of studies with a variety of patient types, medications, and techniques involving preemptive analgesia (the initiation of analgesics before the onset of noxious stimuli with the goal of reducing subsequent pain) are mixed.[64,65] Preemptive studies are difficult to design, and existing studies are difficult to interpret because of measurement, design, and power issues. However, the benefits of preemptive analgesia are well documented in animal studies, and better designed more recent human studies are beginning to suggest a benefit.[63] Since multimodality analgesic therapy (pain interventions aimed at multiple anatomic and pharmacologic sites) and aggressive control of acute pain may improve patient outcomes[65-68] and control of acute pain can minimize the development of chronic pain,[48,49,69,70] preemptive measures should be initiated before a planned noxious event, such as invasive procedures.

Transmission

During transmission, the nociceptive impulse is carried via afferent fibers from the periphery to the spinal cord, then from the spinal cord to the brainstem and thalamus, and finally is it is carried from the thalamus to the cortex of the brain where perception occurs. These three phases of transmission involve different structures and substances of the nervous system. The structures and substances involved in transmission of the nociceptive impulse during these phases are described below.

First the action potential is carried along a primary afferent neuron (also known as a *first order neuron*) through the dorsal nerve root into the dorsal horn of the spinal cord. Messages can be carried via fast, myelinated A-delta fibers or slower, unmyelinated C-fibers. C-fibers are like a tortoise, compared to the hare, the A-delta fibers. Stimulation of A-delta fibers primarily causes an initial sharp, stinging sensation.[39,59] C-fibers are responsible for the second pain that occurs a few seconds later and is described as a dull ache, burning, or throbbing sensation that lasts longer than first pain and covers a wider area.[39] First and second pain may be more noticeable with cutaneous painful stimuli such as a needle stick. If the pain initiates from the deep tissue (e.g., muscle and bone), there is less distinction,[39] and pain transmitted by both types of fibers tends to be perceived as aching, dull, or cramping and may be accompanied by a more prominent autonomic component, such as tachycardia, and diaphoresis.[71]

After entering the spinal root, the first-order neurons divide into branches that ascend or descend a couple of segments before they synapse with second-order neurons in various areas of the laminae in the spinal cord's dorsal horn.[39] Excitatory neurotransmitters such as substance P, glutamate, and tachykinins (neurokinins) are released at the nerve synapse[60,72] and are responsible for transmission of the action potential between the first- and second-order neurons as well as in parts of the brain.[72] Glutamate binds with glutamate and N-methyl-D-aspartate (NMDA) receptors in the spinal cord,[60] facilitating the transmission of pain messages. These excitatory neurotransmitters play a part in central sensitization.[63]

In response to injury, central sensitization occurs in the spinal cord, brainstem, and brain. Song and Carr[63] describe the pathophysiology and related clinical picture of central sensitization in the following way. A-delta and C-fibers evoke slowed synaptic potentials allowing summation of action potentials and progressively longer depolarization in the dorsal horn. Thus, in central sensitization, the central nervous system becomes overresponsive to incoming stimuli. This can continue even after nociceptive messages from the periphery stop, with spontaneous impulses arising in the dorsal horn.[73]

Many physiologic changes can occur during central sensitization. There is an influx of calcium via ion channels;[63] NMDA receptors may become activated by glutamate; and chemicals such as nitric oxide and COX-2 are formed and released resulting in the release of more glutamate, increasing activation of second order neurons.[73] According to Song and Carr,[63] similar to peripheral sensitization, in central sensitization, the receptive fields of the dorsal horn neurons expand into areas associated with surrounding noninjured tissue so that neighboring uninjured areas become painful. In contrast, to peripheral sensitization in central sensitization, nonnociceptive input activates usually latent synapses in the dorsal horn causing nonpainful stimuli transmitted via A-beta fibers (which transmit thermal and touch messages)[74] to be perceived as painful.[63] Thus, similar to peripheral sensitization, central sensitization may become a vicious cycle. Together central sensitization and peripheral sensitization are responsible for the following acute and chronic pain states—hyperalgesia, allodynia, spontaneous pain, referred pain, and sympathetically mediated pain.[63]

With central sensitization, new nerve endings may sprout,[73] and if left unchecked central sensitization may lead to permanent changes in the pain processing system resulting in chronic inflammatory or neuropathic pain. Specifically, glutamate and NMDA receptors play a dominant role in facilitating nociceptive transmission in prolonged pain states.[39] As with peripheral sensitization, preemptive analgesia, or use of analgesic modalities before tissue injury, is believed to prevent central sensitization. This means that less medication may be needed to prevent pain in comparison to treating pain.[63]

Besides excitatory neurotransmitters, inhibitory neurotransmitters such as GABA are also in the brain and spinal cord.[75] Interneurons found in some laminae of the spinal cord are GABA rich, mediating pain in the dorsal horn by synapsing on neurons that contain substance P.[75] GABAergic compounds inhibit nociceptive transmission presynaptically or postsynaptically by binding to receptors on primary afferent and dorsal horn neurons.[57] Baclofen, a GABA agonist, inhibits nociceptive transmission by binding to GABA receptors.[57] Baclofen can produce analgesia for many chronic pain conditions with accompanying muscle spasm.[76]

Nociceptive impulses must transverse a nerve synapse, so transmission can be affected by presynaptic or postsynaptic activity. Neurotransmitters involved in transmitting pain messages may be prevented from binding with the receptor because other substances bind with the receptor, or there may be changes in the amount of neurotransmitter available at the synapse. These are discussed under modulation.

Second-order neurons project towards the brain in bundles called *ascending tracts*.[57] First pain and second pain carried from the lamina to the brain via the evolutionary newer neospinothalamic tract and the primitive paleospinothalamic tract, respectively.[75] Most of the fibers cross over at the level of the spinal cord and ascend to the brain on the side contralateral to the injury. Several of the ascending tracts form the anterior lateral system (ALS). These second-order neurons synapse with third-order neurons in various brain structures such as the thalamus, limbic system, and reticular formation. The third-order neurons carry the nociceptive impulse to the cortex of the brain, where pain is perceived. The intermingling of the tracts and their interaction is responsible for the integration of the many dimensions of the pain experience,[39] which is more fully discussed in the section on perception.

As further evidence of the complexity of the nociceptive system, two dorsal column tracts also ascend ipsilaterally from the spinal cord. These dorsal column tracts appear to play a role in all aspects of pain transmission and may assume the function of contralateral tracts that have been destroyed, which partially explains why cordotomy is not an effective long-term pain control solution.[39] For example, months after undergoing a cordotomy and attaining pain relief, patients may begin to complain of increasing pain.

Several other medications exert their primary effect by preventing or limiting transmission. Local anesthetics given via the intraspinal route prevents transmission of the action potential along the nerves. Along with anticonvulsants, local anesthetics also slow transmission of pain impulses by stabilizing the nerve membrane via sodium channel regulation. Calcium channel blockers such as ziconotide may decrease the depolarization times associated with central sensitization.[77]

Methadone, an opioid that is also an NMDA antagonist, works at opioid as well as the NMDA receptor sites associated with central sensitization to modulate pain by disrupting NMDA receptor activity in chronic inflammatory, neuropathic, and visceral pain states. Because of its dual action, it may be particularly useful in the treatment of neuropathic pain.[78] Other NMDA antagonists such as ketamine may be helpful in intractable chronic pain states.[60] However, since ketamine is an anesthetic, it requires special monitoring and its use by a nurse may be regulated by state nursing boards. It is reserved primarily for incapacitating pain unrelieved by other methods.

Perception

Pain is not perceived until it begins to move from the thalamus to the cerebral cortex. Pain perception is the conscious awareness of an unpleasant sensation along with a negative emotion best described as a threat.[57] This should *not* be misconstrued to suggest that people who are unconscious or sleeping do not feel pain; *nociception still occurs.* Although it has long been thought that pain was not perceived until the nociceptive impulse reached the cerebral cortex via third-order neurons, recent advances suggest awareness of pain is perceived as nociceptive messages are passed on to the brain's cortical area from the thalamus, where reciprocal connections exist with various areas of the central nervous system and where nociceptive messages are integrated and processed.[39] This partially explains the complexity of pain perception and the unique pain experience, which is shaped by the compilation of the numerous interconnections that occur throughout the brain via the second- and third-order neurons. The messages sent via the paleospinothalamic tract (sent via thalamus and hypothalamus) are primarily responsible for emotional and affective responses to pain, whereas messages sent via the spinothalamic tract to the sensory cortex primarily contribute to discriminating location and sensation. The contributions of the major areas of the brain to the pain experience as reported by Pasero and colleagues[60] are described below:

- *Thalamus:* relay station for second- and third-order neurons
- *Reticular system:* autonomic response and biologic alarm
- *Limbic system:* emotional and behavioral response (unconscious memory triggers)
- *Somatosensory cortex:* location and sensory characteristics of pain

Pain stimuli can be interrupted or modified anywhere along the pathway from the periphery to the brain. The converse is also true—for example, anxiety, depression, fear, and negative prior experiences can increase pain perception. Although the cortex primarily provides information about pain location, quality, and intensity, perception is not merely a sensory event because cortical and limbic systems are involved in perception.[57] Therefore social context, environment, culture, and past experience all impact pain perception, resulting in an individualized response.

It is important to understand, from the patient's perspective, the meaning of pain (e.g., a temporary inconvenience verses a life-threatening condition), relative cultural and spiritual perspectives, past pain experiences (including successful and unsuccessful treatments), and the patient's knowledge of others' pain experiences under similar circumstances (e.g., a patient with bony metastasis who had a relative with the same problem but whose pain was not controlled). This information is helpful in understanding the individual pain response and developing effective treatment plans. One also must garner a sense of trust and safety on behalf of the patient. Combined with an understanding of the individual's experience of pain, this may aid in the selection of effective pain interventions and help modulate the pain experience.

The current belief is that there is a finite capacity for the brain to accommodate a limited number of signals.[60] Based on this, cognitive-behavioral strategies can be used to reduce sensory (e.g., sensations, location, and characteristics) and affective (e.g., emotional distress and accompanying autonomic responses) components of pain. Using techniques that require focus such as meditation, distraction, relaxation, breathing exercises, and biofeedback may reduce the number of pain messages reaching the brain, thereby decreasing pain. The effect of these interventions is on the perception of pain, but these interventions work via modulation.

Modulation

During modulation, nociceptive impulses are inhibited or changed.[60] Although modulation traditionally has been portrayed as descending inhibitory messages from the brain that cause attenuation of nociceptive impulses at the dorsal horn of the spinal cord, modulation occurs at multiple levels—the periphery, the spinal cord, brainstem, and brain—and include inhibitory and facilitatory descending pathways.[57] During modulation, efferent nerve fibers carry information back to the site of injury. Visceral and neuropathic chronic pain syndromes are a result of peripheral and central sensitization and facilitatory descending pathway activation. Since efferent fibers pass thru the sympathetic chain ganglia, it is easy to see how the autonomic system and stress can increase pain perception and intensity.[79]

Nociceptive signals may be blocked by neurotransmitters involved in the descending regulation of pain. Inhibitory substances such as endogenous opioids, serotonin, norepinephrine, and GABA are released at nerve synapses and bind with receptors on the primary afferent or dorsal horn neurons to modulate pain via descending inhibitory pathways.[57] In response to pain the body activates a balancing mechanism. Spinal interneurons release inhibitory amino acids such as GABA and neuropeptides such as endogenous opioids, which inhibit nociceptive transmission via presynaptic and postsynaptic mechanisms.[57] Specifically, GABA, endogenous and exogenous opioids, and serotonin—another neurotransmitter that occurs naturally at the receptor site—attempt to balance out the neurotransmitters that transmit pain messages at the synapse. Examples of this balancing act in an attempt to modulate pain are described below.

GABA and serotonin bind with the receptors, preventing binding of some neurotransmitters that facilitate transmission of nociceptive messages to second-order neurons, blocking transmission of at least some nociceptive signals and modulating pain. Conversely, a depletion of serotonin, which occurs during prolonged pain states, facilitates nociceptive message transmission. Endogenous opioids bind to opioid receptors on the primary afferent and prevent the release of neurotransmitters such as substance P.[80] Medications mimic these natural responses. The action of baclofen, a GABAergic agonist, in the management of pain is described in the transmission section. Tricyclic antidepressants modulate pain by increasing serotonin and norepinephrine at the synapse by reducing reuptake of these products, but it may take weeks to months of titration to optimize tricyclic antidepressant dosing for pain. Exogenous opioids also prevent release of substance P,[60] with diffuse pain carried by C-fibers being more sensitive to opioid therapy.[81]

The gate control theory provides a framework for understanding how pain is modulated. It hypothesizes that stimulating nonnociceptive neurons can reduce the transmission of noxious stimuli to the brain at the level of the spinal cord.[82] Theoretically, nonpainful stimuli compete with noxious stimuli to reach the brain, and because nonpainful stimuli are carried on faster nerve fibers (such as A-beta fibers) than noxious stimuli, more nonpainful stimuli get through the gate, and the gate closes to the noxious stimuli. Nonpainful stimuli such as heat, cold, rubbing, or vibration work in this manner.[83] This gate closure is not 100%, so some noxious stimuli may still reach the brain. In the process of closing the gate, it is theorized that some nonpharmacologic pain interventions also may involve neurotransmitters. For example, acupuncture research shows that its effectiveness appears to be related to release of endogenous opioids because its analgesic effects have been partially reversible by naloxone, an opioid antagonist. Transcutaneous electrical nerve stimulation (TENS) may work via similar mechanisms.

In summary, nociceptive input and pain perception can be modulated throughout the body. The variety of modulating mechanisms is in part responsible for wide variations in response to pain.[57] In addition, involvement of areas of the brain responsible for motivation and emotion contribute to variation and supports the belief that pain is not merely a physical sensation.

Pain as a Multidimensional Phenomenon

As a multidimensional phenomenon, pain is reported to have three components: sensory discriminative, motivational affective, and cognitive evaluative.[84] Recent research using functional MRI and PET scanning has provided physical evidence that different parts of the brain are associated with the different dimensions of pain.[85,86] Unfortunately, practitioners tend to primarily focus on the assessment and management of the sensory discriminative dimension of pain. The other dimensions should not be ignored, especially because uncontrolled pain may be a marker for pain that is at least partly attributable to other pain dimensions. Examples of the multidimensional nature of pain include increasing bone pain in an area of known metastasis previously treated by radiation therapy that may signal possible cancer recurrence and include a significant affective or motivational component such as fear, panic, and seeking multiple treatment options to denial and lack of adherence to prescribed medication regimens. Similarly, receiving recent news of a life-threatening diagnosis may mean pain is influenced by a significant affective component, with requests being made for increasing amounts of analgesia to provide sedation and to escape from reality. Management of these scenarios may require interdisciplinary intervention such as from a spiritual counselor, social worker, and/or psychotherapy specialist to achieve adequate pain control.

In summary, nociception is a complex physiologic process. Integration of four basic processes—transduction, transmission, perception and modulation—and permanent physiologic changes and pain resulting from untreated acute pain is responsible for multidimensional individualized dynamic pain experiences. Multiple opportunities exist for modulating pain from physical and psychosocial spiritual perspectives. Use of multiple interventions to prevent and modulate this multidimensional phenomenon presents the best opportunity for modifying the pain experience, providing effective pain control, and preventing chronic pain.

PAIN ASSESSMENT

Because the most common reason for uncontrolled pain in the United States is lack of routine assessment and reassessment of pain and many patients suffer in silence unless asked about their pain,[40] routine screening for pain is imperative. Over a decade ago, federal clinical practice guidelines suggested routine pain assessment every 2 to 4 hours for the first 24 hours postoperatively.[20] Cancer pain assessment also should occur on a routine basis, with each new report of pain, when pain is expected (e.g., with painful procedures or when analgesic action is expected to diminish), suspected (e.g., guarding painful body parts or moaning in a cognitively impaired patient), and postanalgesic intervention. Although assessment should include identifying the cause,[9] effective treatment is imperative regardless of the clinical setting. To facilitate this process, the Agency for Health Care Policy and Research (AHCPR) Cancer Pain Guideline Panel suggests use of the ABCDE mnemonic:

*A*sk about pain regularly and *A*ssess it systematically.

*B*elieve the patient/family in their reports of pain and what relieves it.

*C*hoose pain control options that are appropriate for the individual and the clinical setting.

Deliver timely, logical, and coordinated pain interventions.

Empower patients and their families, ***E***nabling their control to the greatest extent possible.[9]

In 2000 the Joint Commission on Accreditation of Healthcare Organizations (JCAHO) developed the first evidence-based standards, requiring routine screening, assessment, and reassessment of pain,[87] which facilitated guideline implementation by organizations throughout the United States. According to these standards, healthcare organizations are free to determine the frequency of assessment and reassessment. Thus standards vary from institution to institution. Professional organizations have encouraged treating pain as the fifth vital sign.[88] However, assessing pain with each set of vital signs may be unrealistic, burdensome to the patient, and likely to lead to nonadherence. A reasonable compromise is to screen for pain upon admission or presentation to your practice setting when routine vital signs are obtained. Routine screening should be continued on a regular basis as determined by the practice setting (e.g., each treatment visit, pre- and postprocedure, with routine vital signs). Pain screening may be performed by trained healthcare workers such as nursing assistants. Standardized parameters for notification of a nurse or physician are needed (e.g., if pain is greater than 3 on a scale of 0 to 10 or the patient is experiencing more than mild pain), because identification of a pain episode requires a comprehensive pain assessment by a healthcare professional.

Comprehensive Clinical Pain Assessment

A comprehensive clinical pain assessment is imperative to the development of an effective pain management plan. Because pain is a subjective symptom, self-report—the gold standard—should be used whenever possible to assess pain. If the patient cannot self-report, significant others and physical exam are used. The information obtained from a comprehensive assessment provides guidance on the possible source and mechanism of pain the patient is experiencing. It provides robust clues about interventions that are likely to be effective in the management of that pain. Assessment findings guide the nurse in selecting an appropriate intervention from a variety of prescribed options. They also can be used in advocating for an appropriate pain intervention.

A *mnemonic, acronym,* or *modified pain assessment tool* such as the Brief Pain Inventory or McGill Pain Questionnaire, structures the pain assessment and is helpful to ensure that all essential components of the assessment are obtained. Selection should be guided based on the population and the clinical setting. Numerous acronyms and mnemonics are available that delineate the basic components of a pain assessment. Many have been modified, and original sources are often unknown. Some examples are as follows:

- PAIN: (Pattern; Area; Intensity; Nature)
- LIST: (Location; Intensity; Sensation; Timing)[89]
- PQRST

The PQRST mnemonic[90] is detailed below. It is used to guide the practitioner in asking patients questions about their pain.

- **Provoking factors**—What is perceived to be causing the pain and what makes it worse? This helps determine the patient's perceived fears as well as potential causes.
- **Quality**—Words the patient uses to describe characteristics of the pain. These provide information about the possible pain processing mechanisms (see physiology section). Some types of pain are better relieved with certain classes of analgesics or certain nondrug interventions (see treatment sections).
- **Region/radiation/relief**—Where the pain is located, if and where it radiates, and what relieves it. Pain location is often assumed by healthcare professionals based on clinical diagnoses. However, without routinely assessing pain location, important pain diagnoses may be missed (e.g., assuming pain is from a bony metastasis when the patient is actually experiencing chest pain from an evolving myocardial infarction). Changes in location may indicate a new pain problem or increasing complexity of the current pain diagnosis.
  SPECIAL NOTE: *The presence of a new pain does not mean that it should not be treated until a diagnosis is confirmed. The American Pain Society[40] states it is rarely justified to withhold treatment for pain until the cause is determined.*
- **Severity/symptoms/side effects**—Pain severity (or intensity) is determined by using a pain measurement tool several of which are described in detail below. It is useful in determining the appropriate relief strategy. Associated symptoms should include the impact of the pain on other physiologic

processes (e.g., nausea/vomiting), psychologic and physical functioning, and social activities. Side effects pertain to treatment-related side effects.

- **Timing**—Information about onset, frequency, how long it lasts, and times of the day when pain is better or worse are important. Besides helping to identify new pain onset and causative factors, timing data provides information about the length of action of a drug in a particular patient and identifies cyclical increases in pain (e.g., every night, at the end of dose). This information provides guidance useful when adjusting a pain plan of care.

In summary, the use of an acronym, such as PQRST or other pain assessment tools, is an efficient, effective way to organize the critical components of a clinical pain assessment. Used along with clinical information and knowledge of injury and disease, it assists the practitioner in the identification of various pain problems. It also guides the development of a multimodal pain treatment plan with appropriate interventions to ensure safe, effective, and efficient care.

Pain Measurement Tools

A patient self-reported pain intensity score is the gold standard, and patient self-report should be used whenever possible. A variety of reliable, valid pain measurement tools are available for use in the adult population and include the visual analogue scale (VAS), the numerical rating scale (NRS), the verbal descriptor scale, and several FACES scales and are readily available on the web at the Partners Against Pain web page (www.partnersagainstpain.com). Some have been translated into many languages.

Although numerous scales are needed for any given practice environment, select tools that demonstrate reliability and validity in a similar population. Consider tools that are easily integrated into clinical practice—verbal and printed NRS. Some measurement tools are available using several different scales (e.g., 0 to 5, 0 to 10, and 0 to 100). When possible, use the same scale within a practice environment; however, a tool's scaling should not be changed if no evidence supports the modification. For example, the NRS, VAS, and FACES scales may use either 0 to 5 or 0 to 10 scales, but the scale range should not be changed to 0 to 50 without further psychometric testing. A hospital-based radiation oncology department should use the same scales available on the inpatient units. In a particular hospital, the scale for each of these measurement tools should be consistent (e.g., 0–10 for the FACES scale, the NRS, and the VAS). Not all patients are able to use one scale, so it is wise to have several pain measurement tools available within a clinical setting.

Whenever possible, the same pain measurement tool should be used for the same patient for patient ease and to reduce confusion. Although many pain intensity scales used in adults provide approximately equivalent responses,[20,91] results from descriptive scales[91] or faces scales[92] may not be equivalent to results obtained with numerical scales using the same number range. An exception to the rule of using the same pain measurement tool in the same patient should be made when a change in cognitive status requires a change in tool selection.

Because different scales may use different referent points (e.g., 0–5 verses 0–10), verbal and written communications must include the tool and information on the patient's self-reported score. For between institution transfers, reporting the tool's highest possible score is also a necessity. Reporting only a pain score of 5 could lead to interpretation difficulties between the patient and the healthcare professional, and among healthcare professionals, resulting in under- or overmedication. For example, record and report a score of 5/10 on the verbal NRS.

Base patient-specific tool selection on the patient's cognitive ability to understand and relate to the scale. Explain the scale to the patient/family and teach the patient/family the importance of reporting and when to report pain. Verbal and written instructions and diagrams are helpful. Disparities in patient response can be large depending on context, which is compounded by the fact that pain measurement tools may not specify the timeframe or the circumstances under which the patient is to score the pain that is being experienced. Therefore, patients should be given consistent, clear instructions when they are asked to rate their pain. As an example, a recent study showed average pain scores in postoperative orthopedic patients varied from 4.53 ± 2.49 for pain score now, 6.41 ± 2.63 for worst at rest, to 7.70 ± 2.25 for worst pain with movement.[93]

When instructions to rate pain do not specify a time period or context (e.g., movement or rest;

now, worst or best), the exact meaning of the score is unknown. Because pain increases with movement,[93,94] and patients limit movement because of pain,[94] movement-related pain scores are recommended for any patient that experiences pain that varies with activity. This is particularly important because patients with pain scores greater than or equal to approximately 4 or 5 out of 10 experience pain that interferes with function.[13,94] This level of pain puts them at risk for increased morbidity and mortality from pain-related complications discussed earlier.

Even mild and moderately cognitively impaired adults can use self-report pain measurement tools to report pain intensity.[95-99] Cognitively impaired adults who are unable to use a self-report are often able to answer "yes" or "no" when asked whether they are having pain, and this response may be more reliable than scores obtained with a tool. In the rare circumstance that a radiation oncology's self-report of pain is deemed unreliable, an in-depth pain evaluation can be conducted using one of many behavioral tools designed for patients who cannot use a self-report tool because of cognitive impairment. These tools are available at the City of Hope website (www.cityofhope.org/prc/elderly.asp).[100]

Although pain is a subjective experience associated with emotional responses, someone that cannot communicate may still experience pain and be in need of pain-relieving treatment.[46] There has been little testing of pain measurement tools in intubated, sedated patients or in patients suffering from a neurologic insult. Although some nurses rely on vital signs to validate the presence of pain, particularly in the nonverbal population, the literature suggests that heart rate, respiratory rate, pulse rate, and blood pressure may either increase or decrease in response to pain stimuli.[101] In addition, vital signs are not specific for pain. Numerous clinical conditions (e.g., temperature elevation, atherosclerosis, and respiratory illnesses) and other medications used by cancer patients may affect vital signs. It is also unknown how long pain-related autonomic responses last, especially in those who may have limited physiologic reserves.

It is the healthcare provider's responsibility to be alert for signs of pain or the possibility of pain (e.g., painful procedures)[20] in all patients; however, it is imperative in the patient who cannot self-report. The American Society for Pain Management Nursing (ASPMN) has published a position paper with clinical guidelines to guide the assessment of the nonverbal patient that is endorsed by several reputable professional organizations, such as the American Pain Society and the Oncology Nurses Society.[102] Assessment of pain in the cognitively impaired or in a patient that cannot self-report can be enhanced by discussion with significant others and by palpation or performing simple range of motion of known or potential painful sites. Combining these with observations for behavioral pain responses from pain measurement tools is helpful in determining whether a noncommunicative patient may be in pain.

Research on critically ill patients who can self-report suggests behavioral and physiologic pain responses may vary within an individual.[101] Living in a stoic society, it is not surprising that patients attempt to blunt their behaviors in order to hide their pain. However, the extent to which this happens in patients that cannot self-report is unknown. It may be necessary to look for a positive behavioral response during palpation, movement, or range of motion two out of three times or three out of five times to assess whether a patient is experiencing pain. Medicating a patient and looking for changes in behavioral and physiologic responses also may be helpful to determine whether a patient was experiencing pain. Lack of change, however, does not mean the behavioral signs were caused by something other than pain. The analgesic dose may have been inadequate, the tool may lack sensitivity, or the intervention may have been inappropriate (e.g., treating severe pain with acetaminophen).

Pain should be reassessed at frequent intervals. To determine the ideal time interval between assessments, consider the current pain state, the time of analgesic peak effect. For example when managing moderate to severe pain during analgesic titration, pain assessment should be more frequent and based on time of peak effect (Table 31-1). Once pain is controlled, it can be assessed less frequently, with timing based on the half-life of the drug, when analgesic effects are waning.

PAIN MANAGEMENT

In light of the complex nature of pain, the most effective way to manage pain is by using a multimodal approach. This means that multiple pain

Table 31-1 Approximate Time to Peak Effect Table

Route	Peak effect
SHORT-ACTING ANALGESICS	
IV push fentanyl	2–5 min
IV push opioids other than fentanyl	10–20 min
IV opioids over 20 minutes/IM*/SubQ	30 min
IV/IM nonopioid analgesics and NSAIDs	30 min
Oral opioid tablets	45 min–1 hour
Oral liquid opioids	20–30 min
Oral NSAIDs	45 min–1 hour or longer
Transmucosal fentanyl (Actiq)	25–45 min
Rectal nonopioid analgesics, NSAIDs, and opioids	1–2 hours
LONG-ACTING ANALGESICS	
Oral methadone (Dolophine)	2–4 hours
IV methadone over 20 min/IM*/SubQ	30 min–1 hour
Sustained release morphine (MS Contin)	$1^1/_2$–2 hours
Sustained release oxycodone (OxyContin)	45 min–2 hours
Fentanyl patch (Duragesic)	18–24 hours after initial placement

Used with permission from University of Maryland Medical Center: *Pain clinical practice guideline,* 2002, Baltimore, Md.
*Least desired route due to erratic absorption.

management therapies—both pharmacologic and nonpharmacologic—with different mechanisms of action (as described in the physiology of pain section of this chapter) are used to prevent and treat pain. Pain management treatments can be categorized as follows: pharmacotherapy, cognitive therapies, rehabilitative therapies, CAM (complementary alternative methods), and advanced treatment options such as injection and infusion techniques, implantables, and surgery. Because pharmacotherapy is the cornerstone of cancer pain management, it is discussed first.

PHARMACOLOGIC TREATMENT OF PAIN

Individualizing Therapy

The most important principle in pharmacologic management of pain is individualization of therapy. The amount of analgesic required to manage pain of similar severity varies widely.[48,103,104] Medication side effect profiles (e.g., presence of and severity) also vary between individuals.[105,106] Genetics accounts for some differences, with people metabolizing drugs at different rates and some people unable to metabolize certain analgesics (e.g., codeine and ibuprofen).[107-110] The effect of genetics on drug metabolism is fairly stable within an individual. However, other factors that influence drug metabolism may result in wide differences within an individual over time such as (a) food and nutrition (e.g., food-drug interactions and change in protein binding), (b) disease (e.g., renal and liver disease), (c) clinical condition (e.g., shock via change in hepatic blood flow), (d) environmental effects (e.g., smoking and pollutants by changing enzyme activity), and (e) effects of other drugs (e.g., inhibit or increase enzymatic activity required for drug metabolism).[111] All analgesics and adjuvants may be affected by genetic differences or by other factors listed above that affect drug metabolism.

Besides differences in metabolism, the need for individualized therapy is related to the different mechanisms of pain being responsive to different treatments as highlighted in the pathophysiology section. For example, neuropathic pain responds better to differing pharmacologic approaches as compared to nociceptive pain. Specifically, neuropathic pain is less responsive to opioid analgesics than nociceptive pain, with anticonvulsants and tricyclic antidepressants being the cornerstone of therapy for neuropathic pain.

Another reason for individualizing therapy is the recommendation for multimodal therapy in the management of pain. Although analgesics may be used alone, combination therapy is recommended to maximize pain relief. Rational poly pharmacotherapy is the preferred treatment for cancer pain. Therefore, multiple pharmacologic categories are discussed below. First, nonopioids are presented, followed by opioids and then adjuvants. There is a variety of delivery methods available, so treatment modalities such as opioid infusion, IV-PCA, continuous infusion, IV push, and epidural/intrathecal therapy are also discussed. Similar to medication selection, routes of administration require individualization based on treatment goals and patient profile.

Nonopioid Analgesics

Nonopioids include drugs such as acetaminophen, nonselective nonsteroidal antiinflammatory agents (NSAIDs) and selective nonsteroidal agents (COX-2 inhibitors). They are indicated as single drug therapy in the management of mild pain and are often used with opioids in the management of moderate to severe nociceptive pain (e.g., somatic or visceral). All are opioid sparing and result in fewer opioid side effects when used concomitantly with opioids.[66] Their primary mode of action is to reduce prostaglandin activity[112] in the periphery (NSAIDs and COX-2 inhibitors) and/or central nervous system (acetaminophen, NSAIDs, and COX-2 inhibitors). Thus their mechanism of action is different than opioids and their concomitant use with opioids is consistent with rational poly pharmacotherapy. However, when prescribing these nonopioids, patients must be asked and counseled about use of other prescription and over-the-counter nonopioids. Nonopioids are in many over-the-counter colds and cough medications and other preparations and cause toxicity at higher-than-recommended doses.

Acetaminophen, unlike NSAIDs and COX-2 inhibitors, does not reduce inflammation. It produces few if any side effects at analgesic doses, but overdose (a medical emergency) and chronic use can cause liver and sometimes kidney damage. Experts advise that the chronic daily dose be limited to 3 grams per day, particularly in the elderly,[113] despite FDA labeling specifying an upper limit of 4 grams in 24 hours, which is equivalent to 12 Regular Strength or 8 Extra Strength Tylenol. Reduce the dose and use cautiously in patients of advanced age, those who drink more than two alcoholic drinks per day (2500 to 3000 mg suggested), and in those with preexisting liver disease.

Numerous nonselective oral NSAIDs are available in several different classes. These are primarily available as pills, with some are available in liquid or suppository form. When a particular NSAID is ineffective, switching between classes of NSAIDs may result in improved pain relief.[112] Parenteral NSAID (e.g., ketorolac [Toradol]) and oral COX-2 inhibitor (e.g., celecoxib [Celebrex]) choices are limited.

NSAID and COX-2 use may be limited by the potential for GI bleeding and hepatic, hematologic, and renal side effects, regardless of the route of administration.[112] The side effect profile of NSAIDs is purported to be more hazardous than opioids,[105] and the American Pain Society suggests they should be used at the lowest effective dose for the shortest period of time.[40] The elderly in particular are at increased risk of GI bleed.[105,114,115] Concomitant use of a proton pump inhibitor or use of selective COX-2 inhibitors reduce the incidence of major GI bleed.[116] Choline magnesium trisalicylate (Trilisate), an NSAID with platelet-sparing effects, is an alternative for patients at risk for bleeding. Risk for cardiovascular disease is a relative contraindication for the COX-2 drugs.[117-119]

Opioid Analgesics

Opioid therapy is considered to be the major therapeutic approach to patients with cancer and is indicated in the management of moderate to severe pain. The clinician should have knowledge of opioid pharmacology, and a clear grasp of practical guidelines for dosing and expertise in the administration of opioid analgesics is a core competency.[120] Radiation oncology practitioners manage a large number of patients who are currently taking or will be prescribed opioids. Inpatient or outpatient radiation oncology patients receive a number of opioid preparations via a variety of delivery methods. Therefore, familiarity with the various options is critical. The five critical elements to incorporate in a pain management plan are by the mouth, by the clock, by the ladder, for the individual, with attention to detail.[9]

Although opioids continued to be called "narcotics" in some clinical settings, it is a misnomer. "Narcotic" is a legal term that identifies medications with abuse potential and includes medications other than opioids. For example, legally cocaine is a narcotic, but medically it is classified as a local anesthetic, and it has a different mechanism of action than opioids. Calling opioid analgesics "narcotics" reinforces myths and misunderstandings because it emphasizes the potential abuse rather than their clinical efficacy. Switching to the term "opioid" is highly recommended as well as being politically and medically correct.

The 1990 World Health Organization (WHO) analgesic ladder[121] (Figure 31-1) has been used as a key model for analgesic treatment for numerous years. Though considered more an overall operational guide than providing specific pharmacologic information,[122] some suggest modification is needed to include advanced pain therapies (e.g., block techniques and implantable devices) similar to the pyramid diagram used in the AHCPR Cancer Pain Guideline.[123] The modification is likely to be more pertinent to industrialized countries as compared

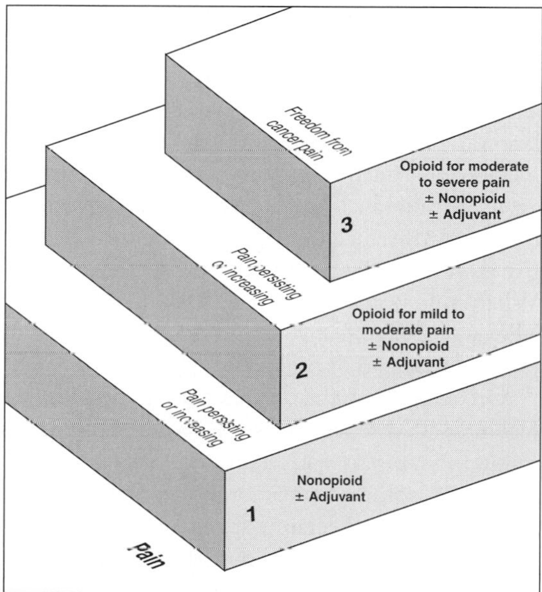

Figure 31-1 World Health Organization Pain Relief Ladder. (Available at www.who.int/cancer/palliative/painladder/en.) If pain occurs, there should be prompt oral administration of drugs in the following order: nonopioids (aspirin, acetaminophen, NSAIDs); then, as necessary, mild opioids (codeine); then strong opioids such as morphine, until the patient is free of pain. To calm fears and anxiety, additional drugs—"adjuvants"—should be used. To maintain freedom from pain, drugs should be given "by the clock," that is every 3 to 6 hours, rather than "on demand." This three-step approach of administering the right drug in the right dose at the right time is inexpensive and 80% to 90% effective. Surgical intervention on appropriate nerves may provide further pain relief if drugs are not wholly effective.

to developing countries because of availability of these progressive techniques. The additional step is estimated to apply to about approximately 10% of cancer patients. Regardless, the WHO ladder offers a successful method of escalating pain medication based on pain severity and has been shown to be effective in managing cancer pain in the majority of patients studied in the United States, Europe, and in developing countries.[124]

Other criticisms of the WHO ladder stem from strict interpretation of the ladder concept, the use of the terms *strong* and *weak opioids*, recommendations in the literature to match the analgesic (NSAID, opioid, and adjuvant) to the type of pain, and the lack of nondrug therapies. First, starting at the lowest rung of the ladder may result in delayed pain relief for those in moderate to severe pain. Second, for most opioids the strength is related to the dose, not to the drug, although combination drug formulations (e.g., opioids with NSAIDs or acetaminophen) and type of opioid (e.g., kappa agonists such as butorphanol) have ceilings beyond which further doses may cause harm without increasing pain relief (also know as a *ceiling effect*). Third, matching the medication to the type of pain is recommended in the literature (e.g., NSAIDs for bone pain, anticonvulsants and/or tricyclic antidepressants for neuropathic pain), however, additional pain relief may be derived from other analgesics such as opioids or NSAIDs on the same or different rungs of the ladder. The necessity of matching the drug to the mechanism of pain has been challenged for some types of pain.[125] However, this was not based on head-to-head comparisons of different treatment modalities or evaluations of multimodal treatment strategies. Clinical anecdotal evidence suggests that with difficult to control pain (e.g., neuropathic pain), the combination of multimodal and mechanism-based treatments is more effective and has an improved side effect profile. Fourth, nondrug therapies is a part of multimodal therapy and can be on any rung of the ladder.

Recognition of the above limitations and tailoring the interventions to the clinical situation means the ladder can still be useful to the practicing clinician. For example, in an opioid naïve (no or limited prior opioid exposure) elderly outpatient with severe pain, mild opioids may be used before stronger opioids. Instead of combination products, single agents in the nonopioid and opioid categories might be prescribed. This allows titration of the opioid without concern for exceeding the maximum dose of the nonopioid if the lower dose is ineffective and side effects are minimal. In contrast, when initially treating pain from a fracture caused by a newly diagnosed bony metastasis, consideration should be given to starting on the rung of the ladder that corresponds to the degree of pain the patient is experiencing, in this case scenario, often moderate to severe. Similarly, when using opioids to treat pain in the opioid tolerant individual (history of current or recent opioid exposure for several days or more), starting at a higher rung of the ladder will most likely be necessary. The WHO analgesic ladder steps and their intended use are described below.

At step 1 of the ladder, when mild pain is reported, nonopiates are used with or without adjuvant analgesics as appropriate. Adjuvants are medications whose primary use is for conditions other than pain, but that have an analgesic effect. Tricyclic antidepressants and anticonvulsants are examples of adjuvants. If nonopiates and adjuvants are not successful in relieving pain, you advance to step 2 of the ladder.

On step 2 of the ladder, indicated for mild to moderate pain, mild opioids are initiated and nonopiates and adjuvants may or may not be continued. "Mild" opioids include codeine (with or without acetaminophen), hydrocodone (combined with acetaminophen or ibuprofen), oxycodone (combined with aspirin or acetaminophen), and propoxyphene (with or without acetaminophen). Tramadol can be included in this rung of the ladder even though it is not a true opioid and is only a weak mu opioid receptor agonist. Similar to other medications listed as mild opioids, its maximum dose is limited by a ceiling effect. Tramadol has unique centrally acting analgesic properties with opioid-like features in combination with a tricyclic antidepressant-like features. Meta-analyses report that tramadol is effective in the management of neuropathic pain, however, additional studies are needed to compare this drug and other conventional treatment.[55,126] It is not considered a controlled substance in the United States, and thus lacks the stigma related to opioids.

Dose escalation of mild opioids is primarily limited because of the ceiling effect of the nonopiate included in the combination product. In order to prevent toxicity, combination products can be safely escalated only until the dose of the nonopioid reaches maximum therapeutic level. Some of the mild opioids have other dosing limitations. Propoxyphene use should be limited to short-term, mild pain because it and its metabolite, norpropoxyphene, both of which have a long half-life accumulate, potentially causing CNS excitation (seizures), cardiac toxicity (arrhythmias), and pulmonary edema, especially in those with renal impairment.[40] Propoxyphene should be used with caution in the elderly, who are at high risk for these toxic effects because of renal insufficiency.[40,113,127] Similarly, tramadol is limited to a maximum of 400 mg per day because of CNS excitation and the potential for seizures.[40] Use of codeine at doses greater than 65 mg parenterally or 1.5 mg/kg orally is not recommended because of the increased side effect profile without incremental increased analgesic effects.[40] Though still used frequently, its antitussive effect may be more valuable than its analgesic effect. Approximately 10% of the population lack the enzymes CYP2 or CYP3 that metabolize codeine into an active pain relieving agent.[40] Individuals unable to metabolize codeine into an active analgesic agent will report ineffective pain control when given codeine preparations. When mild opioids plus or minus nonopioids and adjuvants are ineffective for mild to moderate pain, proceed to step 3 of the ladder.

On step 3 of the ladder, strong opioids are recommended for moderate to severe pain plus or minus nonopioids and adjuvants. Strong opioids include morphine, hydromorphone, fentanyl, oxycodone (without acetaminophen or aspirin), oxymorphone, levorphanol, and methadone, to name a few. Historically, morphine has been considered the "gold standard" based on worldwide experience, ease of dosing, and the availability of numerous formulations. However, wide dosing and side effect variations are increasingly understood to be patient dependent, so drug selection based on patient response is now recommended.[128] Morphine-6 glucuronide, an end metabolite of morphine, is more potent than morphine itself and is responsible for respiratory depression seen in patients with renal failure.[127,129] End metabolites may be responsible for dissociative reactions, myoclonus,[130,131] or delayed onset of nausea/vomiting, especially with prolonged exposure.

Mixed agonists (e.g., nalbuphine [Nubain], butorphanol [Stadol], and pentazocine [Talwin]) and partial antagonists [Buprenex]) are not reviewed because of their ceiling effects and the propensity to precipitate opioid withdrawal and uncontrolled pain when given concomitantly with strong opioids, which are strong mu agonists. Although meperidine is considered a strong opioid, because of its long-acting CNS toxic metabolite, normeperidine, and the potential for seizures, it should not be used for long-term treatment of pain (more than a couple of days). For this reason, many institutions have either removed or restricted its clinical use.[9,40]

With the meperidine restrictions, clinicians are increasingly using hydromorphone (Dilaudid). It has few active metabolites, making it an excellent alternative to morphine, particularly in renal failure patients. The similarity of its name to morphine means that one drug may be confused for the other. Because hydromorphone is more potent than morphine, unintentional overdosing (if hydromorphone is administered using morphine dosing recommendations) or underdosing (if morphine is administered using hydromorphone dosing recommendations) can occur. Equianalgesic doses of these drugs are considerably different, with approximately 1.5 mg of parenteral hydromorphone equivalent to 10 mg of parenteral morphine. Initial parenteral doses should be reduced by $^1/_2$[40] to $^1/_3$ when administered intravenously to minimize untoward side effects from a high peak effect. Another potential dosing error is related to the equivalency of oral hydromorphone. Approximately 1.5 mg of parenteral hydromorphone is equivalent to 7.5 mg of oral hydromorphone. Confusing these doses or writing for the same dose of drug to be given either IV or by mouth may also result in an inadvertent overdose or underdosing event. To minimize errors, the JCAHO suggests educating staff about hydromorphone and morphine mix-ups, limiting the amount of opioid floor stock, and use of sound-alike, look-alike labeling.[132] Other successful interventions include removal of large dose syringes from floor stock and route based upper warning limits requiring pharmacy over-ride.[133] Opioid equivalency ratios are found in Table 31-2.

Oxycodone preparations are also prone to administration errors caused by inadvertent confusion between short- and long-acting formulations. Although there are a variety of brand names for oxycodone, the long-acting formulation brand is named OxyContin. Suggestions to minimize error include special labeling on storage bins, use of sound-alike, look-alike warning labeling, increasing distance between storage areas so they are not next to one another, and use of the brand names along with the generic name. Although OxyContin has received negative press because of illegal diversion; it may be better tolerated, at least in some patients, than long-acting morphine because it has fewer active metabolites.

Oxymorphone, levorphanol, and methadone are less widely used. Of the three, methadone is used most often. Methadone has numerous advantages. It is inexpensive, making it an excellent formulary addition for hospices. It has NMDA receptor activity; although to date no clinical evidence has been shown to support that it is more effective than other opioids in managing cancer-related neuropathic[78] or visceral pain. Methadone also has a long half-life of 23 hours. Unfortunately, its analgesic effect is much shorter, requiring 4-6-hour interval dosing. When administered routinely, methadone accumulates so that doses given today still have an effect on sedation and respirations 4 to 5 days later, placing the patient at risk for respiratory depression. The complex and individualized pharmacokinetics of methadone[134] requires practitioners skilled in methadone use to oversee initial dosing, titration, and monitoring of this drug.[78] Many pain, palliative care, and hospice practitioners have this skill set. Information on half-life and duration of action of the medications is found in Table 31-2.

Fentanyl is more potent than the other opioids discussed. When give intravenously (IV), it is considered a fast-acting opioid, providing analgesic relief within 2 to 3 minutes of administration. When used in single doses, it is eliminated quickly making it an excellent selection for moderate sedation in conjunction with midazolam (Versed), for those rare cases where breakthrough analgesia is not enough to control the pain during positioning. Besides adhering to moderate sedation guidelines, IV fentanyl must be given slowly in small doses to prevent stiff chest syndrome, which makes it difficult for the patient to breathe or to ventilate a patient. Fentanyl has a narrow therapeutic window, with little difference between the dose that provides analgesia and the dose that causes respiratory depression. Prolonged IV administration is not recommended for a variety of reasons. It is

Table 31-2 Opioid Analgesics Used for the Treatment of Persistent Cancer Pain

	Dose (mg) equianalgesic to morphine 10 mg LM*		Half-life†	Duration	
Drug	**PO**	**IM**	**Hours**	**Hours**	**Comment**
Morphine	20–30‡	10	2–3	2–4	Standard for comparison
Morphine CR	20–30	10	2–3	8–12	Various formulations are not bioequivalent
Morphine SR	20–30	10	2–3	24	—
Oxycodone	20	—	2–3	3–4	—
Oxycodone CR	20	—	2–3	12	—
Hydromorphone	7.5	1.5	2–3	2–4	Potency may be greater, that is, hydromorphone:morphine = 3:1, rather than 6.7:1, during prolonged use
Methadone	20	10	12–190	4–12	Although 1:1 ratio with morphine was used in single-dose study, there is a change with chronic dosing, and large dose reduction (75% to 90%) is needed when switching to methadone
Oxymorphone	10	1	2–3	2–4	Available in rectal and injectable formulations
Levorphanol	4	2	12–15	4–6	—
Fentanyl	—	—	7–12†	—	Can be administered as a continuous IV or SQ infusion; based on clinical experience, 100 mcg/hr is roughly equianalgesic to morphine 4 mg/hr
Fentanyl TTS	—	—	16–24	48–72	Based on clinical experience, 100 μg is roughly equianalgesic to morphine 4 mg/hr; a ratio of oral morphine: transdermal fentanyl of 70:1 also may be used clinically

From Derby S, Chin J, Portenoy RK: Systemic opioid therapy for chronic cancer pain: Practical guidelines for converting drugs and routes of administration. *CNS Drugs* 9:99-109, 1998.

*Studies to determine equianalgesic doses of opioids have used morphine by the IM route. The IM and IV routes are considered to be equivalent, and IV is the most common route used in clinical practice.

†Author's note: Length of action varies based on dose and genetics. For example, with continuous infusion, the half life of IV or subcutaneous fentanyl is 7-12 hours compared to 1-3 hours with single dose administration.

‡Although the PO:IM morphine ratio was 6:1 in a single-dose study, other observations indicate a ratio of 2–3:1 with repeated administration.

available in lozenge form. With a rapid onset of action of 15 minutes and the ability for the patient to adjust the dose, it is an excellent choice for the management of breakthrough pain when a patient is unable to tolerate the positioning required for radiation therapy. It is more convenient and less resource intensive than using moderate sedation. The long-acting fentanyl patch is discussed in the transdermal route section.

Although there is no upper dose limit to the majority of strong opioids, dose escalations may be limited by uncontrollable side effects. When side effects cannot be controlled by usual means, anecdotal evidence suggests switching to another opioid may reduce the side effect profile.[135] Maximizing the dose of opioid-sparing nonopioids also may be effective by allowing an opioid dose reduction. Switching the route of administration to one that requires a lower dose for the same analgesic effect also may be beneficial. For example, approximate potency ratios of parenteral to epidural to intrathecal morphine are 10:1:0.1. Although the equivalency ratios for various drugs differ, in general dose reductions are found for other drugs based on route. Usually oral opioids require the largest doses because they are metabolized first in the liver, rendering some of the drug unavailable to provide pain relief (first pass effect), parenteral dosing requires a smaller amount, epidural dosing is still lower, and intrathecal dosing requires the smallest dose.

Opioid Side Effect Management

To improve adherence to prescribed opioid analgesic regimens and maximize the potential for relief, aggressive opioid side effect management is likely to be needed.[7,136,137] Side effect management has not been well studied in the cancer population.[6] Although lack of well designed randomized controlled trials and study and sample heterogeneity prevents metaanalysis,[138] recommendations for the management of opioid side effects is readily available.[7,127,139] Suggestions for the management of opioid side effects are provided in Table 31-3. Additional information is provided below concerning one of the most feared and potentially fatal but rare side effects, respiratory depression.

Although rare,[40,140-143] respiratory depression is one of the opioid side effects most feared by healthcare professionals. Risk does not appear to vary much among administration methods.[142] Tolerance to respiratory depression occurs in the opioid-tolerant patient. Routine monitoring of sedation, which usually precedes respiratory depression, is most often used with IV-PCA (intravenous patient controlled analgesia) and epidural or intrathecal analgesia. However, it should also be used with conventional analgesia,[141,142] in opioid naïve patients or during titration Although there is no uniform agreement in the literature regarding the definition of respiratory depression, the respiratory rate is the most commonly cited parameter. Other hallmarks of respiratory depression include irregular breathing patterns (e.g., periods of apnea usually followed by more rapid breathing), shallow breathing, and a low oxygenation level (pulse oximetry reading of less than 90%). To assess for respiratory depression, the patient's respiratory rate, rhythm, and depth should be assessed for *a full minute before stimulating the patient* (e.g., before calling the patient's name, taking the pulse, or otherwise arousing the patient if asleep). Verbal or physical stimulation may increase respiratory rates, giving a false picture of the patient's true respiratory status. Once left alone and unstimulated, the patient may quickly lapse into respiratory depression, falling asleep even while others are in the room are talking. Although respiratory depression is rare, especially in the opioid-tolerant patient, other anecdotal evidence suggests side effect profiles differ by drug and by patient. These side effects may be reduced by the addition of nonopioids. If side effects persist despite aggressive treatment, opioid rotation or switching the route of administration is suggested.[144-146] A pain or palliative care consult is also recommended.

Delivery Systems

Oral

The oral route is the preferred route for analgesic administration because of its ease of use and the prolonged, steady analgesic effect.[40] Transdermal preparations have similar advantages and can be used when the oral route is contraindicated, but titration is more difficult with long-acting transdermal opioids when patients have rapidly escalating pain. When the oral route is contraindicated and fast onset of action is required, such as with rapid onset, rapidly escalating or severe pain, intravenous, subcutaneous, or buccal routes are recommended. The rectal route is another alternative, but it is generally not preferred by Americans, although it is more acceptable in some countries. New transdermal technologies are in development (transdermal fentanyl PCA patch indicated for acute pain) that may potentially be useful in these circumstances, but are likely to be expensive. Intramuscular administration is recommended only as an immediate intervention in the presence of severe pain when oral administration is contraindicated and IV access is not readily available.[80] Regrettably, a recent secondary data analysis using a self-report pain clinical quality survey found that 10% of acute postoperative pain patients received intramuscular injections,[93] even though this route is discouraged because of erratic absorption.[20]

Because of convenience, patient preference, affordability, flexibility, and ability to attain and maintain a steady blood level with relative ease, oral dosing remains the preferred method of administration for opioids (see Table 31-4). A variety of preparations from pills, capsules, and liquid suspensions allow for individualization. Selection of short-acting versus long-acting opioids is made based on frequency and length of pain episodes.

Table 31-3 Assessment and Management of Opioid-Related Side Effects

- In the presence of uncontrolled side effects, if pain score is 3 out of 10 with movement, consider downward titration, maximizing nonopioid analgesics.
- In the presence of uncontrolled side effects, if pain is uncontrolled, consider switching to another opioid.

Side effect	Assessment	Side effect management/prophylaxis
Constipation*	Monitor bowel elimination pattern	Facilitate normal bowel routine Increase dietary roughage Liberalize fluid intake Increase activity Prophylactic use of a stimulant-laxative plus stool softener (e.g., docusate sodium and senna) is recommended; titrate to effect, but consider dose limitations
Confusion/ hallucinations/ delirium	Monitor for changes in sensorium or bad dreams	Check for other potential causes (e.g., other medications, electrolytes, unrelieved pain) Consider use of long-acting analgesic with minimal active metabolic activity or short-acting analgesics
Myoclonus*	Monitor for uncontrolled muscle jerks	Consider the following: baclofen, diazepam, clonazepam, midazolam, valproic acid, dantrolene
Nausea/vomiting (N/V)	Monitor for N/V (especially nausea with activity, changing positions, or use of PCA button)	Administer antiemetics; consider prophylactic around the clock (ATC) dosing; for patients on chronic opioid therapy, N/V usually resolves after approximately 1 week after opioid initiated but N/V can recur anytime throughout opioid therapy (such as with long-acting morphine) Assess for other potential causes (e.g., concomitant medications)
Pruritus	Observe for itching, especially on trunk or face Assess for rash, which suggests allergic or anaphylactoid reaction	Apply mild local antipyretic (e.g., Sarna lotion) to unbroken skin Maintain cool environment Administer antihistamines; consider ATC administration If rash consider allergy
Respiratory depression[†] (defined as respiratory rate [RR]/min) **< 20 if < 6 months of age** **< 16 if < 2 yr of age** **< 14 if < 8 yr of age** **< 12 if < 16 yr of age** **< 10 if ≥ 16 yr of age**	Monitor RR, especially at peak drug effect (see Table 31-1); observe unstimulated RR for a full minute, assess for change in rate/depth/pattern/quality Monitor for increasing sedation and decreasing RR, which may precede respiratory depression	If not at end of life, reduce dose for increasing/excessive sedation and decreasing RR Stimulate patient, encourage him to breathe Administer naloxone (100 mcg IV push in adults; 3–5 mcg/kg IV push or 100 mcg IV q5min maximum dose in children); because its length of action is shorter than opioids, repeat dosing may be necessary; for patients on long-acting opioids, a naloxone infusion may be needed
Sedation	Monitor sedation level, often the first symptom of opioid accumulation—early recognition and treatment may prevent respiratory depression	Contact physician to report increasing/excessive sedation Check for other causes (e.g., medications) If sedation is not accompanied by changes in respirations, consider the use of caffeine products and/or stimulants (methylphenidate)
Urinary retention	Assess time of last spontaneous void Monitor I&O Assess lower abdominal discomfort Percuss/palpate abdomen	Straight catheter prn as ordered Continuous indwelling catheter as ordered Bethanechol as ordered

Modified with permission from the University of Maryland Medical Center: *Pain clinical practice guideline*, 2002, Baltimore, Md.

*Unlike other side effects, tolerance to this side effect is not known to occur.

[†]Incidence is less than 1%.

PCA, Patient-controlled analgesia; *I&O*, input and output.

Table 31-4 Benefits and Risks of Various Administration Routes

Route	Details	Comments
Oral (PO)	Requires functioning GI tract	Convenient, noninvasive, flexible, less discomfort Slow onset of action, requires patient compliance
Rectal (PR)	Insertion of suppository or solution	Useful for patients who cannot take medications by mouth Absorption may be unpredictable
Intramuscular (IM)	Injection into large muscle	Not recommended due to painful injections, wide fluctuations in drug levels, rapid decline in effect compared with oral administration
Intravenous (IV)	Single, repetitive bolus or patient-controlled analgesia	Most effective for immediate analgesia, permits rapid titration Continuous IV infusion provides steadier drug blood levels, maximizing pain relief and minimizing side effects
Subcutaneous (SC)	Infusion via butterfly needle	Produces steady blood levels, obviates need for GI function Costs less than IV administration Slower onset and offset, lower peak effects than IV administration
Transdermal (TD)	Absorbed through skin, gradual release into systemic circulation	Convenient, noninvasive Provides prolonged, relatively stable analgesia Delayed onset of action with first dose
Oral transmucosal (OT)	Includes sublingual, fentanyl incorporated into a sweet matrix on a stick	Easy, requires little staff supervision, avoids significant liver first-pass effect Some absorption via oral mucosa, some via GI tract Higher drug levels and better bioavailability
Epidural analgesia (EA)	Indwelling catheter is tunneled under the skin or surgically implanted	For acute postoperative pain and chronic pain Permits concomitant use of local anesthetic Greater potency than systemic administration Requires surgical procedure
Intrathecal analgesia (IA)	An indwelling intrathecal catheter is placed for long-term analgesia	Uses include cancer pain and neuropathic pain Single bolus more common for acute pain Provides intense analgesia at lower doses than systemic or epidural administration Can be difficult to titrate drug effect Infection risk Requires surgical procedure
Patient-controlled analgesia (PCA)	Patient controls dosage up to a maximum, usually with epidural or IV administration	Allows patient to manage dynamic changes in pain

Modified with permission from Berry PH, Chapman CR, Covington EC, et al: *Pain: current understanding of assessment, management, and treatments*, Reston, Va, December 2001, National Pharmaceutical Council and the Joint Commission for Accreditation of Healthcare Organizations.
GI, Gastrointestinal.

When pain is continuous or recurs on a regular basis throughout the day, it should be treated prophylactically around the clock. In this case, long-acting opioids are preferred because they help maintain stable blood levels, provide pain relief over time, and are convenient to patients.

Patients are also more likely to adhere to their prescribed dosing schedule when frequent dosing is not burdensome to "normal" life patterns. Short-acting opioids are useful when pain is intermittent, during the first few days of opioid exposure for an opioid-naïve patient, during titration for rapidly escalating pain, or as an addition to long-acting opioid therapy for the treatment of breakthrough pain. The optimum ratio between short- and long-acting drugs has not been determined,[53,147] however, the American Pain Society (APS) suggests using 10% to 15% of the total 24-hour dose administered every 2 hours as the dose of short-acting breakthrough medication.[40] This rule suggests that as long-acting analgesia is increased, the short-acting medication is also increased. Because most long-acting analgesics take a long time to reach peak effect,[40] in most cases short-acting analgesics may be given at the same time as long-acting medications since onset of action and peak effect vary. One exception is long-acting oxycodone (OxyContin), which with its bi-phasic properties releases about one-half of the medication within the first hour, so that onset and peak effect of the medication released in the first phase coincides with the onset and peak effect of other short-acting analgesics taken at the same time.

Breakthrough pain (BTP) can occur suddenly—in bursts—and may last for short periods of time. About one-half to two-thirds of patients with chronic cancer-related pain also experience episodes of breakthrough cancer pain.[148] Pain is considered "breakthrough pain" when it "breaks through" stable, persistent pain that is well controlled with preexisting therapy and may be caused by pain-producing activities or occur spontaneously.[147] Generally, the onset of breakthrough pain is quick, unpredictable, and may last anywhere from seconds to minutes to hours, with the average duration of breakthrough pain in one study of 30 minutes.[148] Provision of preemptive analgesia before radiation therapy may limit the occurrence of BTP and avoid pain-related delays or aborted radiation treatment cycles.

Transdermal/Topical

The transdermal delivery system is easy and convenient for patients, is an attractive alternative to oral medications in the outpatient setting when long-acting opioid treatment is required, and therefore is likely to be used in the radiation oncology patient. Transdermal therapy in general, and "patch" therapy in particular, is becoming more popular for many different drug classes such as analgesics, hormones, cardiovascular agents, local anesthetics, and antidepressants. New transdermal patches are under development or have recently been approved, including a PCA fentanyl button patch. Because a variety of different mechanisms of action for different patches and transdermal medications are available, understanding how the patch delivers, how and when the body absorbs and uses the medication is important. The long-acting transdermal fentanyl patch and topical local anesthetic systems are described below.

Fentanyl is lipophilic. Therefore long-acting transdermal therapy requires placement over subcutaneous tissue with fatty stores. A depot of drug is formed in the subcutaneous fat, which is slowly absorbed into the circulating blood, resulting in a systemic opioid effect; similar to oral and parenteral opioids. If a long-acting transdermal fentanyl patch is placed over bony regions or applied to a cachectic patient with little or no fatty tissue, this delivery system is minimally effective in relieving pain. In comparison to most other long-acting drugs, transdermal fentanyl patch takes 12 to 18 hours before onset of action, and over 24 hours elapses before peak effect. This means analgesia must be provided with another medication via another route until the pain is relieved and makes it a poor selection for treatment of rapidly escalating pain. Decrement of analgesic toxic, and side effects similarly take a prolonged time after patch removal.

In contrast to the transdermal fentanyl patch, topical local anesthetic administered via a patch absorbs directly through the skin, providing analgesia to the local area underneath it, with minimal systemic absorption, within a few hours. Both short- and long-acting preparations (based on length of application time) are available. The short-acting medications are available via patch, solution, or eutectic mixtures and are helpful to manage procedural pain such as IV starts or port access and is often used in the pediatric oncology patient. The long-acting patch is effective for managing neuropathic pain such as postherpetic neuralgia. Anecdotal reports indicate effectiveness in cancer-related and non-cancer related musculoskeletal conditions and peripheral neuropathy. Although all are recommended for use over intact skin, there are anecdotal reports of use of local anesthetic products for the management of wounds in cancer patients, and one meta-analysis found a significant reduction in pain using EMLA (eutectic mixture of local anesthetic) cream for debridement of venous leg ulcers.[149] When used on open wounds, the amount of local anesthetic absorbed systemically is unknown, and the potential for local anesthetic toxicity, which can result in death, should be considered. Dose, time to peak effect, and recommended application time on intact skin varies based on the product, and must be considered when calculating achievement of maximal effect.

Most patch formulations currently on the market use adhesives to promote skin adherence. Skin integrity and signs of adhesive sensitivity must be monitored. Both topical local anesthetic and fentanyl patch systems are affected by heat that will accelerate absorption rates and shorten duration of effect.[150,151] Overdoses have been reported when transdermal fentanyl has been used with heat sources, such as heating pads, saunas, and hot baths.[127] To facilitate constant steady absorption that is not increased by movement, place fentanyl patches on the torso instead of extremities.

Capsaicin is another topical therapy, which provides relief for the management of neuropathic pain. Unfortunately, it causes pain to relieve pain, through the depletion of substance P. Despite skin reactions being one of the more frequently occurring side effects of radiation treatment, relatively few topical therapies have been approved for its management. Additional research is needed.

Buccal Therapy

A few therapies have shown evidence of some effect in managing pain by delivery through the buccal membranes. The fentanyl lozenge discussed previously is one of those methods, although additional analgesia is obtained via absorption through the GI tract. A new effervescent fentanyl tablet is being released. Despite the incidence of mucositis with radiation therapy to the head and neck, few effective treatments have been found via meta-analysis. There is weak evidence for the effectiveness of allopurinol mouthwash, and PCA appears to decrease the duration of pain, but not the severity of pain.[152] The authors note that the data suggest other therapies that may be effective, but more and better-designed randomized clinical trials are needed. Prevention may be an important strategy, with vitamin E reducing the risk of mucositis by 36% in this population and also decreasing pain severity.[153]

Intravenous Opioids

Initial Dose

IV opioid administration is used to manage pain when the oral route is unavailable or the patient is experiencing severe pain and has intravenous (IV) access, such as when an inpatient reports severe BTP after prolonged or difficult positioning during simulation or radiation therapy. The American Pain Society[40] endorses an initial intravenous (IV) dose for a postoperative opioid-naïve intensive care patient of morphine 0.03 mg/kg or an equivalent dose of another similar, short-acting opioid (e.g., hydromorphone). However, no literature supports weight-based opioid dosing in adults and there is little research to draw upon. Another approach is to administer intravenously $^1/_3$ to $^1/_2$ of the parenteral equivalent of short-acting analgesics on an equianalgesic chart. If pain is controlled and no side effects occur, administration of this dose can continue once each hour. Before administering any initial dose, assess the pain level and the sedation and respiratory status. At peak effect of the drug, reassess for pain level and opioid side effects such as sedation, respiratory status, nausea, vomiting, and itching.

Titration

Once an initial dose is determined, titration may be required to determine the optimal dose, the dose with maximum analgesia and minimum side effects. The optimum titration strategy has not been determined. However, short-acting drugs such as morphine and hydromorphone are suggested.[40] Based on recommendations by Edwards and Breed,[154] the American Pain Society suggests repeating an IV dose every 10 minutes until there is a 50% reduction in the patient's self-reported pain score or the patient reports satisfactory relief.[40] Because peak effect of short-acting IV opioids other than fentanyl is about 15 to 20 minutes,[40] patients should be observed carefully for the effects of cumulative dosing. In comparison to other routes, most short-acting IV opioids may be administered more frequently (every 10 minutes; interval is shorter for fentanyl) than that based on peak effect time tables (15 to 20 minutes; interval is shorter for fentanyl), particularly during titration because small doses are given and those doses may not be adequate to reach the minimum effective analgesic concentration. Before repeat administration and at peak effect of the drug, reassess for pain level and opioid side effects such as sedation, respiratory status, nausea, vomiting, and itching. Stretching the interval out between doses or decreasing the dose when using successive doses and 10-minute intervals may minimize the potential for untoward effects.

The character of the pain also should be assessed if the patient does not experience relief. Neuropathic pain may be minimally responsive to opioid therapy, particularly in the short term,[155] and continuing to increase the dose of opioid may put the patient at risk for respiratory depression without providing adequate analgesia.

Patient-Controlled Analgesia

Patient-controlled analgesia (PCA) is an excellent way to individualize dosing for patients receiving analgesics who have the cognitive ability to use specialized analgesic pumps. It can be administered via the intravenous, subcutaneous, or intraspinal route. PCA allows the patient to balance pain and opioid side effects.[156] Identification of the beneficial attributes of PCA therapy compared to other standard treatments (e.g., oral, intramuscular, intravenous) has been difficult because most analgesic study sample sizes are small and studies are not powered to determine clinical superiority or effectiveness.[140,157] Even when individual studies do show superiority of one analgesic technique over another, differences in populations, environment, measurement strategies, drug combinations, and dosing intervals make comparisons between studies difficult. The same issues often prevent the use of meta-analysis or subanalyses of specific populations or drugs.

The most recent meta-analysis comparing IV-PCA to other parenteral therapy (i.e., IM, IV, subcutaneous) found a significant benefit when all pain outcomes were combined and found that IV-PCA patients had fewer pulmonary complications.[142] Some of the benefit of IV-PCA may be related to the decrease in nursing time required to provide analgesia compared to conventional techniques.[158,159] This time-saving feature of IV-PCA is very important in busy clinical settings such as radiation oncology departments where patients are generally seen only daily by radiation technologists, treatment schedules are fixed, and where locating staff to obtain and administer analgesics for breakthrough pain may result in significant delay.

PCA therapy does not preclude the need for a loading dose, titration, or treatment of side effects by a healthcare provider. Despite balancing analgesia and side effects offered by PCA, the patient may still suffer untoward effects such as respiratory depression. When specialized analgesic pumps are programmed to administer a continuous infusion along with the PCA option, the risk of side effects may increase without improving pain relief,[160-163] especially in the opioid-naïve patient. Because of potential risks, frequent monitoring of respiratory rate, sedation, and presence of side effects is required. Monitoring protocols vary from institution to institution. Various PCA monitoring protocols used by numerous American Pain Society Nursing Issues Special Interest Group list serve members is available on the web.[164]

Because PCA is under the patient's control, patients need information on how to use it effectively. Lack of education has been shown to be associated with higher pain ratings[165] with inadvertent or inappropriate use of PCA leading to respiratory depression.[160,166,167] The core elements of patient education include (a) the low risk of addiction, (b) safety mechanisms to prevent overdose, (c) use of PCA button, (d) need to report changes in pain, (e) potential side effects and the need to report them, (f) preemptive use at least 10 minutes (for IV-PCA and 15 for subcutaneous PCA) before activities/procedures that cause pain, (g) time between request to onset of analgesic effect, and (h) time lapse between doses. Repetition of this information and encouragement may be necessary.

Designated authorized controlled analgesia (sometimes referred to as *PCA by proxy*), where someone other than the patient is designated to request a PCA dose by pushing the PCA button, is being used in increasing frequency for patients who cannot interface with the pump based on cognitive age or difficulties. This bypasses the built-in PCA safety feature of the patient becoming too sedated to push the button to receive additional opioid. Pushing of the PCA button by someone other than the patient and without authorization has been associated with respiratory depression and at least one reported death.[160,168] The U.S. Pharmacopoeia med error database contains several untoward incidents where unauthorized family members and healthcare providers pushed patient PCA buttons without permission, leading the JCAHO to issue a sentinel event alert.[168] This alert suggests the following to enhance safety: (a) develop criteria for PCA and nurse-controlled PCA or caregiver-controlled PCA with special attention paid to increased risk factors and special monitoring associated with the latter, (b) monitor patients carefully, (c) provide written instruction and teach families not to push the PCA button, (d) consider signage that indicates *only patients* are to push the PCA button, and (e) caution healthcare professionals about the dangers of administering a PCA dose outside of a PCA by proxy protocol. The American Society of Pain Management Nursing recently released a position statement on authorized and unauthorized PCA dosing that has been endorsed by other groups, outlining how this therapy can be safely used.[169]

Two JCAHO sentinel event alerts pertain to PCA and infusion therapy—the potential for pump free flow and PCA errors regarding concentration and rate.[132,170] All infusion pumps with a risk of free flow need to be removed from service.[170] JCAHO suggests instituting pump double checks to address PCA errors regarding concentration and rate.[170] Standardization of concentrations[171] and pump double checks against the order with initiation, transfer, dosage changes, bag change, and at change of shift decrease errors.[171,172]

Patient factors that may increase the risk of opioid-related respiratory depression with PCA therapy are renal impairment, obstructive sleep apnea, morbid obesity, hypovolemia, increased age (elderly),[143,173-176] and marked liver failure. It is likely that these risk factors are applicable to patients no matter the route of administration. Using opioids without active metabolites such as hydromorphone may decrease this risk, because some active metabolites (i.e., morphine-6 glucuronide) have a greater effect than the parent drug (i.e., morphine) once they accumulate.

Intraspinal Therapies: Epidural/Intrathecal Analgesia

Epidural or intrathecal analgesia provides medication via a catheter or needle administered as a single shot, bolus injections, continuous infusion, patient-controlled analgesia, or any combination thereof. These techniques are also called *intraspinal therapies*. Although used more often in the postoperative population, these therapies are being used increasingly in the management of chronic cancer pain. Compared to best practice, analgesia via catheter technique has been shown to improve pain relief and extend life in cancer patients.[177] Although intraspinal therapies are used most often in patients with difficult-to-control pain who fail conventional treatment or suffer from uncontrollable side effects, catheters may be placed by a pain service, and this technique can be used to facilitate positioning on the radiation oncology table.

Morphine, fentanyl, and hydromorphone are the most commonly administered opioids in the epidural space. Bupivacaine, lidocaine, and ropivacaine are the most commonly administered local anesthetics. For recalcitrant pain problems, other medications including clonidine and ziconotide may be used. The medications may be used alone or in combination; however, a combination of a local anesthetic with an opioid is most common.

The analgesic mechanism of action and potential side effects of intraspinal analgesia vary based on the medications administered. The most common opioid side effects are pruritus, nausea, and vomiting. In general, they are treated in a similar manner as systemic opioid side effects. Motor block and hypotension are among the most frequently occurring local anesthetic side effects, although rates of 3% and less have been reported in large series of patients.[178] Lumbar epidurals have the most frequent incidence for lower extremity motor weakness and risk for fall. When using intraspinal techniques, it important to assess for motor block before weight bearing to minimize falls. When motor block occurs, it is recommended to stop the infusion for 2 hours to see whether the block resolves to rule out treatment-related complications, hematoma or abscess.[178] Hypovolemic patients, such as the cancer patient with persistent emesis or persistent diarrhea from chemotherapy or radiation therapy are at higher risk for hypotension. Because potential side effects include the rare occurrence of respiratory depression (less than 2%),[178] vigilance is necessary. A survey of American Pain Society Nursing Issues Special Interest Group found wide variability in assessment frequency between institutions.[164] Consideration should be given to increasing the frequency of assessments when side effects occur.

One of the rare therapy-related complications associated with intraspinal analgesia is an epidural or subarachnoid hematoma. Iatrogenic or therapeutic coagulopathy is a major risk factor for this complication. Use of this delivery modality in the patient receiving fibrinolytic/thrombolytic therapy (e.g., unfractionated heparin, low molecular weight heparin, anticoagulants, thrombin inhibitors, antiplatelets [NSAIDs], and herbal substances) is not contraindicated, but the decision to initiate needle or catheter placement is made on an individual basis.[179] Timing of needle or catheter insertion and removal is specific to the type of fibrinolytic/thrombolytic therapy administered. To minimize the risk of hematoma in patients receiving fibrinolytic/thrombolytic therapy, catheter insertion and removal requires coordination among the treatment team members, including the pain specialists. So, if the catheter is inadvertently pulled out in a patient receiving any of the medications above, contact the pain service immediately so that corrective measures and frequent assessment can be initiated. A consensus statement by members of The American Society of Regional Anesthesia and Pain Medicine provides guidance based on technique, drug, and route.[180] Abbreviated guidelines are available on the internet at www.asra.com/consensus-statements/2.html.[181]

Epidural or subarachnoid hematoma and abscess, other infrequently occurring therapy-related complications, may present as a motor block. Initial signs may be similar to a local anesthetic block, however, hematoma and abscess may result in permanent paralysis if not detected and treated early. So care providers must be vigilant in assessing for and reporting the presence and extent of motor block. Although no national guidelines exist, a poll of American Pain Society Nursing Issues Special Interest Group list serve members found the majority of respondents assess for motor block every 4 hours.[164] Patients who receive a neuraxial block at or near the time of anticoagulant/antithrombolytic therapy require an increased assessment frequency of at least every 2 hours.[180] Although the epidural space is protective, minimizing the potential for abscess, care should be taken to prevent catheter disconnects during transport and movement by supporting the catheter insertion site in young children as well as securing a catheter loop to the body with tape and preventing tugging on the catheter. If a catheter disconnect occurs, cover the catheter with a sterile gauze and notify the pain service. Do *not* clamp the catheter as it may damage the catheter.

Plexus, Peripheral, and Field Nerve Block Techniques

Local anesthetic plexus, peripheral nerve block, and field block techniques (bolus and continuous infusion) are being used more often to provide regional pain relief. Guidelines for monitoring vary by institution, but should include assessment of pain, medication-related side effects—including motor block or local anesthetic toxicity—and technique-related complications. Side effects and complications are similar to epidural anesthesia, with the exception of urinary retention and sympathetic blockade, which generally do not occur. Abscess and hematoma would occur in the plexus or peripheral nerve associated with the catheter location, instead of in the epidural space. The Neuraxial Anesthesia and Anticoagulation Consensus Statement may be applied to plexus and peripheral techniques, however, it may be more restrictive than necessary.[180]

MANAGEMENT OF PAIN IN OPIOID-TOLERANT PATIENTS

In the radiation oncology setting, patients are in various disease stages and receive a variety of different treatments. During their radiation oncology experience, some patients may experience cancer-related pain for the first time. Individuals who have had little previous exposure to legal or illicit opioids are opioid naïve. In contrast, individuals become opioid tolerant after routine use of opioids for greater than approximately 10 days. Oncology patients currently receiving opioids or with a history (current or recent) of substance abuse are opioid tolerant. This may include individuals who are (a) on chronic opioid therapy for malignant or nonmalignant pain, (b) on methadone maintenance, or (c) abusing opioids.

Tolerance is a state of adaptation in which exposure to a drug induces changes that result in a diminution of one or more of the drug's effects.[182] The good news about tolerance is that tolerance to most opioid side effects occurs. Common side effects of most opioids, such as sleepiness, nausea, itching (not constipation) tend to decrease over time as tolerance to the opioid develops. The bad news is that tolerance to analgesic effects can occur too.

Little is known about the physiologic underpinnings of tolerance. The body's production of endorphins and enkephalins are reported to decrease,[183] reducing the response of the body's own natural pain-relieving substances to acute tissue injury. Evidence also indicates that the opioid receptors change and become less responsive to opioids.[184] Although these are only a few of the physiologic changes that may occur in opioid tolerant individuals,[183] these changes mandate that opioid-tolerant individuals require additional opioid to obtain adequate pain relief. They require a large enough opioid dose to fulfill preexisting opioid requirements, plus additional medication to manage acute pain associated with procedures or injury. In general, opioid-tolerant individuals are able to tolerate faster escalation and larger doses of opioids.[185] The amount of opioid required by an opioid-tolerant patient must be determined on a case-by-case basis.

With tolerance, exposure over time (weeks or months) may change the body's response to the effectiveness of a drug, even if nothing has happened to cause an increase in pain, such as disease progression. This is more common in chronic nonmalignant pain than in cancer pain. With cancer pain, an increase in drug tolerance tends to be due to disease progression. The end result is the same regardless of the cause. When tolerance occurs, the regular drug dose is not as effective in providing relief. When tolerance is suspected, upward adjustment of drug dosing may be required to achieve satisfactory pain relief. Cross-tolerance between opioids occurs, meaning a patient taking any opioid will demonstrate some degree of tolerance to other opioids.[183]

Individuals receiving opioids for 2 weeks or more also develop physical dependence. With repeat exposure to some substances, the body naturally adapts to a higher level of that substance in the blood. When the substance is suddenly unavailable because of its abrupt cessation, a rapid dose reduction, decreasing blood levels, and/or administration of an antagonist,[182] the body recognizes the reduction and a "withdrawal phenomena," or abstinence syndrome, ensues. The symptoms associated with opioid withdrawal are nausea, vomiting, malaise, headache, rhinitis, tremulousness, abdominal cramping, and more.

Besides opioids there are several classes of drugs that can cause physical dependence and withdrawal:

- Benzodiazepines
- Stimulants
- Barbiturates
- Steroids
- Some beta-blockers
- Some antidepressants

Withdrawal can be prevented by gradual reduction in the opioid dose over time so that the body returns to its natural state gradually.

Physical dependence is often mistakenly called *addiction*. Addiction is a medical diagnosis and is defined as a primary, chronic, neurobiologic disease, with genetic, psychosocial, and environmental factors influencing its development and manifestations. It is characterized by behaviors that include one or more of the following: impaired control over drug use, compulsive use, continued use despite harm, and craving.[182] Patients with opioid addictions are opioid tolerant, physically dependent, and may experience withdrawal in the absence of the substance. But, only a *few people* who routinely take opioids are addicted even though they are physically dependent, tolerant, and are at risk of withdrawal.

Individuals with addiction deserve the same quality of pain care as other patients. However, it is difficult to estimate starting doses in patients who have a history of illicit drug use because purity of street drugs varies and different combinations of drugs may be abused. The estimated starting dose in this population is based on clinical judgment, and similar to other opioid tolerant individuals, on patient condition. As in nonaddicted individuals, titration must occur. In nonurgent situations, a pain or palliative care specialist versed in managing pain in substance abusers is highly recommended because these patients usually require a more aggressive pain management plan. Use of a specialist is also likely to reduce the time required to find the optimum regimen. A substance abuse counselor versed in pain management is also an essential addition to the multidisciplinary team for these patients. A 2002 position paper by the American Society for Pain Management Nursing offers treatment recommendations for those actively using, those in recovery, and those on methadone maintenance and is available on the web at www.aspmn.org/Organization/position_papers.htm.[186]

To determine starting dose estimates for patients on chronic opioid therapy, on methadone maintenance therapy, or when switching between opioids or routes in any patient, opioid equianalgesic conversions can be facilitated by using equianalgesic conversion tables or electronic conversion programs.[187-189] The underlying principle of equianalgesic conversion is that various opioids can provide approximately equivalent analgesia, with the amount of opioid required being mathematically calculated depending on the drugs and the routes of administration. Most equianalgesic conversion ratios are based on single dose studies. Few equianalgesic studies use a multiple dose framework or include opioid-tolerant individuals. Those that have identify different conversion factors than those found in single dose studies.[190] Despite the methodology, incomplete cross-tolerance between drugs has been found, resulting in less medication being required than mathematically calculated. Multiple opioid sub-receptors[191] and genetic differences[107,109,110] may partially account for this difference.

Although electronic conversion programs can facilitate estimation of a starting dose, they should not be used indiscriminately. Large differences in calculated doses have been found between programs.[192] Some electronic conversion programs allow for dose reductions for cross-tolerance. Others do not. The majority do not account for chronic dosing and none consider patient condition. Pain and palliative care specialists are well versed in equianalgesic conversions and can provide expert guidance.

Adjuvant Analgesics

Adjuvant analgesics are medications that have a primary indication other than pain but in some conditions provide pain relief.[193] Adjuvants may be used alone or in combination with opioids and nonopioid analgesics to provide pain relief. They can be classified into four groups based on clinical use—multipurpose adjuvant analgesics and adjuvants used for neuropathic pain, bone pain, or visceral pain.[193]

Multipurpose adjuvant analgesics include glucocorticoids.[193] Glucocorticoids such as dexamethasone may exert their action by decreasing edema, anti-inflammatory effects, and directly influencing electrical activity in damaged nerves.[194] They are useful for metastatic bone pain, neuropathic pain, and pain due to CNS tumors. Doses range from a relatively small dose (e.g., dexamethasone 1 to 2 mg twice a day) to a short course of high-dose therapy (e.g., dexamethasone 100 mg, followed by 96 mg per day in divided doses), with the latter being used for pain uncontrolled by opioids.[193] Side effects include dyspepsia, candidiasis, hyperglycemia, edema or cushingoid habitus, weight gain, osteoporosis, and myopathy, which increase with prolonged use. Concomitant administration with nonselective NSAIDs or aspirin is not recommended because of an increased risk of gastroduodenopathy.[195] Rapid withdrawal may exacerbate pain.[40]

Neuropathic pain, one of the most difficult pains to treat, is in general less responsive to opioid therapy than nociceptive pain.[196] Tricyclic antidepressants (TCAs), anticonvulsants, and/or oral local anesthetic drugs are often used to treat neuropathic pain, but there is little consensus on how to best manage it, and there is wide variability in practice.[197] Varying levels of evidence exist for these drugs and no one drug or class of drugs has been found to have a distinct advantage.[125] Evidence for use of the tricyclic antidepressants is the most robust, however, newer therapies may be more tolerable.[55] Although it is likely that drugs with multiple mechanisms of action, such as the TCAs, are needed to treat neuropathic pain, in some instances, TCAs may be contraindicated.[198] In clinical practice it is not unusual to find a patient with neuropathic pain to be using medications from multiple classes of drugs that demonstrate some degree of effectiveness in managing neuropathic pain. This is probably due to neuropathic pain being only partially relieved with existing therapies. Future research needs to focus on optimal dosing, the benefits of combination therapy, and head-to-head comparisons.[55,199,200] The classes of adjuvant drugs that may be effective in managing neuropathic pain are outlined below.

Tertiary amine tricyclic antidepressants such as amitriptyline, doxepin, and imipramine are more effective than the secondary amines such as desipramine and nortriptyline, but are associated with more side effects such as sedation, anticholinergic effects (dry mouth, constipation, and urinary retention), and cardiovascular toxicity. Although selective serotonin uptake inhibitors (SSRIs) such as paroxetine (e.g., Paxil) and fluoxetine (Prozac) are associated with fewer major side effects than are the tertiary and secondary amines, they are less effective in treating neuropathic pain.[200] Side effects of TCA therapy may diminish over time, however, the medication is often given as a single bedtime dose to improve sleep, which is often disrupted in patients with chronic pain. Optimal dosing has not been determined.[55] According to Cherny,[193] starting doses are low (e.g., amitriptyline 10 mg in the elderly or frail to 25 mg in younger patients), with gradual increases equivalent to the starting dose every few days. When the usual effective range is reached (e.g., amitriptyline 75 to 150 mg), slower weekly titration is recommended. Higher does may be given for patients who do not respond and have no dose-limiting side effects. TCAs should not be used in patients with ischemic heart disease, recent myocardial infarction, arrhythmia, and cardiac decompensation.[198]

Meta-analysis suggests there is no difference in efficacy or in adverse events between anticonvulsant drugs and tricyclic antidepressants in the management of neuropathic pain.[200] Gabapentin (Neurontin) is often used off label to treat neuropathic pain, but most of the research is based on weak evidence from open-label trials, and it is suggested that use be restricted to areas for which there is solid evidence—diabetic neuropathy and frequent recurrent migraine headaches.[201] Because gabapentin requires less frequent monitoring than older, well-studied anticonvulsants (e.g., carbamazepine), and there is a great deal of anecdotal evidence regarding its benefit, continued use is likely. A starting dose of gabapentin 300 mg/day on day 1600 mg/day on day 2, and 900 mg/day on day 3 with additional titration to 1800 mg/day to achieve greater efficacy is suggested based on numerous studies.[202] Individualize the dose according to patient response and tolerability with additional titration up to 3600 mg/day needed in some patients. Gabapentin is generally well tolerated. However, there may be some initial sedation. There is beginning evidence that other newer anticonvulsants such as lamotrigine and oxcarbazepine may be effective in the management of neuropathic pain.[203]

Although its use is not supported by meta-analysis,[198] systemic local anesthetic drugs such as mexiletine may be used on occasion to manage neuropathic pain when other medications have been proven to be ineffective. It is usually initiated after a successful trial of IV lidocaine. Mexiletine dosing starts at 100 to 150 mg/day and is increased by a similar amount every few days until the usual maximum dose of 300 mg three times a day is reached.[193] On a rare occasion, a lidocaine drip may be used in patients who are unable to take oral medications, with caution taken to prevent a local anesthetic overdose. No optimum dose has been identified, but doses of 1.5 mg/kg have been effective, and at the high end, doses of 5 mg/kg over 30 minutes are associated with substantial toxicity.[204] Antiarrhythmics such as lidocaine and mexiletine may be contraindicated in patients with electrocardiac abnormalities, reduced left ventricular function, and coronary heart disease.[205] Side effects of systemically administered local anesthetics are similar to epidural administration. In contrast, few side effects have been reported with use of topical lidocaine on intact skin. For small areas of neuropathic pain, a 5% lidocaine patch (Lidoderm) cut to size and placed on the affected area may be effective.[40] It is FDA approved for three patches per day for 12 hours.[206]

Other drugs that are sometimes used for neuropathic pain but that have limited evidence of efficacy are clonidine, baclofen, calcitonin, and ketamine.[207] Calcitonin is suggested as second-line therapy for pain that is uncontrolled by other analgesics or radiation therapy.[208] Baclofen and clonidine are primarily used by pain specialists in selected patients and may be used intraspinally. Only ketamine is thoroughly reviewed here because it is an emerging therapy, one of the few medications with NMDA receptor activity, and it has potential for managing recalcitrant neuropathic and visceral pain problems. No meta-analyses and few randomized controlled clinical trials are available, and many trials do not specifically describe the cause of the neuropathic pain.[209] Hocking and Cousins[209] suggest using ketamine as third-line, short-term therapy for patients' whose pain is unresponsive to conventional therapy.

Ketamine, an anesthetic agent, is primarily used for deep sedation (e.g., when setting orthopedic fractures in the emergency department or for extensive painful dressing changes) and to treat neuropathic pain refractory to other analgesics. When used as an anesthetic agent, it is beyond the scope of nursing practice. Small clinical trials suggest ketamine administered in subanesthetic doses with morphine may help control cancer pain that has a neuropathic component.[210] In these studies, the number of drop-outs due to side effects is high.[211-213] In conjunction with morphine, it is synergistic in cancer patients with decreased responsiveness to high-dose morphine, although this phenomenon may be related to reducing opioid tolerance verses controlling neuropathic pain.[214,215] Ketamine has been found to be beneficial in controlling unclassified acute posttraumatic musculoskeletal pain and chronic neuropathic pain caused by amputation, complex regional pain syndrome, and spinal cord injury.[209,216,217]

Ketamine may be given orally, rectally, transdermally, intranasally, subcutaneously, intramuscularly, intravenously, epidurally, and intrathecally. Equianalgesic doses are not well described.[209,214,218] Caution must be exercised when caring for a person receiving ketamine, because the margin of safety between an analgesic dose and anesthetic dose is narrow. Because of its narrow therapeutic window and its side effect profile, patients receiving ketamine may initially require monitoring in a critical care unit. Ketamine has a myriad of potentially hazardous side effects. It can cause sedation, loss of consciousness,[219] and respiratory depression.[220] Excessive salivation can compromise the airway, so glycopyrrolate (Robinul) should be available. Ketamine is a visual and auditory hallucinogenic and can cause dreams, nightmares, and confusion.[219,220] The prophylactic use of a benzodiazepine may reduce occurrence.[209] Other minor side effects include mood or mental changes, sleep disturbances, and diplopia.[220] Ketamine use should be guided by a pain specialist or palliative care practitioner.

Visceral pain, such as pain from viscus distension and irritation (e.g., bowel distension, capsular distension caused by visceral tumors, radiation cystitis), is a relatively new field of exploration. A review of the most recent cancer pain guideline does not provide guidance for its management. Chronic visceral pain is poorly managed with existing therapies.[221] Because visceral pain is mediated by C-fibers, it may be more sensitive to prostaglandin inhibitors such as NSAIDs. Visceral pain appears to be more sensitive to kappa receptor agonists[222] and other receptor antagonists important to visceral pain processing that have primarily been tested in animal models.[223] Limitations of the mixed opioid agonist antagonists, which have kappa agonist activity, is discussed in the analgesic ladder section. Somatostatin, cholecystokinin, oxytocin, and adenosine modulate the transmission of nociceptive inputs from the gut to the brain and are of clinical pharmacologic interest in the management of visceral pain and discomfort, but their clinical efficacy requires further research.[223] There is preliminary evidence that NMDA receptor antagonists such as ketamine may be helpful in the treatment of chronic hyperalgesia associated with visceral pain, primarily using experimental pain models in healthy volunteers.[224-226] The effect of another NMDA receptor antagonist, methadone, is unknown. The evidence in the literature about managing radiation cystitis is inadequate to justify recommending any particular treatments to guide clinical practice, but suggests areas of future research.[227] Along with the usual analgesic treatments, pain practitioners have used antispasmodics (e.g., belladonna and opium suppositories), anticholinergics, and site-specific analgesics (belladonna and opium suppositories and phenazopyridine [Pyridium]) with varying degrees of success to assist in the management of visceral pain.

DISEASE MODIFYING THERAPIES

Numerous curative or palliative cancer treatments such as chemotherapy, surgery, and radiation therapy are used to manage pain. Curative therapy is usually more aggressive than palliation and may increase patient burden. Therefore the goal of treatment is an important consideration when offering treatments and discussing treatment options with the patient and family. Near the end of life when time becomes increasingly more valuable to the patient and family, treatments and schedules that maximize patient outcomes and minimize patient burden are recommended. Realistic prognostication is extremely helpful in weighing the options. Discussions with patients and families about the options and their benefits are needed. Palliative care specialists are skillful in helping patients and families consider medical options, are familiar with prognostication models, and are an important member of the healthcare team throughout the treatment trajectory.

Selected treatments below provide examples of some nondrug therapies effective for the management of bone metastases, one of the most frequent painful sequelae of disease progression and a common reason for cancer patients to receive a radiation oncology consult. The effect of the interventions discussed is not immediate, so use analgesic therapy as first-line treatment. Because many of these treatments may cause at least an initial increase in pain, proactively develop a pain plan of care with the patient and family that minimizes unnecessary suffering and controls healthcare costs by minimizing trips to the emergency room or hospitalization. Aggressively titrate the analgesic therapy upward and downward to meet the changing pain levels of the pain experienced by the cancer patient using these therapies.

Many of the therapies below are associated with a pain flare, a transient increase in pain experienced as a result of treatment. To manage the flare, titration of short-acting analgesics is recommended. Encourage patients and families to prophylactically fill these prescriptions because some pharmacies do not keep an adequate stock of controlled substances on hand. After patient request, there may be a delay of one to several days to fill a prescription while the pharmacy obtains the medication from a supplier. Obtaining controlled substances during weekends, evenings, and holidays is particularly difficult.

The optimum radiation therapy treatment schedule is unclear.[228] A review of 11 randomized trials found single fraction radiation therapy was as effective as multifraction radiation therapy in controlling bone pain related to metastasis.[228] However, patients receiving single fraction radiation therapy were more likely to have bone fractures and receive additional treatment sessions compared to patients receiving multifraction radiation therapy. A hypofractionated schedule (a lower dose over a shorter period of time) and smaller fields should be considered near the end of life to reduce treatment burden.[7] In one small study, pain flares had an overall incidence of 2% to 14% over the 2-week course of therapy, with 14% having a flare meeting the criteria on day one.[229]

Administration of radiopharmaceuticals such as strontium-89 and samarium-152 may relieve cancer-related bone pain for up to 1 to 6 months.[230] Dosing may be repeated. Treatment may be associated with leukocytopenia and thrombocytopenia and a transient increase in pain 72 hours to 2 weeks after therapy requiring upwards titration of analgesic therapy.[7]

Bisphosphonates inhibit osteoclast activity. They are effective in managing pain in multiple myeloma and other cancers, with breast cancer being frequently studied. Meta-analysis has shown bisphosphonates relieve cancer-related bone pain from multiple myeloma and bone metastases for up to 12 weeks after administration.[231] Bisphosphonate therapy also prevents or delays the onset of skeletal complications associated with breast cancer, reducing the need for palliative radiation.[7] An untoward effect is bone osteonecrosis in some patients.

NONDRUG THERAPIES

A variety of different nondrug treatments are used to manage pain in cancer, including traditional therapies such as educational interventions, hot and cold therapy, rehabilitative treatments such as splints, massage, and cognitive therapies such as relaxation, hypnosis, and imagery. The evidence for the effectiveness of these therapies in managing cancer pain varies. A meta-analysis conducted in the cancer population found small benefits for music therapy. A variety of biobehavioral therapies are effective, especially hypnotic-like therapies such as relaxation, suggestion, and imagery.[232] Some of these therapies, such as massage, have demonstrated additional benefits in addition to the relief of pain.[233] Except in procedural pain, little information is available using meta-analysis for use of these techniques in children.[234] Meta-analysis has found patient education in combination with a pain diary to be effective in managing cancer pain.[235] Other psychoeducational interventions also have been found to be beneficial.[236] The American Pain Foundation recently published a comprehensive public educational booklet called *Treatment Options: A Guide for People Living With Pain*,[237] which has not been tested for its effect, but people living with pain may find it beneficial.

Most nondrug therapies in these categories cause no harm, except perhaps for cost, and can be safely used. Additional evidence for the benefits of some of these treatments may be found for noncancer pain.[20] Brief descriptions and comments about some of these types of nondrug interventions used to manage pain that may be supported by meta-analysis in cancer is found in Table 31-5.

COMPLEMENTARY AND ALTERNATIVE THERAPIES

Complementary and alternative medicine (CAM) therapies are "a group of diverse medical and health care systems, practices, and products that are not presently considered to be part of conventional medicine."[238] They include acupuncture, various mind-body techniques, energy therapies, and chiropractic treatments. According to a recent Stanford University survey, as many as 69% of Americans are using CAM therapies, and many

Table 31-5 Nonpharmacologic Pain Management Strategies

- Consider developmental and cognitive level.*
- Use nonpharmacologics primarily as adjuncts to pharmacologic agents.*

Category	Specific interventions	Comments
Education/instruction	Pain management	Patient/family role, use of pain assessment tool, assess for and remove patient/family barriers
	Sensory and procedural information	Preprocedurally, preoperatively, and during the procedure provide information about: What the patient will hear, see, feel, taste, and smell (use concrete, specific terms such as sharp or dull instead of global terms such as pain) The environment Sequential steps in the procedure Tailor amount of information provided to developmental age
Relaxation	Distraction	Provide diversional activities May cause fatigue if used without analgesia for prolonged periods of time
	Deep breathing	Instruct the patient to "Take a deep breath in....Blow it out"
	Jaw relaxation	Provide specific instruction, such as "make a fist, now let all the tension go" (saying "relax" is ineffective)
	Progressive muscle relaxation*	Teach preoperatively, preprocedurally
	Imagery*	With guided imagery, ask patient to describe a place he finds relaxing When guiding the patient, use information the patient provides about what he would hear, see, feel, taste, and smell in this special place
	Music	Patient-preferred or "easy listening" music
Cognitive interventions	Reframing/positive thinking	Encourage positive thoughts regarding the patient's ability to cope with pain
	Psychotherapy and structured support	Counseling (i.e., social work, pastoral, psychotherapist), support groups
Cutaneous stimulation	Superficial heat or cold	May be helpful in reducing localized pain, inflammation, and/or muscle spasm Use temperature regulated devices for short intervals Protect skin from source; assess skin frequently Do not use on open wounds
	Massage, back rubs, etc.	May be helpful in reducing pain, inflammation, and/or muscle spasm Do not use over open wounds
	Transcutaneous electrical nerve stimulation (TENS)	Referral to physical therapist (PT); consider trial for patients with musculoskeletal or neuropathic (nerve) pain
	Acupuncture	Evidence for effectiveness
Positioning	Position for comfort Immobilization	PT/OT (occupational therapist) referral for splints, positioning devices, activities of daily living aids/devices
Special care to body surfaces Consider for some neuropathic pain problems such as those that elicit an exaggerated response to painful stimuli or those that produce pain to light touch (allodynia)	Substitute soft foam sponge or soft bed linen for terry cloth when bathing	Pat instead of rub (i.e., when washing/drying affected area) Encourage self-care Contact OT to obtain long-handled soft sponge for bathing
	Avoid procedures in affected area	For example, procedures such as BP, venipuncture, IVs
	Bed cradle	Removes covers from feet/legs, which can cause pain if allodynia is present
	Ace wrap/Jobst stocking	Steady light pressure on area of allodynia may be tolerated better than intermittent friction from clothing
Specialty mattress (bed or radiation oncology table)	Special mattress Special beds	Consider for patients with difficult to control pain upon contact with (multiple bony metastases, multiple myeloma, burns)

Modified with permission from the University of Maryland Medical Center: *Pain clinical practice guideline,* 2002.

*Assess patient interest before teaching.

conventional and allopathic doctors are incorporating these therapies into their practices. Thirty-four U.S. medical schools—including Yale and Harvard—now offer courses in complementary and alternative medicine (CAM). People in diverse communities use CAM therapies for the self-treatment of pain. Highest use was noted in suburban areas (82%), with 77% of urban and 58% of rural residents using CAM therapies.[239] Many patients use herbs or food supplements, have acupuncture treatments, or take yoga or Tai-Chi classes, and several of these therapies have moved into mainstream Western medicine.

Most CAM therapies are *holistic;* the focus on the patient as a whole—mind, body, and spirit—steering the body towards wellness and balance. Most treatments are gentle, noninvasive, and rely on the body's ability to heal itself. These treatments (such as acupuncture, various mind-body techniques, energy therapies, and chiropractic) can be used along with mainstream therapies such as non-drug therapies and analgesics to reduce pain, using an integrative approach. Integrative approaches may bring an additional benefit to managing pain. In 1999, the National Institutes of Health opened the National Center for Complementary and Alternative Medicine (NCCAM) to evaluate these methods more thoroughly. NCCAM was created to advance the scientific study of CAM to help answer questions about safety and effect on health promotion/disease prevention and/or management of medical disorders. Evidence of the benefits and safety of CAM therapies is expected to grow. Based on the existing evidence, some CAM therapies have been adopted as important components of nonmalignant pain management. Some of the nondrug therapies such as massage and acupuncture have been integrated into the mainstream such that they are no longer considered CAM therapies, but are now widely accepted nondrug treatments for pain.

Cancer patients in particular have a high use of CAM therapies for pain and other reasons.[240] According to NCCAM, individual studies have found benefits of CAM therapies in managing cancer pain.[240] The NCCAM Clearinghouse has publications and scientific and medical search results on NCCAM therapies available to the public.

There is little evidence for the benefits of CAM using meta-analysis. An exception is acupuncture, which has been cited as an effective treatment for cancer pain[240] for several years. Although a recent meta-analysis on acupuncture had contrary findings, poor quality studies were identified as an issue, and the research team suggested additional, better-designed studies because acupuncture is widely accepted as a method of treatment.[241]

Surprisingly, nearly half of those using complementary and alternative therapies do not tell their healthcare providers about it—either out of embarrassment, fear of being reprimanded, and/or not recognizing the importance of informing their primary care provider. It is vital that patients are encouraged to disclose how they are incorporating CAM approaches into their cancer and/or pain management plan, so that they are used safely, because synergism, potentiation, or counteraction of existing therapies may occur. Foster an environment of trust and inquire about alternative/complementary methods of pain control to facilitate complete disclosure of the patient history. Not asking about or understanding how and why alternative/complementary methods of pain control are used may erect a barrier between you and the patient. Monitoring and educating patients about the risks and benefit of these therapies will then be short of impossible.

SUMMARY

Pain is a frequently occurring phenomenon in cancer patients. Despite numerous advances in pain management, patients continue to suffer from inadequately managed pain. Data suggest patients' outcomes improve when pain is adequately controlled.[25] Complications from uncontrolled pain increase patient morbidity and mortality, may interfere with life-saving treatments, and is responsible for hospital readmissions and prolonged hospital stays. It also affects a patient's function and quality of life, as well as the lives of their loved ones.

Radiation oncology practitioners play an important role in the recognition and successful management of pain for patients in their care. For the radiation therapy patient who is fighting for his life, prompt effective management of pain is vital. An evidence-based review demonstrates numerous drug and nondrug interventions are effective in managing cancer pain.[6] The radiation oncology specialist must have an understanding of pain pathophysiology; pain assessment; various treatment options, their mechanisms of action and principles of use; and must identify and use pain resources to effectively manage pain. Integration of this information into practice is the key to reducing symptom burden and improving quality of life for the radiation oncology patient.

REFERENCES

1. Dickinson E: *The complete poems of Emily Dickinson*, Boston, 1924, Little, Brown. Accessed at Bartleby.com. Accessed June 25, 2000.
2. National Pain Survey: *Fast facts about pain*, American Pain Foundation (website): www.painfoundation.org/page.asp?file=Library/FastFacts.htm. Accessed October 9, 2005.
3. Alliance of State Pain Initiatives: *Pain facts* (website): aspi.wisc.edu/documents/pdf/painfacts.pdf. Accessed November 2, 2006.
4. American Cancer Society: *Cancer facts and figures 2005* (website): www.cancer.org/downloads/STT/CAFF2005 f4PWSecured.pdf. Accessed October 9, 2005.
5. Jemal A, Murray T, Samuels A et al: Cancer statistics, *CA Cancer J Clin* 53(1):5-26, 2003.
6. Carr DB, Goudas LC, Balk EM et al: Evidence report on the treatment of pain in cancer patients, *J Natl Cancer Inst Monogr* (32):23-31, 2004.
7. Miaskowski C, Cleary J, Burney R et al: *Guideline for the management of cancer pain in adults and children*, Glenview, Ill, 2005, American Pain Society.
8. Cleeland CS, Gonin R, Baez L et al: Pain and treatment of pain in minority patients with cancer: the Eastern Cooperative Oncology Group Minority Outpatient Pain Study, *Ann Intern Med* 127(9):813-816, 1997.
9. Jacox A, Carr DB, Payne R et al: *Management of cancer pain, Clinical practice guidelines No. 9.* AHCPR Publication No. 94-0592, Rockville, Md, 1994, US Department of Health and Human Services, Public Health Service.
10. Lyne ME, Coyne PJ, Watson AC: Pain management issues for cancer survivors, *Cancer Pract* (10 suppl 1): S27-S32, 2002.
11. Campa JHI, Payne R: Pain syndromes due to cancer treatment. In Patt RB, editor: *Cancer pain,* Philadelphia, 1993, JB Lippincott, pp 41-56.
12. Burrows M, Dibble SL, Miaskowski C: Differences in outcomes among patients experiencing different types of cancer-related pain, *Oncol Nurs Forum* 25(1):35-48, 1998.
13. Serlin RC, Mendoza TR, Nakamura Y et al: When is cancer pain mild, moderate or severe? Grading pain severity by its interference with function, *Pain* 61(2): 277-284, 1995.
14. Cleeland CS: The impact of pain on the patient with cancer, *Cancer* 54(suppl 11):2635-2641, 1984.
15. Ferrell BR, Wisdom C, Wenzl C: Quality of life as an outcome variable in the management of cancer pain, *Cancer* 63(suppl 11):2321-2327, 1989.
16. Ferrell BR, Rhiner M, Cohen MZ et al: Pain as a metaphor for illness: impact of cancer pain on family caregivers, part 1, *Oncol Nurs Forum* 18(8):1303-1309, 1991.
17. Ferrell BR, Cohen MZ, Rhiner M et al: Pain as a metaphor for illness: family caregivers' management of pain, part 2, *Oncol Nurs Forum* 18(8):1315-1321, 1991.
18. Miaskowski C, Kragness L, Dibble S et al: Differences in mood states, health status, and caregiver strain between family caregivers of oncology outpatients with and without cancer-related pain, *J Pain Symptom Manage* 13(3):138-147, 1997.
19. Miaskowski C, Zimmer EF, Barrett KM et al: Differences in patients' and family caregivers' perceptions of the pain experience influence patient and caregiver outcomes, *Pain* 72(1-2):217-226, 1997.
20. Acute Pain Management Guideline Panel: *Acute pain management: operative or medical procedures and trauma. Clinical practice guideline.* Publication No. 92-0032, Rockville, Md, 1992, Agency for Health Care Policy and Research, US Department of Health and Human Services, Public Health Service.
21. Page GG: The medical necessity of adequate pain management, *Pain Forum* 5(4):227-233, 1996.
22. Sibbald W, Gill R: The philosophy and economics of pain management. In Hamill RJ, Rollingson JC, editors: *Handbook of critical care pain management,* New York, 1994, McGraw-Hill, pp 3-9.
23. Page G: *Acute pain and immune impairment*, International Association for the Study of Pain (website): http://iasp-pain.org/PCU05-1.pdf. Accessed October 22, 2005.
24. Macfarlane GJ, McBeth J, Silman AJ: Widespread body pain and mortality: prospective population based study, *BMJ* 323(7314):662-665, 2001.
25. Lewis KS, Whipple JK, Michael KA et al: Effect of analgesic treatment on the physiological consequences of acute pain, *Am J Hosp Pharm* 51(12):1539-1554, 1994.
26. Chang CH, Jiang CC: Evaluation of critical postoperative situations in orthopedic patients, *J Formosan Med Assoc* 96(12):990-995, 1997.
27. Carr DB, Goudas LC: Acute pain, *Lancet* 353(9169): 2051-2058, 1999.
28. Grant M, Ferrell BR, Rivera LM et al: Unscheduled readmissions for uncontrolled symptoms: a health care challenge for nurses, *Nurs Clin North Am* 30(4):673-682, 1995.
29. Duggleby W, Lander J: Cognitive status and postoperative pain: older adults, *J Pain Symptom Manage* 9(1):19-27, 1994.
30. Egbert AM, Parks LH, Short LM et al: Randomized trial of postoperative patient-controlled analgesia vs intramuscular narcotics in frail elderly men, *Arch Intern Med* 150(9):1897-1903, 1990.
31. Williams MA, Campbell EB, Raynor WJJ et al: Predictors of acute confusional states in hospitalized elderly patients, *Res Nurs Health* 8(1):31-40, 1985.
32. Carroll KC, Atkins PJ, Herold GR et al: Pain assessment and management in critically ill postoperative and trauma patients: a multisite study, *Am J Crit Care* 8(2):105-117, 1999.
33. Dasta J, Fuhrman T, McCandles C: Use of sedatives and analgesics in a surgical intensive care unit: a follow-up and commentary, *Heart Lung* 24(1):76-78, 1995.
34. Puntillo K, Schell H, Cohen N: Knowledge of critical care physicians and nurses about analgesics, sedatives, and neuromuscular blocking agents: extensive, but insufficient, *Crit Care Med* 27(1S):101A, 1999.

35. Puntillo K: Pain experiences of intensive care unit patients, *Heart Lung* 19(5 pt 1):526-533, 1990.
36. Tittle M, McMillan SC: Pain and pain-related side effects in an ICU and on a surgical unit: nurses' management, *Am J Crit Care* 3(1):25-30, 1994.
37. Sun X, Quinn T, Weissman C: Patterns of sedation and analgesia in the postoperative ICU patient, *Chest* 101(6):1625-1632, 1992.
38. Stannard D, Puntillo K, Miaskowski C et al: Clinical judgment and management of postoperative pain in critical care patients, *Am J Crit Care* 5(6):433-441, 1996.
39. Blakely WP, Page GG: Pathophysiology of pain in critically ill patients, *Crit Care Nurs Clin North Am* 13(2): 167-179, 2001.
40. American Pain Society: *Principles of analgesic use in the treatment of acute pain and cancer pain*, ed 5, Glenview, Ill, 2003, American Pain Society.
41. Dahl JL: Pain: impediments and suggestions for solutions, *J Natl Cancer Inst Monogr* (32):124-126, 2004.
42. Gordon DB, Pellino TA, Miaskowski C et al: A 10-year review of quality improvement monitoring in pain management: recommendations for standardized outcome measures, *Pain Manag Nurs* 3(4):116-130, 2002.
43. IASP Task Force on Taxonomy: *Classification of chronic pain*, ed 2, Seattle, 1994, International Association for the Study of Pain.
44. Merskey H: Classification of chronic pain: description of chronic pain syndromes and definitions of pain terms, *Pain* 3(S):S217, 1979.
45. McCaffery M: *Nursing practice theories related to cognition, bodily pain, and non-environment interactions*, Los Angeles, 1968, UCLA Student Store.
46. International Association for the Study of Pain: Pain terms: a list with definitions and notes on usage, *Pain* 6(3):249, 1979.
47. McCaffery M, Beebe A: *Pain: clinical manual for nursing practice*, St Louis, 1989, Mosby.
48. Cousins MJ: John J. Bonica distinguished lecture. Acute pain and the injury response: Immediate and prolonged effects, *Reg Anesth* 14(4):162-179, 1989.
49. Desbiens NA, Wu AW, Alzola C et al: Pain during hospitalization is associated with continued pain six months later in survivors of serious illness, *Am J Med* 102(3):269-276, 1997.
50. Brookhoff D: *Chronic pain: 1. a new disease?* (Alexander DeLuca and Addiction, Pain & Public Health websites): www.doctordeluca.com/Library/Pain/CP1NewDisease2K.htm. Accessed November 15, 2006.
51. Ashburn MA, Lipman AG: Pain in society. In Lipman AG, editor: *Pain management for primary care clinicians*, Bethesda, Md, 2004, American Society of Health-System Pharmacists, 1-11.
52. Bonica J: History of pain concepts and therapies. In Bonica J, editor: *The management of pain*, Philadelphia, 1990, Lea & Febiger, pp 2-17.
53. Zeppetella G, Ribeiro MD: Opioids for the management of breakthrough (episodic) pain in cancer patients, *Cochrane Database Syst Rev* (1):CD004311, 2006.
54. Fakata KL, Miaskowski C, Lipman AG: Chronic malignant pain. In Lipman AG, editor: *Pain management for primary care clinicians*, Bethesda, Md, 2004, American Society of Health-System Pharmacists, pp 139-151.
55. Sindrup SH, Jensen TS: Efficacy of pharmacological treatments of neuropathic pain: an update and effect related to mechanism of drug action, *Pain* 83(3):389-400, 1999.
56. Watkins LR, Maier SF: *Neuropathic pain: the immune connection*, International Association for the Study of Pain (website): http://iasp-pain.org/PCU04-1.pdf. Accessed October 22, 2005.
57. American Pain Society: *Pain: current understanding of assessment, management and treatments—Continuing Education offering*, American Pain Society (website): www.ampainsoc.org/ce/npc/I/b_definitions.htm. Accessed February 16, 2005.
58. Scholz J, Woolf CJ: Can we conquer pain? *Nat Neurosci* 5(suppl):1062-1067, 2002.
59. Fields HL: *Pain*, New York, 1987, McGraw-Hill.
60. Pasero C, Paice JA, McCaffery M: Basic mechanisms underlying the causes and effects of pain. In McCaffery M, Pasero C, editors: *Pain: clinical manual*, St Louis, 1999, Mosby, pp 15-34.
61. Levine JD, Reichling DB: Peripheral mechanisms of inflammatory pain. In Wall PD, Melzack R, editors: *Textbook of pain*, Philadelphia, 1999, Churchill Livingstone, pp 59-84.
62. *Untitled* (FA Davis website): www.fadavis.com/related_resources/27_1885_654.pdf. Accessed October 20, 2005.
63. Song S-O, Carr DB: *Pain and memory*, International Association for the Study of Pain (website): www.iasp-pain.org/PCU99a.html. Accessed October 22, 2005.
64. McQuay HJ: Pre-emptive analgesia: a systematic review of clinical studies, *Ann Med* 27(2):249-256, 1995.
65. Ochroch EA, Mardini IA, Gottschalk A. What is the role of NSAIDs in pre-emptive analgesia? *Drugs* 63(24): 2709-2723, 2003.
66. Kehlet H: Balanced analgesia: a prerequisite for optimal recovery, *Br J Surg* 85(1):3-4, 1998.
67. Kehlet H, Werner M, Perkins F: Balanced analgesia: what is it and what are its advantages in postoperative pain? *Drugs* 58(5):793-797, 1999.
68. Kehlet H, Holte K: Effect of postoperative analgesia on surgical outcome, *Br J Anaesth* 87(1):62-72, 2001.
69. Bach S, Noreng MF, Tjellden NU: Phantom limb pain in amputees during the first 12 months following limb amputation, after preoperative lumbar epidural blockade, *Pain* 33(3):297-301, 1988.
70. Katz J, Jackson M, Kavanagh BP et al: Acute pain after thoracic surgery predicts long-term post-thoracotomy pain, *Clin J Pain* 12(1):50-55, 1996.
71. Marchettini P, Simone DA, Caputi G et al: Pain from excitation of identified muscle nociceptors in humans, *Brain Res* 740(1-2):109-116, 1996.
72. Hopely L, van Schalkwyk J: *Pain physiology*, Anaesthetist.com (website): www.anaesthetist.com/icu/pain/pain_how.htm. Accessed on January 29, 2006.
73. Edwards AD: Physiology of pain. In St Marie B, editor: *Core curriculum for pain management nursing*, Philadelphia, 2002, WB Saunders, pp 121-145.
74. Melzack R, Wall PD: The gate control theory of pain. In Soulairac A, Cahn J, Carpentier J, editors: *Pain: Proceedings*

of the International Symposium on Pain, London, 1968, Academic Press, pp 11-31.

75. Hopely L, van Schalkwyk J: *Pain physiology*, Anaesthetist.com (website): www.anaesthetist.com/icu/pain/pain3.htm. Accessed January 29, 2006.
76. Portenoy RK: Basic mechanisms. In Portenoy RK, Kanner RM: *Pain management: theory and practice*, Philadelphia, 1996, FA Davis, pp 19-39.
77. Miljanich GP: Ziconotide: neuronal calcium channel blocker for treating severe chronic pain, *Curr Med Chem* 11(23):3029-3040, 2004.
78. Nicholson AB: Methadone for cancer pain, *Cochrane Database Syst Rev*, 2004 2:CD003971.
79. Hare BD, Viotanik S, Lipman AG: Pathophysiology of pain. In Lipman AG, editor: *Pain management for primary care clinicians*, Bethesda, Md, 2004, American Society of Health-System Pharmacists, pp 13-25.
80. McCaffery M, Pasero C: *Pain clinical manual*, ed 2, St Louis, 1999, Mosby.
81. Wallace K: The pathophysiology of pain, *Crit Care Nurs Q* 15(2):1-13, 1992.
82. Melzack R: Recent concepts of pain, *J Med* 13(3): 147-160, 1982.
83. Hilbers SM, Gennaro S: *Nonpharmacologic pain relief*, vol 5, New Jersey: Continuing Professional Education Center, Inc., 1986, NAACOG Update Series.
84. Melzack R, Casey KL: Sensory, motivational, and central control determinants of pain: a new conceptual model. In Kenshalo D, editor: Springfield, Ill, 1968, Charles C Thomas.
85. Ingvar M, Hsieh J: The image of pain. In Wall PD, Melzack R, editors: *Textbook of pain*, Philadelphia, 1999, Churchill Livingstone, pp 215-233.
86. Tolle T, Kaufmann T, Siessmeier T et al: Region-specific encoding of sensory and affective components of pain in the human brain: a positron emission tomography correlation analysis, *Ann Neurol* 45(1):40-47, 1999.
87. *Comprehensive accreditation manual for hospitals: the official handbook (CAMH)*, Oakbrook Terrace, Ill, 2000, Joint Commission on Accreditation of Healthcare Organizations.
88. *Pain the 5th vital sign*, American Pain Society (website): www.ampainsoc.org/advocacy/fifth.htm. Accessed February 18, 2005.
89. Brown M: *LIST acronym*, 2003.
90. Original author unknown revised University of Maryland Medical Center: *PQRST mnemonic*. 2000.
91. Jensen M, Karoly P, Braver S: The measurement of clinical pain intensity: a comparison of six methods, *Pain* 27(1):117-126, 1986.
92. Herr KA, Mobily PR, Kohout FJ et al: Evaluation of the Face Pain Scale for use with the elderly, *Clin J Pain* 14(1):29-38, 1998.
93. Kaiser K: *The relationship of patient characteristics and process of care characteristics to post-operative pain outcomes in the orthopedic patient*, 1, Baltimore, 2004, University of Maryland.
94. Stanik-Hutt JA, Soeken KL, Belcher AE et al: Pain experiences of traumatically injured patients in a critical care setting, *Am J Crit Care* 10(4):252-259, 2001.
95. Chibnall JT, Tait RC: Pain assessment in cognitively impaired and unimpaired older adults: a comparison of four scales, *Pain* 92(1-2):173-186, 2001.
96. Feldt KS, Ryden MB, Miles S: Treatment of pain in cognitively impaired compared with cognitively intact older patients with hip-fracture, *J Am Geriatr Soc* 46(9):1079-1085, 1998.
97. Taylor LJ, Harris J, Epps CD et al: Psychometric evaluation of selected pain intensity scales for use with cognitively impaired and cognitively intact older adults, *Rehabil Nurs* 30(2):55-61, 2005.
98. Taylor LJ, Herr K: Pain intensity assessment: a comparison of selected pain intensity scales for use in cognitively intact and cognitively impaired African American older adults, *Pain Manag Nurs* 4(2):87-95, 2003.
99. Ware LJ, Epps CD, Herr K et al: Evaluation of the Revised Face Pain Scale, Verbal Descriptor Scale, Numeric Rating Scale, and Iowa Pain Thermometer in older minority adults, *Pain Manag Nurs* 7(3):117-125, 2006.
100. *State of the art review of tools for assessment of pain in nonverbal older adults*, City of Hope (website): www.cityofhope.org/prc/elderly.asp. Accessed November 11, 2006.
101. Puntillo KA, Miaskowski C, Kehrle K et al: Relationship between behavioral and physiological indicators of pain, critical care patients' self-reports of pain, and opioid administration, *Crit Care Med* 25(7):1159-1166, 1997.
102. Herr K, Coyne PJ, Key T et al: Pain assessment in the nonverbal patient: position statement with clinical practice recommendations, *Pain Manag Nurs* 7(2):44-52, 2006. Accessed at *Pain Management Nursing* website: www.aspmn.org/Organization/documents/NonverbalJournalFINAL.pdf. Accessed October 9, 2006.
103. Kuhn S, Cooke K, Collins M et al: Perceptions of pain relief after surgery, *BMJ* 300(6741):1687-1690, 1990.
104. Tamsen A, Hartvig P, Dahlstrom B et al: Patient controlled analgesic therapy in the early postoperative period, *Acta Anaesthesiol Scand* 23(5):462-470, 1979.
105. AGS Panel on Persistent Pain in Older Persons: The management of persistent pain in older persons, *J Am Geriatr Soc* 50(suppl 6):S205-S224, 2002.
106. Zun LS, Downey LV, Gossman W et al: Gender differences in narcotic-induced emesis in the ED, *Am J Emerg Med* 20(3):151-154, 2002.
107. Fagerlund T: No pain relief from codeine…? An introduction to pharmacogenomics, *Acta Anaesthesiol Scand* 45(2):140-149, 2001.
108. Walker J, Carmody J: Experimental pain in healthy human subjects: gender differences in nociception and in response to ibuprofen, *Anesth Analg* 86(6):1257-1262, 1998.
109. Wolf CR, Smith G: Pharmacogenetics, *Br Med Bull* 55(2):366-386, 1999.
110. Wolf CR, Smith G, Smith RL: Science, medicine, and the future: pharmacogenetics, *BMJ* 320(7240):987-990, 2000.
111. Streetman DS: Metabolic basis of drug interactions in the intensive care unit, *Crit Care Nurs Q* 22(4):1-13, 2000.
112. Lee VC, Rowlingson JC, Hamill RJ: Nonsteroidal analgesic and anti-inflammatory agents. In Hamill RJ, Rollingson JC, editors: *Handbook of critical care pain management*, New York, 1994, McGraw-Hill, pp 103-115.
113. St Marie B, Loeb JL: Gerontologic pain management. In St Marie B, editor: *Core curriculum for pain management nursing*, Philadelphia, 2002, WB Saunders, pp 417-426.

114. Elias M: Gastropathy and NSAIDs, *Anesthesiology* 93(2):587, 2000.
115. Scapa E, Horowitz M, Waron M et al: Duodenal ulcer in the elderly, *J Clin Gastroenterol* 11(5):502-506, 1989.
116. Mamdani M, Rochon PA, Juurlink DN et al: Observational study of upper gastrointestinal haemorrhage in elderly patients given selective cyclo-oxygenase-2 inhibitors or conventional non-steroidal anti-inflammatory drugs, *BMJ* 325(7365):624, 2002.
117. Bresalier RS, Sandler RS, Quan H et al: *Cardiovascular events associated with rofecoxib in a clinical trial for colorectal adenoma chemoprevention* (serial online): www.nejm.org. Accessed February 16, 2005.
118. Nussmeier NA, Whelton AA, Brown MT et al: *Complications of the COX-2 inhibitors parecoxib and valdecoxib after cardiac surgery* (serial online): www.nejm.org. Accessed February 16, 2005.
119. Solomon SD, McMurray JJV, Pfeiffer MA et al: *Cardiovascular risk associated with celecoxib in a clinical trial for colorectal adenoma prevention* (serial online): www.nejm.org. Accessed February 16, 2005.
120. Portenoy RK, Lesage P: Management of cancer pain, *Lancet* 353(9165):1695-1700, 1999.
121. *WHO's pain relief ladder,* World Health Organization (website): www.who.int/cancer/palliative/painladder/en/. Accessed October 9, 2005.
122. Gabriel SE: *Cancer pain relief: with a guide to opioid availability*, ed 2, Geneva, 1996, World Health Organization.
123. Jacox AK, Bausell BR, Mahrenholz DM: Patient satisfaction with nursing care in hospitals, *Outcomes Manag Nurs Pract* 1(1):20-28, 1997.
124. Jadad AR, Browman GP: The WHO analgesic ladder for cancer pain management: stepping up the quality of its evaluation, *JAMA* 274(23):1870-1873, 1995.
125. McCleane G: Pharmacological strategies in relieving neuropathic pain, *Expert Opin Pharmacother* 5(6):1299-1312, 2004.
126. Dühmke RM, Cornblath DD, Hollingshead JRF: Tramadol for neuropathic pain, *Cochrane Database Syst Rev* (2):CD003726, 2004.
127. Pasero C, Portenoy R, McCaffery M: Opioid analgesics. In McCaffery M, Pasero C, editors: *Pain clinical manual,* St Louis, 1999, Mosby, pp 161-299.
128. *Management of cancer pain—opioid analgesics section* (Pain management online series 11): www.ama-cmeonline.com/pain_mgmt/module11/05opio/02_01.htm. Accessed October 25, 2005.
129. Kurella M, Bennett WM, Chertow GM: Analgesia in patients with ESRD: a review of available evidence, *Am J Kidney Dis* 42(2):217-228, 2003.
130. Faura CC, Moore RA, Horga JF et al: Morphine and morphine-6-glucuronide plasma concentrations and effect in cancer pain, *J Pain Symptom Manage* 11(2):95-102, 1996.
131. Lawlor PG: The panorama of opioid-related cognitive dysfunction in patients with cancer: a critical literature appraisal, *Cancer* 94(6):1836-1853, 1915.
132. JCAHO: *Sentinel event alert—high alert medications and patient safety,* Joint Commission on Accreditation of Healthcare Organizations (website): www.jcaho.org/about+/news+letters/sentinel+event+alert/sea_11.htm. Accessed February 27, 2005.
133. Kaiser K, Diep L: *Unpublished work*, 2005.
134. Inturrisi CE, Colburn WA, Kaiko RF et al: Pharmacokinetics and pharmacodynamics of methadone in patients with chronic pain, *Clin Pharmacol Ther* 41(4): 392-401, 1987.
135. Quigley C: Opioid switching to improve pain relief and drug tolerability, *Cochrane Database Syst Rev* (3): CD004847, 2004.
136. Du Pen SL, Du Pen AR, Polissar N et al: Implementing guidelines for cancer pain management: results of a randomized controlled clinical trial, *J Clin Oncol* 17(1):361-370, 1999.
137. Miaskowski C, Dodd MJ, West C et al: Lack of adherence with the analgesic regimen: a significant barrier to effective cancer pain management, *J Clin Oncol* 19(23):4275-4279, 2001.
138. McNicol E, Horowicz-Mehler N, Fisk RA et al: Management of opioid side effects in cancer-related and chronic noncancer pain: a systematic review, *J Pain* 4(5):231-256, 2003.
139. Cherny N, Ripamonti C, Pereira J et al: Strategies to manage the adverse effects of oral morphine: an evidence-based report, *J Clin Oncol* 19(9):2542-2554, 2001.
140. Liu S, Carpenter RL, Neal JM: Epidural anesthesia and analgesia: their role in postoperative outcome, *Anesthesiology* 82(6):1474-1506, 1995.
141. Rawal N: Epidural and spinal agents for postoperative analgesia, *Surg Clin North Am* 79(2):313-344, 1999.
142. Walder B, Schafer M, Henzi I et al: Efficacy and safety of patient-controlled opioid analgesia for acute postoperative pain: a quantitative systematic review, *Acta Anaesthesiol Scand* 45(7):795-804, 2001.
143. Macintyre PE: Safety and efficacy of patient-controlled analgesia, *Br J Anaesth* 87(1):36-46, 2001.
144. Enting RH, Oldenmenger WH, van der Rijt CC et al: A prospective study evaluating the response of patients with unrelieved cancer pain to parenteral opioids, *Cancer* 94(11):3049-3056, 2002.
145. McNamara P: Opioid switching from morphine to transdermal fentanyl for toxicity reduction in palliative care, *Palliat Med* 16(5):425-434, 2002.
146. Mercadante S: Opioid rotation for cancer pain: rationale and clinical aspects, *Cancer* 86(9):1856-1866, 1999.
147. Mercadante S, Radbruch L, Caraceni A et al: Episodic (breakthrough) pain: consensus conference of an expert working group of the European Association for Palliative Care, *Cancer* 94(3):832-839, 2002.
148. Portenoy RK, Hagen NA: Breakthrough pain: definition, prevalence and characteristics, *Pain* 41(3):273-281, 1990.
149. Briggs M, Nelson EA: Topical agents or dressings for pain in venous leg ulcers, *Cochrane Database Syst Rev* (1): CD001177, 2003.
150. Argoff CE, Galer BS, Jensen MP et al: Effectiveness of the lidocaine patch 5% on pain qualities in three chronic pain states: assessment with the Neuropathic Pain Scale, *Curr Med Res Opin* 20(suppl 2):S21-S28, 2004.
151. Young-Chang P, Wasa U: Warm steaming enhances the topical anesthetic effect, *Anesth Analg* 98(4):982-985, 2004.
152. Worthington HV, Clarkson JE, Eden OB: Interventions for treating oral mucositis for patients with cancer receiving treatment, *Cochrane Database Syst Rev* (2): CD001973, 2004.

153. Ferreira PR, Fleck JF, Diehl A et al: Protective effect of alpha-tocopherol in head and neck cancer radiation-induced mucositis: a double-blind randomized trial, *Head Neck* 26(4):313-321, 2004.
154. Edwards TD, Breed R: Treatment of postoperative pain in the post anesthesia care unit, *Anesthesiol Clin North Am* 92:665, 1990.
155. Eisenberg E, McNicol E, Carr DB: Opioids for neuropathic pain, *Cochrane Database Syst Rev* (3):CD006146, 2006.
156. Chumbley GM, Hall GM, Salmon P: Why do patients feel positive about patient-controlled analgesia? *Anaesthesia* 54(4):386-389, 1999.
157. Moore RA, Gavaghan D, Tramer MR et al: Size is everything—large amounts of information are needed to overcome random effects in estimating direction and magnitude of treatment effects, *Pain* 78(3):209-216, 1998.
158. Choiniere M, Rittenhouse BE, Perreault S et al: Efficacy and costs of patient-controlled analgesia versus regularly administered intramuscular opioid therapy, *Anesthesiology* 89(6):1377-1388, 1998.
159. Colwell CW Jr, Morris BA: Patient-controlled analgesia compared with intramuscular injection of analgesics for the management of pain after an orthopaedic procedure, *J Bone Joint Surg* 77(5):726-733, 1995.
160. Looi-Lyons LC, Chung FF, Chan VW et al: Respiratory depression: an adverse outcome during patient controlled analgesia therapy, *J Clin Anesth* 8(2):151-156, 1996.
161. Hansen LA, Noyes MA, Lehman ME: Evaluation of patient-controlled analgesia (PCA) versus PCA plus continuous infusion in postoperative cancer patients, *J Pain Symptom Manage* 6(1):4-14, 1991.
162. Parker RK, Holtmann B, White PF: Patient-controlled analgesia: does a concurrent opioid infusion improve pain management after surgery? *JAMA* 266(14):1947-1952, 1991.
163. Parker RK, Holtmann B, White PF: Effects of a nighttime opioid infusion with PCA therapy on patient comfort and analgesic requirements after abdominal hysterectomy, *Anesthesiology* 76(3):362-367, 1992.
164. Kaiser K: *American Pain Society Nursing Issues Special Interest Group List Serve Survey on Epidural and PCA Monitoring* (Karen Kaiser website): http://home.comcast.net/~kaiser/mywebpages/EPIDURAL-PCA.doc. Accessed February 25, 2005.
165. Chumbley GM, Hall GM, Salmon P: Patient-controlled analgesia: an assessment by 200 patients, *Anaesthesia* 53(3):216-221, 1998.
166. Farmer M, Harper NJ: Unexpected problems with patient controlled analgesia, *BMJ* 304(6826):574, 1992.
167. Johnson T, Daugherty M: Oversedation with patient controlled analgesia, *Anaesthesia* 47(1):81-82, 1992.
168. *Sentinel event alert—patient controlled analgesia by proxy*, Joint Commission on Accreditation of Healthcare Organizations (website): www.jcaho.org/about+us/news+letters/sentinel+event+alert/sea_33.htm. Accessed February 27, 2005.
169. *Authorized and unauthorized ("PCA by proxy") dosing of analgesic infusion pumps,* American Society of Pain Management Nursing (website): www.aspmn.org/Organization/documents/PCAbyProxy-final-EW_004.pdf. Accessed September 11, 2006.
170. *Sentinel event alert—infusion pumps: preventing future adverse events,* Joint Commission on Accreditation of Healthcare Organizations (website): www.jcaho.org/about+us/news+letters/sentinel+event+alert/sea_15.htm. Accessed February 27, 2005.
171. Kaiser K, Armstrong L: *Unpublished work*, 2003.
172. Dunwoody C: *Personal communication*, 2002.
173. Etches RC: Respiratory depression associated with patient-controlled analgesia: a review of eight cases, *Can J Anaesth* 41(2):125-132, 1994.
174. Richtsmeier AJ Jr, Barnes SD, Barkin RL: Ventilatory arrest with morphine patient-controlled analgesia in a child with renal failure, *Am J Ther* 4(7-8):255-257, 1997.
175. Sidebotham D, Dijkhuizen MR, Schug SA: The safety and utilization of patient-controlled analgesia, *J Pain Symptom Manage* 14(4):202-209, 1997.
176. Van Dercar DH, Martinez AP, De Lisser EA: Sleep apnea syndromes: a potential contraindication for patient-controlled analgesia, *Anesthesiology* 74(3):623-624, 1991.
177. Smith TJ, Staats PS, Deer T et al: Randomized clinical trial of an implantable drug delivery system compared with comprehensive medical management for refractory cancer pain: impact on pain, drug-related toxicity, and survival, *J Clin Oncol* 20(19):4040-4049, 2002.
178. Wheatley RG, Schug SA, Watson D: Safety and efficacy of postoperative epidural analgesia, *Br J Anaesth* 87(1):47-61, 2001.
179. Horlocker TT, Wedel DJ, Benzon H et al: Regional anesthesia in the anticoagulated patient: defining the risks, *Reg Anesth Pain Med* 29(2S):1-12, 2004.
180. Horlocker TT, Wedel DJ, Benzon H et al: Regional anesthesia in the anticoagulated patient: defining the risks (the Second ASRA Consensus Conference on Neuraxial Anesthesia and Anticoagulation), *Reg Anesth Pain Med* 28(3):172-197, 2003.
181. *Second ASRA Consensus Conference on Neuraxial Anesthesia and Anticoagulation,* American Society of Regional Anesthesia and Pain Medicine (website): www.asra.com/consensus-statements/2.html. Accessed February 25, 2005.
182. The American Society of Addiction Medicine, the American Pain Society: *Consensus statement on the definitions related to the use of opioids for the treatment of pain* (website): www.asam.org/ppol/Opioid%20Definition%20C%2002.htm. Accessed November 12, 2006.
183. Stimmel B: *Pain and its relief without addiction*, New York, 1997, Hayworth Medical.
184. Kosten TR, George TP: *The neurobiology of opioid dependence: implications for treatment,* Science and Practice Perspective (website): http://165.112.78.61/PDF/Perspectives/vol1no1/03Perspectives-Neurobio.pdf. Accessed February 19, 2005.
185. Foley KM: Misconceptions and controversies regarding the use of opioids in cancer pain, *Anticancer Drugs* 6(suppl 3):4-13, 1995.
186. American Society for Pain Management Nursing: *Pain management for the person with addictive disease* (website): www.aspmn.org/Organization/position_papers.htm. Accessed January 22, 2005.
187. *Tools for health care providers: drug conversion calculator,* Hypermedia Assistant for Cancer Pain Management (website): www.painresearch.utah.edu/cancerpain/provtoolsF.html. Accessed February 19, 2005.

188. Sidney Kimmel Cancer Center: *Hopkins Opioid Program (HOP)* (website): www.hopkinskimmelcancercenter.org/specialtycenters/hop_login.cfm?facilityid=27. Accessed February 19, 2005.
189. Software.net web page CG: *Opioid calculator,* Cynergy (website): www.software.net/dr/v2/ec_MAIN.Entry24?SP=10024&PN=14&XID=56498&Search_String=cynergy. Accessed February 19, 2005.
190. Gammaitoni AR, Fine P, Alvarez N et al: Clinical application of opioid equianalgesic data, *Clin J Pain* 19(5):286-297, 2003.
191. Pasternak GW: Multiple opiate receptors: deja vu all over again, *Neuropharmacology* 47(suppl 1):312-323, 2004.
192. Blenko J: *Comparison of electronic equianalgesic conversion programs*, 2002.
193. Cherny NI: The management of cancer pain. In Melzack R, Wall PD, editors: *Handbook of pain management: a clinical companion to Wall and Melzack's textbook of pain,* Philadelphia, 2003, Churchill Livingstone, pp 641-666.
194. Devor M, Govrin-Lippmann R, Raber P: Corticosteroids suppress ectopic neural discharge originating in experimental neuromas, *Pain* 22(2):127-137, 1985.
195. Ellershaw JE, Kelly MJ: Corticosteroids and peptic ulceration, *Palliat Med* 8(4):313-319, 1994.
196. Namaka M, Gramlich CR, Ruhlen D et al: A treatment algorithm for neuropathic pain, *Clin Ther* 26(7):951-979, 2004.
197. Chong MS, Bajwa ZH: Diagnosis and treatment of neuropathic pain, *J Pain Symptom Manage* 25(suppl 5): S4-S11, 2003.
198. Sindrup SH, Jensen TS: Pharmacologic treatment of pain in polyneuropathy, *Neurology* 55(7):915-920, 2000.
199. McQuay H, Carroll D, Jadad AR et al: Anticonvulsant drugs for management of pain: a systematic review, *BMJ* 311(7012):1047-1052, 1995.
200. McQuay HJ, Tramer M, Nye BA et al: A systematic review of antidepressants in neuropathic pain, *Pain* 68(2-3): 217-227, 1996.
201. Mack A: Examination of the evidence for off-label use of gabapentin, *J Manag Care Pharm* 9(6):559-568, 2003.
202. Backonja M, Glanzman RL: Gabapentin dosing for neuropathic pain: evidence from randomized, placebo-controlled clinical trials, *Clin Ther* 25(1):81-104, 2003.
203. Chandramouli J: Newer anticonvulsant drugs in neuropathic pain and bipolar disorder, *J Pain Palliat Care Pharmacother* 16(4):19-37, 2002.
204. Mao J, Chen LL: Systemic lidocaine for neuropathic pain relief, *Pain* 87(1):7-17, 2000.
205. Fields HL: Peripheral neuropathic pain: An approach to management. In Melzack R, Wall PD, editors: *Handbook of pain management: a clinical companion to Wall and Melzack's textbook of pain,* Philadelphia, 2003, Churchill Livingstone, pp 581-589.
206. *Valdecoxib* (website): www.nlm.nih.gov/medlineplus/druginfo/medmaster/a602011.html. Accessed March 4, 2005.
207. Lipman AG: Analgesic drugs for neuropathic and sympathetically maintained pain, *Clin Geriatr Med* 12(3): 501-515, 1996.
208. Martinez MJ, Roqué M, Alonso CP et al: Calcitonin for metastatic bone pain, *Cochrane Database Syst Rev* (3): CD003223, 2003.
209. Hocking G, Cousins MJ: Ketamine in chronic pain management: an evidence-based review, *Anesth Analg* 97(6):1730-1739, 2003.
210. Bell R, Eccleston C, Kalso E: Ketamine as an adjuvant to opioids for cancer pain, *Cochrane Database Syst Rev* (1): CD003351, 2003.
211. Hostetler MA, Auinger P, Szilagyi PG: Parenteral analgesic and sedative use among ED patients in the United States: combined results from the National Hospital Ambulatory Medical Care Survey (NHAMCS), 1992-1997, *Am J Emerg Med* 20(3):139-143, 2002.
212. Kannan TR, Saxena A, Bhatnagar S et al: Oral ketamine as an adjuvant to oral morphine for neuropathic pain in cancer patients, *J Pain Symptom Manage* 23(1):60-65, 2002.
213. Power I, Barratt S: Analgesic agents for the postoperative period: nonopioids, *Surg Clin North Am* 79(2):275-295, 1999.
214. Mercadante S: Ketamine in cancer pain: an update, *Palliat Med* 10(3):225-230, 1996.
215. Wiesenfeld-Hallin Z: Combined opioid-NMDA antagonist therapies: what advantages do they offer for the control of pain syndromes? *Drugs* 55(1):1-4, 1998.
216. Gurnani A, Sharma PK, Rautela RS et al: Analgesia for acute musculoskeletal trauma: low-dose subcutaneous infusion of ketamine, *Anaesth Intensive Care* 24(1):32-36, 1996.
217. Kvarnstrom A, Karlsten R, Quiding H et al: The analgesic effect of intravenous ketamine and lidocaine on pain after spinal cord injury, *Acta Anaesthesiol Scand* 48(4):498-506, 2004.
218. Benitez-Rosario MA, Feria M, Salinas-Martin A et al: A retrospective comparison of the dose ratio between subcutaneous and oral ketamine, *J Pain Symptom Manage* 25(5):400-402, 2003.
219. *Ketamine* (website): www.nlm.nih.gov/medlineplus/druginfo/uspdi/203043.html. Accessed March 5, 2005.
220. Subramaniam K, Subramaniam B, Steinbrook RA: Ketamine as adjuvant analgesic to opioids: a quantitative and qualitative systematic review, *Anesth Analg* 99(2): 482-495, 2004.
221. Blackshaw LA, Gebhart GF: The pharmacology of gastrointestinal nociceptive pathways, *Curr Opin Pharmacol* 2(6):642-649, 2002.
222. Gebhart GF: Descending modulation of pain, *Neurosci Biobehav Rev* 27(8):729-737, 2004.
223. Bueno L, Fioramonti J, Delvaux M et al: Mediators and pharmacology of visceral sensitivity: from basic to clinical investigations, *Gastroenterology* 112(5):1714-1743, 1997.
224. Weixler D, Hartmann W: Intravenous S-+-ketamine for treatment of visceral pain in the final phase [German], *Wien Med Wochenschr* 156(9-10):318-323, 2006.
225. Kuiken SD, van den Berg SJ, Tytgat GN et al: Oral S(+)-ketamine does not change visceral perception in health, *Digest Dis Sci* 49(11-12):1745-1751, 2004.
226. Willert RP, Woolf CJ, Hobson AR et al: The development and maintenance of human visceral pain hypersensitivity is dependent on the N-methyl-D-aspartate receptor, *Gastroenterology* 126(3):683-692, 2004.

227. Denton AS, Clarke NW, Maher EJ: Non-surgical interventions for late radiation cystitis in patients who have received radical radiotherapy to the pelvis, *Cochrane Database Systematic Rev* (3):CD001773, 2002.
228. Sze WM, Shelley M, Held I et al: Palliation of metastatic bone pain: single fraction versus multifraction radiotherapy, *Cochrane Database Syst Rev*, 2002.
229. Chow E, Ling A, Davis L et al: Pain flare following external beam radiotherapy and meaningful change in pain scores in the treatment of bone metastases, *Radiother Oncol* 75(1):64-69, 2005.
230. Roqué M, Martinez MJ, Alonso CP et al: Radioisotopes for metastatic bone pain, *Cochrane Database Syst Rev* 4: CD003347, 2003.
231. Wong R, Wiffen PJ: Bisphosphonates for the relief of pain secondary to bone metastases, *Cochrane Database Syst Rev* (2):CD002068, 2002.
232. Mundy EA, Du Hamel KN, Montgomery GH: The efficacy of behavioral interventions for cancer treatment-related side effects, *Semin Clin Neuropsychiatry* 8(4): 253-275, 2003.
233. Fellowes D, Barnes K, Wilkinson S: Aromatherapy and massage for symptom relief in patients with cancer, *Cochrane Database Syst Rev* (2):CD002287, 2004.
234. Maikler VE: Pharmacologic pain management in children: a review of intervention research, *J Pediatr Nurs* 13(1):3-14, 1998.
235. Allard P, Maunsell E, Labbe J et al: Educational interventions to improve cancer pain control: a systematic review, *J Palliat Med* 49(2):191-203, 2001.
236. Devine EC, Westlake SK: The effects of psychoeducational care provided to adults with cancer: meta-analysis of 116 studies, *Oncol Nurs Forum* 22(9):1369-1381, 1995.
237. *Treatment options: a guide for people living with pain*, American Pain Foundation (website): https://secure2.convio.net/apf/site/SSurvey?ACTION_REQUIRED=URI_ACTION_USER_REQUESTS&SURVEY_ID=1780. Accessed November 12, 2006.
238. *What is complementary and alternative medicine?* National Institutes of Health National Complementary and Alternative Medicine (website): http://nccam.nih.gov/health/whatiscam/. Accessed November 17, 2006.
239. Vallerand AH, Fouladbakhsh JM, Templin T: The use of complementary/alternative medicine therapies for the self-treatment of pain among residents of urban, suburban, and rural communities, *Am J Public Health* 93(6):923-925, 2003.
240. *Cancer and complementary and alternative medicine in cancer,* National Institutes of Health National Complementary and Alternative Medicine (website): http://nccam.nih.gov/health/camcancer/. Accessed November 17, 2006.
241. Lee H, Schmidt K, Ernst E: Acupuncture for the relief of cancer-related pain—a systematic review, *Eur J Pain* 9(4):437-444, 2005.

Chapter 32

Mucositis

Mary Ellyn Witt

Oral mucositis has been a major consequence of radiation therapy and has been used to guide therapy since the founding of radiation therapy in the beginning of the 20th century.

Samuel Hellman, MD

Mucositis has been a recognized side effect of cancer therapy for more than 75 years. Oral mucositis is an inflammatory, ulcerative process resulting from the systemic effects of cytoxic chemotherapy and the local effects of radiation therapy.[1,2] Approaches to managing mucositis have evolved as scientific knowledge has grown and the desire to treat with evidence-based practice has matured.

The incidence of oral mucositis depends on patient characteristics and treatment regimens. Populations at highest risk include patients treated for head and neck cancer and patients undergoing intensive high-dose chemotherapy for bone marrow transplant.[2] Thirty-three studies on head and neck cancer were reviewed by Trotti and colleagues,[3] and the mean incidence for mucositis was 80%.

Oral mucositis is a multifaceted problem that can cause pain, infection, and debilitation and lead to a decrease in one's quality of life.[3] This common side effect may result in a modification in treatment, which may decrease the effectiveness of the therapeutic regimen. It can be a clinical burden to patients and caregivers and an economic burden to families and third-party payors.[4]

Oncology nurses are at the forefront of delivering the majority of care for treatment-related side effects required by patients with oral mucositis. The nurses' responsibilities include toxicity grading, symptom management, and educating patients, caregivers, and fellow staff.[5]

PATHOPHYSIOLOGY OF MUCOSITIS

The oral cavity is a complex environment that consists of three distinctly different types of mucosa. These include the following:

- *Lining mucosa.* This mucosa is the most abundant and is located on the inner aspects of the cheeks and lips, ventral tongue, and soft palate. Lining mucosa is distributed over loose connective tissue. It consists of nonkeratinizing squamous epithelium and is susceptible to trauma.
- *Specialized mucosa.* This mucosa is found on the dorsal tongue and consists of numerous papillae that contain sensory nerve endings for taste.
- *Masticatory mucosa.* This mucosa is characterized by a tough, keratinizing surface and is tightly bound to bone.

The submucosa is located throughout the oropharynx and beneath all types of oral mucosa This layer contains inflammatory cells, the extracellular matrix, and the blood and nerve supply to the mucosa.[6]

Tasks of everyday living, such as chewing, swallowing, coughing, and sneezing cause the lining of the oral mucosa to slough. Continuity and integrity of the normal mucosa depends on the tissue's ability to be continuously nourished and replaced. In general, it requires approximately 2 weeks for cells to progress from their stem source to the surface.[6]

Historically, it was believed that mucositis was caused by radiation and chemotherapy nonselectively damaging rapidly dividing cells. Damage to the epithelium led to the loss of the renewal capacity of the epithelium, which lead to cell death, atrophy, and consequent ulceration.[7] Research reported by Sonis explains that mucositis is not just a problem with epithelium damage. Radiation-induced injury to the epithelium of blood vessels is an early event in the development of mucositis. In addition, selected proteins associated with tissue injury (cytokines) are elevated in patients with mucositis. Suppression of these proteins may be associated with a reduction of mucositis. The interactions among the various mucosal components, including those influenced by the oral environment, collectively lead to mucositis.[6,7]

The degree and duration of mucositis in patients treated with radiation therapy is related to the radiation source, cumulative dose, dose intensity, and effects of combination chemotherapy.

In standard 2-Gray (Gy) daily fractionated radiation therapy programs, mucosal erythema occurs within the first week of treatment. Patchy or confluent pseudomembranous radiation-induced mucositis peaks during the fourth to fifth week of therapy. Less severe mucositis is noted in programs with daily radiation doses lower then 2 Gy; however, in accelerated radiation therapy programs mucositis peaks within 3 weeks.[8]

Mucosal injury can be viewed as having five phases: initiation, upregulation and generation of messenger signals (damage response), signaling and amplification, ulceration, and healing. Although the model described seems linear, injury occurs very quickly in all tissues (Table 32-1).[7,9]

Initiation

The action of radiation and chemotherapy result in oxygen changes at the cellular level. These free-oxygen radicals can alter DNA, proteins, and membrane phospholipids. This results in the changes to blood vessels and tissues that hallmark the initiation phase of mucositis.[7,10]

Damage Response

Once initiation has occurred, a number of biologic switches are turned on during the upregulation and message-generating phase. Transcription factors, such as necrosis factor–kappa beta (NF-κβ), upregulate genes that control the synthesis of proteins. Among the proteins generated are compounds called *cytokines*. Cytokines target epithelium, endothelium, and connective tissue and produce tissue injury. Concurrently, radiation and chemotherapy are capable of activating enzymes that produce increased rates of cell death. As a result, the mucosa is significantly targeted by a broad array of messages that result in damage and death of the controlling cells of the epithelium. The mucosa starts to thin, becomes erythematous, and begins to feel painful to the patient.[6]

Signaling and Amplification

Proinflammatory cytokines play an indirect role in amplifying mucosal injury. Specific cytokines, especially tumor necrosis factor X, and other mediators react to the damage and create additional proinflammatory changes. This stage occurs below the mucosa layer and damage may continue after radiation and chemotherapy is completed.[6,7,9]

Ulceration

This is the most clinically obvious and dangerous phase for patients. Neuronal endings are exposed, creating significant pain. Colonization of the ulcers occurs and causes release of cell wall products that penetrate into adjoining tissue. These products act as toxins and stimulate inflammatory cells that accumulate beneath the ulcer. Additional damaging cytokines are generated. In the case of the neutropenic patient, bacteria may invade submucosa, penetrate vascular walls, and produce bacteremia and sepsis.[6]

Healing

The healing phase starts with a signal for the extracellular matrix to initiate repair. New messenger molecules direct the epithelium to divide, migrate, and differentiate into new healthy mucosa. After the healing phase, the oral mucosa appears normal, but the mucosal environment has been significantly altered. Such altered mucosa increases the risk of future episodes of oral mucositis with subsequent anticancer therapy.[6,7]

PREVENTION, RISK FACTORS, AND INFECTION

Cancer treatment–related mucositis is one of the areas of oncology nursing in which evidence-based practice is an important endeavor. Historically, nurses have taken diverse approaches to assess and manage mucositis. In the past 10 years, nurses, along with other professionals, have been challenged to become involved in studies that focus on prevention of mucositis.[11,12] More than 100 studies have been published on methods for preventing mucositis.[13]

All of the interventions for prevention have one of the following biologic effects : (1) attempt to alter the exposure of oral mucosa to chemotherapy and radiation therapy, (2) provide protection of mucosal proliferating cells, (3) enhance mucosal epithelial maturation and healing, (4) reduce the inflammatory response and oral bacteria load.[12] The Cochrane Database of Systemic Reviews perused 109 studies. Of those, 57 were excluded for lack of useful information. The 52 useable studies included 3594

Table 32-1 Phases of Mucositis

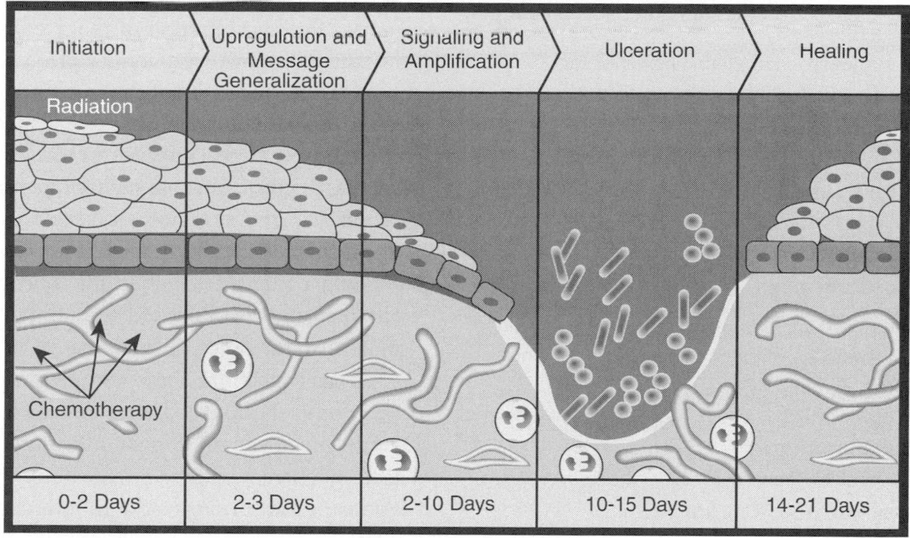

Phase	Biologic actions
Phase 1: Initiation	Damage to DNA causes cell death Generation of reactive oxygen species Stimulation of transcription factors
Phase 2: Upregulation and message generation	Activation of transcription factors nuclear factor-kappa beta (NF-κβ) greater than proinflammatory cytokines Angiogenesis Fibroblast breakdown: macrophages to metalloproteinases to tissue injury or production of tumor necrosis factor-alpha (TNF-α)
Phase 3: Signaling and amplification	Direct damage continues TNF-α activates NF-κβ Feedback loop amplifies effects
Phase 4: Ulceration	Ulceration from epithelium to submucosa Pseudomembrane over ulcer Bacterial colonization Bacterial wall products activate macrophages Macrophages stimulate proinflammatory cytokines
Phase 5: Healing	Signal from extracellular matrix Migration and proliferation Layering of cells Normal flora is established

From Cawley MM, Benson LM: *Clin J Oncol Nurs* 9(5):586, 2005.

randomized patients. Interventions evaluated were acyclovir, allopurinol mouth rinse, amifostine, antibiotic pastille or paste, benzydamine, camomile, chlorhexidine, clarithromycin, folinic acid, glutamine, GM-CSF (granulocyte-macrophage colony-stimulating factor), hydrolytic enzymes, ice chips, oral care, pentoxifyline, povidone, prednisone, propantheline, prostaglandin, sucralfate, and Traumeel™. Of the 21 interventions included in trials, nine showed some evidence of preventing or reducing the evidence of mucositis.[13] Table 32-2 provides a summary of interventions for which there was more than one trial and a significant difference as compared to placebo or no treatment.

Table 32-2 Interventions for Mucositis

Agent	Effects on mucositis prevention
Allopurinol mouth rinse	Unreliable evidence for reduction in severity
Amifostine	Minimal benefit in reducing mucositis
Antibiotic	Moderate benefit
GM-CSF	Prevented mucositis
Hydrolytic enzymes	Reduced the severity
Ice chips	Prevented mucositis
Povidone	Weak evidence for prevention
Oral care products	Weak evidence for prevention

Data from McGuire D, Rubenstein E, Peterson D: *Semin Oncol Nurs* 20(1):59-66, 2004 and Worthington HV, Clarkson JE, Eden OB: *Cochr Rev*, Issue 4, Article No. CD000978, 2006.
GM-CSF, Granulocyte-macrophage colony-stimulating factor.

Reducing risk factors can reduce the severity of mucositis. Mucositis will be enhanced and prolonged in patients who have preexisting poor oral or dental hygiene or poor-fitting dentures.[14,15] There is no evidence-based practice to support these as risk factors. However, it stands to reason that the rubbing effect of poor-fitting dentures or unhealthy teeth creates a more conducive environment for the patient to experience mucositis. Poor dental health will also increase a patient's risk for infection.[2]

Spicy foods, citrus, use of oxygen, smoking tobacco, chewing tobacco, drinking alcohol, and use of mouthwashes with alcohol are risk factors for enhancing and prolonging mucositis.[14,15] Tobacco is an irritant to the oral mucosa, and alcohol dries the oral mucosa. Patients may require intervention to overcome the addictive properties associated with the use of alcohol and tobacco. All of these described irritants should be avoided during treatment and recovery phases of care.

Other factors influencing an individual's risk of developing oral mucositis include defects of certain metabolic enzymes and DNA-repair mechanisms, deficiencies of folic acid and vitamin B_{12}, or delayed elimination of antineoplastic agents because of impaired renal or hepatic function. Xerostomia contributes to mucositis secondary to the decreased production and reduced buffering capacity of saliva, an increase in the viscosity and acidity of saliva, and reduced oral IgA levels favoring the growth of infectious oral flora.[8]

The most severe and life-threatening complication of oral mucositis is infection. An intact oral mucosa limits infiltration of many compounds into the epithelium by maintaining a physical and chemical blockade and reduces the levels of oral microorganisms colonizing the mucosa by shedding of the surface layer. If the integrity of the oral mucosa is broken, microorganisms, including those from the patient's normal oral flora, are provided a portal of entry into the body and eventually the blood stream. When a patient has significant mucositis, coupled with neutropenia or limited potential to fight microorganisms, the outcome could be life threatening.[2]

Fungal infections account for the most common infections of damaged oral mucosa. Candidiasis is the predominant fungal infection, manifesting itself by characteristic white coats or erythematous lesions in the corners of the mouth and on the soft palate and tongue. Aspergillosis and mucormycosis, characterized by painful oral ulcerations, which may invade the orofacial skeleton, are observed less often. Prophylactic use of various antifungal agents is recommended in patients who are likely to develop prolonged granulocytopenia.[8] Kostler and colleagues[8] reviewed four studies, published between 1977 and 1992, using polyene antifungal agents, such as nystatin, as topical prophylaxis. These agents were found to have little benefit in most clinical trials. There is now ample evidence to indicate that prophylactic use of azole agents such as fluconazole and clotrimazole, absorbed either fully or partially through the gastrointestinal tract, reduce the clinical signs of oral candidiasis. Soysa and colleagues[16] reviewed five studies, published between 1994 and 2000, that supported fluconazole as being the drug of choice in preventing and treating oral candidiasis.

Second to fungi, viruses, particularly herpes simplex virus type I (HSV) and varicella zoster virus (VZV), represent the most common pathogens aggravating oral mucositis. Oral infections are characterized by grouped small vesicles that tend to burst and leave behind painful ulcers. Topical and systemic acyclovir treatment is effective in the management of oral herpetic infections and for preventing oropharyngeal shedding of the herpetic virus.[8]

The oral mucosa is colonized by a variety of potentially pathogenic microorganisms, especially gram-positive cocci and gram-negative opportunistic bacteria. Disturbed integrity of the oral epithelial barrier, leukopenia, changes in salivary flow, and composition, and a shift of the oral microflora to an abundance of gram-negative organisms—particularly in patients with periodontal disease—favor the emergence of oral infections. The necessity of antimicrobial agents for the prophylaxis and treatment of oral mucositis has become the standard of care.[8] Oral mucositis affects the quality of life for patients undergoing treatment for cancer. Though prevention of oral mucositis is difficult, attempts to decrease its associated risk factors and aggressively treating infections may influence overall patient outcome.

MEASUREMENT TOOLS

From routine patient care to sophisticated clinical research settings, the importance of being able to describe precisely, classify objectively, and reliably measure the severity of mucosal damage cannot be overestimated. The mucositis scoring system should be objective, validated, and reproducible.[7] Use of valid and reliable instruments is necessary to measure specific changes in the oral cavity so that the effectiveness of interventions can be clearly articulated. In addition, use of tools that are not valid and reliable limits the ability to compare outcomes between interventions.[17]

Numerous members of the healthcare team can conduct oral assessments. Oral assessment needs to be preceded by thorough training, requires attention to detail, and must be performed consistently.[17]

Timing of assessment is important. The performance of oral hygiene before an oral assessment and the quality of that oral care may influence the findings. Timing of interventions for pain will influence reports of pain intensity, which if included in the oral assessment, will affect the results. If assessment is too infrequent, it may not identify important changes as mucositis develops and resolves. If done too frequently, it may result in excessive patient burden and data.[17]

Appropriate lighting is critical to adequately view all areas of the oral cavity. Halogen light sources are the standard in research studies. Halogen light sources are preferred because they provide consistent intensity and color. Individuals performing regular assessment can use an otoscope or a flashlight. Keep in mind, a flashlight can vary in intensity and may distort the color of the oral tissues.[7,17] A tongue blade, dental mirror, and gauze provide assistance in visualization. The gauze can be wrapped around the tongue to allow retraction from side to side. Mucosal pain or a sensitive gag reflex may limit visualization.[17]

Choosing which oral assessment guide to use can be complicated. Since the 1970s more then 10 mucositis scales have been developed, all of which have been validated in research studies.[7] Most assessment guides do not assess for level of pain or infection. A thorough assessment must account for these two factors. Eiler's scale (Table 32-3) is a global scale that can reflect clinical status and outcome. This scale is suitable for nursing care decision making.[7]

Selection of the correct measurement instrument is essential for research and routine use. The knowledge, skills, and abilities required to perform assessment must be considered when choosing the assessment guide. Most important, the primary goal of oral assessment is to assist in developing comprehensive oral care protocols to improve the patient's functional status, control pain, promote nutrition, identify the presence of infection, and assess progress of oral changes.[18]

TREATMENT RECOMMENDATIONS

Patients experiencing mucositis deal with discomfort and pain and are at risk for infection, weight loss, malnutrition, and cancer treatment interruptions or delays. Even though we are unable to prevent mucositis, nursing goals revolve around patient comfort, prevention of infection, and maintaining nutrition.

Shih and colleagues[19] reviewed more then 50 published papers aimed at reduction of radiation-induced mucositis. The most often studied recommendations included the use of antimicrobials, coating agents, antiinflammatory agents, and the use of cytokinine granulocyte-macrophage colony-stimulating factor. These four recommendations are reviewed here using evidence-based criteria.

Antimicrobial agents include hydrogen peroxide, antibiotic lozenges, benzydamine, and chlorhexidine.[19,20] Hydrogen peroxide is no longer a valued recommendation for treatment of mucositis. Peroxide has an antibacterial effect and is effective in cleaning and debriding the mouth. Contraindications for peroxide mouthwashes include the unpleasant taste, exacerbation of dryness, and the

Table 32-3 Oral Assessment Guide

Category	Type of assessment	Methods of measurement	Numerical and descriptive ratings		
			1	2	3
Voice	Listening	Converse with patient	Normal	Deeper or raspy	Difficulty or pain with talking
Swallowing	Observation	Ask patient to swallow To test gag reflex, gently place tongue blade on back of tongue and depress	Normal	Some pain with swallowing	Unable to swallow
Lips	Observation Palpation	Observe and feel tissue	Smooth, pink, and moist	Dry or cracked	Ulcerated or bleeding
Tongue	Observation Palpation	Observe and feel tongue	Pink and moist, with papillae	Coated, loss of papillae, or a shiny appearance with or without redness	Blistered or cracked
Saliva	Observation	Insert tongue blade into mouth touching center of the tongue and floor of the mouth	Watery	Thick or ropey	Absent
Mucous membranes	Observation	Observe appearance of tissue	Pink and moist	Red or coated (whiteness without ulceration)	Ulceration
Gingiva	Observation	Gently press tissue with tip of tongue blade	Pink, stippled, and firm	Edematous with or without redness	Spontaneous bleeding or bleeding with pressure
Teeth, dentures, or denture-bearing areas	Observation	Observe appearance of teeth, dentures, and denture-bearing area	Clean, with no debris	Plaque or debris in localized areas, such as between teeth	Plaque or debris generalized along gum line or denture-bearing area

From June Eilers, PhD, APRN, BC; The Nebraska Medical Center, Omaha, Nebr.

possibility of the patient experiencing burns, stinging, pain, and nausea. Peroxide use will disrupt the normal flora of the mouth and predispose the patient to fungal superinfections.[21]

The use of antibiotic lozenges was reviewed in three different articles. Kostler and colleagues[8] reviewed three studies in which lozenges were used with radiation patients. These three studies were published in the 1990s.[22-24] The lozenges in all three studies contained polymyxin, tobramycin, and amphotericin. Their conclusion stated that the use of antibiotic lozenges reduced the incidence or discomfort of mucositis.[8] Two of the three antibiotic lozenge studies were again reviewed by Shih and colleagues[19] and Kwong.[12] They agree that the research by Symonds[23] demonstrated an improvement in reduction of severity of mucositis. In reviewing, the research by Okuno,[24] Shih and colleagues,[19] and Kwong[12] agrees that the lozenges showed no objective difference.

Benzydamine hydrochloride is a nonsteroidal drug that has shown topical antiinflammatory, analgesic, anesthetic, and antimicrobial activities. Benzydamine inhibits the chemical mediators of inflammation, including prostaglandins, serotonin, histamine, and acetylcholine. The mechanism of action is believed to be the stabilization of cellular and intracellular membranes through inhibition of platelet aggregation and degranulation of leukocytes.[19,25]

Epstein and colleagues[25] published data on a multicentered, randomized, double-blind, placebo-controlled trial that compared the effect of benzydamine 0.15% with a placebo mouthwash in regard to mucositis severity, mouth pain, weight loss, use of analgesic, and enteral nutrition support in 172 patients with head and neck irradiation. In this study, the benzydamine group experienced significant reduction of erythema and ulceration and the use of systemic analgesic during conventional irradiation as compared with the control group. Kostler and colleagues[8] reviewed three additional studies comparing benzydamine with placebo, and all three studies demonstrated a reduction in mucositis symptoms.

Chlorhexidine is a bisbiguanide that is used to control plaque-dependent oral disease and is effective against gram-positive and gram-negative bacteria, as well as yeast and fungal organisms.[19] Kostler and colleagues[8] reviewed three studies and Shih and colleagues[19] reviewed two of the same studies in patients using chlorhexidine versus placebo. Both reviews concluded that there was no significant difference in the chlorhexidine group.

Coating agents have cytoprotective functions that facilitate mucosal healing and cell regeneration. The most common coating agent is sucralfate suspension.[19] Sucralfate is a sucrose aluminum hydroxide compound that forms a gel-like webbing over tissues, serving as a type of bandage, acting through a topical protectant effect. Sucralfate must be used 4 times a day (swish and swallow) in order to provide a continuous protective layer.[26]

Shih and colleagues[19] reviewed eight double-blind, randomized trials that have investigated the efficacy of sucralfate rinse in reducing radiation-induced mucositis. These studies were published between 1991 and 1999. Seven studies demonstrated that no significant differences in the severity of mucositis oral pain or other associated symptoms existed when sucralfate was compared with placebo. Kostler and colleagues[8] also reviewed eight studies comparing sucralfate in radiation patients. The studies they reviewed were published from 1988 through 2000. They concluded that sucralfate seems to have little—if any—benefit when compared with standard oral hygiene and symptomatic treatment of oral mucositis.

Dodd and colleagues[27] published a study in 2003 that compared sucralfate versus salt and baking soda mouthwashes. There was no significant difference found between the time of onset, rating of pain, or the time to healing. In their conclusion, they stated that because there is no significant difference between the two mouthwashes, use of the less costly salt and baking soda is prudent and cost effective.

The theory behind antiinflammatory rinsing agents is based on the hypothesis that these agents could decrease the inflammatory process, minimize microbial infection, or protect the oral mucosa from radiation damage. Shih and colleagues[19] reviewed four studies, published from 1990 through 1998, that used various antiinflammatory agents. The four agents studied included: hydrocortisone, kamillosan liquidum oral rinse, prostaglandin E1, and corticosteroid. The conclusion was that although the use of antiinflammatory agents to reduce the severity of mucositis makes sense from a theoretical perspective, none of the studies conducted to date, using these agents, produced significant results.

Granulocyte-macrophage colony-stimulating factor (GM-CSF) in a mouth rinse or given subcutaneously enhances the proliferation of endothelial cells and keratinocytes in the basal epithelium.[28] Several studies have been published that investigated the efficacy of cytokine-like agents in managing mucositis.

Shih and colleagues[19] reviewed three studies of patients receiving radiation and daily subcutaneous injections of GM-CSF. Most of the patients in the three studies completed treatment with only grade 1 or grade 2 mucositis and were able to tolerate oral intake. Unfortunately, for some patients, the side effects of the GM-CSF resulted in patients dropping out of the study. Side effects included local skin reaction, fever, bone pain, and nausea.

The use of granulocyte-macrophage colony-stimulating factor in mouthwash was reviewed in two studies by Shih and colleagues.[19] The patients using the GM-CSF mouthwash had less severe mucositis and used less pain medication. GM-CSF mouthwash is expensive; this may be an issue when recommending it to patients.

Box 32-1 Management of Patients Who May Develop Mucositis From Radiation Therapy

1. Schedule dental evaluation for optimal care of existing teeth or necessary dental extractions before treatment begins.
2. Avoid irritants such as hot, spicy, and course foods; citrus; smoking tobacco; and chewing tobacco.
3. Avoid drinking alcoholic beverages and using mouthwashes that include alcohol.
4. Because mechanical cleansing with a toothbrush may cause microtraumas, which may promote infection, foam brushes and rinsing solutions are recommended.
5. A safe, cost-effective rinsing solution is saline. Combine ½ tsp salt in 1 cup of warm water. Mouth should be rinsed after every meal, or at least every 4 hours.
6. Oral prosthetic devices can increase irritation to the mucosa. Use prosthetic device only when necessary.
7. Maintain hydration. Encourage fluid intake of greater than 3 L/day.
8. Maintain a diet high in calories and protein. Nutrition supplemental drinks are encouraged.
9. Administration of pilocarpine, artificial saliva, or amifostine may improve xerostomia and its long-term effects on the oral mucosa.

Data from Kostler W, Hejna M, Wenzel C, et al: *CA Cancer J Clin* 51(5):290-315, 2001; Berendt M, Agostino S: Alteration in nutrition. In Itano J, Taoka K, editors: *Core curriculum for oncology nursing*, St Louis, 2005; Mosby; Shih A, Miaskowski C, Dodd M, et al: *Oncol Nurs Forum* 29(7):1063-1080, 2002; Witt ME: Head and neck site-specific management. In Watkins-Bruner D, Haas M, Gosselin-Acomb TK, editors: *Manual for radiation oncology nursing practice and education*, Pittsburgh, 2005, Oncology Nursing Society; Velez I, Tamara L, Mintz S: *Quintessence Int* 35(2):129-136, 2004; Dodd M, Miaskowski C, Greenspan D, et al: *Cancer Invest* 21(1):21-33, 2003.

The number of products and approaches for treating mucositis is endless. The review of evidence-based practice points in the direction that patients may benefit from the use of benzydamine mouthwash or the cytokinine-like products. The studies on the cytokines are still small and need further investigation. Whether the management team chooses to use a specific product or normal saline or baking soda mouth rinses, some general guidelines should be followed for every patient to enhance comfort and prevent complications (Boxes 32-1 and 32-2).

Box 32-2 Interventions for Mouth and Throat Tenderness

1. Follow recommendations in Box 32-1.
2. Perform daily oral assessment. Evaluate for possible infection. Bacterial, fungal, and viral infections should be treated with appropriate medication.
3. Assess weight biweekly and hydration daily. Feeding tube may be necessary if aspiration, hydration, or rapid weight loss is a concern.
4. Assess pain on a daily basis. When lesions are confined to a limited area, topical anesthetic is recommended. Systemic pain medication should be considered when topical anesthetic is ineffective.

Data from Berendt M, Agostino S: Alteration in nutrition. In Itano J, Taoka K, editors: *Core curriculum for oncology nursing*, St Louis, 2005, Mosby; Shih A, Miaskowski C, Dodd M, et al: *Oncol Nurs Forum* 29(7):1063-1080, 2002; Witt ME: Head and neck site-specific management. In Watkins-Bruner D, Haas M, Gosselin-Acomb TK, editors: *Manual for radiation oncology nursing practice and education*, Pittsburgh, 2005, Oncology Nursing Society.

PAIN MANAGEMENT

Mucositis pain impairs adequate nutritional and liquid intake, affects the quality of life, and may result in serious clinical complications.[29] Oral mucositis pain results from injury to tissues that affects and activates nociceptive receptors at the site of injury. The associated pain has a limited duration and the pain resolves when underlying tissue damage heals. When pain is present, pain management must be individualized and the goals communicated to the patient, caregivers, and staff.[30]

Patients should be instructed on basic oral care and minimizing mucosal damage. The goal of basic oral care is to maintain oral health, prevent tissue damage, reduce tissue irritation, maintain tissue stability, maintain hydration and nutrition, and promote comfort. Meticulous oral care will also reduce bacterial dental plaque levels, which will decrease gingival inflammation and oral microbal colonization.[30]

When mucositis pain is present, assessment of the oral cavity and a formal pain assessment should be performed at least daily. Documentation should include an assessment of pain intensity, changes in the grading of mucositis, assessment for infection, changes in nutrition and hydration, response to pain management, and patient's compliance with oral care regimen. Assessment and documentation is the only valid way to evaluate the patient's response to the suggested management.

Many products have been presented in both the prevention and treatment sections of this chapter. This section on topical and systemic pain management addresses only pain medications.

The oral mucosa is easily accessible for topical application of medication that may produce local effects with little risk of systemic effects. Topical anesthetics have been used over the years for managing mucositis pain, but there have been very few controlled clinical trials to determine the effectiveness of these. One commonly used agent, topical lidocaine, may sting with initial application, but is followed by anesthesia lasting 15 to 30 minutes. Lidocaine also will anesthetize the taste receptors and when the posterior oropharyngeal area is anesthetized, the gag reflex can be suppressed.[30]

Cerchietti and colleagues[29] published a study that compared topical morphine solution and a mouthwash that combined lidocaine, diphenhydramine, and magnesium aluminum hydroxide for patients receiving chemoradiotherapy for head and neck cancer. The morphine group used an oral rinse of 2% morphine solution, every 3 hours, 6 times a day. The duration of severe pain and intensity of pain was significantly lower in the morphine group. The study also concluded that the anesthetic cocktail relieved oral pain, but the relief was short-lived, initiated or intensified oral discomfort (viscous saliva, dry mouth), and prevented taste perception, which can all interfere with food intake. The study had only 26 patients, thus more research would be needed to validate this recommendation.

Systemic pain management for mucositis should be governed by prevailing clinical practice guidelines, such as those promulgated by the World Health Organization (WHO). One of the central recommendations of the WHO Pain Management Ladder is that pain medication of appropriate potency needs to be administered on a time-contingent basis rather than delaying doses until the patient experiences increasing pain. Medication on the first step of the ladder includes nonopioid analgesics. Nonsteroidal antiinflammatory drugs (NSAIDs) should be used with caution in patents with thrombocytopenia or when concerned that a fever may be suppressed and thus mask an infection. When the first step fails to provide adequate pain relief, the patient is escalated to the second step of the ladder, which recommends the administration of mild or weak opioid analgesics. Finally, when the second step fails to adequately control pain, the patient is moved to the third step of the ladder, which uses potent opioid analgesics. Depending on the individual patient population, numerous routes may be considered including oral (often liquid and not pill form), rectal, transdermal, and various intravenous or subcutaneous approaches.[19,30-32]

A variety of complementary strategies for managing pain are available. Research published on complementary studies focused on pain and nausea, but few actually focused on oral mucositis pain. Syrjala and colleagues[33] concluded that relaxation and imagery were shown to be useful in oral mucositis pain.[33] Patients can be offered hypnosis, counseling, distraction, and acupuncture.

At this time, there is little evidence-based practice to support that these techniques specifically aid in the relief of pain associated with oral mucositis. An inexpensive and easily available suggestion for pain relief also may include offering patients ice chips for their mouth.[30]

NOVEL THERAPIES

Mucositis management had been typically empirically based because of limited data relative to the pathobiology of the lesion. Advances in the 1990s have reformed this approach. Thus investigators have been able to design clinical trials that are now based on selected mechanism of mucosal injury and repair.[34] Newer approaches for treatment, based on evidence-based practice are discussed below.

Amifostine is an antioxidant delivered either subcutaneously or intravenously.[34] It is a radioprotectant able to enhance the tolerance of normal tissues to a given dose of radiation. Its cytoprotective mechanism involves DNA protection, repair acceleration, and antioxidant function.[35]

Most of the research with amifostine has been conducted in patients with head and neck cancer. Such reports support its benefit with xerostomia, but do not conclusively indicate a clear benefit to using amifostine to decrease the incidence or severity of mucositis. Brizel and colleagues[36] reported a xerostomia benefit for patients, but amifostine did not diminish the severity of acute mucositis. Suntharalingam and colleagues[37] reported an evaluation of 17 head and neck patients receiving amifostine. No patients experienced grade IV mucositis, but 40% experienced grade III. Kostler and colleagues[8] reported on three additional studies using amifostine. They concluded that there was a reduction in the incidence and severity of mucositis, but there were inconsistencies regarding the tolerability of the drug. Side effects include nausea, headaches, and hypotension, but these side effects are more common when amifostine is delivered intravenously.[34]

Glutamine is a nonessential amino acid and well-known protector of the bowel from radiation-induced mucosal injury.[8] Huang and colleagues[38] reported a randomized trial of 17 patients receiving radiation to their oral cavity. Patients were randomized to glutamine mouthwashes or placebo. The glutamine group demonstrated a significant reduction of the incidence, severity, and duration of oral mucositis. Further studies on this approach are needed.

Gelclair is a concentrated oral gel that contains the barrier-forming ingredients polyvinylpyrrolidone and sodium hyaluronate. When rinsed in the mouth, it forms an adherent barrier over the oral mucosa, shielding the mucosa from over stimulation. It does not contain alcohol or an anesthetic base and does not sting on application. This product is growing in popularity within the radiation oncology community. Support of this product with evidence-based practice is limited. Innocenti and colleagues[39] published preliminary findings from an open pilot study with hospice patients. After 1 week of using Gelclair, 87% of patients reported overall improvement from baseline scores related to pain with swallowing food, liquids, and saliva.[39]

Low-intensity laser therapy may improve wound healing and accelerate the replication of cells. Most studies involved chemotherapy patients.[26] Bensadoun and colleagues[40] reported their study done on radiation-induced mucositis. Thirty patients were randomized to low-energy laser light or placebo light. Laser was capable of reducing the severity and duration of oral mucositis. Patients received laser treatments everyday that they received radiation, and it had to be performed by someone experienced with this technique.[40]

Advances in molecular modeling of oral mucositis have permitted evidence-based design of new clinical trials. Before new agents and approaches are adopted into practice, it is important that research proceed beyond phase II trials to randomized clinical studies in the radiation therapy population.[34]

SUMMARY

The side effect of mucositis has been a patient management issue for over 75 years. Deciding whether to stop treatment with orthovoltage accelerators has historically been based on skin reactions and mucositis. The very first article on mucositis published in the Oncology Nursing Forum, "Patient care evaluation: a comparison of current practice and nursing literature for oral care of persons receiving chemotherapy," was published in Spring, 1982.[41] The role of the nurse has always been to enhance patient comfort when mucositis starts.

As time progressed, the role of the radiation oncology nurse became more sophisticated. The refinement of assessment skills, the application of nursing research, and time spent with patients to teach and reinforce an oral care regimen has improved the patient's quality of life and decreased treatment-related complications. The nurse's role as teacher goes beyond what is done at the bedside. Educating one another and participating in research on mucositis also should be a part of the oncology nurse's role now and in the future.

REFERENCES

1. Avritscher EB, Cooksley CD, Elting LS: Scope and epidemiology of cancer therapy-induced oral and gastrointestinal mucositis, *Semin Oncol Nurs* 20(1):3-10, 2004.
2. Brown C, Wingard J: Clinical consequences of oral mucositis, *Semin Oncol Nurs* 20(1):16-21, 2004.
3. Trotti A, Bellm L, Epstein J et al: Mucositis incidence, severity and associated outcomes in patients with head and neck cancer receiving radiotherapy with or without chemotherapy: a systemic literature review, *Radiother Oncol* 66(3):253-262, 2003.
4. Elting L, Cooksley C, Chambers M et al: The burdens of cancer therapy, *Cancer* 98(7):1531-1539, 2003.
5. Professional Cancer Consultants: Current Topics in Oncology—*Management of oral mucositis: 2004 in review* (website): http://professional.cancerconsultants.com. Accessed on 3/29/05.
6. Sonis S: Pathobiology of mucositis. *Semin Oncol Nurs* 20(1):11-15, 2004.
7. Sonis S, Elting L, Keefe D et al: Perspectives on cancer therapy-induced mucosal injury, *Cancer* 100(9 suppl): 1995-2025, 2004.
8. Kostler W, Hejna M, Wenzel C et al: Oral mucositis complicating chemotherapy and/or radiotherapy: options for prevention and treatment, *CA Cancer J Clin* 51(5):290-315, 2001.
9. Cawley MM, Benson LM: Current trend in managing oral mucositis, *Clin J Oncol Nurs* 9(5):584-592, 2005.

10. Gate L, Paul J, Nguyen-Ba G et al: Oxidative stress induced in pathologies: the role of antioxidants, *Biomed Pharmacother* 53(4)169-180, 1999.
11. McGuire D, Rubenstein E, Peterson D: Evidence-based guidelines for managing mucositis, *Semin Oncol Nurs* 20(1):59-66, 2004.
12. Kwong K: Prevention and treatment of oral mucositis following cancer therapy, *Cancer Nurs* 27(3):183-205, 2004.
13. Clarkson J, Worthington H, Eden O: Interventions for preventing oral mucositis for patients with cancer receiving treatment, *Cochrane Rev*, Issue 4, Article No. CD000978, DOI: 10.1002/14651858.CD000978.pub2, 2006.
14. Maher K: Radiation therapy: toxicities and management. In Yarbo CH, Frogge MH, Goodman M et al, editors: *Cancer nursing: principles and practice*, Sudbury, Mass, 2000, Jones and Bartlett, pp 323-351.
15. Berendt M, Agostino S: Alteration in nutrition. In Itano J, Taoka K, editors: *Core curriculum for oncology nursing*, St Louis, 2005, Mosby, pp 277-317.
16. Soysa N, Samaranayake L, Ellepola A: Cytotoxic drugs, radiotherapy, and oral candidiasis, *Oral Oncol* 40(10), 971-978, 2004.
17. Eilers J, Epstein J: Assessment and measurement of oral mucositis, *Semin Oncol Nurs* 20(1):22-29, 2004.
18. Hyland S: Assessing the oral cavity. In Frank-Stromberg M, Olsen SJ, editors: *Instruments for clinical health-care research*, Boston, 1997, Jones and Bartlett, pp 519-527.
19. Shih A, Miaskowski C, Dodd M et al: A research review of the current treatments for radiation induced oral mucositis in patients with head and neck cancer, *Oncol Nurs Forum* 29(7):1063-1080, 2002.
20. Witt ME: Head and neck site-specific management. In Watkins-Bruner D, Haas M, Gosselin-Acomb TK, editors: *Manual for radiation oncology nursing practice and education*, Pittsburgh, 2005, Oncology Nursing Society, pp 86-97.
21. Miller M, Kearney N: Oral care for patients with cancer: a review of the literature, *Cancer Nurs* 24(4):241-254, 2001.
22. Spijkervet FK, Van Saene HK, Van Saene JJ et al: Effect of selective elimination of the oral flora on mucositis in irradiated head and neck cancer patients, *J Surg Oncol* 46(3):167-173, 1991.
23. Symonds RP, McIlroy P, Khorrami J et al: The reduction of radiation mucositis by selective decontamination antibiotic pastilles: a placebo-controlled double-blind trial, *Br J Cancer* 74(2):312-317, 1996.
24. Okuno SH, Foote RL, Loprinzi CL et al: A randomized trial of non-absorbable antibiotic lozenge given to alleviate radiation-induced mucositis, *Cancer* 79(11):2193-2199, 1997.
25. Epstein J, Silverman S, Paggiarino D et al: Benzydamine HCl for prophylaxis of radiation-induced oral mucositis, *Cancer* 92(4):875-885, 2001.
26. Velez I, Tamara L, Mintz S: Management of oral mucositis induced by chemotherapy and radiotherapy: an update, *Quintessence Int* 35(2):129-136, 2004.
27. Dodd M, Miaskowski C, Greenspan D et al: Radiation induced mucositis: a randomized clinical trial of micronized sucralfate versus salt and soda mouthwashes, *Cancer Invest* 21(1):21-33, 2003.
28. Biron P, Sebban C, Gourmet R et al: Research controversies in management of oral mucositis, *Support Care Cancer* 8(1):68-71, 2000.
29. Cerchietti L, Navigante A, Bonomi M et al: Effect of topical morphine for mucositis-associated pain following concomitant chemoradiotherapy for head and neck carcinoma, *Cancer* 95(10):2230-2236, 2002.
30. Epstein J, Schubert M: Managing pain in mucositis, *Semin Oncol Nurs* 20(1):30-37, 2004.
31. Meuser T, Pietruk C, Radbruch L et al: Symptoms during cancer pain treatment following WHO guidelines: a longitudinal follow-up study of symptom prevalence, severity and etiology, *Pain* 93(3):247-257, 2001.
32. Haas M, Kuehn E: Head and neck cancers. In Watkins-Bruner D, Moore-Higgs G, Haas M, editors: *Outcomes in radiation therapy*, Boston, 2001, Jones and Bartlett, pp 195-213.
33. Syrjala K, Donaldson G, Davis M et al: Relaxation and imagery and cognitive behavior training can reduce pain during cancer treatment: a controlled clinical trial, *Pain* 63(2):189-198, 1995.
34. Peterson D, Beck S, Keefe D: Novel therapies, *Semin Oncol Nurs* 20(1):53-58, 2004.
35. Koukourakis M: Amifostine in clinical oncology: current and future use, *Anticancer Drugs* 13(3):181-209, 2002.
36. Brizel D, Wasserman T, Henke M et al: Phase III randomized trial of amifostine as a radioprotector in head and neck cancer, *J Clin Oncol* 18(19):3339-3345, 2000.
37. Suntharalingam M, Jaboin J, Taylor R et al: The evaluation of amifostine for mucosal protection in patients with advanced loco-regional squamous cell carcinoma of the head and neck (SCCHN) treated with concurrent weekly carboplatin, paclitaxel, and daily radiotherapy (RT), *Semin Oncol* 31(6 Suppl 18):2-7, 2004.
38. Huang EY, Leung SW, Wang CJ et al: Oral glutamine to alleviate radiation induced oral mucositis: a pilot randomized trial, *Int J Radiat Oncol Biol Phys* 46(3):535-539, 2000.
39. Innocenti M, Moscatelli G, Lopez S: Efficacy of Gelclair™ in reducing pain in palliative care patient with oral lesions, *J Pain Sympt Manage* 24(5):456-457, 2002.
40. Bensadoun RJ, Franquin JC, Ciais G et al: Low-energy He/Ne laser in the prevention of radiation-induced mucositis, *Support Care Cancer* 7(4):244-252, 1999.
41. Hart CN, Rasmussen D: Patient care evaluation: a comparison of current practice and nursing literature for oral care of persons receiving chemotherapy, *Oncol Nurs Forum* 9(2):22-27, 1982.

Chapter 33 Nutrition Through the Continuum of Cancer Care

Sandra L. Luthringer

Nutrition plays a role in all phases of cancer, from prevention to treatment and end-of-life issues. The relationship between nutrition and cancer has been recognized for years. Scientific interest in nutrition and cancer began about 35 years ago when the National Cancer Act of 1971 required that the National Cancer Institute (NCI) investigate the relationship between nutrition and cancer. Since that time, many reports have been issued, and the relationships between diet and cancer have been confirmed.[1] Today, the American Cancer Society (ACS) estimates that about one-third of cancer deaths in the United States each year are the result of nutrition and physical activity factors, including obesity.[2] The landmark 1997 report, *Food, Nutrition and the Prevention of Cancer: a Global Perspective*, published by the American Institute and the World Cancer Research Fund, documented that good nutrition is vital in cancer prevention strategies and estimated that 30% to 40% of cancers are directly linked to diets and related factors, such as maintaining a healthy weight and staying physically active.[1] Researchers continue to seek the answers to many of the questions still remaining regarding the impact that nutritional support has on cancer prevention and cancer treatments and survivorship.

SCREENING AND ASSESSMENT

Nutritional screening is the process of identifying risk factors known to be associated with specific nutritional problems. Its main purpose is to identify those individuals who are likely to be at the most nutritional risk. The nutritional status of a patient can play an important role in determining not only the risk of developing cancer but also the risk of therapy-related toxicities and medical outcomes.[3] Whether the goal of cancer treatment is curative or palliative, early detection of nutritional problems and prompt intervention are essential. Preventing or correcting nutritional deficiencies can minimize malnutrition-related morbidity and improve quality of life. Nutrition screening and assessment should be interdisciplinary and include all members of the healthcare team. Physicians, nurses, dietitians, social workers, therapists, and other support staff should all be involved in the management of patients' nutrition throughout their course of care. Nutrition assessment has three goals[4]:

- To identify patients who have, or are at risk of developing, protein/energy malnutrition or deficiencies of specific nutrients
- To quantify a patient's risk of developing malnutrition-related medical complications
- To monitor the adequacy of nutritional therapy

Screening and Assessment Tools

A number of screening and assessment tools are currently available to assist healthcare members in identifying high-risk patients. For a tool to be effective it must be easy to use, cost-effective, validated for use with the targeted patient population, reliable, sensitive, specific, and include an action plan for intervention.[5] Examples of some nutrition assessment tools include the Mini Nutritional Assessment (MNA), Subjective Global Assessment (SGA), the Prognostic Nutrition Index (PNI), anthropometric analysis tools such as the Bioelectrical Impedance Analysis (BIA) and body mass index (BMI), and various institution-specific guidelines. Unfortunately, none of these tools contains all of the necessary characteristics as described above. Many do not take into consideration specific cancer symptoms that have an impact on nutritional status. Most are not validated for use in the oncology population, and some involve costly laboratory studies.[6] Another tool, the scored Patient-Generated Subjective Global Assessment

(PG-SGA) is an easy-to-use and inexpensive approach for identifying individuals at nutritional risk; it has been validated in the oncology setting. The tool can be used to triage patients to a dietitian for more extensive medical nutrition therapy. This assessment tool, developed by Faith Ottery, MD, PhD, includes tables and worksheets and allows for part of the assessment to be patient or family driven. Questions concerning weight changes, appetite and food intake, activity, and specific nutrition impact symptoms are completed by the patient or family. A member of the healthcare team such as a nurse, physician assistant, or registered dietitian then completes the assessment with an analysis of the diagnosis, metabolic demand of the patient, and a physical exam to determine nutritional status. Many studies have demonstrated its usefulness in all oncology settings, including hospitals, outpatient clinics, home care, and hospice settings to provide a global assessment of the patient's nutritional status and identify nutrition impact symptoms that can adversely affect quality of life.[3,7,8] Nutritional problems are commonly addressed reactively rather than proactively, which has led to patients being offered interventions only when they are moderately to severely malnourished.[9,10] The PG-SGA can provide the healthcare team with a tool to identify nutritional concerns early in the diagnostic phase and to support the patients throughout the course of treatment (Figures 33-1 and 33-2).

NUTRITIONAL CHALLENGES FOR PATIENTS DURING TREATMENT

Nutrition Impact Symptoms

Nutritional support during radiation therapy is vital, and intervention is based on managing the symptoms that occur during and after treatment. The side effects of radiation therapy are specific to the area irradiated, total dose, duration, and whether the radiation is given in combination with another form of treatment, such as chemotherapy. The effect of radiation therapy on healthy tissue within the treatment field can produce many nutrition-related symptoms that may interfere with food ingestion, digestion, or absorption. Some of these side effects can be acute, developing around the second or third week of treatment and resolving within several weeks after the completion of therapy. Others, however, can be chronic and continue or even occur after treatment has been completed, such as taste and saliva changes resulting from head and neck radiation or radiation enteritis from treatment to the pelvis. Individuals receiving radiation therapy to any part of the gastrointestinal (GI) tract are more susceptible to nutrition-related side effects, with patients whose cancers involve the head and neck, lung, esophagus, pelvis, colorectal area, or pancreas being at the highest risk.[11] These nutrition impact symptoms, the symptoms that impede oral intake, are listed in Table 33-1.[11-16]

As mentioned previously, optimal nutrition can improve the clinical course, outcome, or quality of life of patients undergoing treatment for cancer. Dietary modifications based on nutrition impact symptoms continue to be appropriate standards of care for patients receiving radiation therapy. Table 33-2 offers a summary of suggested dietary modifications to help overcome the variety of symptoms that are typical to many cancer patients receiving radiation therapy.[11-16]

Cancer-Induced Weight Loss

Although many of these nutrition impact symptoms can be lessened by dietary modifications, treatment for the anorexia-cachexia syndrome is not so straightforward. Cancer cachexia is a common problem in cancer patients; it impinges on patient quality of life and impacts morbidity and mortality. Whereas anorexia is defined only as the loss of desire to eat, cachexia is more complex and multifactorial. The syndrome is characterized by progressive wasting of skeletal muscle mass and adipose tissue, immune dysfunction, and alterations in metabolic function. Although anorexia commonly accompanies the cachexia syndrome, the degree of weight loss cannot completely be attributed to the reduced food intake, and muscle wasting is often observed in patients with a normal intake of food. In recent years, much research has been published to identify the pathogenesis of this cancer-induced weight loss, and specific cytokines and tumor-derived factors have been identified.[17] With this research now comes advances in treatment options for patients. A team approach using both nutritional counseling and pharmacologic approaches should be considered.[18]

Supplementing the Diet

Many patients are not able to obtain the calories and protein necessary to prevent weight loss and muscle

(Text continued on p. 581.)

Scored Patient-Generated Subjective Global Assessment (PG-SGA)

Patient ID information

History (Boxes 1-4 are designed to be completed by the patient.)

1. Weight *(See Worksheet 1)*

In summary of my current and recent weight:

I currently weigh about ________ pounds
I am about ________ feet ________ tall

One month ago I weighed about ________ pounds
Six months ago I weighed about ________ pounds

During the past two weeks my weight has:
☐ decreased(1) ☐ not changed(0) ☐ increased(0)

Box 1 ☐

2. Food Intake: As compared to my normal intake, I would rate my food intake during the past month as:
☐ unchanged(0)
☐ more than usual(0)
☐ less than usual(1)
☐ I am now taking:
- ☐ *normal food* but less than normal amount(1)
- ☐ little solid food(2)
- ☐ only liquids(3)
- ☐ only nutritional supplements(3)
- ☐ very little of anything(4)
- ☐ only tube feedings or only nutrition by vein(0)

Box 2 ☐

3. Symptoms: I have had the following problems that have kept me from eating enough during the past two weeks (check all that apply):
☐ no problems eating(0)
☐ no appetite, just did not feel like eating(3)
☐ nausea(1) ☐ vomiting(3)
☐ constipation(1) ☐ diarrhea(3)
☐ mouth sores(2) ☐ dry mouth(1)
☐ things taste funny or have no taste(1) ☐ smells bother me(1)
☐ feel full quickly(1)
☐ problems swallowing(2) ☐ fatigue(1)
☐ pain; where?(3) ____________
☐ other**(1) ____________________

**Examples: depression, money, or dental problems

Box 3 ☐

4. Activities and Function: Over the past month, I would generally rate my activity as:
☐ normal with no limitations(0)
☐ not my normal self, but able to be up and about with fairly normal activities(1)
☐ not feeling up to most things, but in bed or chair less than half the day(2)
☐ able to do little activity and spend most of the day in bed or chair(3)
☐ pretty much bedridden, rarely out of bed(3)

Box 4 ☐

Additive Score of the Boxes 1-4 ☐ **A**

The remainder of this form will be completed by your doctor, nurse, or therapist. Thank you.

5. Disease and its relation to nutritional requirements *(See Worksheet 2)*
All relevant diagnoses (specify) ____________________
Primary disease stage (circle if known or appropriate) I II III IV Other ____________
Age ________

Numerical score from Worksheet 2 ☐ **B**

6. **Metabolic Demand** *(See Worksheet 3)*

Numerical score from Worksheet 3 ☐ **C**

7. **Physical** *(See Worksheet 4)*

Numerical score from Worksheet 4 ☐ **D**

Global Assessment *(See Worksheet 5)*
☐ Well-nourished or anabolic (SGA-A)
☐ Moderate or suspected malnutrition (SGA-B)
☐ Severely malnourished (SGA-C)

Total PG-SGA score
(Total numerical score of A+B+C+D above) ☐
(See triage recommendations below)

Clinician Signature ____________________ RD RN PA MD DO Other ________ Date ____________

Nutritional Triage Recommendations: Additive score is used to define specific nutritional interventions including patient & family education, symptom management including pharmacologic intervention, and appropriate nutrient intervention (food, nutritional supplements, enteral, or parenteral triage). First line nutrition intervention includes optimal symptom management.

0-1 No intervention required at this time. Re-assessment on routine and regular basis during treatment.
2-3 Patient & family education by dietitian, nurse, or other clinician with pharmacologic intervention as indicated by symptom survey (Box 3) and laboratory values as appropriate.
4-8 Requires intervention by dietitian, in conjunction with nurse or physician as indicated by symptoms survey (Box 3).
≥9 Indicates a critical need for improved symptom management and/or nutrient intervention options.

Figure 33-1 Scored Patient-Generated Subjective Global Assessment (PG-SGA).

Worksheets for PG-SGA Scoring

Boxes 1-4 of the PG-SGA are designed to be completed by the patient. The PG-SGA numerical score is determined using 1) the parenthetical points noted in boxes 1-4 and 2) the worksheets below for items not marked with parenthetical points. Scores for boxes 1 and 3 are additive within each box and scores for boxes 2 and 4 are based on the highest scored item checked off by the patient.

Worksheet 1 – Scoring Weight (Wt) Loss

To determine score, use 1 month weight data if available. Use 6 month data only if there is no 1 month weight data. Use points below to score weight change and add one extra point if patient has lost weight during the past 2 weeks. Enter total point score in Box 1 of the PG-SGA.

Wt loss in 1 month	Points	Wt loss in 6 months
10% or greater	4	20% or greater
5-9.9%	3	10-19.9%
3-4.9%	2	6-9.9%
2-2.9%	1	2-5.9%
0-1.9%	0	0-1.9%

Score for Worksheet 1 ☐
Record in Box 1

Worksheet 2 – Scoring Criteria for Condition

Score is derived by adding 1 point for each of the conditions listed below that pertain to the patient.

Category	Points
Cancer	1
AIDS	1
Pulmonary or cardiac cachexia	1
Presence of decubitus, open wound, or fistula	1
Presence of trauma	1
Age greater than 65 years	1

Score for Worksheet 2 = ☐
Record in Box B

Worksheet 3 – Scoring Metabolic Stress

Score for metabolic stress is determined by a number of variables known to increase protein & calorie needs. The score is additive so that a patient who has a fever of >102 degrees (3 points) and is on 10 mg of prednisone chronically (2 points) would have an additive score for this section of 5 points.

Stress	none (0)	low (1)	moderate (2)	high (3)
Fever	no fever	>99 and <101	≥101 and <102	≥102
Fever duration	no fever	<72 hrs	72 hrs	>72 hrs
Corticosteroids	no corticosteroids	low dose (<10mg prednisone equivalents/day)	moderate dose (≥10 and <30mg prednisone equivalents/day)	high dose steroids (≥30mg prednisone equivalents/day)

Score for Worksheet 3 = ☐
Record in Box C

Worksheet 4 – Physical Examination

Physical exam includes a subjective evaluation of 3 aspects of body composition: fat, muscle, & fluid status. Since this is subjective, each aspect of the exam is rated for degree of deficit. Muscle deficit impacts point score more than fat deficit. Definition of categories: 0=no deficit, 1+=mild deficit, 2+=moderate deficit, 3+=severe deficit. Rating of deficit in these categories are *not* additive but are used to clinically assess the degree of deficit (or presence of excess fluid).

Fat Stores:				
orbital fat pads	0	1+	2+	3+
triceps skin fold	0	1+	2+	3+
fat overlying lower ribs	0	1+	2+	3+
Global fat deficit rating	**0**	**1+**	**2+**	**3+**
Muscle Status:				
temples (temporalis muscle)	0	1+	2+	3+
clavicles (pectoralis & deltoids)	0	1+	2+	3+
shoulders (deltoids)	0	1+	2+	3+
interosseous muscles	0	1+	2+	3+
scapula (latissimus dorsi, trapezius, deltoids)	0	1+	2+	3+
thigh (quadriceps)	0	1+	2+	3+
calf (gastrocnemius)	0	1+	2+	3+
Global muscle status rating	**0**	**1+**	**2+**	**3+**

Fluid Status:				
ankle edema	0	1+	2+	3+
sacral edema	0	1+	2+	3+
ascites	0	1+	2+	3+
Global fluid status rating	**0**	**1+**	**2+**	**3+**

Point score for the physical exam is determined by the overall subjective rating of total body deficit.

No deficit	score = 0 points
Mild deficit	score = 1 point
Moderate deficit	score = 2 points
Severe deficit	score = 3 points

Score for Worksheet 4 = ☐
Record in Box D

Worksheet 5 – PG-SGA Global Assessment Categories

	Stage A	Stage B	Stage C
Category	Well-nourished	Moderately malnourished or suspected malnutrition	Severely malnourished
Weight	No wt loss **OR** Recent non-fluid wt gain	~5% wt loss within 1 month (or 10% in 6 months) **OR** No wt stabilization or wt gain (i.e., continued wt loss)	>5% wt loss in 1 month (or >10% in 6 months) **OR** No wt stabilization or wt gain (i.e., continued wt loss)
Nutrient intake	No deficit **OR** Significant recent improvement	Definite decrease in intake	Severe deficit in intake
Nutrition impact symptoms	None **OR** Significant recent improvement allowing adequate intake	Presence of nutrition impact symptoms (Box 3 of PG-SGA)	Presence of nutrition impact symptoms (Box 3 of PG-SGA)
Functioning	No deficit **OR** Significant recent improvement	Moderate functional deficit **OR** Recent deterioration	Severe functional deficit **OR** Recent significant deterioration
Physical exam	No deficit **OR** Chronic deficit but with recent clinical improvement	Evidence of mild to moderate loss of SQ fat &/or muscle mass &/or muscle tone on palpation	Obvious signs of malnutrition (e.g., severe loss of SQ tissues, possible edema)

Global PG-SGA rating (A, B, or C) = ☐

Figure 33-2 Worksheets for Patient-Generated Subjective Global Assessment (PG-SGA) Scoring.

Table 33-1 Nutritional Effects of Radiation Therapy

Site	Acute side effects	Chronic side effects	Interventions
ABDOMINAL REGION			
Stomach, liver, pancreas, bile duct, small intestine	Nausea, vomiting	Gastrointestinal ulceration, perforation	Antiemetic medications before radiation therapy and meals; small frequent meals; avoid foods with strong odor; liquids between meals; low fat diet
	Enteritis, malabsorption	Intestinal fistula, fibrosis, necrosis, obstruction	Pancreatic enzymes; low-fat, low-residue, low-lactose diet; tube feeding with elemental formula or TPN if high output from fistula
HEAD AND NECK REGION			
Tongue, soft and hard palate, tonsils, pharynx, nasopharynx mandible	Mucositis	Oropharyngeal ulcers	Oral anesthetics; good oral care; avoid temperature extremes; avoid irritants
	Xerostomia	Xerostomia	Moist foods; artificial saliva; extra fluids with meals
	Dysgeusia	Dysgeusia	Determine specific aberrations—emphasize use of acceptable seasonings and flavors; tart foods may help
	Dental caries	Dental caries	Good oral care; topical fluoride; avoid sticky, sugary foods
	Viscous saliva		Pureed or liquid diet; limit milk products; avoid oily, greasy, or dry foods; increase fluid intake
		Osteoradionecrosis	Pureed/liquid diet if able to tolerate—TPN/ tube feedings
		Fistula	Depending on location may need tube feeding until healed or surgery
		Trismus	Depends on severity—liquids may be tolerated; may need tube feeding
MEDIASTINAL REGION			
Esophagus, thorax, thyroid, thoracic, cervical spine	Esophagitis, dysphagia	Esophagitis, esophageal stricture, fibrosis	Adjust texture of foods; avoid irritants; adjust liquids as needed for dysphagia; dilation for stricture; tube feeding for dysphagia
PELVIC REGION			
Bladder, prostate, colon, rectum, male and female sexual organs	Colitis, cystitis, diarrhea	Chronic colitis, proctitis	Low-residue, low-lactose diet; avoid irritants; antidiarrheal medications; increase soluble fiber
		Radiation enteritis	Low-residue, lactose-reduced, low-fat diet; bowel rest with elemental formula or TPN; glutamine supplement

Data from Luthringer SL: Nutrition concerns with the radiation therapy patient. In Molseed L, McCallum PD, Elliott L, editors: *The clinical guide to oncology nutrition*, ed 2, Chicago, Ill, 2005, The American Dietetic Association; Eldridge B, Hamilton KK: *Management of nutrition impact symptoms in cancer and educational handouts*, ed 2, Chicago, Ill, 2004, American Dietetic Association; *Nutrition in cancer care (PDQ®)*, Bethesda, Md, 2005, National Cancer Institute, updated March 30, 2005 (website): www.cancer.gov/cancerinfo/pdq/supportivecare/nutrition/healthprofessional. Accessed April 15, 2005; Kogut VJ, Luthringer SL, editors. *Nutritional issues in cancer care*, Pittsburgh, Penn, 2005, Oncology Nursing Society; American Cancer Society: *Nutrition for the person with cancer: a guide for patients and families*, ACS publication No. 9410-HCP, Atlanta, Ga, 2002, ACS; National Cancer Institute: *Eating hints for cancer patients before, during and after treatment*, NIH publication No. 03-2079, Bethesda, Md, 2003, NIH.

TPN, Total parenteral nutrition.

Table 33-2 Nutrition Impact Symptoms and Nutrition Intervention

Symptom	Nutritional intervention
Anorexia	Determine specific factors contributing to symptom such as pain, constipation, GI symptoms and treat appropriately
	Encourage small frequent feedings
	Encourage nutrient dense foods and add protein and calories to favorite foods using extra butter, margarine, cheese, and nonfat dry milk powder
	Evaluate anorexic affects of other medications
	Drink nutrient-dense beverages between meals to avoid feeling too full with meals
Constipation	Consider pharmacologic therapy with appetite-enhancing medications
	Eat at regular intervals throughout the day
	Increase fluid intake
	Increase dietary fiber
	Try hot beverages as a bowel stimulant
	Increase physical activity as tolerated
Diarrhea	Establish an appropriate bowel program including the regular use of pharmacologic agents
	Assess severity including hydration status and associated symptoms
	Consider diagnostic evaluation including stool analysis if diarrhea not treatment-related and manage appropriately
	Verify that diarrhea is not related to impaction, especially in patients on narcotic medications
	Try prophylactic glutamine supplementation—optimal dose 10 g TID
	Drink adequate fluid intake—at least 1 cup of fluid for each loose bowel movement added to usual intake
	Replace fluid with sodium and potassium—containing fluids such as broth, sports drinks with less than 15 g of carbohydrate per serving
	Drink clear liquids or BRAT (bananas, rice, applesauce, toast) diet for 24–48 hours until symptoms improve
	Minimum to low residue diet for maintenance to control frequency with increased intake of foods high in soluble fiber (bananas, oatmeal, white rice, applesauce and noodles)
	Restrict lactose if enteritis or small bowel is in radiation therapy field
Dysphagia	Assure adequate pharmacologic treatment is being used
	Modify diet consistency and follow swallowing techniques provided by the speech pathologist
	Eat softer, moist, or pureed foods
	Use commercially available food thickeners, tapioca, instant mashed potatoes, or infant rice cereal to thicken liquids
	Avoid breads, cakes, dry cookies and crackers unless taken with plenty of liquids
Early satiety	Consider feeding tube if unable to obtain adequate nourishment orally
	Eat small, frequent, nutrient-dense meals and snacks
	Add protein and calories to favorite foods using extra butter, margarine, cheese, nonfat dry milk powder
	Try high-calorie/high-protein liquid drinks, which may be better tolerated than solid foods
	Keep nutrient-dense snacks available and snack frequently
	Capitalize on the times when feeling the best
Esophagitis	Try pharmacologic treatment with medications that increase digestive motility
	Eat soft, moist foods with extra sauce, dressings and gravies
	Avoid acidic foods like tomatoes, citrus foods, carbonated beverages, and alcohol
	Avoid spicy foods
	Avoid dry, coarse, or rough foods
	Rinse mouth and gargle frequently with mild saline solution
	Avoid alcohol-based mouthwashes
	Try pharmacologic treatment to coat or numb esophagus before eating
	Consider feeding tube if unable to obtain adequate nourishment orally

(continued)

Table 33-2 Nutrition Impact Symptoms and Nutrition Intervention—cont'd

Symptom	Nutritional intervention
Fatigue	Recognize that fatigue is defined by the person experiencing it Assess for treatable causes of fatigue such as anemia, infection, pain, neutropenia, depression, medication side affects and manage appropriately Educate patient as to potential side affects of treatment and how to manage them appropriately Maintain optimal nutritional status Encourage light exercise unless contraindicated by medical condition Encourage assistance with housework and meal preparation
Lactose intolerance	Use a lactase enzyme supplement to help digest dairy products or use dairy products already treated with lactase enzyme Substitute milk with non-dairy beverage, soy, or rice milk
Mucositis	Prevention is key—good oral hygiene with frequent mouth rinses is important (avoid alcohol-based products) Treat oral lesions pharmacologically as appropriate (antifungal meds if needed) Consider using oral topical agents and anesthetics such as viscous lidocaine and institution-specific mouth rinses that are combinations of nystatin, Maalox, diphenhydramine, hydrocortisone, viscous lidocaine Adjust texture/temperature as tolerated Avoid carbonated beverages Avoid caffeine/alcohol/tobacco products Avoid other irritants (acidic, spicy foods) Try ice chips before and during bolus infusion of 5-FU because this causes vasoconstriction in oral mucosa and may minimize mucosal damage Try oral glutamine supplementation—optimal dose is 10 g TID Consider feeding tube if unable to obtain adequate nourishment orally
Nausea/ vomiting	Provide optimal antiemetic medication for planned therapy Use relaxation techniques for anticipatory vomiting Evaluate other factors possibly contributing to vomiting such as constipation, brain metastasis, other medications Eat small, frequent, low-fat meals with minimal odors Try dry, starchy and/or salty foods such as pretzels, saltines, potatoes, noodles, cereals Try room temperature or cold foods Sip on ginger ale, tea or candied dried ginger Avoid favorite foods until symptoms resolve Eat clear liquids such as broth, gelatin, juice drinks on chemotherapy day because these may be better tolerated than solid food
Taste alterations	Identify specific taste sensations altered and correlate findings with specific selections such as adding seasonings/flavorings or substituting specific food group with items of comparable nutrient content (fish, poultry, legumes in place of meats) and avoid offending foods Clear palate before meals by brushing teeth, gums, oral cavity and rinsing with baking soda and salt water rinses. Use plastic utensils for metallic taste Include foods that have a pleasing taste Avoid cigarette smoking Suck on fruit-flavored candies or chew gum between meals Eat tart foods such as sherbet, Italian ices, sorbet because they may be better tolerated than sweet foods Add lemon, lime vinegar, or salt to foods that are too sweet Try marinades and spices to mask strange tastes Avoid canned food products if metallic taste is problematic Eat foods that do not need to be heated up because they are better tolerated than cooked foods with more prominent odors and flavors; try eating cold foods like sandwiches, cottage cheese, yogurt, etc

Table 33-2 Nutrition Impact Symptoms and Nutrition Intervention—cont'd

Symptom	Nutritional intervention
Xerostomia	Try tart foods to stimulate saliva Sip on liquids or suck on ice chips throughout the day Avoid caffeine, alcohol, and tobacco products Try using a cool mist humidifier at bedtime Try drinking through a straw Rinse mouth frequently with mild saline solution Add extra sauces and gravies to foods

Data from Luthringer SL: Nutrition concerns with the radiation therapy patient. In Molseed L, McCallum PD, Elliott L, editors: *The clinical guide to oncology nutrition*, ed 2, Chicago, Ill, 2005, The American Dietetic Association; ; Eldridge B, Hamilton KK: *Management of nutrition impact symptoms in cancer and educational handouts*, ed 2, Chicago, Ill, 2004, American Dietetic Association; *Nutrition in Cancer Care (PDQ®)*, Bethesda, Md, 2005, National Cancer Institute, updated March 30, 2005 (website): www.cancer.gov/cancerinfo/pdq/supportivecare/nutrition/healthprofessional. Accessed April 15, 2005; Kogut VJ, Luthringer SL, editors: *Nutritional issues in cancer care*, Pittsburgh, Penn, 2005, Oncology Nursing Society; American Cancer Society: *Nutrition for the person with cancer: a guide for patients and families*, ACS publication No. 9410-HCP, Atlanta, Ga, 2002, ACS; National Cancer Institute: *Eating hints for cancer patients before, during and after treatment*, NIH publication No. 03-2079, Bethesda, Md, 2003, NIH.

TID, Titrated initial dose; *5-FU*, 5-fluorouracil.

wasting from their usual diets or by way of the suggested modifications. In such cases, nutritional supplements are often recommended. These supplements are high in protein and calories and have extra vitamins and minerals. They come in a variety of forms such as liquid, powders, or puddings, and most are lactose free for those patients who are sensitive to the lactose in dairy products. The most common supplements are similar to a milkshake in texture and flavor, but some clear, liquid juice-drink flavored supplements are available as well. Most of these commercial supplements are readily available in drugstores or supermarkets. Over 100 different supplements are available today, many of which are specialized to meet the needs of patients with a particular disease or metabolic condition. The most popular formulas for use with oncology patients are listed in Table 33-3.

Enteral Nutrition

Every attempt should be made to provide adequate nutrition by eating solid foods or a modified diet such as soft or liquid foods, but in some instances, enteral nutrition provided by way of a feeding tube is necessary. Head and neck cancer patients and patients with esophageal cancer often require enteral nutrition support to help meet their high nutritional demands. They often have functioning digestive systems but are unable to swallow foods or liquids because of the presence of tumor or severe symptoms from the treatment that make swallowing too difficult. Numerous studies have demonstrated the benefit of enteral feedings in this and selected other groups of patients.[19] It is best to initiate the tube feedings in the beginning phase of treatment planning so that breaks in treatment do not occur while the feeding tube is being inserted and protein and calorie deficits resulting in significant weight loss during and after treatment are prevented.

There are various methods of tube feedings, each requiring the tube to be inserted into a different part of the digestive tract.

- **Nasogastric (NG) tube feedings**—use a feeding tube that is inserted through the nose, into the esophagus, and then rests in the stomach. This method is used when the tube feedings are expected to be short term.
- **Gastrostomy tube feedings**—tubes are placed either surgically through the abdominal wall and into the stomach or by the aid of a flexible scope (percutaneous endoscopic gastrostomy—PEG) that is placed down the throat and assists in guiding the placement of the tube through the wall of the stomach. This tube is used when tube feedings are expected to last longer than 2 weeks.
- **Jejunostomy (J) tube feedings**—used when it is necessary to bypass the stomach for feeding. This tube is surgically placed through an opening in the abdominal wall; the tube rests in part of the small intestine or in the jejunum.

Table 33-3 Oral Nutritional Supplements

Oral supplements commonly available	Oral supplements appropriate for diabetics	Oral supplements that are good alternatives for creamy shakes	Oral supplements specific for cancer-associated weight loss	Alternative supplements available
The following are milkshake drinks used to provide additional calories and nutrients to the diet They come in a variety of flavors Most are available in powder form or ready to drink Some have added fiber or additional protein added Some are milk-based; most are lactose free They range in calorie levels from 250 to 400 calories per serving Most are readily available in retail stores but some require special ordering; most companies offer direct ordering with home delivery	The following are milkshake drinks used to provide additional calories and nutrients to the diet They are specially formulated to contain less carbohydrate and more fiber than standard oral supplements so they are appropriate for people with diabetes Most are readily available in retail stores but some require special ordering; most companies offer direct ordering with home delivery	The following products are clear liquid in nature, contain no fiber or fat and are easily digested They come in a variety of flavors They range in calorie levels from 160 to 300 calories per serving Some are available in retail stores, but most require special ordering; most companies offer direct ordering with home delivery	The following products are designed specifically for cancer patients with tumor-induced weight loss and cachexia They contain an omega-3 fatty acid and amino acid blends that may help build muscle and promote weight gain in cancer patients They are available in a variety of flavors Require special ordering from pharmacy or direct ordering from the company with home delivery	There are many other products that can be very useful to help add nutrients to one's diet Pediatric formulas are also available but not listed Individual nutrients currently used for specific symptoms associated with cancer treatments are also available but not listed Most of these products are not available in retail stores but can be special ordered or are available through the companies home delivery programs
Boost, Boost Plus, Boost High Protein, Boost with Fiber Carnation Instant Breakfast powder Carnation Instant Breakfast ready-to-drink Carnation Instant Breakfast VHC Ensure and Ensure Plus Scandishake Variety of store brands and generic products are available, such as Equate, which are similar in nutritional value	Carnation Instant Breakfast with no sugar added Choice DM beverage Glucerna ShakeNutren Glytrol	Boost Breeze Carnation Instant Breakfast Juice Drink Enlive Resource Fruit Beverage	Resource Support Prosure Shake	Boost Pudding Ensure Nutrition and Energy Bars Ensure Pudding Resource Benecalorie Resource Beneprotein Nestle Additions

Many formulas are available to choose from to deliver the best nutrition to the patient. A patient's medical condition and nutritional needs will help determine which formula is best suited for that patient because many disease-specific formulas are now available. A registered dietitian should be consulted to help assess the specific nutritional needs of the patient.

Scheduled delivery of the formula through the tube depends on the patient's home care needs, medical condition, tolerance to tube feedings, and location of the tube feeding. Bolus, intermittent, continuous drip, and cyclic administration are the four main methods of delivery.

- **Bolus**—involves the rapid delivery of formula several times a day through the tube with the use of a syringe or funnel.
- **Intermittent**—allows for the feedings to be provided over a short time period several times per day. Gravity drip method is most often used.
- **Continuous drip**—a pump is used to regulate the flow of the formula through the tube. This method is generally used with jejunostomy tube feedings, because rapid delivery of formula into the small intestine is not generally tolerated well by the patient.
- **Cyclic**—continuous drip with the use of a pump, for only part of the day or night, provides the nourishment that is necessary and offers the flexibility of intermittent feedings.

Although tube feedings are generally considered to be safe, occasionally a problem may arise. Table 33-4 lists some of the common problems, how to prevent them, and some possible solutions.

NUTRITIONAL SUPPORT IN ADVANCED CANCER

Palliative Care

The focus of care in patients with advanced cancer is palliation of symptoms, establishing a sense of well-being, and maintaining quality of life.[20] Common side effects seen in patients with advanced disease include pain, anorexia, early satiety, constipation, and weakness. Modifications in meals and eating patterns can be made to meet the ever-changing needs of these challenged individuals. Identifying and treating symptoms early and educating the family can help ease much of the tension that surrounds mealtimes. Some helpful suggestions include letting the patient be in control and not force feeding meals, monitoring likes and dislikes, because tastes and preferences change frequently, and offering smaller, more frequent snacks throughout the day in place of larger more structured meals.[12]

Hospice and End-of-Life Care

When palliative care progresses to hospice care, the nutrition intervention must be modified. Providing comfort for the patient becomes the priority. As much as families often think that nutritional support will make the patient stronger, there is insufficient evidence to support the role of aggressive nutrition intervention in terminal illness. Some research reports that the addition of nutritional support may actually decrease the patient's quality of life, comfort, and overall outcome. In terminally ill cancer patients, hunger is rarely expressed and feelings of discomfort are identified when patients eat only to please their families. Thirst, however, is one of the few symptoms that patients continue to experience, which reinforces the continued need for comfort measures of adequate fluid intake and regular mouth care.[21]

Studies show that there may be a limited role for enteral or parenteral nutrition support in sustaining life or improving well-being at the end of life.[22] Many ethical and legal implications surround the decision of whether or not to continue feeding terminally ill patients. The position of the American Dietetic Association is to develop both clinical and ethical criteria for nutrition and hydration. Members of the healthcare team, including a registered dietitian, should establish these criteria, and recommendations should be made on a case-by-case basis. Each patient is unique, and the plan of care should be reassessed on a continued basis for each individual, keeping in mind the growing support in the literature that neither nutrition nor hydration in terminal patients increases comfort or quality of life.[23]

PHARMACOLOGIC OPTIONS

Appetite Stimulants

Although dietary modifications are helpful in treating and preventing many nutrition-related symptoms associated with cancer and its treatment, especially the reversible symptoms such as diarrhea, constipation, nausea, and mucositis, nutritional therapy alone is often not enough to

Table 33-4 Common Enteral Feeding Problems

Problem	Possible cause	Management
Aspiration	Altered gag reflex Poor gastric emptying Vomiting or reflux	Stop tube feedings immediately until further assessment of patient's status When tube feedings restart, keep head of bed elevated greater than 30 degrees, and check stomach residuals Check tube placement Change to continuous pump feedings if on bolus or intermittent gravity drip feedings Consider jejunostomy tube
Bloating/fullness	Constipation Delayed gastric emptying Tube feeding formula Rate of feeding too high Cold formula	Decrease volume of formula and increase frequency of feedings Consider changing to continuous pump feedings Feed sitting up in a chair; if in bed, keep head of bed elevated Follow prescribed antiemetic regimen if nauseated Follow prescribed bowel program if constipated Consider metoclopramide (Reglan) to aid in stomach emptying
Clogged tubes	Kink or bend in the tube Medication build-up Formula too thick Not flushing tube regularly	Always flush the feeding tube before and after each feeding and before and after administration of medications Water is the best liquid to flush tube with Use of acidic juices may cause the protein in the tube feeding to curdle, which will make the clog worse
Constipation	Inadequate water Inadequate or excessive fiber in tube feeding formula Inactivity Medications, especially pain medications	Increase water flushes for adequate hydration Follow prescribed bowel program to include stool softeners Increase activity as tolerated Change formula to higher fiber formula if not currently using one
Dehydration	Inadequate water intake Diarrhea Fever	Increase water flushes for adequate hydration Consider more dilute formula Medical attention
Diarrhea	Tube feedings given too quickly Tube feeding formula too concentrated Tube feeding formula volume too high Medications Related to tube feeding administration	Consider antidiarrheal medications Reduce rate of delivering formula, change to gravity or continuous drip if bolus fed Reduce volume of formula and gradually increase as tolerated Change tube feeding formula to one that is less concentrated Change tube feeding formula to one that contains fiber Make certain that all opened formula is kept refrigerated Change feeding set and syringe daily and make certain that hands and work areas are cleaned well
Nausea/vomiting	Illness Tube not in correct position	Stop delivery of formula if vomiting Check for tube position and placement Consider changing formula when tube feedings restart Keep elevated when receiving tube feedings

Data from Novartis Medical Nutrition: *At home living with tube feeding*, Minneapolis, Minn, 2005, Novartis Medical Health, Inc; Kagan SH, Sweeney-Cordes E: Head and neck cancers. In Kogut VJ, Luthringer SL, editors: *Nutritional issues in cancer care*, Pittsburgh, Penn, 2005, Oncology Nursing Society, pp 113-114.

improve appetite. Pharmacologic intervention for cancer-related weight loss falls into four main categories: (1) drugs to treat symptoms that interfere with adequate nutrition, such as antiemetics and digestive aides, (2) appetite stimulants, such as corticosteroids, progestational agents, cannabinoids, and some antihistamines, (3) drugs that affect metabolism or specific inflammatory responses such as melatonin, thalidomide, and eicosapentaenoic acid, or EPA, and (4) anabolic steroids such as oxandrolone.[24] It is important to remember that although many of these therapies have some value, more research is needed before they become standard treatment. Intervention should be chosen based on the patient's treatment goals and his or her prognosis. Careful evaluation of the patient's symptoms and correction of reversible symptoms should be completed before considering these forms of pharmacologic treatments.[25]

Specialized Nutrients

Although dietary modifications can minimize many of the common nutrition impact symptoms, prevention of symptoms is the ultimate goal. Specific nutrients that may reduce the toxicity from treatment are being researched. The amino acid glutamine may prevent or minimize mouth sores and mucositis, a common side effect of radiation therapy to the head and neck area, and may prevent or minimize diarrhea, common to patients receiving radiation therapy to the pelvic region.[26] Although further studies are needed, clinical trials using zinc sulfate as a supplement during radiation therapy to the head and neck area have shown some promise in expediting the return of the sense of taste—with loss of taste being a symptom common to this population of patients.[27] Omega-3 fatty acids, specifically eicosapentaenoic acid (EPA) and docosahexaenoic acid (DHA), have been shown in studies to reverse the weight loss and cachexia in patients. Liquid nutritional supplements containing EPA and/or DHA may be beneficial to patients with tumor-induced weight loss.[17]

COMPLEMENTARY AND ALTERNATIVE TREATMENTS

The National Cancer Institute defines complementary and alternative medicine (CAM) as a group of diverse medical and healthcare systems, practices, and products that are not presently considered to be part of conventional medicine. Complementary medicine is used together with conventional treatments, whereas alternative medicine is used in place of evidence-based treatments.[28] Various studies have reported that CAM use among cancer patients is quite high, with approximately 60% of patients reporting at least one CAM therapy as part of their cancer treatment program.[29] Many alternative therapies are marketed as nontoxic, safe, and "natural," making the patient and their families vulnerable to accepting these therapies as an alternative to conventional treatments and to the many side effects that go along with them. These treatments give patients and their families hope and allow them the ability to take an active role in their care. Some of the most common forms of CAM include spiritual prayer, relaxation, massage, imagery, yoga, herbal medicines, and special diets. When combined with standard cancer treatment, many of these therapies have shown benefit in relieving stress, nausea, and pain, thus improving the quality of life, but some therapies can be harmful. Many CAM diet regimens are nutritionally incomplete in their balance of protein, carbohydrates, fats, and other nutrients. For this reason, special diets that patients want to follow should be evaluated and adjustments recommended. The most common "self-prescribed" form of CAM is nutrient or herbal supplementation. Consumers rarely think herbal and vitamin supplementation can produce potential harm because they are sold over the counter without the need for a physician prescription. However, vitamins and herbal products can compromise the safety and efficacy of the anticancer treatments that have been prescribed. The current lack of regulation on dietary supplements has led to misleading health claims for consumers. Only a few of the many, many herbal and botanical supplements available have been studied to evaluate their effectiveness as a cancer treatment. The lack of research and reliable information about the functions of these supplements, their therapeutic doses, toxicity levels, and interaction with chemotherapy and radiation therapy are all cause for concern. For these reasons, it is always advisable for healthcare providers to question patients in regard to their use of dietary supplements during cancer treatments and to provide them with the most current recommendations regarding their use.[20] Although not all herbal and vitamin supplements are harmful, it is important to note that some may be contraindicated during radiation and chemotherapy. High-dose antioxidant vitamins, namely vitamins A, C, E, and selenium, when taken in the form of supplements, should be avoided during radiation therapy, because some research indicates that these vitamins may interfere with the radiation's ability to cause damage to the cells.[30] In a 2004 study by Wernecke and colleagues,[31] over 47% of 318 patients in the study took herbal and vitamin supplements. The study found that overall, 18 people, or 11%, took more than the recommended dosage of the supplement. Health warnings were given to 20, a little over 12%, of these patients when the use of their supplements was identified as interfering with their treatment.[31] Of the 15 best-selling herbal remedies used in the United States, 9 were identified as being a risk for negative interactions with specific anticancer medications, including the most popular herbs, echinacea, ginseng, and St. John's wort.[32] As research in this field continues, it is important for health practitioners to identify the potential risks of CAM and equally important for patients to be encouraged to disclose their use. The most prudent advice to patients is to include in their diet foods that are rich in antioxidant vitamins and avoid excessive supplementation until more research is available. Table 33-5 lists some potentially harmful herbals.[12,13,32,33]

NUTRITION AND CANCER PREVENTION

It is well documented that the dietary practices followed by individuals can either promote health or play a major role in the development of diseases. Over the years, nutrition and diet guidelines have been developed to help improve the health of Americans. The United States Department of Agriculture (USDA) has developed the most commonly used set of nutrition guidelines, called the *Dietary Guidelines for Americans.* These guidelines feature recommendations that support good overall health and were recently updated to reflect the most current research.[34] The guidelines encompass the more specific dietary advice for cancer prevention that was previously established by the American Cancer Society (ACS)[20] and by the American Institute for Cancer Research (AICR).[35] Although these guidelines were created for healthy

Table 33-5 Herbs Identified as Having Potential for Interacting With Cancer Therapy

Herbal	Possible interactions
Black cohosh	May interact with antiestrogen therapy
Chamomile	May increase bleeding time and affect platelet count
Dong quai	May increase effects of warfarin, used to thin blood
Echinacea	May interfere with some chemotherapy medications
Garlic	May increase bleeding time, interacts with some chemotherapy medications
Gingko	May increase bleeding time and interfere with chemotherapy medications, especially the alkylating agents
Ginseng	May affect platelets and blood coagulation
	Should be avoided in women with estrogen receptor–positive breast and endometrial cancers
	Interferes with several chemotherapy medications
Grape seed	Use with caution with chemotherapy agents
Kava	Avoid with liver disease or with drugs that are toxic to the liver
Ma Huang (ephedra)	Increases toxicity with blood pressure medications, caffeine, and antidepressants
St. John's wort	Avoid with ALL types of chemotherapy
Valerian	Use with caution with some chemotherapy medications
Yohimbe	Decreases the effect of antidepressants, antihypertensives, and other medications
Soy supplements	Supplements (not foods) should be avoided with estrogen receptor–positive breast or endometrial cancers or with antiestrogen therapy

Data from Eldridge B, Hamilton KK: *Management of nutrition impact symptoms in cancer and educational handouts*, ed 2, Chicago, 2004, American Dietetic Association; *Nutrition in Cancer Care (PDQ®)*, Bethesda, Md, 2005, National Cancer Institute, updated March 30, 2005 (website): www.cancer.gov/cancerinfo/pdq/supportivecare/nutrition/healthprofessional. Accessed April 15, 2005; Kong Q, Lillehei KO: *Med Hypotheses* 51(5):405-409, 1998; Wernecke U, Earl J, Seydel C, et al: *Br J Cancer* 90:408-413, 2004.

individuals, they can be modified to focus on specific medical conditions such as cancer, and many patients can benefit from following these recommendations during and after treatment.

Key recommendations in the 2005 version of *Dietary Guidelines for Americans* include the following:

- Consume adequate nutrients within caloric needs.
- Maintain body weight in a healthy range.
- Engage in regular physical activity.
- Consume a variety of fruits, vegetables, whole grains, and low-fat dairy products each day.
- Consume less fat, keeping trans-fatty acid consumption as low as possible.
- Choose fiber-rich fruits, vegetables, and whole grains often.
- Consume less high-sodium foods and more potassium-rich foods.
- Those who choose to drink alcoholic beverages should do so sensibly and in moderation, keeping in mind that certain individuals should avoid alcohol entirely.
- Keep food safety in mind during the preparation, storing, and serving of foods.

Although these guidelines were established to foster healthy eating habits in Americans for the prevention of disease, the importance of maintaining a healthy diet and lifestyle extends through the continuum of care. Although research is not specific regarding the role that nutrition plays in the prevention of secondary cancers and cancer recurrence, it is generally accepted that after treatment individuals should follow the established cancer prevention dietary recommendations. Research is abundant regarding the role of dietary intake, specifically a diet consisting of plenty of fruits and vegetables, low-fat food choices, and high-fiber foods, along with a balance in calories, to promote a healthy weight in an effort to prevent many cancers including prostate, breast, colon, and lung cancers.

SUMMARY

It is clear that nutrition plays a key role in the prevention, treatment, and survivorship of cancer patients. Treatment side effects from surgery, radiation therapy, and/or chemotherapy can be minimized, or prevented with early nutritional intervention. The team approach to care, including assessing and addressing the nutritional needs of the patient, can lead to an improved outcome and quality of life for the patient.

REFERENCES

1. *Food, nutrition and the prevention of cancer: a global perspective*, Washington, DC, 1997, World Cancer Research Fund and American Institute for Cancer Research.
2. Jemal A, Murray T, Ward E et al: Cancer statistics, 2005, *CA Cancer J Clin* 55(1):10-30, 2005.
3. McMahon K, Decker G, Ottery FD: Integrating proactive nutritional assessment in clinical practices to prevent complications and cost, *Semin Oncol* 25(2 suppl 6):20-27, 1998.
4. Klein S, Kinney J, Jeejeebhoy K et al: Nutrition support in clinical practice: review of published data and recommendations for future research directions, *Am J Clin Nutr* 66(3):683-706, 1997.
5. Arrowsmith H: A critical evaluation of the use of nutrition screening tools by nurses, *Br J Nurs* 8(22):1483-1490, 2000.
6. *Appetite stimulation and weight loss: re-thinking your approach to early intervention*, Newark, NJ, 2003, University of Medicine and Dentistry of New Jersey.
7. Bauer J, Capra S, Ferguson M: Use of the scored patient-generated subjective global assessment (PG-SGA) as a nutrition assessment tool in patients with cancer, *Eur J Clin Nutr* 56(8):779-785, 2002.
8. Isenring E, Bauer J, Capra S: The scored patient-generated subjective global assessment (PG-SGA) and its association with quality of life in ambulatory patients receiving radiotherapy, *Eur J Clin Nutr* 57(2):305-309, 2003.
9. Ottery FD, Bender F, Kasenic S: The design and implementation of a model nutritional oncology clinic, *Oncology Issues, Integrating Nutrition Into Your Cancer Program* 17(2):2-6, 2002.
10. Ottery FD: Supportive nutritional therapy to prevent cachexia and improve quality of life, *Semin Oncol* 22(2 suppl 3):98-111, 1995.
11. Luthringer SL: Nutrition concerns with the radiation therapy patient. In Molseed L, McCallum PD, Elliott L, editors: *The clinical guide to oncology nutrition*, ed 2, Chicago, Ill, 2006, The American Dietetic Association, pp 88-93.
12. Eldridge B, Hamilton KK: *Management of nutrition impact symptoms in cancer and educational handouts*, ed 2, Chicago, Ill, American Dietetic Association, 2004.
13. National Cancer Institute: *Nutrition in Cancer Care (PDQ®)* (website): www.cancer.gov/cancerinfo/pdq/supportivecare/nutrition/healthprofessional. Accessed April 15, 2005.
14. Kogut VJ, Luthringer SL, editors: *Nutritional issues in cancer care*, Pittsburgh, 2005, Oncology Nursing Society.
15. *Nutrition for the person with cancer: a guide for patients and families* (publication no. 9410-HCP), Atlanta, American Cancer Society, 2002.
16. *Eating hints for cancer patients before, during and after treatment* (NIH publication no. 03-2079), Bethesda, Md, 2003, National Cancer Institute.
17. Laviano A, Meguid MM, Inui A et al: Therapy insight: cancer anorexia-cachexia syndrome...when all you can eat is yourself, *Nat Clin Pract Oncol* 2(3):158-165, 2005.

18. Strasser F, Bruera ED: Update on anorexia and cachexia, *Hematol Oncol Clin North Am* 16(3):589-617, 2002.
19. Piazza-Barnett R, Matarese LE: Enteral nutrition in adult medical/surgical oncology. In McCallum PD, Polisena CG, editors: *The clinical guide to oncology nutrition*, Chicago, Ill, 2000, The American Dietetic Association, pp 106-118.
20. Brown J, Byers T, Thompson K et al: Nutrition during and after cancer treatment: a guide for informed choices by cancer survivors, *CA Cancer J Clin* 51(3):153-187, 2001.
21. Sutton LM, Demark-Wahnefried W, Clipp EC: Management of terminal cancer in elderly patients, *Lancet Oncol* 4(3):149-157, 2003.
22. Billings JA: Recent advances in palliative care, *BMJ* 321(7260):555-558, 2000.
23. American Dietetic Association: Position of the American Dietetic Association: ethical and legal issues in nutrition, hydration, and feeding, *J Am Diet Assoc* 102(5):716-726, 2002.
24. Von Roenn JH: Pharmacologic interventions for cancer-related weight loss, *Oncology Issues, Integrating Nutrition Into Your Cancer Program* 17(2):18-21, 2002.
25. Murphy S, Von Roenn JH: Pharmacological management of anorexia and cachexia. In McCallum PD, Polisena CG, editors: *The clinical guide to oncology nutrition*, Chicago, Ill, 2000, The American Dietetic Association, pp 127-133.
26. Savarese DM, Savy G, Vahdat L et al: Prevention of chemotherapy and radiation toxicity with glutamine, *Cancer Treat Rev* 29(6):501-513, 2003.
27. Ertekin MV, Koc M, Karslioglu I et al: Zinc sulfate in the prevention of radiation-induced oropharyngeal mucositis: a prospective, placebo-controlled, randomized study, *Int J Radiat Oncol Biol Phys* 58(1):167-174, 2004.
28. National Cancer Institute: *Complementary and alternative medicine in cancer treatment: questions and answers* (website): http://www.cancer.gov/cancertopics/factsheet/therapy/CAM. Accessed November 22, 2006.
29. Richardson MA, Sanders T, Palmer JL et al: Complementary/alternative medicine use in a comprehensive cancer center and the implications for oncology, *J Clin Oncol* 18(13):2505-2514, 2000.
30. Kong Q, Lillehei KO: Antioxidant inhibitors for cancer therapy, *Med Hypotheses* 51(5):405-409, 1998.
31. Wernecke U, Earl J, Seydel C et al: Potential health risks of complementary alternative medicine in cancer patients, *Br J Cancer* 90(2):408-413, 2004.
32. Sparreboom A, Cox MC, Acharya MR et al: Herbal remedies in the United States: potential adverse interactions with anticancer agents, *J Clin Oncol* 22(12):2489-2503, 2004.
33. Sparreboom A, Cox MC, Acharya MR et al: Herbal remedies in the United States: potential adverse interactions with anticancer agents. *J Clin Oncol* 2004 Jun 15;22(12):2489-2503.
34. US Department of Agriculture, US Department of Health and Human Services: *Dietary guidelines for Americans 2005* (website): www.healthierus.gov/dietaryguidelines. Accessed May 6, 2005.
35. American Institute for Cancer Research: Simple steps to prevent cancer (website): http://www.aicr.org/site/PageServer?pagename=pub_ss_prevent_cancer. Accessed November 22, 2006.

Chapter 34

Radiation-Induced Nausea, Vomiting, and Diarrhea

Constance Engelking, Rita J. Wickham, and Carmel Sauerland

Nausea, vomiting, and diarrhea are three radiation-induced gastrointestinal (GI) symptoms that can produce both physical and emotional distress and life-threatening consequences if identified late or inadequately managed. Serious physical effects include dehydration and electrolyte imbalances whereas psychosocial effects are associated with dependency, interruptions in interpersonal relationships, and altered perception of body image and sexuality. At moderate to severe levels, these symptoms also can cause treatment delays and discontinuation of treatment that may ultimately interfere with tumor response.[1]

GI symptoms commonly occur in up to 100% of patients undergoing radiation that targets and exerts local effects on organs and tissues within the abdominal and lower thoracic radiation fields including the following:

- Abdominopelvic radiation used to treat genitourinary, gynecologic, and gastrointestinal cancers
- Lower thoracic and lumbosacral irradiation used in the treatment of spinal tumors and cord compression
- Hemibody and total body irradiation (TBI) used as conditioning for allogeneic stem cell transplantation[2,3]

Symptom occurrence, character, and severity depends on radiation dose rate, field location and size, technique (e.g., teletherapy versus brachytherapy; cobalt versus linear accelerator with three-dimensional [3D] conformal treatment planning; intensity modulated radiation), treatment protocol (e.g., radiation in combination regimen with chemotherapy), and presence of related comorbid conditions or other host factors.[1-3] Management of GI effects is changing in response to the maturation of data related to efficacy of traditional approaches and to the integration of newer antidiarrheal and antiemetic agents into patient care.[4,5]

Nurses caring for patients undergoing radiation with the potential to produce these distressing symptoms need to understand their underlying mechanisms and be aware of effective interventions for preventing, minimizing, and managing associated discomfort and life-threatening consequences.[1,3,6] To assist clinicians in caring for patients experiencing these symptoms, published guidelines detailing accepted and evidence-based interventions for assessment, pharmacologic, and nonpharmacologic management are available in the literature[1,4,7,8] and on the internet (www.nccn.org).

NAUSEA AND VOMITING

Nausea and vomiting (N&V) are less common after radiation therapy (RT) than chemotherapy. Nonetheless, 40% to 80% of all patients treated with RT experience prolonged N&V (radiation-induced nausea and vomiting [RINV]) that may affect quality of life (QOL) and decrease a patient's willingness and ability to continue RT.[9,10] Furthermore, patients who received fractionated RT to the abdomen over several weeks often experienced diarrhea and anorexia and RINV.[11] Patients found these symptoms to be highly inconvenient and to have a significant and prolonged effect on their QOL.

RINV is also a major problem because many nurses and physicians are not familiar with the risks for RINV or current management guidelines. For instance, only 33% of 102 RT oncologists surveyed reported they prescribed *any* antiemetic for patients undergoing RT.[10] Only 26% would prescribe a recommended antiemetic (a serotonin antagonist) for patients undergoing TBI. Another study was done to examine the incidence and patterns of RINV in more than 900 patients, to identify risk factors predicting RINV and to evaluate antiemetics used in RT clinical practice.[12] Only 14% of patients were given antiemetics; 5% were prophylactically prescribed and 9% were symptomatically given. Radiation oncologists largely preferred a 'wait and see' strategy and usually reserved serotonin antagonists for rescue/symptomatic treatment of RINV.

Many radiation oncologists still prescribe older, less effective antiemetics such as metoclopramide because of costs.[13] Prescribing older antiemetics by habit rather than more 'expensive' newer antiemetics may actually increase nursing care costs and decrease survival in patients unable to continue with RT. Therefore, prophylaxis with effective antiemetics is better than treating breakthrough RINV on an as needed (prn) basis in terms of drug and nursing costs, particularly because RINV is more difficult to control after it starts than before.

Definitions and Presentation

Acute RINV often begins suddenly, about 90 minutes after RT, and persists for about 5 hours.[13] However, RT is typically administered in fractionated (divided) doses for up to 6 or 8 weeks. Repeated days of unmanaged RINV may lead to cumulatively worsening symptoms, which can become intractable and may limit further RT. Compounding the problem, many patients receiving RT as outpatients develop RINV after they go home.

Risk Factors

Treatment- and patient-related factors influence the risk for RINV (Table 34-1). Treatment factors include large dose (single or total fractionated), volume of tissue radiated, site treated, and concomitant chemotherapy. The risk for RINV ranges from none in the lower extremities to almost 100% after total body irradiation (TBI).[10,14] RINV is most common in patients receiving RT for tumors in the upper abdomen (e.g., lymphomas, Hodgkin's disease, pancreatic, gastric, gallbladder). Large RT fractions are the most likely to be associated with RINV; these include TBI, a large treatment area in the upper abdomen, or hemibody RT (rarely used for pain control). RT to the lower abdomen, pelvis, upper chest, and brain are less likely to cause RINV, whereas few patients receiving RT for tumors of head and neck or in an extremity develop RINV at all.[12] Many tumors are now treated with regimens including chemotherapy and RT administered at the same time. Emetogenic chemotherapy administered previously or simultaneously further increases risk for and severity of RINV.[12] Some patient-related factors associated with N&V from chemotherapy also may increase RINV risk. These factors include female gender, age less than 55 years, low or no chronic alcohol intake, and perhaps, anxiety.[3]

Pathophysiology

General Theories

Pathophysiologic mechanisms differ for nausea and vomiting. Vomiting is a protective reflex that serves to rid the body of accidentally ingested oral toxic substances. The body may incorrectly interpret endogenous hormones or electrolyte abnormalities or iatrogenic agents—such as chemotherapy agents and other drugs, anesthesia, and radiation—as toxic and therefore may induce N&V.[14] These symptoms may occur independently, consecutively, or concomitantly. The pathophysiology of vomiting is much better understood than the processes leading to nausea. Vomiting occurs when a group of neurons in the brainstem, collectively termed the *vomiting center* (VC), are stimulated. Afferent signals from other central nervous system (CNS) or peripheral sites carry the message to vomit to the VC. CNS sites that can be stimulated to in turn activate the VC include the chemoreceptor trigger zone (CTZ) that lies near the VC in the brainstem. The CTZ, which receives chemical and neural signals from other CNS sites, peripheral sites, and the bloodstream, plays some role in drug-induced (and perhaps RT-induced) N&V. Other areas of the brain send vomiting messages to the VC. These are the vestibular apparatus, the cortex, and the limbic region, which are involved with N&V related to motion sickness or middle-ear infections and anticipatory N&V. The most important peripheral sites where vomiting stimuli initiate are at vagal nerve endings in the upper GI tract. GI mechanoreceptors and bloodstream receptors also might be involved in cases of nausea and vomiting from obstruction or compression, electrolyte or hormone abnormalities, and some drug reactions.

Several neurotransmitters and neuroreceptors are involved in the onset of N&V. Neurotransmitters include dopamine, histamine, acetylcholine, endocannabinoids, serotonin (5-HT), and substance P. Corresponding receptors are the dopamine 2 (D_2), histamine 1 (H_1), muscarinic cholinergic (M), cannabinoid 1 (CB_1), serotonin 3 and 4 (5-HT_3 and 5-HT_4), and the neurokinin 1 (NK_1). It is important to recognize the complexity of N&V in order to understand that no single antiemetic will alleviate

Table 34-1 Risk for Radiation-Induced Nausea and Vomiting

Risk classification	Site	Antiemetic recommendations—each day of treatment	Example
High (90%)	Total body irradiation Total nodal irradiation	Prophylaxis with a 5-HT_3 antagonist	Ondansetron (Zofran) 8 mg PO bid or tid or Granisetron (Kytril) 2 mg PO + treat breakthrough RINV
Moderate (60%–90%)	Upper hemibody irradiation Upper abdomen Whole abdomen	Prophylaxis with a 5-HT_3 antagonist Corticosteroid	Ondansetron (Zofran) 8 mg PO bid or tid or Granisetron (Kytril) 2 mg PO or Dexamethasone 2 mg tid + treat breakthrough RINV
Moderate (60%–90%)	Upper hemibody irradiation Upper abdomen Whole abdomen	Prophylaxis with a 5-HT_3 antagonist Corticosteroid	Ondansetron (Zofran) 8 mg PO bid or tid or Granisetron (Kytril) 2 mg PO or Dexamethasone 2 mg tid + treat breakthrough RINV
Low (30%–60%)	Lower hemibody irradiation Lower thoracic region Pelvis	Prophylaxis or rescue with a 5-HT_3 antagonist	Ondansetron (Zofran) 8 mg PO bid or tid or Granisetron (Kytril) 2 mg PO
Minimal (<30%)	Head, neck Extremities Extra-abdominal areas	Rescue with a dopamine antagonist or a 5-HT_3 antagonist	Metoclopramide (Reglan) 10 mg PO tid or Ondansetron (Zofran) 8 mg PO once-tid

Data from NCCN clinical practice guidelines in oncology—antiemesis, vol 2, 2006 (website): www.nccn.org/professionals/physician_gls/PDF/antiemesis.pdf; Feyer R, Maranzano E, Molassiotis A, et al: *Support Care Cancer* 13(2):122-128, 2005; National Cancer Institute: *Nausea and vomiting,* 2006 (website): www.nci.nih.gov/cancerinfo/pdq/supportivecare/nausea/healthprofessional#Section_3; Kirbride P, Bezjak A, Pater J, et al: *J Clin Oncol* 18(9):1960-1966, 2000.
bid, twice daily; *tid,* three times daily.

nausea and/or vomiting in every instance. A basic understanding of pathophysiologic mechanisms also aids in understanding why one or more anti-emetics might or might not be useful.[14]

Radiation-Induced Nausea and Vomiting

Most knowledge about N&V has been generated from chemotherapy-related N&V. Less is known about RINV, but the mechanisms of both are probably somewhat similar. This seems most certain when comparing RINV in patients after epigastric or abdominal RT to N&V in patients after chemotherapy. In both instances, peripheral mechanisms play a key role. As mentioned, vomiting is the body's response to what would usually be oral ingestion of a noxious substance. When this happens, enterochromaffin cells in the GI tract are stimulated to release serotonin (5-HT). Subsequently, 5-HT acts as an agonist and binds to corresponding 5-HT_3 neural receptors along the vagus nerve, with transmission of the vomiting impulse to the VC in the CNS. Abdominal RT and some chemotherapy drugs damage or otherwise stimulate the enterochromaffin cells with 5-HT release and binding to the vagus nerve. RT to other sites may involve other neurotransmitters, which probably play similar roles at their corresponding receptors and act as *agonists* to cause N&V.

Prevention and Management

Patient Assessment

Initial assessment focuses on establishing a baseline for later comparison and identification of patient-specific factors to project risk for N&V. Reaching agreement between clinician and patient as to what constitutes N&V is essential to accurate evaluation. In addition, investigating the patient's past experience with radiation and/or chemotherapy can facilitate understanding of patient misconceptions, potential compliance issues, and formulating an effective intervention plan. To develop an accurate representation of the patient's profile, several factors should be addressed including (1) the nature of radiation prescribed, (2) whether or not the treatment regimen includes emetogenic chemotherapy, and (3) the presence of other host-related medical factors that could influence occurrence and severity of N&V. Other factors that have been identified to increase chemotherapy nausea and vomiting experience are age (less than 50 years of age), gender (females),[15] history of motion sickness,[16] feeling of warmth during or after chemotherapy, people who are alcohol naïve, and those with high anxiety.[17]

Patients can be categorized into a high, moderate, low, or minimal risk category based on analysis of the factors presented. Table 34-2 outlines questions to be considered in projecting risk. An appropriate prevention plan along with intensity of monitoring and support can then be customized to the patient based on his or her risk categorization. In addition to the history intake, a physical exam and laboratory testing before the initiation of therapy should be performed to establish baseline data for later comparison.

Monitoring during treatment should take place on a regular basis, usually weekly. Assessment parameters include the severity and pattern of nausea, frequency of vomiting, compliance with and response to prevention and management measures, and assessment for any side effects from prevention or treatment medications. In addition, a thorough review of the effect N&V is having on the patient is warranted: Is there a loss of appetite

Table 34-2 Questions for Projecting Risk and Severity of Nausea and Vomiting

Risk factors	Cue questions
Treatment regimen	Radiation therapy prescription?
	Does field include abdomen and pelvis?
	Is it total or hemibody irradiation?
	What is total dose prescribed?
	Is it a fractionated technique?
	How will therapy be delivered (teletherapy, brachytherapy, conformal, or intensity-modulated technique)?
	Multimodal regimen?
	Will emetogenic chemotherapy be a part of the regimen?
	If yes, what agents, dosages, and administration schedule?
Comorbid conditions	Is the patient experiencing or likely to experience any of the following?
	Hypercalcemia
	Hyponatremia
	Hyperglycemia
	Constipation
	Increased intracranial pressure
	Oral cavity infection
Influencing host factors	Age (less than 50 years of age) and gender (females)?
	Negative past experiences with nausea and vomiting?
	History of motion sickness or feeling of warmth during or after previous chemotherapy?
	Alcohol naïve and high anxiety?

Data from Marchioro G, Azzarello G, Viviani F, et al: *Oncology* 59(2):100-104, 2000; Grant M, Kravitz K: *Semin Oncol Nurs* 16(2):113-121, 2000; Eckert RM: Understanding anticipatory nausea, *Oncol Nurs Forum* 28(10), 2001 (online serial): www.ons.org/publications/journals/ONF/Volume28/Issue10/28101553.asp#top.

(weekly weight)? Are there signs of dehydration? If so, electrolytes should be assessed. And are the symptoms interfering with the patient's quality of life? A thorough assessment along with timely interventions can assist in maintaining a patient on the treatment course. Older patients may require more frequent monitoring.[18] The treatment plan and the side effects from the medications could influence efficacy and safety in the elderly population and, therefore, need to be part of the ongoing assessment.[19]

The best way to obtain the above information is by encouraging the patient and/or care provider to keep a diary or log of the patient's experience. Many diary formats exist related to the chemotherapy experience that could easily be adapted for those undergoing radiation. One example is the MAT antiemesis tool developed by the Multinational Association of Supportive Care in Cancer.[20] This tool can be used by the nurse not only to determine an individual patient's status but also to track outcomes in subgroups of patients receiving this type of treatment. This tool uses a 0 to 10 visual analog scale similar to the one used for pain assessment.

The National Cancer Institute (NCI) toxicity grading scale grades nausea and vomiting independently on scales of 1 to 5 (Table 34-3).[21] Many facilities use a modified NCI scale that fits with the culture, policies, and procedures of their particular organization. For example, Moore and Knobf[22] use a 0 to 3 scale for nausea where 0 = none, 1 = mild, 2 = moderate, and 3 = severe. Vomiting is assessed according to the number of episodes experienced in a 24-hour period. Relief is graded as acceptable or unacceptable. It is clear that only one grading scale should be used at a facility by both radiation oncologists and nurses to allow for clear communication about the patient's status. It is important that assessments continue posttreatment because the side effects may continue for several weeks after treatment has been completed.

Management

There is very little research that has evaluated antiemetics for RINV, and oncology practitioners generally assume that antiemetics useful for N&V from chemotherapy—particularly serotonin (5-HT_3) antagonists and dopamine (D_2) antagonists—will be similarly helpful for RINV. Ondansetron (Zofran) and granisetron (Kytril) are the 5-HT_3 antagonists available in the United States that have been studied for RINV. Both are available in oral and IV formulations and are generally well tolerated. A major adverse effect of 5-HT_3 antagonists, particularly when they are taken for many days in a row, is constipation. Unmanaged constipation can progress to obstipation, severe discomfort, and increasing nausea. Metoclopramide, which has 5-HT_3-antagonistic and D_2 antagonist effects, is another useful antiemetic for RINV. Phenothiazines, such as prochlorperazine (Compazine), are also D_2 antagonists that **may** successfully counter RINV. Dexamethasone has been used as an antiemetic for chemotherapy and postanesthesia N&V and is also useful in patients at high risk for RINV, such as those receiving RT to the upper abdomen.[23]

According to the current standard of care, it is unacceptable to *not* treat RINV with effective antiemetics.[24] Nurses can be patient advocates by recog-

Table 34-3 NCI Common Toxicity Criteria for Nausea and Vomiting

	Grade			
	1	2	3	4
Nausea	Loss of appetite without alteration in eating habits	Oral intake decreased without significant weight loss, dehydration or malnutrition; IV fluids indicated for <24 hours	Inadequate oral caloric or fluid intake; IV fluids, tube feeding, or TPN indicated for >24 hours	Life threatening consequences
Vomiting	1 episode in 24 hours	2–5 episodes in 24 hours; IV fluids indicated for <24 hours	>6 episodes in 24 hours; IV fluids or TPN indicated for >24 hours	Life threatening consequences

Adverse Events: Nausea; Vomiting. Modified based on Cancer Therapy Evaluation Program, National Cancer Institute Common Terminology Criteria for Adverse Events v3, DCTD, NCI, NIH, DHHS. June 10, 2003, NIH Publication #03-5410. http://ctep.cancer.gov/reporting/ctc.html.

nizing high-risk individuals, particularly those undergoing TBI or RT to the chest or abdomen. The current published guidelines classify the likelihood of RINV from minimal to high RT according to site treated (see Table 34-1).[9,21] However, these classification schemas do not consider patient risk factors,[25] which could increase overall risk in given patients. The most detailed guideline for RINV has been published by the National Comprehensive Cancer Network (NCCN), an alliance of 19 cancer centers in the United States, which recommends prophylaxis for patients receiving TBI or RT to the upper abdomen, as well as those receiving chemotherapy with RT.[21]

DIARRHEA

Diarrhea, like N&V, is a cancer treatment–induced symptom with potential to dramatically affect activities of daily living, physiologic and emotional well-being. The consequences of unrecognized and undertreated diarrhea are numerous; key physical consequences include dehydration, electrolyte disturbances, altered skin integrity, intestinal hemorrhage, proctitis and anal or rectal fissuring, malnutrition, abdominal pain and discomfort, impaired sleep patterns, and decreased performance levels. Emotional consequences can affect both patient and family members; these include anxiety and fear, altered body image and subsequent social isolation, perceived loss of personal control, diminished self-esteem, disrupted personal relationships, altered role function, and caregiver burden.[2,26-29]

Though it may be life-threatening and can significantly impair quality of life, cancer treatment–induced diarrhea (CTID) has received surprisingly little attention in the clinical literature and, with the exception of radiation nurses, given little attention by the oncology nursing community. In a rare study of nursing perceptions, knowledge, and skills related to CTID, of 1288 oncology nurses surveyed about their clinical practice experiences with disease and treatment-related diarrhea, radiation oncology nurses perceived radiation therapy as being more influential as a cause of diarrhea in their patients than did nurses from all other practice settings ($n = 93$; $p < 0.001$). This finding suggests that oncology nurses who care for patients undergoing radiation therapy, but who do not subspecialize in radiation oncology may need information about radiation-induced diarrhea and the impact of combined modality therapy in their patients.[6] Radiation oncology nurses can be instrumental in providing that education to their colleagues and to patients and their families.

Definitions and Presentation

Diarrhea is a complex clinical consequence of RT that may be acute or chronic in nature and is heightened in patients who undergo multimodal therapies or who are experiencing comorbid conditions. In general, diarrhea is defined as an abnormal increase in stool liquidity and frequency. Stools considered diagnostic for diarrhea:

- Weigh more than 200 g
- Contain 70% to 90% water
- Occur in volumes greater than 300 mL and/or
- Occur more frequently than two to three per day

Diarrhea has also been simply described as stool that conforms to the shape of its container.[2,30] Because bowel patterns can vary significantly among individuals, it has been suggested that the definition be broadened to state that stool losses must be significant enough to constitute a change in the patient's normal bowel habits in order to be classified as diarrhea.[31-33]

Radiation therapy–induced diarrhea (RTID) presents as high frequency stooling (more than 6 episodes/day) with stool volume that, although variable, is generally less than 1 liter/day. RTID is typically associated with anemia and hypoalbuminemia resulting from cumulative blood and protein losses through the bowel wall.[2,26,27] Patients experiencing RTID also can present with anorexia, nausea and vomiting, abdominal cramping, tenesmus, and rectal bleeding.[34]

RTID can present early (within hours of initial treatment), shortly after therapy has been initiated (2 to 3 weeks) or late (months to years after therapy).[34] Onset varies from patient to patient, but generally begins after a total dose in the range of 10 Gy to 30 Gy. Patients receiving 35 Gy to 50 Gy can develop injury to the small intestine resulting in severe diarrhea unresponsive to dietary and pharmacologic interventions.[32,35,36]

Risk Factors

RTID is reported to occur in 50% to 70% of patients undergoing pelvic radiation, with 18% to 20% of patients experiencing diarrhea at grade 3 to 4 severity levels. The addition of chemotherapy, particularly fluoropyrimidines and topoisomerase inhibitors, to RT increases both incidence rates (i.e., 60% to 80%) and severity levels (i.e., 35% grade 3 or higher).[4,37,38] Other factors that can potentially increase diarrhea risk and severity include radiation dosage and type of radiation techniques including the fractionation schedule.[1] Reported incidence of peri- and posttreatment diarrhea in patients undergoing abdominoperineal radiation is 20% to 49%.[6] Incidence and severity are directly related to the radiation dose rate and the volume of bowel in the radiation field. Whole abdomen and full pelvis fields are most often associated with diarrhea.[36] Comorbidities such as a history of colitis, ileitis, irritable bowel syndrome, or previous abdominal surgeries heightened risk of diarrhea occurrence and severity and the probability that symptoms will occur at lower dose rates.[2,36]

Chronic ischemic radiation enteritis, occurring in 5% to 15% of patients undergoing abdominoperineal radiation, has a median onset of 8 to 12 months and may occur as late as 15 years after radiation.[1] This late effect is the result of mucosal atrophy, fibrosis, and vascular insufficiency secondary to damaged endothelial cells in the blood vessels and connective tissues. These changes ultimately produce osmotic and/or malabsorptive types of diarrhea.[26,27,32,35,39,40] The dose-limiting structure with abdominopelvic radiation is the small intestine because it is the most sensitive to late radiation effects.[41]

Overall morbidities associated with neoadjuvant and adjuvant chemoradiotherapy in patients treated for rectal cancer are significant and include small bowel obstruction (5% to 10%), radiation enteritis (4%) and rectal stricture formation (5%).[42] In one study (n = 100), patients treated with postoperative adjuvant chemoradiotherapy for stages B2 and C rectal carcinoma were surveyed 2 to 5 years after treatment to determine patterns of long-term effects on bowel function. The chemoradiotherapy group had more frequent bowel activity and symptoms than did the untreated group including bowel movements per day (median 7 versus median 2, $p < 0.001$); clustering of bowel movements (42% versus 3%, $p < 0.001$), nighttime movements (46% versus 14%, $p < 0.001$), fecal incontinence (17% versus 0%, $p < 0.001$), wore an incontinent pad (41% versus 10%, $p < 0.001$) and were unable to defer defecation for more than 15 minutes (78% versus 19%, $p < 0.001$). In addition, the treated group had stool of liquid consistency, regularly used antidiarrheal medications, had perianal skin irritations, were unable to differentiate stool from gas, and needed to repeat defecation within 30 minutes of a bowel movement.[43] In another study (n = 171) patients who had undergone curative high dose (5 × 5 Gy) preoperative radiation therapy, fecal incontinence, urgency, and emptying difficulties were all higher in the treated group for at least 5 years posttreatment. Further, 30% of the treated group reported experiencing impaired social life secondary to bowel dysfunction versus 10% of patients undergoing surgery alone.[44]

The effects of pelvic radiation therapy on bowel, bladder, and sexual functioning in patients treated for prostate cancer were evaluated using a confidential questionnaire (n = 192). Moderate alterations in bowel function were reported by 25% of respondents whereas 11% reported severe changes. The most frequent complication related to bowel function noted by respondents was rectal urgency (20%). No correlation between technical factors such as treatment volumes and total dose rate and symptom severity could be documented.[45]

Pathophysiology

Two principal mechanisms ensure the balanced transport of intestinal fluid and electrolytes: (1) *secretion* that takes place in the crypt cells and (2) *absorption* that occurs in the enterocytes lining the intestinal villi. Changes in one or both of these mechanisms can disrupt the ratio between intestinal secretion and absorption. Diarrhea results when the total secretion of fluid and electrolytes overwhelms the absorptive capacity of the bowel.[2,3,36]

CTID is categorized according to discrete pathophysiologic mechanisms and clinical presentations (Table 34-4). Acute RTID is classified as *exudative* or *inflammatory diarrhea,* which is characterized by the discharge of mucus, serum proteins, and blood in the bowel lumen resulting from radiation injury.[2,26,27,33,36] Other types of diarrhea experienced by patients after radiation therapy are a result of concomitant treatments or malignant disease and include osmotic, malabsorptive, and dysmotility-associated diarrhea. Accurate categorization of the underlying causes of and mechanisms responsible for producing diarrhea is essential to formulating effective treatment recommendations but is difficult because these etiologies overlap in patients with cancer.[26,27]

Table 34-4 Types of Diarrhea, Pathophysiologic Mechanisms, Etiologies, and Clinical Presentations

Type of diarrhea	Pathophysiologic mechanisms	Etiologies	Clinical presentation
Osmotic	Mechanical disturbance Characterized by large volume influx of fluid and electrolytes into intestinal lumen, which overwhelms absorptive capacity of bowel Osmotic forces responsible for drawing substrates across the intestinal epithelium are interrupted by direct contact with hyperosmolar stimuli	*Ingestion of hyperosmolar preparations and substances:* *Nonabsorbable solutes* (sorbitol, magnesium-based antacids, etc) *Enteral feeding solutions* *Intestinal hemorrhage:* Intraluminal blood acts as an osmotic substance	Large watery stools that resolve when the causative agent is withdrawn
Malabsorptive	Combined disturbance of mechanical and biochemical mechanisms responsible for mediating the absorptive process Secondary to factors that alter luminal and mucosal integrity and nature; ↓ in available mucosa or membrane permeability disrupts enterohepatic circulation of bile salts; unabsorbed osmotically active substances can then enter the colon and exert direct bowel stimulatory effects	*Enzyme deficiencies* that prevent complete digestion of fats: *Lactose intolerance* *Pancreatic insufficiency* 2° to obstruction by cancer or pancreatectomy *Morphologic/structural changes* resulting in ↓ absorptive capacity *Surgical resection* of intestine *Mucosal changes* that alter membrane permeability	Large volume, foul-smelling steatorrheic stools
Secretory	Primarily biochemical disturbance with mechanical responses. Characterized by intestinal hypersecretion stimulated by an array of endogenous mediators that exert a primary effect on intestinal transport of water and electrolytes resulting in an accumulation of intestinal fluids	*Endocrine tumors* can produce excessive quantities of peptide secretagogues VIPoma, carcinoid gastrinoma, insulinoma, glucagonoma *Enterotoxin-producing pathogens* irritate bowel wall thus stimulating intestinal secretion Associated with antibiotic-induced change in the microbial flora that permit growth of *Clostridium difficile* *Acute intestinal GVHD:* Mucosal damage stimulates the release of hormones; thus volume of diarrhea corresponds to extent of damage *Short gut syndrome* has both malabsorptive and secretory components	Large volume watery stool (> 1000 cc/day) that persists despite fasting; osmolality equals plasma concentration

Table 34-4 Types of Diarrhea, Pathophysiologic Mechanisms, Etiologies, and Clinical Presentations—cont'd

Type of diarrhea	Pathophysiologic mechanisms	Etiologies	Clinical presentation
Exudative	Characterized by the discharge of mucus, serum protein, and blood into the bowel; associated with hypoalbuminemia and anemia Occurs in response to inflammation and ulceration of the bowel mucosa	*Radiation to bowel mucosa:* Incidence and severity dose dependent; acute effects due to depletion of crypt stem cells whereas late or chronic radiation enteritis is 2° to mucosal atrophy and fibrosis *Opportunistic infection:* Bacteria (e.g., normal flora) invade altered bowel mucosa; neutropenic typhlitis an extension of this process in which intramural infection leads to edema, bowel thickening, possible perforation	Variable volume (< 1000 mL/day) but high frequency (> 6 stools/day) stooling associated with hypoalbuminemia and anemia from cumulative protein and blood loss
Dysmotility-associated	Mechanical disturbance characterized by deranged intestinal motility resulting in rapid transit of stool through the small and large intestine Peristaltic dysfunction (enhancement or suppression) in response to alterations in a variety of mechanical stretch or neural stimuli	*Clinical problems* such as irritable bowel syndrome or narcotic withdrawal syndrome *External factors* such as ingestion of peristaltic stimulants (food, fluid, or medication) or psychoneuroimmunologic effects of stress, anxiety, and fear	Frequent small semisolid to liquid stools of variable volume and frequency
Chemotherapy-induced	Combination of mechanical and biochemical disturbances stimulated by chemotherapeutic effects on the bowel mucosa Characterized by cascade of events beginning with mitotic arrest of intestinal epithelial crypt cells, followed by superficial necrosis and extensive inflammation of the bowel wall; resulting in production of mucosal and submucosal factors (leukotrienes, cytokines, free radicals), which subsequently stimulate the oversecretion of intestinal water and electrolytes; destruction of brush border enzymes responsible for carbohydrate and protein digestion further contributes to excess gut wall secretion; the influx of fluid overwhelms the absorptive capacity of the bowel resulting in diarrhea	*Chemotherapy-induced gut wall toxicity*; although an array of agents are associated with diarrhea, the most common agents include: Fluoropyrimidines (e.g., 5-fluorouracil) Topoisomerase inhibitors (e.g., CPT-11)	Frequent watery to semisolid stools with onset occurring within 24 to 96 hours post-chemotherapy administration

From Rutledge D, Engelking C: Cancer-related diarrhea: selected findings of a national survey of oncology nurse experiences, *Oncol Nurse Forum* 5: 861-873, 1998.

Radiation produces inflammatory changes in the bowel wall that can progress to microulcerations, which eventually coalesce into larger lesions that disrupt the intestinal mucosal lining. Specific morphologic changes in the mucosa include sloughing and denuding of the epithelial surface and shortening of intestinal villi; these effects reduce absorptive capacity by decreasing the total mucosal surface area available for the balanced transport of fluid and electrolytes.[2,33] Acute radiation-induced enterocolitis results from depletion of mitotically active intestinal crypt stem cell (crypt cells are responsible for epithelial cellular replacement). In contrast, late or chronic enteritis is produced by atrophy of the mucosa induced by injury to less mitotically active vascular endothelial and connective tissue cells.[33]

Injury to capillary endothelium interferes with blood supply to the mucosa, further contributing to mucosal disruption and presenting risk for invasion by intestinal microbes and sepsis. Suspending or reducing radiation when symptoms become significant is warranted to prevent life-threatening effects. Crypt mitosis returns to normal within 3 days. However, complete histologic recovery can takes as long as 6 months.[34]

Chronic effects usually manifest after 6 to 24 months and are caused mostly by obliterative arteritis and thromboses of vessels; the result is ischemia or necrosis. Malabsorption of fats, carbohydrates, and protein each play a role in the production of postradiation diarrhea. Fat malabsorption reduces bile salt absorption in the terminal ileum, thus leading to the inhibition of water reabsorption and heightened peristalsis.[33,41]

Prevention and Management

Patient Assessment

Establishing an effective diarrhea management plan requires a comprehensive patient history to ascertain risk factors for RTID occurrence and severity, development of a clear picture of the current clinical presentation, and a focused physical examination. History taking should include questions that (1) elucidate past and current medical conditions or treatments that could influence bowel function, (2) establish baseline bowel elimination pattern and function, and (3) profile currently altered bowel pattern. Specific parameters for history taking are outlined in Table 34-5.

Criteria for the optimal assessment of diarrhea include stool consistency grading using graphic illustrations if possible, measuring liquid stool by volume rather than episodes, onset and duration of diarrhea in relation to potential causative factors, identification of accompanying symptoms, presence of perianal or peristomal skin impairment graded according to severity, patient report of self-care interventions and their efficacy, and the effect of diarrhea on patient performance levels and functional ability. Incorporating these parameters into an expanded assessment help to develop a clearer picture of the patient's diarrhea experience.[2,46] Although the NCI Common Toxicity Criteria for diarrhea (Table 34-6) is a useful and commonly used tool for grading diarrhea severity, a number of these parameters are not included in this grading scale.[20,46]

Additional tools for measurement and characterization of diarrhea rely heavily on clinician interpretation of patient self-report (Box 34-1).

Focused physical examination should include auscultation for bowel sounds (i.e., normal, hyperactive, or absent), abdominal palpation, and rectal examination to rule out fecal impaction and obstruc-

Box 34-1 Additional Diarrhea Assessment Tools

- *Diarrhea Self-Report Questionnaire:* A three-part self-report questionnaire addressing stool form (consistency) with pictorial grading across six categories, stool frequency, and diarrhea morbidity grading from the patient's perspective and including a scoring technique.[56]
- *Bowel Movement Consistency Schema:* A continence history tool that includes a 10-point pictorial scale with stool consistency graphics ranging from "watery" to "hard and dry."[57]
- *Incontinence Scoring System:* A scoring schema addressing the type and frequency of incontinent episodes and the impact of incontinence on lifestyle.[58]
- *Functional Alterations due to Changes in Elimination (FACE):* A 15-item Likert-type self-rating scale designed to measure intrusion on daily functioning caused by changes in elimination as measured by two subscales (changes in urinary function and changes in bowel function).[41]
- *Cognitive Scale for Functional Bowel Disorders:* A 25-item scale examining psychosocial factors associated with functional bowel disorders.[59]

Table 34-5 Diarrhea Risk Assessment

Risk factors	Cue questions
Usual patterns	Normal bowel elimination pattern and stool character (e.g., defecation frequency and timing, stool consistency)? Normal dietary pattern and habits (e.g., eating schedule and food types)? Usual fluid intake pattern (e.g., volume and schedule)? Factors that typically influence bowel pattern?
Past history	Had previous abdominopelvic surgery; bowel resection with or without diversion? *If yes,* how much and which segment of bowel resected? Had previous diarrhea-inducing cancer therapies (e.g., concurrent chemoradiotherapy with fluoropyrimidines or topoisomerase inhibitor, use of selected cytoprotectants, chemotherapy, and high radiation dosage levels, large volume radiation field and location)? Pattern of using laxatives and other over-the-counter medications including use of herbal remedies and botanicals? History of recent travel outside of the country or family members with diarrhea?
Comorbid conditions	Preexisting bowel conditions such as irritable or inflammatory bowel syndromes (colitis, diverticulosis, lactose intolerance) Presence of abdominal or gastrointestinal tumor associated with hormonal hypersecretion (e.g., VIPoma), gastric enzyme production, or impairment of bowel function (e.g., colorectal or other abdominal tumor)? *If yes,* what are specific tumor locations (e.g., primary and metastatic sites)?
Planned therapy	Anticipated plan for supportive care plan that may induce or exaggerate diarrhea (e.g., nutritional support products, antibiotic therapy)?
Clinical manifestations	Recent change in pattern of bowel function, stool frequency, or character (e.g., frequency, amount, character, time of day, incontinence)? Onset and duration of diarrhea; response to home remedies or prescribed medication/treatment plan; aggravating and alleviating factors? Presence of associated abdominal pain or cramping (intermittent or continuous and intensity)? Presence of other coexisting signs and symptoms (e.g., fever, flatus, incontinence, urgency, nocturnal stool, dehydration)?

Data from Engelking C: Diarrhea. In Yarbro CJ, Frogge MH, Goodman M, editors: *Cancer symptom management,* ed 3, Boston, 2004, Jones and Bartlett, pp 528-557; Kornblau S, Benson AB, Catalano R, et al: *J Pain Symptom Manage* 19(2):118-129, 2000.

Table 34-6 NCI Common Toxicity Criteria for Diarrhea

	Grade			
	1	2	3	4
Diarrhea without colostomy	Increase of <4 stools/day over pretreatment	Increase of 4–6 stools/day, or nocturnal stools	Increase of ≥7 stools/day or incontinence; or need for parenteral support for dehydration	Physiologic consequences requiring intensive care; or hemodynamic collapse
Diarrhea with colostomy	Mild increase in loose, watery colostomy output compared with pretreatment	Moderate increase in loose, watery colostomy output compared with pretreatment, but not interfering with normal activity	Severe increase in loose, watery colostomy output compared with pretreatment, interfering with normal activity	Physiologic consequences, requiring intensive care; or hemodynamic collapse

Adverse Events: Diarrhea. Modified based on Cancer Therapy Evaluation Program, Common Terminology Criteria for Adverse Events v3.0, DCTD, NCI, NIH, DHHS. June 10, 2003, NIH Publication #03-5410. http://ctep.cancer.gov/reporting/ctc.html.

tion. Determination of hydration status (e.g., thirst level, vein filling and emptying times, skin turgor and resiliency, degree of mucosal moisture, intake and output comparisons, urine specific gravity and osmolality, orthostatic blood pressure, weight) is critical to identifying and preventing progression of dehydration and electrolyte imbalances to severe levels. Stools must be inspected visually to ascertain consistency, color, odor, and presence of blood, mucus, or pus. Perianal and peristomal areas also must be inspected to identify disruptions in skin integrity and the presence of hemorrhoids or proctitis.

Laboratory and diagnostic evaluation should be employed from least to most invasive testing with a primary focus on using objective measures to distinguish between infectious and noninfectious etiologies for diarrhea. Complete blood count will help to rule out infection and determine the effect of bleeding. Serum chemistry profile will identify electrolyte abnormalities and help to establish the severity of dehydration and protein/calorie malnutrition (i.e., hypoalbuminemia). Stool analyses should be employed to rule out infectious causes (e.g., presence of blood, fecal leukocytes, bacteria such as *Clostridium difficile*, ova and parasites). Radiographic examination, endoscopic exploration, and biopsy are more invasive and should be reserved for clinical situations in which diarrhea is persistent and refractory to antidiarrheal interventions or to rule out conditions requiring tissue diagnosis (e.g., GVHD).[2,36]

Indicators useful in determining whether diarrhea is acute or chronic are not well established although these categories are associated with time dimensions, relief patterns, severity, impact on functionality and quality of life, and patient population.

The multifactorial nature of diarrhea and the tendency of patients to underreport its occurrence produce numerous challenges to accurate measurement of the experience and the effect of diarrhea management interventions. Existing instruments tend to be simple, superficial, and unidimensional. They neither take into account the broad impact of this clinical problem on physical and psychosocial well-being of patients nor target the evaluation to a patient's unique characteristics (which determine feasibility of available management approaches and have bearing on overall outcomes). Defining the experience, distinguishing among causative factors, and determining whether it is an acute or chronic phenomenon are the most difficult assessment challenges to be overcome. Radiation oncology nurses can be instrumental in addressing this issue by using available tools and developing and testing new tools that have relevance to their practice settings.[26,27,36]

Management

An array of traditional pharmacologic and nonpharmacologic interventions are available to manage RTID. Some newer approaches involve novel applications of traditional drugs, pretreatment preventive regimens, and multiagent combination regimens; innovative supportive care strategies also are reported. However, there is limited definitive scientific evidence to support many of these management approaches, and practice standards are only beginning to emerge. In the absence of data, anecdotal observations have led to integration of these interventions into routine clinical care rendering them "state-of-the-art" management.[26,27,36]

There are no published standards of care for RTID management. Most recently, however, general CTID clinical practice guidelines have been recommended by a special panel of clinicians (Figure 34-1). These guidelines are organized to offer management options based on whether diarrhea is uncomplicated (grades 1 to 2 without complicating signs or symptoms) or complicated (grades 3 to 4 or grades 1-2 with one or more complicating signs or symptoms such as cramping, nausea and vomiting, decreased performance status, fever with or without sepsis, neutropenia, frank bleeding, and dehydration). The guidelines mention RT as well as chemotherapy and include assessment parameters and pharmacologic and nonpharmacologic interventions.[4]

Pharmacologic Management

Key agents used for diarrhea management include intraluminal agents, intestinal transit inhibitors, antisecretory agents, and ammonium resins (Table 34-7). Patients with uncomplicated RTID, regardless of its etiology (i.e., either chemotherapy or radiation therapy), are managed on an outpatient basis with standard doses of loperamide and dietary modification until resolution of diarrhea. Second-line agents may be trialed in those patients who are refractory to loperamide. Dietary modification, rehydration, and oral antibiotics are prescribed on an as required basis. Hospitalization, parenteral fluids, and antibiotics and octreotide are recommended for patients with complicated diarrhea.

The current gold standard for management of RTID is synthetic opioids; the most commonly prescribed are loperamide (Lomotil) and diphenoxylate (Imodium). These agents act by binding to opiate receptors in the smooth muscle of both small and large intestine to increase tone and decrease motility, resulting in enhanced fluid absorption. Loperamide is superior to diphenoxylate in both safety and efficacy, is inexpensive, and readily available in community pharmacies. A small randomized clinical trial (n = 61) conducted in patients experiencing grades 2 to 3 diarrhea found octreotide (100 mcg tid) to be significantly more effective than diphenoxylate (10 mg/day) with diarrhea resolving within 3 days in 61% of patients versus 14% of patients treated with diphenoxylate.[47] However, octreotide requires injection and is considerably more expensive than the oral synthetic opioids, but may be an option for those patients refractory to the opioids.

Other antidiarrheal agents from a variety of drug classes also have been used to prevent or manage RTID, including nonsteroidal antiinflammatory agents, ammonium resins, glucocorticoids, thiols, salicylates, and sucralfate. Many of these pharmacologic interventions are under investigation. Sucralfate and the salicylates have been a focus of prevention studies in the recent past. Sucralfate has previously been considered effective in ameliorating diarrhea during pelvic irradiation, but recent conflicting data has raised questions about its use. In one double-blind randomized trial, dose granules of sucralfate or placebo were administered 2 weeks after radiation and continued for a 6-week period. Patients receiving sucralfate experienced fewer problems with acute and chronic bowel distress and had lower loperamide consumption than did the placebo group without adverse effects.[48] In contrast, the results of a more recent randomized study of patients receiving pelvic radiation demonstrated that compared to placebo, patients in the sucralfate-treated group (n = 123) experienced moderate to severe diarrhea more frequently (53% versus 41%), had more fecal incontinence (34% versus 16%), and required protective clothing more often (23% versus 8%). In addition, the occurrence and severity of nausea and vomiting was higher in those who were treated with sucralfate.[37] The rationale for application of salicylates is based on the theory that prostaglandin release plays a role in producing RTID. Benson and colleagues[4] recommend that sulfasalazine should be used only within the context of a clinical trial, and further state that there is currently no scientific evidence to support preventive measures for RTID. More study will be necessary to resolve these debates and identify effective prophylaxis for RTID.

Nonpharmacologic Management

Drug therapy alone is rarely sufficient to completely eradicate RTID; nonpharmacologic interventions must accompany antidiarrheal medications to maximize effectiveness of the management plan. Incorporating a variety of supportive care interventions and customizing those interventions to the individual will speed restoration of and help to maintain patients' usual bowel elimination patterns while at the same time providing for patient safety, comfort, and dignity.

Fluid and electrolyte replacement will maintain homeostasis when diarrhea is severe enough to produce significant fluid loss (more than 1 L unreplaced) and the patient is exhibiting indicators of electrolyte imbalance, in particular hypokalemia and hypomagnesemia. Oral rehydration solutions (e.g., Pedialyte, Gatorade) are effective for patients who can tolerate oral intake. Those replacing fluids orally should be instructed to vary the type of fluids ingested to avoid water intoxication. For patients exhibiting indicators of obstruction (e.g., vomiting, toxic fluid volume deficit) or cannot tolerate high-volume intake of glucose-electrolyte solutions, parenteral replacement in hospital, radiation, or infusion center is appropriate.[1,36]

Dietary modifications are directed at stopping diarrhea or, when that is not feasible, reducing its severity. Dietary intake should be modified to be:

- Low residue (i.e., avoidance of fresh raw vegetables, dried legumes, whole grain breads and cereals, nuts, high-fat spreads or dressings, fried or fatty meats, candied fruits or coconut)
- Low lactose or lactose-free (i.e., no diary products including milk, cheese, butter, yogurt, ice cream)
- Low in fat content (i.e., excludes oily or fried foods and rich desserts)
- High in foods that will build stool consistency (i.e., rice, pectin-containing foods)
- Free of bowel irritants (caffeine-containing food and fluids—coffee, tea, or alcohol; pickles and relishes; chocolate; spicy or rough foods).

One randomized trial evaluated the health-related quality of life effects of a low-fat and low-lactose diet on women undergoing pelvic

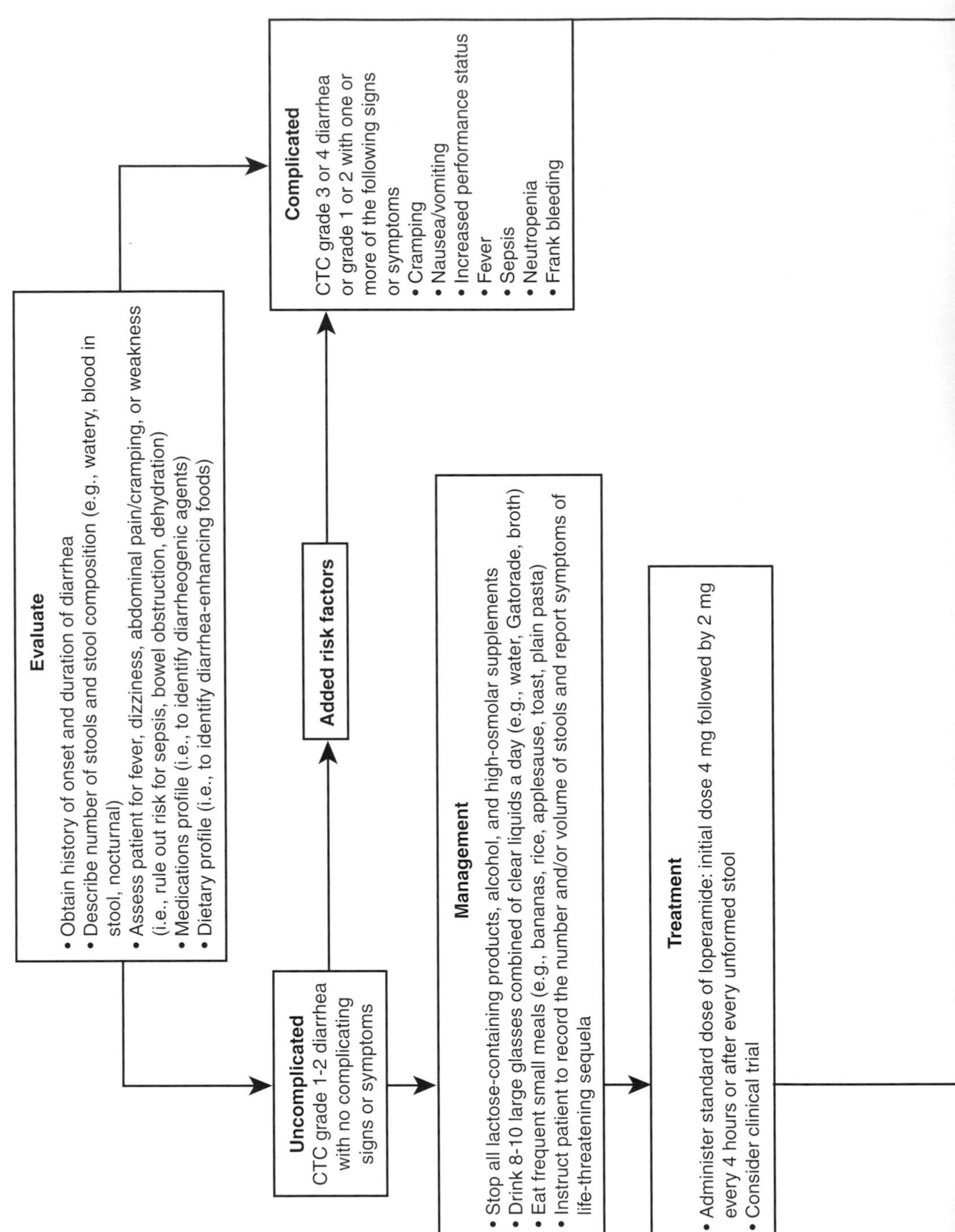

Figure 34-1 Guidelines for Managing Diarrhea Caused by Cancer Treatment.
From Benson AB, Ajani JA, Catalano RB, et al: J Clin Oncol 22(17):2918-2926, 2004.

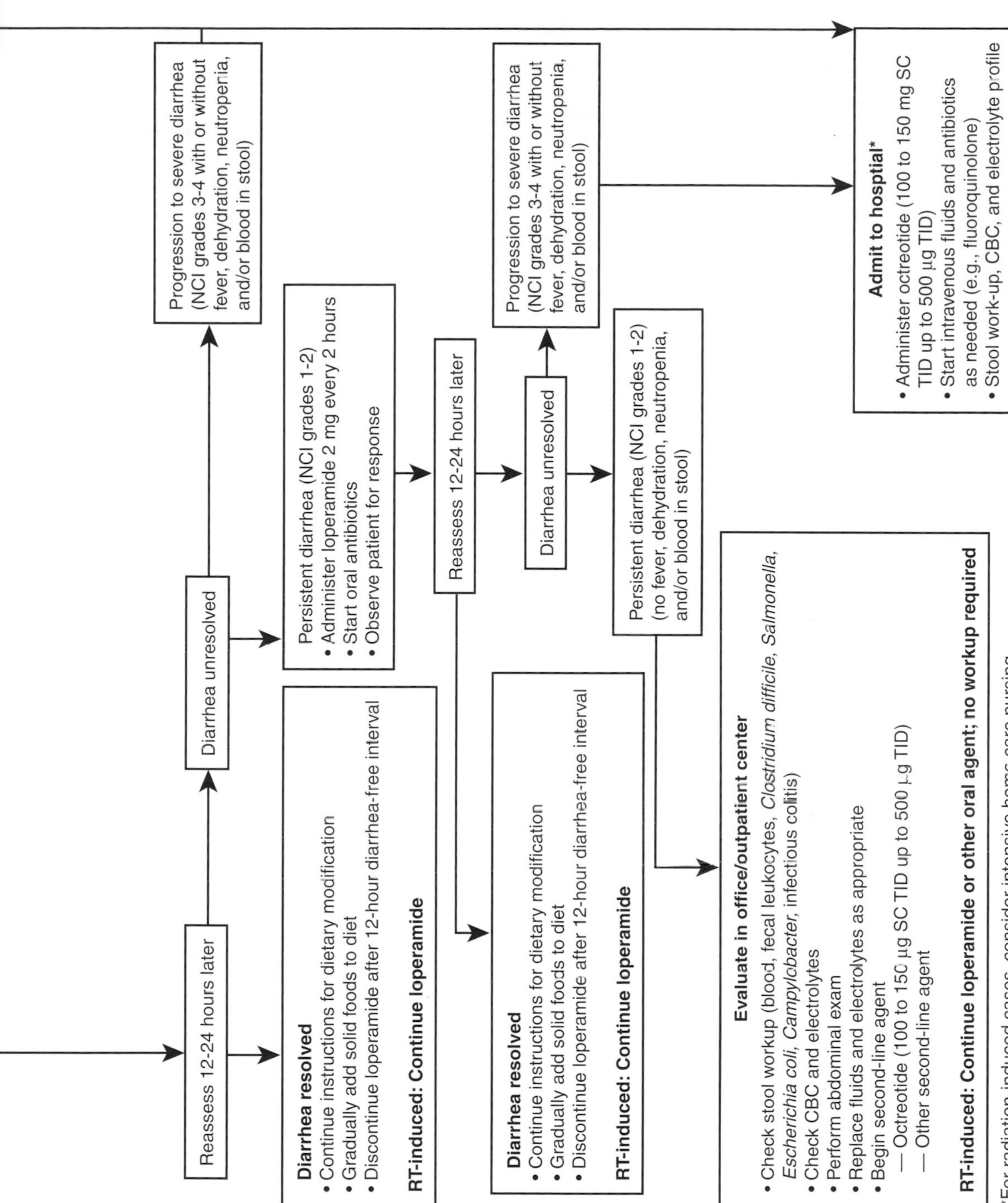

*For radiation-induced cases, consider intensive home care nursing

Table 34-7 Pharmacologic Options for Radiation-Induced Diarrhea

Drug class	Agents	Mechanism	Comment
INTRALUMINAL AGENTS			
Adsorbents	Clays, activated charcoal, cholestyramine, mucilloid preparations	Control diarrhea mechanically by forming stool bulk, absorbing water, producing a protective barrier between luminal contents and intestinal wall	Common over-the-counter antidiarrheal agents Agents are difficult to ingest, can create uncomfortable bloating sensations Have limited efficacy in controlling persistent or moderate-to-severe diarrhea
Absorbents	Psyllium derivatives, kaolin and pectate, bismuth		
INTESTINAL TRANSIT INHIBITORS			
Anticholinergics	Atropine sulfate, scopolamine, belladonna preparations	Act as local antispasmodics to provide temporary reduction in gastric secretion and peristalsis	Effective for painful cramping with diarrhea but side effects (blurred vision, urinary retention, and mucosal drying) that are uncomfortable and limit performance
Opiate agonists	Synthetic: Loperamide, diphenoxylate Traditional: Paregoric, codeine, tincture of opium	Bind smooth muscle of bowel slowing intestinal motility and increasing fluid absorption	Synthetic opioids current gold standard; loperamide considered most efficacious and better tolerated Diphenoxylate is a meperidine congener associated with more CNS side effects and is not recommended for children under 12 years or in patients with advanced liver disease; reserved for special clinical situations such as refractory diarrhea or when patients are experiencing pain and could benefit Traditional opioids associated with undesirable side effects including sedation, constipation; can serve as second-line therapy
ANTISECRETORY AGENTS			
Synthetic somatostatin analogue	Octreotide acetate	Prolongs intestinal transit time by up to fourfold increase and regulates intestinal water and electrolyte transport by inhibiting gastrointestinal secretogogues responsible for altering transport and absorption balance	Available as short- or long-acting subcutaneous or intravenous formulations Expensive agent when administered on an outpatient basis; should be reserved for special clinical situations (refractory diarrhea, TBI, or GVHD-associated diarrhea)

Table 34-7 Pharmacologic Options for Radiation-Induced Diarrhea—cont'd

Drug class	Agents	Mechanism	Comment
Glucocorticoids		Exert antisecretory effect on intracellular proteins that inhibit action of certain enzymes blocking release of transmitter substances that stimulate secretogogues implicated in diarrhea production after bowel wall injury	
Ammonium resin	Cholestyramine	Minimizes choleric diarrhea (i.e., caused by passage of unreabsorbed bile salts into the colon) by binding bile salts in the terminal ileum before they pass through to the colon	Inhibits absorption of many drugs interfering with other aspects of the patient's treatment plan; can result in constipation and phenylketonuria

Data from Engelking C: Diarrhea. In Yarbro CJ, Frogge MH, Goodman M, editors: *Cancer symptom management,* ed 3, Boston, 2004, Jones and Bartlett, pp 528-557; Benson AB, Ajani JA, Catalano RB, et al: *J Clin Oncol* 22(14):2918-2926, 2004; Cascinu S: *Crit Rev Oncol Hematol* 18(1):37-50, 1995; Engelking C, Sauerland C: Maintenance of normal elimination. In Watkins-Bruner D, Moore-Higgins G, Haas M, editors: *Outcomes in radiation therapy,* Boston, 2001, Jones and Bartlett, pp 530-562; Dow K, Hilderly KL, editors: *Nursing care in radiation oncology,* Philadelphia, 1992, WB Saunders.

CNS, Central nervous system; *TBI,* total body irradiation; *GVHD,* graft-versus-host disease.

radiation therapy for gynecologic malignancy (n = 143) using the 36-item EORTC Core Quality of Life Questionnaire. Fewer women in the intervention group experienced diarrhea than in the control group (23% versus 48%; $p < 0.01$), and the dietary modification did not appear to interfere with emotional and social functioning.[49]

Skin care measures may be necessary to combat the causative effects of diarrhea. Liquid or diarrheal stools contain acids that can be irritating to exposed skin in perianal, peristomal, buttocks, and thighs. Repeated exposures to stool and the friction of wiping the area clean can result in irritation and excoriation. Treating the area with protective skin barriers such as petroleum jelly, desitin ointment, or other moisture barrier products can help to minimize skin impairment. Cleansing after each exposure is also important, but the area should be patted rather than rubbed dry, and when possible, periods of air-drying can be restorative.[2]

EDUCATING PATIENTS AND FAMILY MEMBERS

Providing accurate and pertinent information to enable self-management by patients and their family members is a critical role of oncology nurses.[50] Timely intervention to prevent treatment interruption and ensure completion of therapy is key to positive outcomes. Clarifying definitions and perceptions with patients and their caregivers as to what their perceptions are concerning what constitutes RINV and RTID and open discussion of their associated concerns, fears, and fantasies are important to developing management plans that will be effective and with which patients can easily comply.

The goal of patient education is to empower patients and their family with information that will allow personal control and a sense of support. Education plans need to be customized to the individual to encourage compliance and must encompass all possible risk factors, to ensure patient awareness of consequences of therapy and an understanding of how important it is to let staff know if they are having difficulty (even when they are in the low-risk category for symptoms).

Nausea and Vomiting

If the patient is at high or moderate risk of experiencing nausea, interventions should focus on prevention. The patient and/or caregiver need to understand the goal of the intervention and how the timing of medication administration will effect achievement of that goal. Because the oral route is preferred, antiemetics being administered as premedications must be taken at least 1 hour before treatment. Those using prn antiemetics to manage RINV associated with a particular pattern (i.e., onset of nausea 1 to 3 hours after treatment) also should be instructed to time the medication to achieve the best benefit. Patients should be instructed to keep well hydrated. If they have trouble drinking, Jell-o and frozen ices should be encouraged to maintain hydration. Eating small, frequent light meals also may be helpful. Ethnic/cultural influences have to be taken into consideration when reviewing eating and drinking habits and patterns. Helping the patient understand that changes to their dietary pattern could prevent or minimize the symptom is essential. Also important is exploring whether the patient knows traditional remedies they may use to treat nausea.

The addition of nonpharmacologic interventions to the plan, such as antianxiety activities such as relaxation and distraction techniques and acupuncture, also should be discussed with patients who indicate an interest in exploring these strategies.[51,52] Patients who report using these techniques in other dimensions of their lives are likely to be amenable and skilled at integrating these approaches. Exposure to fresh air also may be helpful.[16]

Diarrhea

Patients who are at risk of developing RTID should be informed of when to expect onset, so they can be prepared to implement the appropriate self-care measures. Currently, there are no reliable preventive measures. However, early intervention can help minimize diarrhea severity and duration and prevent secondary complications such as dehydration. Education should begin by arriving at a common definition of what constitutes diarrhea to set the stage for accurate communication about the symptom—among patient, caregiver, nurse, and physician. Patients need to be instructed on recording bowel activity, timing, frequency, consistency, and presence or absence of coexisting symptoms such as abdominal pain or fever, from the beginning of treatment so changes can be identified early. Reinforcing instructions regarding the discontinuation of diarrhea-producing medications during periods of RTID is critical, especially for older individuals who may routinely take laxatives or stool softeners.[53]

Patients and their caregivers need clear instruction on what, how much, and when to self-administer antidiarrheal agents. For example, antidiarrheals are often taken after each episode of diarrhea for a maximum number of tablets within a 24-hour period. Patients need to know when to start and stop the drug.

Nonpharmacologic interventions focus on dietary modifications, skin care, and stress reduction. Several dietary changes could help reduce the degree of diarrhea, such as serving foods and drinks at room temperature; instructing patients to avoid caffeinated drinks and spicy, fried, or fatty foods; eating low-fiber foods, and eating small, frequent meals.[54] Encouraging the consumption of foods high in pectin such as bananas, avocados, and plain applesauce,[55] also may be helpful. Daily hydration should be stressed. Hydrating liquids such as water, Gatorade, or bouillon or gelatin are encouraged.

Proper perineal skin care is imperative in preventing skin breakdown and decreasing the risk for more serious side effects such as infection. Nonalcohol-containing moist wipes or very soft toilet paper (i.e., those containing lotion) can be used instead of traditional toilet paper. The use of mild soap and patting the area dry instead of rubbing also can help maintain skin integrity. Moisture barrier ointments such as those used on infants to prevent diaper rash can be used as long as the skin is intact and provided the area is not in the radiation field. If the area is in the radiation field, patients should follow the radiation oncologist's advice. These interventions should be implemented at the beginning of treatment before diarrhea even starts. The patient/caregiver should be instructed to report any signs of skin breakdown. At that point, special skin products maybe required, and patients should be encouraged to cleanse by irrigating the area instead of scrubbing and increasing the irritation.

Patients/caregivers also should be instructed to report red flag symptoms including fever, excessive thirst, dizziness, severe abdominal cramping, bloody stools, and diarrhea that is not responding to prescribed interventions.[36] The patient and/or caregiver should understand that these symptoms require immediate attention to avoid life-threatening consequences. The patient and/or caregiver should clearly understand whom to call and have easy access to the number(s).

Teaching/Learning Approaches

Patient information can be provided in writing, by means of audiovisual technologies and/or by computer. Selecting among teaching techniques relies heavily on the findings of initial patient assessment of preferred learning styles and special needs. Among the internet resources that provide patient education materials are the American Cancer Society (www.cancer.org), National Cancer Institute (www.nih.gov), National Comprehensive Cancer Network (www.nccn.org), the Oncology Nursing Society (www.ons.org), and Cancer Care (www.cancercare.org).

Encouraging the patient to keep a log of the symptoms, timing of the symptoms, and effectiveness of intervention will help the patient and the healthcare provider gain a better sense of what truly is happening and how effective or ineffective the current treatment plan is. It removes the burden of trying to remember each day's events and provides the opportunity to identify patterns.

SUMMARY

Nausea, vomiting, and diarrhea are commonly occurring GI side effects that can be anticipated in patients undergoing abdominopelvic RT, hemibody RT, and TBI. Recognition of risk for occurrence and early intervention can oftentimes minimize severity and occasionally prevent occurrence. Empowering patients to identify and self-manage these symptoms by providing anticipatory guidance and information places them in a position of control and promotes early identification and intervention, thus facilitating prevention of secondary complications that may be more serious and can delay or even cause discontinuation of anticancer treatment.

REFERENCES

1. Bruner DW, Haas ML, Gosselin-Acomb TK: *Manual for radiation oncology nursing practice and education*, ed 3, Pittsburgh, 2005, Oncology Nursing Society.
2. Engelking C: Diarrhea. In Yarbro CJ, Frogge MH, Goodman M, editors: *Cancer symptom management*, ed 3, Boston, 2004, Jones and Bartlett, pp 528-557.
3. Wickham R: Nausea and vomiting. In Yarbro CJ, Frogge MH, Goodman M editors: *Cancer symptom management*, ed 3, Boston, 2004, Jones and Bartlett, pp 187-207.
4. Benson AB, Ajani JA, Catalano RB et al: Recommended guidelines for the treatment of cancer treatment-induced diarrhea, *J Clin Oncol* 22(14):2918-2926, 2004.
5. *NCCN clinical practice guidelines in oncology-antiemesis, V. 2.2006* (website): www.nccn.org/professionals/physician_gls/PDF/antiemesis.pdf. Accessed June 19, 2006.
6. Rutledge D, Engelking C: Cancer-related diarrhea: selected findings of a national survey of oncology nurse experiences, *Oncol Nurs Forum* 25(5):861-873, 1998.
7. Gralla RJ, Osoba D, Kris MG: Recommendations for the use of antiemetics: evidence-based clinical practice guidelines. American Society of Clinical Oncology, *J Clin Oncol* 17(9):2971-2994, 1999.
8. Wadler S, Benson AB, Engelking C et al: Recommended guidelines for the treatment of chemotherapy-induced diarrhea, *J Clin Oncol* 16(9):3169-3178, 1998.
9. Feyer R, Maranzano E, Molassiotis A et al: Radiotherapy-induced nausea and vomiting (RINV): antiemetic guidelines, *Support Care Cancer* 13(2):122-128, 2005.
10. Goldsmith BJ: Antiemetic patterns of care for radiotherapy-induced nausea and vomiting (Abstract 2975), *Proceedings 2003 ASCO Annual Meeting,* Alexandria, Va.
11. Franzen L, Nyman J, Hagberg H et al: A randomized placebo-controlled study with ondansetron in patients undergoing fractionated radiotherapy, *Ann Oncol* 7(6): 587-592, 1996.
12. The Italian Group for Antiemetic Research in Radiotherapy: Radiation-induced emesis: a prospective observational multicenter Italian trial, *Int J Radiat Oncol Biol Phys* 44(3):619-625, 1999.
13. Horiot JC: Blueprint for the control of radiation-induced nausea and vomiting: introduction, *Acta Oncol* 43 suppl 15:3-4, 2004.
14. Wickham R: Nausea and vomiting: palliative care issues across the cancer experience, *Oncol Support Care* 1(4): 44-57, 2003.
15. Marchioro G, Azzarello G, Viviani F et al: Hypnosis on the treatment of anticipatory nausea and vomiting in patients receiving cancer chemotherapy, *Oncology* 59(2):100-104, 2000.
16. Grant M, Kravitz K: Symptoms and their impact on nutrition, *Semin Oncol Nurs* 16(2):113-121, 2000.
17. Eckert RM: Understanding anticipatory nausea [online exclusive], *Oncol Nurs Forum* 28(10), 2001 (website): www.ons.org/publications/journals/ONF/Volume28/Issue10/28101553.asp#top. Accessed February 10, 2006.
18. Haas ML: Utilizing geriatric skills in radiation oncology, *Geriatr Nurs* 25(6):355-360, 2004.
19. Gridelli C, Aapro M: Factors influencing the choice of 5-HT3-receptor antagonist antiemetics: focus on elderly cancer patients. *Support Care Cancer* 2(7):487-496, 2004.
20. Multinational Association of Supportive Care in Cancer: *A quick guide to MASCC antiemesis tool (MAT),* 2004 (website): www.mascc.org/index.php?load=pro_study_groups&page_id=83. Accessed February 10, 2006.
21. National Cancer Institute: *Nausea and vomiting,* 2006 (website): www.nci.nih.gov/ cancerinfo/pdq/supportivecare/nausea/healthprofessional#Section_3. Accessed February 9, 2006.
22. Moore JM, Knobf MT: A nursing flow sheet for documentation of ambulatory oncology, *Oncol Nurs Forum* 18(5):933-939, 1991.
23. Kirbride P, Bezjak A, Pater J et al: Dexamethasone for the prophylaxis of radiation-induced emesis: a National Cancer

Institute of Canada Clinical Trials Group phase III study, *J Clin Oncol* 18(9):1960-1966, 2000.
24. Horiot JC: Prophylaxis versus treatment: is there a better way to manage radiotherapy-induced nausea and vomiting? *Int J Radiat Oncol Biol Phys* 60(4):1018-1025, 2004.
25. Feyer P: The importance of simple, easy-to-follow anti-emetic guidelines, *Acta Oncol* 43 suppl 15:5-8, 2004.
26. Engelking C, Rutledge FN, Ippoliti C et al: Cancer-related diarrhea: a neglected cause of symptom distress, *Oncol Nurs Forum* 25(5):859-860, 1998.
27. Engelking C, Rutledge D: Cancer treatment-related diarrhea: selected findings of a national survey of oncology nurse experiences, *Oncol Nurs Forum* 5(2):861-873, 1998.
28. Engelking C, Wickham R, Iwamoto R: Cancer-related gastrointestinal symptoms: dilemmas in assessment and management, *Dev Support Cancer Care* 1(1):3-10, 1996.
29. Jensen LL: Fecal incontinence: evaluation and treatment. *J Wound Ostomy Continence Nurs* 24(5):277-282, 1997.
30. Bhandari R, Burakoff R: A pharmacological approach to secretory diarrhea, *Gastroenterologist* 3(1):67-74, 1995.
31. Fruto LV: Current concepts: management of diarrhea in acute care, *J Wound Ostomy Continence Nurs* 21(5):199-205, 1994.
32. Martz CH: Diarrhea. In Groenwald SH, Frogge MH, Goodman M et al, editors: *Cancer symptom management*, Boston, 1996, Jones and Bartlett, pp 498-520.
33. Mercadante S: Diarrhea in terminally ill patients: pathophysiology and treatment. *J Pain Symptom Manage* 10(4): 298-309, 1995.
34. Vasudeva R, Elraie K: *Intestinal radiation injury*, (website): www.emedicine.com/med/topic1184.htm. Accessed June 20, 2006.
35. Cascinu S: Drug therapy in diarrheal diseases in oncology and hematology patients, *Crit Rev Oncol Hematol* 18(1): 37-50, 1995.
36. Engelking C, Sauerland C: Maintenance of normal elimination. In Watkins-Bruner D, Moore-Higgins G, Haas M, editors: *Outcomes in radiation therapy*, Boston, 2001, Jones and Bartlett, pp 530-562.
37. Martenson JA, Bollinger JW, Sloan JA et al: Sucralfate in the prevention of treatment-induced diarrhea in patients receiving pelvic radiation therapy: a North Central Cancer Treatment Group phase III double-blind placebo-controlled trial, *J Clin Oncol* 18(6):1239-1245, 2000.
38. Saverese DM, Savy G, Vahdat L et al: Prevention of chemotherapy and radiation toxicity with glutamine, *Cancer Treat Rev* 29(6):501-513, 2003.
39. Levy MH: Constipation and diarrhea in cancer patients, *Cancer Bull* 43:412-422, 1992.
40. Sedgwick DM, Howard GC, Ferguson A: Pathogenesis of acute radiation injury to the rectum, *Int J Colorectal Dis* 9(1):23-30, 1994.
41. Bruner DW, Bucholtz JD, Iwamoto R et al: *Manual for radiation oncology nursing practice and education*, Pittsburgh, 1998, Oncology Nursing Press.
42. Ooi BS, Tjandra JJ, Green MD: Morbidities of adjuvant chemotherapy and radiotherapy for resectable rectal cancer: an overview, *Dis Colon Rectum* 42(3):403-418, 1999.
43. Kollmorgen CR, Meagher AP, Wolff BG et al: The long-term effect of adjuvant postoperative chemoradiotherapy for rectal carcinoma on bowel function, *Ann Surg* 220(5): 676-682, 1994.
44. Dahlberg M, Glimelius B, Graf W et al: Preoperative irradiation affects functional results after surgery for rectal cancer: results from a randomized study, *Dis Colon Rectum* 41(5):543-549, 1998.
45. Crook J, Esche B, Futter N: Effect of pelvic radiotherapy for prostate cancer on bowel, bladder, and sexual function: the patient's perspective, *Urology* 47(3):387-394, 1996.
46. Kornblau S, Benson AB, Catalano R et al: Management of cancer treatment-related diarrhea: issues and therapeutic strategies, *J Pain Symptom Manage* 19(2):118-129, 2000.
47. Yavuz MN, Yavuz AA, Ilis E et al: A randomized study of the efficacy of octreotide versus diphenoxylate on radiation-induced diarrhea (Abstract 2370), *Proc Am Soc Clin Oncol* 19:602, 2000.
48. Henriksson R, Franzen L, Littbrand B: Effects of sucralfate on acute and late bowel discomfort following radiotherapy of pelvic cancer, *J Clin Oncol* 10(6):969-975, 1992.
49. Bye A, Ose T, Kaasa S: Quality of life during pelvic radiotherapy, *Acta Obstet Gynecol Scand* 74(2):147-152, 1995.
50. Hilderley LJ: Radiation therapy. In Gates RA, Fink RM, editors: *Oncology nursing secrets*, ed 2, Philadelphia, 2001, Hanley and Belfus, pp 39-43.
51. Finley J: Management of cancer cachexia, *AACN Clin Issues* 11(4):590-603, 2000.
52. Zakim L: Acupuncture for side effects of chemoradiation therapy in cancer patients, *Semin Oncol Nurs* 21(3): 190-195, 2005.
53. Tuchmann L, Engelking C: Cancer-related diarrhea. In Gates RA, Fink RM, editors: *Oncology nursing secrets*, ed 2, Philadelphia, 2001, Hanley and Belfus, pp 310-322.
54. Kuck A, Ricciardi E: Alterations in elimination. In Itano JK, Taoka KN, editors: *Core curriculum for oncology nursing*, ed 4, St Louis, 2005, WB Saunders, pp 318-344.
55. Hogan C: The nurse's role in diarrhea management, *Oncol Nurs Forum* 25(5):879-886, 1998.
56. Mertz HR, Beck CK, Dixon W et al: Validation of a new measure of diarrhea, *Dig Dis Sci* 40(9):1873-1882, 1995.
57. Pearson BD, Kelber S: Urinary incontinence: treatments, interventions and outcomes, *Clin Nurse Spec* 10(4):177-182, 1996.
58. Rothenberger DA: Anal incontinence. In Cameron JL, editor: *Current surgical therapy*, ed 3, Philadelphia, 1989, BC Decker, pp 185-194.
59. Toner BB, Stuckless N, Ali A et al: The development of a cognitive scale for functional bowel disorders, *Psychosom Med* 60(4):492-497, 1998.
60. Dow K, Hilderly KL, editors: *Nursing care in radiation oncology*, Philadelphia, 1992, WB Saunders.

Chapter 35

Sexuality and Sexual Dysfunction

Judith A. Shell

Individuals who are considered to be physically disabled through an illness such as cancer frequently suffer social discrimination in a society that places great emphasis on physical appearance. The "body beautiful" is America's ideal, and a healthy individual's unconscious body image may be threatened by the appearance of someone with a physical impairment related to illness or its treatment (e.g., hair loss or skin changes), and in turn, will react negatively to that individual. Quite naturally, one takes unto her/himself the attitudes of others toward her/his personal self, because one's character consists of attitudes, values, and the behaviors ascribed by society.

Our sexuality, a primary part of being human, is present from birth until death and is a part of all of the activities in which a person engages: relationships, socialization, work, telephone conversations, the decoration of one's home, expressions of affection, child rearing, watching a movie together, or walking down the street. It is an expression of one's personality and is evident in everyday interactions (Box 35-1). Differentiation and clarification among the many meanings associated with the term "sexuality" is important because phraseology such as "sexual intercourse," "sex act," and "sex" are often used synonymously with "sexuality." More than just the physical aspect of sexual expression, sexuality embraces the essence of maleness and femaleness and integrates the somatic, emotional, intellectual and social aspects of the sexual being to enrich and enhance personalities, communication, and love.[1]

Lauman, Paik, and Rosen[2] reported on rates of sexual dysfunction in a national probability sample of normal, healthy people and found that 43% of women and 31% of men experienced some element of dysfunction. Given these facts related to healthy individuals, it is understandable that cancer can and does impact an individual's sexuality and may include issues such as self-esteem, self-image, and feelings of adequacy and competency. Along with sociocultural partiality and personal beliefs and values, physical disease and illness introduces yet another faction the clinician must keep in mind. For some people, the mere process of being ill may cast doubt on their sexual identity and response, which may reflect on their sense of adequacy. Even with newer therapies and techniques, somewhere between 10% and 90% of cancer survivors continue to report sexual difficulties depending on diagnosis, gender, and treatment.[3] Premorbid factors may be present as well, such as increased age, gender, anxiety and depression, and/or other chronic diseases (diabetes, hypertension) that may exacerbate sexuality dilemmas created by the cancer diagnosis and its treatment.

SEXUAL REHABILITATION

Sexual rehabilitation for cancer survivors has taken on new importance in the past 20 years, and although sexuality remains a sensitive issue, attitudes are beginning to change regarding the care for sexual side effects from cancer and its treatment. There is better education concerning human sexuality, society is more receptive to being educated, and there is an increased demand for open discussion of sexuality issues.[4] Research in this area has promoted and increased the knowledge of how people function sexually, how cancer will affect these complex mechanisms can be more precisely predicted, and the prevention and/or reduction of potentially devastating side effects is often possible.[5-12] (See Table 35-1 for the normal physiological sexual response cycle.) However, there remains a paucity of evidence-based research in relation to interventions for the most common sexual side effects.[12]

Once a cancer diagnosis has been made and the type of treatment is ascertained, it is crucial to advise the patient and partner on how their

Box 35-1 Interactions Between Sexuality, Personality, and Activities of Daily Living

- Physical acts of sex are only a part of one's sexuality.
- Sexuality is an integral part of everyone's personality and is expressed in all that we do.
- People have a right to one's own beliefs and convictions about sexuality.
- Sexual energy is always with us.
- Sexual energy is a kind of power one has to influence others and make a difference in the world.
- Body ownership and self-knowledge help to create healthy intimacy boundaries.
- Every person is the sole owner of his or her body.
- Sexual fantasies, feelings, and thoughts are natural.
- Guilt and shame are not part of a healthy sexuality.

sexuality and intimate relationship may be impacted. Patients and partners may need questions answered related to physical ability, health risks, and other personal concerns; therefore, education about the patient's particular cancer and/or treatment and other related medical issues may help put troubled minds at ease. Individuals/couples may have to adjust emotionally to changes in sexual behavior, and this may leave the patient wondering about his/her ability to function as a man or woman. Couples may need encouragement to seek therapeutic counseling for the many emotional issues that can arise; this may help to minimize possible resentment toward the illness and the patient.

Once a therapeutic relationship has been established between patient and clinician, the patient may begin to feel more comfortable discussing sexuality issues; however, initially anxiety may still be present and these concerns may be disguised as talk with the clinician about parenting, relationship, or other social situations. Another stumbling block may be a dubious attitude toward sexuality and illness that may prevail among clinicians, and although they feel a sense of responsibility to address the patient's sexual concerns, the clinician may feel discomfort with this role. Not only can clinicians harbor certain stereotypes, they also tend to focus on sexual *pathology* rather than on the concept of sexual *health*.

One other situation that may be uncomfortable for the patient is his or her sexual orientation and whether or not to disclose this to healthcare providers. Information about whether the client is gay or lesbian may be missed because the clinician does not ask the right questions as a result of inexperience or insensitivity.

It is essential to remember that not all individuals have partners, and if they do, they may not be of the opposite sex. The assumption that all people are in heterosexual relationships can be detrimental to both the gay/lesbian/bisexual patient and his or her partner. Fields and Scout[13] speak to the issue of a 42-year-old woman who had waited to have her first Pap smear until age 42 because of "multiple bad experiences with doctors—" the cost to her was a large ulcerated cervical tumor and a diagnosis of cervical cancer." One study explained that over 25% of lesbians who "came out" to their physicians, felt their healthcare was negatively affected.[14] If the partner is excluded from being a part of the treatment process because of provider ignorance, the patient may have greater difficulty with decision-making, and the disgruntled couple may show little or no affection toward each other during office visits or hospitalizations. Whether a couple is gay or straight, they will most likely be nervous and worry about each other and want to be protective during their cancer experience. It is most important, then, to focus on an assessment of the patient/partner's strengths and resources, even in the midst of the cancer crisis, and to provide subsequent counseling and interventions as needed.

PSYCHOSEXUAL ISSUES, SEXUAL FUNCTION, AND CANCER

A person's sexual expression will vary throughout the life cycle, and interference with the psychosexual stages of development by an event such as cancer may cause sexual dysfunction. Awareness of these stages in normal development will enhance the clinician's ability to promote sexual function during and after treatment for cancer. If the patient is young and just beginning to embark upon relationship and career, his or her focus will probably be one of courtship, marriage, and procreation. The patient's sexuality interests will be much different from those of a middle age or older group of patients who now envision their sexuality

Table 35-1 Normal Physiologic Sexual Response Cycle*

Changes in females	Changes in males	Changes in both genders
EXCITEMENT PHASE		
Moving from unaroused to aroused state		
Pelvic vasocongestion	Erection of penis	Sex flush
Vaginal lubrication and expansion	Elevation of testes closer to body	Increase in muscle tension
Swelling of breasts, external genitalia, and clitoris	Swelling of the testes	Increased heart rate and blood pressure
Vagina secretes clear liquid to lubricate	Scrotal skin thickens	
Upper ⅔ of vagina expands	Nipples become erect	
Vagina lengthens and opens like a balloon		
Uterus elevates and moves upward		
Labia majora flattens and moves apart for exposure		
PLATEAU STAGE		
Physiologic preparation for intercourse		
Greater vasocongestion	Penis becomes larger	Increased sex flush in some men, women
Clitoris elevates or retracts under clitoral hood	Testicles swell 50% beyond size and pull closer to body	Greater voluntary, involuntary muscle tension
Swelling of tissues around the outer ⅓ of the vagina	Pre-ejaculatory emission from Cowper's gland (drops of fluid may contain active sperm)	Hyperventilation
Vagina entrance becomes smaller		Further increase in heart rate
Color of inner labia change color		Elevation in blood pressure
ORGASM PHASE		
An intense sensation occurring at peak of sexual arousal, followed by release of sexual tension		
Physiologically, no difference between male and female	Male orgasm is actually 2 phases	
	1st stage: Vas deferens, seminal vesicles, and prostate contract, force ejaculate in bulb at base of urethra	Physiologically the same in male and female
	2nd stage: Urethra bulb and penis contract rhythmically, forcing out semen	Series of rhythmic contractions of pelvic organs
		Sharp increase in blood pressure, heart rate, and respiration
REFRACTORY PERIOD (MALES ONLY)		
	Period immediately after orgasm when a man cannot be sexually stimulated	
	Young teenage male = 1–2 minutes	
	Men >30 yr—can extend 1–2 hours or more	
	Men >50 yr—can take up to 24 hours	
RESOLUTION PHASE		
Period of involuntary relaxation—returns person to unaroused state		
		Extra blood drains away from sexual tissues
		Return to normal heart rate, blood pressure, and breathing

Data from Masters WH, Johnson VE: *Human sexual response,* New York, 1966, Harper Perennial.

*Masters and Johnson's sexual response cycle only focuses on the physiologic features of arousal.[85] They completely ignored the emotional side (desire and passion), the cognitive side (thoughts, perceptions, evaluations), and the unique experience of the individual.

and intimate sexual relationship to be one of physical nearness, intimate communication, pleasure seeking and companionship.

Upon learning of the uncertain prognosis associated with a cancer diagnosis, initially patients may fear for their life, however, once they are confident of survival, fear often reverts to anxiety over quality of life and whether it will be "normal." Questions arise about whether participation will be possible in areas such as work, recreation, and travel; couple relationship; and parenting. Will they be able to function in social activities that are usually taken for granted? Financial hardships may arise in conjunction with office visits, tests, meals away from home, and childcare. Treatment effects may curtail energy, cause discomfort and debilitation. Consequently, all of these limitations will impact self-concept, self-esteem, body image, and level of sexual interest, ability, and adjustment.

In the American culture, extreme importance is placed on relationship with others and one's ability to relate sexually. Patients may decide to isolate themselves, they may proclaim a disinterest in sex to protect their dignity, or they may even reject their partner in the expectation of being rejected themselves. If the patient is considering initiating a new relationship, they must decide when and how to account for their illness and the treatment course. If they provide too much information before a bond is created, it may increase their chance of rejection. As well, patients often overlook their own positive attributes, the aspects of sexuality that remain normal, and they forget to emphasize the positive aspects of the experience: learning to reprioritize and to "stop and smell the roses."

RADIATION THERAPY AND SEXUALITY

Treatment with radiation therapy can be used alone or in combination with other therapies in an attempt to achieve a cure or for palliation from consequences of the cancer itself.

Although early side effects usually occur within about 2 weeks and subside about 2 to 3 weeks after therapy completion, many patients complain of fatigue after several months, and late reactions can occur years later.[15] Whether early or late, Iwamoto[15] explains that, "because radiation therapy has its greatest effect on rapidly dividing cells, the epithelial tissues, such as mucous membranes and the skin, are most susceptible to its effects."

The patient may experience a change in sexual capability and body image as a result of various side effects from radiation therapy. Skin changes resulting from erythema (a reddening of the skin), dry flaky skin, or moist desquamation (blisters that can form ulcers), or loss of hair in the irradiated area (head, axilla, pubic) can foster a negative body image. Depending on the area and amount of bone marrow irradiated, patients can experience a decrease in white and red blood cell and platelet counts, predisposing them to malaise and weakness, infection, and bleeding. A negative indirect effect on sexual function can occur due to acute effects such as fatigue and nausea. Soft tissue damage to the rectum, bladder, and vagina and prostate, which results in proctitis, cystitis, vaginal stenosis, and erection difficulty, will directly effect sexual functioning. Because of the varied side effects attributed to radiation therapy, it is well advised to explore individual cancers and ascertain the site-specific effects that may impact the patient's sexuality and intimate sexual relationship.

Schover, Montague and Lakin[16] define sexual rehabilitation as, "remediating the emotional impact of cancer on body image, relationship satisfaction, and reproductive capacity." Therefore, this chapter explores the effects that radiation therapy has on sexual function in the cancer survivor and relates best evidence-based practice to manage the body's response and restore a healthy sense of femininity and masculinity.

SEXUALITY ISSUES IN SITE-SPECIFIC CANCERS

Brain Tumors

Although the outlook for many cancers has improved dramatically over the past several decades, the treatment success for brain tumors is not one of them. The median survival for those patients with malignant gliomas is about 1 year, and this is with surgery, 55 Gy to 60 Gy of fractionated external beam radiation therapy, and chemotherapy.[17] Age, functional status, and tumor grade remain important prognostic factors, and because prognosis is poor, reduction of treatment-related toxicity and improved quality of life are of utmost importance.[18]

The symptoms associated with brain tumors often vary and can include headaches and seizures, nausea and vomiting, vision changes and slurred speech, motor function disabilities, and changes in mental status. Hair loss is also a traumatic insult to body image when it begins to occur after 2500cGy to 3000cGy.[15] Although none of these effects are directly related to sexual function, they are most definitely related in a secondary manner. It is well known that brain cancer and its treatment create emotional, behavioral, and cognitive changes, and in particular, the focus of cognitive changes has centered around the effects of cranial radiation.[15] However, recent research describes cognitive impairment in patients who have received systemic chemotherapy[19] as well, but Martin[20] reports that these changes are particularly noticeable in brain tumor patients. Although clinical studies have usually looked at survival as a primary end point, cognitive function related to the quality of life of patient and partner also must be entertained.[21] Few studies have addressed adult brain tumor patients and their psychosocial function, which should include their sexual function.[21,22] According to Scheibel, Meyers, and Levin[23] who studied 245 patients with malignant gliomas, patients will frequently experience memory loss and poor verbal fluency and verbal learning, especially if they have left hemisphere tumors. Pringle, Taylor and Whittle[24] noted that more women with left-sided brain tumors experienced more depression when scored preoperatively according to the Hospital Anxiety and Depression scale. Although this is obviously frustrating for the patient, the caregiver also must adjust emotionally to a loved one who shows decline in neurocognitive skills such as attention, memory, and most troubling, personality changes. Improvement in the ability to function may be realized through cognitive, behavioral, and vocational rehabilitation, and/or medical management with antidepressants or stimulant medication.[21] Although an intimate sexual relationship may no longer be possible, the couple may be able to enjoy emotional closeness and physical touching for a longer period of time using some of these rehabilitation techniques. The clinician can therefore be supportive of healthy sexual function by encouraging improved treatment choices and the provision of informed care decisions for patients with changing levels of cognitive functioning and care needs.

Breast Cancer

Treatment for breast cancer may entail either mastectomy or breast-conserving surgery with subsequent radiation therapy. The sexuality and body image concerns for the woman who must endure mastectomy are different than those for the woman who endures removal of a segment of the breast or the lump alone; however, it has been documented that there is little difference in overall sexual function between women receiving these various treatment options.[25-29] The literature reveals no direct long-term sexual side effects, specifically from radiation therapy, in breast cancer survivors, although lymphedema may be a result of surgery and radiation combined and this may affect body image.[30]

It is possible that a skin reaction, fatigue, and nausea, which usually occur within 2 to 3 weeks during radiation therapy, will impact sexual function and desire.[31] A skin reaction can influence body image and desirability because it may be necessary for a woman to go without a brazier during treatment and a dressing may be necessary if a severe reaction occurs. Assistance may be needed from the spouse/partner. The skin in the radiated area also turns a darker color and can remain so for several months to years.[31] This also can be embarrassing for men who wish to wear no shirt or women who may want to wear low-neck clothing or for both genders when wearing a bathing suit. Patients are always discouraged from allowing direct sunlight on the radiated area, and this can be frustrating to those who frequent the outdoors.

Women who have had mastectomy will often choose to have reconstruction done, and this may be accomplished by either autologous reconstruction or with an expander and implant. Many of these women go on to have radiation therapy after reconstruction. One study with 48 breast cancer patients revealed a better cosmetic outcome with fewer complications for those women who had reconstruction with a transverse rectus abdominis myocutaneous (TRAM) flap (n = 30) than those who had expander and implant (E/I) reconstruction (n = 18), either before or after radiation therapy.[32] A complication rate of 53% was reported in the E/I group whereas only 12% was reported for those who had TRAM reconstruction. The author's conclusion was that tolerance and cosmetic outcome depended on the type of reconstruction used.[32]

All treatments for breast cancer will have some impact on sexuality and sexual health; however, multiple studies show that chemotherapy is generally associated with poorer sexual functioning than is radiation therapy.[33,34] In one study that examined the predictors of sexual health in 1134 women who had survived breast cancer, it was found that vaginal dryness, past chemotherapy use, and having a new partner since the diagnosis were the most significant predictors of sexual dysfunction.[35] The most prominent indicators of sexual interest were good mental health and body image, and sexual satisfaction was related to the quality of the partnered relationship and whether or not the partner had sexual problems.[35] Gantz[35] explains that, "...we can assure breast cancer survivors that after the acute phase of cancer treatment they can expect to function well, and exhibit levels of physical, emotional, and social well-being that are similar to age-matched healthy women and are superior to those seen for patients with other chronic diseases."

Colorectal Cancer

Once again, there is no specific research in the literature regarding colorectal cancer and sexual side effects from radiation therapy. Sexuality issues in this disease stem primarily from surgery, particularly in males, and whether or not stoma placement is necessary.[36-39] Radiation therapy to the lower pelvic/rectal area in doses used to cure rectal cancer can cause fibrosis of soft tissue along with nerve damage.[40] This can be particularly devastating to men if there is damage to nerves and blood vessels responsible for sexual function (erection or ejaculation). Radiation-induced constriction of blood vessels that results in atherosclerosis and a decreased blood supply to the penis is thought to effect erectile function.[41] Both men and women may be affected if there are incontinence problems. For more information about the side effects from radiation to the pelvis, see the Gynecologic (GYN) and Prostate Cancer sections of this chapter.

Gynecologic Cancer

Gynecologic (GYN) malignancies include cervical, endometrial, ovarian, vaginal, and vulvar cancers, and treatment can include surgery, chemotherapy, and/or radiation therapy. However, radiation therapy is most commonly used to treat cancers of the cervix and endometrium. Damage from radiation therapy to the female pelvis can impede sexual function in two forms; one is through premature ovarian failure and the other is by causing damage to the epithelium in the vaginal canal.

As the abdominal dose escalates above 1.5 Gy, amenorrhea can occur with ensuing premature menopause.[16] Depletion of estrogens and androgens will cause young women to experience what their older counterparts have already been through, including troublesome hot flashes, mood swings, vaginal thinning, and decreased vaginal lubrication.[16] As a result, dyspareunia often follows that may influence a decrease in sexual arousal and intercourse will no longer be pleasurable. Another concern is precipitated during abdominal radiation for such diseases as Hodgkin's lymphoma or cervical cancer. The ovaries, which do not need to be treated, are in the radiation field, but they may be moved to the midline behind the uterus to protect their function; results for this technique are questionable.[42]

Ovarian ablation with direct irradiation affects not only the vaginal tissues but also permanently destroys "the basal cell layer of the vaginal epithelium, the endothelium of small vessels in the genital area, and the fibroblasts of the connective tissues in the subepithelium."[37] Consequently, fibrosis can occur, which again produces dyspareunia, possible vaginal ulcerations, postcoital bleeding, and irritation.[16] Long-term radiation sequelae include occasional fistulas, vaginal shortening, stenosis and dryness, and insufficient vaginal elasticity.[43] Although women complain about many of the aforementioned sexual dysfunctions, it is not particularly clear whether there are fewer of these side effects with radiation therapy or with hysterectomy. Flay and Matthews[44] showed that the most frequently reported reason for decreased sexual functioning in women with cervical cancer was the complaint of vaginal shortening. This was more common in women who had undergone surgery and radiation than in those who received radiation alone. Sexual dysfunction was also a result of dyspareunia and concerns about vaginal bleeding.[44] Another study compared the sexual side effects of treatment (surgery or radiation therapy) and demonstrated that the type of treatment received was *not* associated with the prevalence of specific vaginal changes that affected sexual functioning.[45] Approximately 25% of these women reported vaginal changes up to 5 years after treatment, and about the same number reported moderate to severe levels of psychologic distress associated with vaginal changes.[45] These conflicting data make it difficult for the clinician and physician when they counsel women with cervical cancer in relation to sexual side effects and what specific changes can be anticipated in their bodies and their sexuality.

Andersen and Golden-Kreutz[46] reported that women who have endured GYN cancer experience significantly less frequent vaginal intercourse during the early months of recovery, and this remains low throughout the first posttreatment year. There are noticeable changes in physical sensation, sexual behaviors, and quality of the sexual response.[46] A negative focus on the part of their body that encountered change is often maintained. Each woman will respond uniquely to changes that occur with treatment; a perceived shortening of the vagina may be mildly upsetting to one woman whereas devastating to another.[47]

Head and Neck Cancer

Head and neck cancer can be particularly destructive physically and emotionally because it is often readily visible and the side effects from treatment, particularly radiation therapy, can be devastating to quality of life. One of the most prominent complaints is dysphasia, and although this does not directly affect sexual function, it has an indirect affect on sexuality because it impacts self-esteem and self-image. If patients are unable to swallow, a gastrostomy or other feeding tube may need to be placed, and this type of unnatural method of food intake can be psychologically isolating. Mealtimes are known to be occasions when families get together to share the events of the day; in other settings they also may be designed as romantic preludes (flowers, candles, and music) that often lead to an intimate encounter for couples. Although this may seem like an insignificant issue, when combined with other ramifications of treatment such as an uncomfortable and/or dry mouth, lack of the ability to taste, fatigue, and obvious skin changes, patients have described feelings of anger, frustration, lack of self-esteem, and little self-confidence.[37,48] A recent retrospective study with 73 head and neck cancer patients revealed that dysphagia created increased morbidity and was correlated with anxiety, depression, and a diminished quality of life. In an effort to improve mood status and physical goodness, Nordgren and colleagues[49] encouraged "a team approach involving nutritional support, physical therapy, speech rehabilitation, pain management, and psychological counseling."

Another bewildering problem in this population is xerostomia. Although patients treated for head and neck cancer have difficulty with swallowing problems and social eating, pain, and hoarseness, they also can have treatment-related side effects such as dyspnea, sticky thick saliva, and particularly xerostomia (dry mouth). One prospective study with 36 patients reported that a parotid-sparing intensity-modulated radiation therapy (IMRT) technique reduced the incidence and intensity of xerostomia when compared with conventional radiation therapy.[50] Because of the reduced xerostomia with the IMRT method, patients reported that eating, communication, pain, and emotion (the quality of life domains that were assessed) improved significantly over standard radiation therapy at 1 year after treatment finished.[50] Given the aforementioned disease and treatment consequences, a sexual relationship will most likely be compromised due to weakness, fatigue, and cachexia that may result in a poor body image and decreased libido and sexual expression, along with pain, disfigurement, and simply the interference with the usual means of sexual expression. However, with some of the newer radiation techniques that have become available to these patients, they have an increased probability of preserving not only a better quality of life, but more precisely, a better quality of their sexual self-esteem.

Lung Cancer

Even though the 1- and 5-year survival rates have increased in the past $2\frac{1}{2}$ decades, lung cancer remains one of the most deadly forms of this disease. The treatment for lung cancer often includes radiation therapy along with possible surgery and chemotherapy. Simply the diagnosis and treatment themselves create tremendous tension and strain; however, the other stressors in relation to the possible spread of malignancy, an uncertain prognosis, psychosocial issues, and emotional distress are all factors that necessitate lifestyle adjustments.[51]

Although the systemic side effects that chemotherapy causes are well known, radiation therapy also can cause a reaction in the skin that results in embarrassing darkened color changes, along with fatigue and weakness, especially when radiation is used in conjunction with chemotherapy. These effects can permeate body image and affect self-esteem in a negative manner. While treatment is ongoing and even after completion, the sense of femininity or masculinity a person feels also may be hindered simply because comforting drugs being used, such as narcotics and antinausea medication, can influence the sexual response cycle. As the patient becomes more debilitated, the satisfaction of intimate pleasure can be expressed through increased closeness, both physically and emotionally.[51]

There is little research literature relative to sexuality and lung cancer and none specific to radiation therapy alone. One Canadian study examined psychiatric illness and psychosocial concerns in 52 male (75%) and female (25%) lung cancer patients; 94% were 50 years of age or over. One of 20 outcome measures (loss of libido) was related to the patients' sexuality.[52] In regard to sexuality concerns, 25 patients (48%) acknowledged loss of libido; this was severe in 27%.[52] Sarna[53] studied a group of 69 women with lung cancer who reported a greater disturbance in their quality of life than did women with other cancers, particularly those with recurrent lung disease. They had greater psychologic distress, greater marital dysfunction, and a 38% decrease in sexual activity; many were no longer interested in sex and did not feel sexually attractive.[53]

Prostate Cancer

Several standard treatment options for prostate cancer include external beam radiation therapy (EBR) and radical prostatectomy, brachytherapy (BT) and cryotherapy, and observation.[54-56] Traditionally, factors that determine treatment choice are not only tumor stage but also the patient's age, possible comorbidities, and the urologist's and patient's preferences.[54] Presently, more clinical trials are including quality of life issues, including sexual function, and more frequently, quality of life has become a decision-making factor.

When sexual function is evaluated in this population, the National Institute of Health recommends that the term *erectile dysfunction (ED)* rather than impotence be used because it is more precise in describing the side effect. ED is defined as the recurrent inability to achieve and maintain an erection adequate enough for satisfactory sexual intercourse.[57] However, during a sexual function assessment, other elements should be included such as the quality (firmness) of the erection, ability to ejaculate, libido, interest in sex, the presence of an interested partner, and satisfaction with their own sexual lifestyle. Although organic factors are notably important, personal and psychologic factors can play a role in irradiated men as well.

The etiology of ED in irradiated men has not been well determined, but Zelefsky and Eid[58] evaluated 38 patients after they received EBR or with iodine-125 (^{123}I). They concluded that predominantly ED was arteriogenic due to a disruption of the arteriolar system that supplies the corporal muscles. Although other unknown factors might have played a role, they also reported that comorbidity, hormonal manipulation, smoking, and age had no influence on the type of dysfunction observed.[58] Many EBR prospective studies have been conducted with varying rates of ED reported—from 7% to 72%—and the time component (i.e., time since radiation therapy) was found to be relevant.[59-63] Other factors had no predictive value for sexual dysfunction after EBR: factors such as tumor stage, comorbidity, radiation dose, and transurethral resection of the prostate before EBR. However, a younger age and functional erections before EBR were good prognostic factors[63] A relationship was also shown between sexual function and the size of the radiation field; a smaller field related to better sexual function.[60]

In brachytherapy studies using ^{125}I or palladium-103 (^{103}Pd), ED rates were from 2% to 51%. Those on the higher end (toward the 50% mark) were those in whom brachytherapy was combined with EBR.[64-68] In an updated metaanalysis done by Robinson and colleagues[69] looking at rates of erectile function after treatment for prostate cancer, their "findings showed statistically significant differences in the probabilities for erectile function among the evaluated treatments, with brachytherapy showing the highest probability. Brachytherapy plus EBRT and EBRT alone were tied for second, followed by nerve-sparing radical prostatectomy, standard radical prostatectomy, and finally cryotherapy."[69] They also stated that various radiation techniques (three-dimensional conformal radiation therapy) may decrease the dose to the bulb of the penis, which correlates positively with sustained erectile ability after treatment.[69,70] However, controversy exists in the literature relative to potency preservation and dose to the proximal penis.[71]

Although ED is the usual sexual function concern in irradiated prostate cancer patients, ejaculatory disorder also has been noted in patients both with EBR and BT and ranges from a reduction or absence of ejaculate volume to painful ejaculation and hemospermia.[72,73] Helgason and colleagues[73] also reported that these men experienced a decreased intensity of orgasm, decreased frequency and rigidity of erections, and a decreased importance of sex.[73] Another troublesome side effect of EBR or BT is urinary incontinence; reported incidence is between 5% to 26% and 0% to 40%, respectively.[74,75] Although the exact mechanism of incontinence is not well defined, urinary leakage is thought to be caused by tissue damage and a decreased urethral closing related to dry, thin, and fibrosed tissue. This often necessitates the use of a protective pad, something that men have never been accustomed to wearing. Herr[74] contends that men believe urinary incontinence to be even more disabling and disruptive than ED.

Testicular Cancer

Treatment for early-stage testicular cancer (seminoma) usually requires orchiectomy followed by radiation therapy to the para-aortic and pelvic lymph nodes, whereas chemotherapy and retroperitoneal lymphadenectomy is required treatment for nonseminomatous testicular cancer.[76,77] Arai and colleagues[78] revealed numerous elements of sexual dysfunction in irradiated men comprising loss of sexual desire, erectile problems, less intense orgasms, premature or inability to ejaculate, and a reduced semen volume, but only 8% of those men reported a decrease in sexual satisfaction after treatment completion compared to before treatment commenced. Another frequently cited study done more than a decade ago showed that 87 men with seminomatous testicular cancer who were irradiated experienced more fertility distress, more performance distress, but not more overall desire distress than matched controls.[79] Although radiation for testicular cancer can cause sexual difficulties, Incrocci and colleagues,[80] in their study with 123 seminoma patients, found that, "interest in sex, satisfaction with sexual life, and erectile difficulties were not different from healthy age-matched controls."[77]

During radiation treatment, the remaining testicle is carefully shielded to prevent radiation scatter from damaging the capacity for spermatogenesis.[81] Fertility is usually protected if radiation is less than 2cGy, and in one study, no genetic abnormalities were noted in children conceived within a mean period of 32 months after radiation ended.[82] Men who have lost one testicle to cancer may have issues with body image and will most likely be interested in information regarding placement of a prosthesis. Some studies have reported a positive increase in body image after placement of a testicular prosthesis, which is a simple procedure with few complications.[80,83]

CLINICIAN RESPONSIBILITY TO INITIATE SEXUALITY DISCUSSION

The clinician can facilitate sexual health not only by providing information when the patient presents with a question or problem, but also by promoting sexual function through assessment, education, and intervention. Throughout treatment and after treatment, education should be offered to all patients and conveyed in diverse fashions—through written, verbal, and visual aids—to promote gentle encouragement and knowledge. One significant objective in this instance should be to focus on the characteristics that will remain intact after treatment, because patients often tend to focus on what they will loose.

The therapeutic approach will vary depending on the problem encountered and may be as simple as listening to the frustration of a dry mouth, which impedes oral sex, or an embarrassing skin reaction of the irradiated breast, or as complicated as restructuring an entire relationship. Referral to a psychotherapist would be the most beneficial for the later problem. An erection or lubrication problem or a question about position during intercourse may lead to the healthcare provider giving a response that includes discussion of suggested "sexual tasks" such as, nondemand pleasuring (sensate focus), dispelling the fear of failure, distracting obsessive thoughts, or permission to be "selfish." A thorough assessment will provide the foundation for an appropriate discussion about sexuality, sexual behaviors, and/or specific sexual performance issues. For various therapeutic assessment principles see Box 35-2.

INTERVENTIONS FOR RADIATION-INDUCED SIDE EFFECTS

As an integral part of every patient's recovery, the clinician must help enhance sexual function by addressing sexuality, but this may be difficult, at best, particularly if the patient is young or old, single or widowed. This is especially true because

Box 35-2 Principles of a Therapeutic Assessment Technique

1. Present a positive, relaxed, and professional demeanor.
2. Provide a private, confidential, and professional atmosphere.
3. Be sensitive to feelings.
4. Expect the patient's anxiety to rise during a discussion about sexuality.
5. Provide accurate positive information to help decrease anxiety.
6. Assess the following:
   - Pre-disability experiences and perceptions about sexuality and sexual behaviors and experiences/perceptions since the onset of cancer
   - Sexual preference (e.g., heterosexual, gay/lesbian, bi-sexual)
   - Is there a disabling condition and what is the effect on motor and sensory function, communication, cognition, fertility; include related physical problems such as pain, spasticity, decreased endurance, and bowel/bladder function
   - History of surgery and/or chemotherapy along with the presence of other significant medical conditions
   - Medications: other than hormones and chemotherapy
   - Presence or absence of a partner
   - Intrapersonal, interpersonal, and psychosocial factors that may enhance or interfere with a sexual relationship

society usually views sexuality and a sexual relationship as belonging only to men and woman who are in a committed heterosexual relationship, and who are without disability of any kind. "Activities that may help nurses deal with these issues include assessing personal value systems, biases towards other's values, and attitudes related to patient's sexual preferences."[84] All patient's, regardless of age or health status, perceive themselves as sexual beings and look for reassurance of their femininity or masculinity and their ability to function sexually, which enhances their sense of self-worth. Patients continue to fear that they will be radioactive, burned, or scarred, and although side effects can be irritating, uncomfortable, and disruptive to sexual activity, it is important to educate them concerning interventions that are helpful and reassuring (Box 35-3). Early side effects from radiation therapy that may hamper sexuality or a relationship usually begin to occur within about 2 weeks into treatment and may not subside until about 2 to 3 weeks after therapy completion; late reactions can occur years later.[15]

Clinicians can take many pathways to intercede on behalf of their patients. Speaking to the patient and partner "proactively" by giving them accurate information about what to expect during and after radiation treatments will allow them to anticipate changes and to cope more effectively. Often, merely talking with a patient and partner will help to validate their concerns and provide reassurance that behaviors, feelings, and fantasies are appropriate and acceptable. Encouraging open, honest communication with a shift away from body defects and toward the positive attributes that remain promotes a loving relationship and positive self-esteem. Finally, by counseling and educating them to be aware of and appreciate the many alternative ways to express their sexuality and sexual being through their own values, clinicians can emphasize the pleasure that can be derived from the closeness of a tender moment, the reassurance of an embrace, or simply enjoying a relaxing walk together hand in hand around a lake.

SUMMARY

Providing the patient and partner with a thorough education about the nature of radiation therapy and the changes they can expect relative to their sexuality and sexual function is of vital importance. The ability to emotionally and physically cope with these changes will be more positive if information is provided initially and reinforced throughout treatment. Although sexual function may be influenced and altered, it cannot be destroyed by the illness or the environmental factors related to treatment; sexuality is part of who one is as a man or woman. Reassurance can be provided to the patient and partner by encouragement and education about the many means of sexual expression that can bring pleasure and satisfaction to an intimate relationship. However, "the nurse must guard against expectations that could be threatening to the couple. Sex should not be an "all" or "nothing" experience; too much enthusiasm for exploring alternative methods of sexual expression may be too overwhelming for the patient and partner."[98] Oncology clinicians are privileged to have the kind

Box 35-3 Nursing Interventions for Radiation Side Effects to Enhance Sexuality

GENERAL "EMOTIONAL" INTERVENTIONS

- ALWAYS PRACTICE SAFE SEX
- Promote increased communication between partners about activities of daily living, their relationship, and their feelings and affection for one another.
- Foster the development of increased intimacy in a relationship rather than thinking only about sex. This promotes affection and actually whets the appetite for lovemaking.
- Foster the development of a comfort with sensuality and the value of sensual touching, rather than only making love with sexual intercourse as the end result.
- Inspire a realistic expectation about sexual performance, and eliminate the perspective that sexual desire must remain as strong as it was at the inception of the relationship.
- Time must be carved out for fun and companionship—to play together, laugh, travel, listen to music, communicate, and be emotionally available.

GENERAL "PHYSICAL" INTERVENTIONS

- Patients receiving radiation to the pelvis or mediastinum may experience anemia, neutropenia, or thrombocytopenia. They should be cautioned against oral, vaginal, and anal manipulation if counts are very low. As well, if fatigue occurs from anemia, a supine or side-lying position for intercourse will use less energy. (See Schover's *Sexuality and Cancer: for the Woman/Man Who Has Cancer and Her/His Partner*).[86,87] A nap may also be helpful.
- Emphasize the importance of contraception during radiation therapy. Encourage sperm banking if the testicular area will be radiated. If quality or quantity of preserved sperm is too low for intrauterine insemination, in vitro fertilization or intracytoplasmic sperm injection (ICSI) may be used. ICSI is a new technique whereby a single sperm is isolated and injected into the egg, it is cultured until an embryo develops, and then is transferred to the uterus.[88] Women who receive radiation to the abdominal area may undergo in vitro fertilization and cryopreserve embryos for future pregnancies. If unmarried, they may wish to freeze harvested mature oocytes for future fertilization in the laboratory.[89]
- Skin reactions can be painful and create a self-conscious attitude. If a reaction occurs in the perineum, the patient can be encouraged to take frequent lukewarm sitz baths and expose the area to air several times per day. For early skin reactions, flucinonide (Lidex) 0.05% or Biafine may be used, and in later stage skin reactions, Silvadene cream (sometimes mixed with Desitin cream to promote adherence to the skin) or Rādx (with lidocaine) may be used. After urinating or having a bowel movement, cleanse the area with cotton balls soaked in warm water and pat area dry with cotton balls as well. Discourage toilet paper since many are instilled with perfumes or other products.

INTERVENTIONS FOR RADIATION TO THE UPPER BODY

- If the patient enjoys oral sex, a dry mouth from xerostomia may be very irritating. This can be relieved with artificial saliva (e.g., Moi-Stir, Xerolube), citric acid (i.e., sugar-free lemon drops) may also help stimulate saliva to lubricate the mucous membrane. Sugarless mints will help to freshen breath.
- Acupuncture may stimulate salivary flow, but this method is experimental.[90]
- Pilocarpine 15 mgm may stimulate the flow of saliva. This may be increased by 5-mgm increments at week 5 and week 9. This intervention is usually started about 3 to 4 months after completion of radiation therapy.[90]
- Candles, may enhance ambience, however, fragrance may not be appreciated since the patient may have a decreased sense of smell.
- Tracheostomy sites may become irritated and sore; a cover may enhance body image and can be obtained from Byram Health Care Center, Inc., Greenwich, Conn., 800-354-4054.
- Dyspnea may be increased with radiation to the head and neck or lung area, therefore sexual closeness which does not necessarily lead to intercourse will allow the patient to feel "alive" without hampering oxygen intake. This is especially nice since patients can enjoy closeness and they don't feel that they are being treated like an invalid.
- To prevent bronchospasm, decrease or eliminate environmental irritants like perfumes, colognes, and hairsprays.
- Avoid long, slow kisses on the mouth because patients can become fearful of not getting enough oxygen.

(continued)

Box 35-3 Nursing Interventions for Radiation Side Effects to Enhance Sexuality—cont'd

- To reduce exertion during sexual activity, encourage the use of a waterbed; movement can be created without effort.
- Non-performance closeness and touching such as soft caressing or light massage with oils or creams is sensual and helps reduce discomfort. Other activities may include a warm bubble bath with candlelight, romantic music and some wine (in plastic glasses).
- To conserve energy, partners can be sexual with mutual masturbation and watching erotic videos.
- If a woman is receiving radiation treatment for breast cancer and a skin reaction has occurred that is unsightly, she can camouflage the wound by wearing a camisole or fancy short nightgown that enhances femininity.
- The couple may wish to try other positions for intercourse that do not enhance a direct view of the treated breast. A side-lying or rear entry position is recommended. (See Schover's *Sexuality and Cancer: for the Woman/Man Who Has Cancer and Her/His Partner*).[87]
- The patient may wish to make love by candlelight or to replace a white light bulb in a lamp with a red one to enhance the ambiance.
- Many women derive great pleasure from manipulation, touching or sucking on the breast. Inform her that she will not cause a cancer in the other breast while enjoying this kind of stimulation. If the treated breast will be reconstructed, it is important that she know there will be little to no sensation in that breast. Many men enjoy manipulation of the breast nipples during love-making and he can receive the same information.
- If the stomach is in the radiation field and nausea occurs, plan a sexual interlude after antiemetics have taken effect. Also cut down on alcohol intake.

INTERVENTIONS FOR RADIATION TO THE LOWER BODY

For Men and Women

- Radiation may cause intermittent cramping and diarrhea, which can be embarrassing. A low-residue diet along with medications like Pepto-Bismol, Kaopectate, Lomotil or Imodium will help to control this effect.
- Proctitis, which is aggravated by the diarrhea may be eased by sitz baths or the use of Proctofoam or Annusol (HC) suppositories.
- Urinary incontinence may be managed by pelvic muscle strengthening exercises (Kegel), bladder habit re-training and scheduled toileting, fluid management, medications (Oxybutynin and Tolterodine), and surgical techniques (AMS Sphincter 800 Urinary Prosthesis, bladder suspension, collagen injections, pessary supports, vaginal cones, urethral plugs).[91,92]
- The bladder should be emptied before intercourse if incontinence is a problem. If an accident should occur, remind the partner that urine is sterile and can be washed off easily, perhaps in the shower together.

For Men

- Partners may need to be reminded that cancer cannot be transmitted through sexual activity (ejaculated sperm), and if radiation therapy is being used, they will not be contaminated.
- If the man has had a brachytherapy implant, intercourse can continue with a condom 2 weeks after the procedure. Condoms should be worn to protect the partner from a seed that could be passed in the ejaculate. Semen may also be dark brown in color due to some bleeding and will resolve in time. He may also experience painful ejaculation for 6 months or more.[93,94]
- If impotence is a problem, there are several possible remedies:
  - Vacuum devices: a cylindrical tube is placed over the penis, a vacuum is created, an erection occurs, a soft rubber O-ring is placed on the base of the penis and the vacuum tube is removed and intercourse is possible.[95]
  - Vasoactive agents: MUSE (Medicated Urethral System for Erection), a urethral suppository, or alprostadil, an injection into base of the penis. Dose starts at 125 mcg and comes in increments of 250, 500, 1000 mcg. A tiny 3/8-inch needle is used to inject medication into the base of penis.[96]
  - Oral medication: sildenafil (Viagra), vardenafil (Levitra), or tadalafil (Cialis): oral medications that dilate blood vessels to enhance inflow to the corpus cavernosum. It does not increase desire. In brachytherapy-induced erectile dysfunction (ED), sildenafil is started at 50 mg 1 hour before intercourse; if not effective in three doses, it's increased to 100 mg for three doses. If still not effective, drug is discontinued.[97]

Box 35-3 Nursing Interventions for Radiation Side Effects to Enhance Sexuality—cont'd

- Penile prostheses: Semi-rigid implants are paired silicone-covered malleable metal rods placed in the corpora cavernosa; self-contained inflatable prosthesis are paired silicone cylinders that have a pump at the prosthesis tip and a reservoir within the shaft that transfers fluid so the cylinders become firm; inflatable penile prostheses are soft paired silicone inner tubes filled with solution that comes from a reservoir placed under the glans penis. When more fluid is pumped into the inner tubes, the erection becomes larger and firmer.[92]
- Arousal may be stimulated through use of erotic books, pictures, or videos.
- Stimulation may also occur with long periods of foreplay that include a change in environment (an inexpensive motel or house sitting for a friend), a romantic dinner, and showering together.
- Mutual masturbation may help the patient reach orgasm and ejaculation if erection is not possible. By inserting a partially erect penis into the vagina and flexing the perineal muscles, a female partner may help with an erection.
- If the patient has been radiated for testicular cancer, normal sexual desire and pleasurable sensations will most likely continue. If testosterone levels are decreased, hormone replacement therapy may be necessary after treatment is finished.
- A man may be embarrassed after the loss of a testicle; silicone gel-filled implants are available which cause few complications and create better body image.[83]

For Women

- Encourage the woman to continue intercourse during treatment until it becomes uncomfortable, and then resume when the vagina is healed. This helps prevent adhesions and shortening of the vagina. Semen can cause vaginal burning when the vagina becomes irritated from radiation; therefore, the man should try to withdraw before ejaculation or use a condom.[98]
- If the woman does not have a partner, she should be encouraged to use a dilator (they come in sizes from extra small to large) three times per week for 15 minutes at a time. They should also be used while the woman cannot tolerate intercourse. Sensitivity must be used when explaining dilator use.[99]
- A water-soluble lubricant must be used for intercourse or when using a dilator since the ability of the vagina to lubricate will be damaged from the radiation. A lubricant can be applied either privately or as part of foreplay. Lubricants include Astroglide, Slippery-Stuff, KY jelly products and others. They are obtained at any local drugstore or supermarket. Replens is another product that is a vaginal moisturizer and can be applied on a daily basis especially in women who have had total body radiation.[9]
- Alternatives to intercourse must be provided and encouraged even if intercourse is possible. These include nudity and cuddling with general pleasuring, autoeroticism and mutual masturbation, oral-genital stimulation, anal love play, and fantasy with DVD or videos. The Kama Sutra created by the Sinclair Intimacy Institute is a good choice and they can be reached by going to www.BetterSex.com.
- Vaginal estrogen products that decrease dryness and irritability are an option and several are on the market such as Estrace (a vaginal cream), Vagifem tablets, and the Estring. The tablets and Estring are the least absorbed systemically.
- Kegel exercises (tensing and relaxing the pelvic muscles) will help to relieve tension, increase elasticity, reduce urinary incontinence, and decrease dyspareunia.
- During sexual activity, the hips may be elevated to improve stimulation. If rear entry is preferred, the thighs may be adducted and lubricated to emulate a deeper vaginal barrel. More control is afforded in the female superior position but may not be as comfortable.[100]

of caring relationship with their patients that fosters discussion of the patient's most intimate issues. As this relationship becomes firmly established, there is often the expectation that the clinician will be knowledgeable and able to guide patient and partner through decisions and appropriate interventions; these interventions will bring hope, enhance body image, and instill confidence through an increased sense of self-esteem.

REFERENCES

1. *Education and trends in human sexuality: the training of health care professionals*, Technical Report Series no. 572, Geneva, 1976, World Health Organization.
2. Lauman EO, Paik A, Rosen RC: Sexual dysfunction in the United States: prevalence and predictors, *JAMA* 281(6):537-544, 1999.
3. Syrjala KL, Schroeder TC, Abrams JR et al: Sexual function measurement and outcomes in cancer survivors and matched controls, *J Sex Res* 37(3):213-226, 2000.

4. Shell JA: Impact of cancer on sexuality. In Otto SE, editor: *Oncology Nursing*, ed 4, St Louis, 2001, Mosby, pp 973-999.
5. Gantz PA, Rowland JH, Desmond K et al: Life after breast cancer: understanding women's health-related quality of life and sexual functioning, *J Clin Oncol* 16(2):501-514, 1998.
6. Jonker-Pool G, van Basten JP, Hoekstra HJ et al: Sexual functioning after treatment for testicular cancer: comparison of treatment modalities, *Cancer* 80(3): 454-464, 1997.
7. Lamb MA: Effects of cancer on the sexuality and fertility of women, *Semin Oncol Nurs* 11(2):120-127, 1995.
8. Little FA, Howard GC: Sexual function following radial radiotherapy for bladder cancer, *Radiother Oncol* 49(2):157-161, 1998.
9. Loprinzi CL, Abu-Ghazaleh S, Sloan JA et al: Phase III randomized double-blind study to evaluate the efficacy of a polycarbophil-based vaginal moisturizer in women with breast cancer, *J Clin Oncol* 15(3):969-973, 1997.
10. Carmack Taylor CL, Basen-Engquist K, Shinn EH et al: Predictors of sexual functioning in ovarian cancer patients, *J Clin Oncol* 22(5):881-889, 2004.
11. Jenkins R, Schover LR, Fouladi RT et al: Sexuality and health-related quality of life after prostate cancer in African-American and white men treated for localized disease, *J Sex Marital Ther* 30(2):79-93, 2004.
12. Shell JA: Evidence-based practice for symptom management in adults with cancer: sexual dysfunction, *Oncol Nurs Forum* 29(1):53-66, 2002.
13. Fields B, Scout: Addressing the needs of lesbian patients, *J Sex Educ Ther* 26(3): 182-188, 2001.
14. Lehmann J, Lehmann C, Kelly P: Development and health care needs of lesbians, *J Women's Health* 7(3): 379-387, 1998.
15. Iwamoto R: Radiation therapy. In Otto SE, editor: *Oncology Nursing*, ed 4, St Louis, 2001, Mosby, pp 606-637.
16. Schover LR, Montague DK, Lakin MM: Sexual problems. In DeVita VT, Hellman S, Rosenberg SA, editors: *Cancer: principles and practices of oncology*, ed 5, Philadelphia, 1997, Lippincott-Raven, pp 2857-2871.
17. Halperin EC, Herndon J, Schold SC et al: A phase III randomized prospective trial of external beam radiotherapy, mitomycin C, carmustine, and 6-mercaptopurine for the treatment of adults with anaplastic glioma of the brain, *Int J Radiat Oncol Biol Phys* 34(4):793-802, 1996.
18. Curran WJ Jr, Scott CB, Horton J et al: Recursive partitioning analysis of prognostic factors in three radiation therapy oncology group malignant glioma trials, *J Natl Cancer Inst* 85(9):704-710, 1993.
19. Carlson RH: "Chemo brain": cognitive loss confirmed in adult cancer patients receiving systemic chemotherapy, *Oncol Times* 22:35, 2000.
20. Martin GA: Commentary on "psycho-social and neuro-psychiatric aspects of patients with primary brain tumors" by Michael Weitzner, *Cancer Invest* 17(2):296-297, 1999.
21. Weitzner MA, Meyers CA: Cognitive functioning and quality of life in malignant glioma patients: a review of the literature, *Psychooncology* 6(3):169-177, 1997.
22. Lovely MP: Quality of life of brain tumor patients, *Semin Oncol Nurs* 14(1):73-80, 1998.
23. Scheibel RS, Meyers CA, Levin VA: Cognitive dysfunction following surgery for intracerebral glioma: influence of histopathology, lesion location, and treatment, *J Neurooncol* 30(1):61-69, 1996.
24. Pringle AM, Taylor R, Whittle IR: Anxiety and depression in patients with an intracranial neoplasm before and after tumour surgery, *Br J Neurosurg* 13(1):46-51, 1999.
25. Gantz PA, Rowland JH, Desmond K et al: Life after breast cancer: understanding women's health-related quality of life and sexual functioning, *J Clin Oncol* 16(2):501-514, 1998.
26. Schover LR: Sexuality and body image in younger women with breast cancer, *J Nat Cancer Inst Monogr* (16): 177-182, 1994.
27. Wilmoth MC, Townsend, JA: A comparison of the effects of lumpectomy versus mastectomy on sexual behaviors, *Cancer Pract* 3(5):279-285, 1995.
28. Wilmoth MC, Ross JA: Women's perception: breast cancer treatments and sexuality, *Cancer Pract* 5(6):353-359, 1997.
29. Schover L, Yetman R, Tuason L et al: Comparison of partial mastectomy with breast reconstruction on psycho-social adjustment, body image, and sexuality, *Cancer* 75(1):54-64, 1995.
30. Wilmoth MC, Brunner DW: Integrating sexuality into cancer nursing practice, *Oncol Nurs Updates* 9(1):1-14, 2002.
31. Wilmoth MC, Botchway P: Psychosexual implications of breast and gynecologic cancer, *Cancer Invest* 17(8): 631-636, 1999.
32. Tallet AV, Salem N, Moutardier V et al: Radiotherapy and immediate two-stage breast reconstruction with a tissue expander and implant: complications and esthetics, *Int J Radiat Oncol Biol Phys* 57(1):136-142, 2003.
33. Meyerowitz BE, Desmond KA, Rowland JH et al: Sexuality following breast cancer, *J Sex Marital Ther* 25(3):237-250, 1999.
34. Yurek D, Ferrar W, Andersen BL: Breast cancer surgery: comparing surgical groups and determining individual differences in postoperative sexuality and body change stress, *J Consult Clin Psychol* 68(4):697-709, 2000.
35. Gantz PA, Desmond KA, Belin TR et al: Predictors of sexual health in women after a breast cancer diagnosis, *J Clin Oncol* 17(8):2371-2380, 1999.
36. Mancini R, Cosimelli M, Filippini A et al: Nerve-sparing surgery in rectal cancer: feasibility and functional results, *J Exp Clin Cancer Res* 19(1):35-40, 2000.
37. Monga U: Sexuality in cancer patients, *Arch Phys Med Rehab* 9(2):417-442, 1995.
38. Turnbull GB: *Intimacy, sexuality, and an ostomy*, Irvine, Calif, 2001, United Ostomy Association.
39. Sprunk E, Alteneder RR: The impact of an ostomy on sexuality, *Clin J Oncol Nurs* 4(2):85-88, 2000.
40. Gantz PA, Litwin MS, Meyerowitz BE: Sexual problems. In DeVita VT, Hellman S, Rosenberg SA, editors: *Cancer: principles and practices of oncology*, ed 6, Philadelphia, 2001, Lippincott-Raven.
41. Banker FL: The preservation of potency after external beam irradiation for prostate cancer, *Int J Radiat Oncol Biol Phys* 15(1):219-220, 1988.
42. Feeney DD, Moore DH, Look KY et al: The fate of the ovaries after radical hysterectomy and ovarian transposition, *Gynecol Oncol* 56(1):3-7, 1995.

43. Lamb MA: Effects of cancer on the sexuality and fertility of women, *Semin Oncol Nurs* 11(2):120-127, 1995.
44. Flay LD, Matthews JHL: The effects of radiotherapy and surgery on the sexual function of women treated for cervical cancer, *Int J Radiat Oncol Biol Phys* 31(2): 399-404, 1995.
45. Bergmark K, Avall-Lundqvist E, Dickman PW et al: Vaginal changes and sexuality in women with a history of cervical cancer, *N Engl J Med* 340(18):1383-1389, 1999.
46. Andersen BL, Golden-Kreutz DM: Sexual self-concept for the woman with cancer. In Baider L, Cooper CL, Kaplan De-Nour D, editors: *Cancer and the family*, Chichester, NY, 1996, John Wiley & Sons, pp 311-334.
47. Andersen BL, LeGrand J: Body image for women: conceptualization, assessment, and a test of its importance to sexual dysfunction and medical illness, *J Sex Res* 28(5):457-478, 1991.
48. Nguyen NP, Frank C, Moltz MS et al: Impact of dysphagia on quality of life after treatment of head-and-neck cancer, *Int J Radiat Oncol Biol Phys* 61(3):772-778, 2005.
49. Nordgren M, Abendstein H, Jannert M et al: Health-related quality of life five years after diagnosis of laryngeal carcinoma, *Int J Radiat Oncol Biol Phys* 56(5):1333-1343, 2003.
50. Lin A, Kim HM, Terrell JE et al: Quality of life after parotid-sparing IMRT for head-and-neck cancer: a prospective longitudinal study, *Int J Radiat Oncol Biol Phys* 57(1):61-70, 2003.
51. Shell JA: *The longitudinal effects of cancer treatment on sexuality in individuals with lung cancer.* Unpublished doctoral dissertation, Michigan State University, East Lansing, Mich, 2002.
52. Ginsberg M, Quirt C, Ginsberg A et al: Psychiatric illness and psychosocial concerns of patients with newly diagnosed lung cancer, *Can Med Assoc* 5(6):701-708, 1995.
53. Sarna L: Women with lung cancer: impact on quality of life, *Qual Life Res* 2(1):13-22, 1993.
54. American Urological Association, Prostate Cancer Clinical Guidelines Panel: *Report on the management of clinically localized prostate cancer*, Baltimore, Md, 1995, American Urological Association.
55. Stokes S: Comparison of biochemical disease-free survival of patients with localized carcinoma of the prostate undergoing radical prostatectomy, transperineal ultrasound-guided radio-active seed implantation, or definite external beam irradiation, *Int J Radiat Oncol Biol Phys* 47(1):129-136, 2000.
56. Saliken J, Donnelly B, Brasher P et al: The outcome and safety of TRUS-guided percutaneous cryotherapy for localized prostate cancer, *J Vasc Interv Radiol* 10(2 pt 1):199-208, 1999.
57. NIH Consensus Conference: impotence. NIH Consensus Development Panel on Impotence, *JAMA* 270(1):83-90, 1993.
58. Zelefsky MJ, Eid JF: Elucidating the etiology of erectile dysfunction after definitive therapy for prostatic cancer, *Int J Radiat Oncol Biol Phys* 40(1):129-133, 1998.
59. Borghede G, Sullivan M: Measurement of quality of life in localized prostatic cancer patients treated with radiotherapy: development of a prostate cancer-specific module supplementing the EORTC QLQ-C30, *Qual Life Res* 5(2):212-222, 1996.
60. Beard CJ, Propert KJ, Rieker PP et al: Complications after treatment with external-beam irradiation in early-stage prostate cancer patients: a prospective multiinstitutional outcomes study, *J Clin Oncol* 15(1):223-229, 1997.
61. Borghede G, Hedelin H: Radiotherapy of localized prostate cancer: analysis of late treatment complications—a prospective study, *Radiother Oncol* 43(2):139-146, 1997.
62. Turnmer SL, Adams K, Bull CA et al: Sexual dysfunction after radical radiation therapy for prostate cancer: a prospective evaluation, *Urology* 54(1):124-129, 1999.
63. Beckendorf V, Hay M, Rozen R: Changes in sexual function after radiotherapy treatment of prostate cancer, *Br J Urol* 77(1):118-123, 1996.
64. Kaye KW, Olson DJ, Payne JT: Detailed preliminary analysis of iodine-125 implantation for localized prostate cancer using percutaneous approach, *J Urol* 153(3 pt 2):1020-1025, 1995.
65. Stock RG, Stone NN, Iannuzzi C: Sexual potency following interactive ultrasound-guided brachytherapy for prostate cancer, *Int J Radiat Oncol Biol Phys* 35(2): 267-272, 1996.
66. Zelefsky MJ, Wallner KE, Ling CC et al: Comparison of the 5-year outcome and morbidity of three-dimensional conformal radiotherapy versus transperineal permanent iodine-125 implantation for early-stage prostatic cancer, *J Clin Oncol* 17(2):517-522, 1999.
67. Sharkey J, Chovnick SD, Behar RJ: Minimally invasive treatment for localized adenocarcinoma of the prostate: review of 1048 patients treated with ultrasound-guided palladium-103 brachytherapy, *J Endourol* 14(4):343-350, 2000.
68. Merrick GS, Butler WM, Galbreath RW et al: Erectile function after permanent prostate brachytherapy, *Int J Radiat Oncol Biol Phys* 52(4):893-902, 2002.
69. Robinson JW, Moritz S, Fung T: Meta-analysis of rates of erectile function after treatment of localized prostate carcinoma, *Int J Radiat Oncol Biol Phys* 54(4):1063-1068, 2002.
70. Fisch B, Pickett B, Weinberg V et al: Dose of radiation received by the bulb of the penis correlates with risk of impotence after three-dimensional conformal radiotherapy for prostate cancer, *Urology* 57(5):955-959, 2001.
71. Selek U, Cheung R, Mingfwu L et al: Erectile dysfunction and radiation dose to penile base structures: a lack of correlation, *Int J Radiat Oncol Biol Phys* 59(4):1039-1046, 2004.
72. Arterbery VE, Frazier A, Dalmia P: Quality of life after permanent prostate implant, *Surg Oncol* 13(3):461-464, 1997.
73. Helgason AR, Fredrikson M, Adolfsson J et al: Decreased sexual capacity after external radiation therapy for prostate cancer impairs quality of life, *Int J Radiat Oncol Biol Phys* 32(1):33-39, 1995.
74. Herr HW: Quality of life in prostate cancer patients, *CA Cancer J Clin* 47(4):207-217, 1997.
75. Gelblum DY, Potters L, Ashley R et al: Urinary morbidity following ultrasound-guided transperineal prostate seed implantation, *Int J Radiat Oncol Biol Phys* 45(1):59-67, 1999.

76. Giacchetti S, Raoul Y, Wibault P et al: Treatment of stage I testis seminoma by radiotherapy: long-term results—a 30 year experience, *Int J Radiat Oncol Biol Phys* 27(1):3-9, 1993.
77. Incrocci L, Hop WCJ, Wijnmaalen A et al: Treatment outcome, body image, and sexual functioning after orchiectomy and radiotherapy for state I-II testicular seminoma, *Int J Radiat Oncol Biol Phys* 53(5):1165-1173, 2002.
78. Arai Y, Kawakita M, Okada Y et al: Sexuality and fertility in long-term survivors of testicular cancer, *J Clin Oncol* 15(4):1444-1448, 1997.
79. Rieker PP, Fitzgerald EM, Kalish LA et al: Psychosocial factors, curative therapies and behavioral outcomes, *Cancer* 64(11):2399-2407, 1989.
80. Incrocci L, Bosch JL, Slob AK: Testicular prostheses: body image and sexual functioning, *BJU Int* 84(9): 1043-1045, 1999.
81. Stempkowski L: The young adult with testicular cancer. In Whedon MB, editor: *Quality of life: a nursing challenge*, vol 4, Meniscus Educational Institute, 1997, Bala Cynwyd, pp 15-21.
82. Malas S, Levin V, Sur R et al: Fertility in patients treated with radiotherapy following orchidectomy for testicular seminoma, *Clin Oncol (R Coll Radiol)* 6(6):377-380, 1994.
83. Adshead J, Khoubehi B, Wood J et al: Testicular implants and patient satisfaction: a questionnaire-based study of men after orchidectomy for testicular cancer, *BJU Int* 88(6):559-562, 2001.
84. Shell J: Do you like the things that life is showing you? The sensitive self-image of the person with cancer, *Oncol Nurs Forum* 22(6):907-911, 1995.
85. Masters WH, Johnson VE: *Human sexual response*, New York, 1966, Harper Perennial.
86. Schover LR: *Sexuality & cancer: for the man who has cancer and his partner*, Atlanta, 2001, American Cancer Society.
87. Schover LR: *Sexuality & cancer: for the woman who has cancer and her partner*, Atlanta, 2001, American Cancer Society.
88. Leonard M, Hammelef K, Smith GD: Fertility considerations, counseling, and semen cryopreservation for males prior to the initiation of cancer therapy, *Clin J Oncol Nurs* 8(2):127-131, 2004.
89. Schover LR: Cancer patient survey: more information on reproduction needed, *Oncologistics* 3(third quarter):20-27, 2003.
90. Berk LB, Shivnani AT, Small W: Pathophysiology and management of radiation-induced xerostomia, *J Support Oncol* 3(3):191-200, 2005.
91. Smith DB: Urinary continence issues in oncology, *Clin J Oncol Nurs* 3(4):161-167, 1999.
92. American Medical Systems Products, Minnetonka, Minn. Penile prostheses for the treatment of erectile dysfunction (impotence). 8/1/01. Info@visitams.com.
93. Cash JC, Dattoli MJ: Management of patients receiving transperineal palladium-103 prostate implants, *Oncol Nurs Forum* 24(8):1361-1367, 1997.
94. Wallner K, Blasko J, Dattoli M: *Prostate brachytherapy made complicated*, Seattle, 1997, Smart Medicine Press.
95. Lewis J: Nursing management for patients using external vacuum devices: a unique opportunity, *Urol Nurs* 13(3): 80-85, 1993.
96. Crenshaw TL, Goldberg JP: *Sexual pharmacology: drugs that affect sexual functioning*, New York, 1996, Norton.
97. Stipetich RL, Abel LJ, Blatt HJ et al: Nursing assessment of sexual function following permanent prostate brachytherapy for patients with early-stage prostate cancer, *Clin J Oncol Nurs* 6(5):271-274, 2002.
98. Shell JA: Sexuality for patients with gynecologic cancer. In Loudermilk D, editor: *NAACOG's clinical issues in perinatal and women's health nursing*, Philadelphia, 1991, JB Lippincott, pp 54-66.
99. Gosselin TK, Waring JS: Nursing management of patients receiving brachytherapy for gynecologic malignancies, *Clin J Oncol Nurs* 5(2):59-63, 2001.
100. Shell JA: Sexual functioning: body image. In Dow KH, editor: *Nursing care of women with cancer*, St Louis, 2006, Mosby.

Unit VII

Dimensions of Clinical Practice

Chapter 36

Nursing Research and Clinical Trials

Norissa Walter Honea

Research in oncology has led to remarkable improvements in outcomes for patients undergoing cancer therapy. Great strides in technology provide more sophisticated imaging, as well as precision in treatment planning and delivery of radiation dose. Many of these improvements are resulting in longer disease-free survival and reduction in toxicity to surrounding normal tissues. Although people with cancer are living longer thanks to research results from clinical trials for cancer treatment, nursing research aims to describe, explain, predict, and influence or control patient responses to cancer diagnosis, disease, and treatment. This chapter aims to shed light on these developments and their importance to clinicians in radiation oncology.

NURSING RESEARCH

A Place In History

As nurses in a basic nursing program, many learned how Florence Nightingale changed the world for the soldiers in her care. Her 'wild' ideas about disease transmission lead to a drastic reduction in mortality (from 42% to 2%) during the Crimean War. First, she theorized the concepts of health and the relationship to fresh air, light, clean water, clean bandages. She kept meticulous notes to record her interventions and outcomes. Originally published in 1860, her compiled data from 14 years of observation and thoughts are titled, "Notes on Nursing".[1] The results of this data allowed her to show improvements in outcomes and to influence the military in their practice towards the soldiers who were wounded during the war and to influence society to recognize the need for testing of public water and improving sanitation.

Other key developments occurred relative to the importance of nursing research through the last century and into this one. In the early 1900s, nursing research was aimed at nursing education and improvements in nursing curriculum. As the decades passed, more focus was placed on patient care delivery and then on quality of life for patients. The American Nurses Association (ANA) began a study of nursing functions and activities in 1950. Dissemination of those research results led to the development of ANA statements on nursing functions, standards, and qualifications for professional nurses published in 1959.[2] Nursing scholars developed conceptual models and theories during the 1960s and 1970s. New journals emerged to disseminate the works related to these theories; among these were a number of specialty nursing journals, including the *Oncology Nursing Forum* and *Cancer Nursing*. More journals arrived on the scene in the 1980s. In 1983 the *Annual Review of Nursing Research* had its debut, and *Seminars in Oncology Nursing* was launched in 1985. The National Institute for Nursing Research (NINR), formed in 1986 as the National *Center* for Nursing Research and then later renamed as an *Institute*, brought visibility and funding opportunities for nursing research that continue into the twenty-first century. Research results have been disseminated by publication of journal articles, conference presentations, abstracts, and posters promoting evidenced-based practice. These forums have highlighted the state of the science on nursing knowledge in a variety of areas.

Defining the Nursing Profession

Burns and Grove[2] assert that nursing research must focus on issues germane to nurses in order to "develop a unique body of knowledge for practice." The ANA[3] provides the following definition of nursing:

Nursing is the protection, promotion, and optimization of health and abilities, prevention of illness and injury, alleviation of suffering through the diagnosis and treatment of human response, and advocacy in the care of individuals, families, communities, and populations.

Nursing knowledge gained through scientific investigations answer *what, why*, and *how* types of questions nurses ask in their efforts to understand and/or improve human responses to actual or potential health problems such as diagnosis of disease and treatment effects.[2] This knowledge is along a continuum of concrete to abstract thought, where concrete thinking is limited by an experience that is observed in time and space. Abstract thought processes of introspection, intuition, and reasoning enable scientific findings to be developed into theories. A blending of science and theories into an integrated body of knowledge, guided by a philosophical framework is applied to nursing practice.[2] Quantitative methods use numbers in statistical tests that can be analyzed objectively to describe, compare, correlate, and make predictions. Abstract thinking looks for meaning, patterns, relationships, and philosophical implications to understand the 'big picture' from another's perspective. Qualitative methods employ words, text as language, with concern for finding subjective meaning and discovery within individual, historical, social, or cultural contexts. Scientific research conducted using quantitative or qualitative methods can employ methods in concert with each other.

Evidence-based practice (EBP) is a process clinicians use to make clinical decisions using the best research evidence available along with clinical expertise and patient preference.[4] Using EBP involves (1) clearly identifying the problem based on current nursing knowledge and practice; (2) reviewing relevant research from the literature; (3) critically evaluating the research evidence for scientific merit; and (4) choosing interventions justified as the most valid evidence.[4] Research utilization is the use of evidence, demonstrated by a change in practice, to enhance outcomes of care.[4] Chapter 38 discusses EBP more fully.

The National Institute for Nursing Research (NINR) Congressional Justification Report for their 2006 budget focuses on nursing research that addresses important national health concerns. Nursing research priorities aim at self-management and quality of life for children, adolescents, and understudied populations with chronic diseases. Additional priorities include health risk behavior change, improving care of dying and quality of life at the end-of-life, translating genetics/genomic research into clinical practice, managing symptom clusters in people with cancer and HIV/AIDS, and reducing health disparities among minority and underserved women.[5]

Research in Radiation Oncology

The Oncology Nursing Society (ONS), incorporated in 1973, was the first professional nursing organization dedicated to the field of oncology nursing. ONS surveys its membership every 4 years to determine research priorities and has done so since 1981. Grant and Stromborg[6] published results of the first ONS survey of members' research activities where respondents described data collection for medical research as the most frequent activity performed. In 1985, McGuire and colleagues[7] found that survey respondents participated in other research activities such as literature reviews and proposal development and more nurse-directed research.[7,8] Results from subsequent ONS surveys served to delineate priorities for nursing research for the society. Symptom management, quality of life (QOL), pain, cancer risk reduction, screening and detection, economic/cost issues, end-of-life/palliative care, and patient education, research utilization and evidenced-based practice, and coping and stress management have consistently been in the top 10 priorities over the past 2 decades.[9-12]

The Radiation Nursing Special Interest Group (SIG) of ONS, chartered in 1989 as one of the first 11 SIGs, organized to provide a network of support, foster professional development, and develop guidelines for patients undergoing radiation therapy (RT).[13] Today, with more than 390 members, it is one of the largest ONS SIGs.

Providing further evidence of the value of clinicians specializing in RT, clinicians became eligible to join the American Society for Therapeutic Radiology and Oncology (ASTRO), a professional organization formed in 1958 for physicians, physicists, scientists, and therapists, further supporting the growth in professionalism of radiation oncology nursing. The Committee on Nursing within ASTRO formed in 1996 to promote excellence in patient care and advance oncology nursing practice by disseminating results of scientific nursing research and provide opportunities for nursing educational and professional development.[14]

Commitment to providing a scientific foundation for nursing practice through research can be seen in the broadening range of studies over the past 2 decades. Grant[8] summarized nursing research in RT for the first decade. Dow[15] then summarized RT nursing research through 1996, followed by Shepard and Kelvin who summarized the studies through early 1999.[14,15]

Early studies described the staff nurse role in radiation departments; patient descriptions of the radiation experience; patient self-care, side effects, and clinical care, late effects, quality of life (QOL), and functional status responses to RT.[8] Later studies examined information needs of those who were undergoing radiation therapy. Intervention studies evaluated various patient educational methods aimed at meeting information needs. Nutritional needs, skin care management, fatigue, coping and comfort, and late effects and survivorship issues were the focus of many studies in the 1990s.[14,15] Identification of relevant studies can be found in the Cumulative Index to Nursing and Allied Health Literature (CINAHL) and PubMed databases and in research abstracts from oncology meetings. Because this entire textbook covers cumulative knowledge in radiation oncology nursing, a synopsis of selected published studies related to radiation oncology nursing research from 1999 to 2005 is found in the next section. The studies primarily relate to nursing roles and staffing, information needs, coping, treatment effects and symptom management, and QOL.

Nursing Roles and Staffing in Radiation

A descriptive study by Moore-Higgs and colleagues[16] examined the role and responsibilities of licensed nursing personnel within ONS membership and the RT SIG who indicated they worked in radiation oncology centers in North America. Returned surveys totaled 284 of the 500 that were sent to ONS members. The majority of the returned surveys (92%) came from RT SIG members. Three surveys were deemed ineligible because the nurses indicated they no longer worked in radiation. The survey instrument was developed by the RT SIG subcommittee whose goal was to describe the current roles and responsibilities of licensed nurses. Study respondents returned a six-page, self-administered questionnaire with both fixed-choice and open-ended questions about demographic and professional characteristics, practice setting and employment characteristics, and responsibilities for administrative, clerical, clinical, education, and research functions.

Respondents were primarily female (94%), aged 40 to 49 years (46%) with a bachelor's or master's degree as the highest level of education (58%) and were oncology certified nurses (68%) in staff nurse (51%) or clinician positions (12%) working 40 or more hours per week (80%). More than half had been working in radiation for more than 5 years (64%) with nearly a third having more than 10 years experience. Practice settings were primarily community-based hospital facilities (49%), including both private practice freestanding and hospital-based settings, and academic practice settings represented by generally urban (51%) or suburban (34%) communities. Group practice physicians employed the majority of respondents (70%). Only 22% reported having a nurse as their immediate supervisor (18% of respondents indicated their title was nurse supervisor or manager).

Administrative activities reported were supervision of other staff, writing nursing and/or non-nursing policies and procedures, checking emergency equipment, medication monitoring, and quality improvement studies. Clerical responsibilities dealt with scheduling procedures, writing orders, and third-party payment documents, as well as requesting films and records for new patient evaluations. Almost half indicated they had responsibility for completing disability or insurance forms (49%). Coordinating schedules between radiation and chemotherapy were reported by staff nurses, nurse managers, and advanced practice nurses (APN). Staff nurses reported a variety of administrative, clerical, patient care/clinical, and research activities. Traditional patient care responsibilities of the clinicians in RT departments include escorting patients to exam rooms, cleaning instruments, stocking supplies, obtaining vital signs, completing initial nursing assessment, detailed history, physical exam, monitoring patients during sedation, administering IV fluids, performing telephone triage, obtaining consents, assessing and managing symptoms, and providing patient education. Patient education activities regularly performed by staff nurses, nurse managers, and APNs included teaching about radiation procedures (98%, 80%, 92%), side effects (98%, 92%, 93%), and counseling for social service needs (70%, 59%, 70%). The patient education role was strongly demonstrated in this study. Although the majority of respondents reported no participation in clinical research activities, those who did performed data management activities and coordinated follow-up exams and studies as their primary tasks. APNs reported spending more time in research activities than staff nurses or nurse managers (6%, 2%, and 2%, respectively). Limitations of the study were that the survey was sent only to ONS members who reported working in radiation oncology, which may not represent the true number of clinicians working in radiation oncology across the United States and Canada. The instrument limited responses to "yes" or "no" for a number of tasks chosen by the committee, which did not allow for other activities that may have been performed in individual practices. Additionally, with regard to category labels (e.g., administrative, clerical, research, or patient care tasks) in the questions about percentage of time spent performing tasks, respondents were left to interpret what was meant by the labels and could consider certain tasks differently with regard to administrative and clerical.

Information Needs and Coping

Christman, Oakley, and Cronin[17] conducted a prospective descriptive study in which they interviewed women undergoing radiation therapy (brachytherapy or external beam RT) for uterine cancer to ascertain their symptom experience. The study was necessary to develop preparatory intervention guided by self-regulation theory, which asserts that mental images of stressful experiences guide coping efforts.[18-20] The schema is from a description of concrete, objective features of a stressful experience that help patients focus more on objective aspects of the experience rather than the subjective, emotional reactions.

Women aged 49 to 52 years, with stage I–IIB disease and high functional status (Karnofsky performance status [KPS] of 80% or more), underwent weekly interviews during RT and at 2 and 4 weeks posttreatment to document symptom experiences. Symptoms most frequently reported were sleep disorder, fatigue, diarrhea, anorexia, nausea, urinary complaints, and vaginal discharge. However, symptom reports apparently determined that incidence of urinary frequency and burning increased with brachytherapy, and a greater incidence of vaginal discharge and irritation were found in those who were preoperative.

Stage of cancer, operative status, and timing of brachytherapy were found to influence respondent reports of symptoms. The most meaningful differences in symptom reports were related to operative status with a gradual decrease over the 3 months after treatment. Previous reports of patients who received concrete objective information while they underwent RT, maintained more of their usual activities than those who did not. In this study, the severity of the symptoms was associated with a disruption in usual activities and whether symptoms caused emotional distress.[17]

Velji and Fitch[21] conducted interviews with 10 women aged 36 to 75 years, receiving low-dose brachytherapy for cervical or endometrial cancer. These researchers began from the assumption that brachytherapy would be a very difficult treatment, that reactions to treatment would be shaped by having cancer in a gynecologic organ and by having had previous treatment. Also assumed were that their respondents' experiences were influenced by the dimensions of the brachytherapy, which included isolation, immobility; limited contact with care providers, perceptions of being radioactive, and altered bodily functions. Interviews started with an open-ended question asking women to describe in their own words what the brachytherapy experience was like for them. Specific questions were asked as follow up for clarifications about the content. Verbatim transcripts were analyzed using a specific method as a guide. Researchers identified three main themes from this study. These were (a) women's experiences with brachytherapy were embedded within the complete context in which treatment was given, shaped by personal, environmental, and treatment-related factors; (b) the discomfort experienced during brachytherapy was perceived as a totality of symptoms, including but not limited to pain; and (c) the brachytherapy experience was characterized by an intense focus on time and tensions embedded in issues related to time.[21] Rich descriptive quotes from respondents were reported to allow the reader an elaborated example from the themes. Although three main themes were identified, the authors stated the women also spoke of what helped them get through treatment: prayer and faith in God, rationalized benefits of treatment, social support and open communication, and support of care providers.[21]

Long[22] explored the meanings and experiences of 20 individuals undergoing RT for cancer or brain tumor. How these patients interpreted the meanings of their experience within the context of an intensive course of radiation therapy was the aim of the study so findings could be related to clinicians in the radiation oncology setting. The main theme of *Being Informed* emerged from the interviews. Often reported as inadequate or did not meet the needs of individuals in the study were reports about information and preparation for RT. Participants suggested that healthcare providers did not address their preformed misconceptions about RT (from experiences of others and media), supporting literature elsewhere suggesting difficult communication between patients and providers.[22] Participants continued to adopt the 'sick' role even though they attend treatments as an outpatient and are required to manage their own care. Participant coping styles varied and were not clearly identified or assisted by relevant health personal.[22] Glimpses into the experiences of those who participated in the interviews provide helpful information, yet it is not possible to draw conclusions that all patients undergoing RT share common themes with these participants.

A three-group randomized clinical trial with a sample of 76 adults (Mean age = 55 yrs; 68% women, 92% Caucasian) who had gynecologic, head and neck, or lung cancer—all receiving RT with a curative intent—was conducted by Christman and Cain.[23] Effects of concrete objective information (COI) and relaxation instruction (RI) and the role of symptom uncertainty and body awareness to the intervention effects were examined at week 3 of RT and 2 and 4 weeks after RT. Study hypotheses were as follows: (1) Patients receiving COI would report maintaining more of their usual activities than those who do not receive the information. (2) Patients receiving RI would report less emotional distress than those who do not receive the instruction. (3) The effects of both interventions would be greater in patients who report more awareness of bodily sensations than those who report less awareness. (4) Uncertainty about symptom experienced would help to explain why COI is effective. Research variables were intervention group (COI, RI, control), social, household, and recreational activities measured by the 18 visual analog scales (VAS) from the Sickness Impact Profile (SIP); anxiety, depression, and anger using the Profile of Mood States (POMS) instrument; body awareness measured using a subscale of the Body Consciousness Questionnaire; symptoms and symptom uncertainty.

Interventions for women having RT for gynecologic cancer, that is, COI messages describing what patients usually hear, see, feel during RT, used symptom descriptors from the study previously described by Christman and colleagues.[17] Descriptors were different for preoperative and postoperative women. Descriptors for patients with head and neck or lung cancer were symptoms that were described by King and colleagues in 1985 as well as those described by Johnson et al. were incorporated into the COI messages.[24,25] Each professionally audio-recorded COI message also incorporated symptom changes expected across the treatment experience as they related to RT. Adapted from progressive relaxation technique, RI audio-recordings given to participants during first week of RT included an introduction to relaxation and focused on progressive and systematic relaxation of all muscle groups. A shortened version of the tape was given to participants during the last week of treatment. It also included a suggestion for how relaxation might be helpful in dealing with daily life events. Control group participants received professionally recorded tapes with general information from the NIH booklet *Radiation Therapy and You.* The second message included general information about follow-up care.

Participants were asked at 4 weeks after treatment to indicate whether they had used any of the coping strategies since beginning RT. More of the patients from the RI group reported use of a relaxation method than those from the other two groups. Repeated measures analysis of covariance indicated that the only effect on emotional distress was for the covariate of preintervention distress. In week 3 of treatment, participants from both the COI and RI groups reported more social activity than those from the control group. Neither of the intervention groups differed from the control group at the posttreatment measurement times with regard to social activity. People who scored high in body awareness indicated greater household activity within the RI group compared to the control group, although only during week 3 of treatment, and no differences were found between the intervention and control groups at the time of posttreatment measurements. Preparatory information that described typical experiences, including symptom experiences, helped patients form a mental representation that reduced uncertainty about their own symptom experiences and aided focus on positive coping skills. Findings from this study support the positive effects of COI on functional status and suggest that RI may improve functional status during RT.[23]

Treatment Effects and Symptom Management

Treatment effects can be acute, as noted, during treatment or shortly after RT. Late treatment effects may manifest weeks, months, to years after RT and depend on the site, dose, and type of RT delivered (external beam versus brachytherapy). Nursing assessment for actual and potential treatment-related toxicity is a key function of clinicians. The clinician keeps in mind that symptoms or treatment effects are aggravated with the use of concomitant chemotherapy or biotherapy.

Fatigue, noted as the most common side effect of radiation for over 25 years, is one side effect that clinicians still grapple with understanding as they assist patients who experience fatigue because of radiation therapy.[24,26-31] Lovely, Miaskowski, and Dodd[32] conducted a descriptive study to evaluate fatigue and QOL in patients with glioblastoma multiforme (GBM), a malignant brain tumor. Sixty patients who could read, write, and understand English completed surveys for this study at both baseline (after diagnosis and surgery), and again within 2 weeks of completing radiation therapy. In comparing results from baseline to post RT, they found significant increases noted in the fatigue subscale score of the POMS instrument. In correlating fatigue and QOL subscales from the Multidimensional QOL Scale—Cancer, Version 2, they found that higher levels of fatigue were associated with poorer QOL for the physical, interpersonal, and psychosocial well-being and symptom management, but not with nutritional well-being. This was actually the first study to show the increase in fatigue in patients with GBM after radiation.

Mangan and Mood[33] also looked at the multidimensionality of the fatigue experience of patients receiving radiation for a variety of a disease sites. They recruited 384 subjects from two urban, university-affiliated outpatient radiation clinics in the Midwest for their corollary study to a parent study from 1995 to 1999. They looked at baseline hemoglobin; health state measured by proxy from the Functional Assessment of Cancer Therapy (FACT) tool, global symptom distress measure with Mood's Symptom Scale, and mood disturbance measured using POMS. Fatigue characteristics of presence, onset, duration, and severity of distress were measured at five time periods, (1) baseline, (2) at 2 weeks, and (3) final week of treatment, and then again at (4) 1 month and (5) 3 months after treatment. No significant between-group differences were found with regard to variables of interest, so subjects from different groups were pooled for analysis. Onset of fatigue was widely variable, with the average at about halfway through week 2 of treatment. The investigators reported that 20% of their subjects reported fatigue started or worsened from the very first treatment day. Reports of fatigue duration were 1 to 78 days. Severity of fatigue was greater at the end of treatment than earlier in the course. They did find that those who reported earlier *onset* of fatigue, greater distress from fatigue, and the longer duration of fatigue were more highly correlated with global symptom distress and mood disturbance. A significant difference was noted in the mean *duration* of fatigue where women with gynecologic cancer had a longer duration than men treated for prostate cancer. However, regarding severity of *distress* from fatigue, those treated for lung cancer reported greater distress than those treated for prostate cancer. A later onset of fatigue correlated with more positive health status.

An interesting study conducted by Sarna and Conde[34] used wrist actigraph monitors on adult subjects undergoing radiation therapy for breast, chest, or abdominal areas over a 6-week course. The wrist actigraph monitors were worn for 72 hours (placed on Monday, removed on Friday) during the second and fifth weeks of treatment. Subjects kept a daily diary of their physical activity prior to bedtime during this time. The POMS vigor-activity and fatigue-inertial subscales were used to assess subjects' perceptions of their levels of activity and fatigue. Additionally, a Linear Analogue Scale—Fatigue was used daily for self-assessment of fatigue during the study period. The Symptom Distress Scale, a self-report tool, indicated the degree of discomfort from a number of cancer and treatment-related symptoms. Subjects were instructed to record on this tool on Mondays and Fridays during the study period. Seven of eight subjects completed all measures at both study periods. The researchers found that activity recorded by the actigraph monitors increased by the end of the week and correlated with the POMS

Vigor-Activity subscales for both weeks of study. Interestingly, subjects reported lower levels of fatigue as measured by the POMS fatigue-inertia subscales and the Linear Analogue Scale—Fatigue at the end of each study interval. In this small sample, no direct relationship was found regarding perception of fatigue and the total dose of radiation.[34]

Although multiple symptoms often appear together as a cluster, they may be difficult to tease apart. Some have explored the relationship between fatigue and nutritional status.[35] In her concept analysis, Armstrong[36] defined *symptom experience* "as the perception of frequency, intensity, distress, and meaning occurring as symptoms are produced and expressed." Many previous nursing research studies focused on individual symptoms rather than clusters of symptoms occurring simultaneously.

Shih and colleagues[37] conducted an extensive literature review of research studies from 1966 to 2001 of treatments for radiation-induced oral mucositis, the most common complication among patients with head and neck cancer. From their investigations, the researchers found over 50 such articles and were able to categorize the treatments as antimicrobial, coating, antiinflammatory, or cytokine-like agents. They noted that many of the studies had small samples and used inconsistent methods to evaluate the extent and severity of mucositis. Although many strategies and products appear promising, lack of consistent results makes it difficult to generalize or make specific conclusions about the effectiveness of any one type of agent.

As pelvic RT is employed for prostate and gynecologic cancers, diarrhea is a common complication for these patients. Murphy and colleagues[38] found in their randomized pilot study of 60 patients that the bulking agent psyllium was beneficial in reducing the severity and incidence of radiation-induced diarrhea, although results did not reach statistical significance. Their newly designed tool (patient diary) to measure the frequency and texture of stools and the use of antidiarrheal medications lacked validity and reliability and perhaps did not adequately reflect their intended construct. The clinical significance was enough for these researchers to recommend further investigation with larger samples.

Due to limited time in the clinical setting to assess in depth the patient symptom and QOL experience, Berry and colleagues[39] developed and pilot-tested a computerized assessment tool during a 15-month period in 2001 to 2002, with 45 women and 56 men receiving outpatient RT. Six clinicians from the RT department participated in standing focus groups in the tool development process, recommending brevity, flexibility, and simplicity as priorities. The main research variables were pain intensity, symptoms, QOL, and demographics. Computerized versions of the 0 to 10 Pain Intensity Numerical Scale, Symptom Distress Scale, and Short Form-8 (SF-8) were tested. Although less than half the subjects reported using a computer with any regularity, it took on average, less than 8 minutes for subjects to complete the computerized form. More often reported were moderate to high levels of distress for fatigue, pain, and emotional issues. The ease with which the computerized tool was completed could make it quite feasible in many RT departments, with the caveat that the program can be programmed to direct the respondent for further evaluation and coordination of care.

A companion study, conducted by Mullen, Berry, and Zierler[40] as part of the larger study to determine the acceptability of the computerized tool by patients and the usability of the information (output) by the healthcare providers. Six preassessment items and 10 postassessment items used Likert-type responses. Total scores were not calculated. Preassessment questions asked about attitudes towards computers, paper-and-pencil surveys, computer questionnaires, and face-to-face interviews. Seven of the postassessment items asked about the experience of using the computerized program (ease, enjoyable, understandable, helpful, whether they liked the program, amount of time to complete was acceptable, and overall satisfaction with the program). Three additional questions were designed to draw out preferences of interview method comparing computer, written, and face-to-face interviews. Clinician usability was computed by four written questions using Likert-type responses as well (had the tool been viewed before the patient encountered it, was graphic display of results useful). Comparisons were made between pre- and postassessment responses. Results indicated a significantly negative correlation between age and computer use. All the respondents who reported they never used a computer were over age 54 years. Of the 45 patient participants, 62% indicated they liked computers, 18% were neutral, 9% did not like, and 11% did not respond. Of the 39 respondents, 41% signified they liked paper-pencil surveys, 54% liked computer questionnaires, and 65% liked face-to-face interviews. None of the 33 respondents reported having much difficulty with the program, reporting an average of 10 minutes to complete as indicated by the postassessment survey in which 70% indicated they were satisfied with the computer program. Due to the small sample size and variation in clinician background, differences in groups were not calculated, but nurses/nurse practitioners gave the most favorable reports on the utility of the graphic form of patient data, and overall, the computer-generated graphics were helpful (>70%) to identify areas of concern, guide clinical interactions, promote communication, and identify areas of patient need. Results cannot be generalized; however, they do provide an alternate means for generating patient information about QOL and symptom experience in a busy RT setting by using technology to alert healthcare providers of patient concerns and needs.

Quality of Life

Ward-Smith, Wittkopp, and Sheldon[41] examined quality of life (QOL) among men treated with brachytherapy for prostate cancer. A sample of 58 men, age ranging from 52 to 82, who chose to undergo brachytherapy for localized prostate cancer completed a series of self-evaluated QOL measures using the Functional Assessment of Cancer Therapy—Prostate (FACT-P) survey at baseline, and at 3, 6, and 12 months after treatment. The FACT-P was designed to measure health-related QOL for functional well-being, social well-being, physical well-being, emotional well-being, and specific prostate concerns in patients with prostate cancer. They found changes in the subscales of emotional well-being and specific prostate concerns. Emotional well-being scores varied from pretreatment to 12 months after RT. Specific prostate concerns varied from baseline to 3 months after RT indicating concerns dissipate over time.

Overcash[42] used narrative research to understand the QOL of older women with breast cancer. Her sample of 12 women undergoing active treatment (chemotherapy, n = 3; RT, n = 4, or hormonal, n = 8; [some combinations for hormonal/RT]) for breast cancer included women who were at least 70 years old. Most of the women in her sample had metastatic disease. The respondents were asked to reflect on their life experiences before the cancer diagnosis, as well as during and after diagnosis and treatment. Verbatim transcripts were analyzed using specific criteria to answer the following research question, "What are the elements affecting QOL of women aged 70 or older who are currently undergoing treatment for breast cancer?"[42] The criteria used were a recurrence of ideas within the narratives, repetition, and forcefulness (cues that reinforce the concept). Eight major themes (from 30) emerged from the data. They included (1) importance of God, (2) importance of positive attitude, (3) no alteration in lifestyle, (4) physician trust, (5) caregiver to others, (6) need to protect family, (7) importance of health, and (8) importance of family. The authors stated there was a great amount of variation among the eight multidimensional themes because respondents designated their own different meanings for the same terms. Nursing implications point to the ability to detect and realize the cultural and personal uniqueness of the individuals in everyday practice. Careful attention to maintaining and supporting the functional ability and resources for the elderly is desired, with de-emphasis on the stereotype of elderly as frail, ill, or dependent. Interviewing patients can fill in the data gaps not always captured with quantitative gathering and may have a therapeutic value.

In a study of 23 consecutive subjects, aged 40 to 73 years, with non–small cell lung cancer (NSCLC) scheduled to receive curative RT, John examined perceptions of QOL over four measurement periods.[43] Roy's Adaptation Model was used as the conceptual framework for the study that conceptualizes the individual as an adaptive biopsychosocial responsive being with adaptive or ineffective coping mechanisms to deal with various stimuli in a changing environment. Coping with cough, dyspnea, hemoptysis, emotional effects of diagnosis and treatment, and the physical consequences of treatment are all stimuli to which one must respond. Subjects completed the self-report FACT-L (for lung cancer) instrument of 28 Likert-type questions, comprised of subscales for physical well-being, social/family well-being, relationship with doctor, emotional well-being, and functional well-being. Higher scores indicate greater satisfaction with QOL and range from 0 to 148. Surveys were completed pre-RT, during the fourth week of treatment, at the end of RT and at posttreatment follow-up for comparisons to answer the research question, "Do perceptions of QOL change over time in patients with NSCLC receiving RT?"[43] Results of the repeated measures analysis of variance indicated subjects rated significantly lower QOL scores during RT and significantly higher 1-month post-RT. These were consistent with other studies of QOL in people with NSCLC that indicated improvement in QOL from the start of treatment.[44,45] Implications for nursing practice include patient education about expected treatment side effects and their management; assessment of patient's coping skills, adaptation, and QOL through RT; anticipation of needs; and providing appropriate intervention strategies.

Looking Back, Looking Forward

The importance of generating public awareness about the contributions nursing research makes to patient outcomes is a strategic goal of ONS.[46] Clinicians in the radiation oncology specialty can help generate that awareness. Reading professional journals, attending nursing research conferences, both venues for dissemination of research findings, 'provide a forum for scholarly exchange related to the foundation and advancement of cancer nursing science and practice,' and give birth to new ideas and directions for study.[47] Nursing research priority assessment by the NINR, ONS, and others, yields great opportunity to provide direction and potential funding. Nursing research projects with nursing interventions may lead to changes in patient's symptom experience, function, safety, emotional distress, and/or cost.[46] A listing of resources for oncology nursing research is provided in Box 36-1.

Box 36-1 Resources for Nursing Research

American Nurses Association
www.ana.org

Eastern Nursing Research Society
www.enrs-go.org

Midwest Nursing Research Society
www.mnrs.org

National Institute for Nursing Research
www.nih.gov/ninr

Oncology Nursing Society
www.ons.org

Sigma Theta Tau International Honor Society of Nursing
www.nursingsociety.org

Southern Nursing Research Society
www.snrs.org

University of Minnesota Evidence-Based Nursing
http://evidence.ahc.umn.edu/ebn.htm

Western Institute of Nursing
www.ohsu.edu/son/win

CLINICAL TRIALS

Cancer clinical trials are research studies that involve people in an effort to answer scientific questions that improve how cancer is prevented, diagnosed, or treated. These trials can be treatment trials, prevention trials, early-detection or screening trials, diagnostic trials, and quality of life and supportive care studies. Clinical trials in oncology provide the basis for what becomes "standard of care" for prevention, detection, treatment of cancer, or supportive measures during treatment. Those who participate in clinical trials pave the way for future patients who develop cancer. The more who participate, the sooner the critical questions can be answered.

National Cancer Institute

"The mission of the National Cancer Institute (NCI) is to eliminate the suffering and death due to cancer....through a process of discovery, development and delivery."[48] The Clinical Trials Program is the largest collaborative research activity of the NCI. The NCI established the Clinical Trials Cooperative Group Program in 1955, now with over 1700 participating institutions that collectively enroll more than 22,000 new cancer patients/subjects annually. Cooperative groups are listed in Box 36-2.[48]

Through the testing of interventions to prevent, detect, and treat cancer, the NCI supports more than 1300 clinical trials each year, aiding more than 200,000 people in the process. Currently, nearly 95% of children with cancer participate in clinical trials, yet only about 3% of adults with cancer participate.

Patient and provider barriers contribute to this low percentage of adult participation in cancer clinical trials. Patients may not know about or have access to a clinical trial. They may be afraid or

Box 36-2 Websites of NCI Clinical Trials Cooperative Groups

American College of Radiology Imaging Network
www.acrin.org

American College of Surgeons Oncology Group
www.acosog.org

Cancer and Leukemia Group B
www.calgb.org

CureSearch: Children's Oncology Group
www.childrensoncologygroup.org

Eastern Cooperative Oncology Group
www.ecog.org

European Organization for Research and Treatment of Cancer
www.eortc.be/default.htm

Gynecologic Oncology Group
www.gog.org

National Cancer Institute of Canada, Clinical Trials Group
www.ctg.queensu.ca

National Surgical Adjuvant Breast and Bowel Project
www.nsabp.pitt.edu

North Central Cancer Treatment Group
http://ncctg.mayo.edu

Radiation Therapy Oncology Group
www.rtog.org

Southwest Oncology Group
www.swog.org

NCI, National Cancer Institute.

suspicious of research stemming from knowledge of historical unethical conduct, misuse or fraud related to research in the past. Patients may not be able to afford to participate in a clinical trial because of travel or time constraints dictated by a protocol. Additionally, some patients may not wish to go against what they feel their physician wishes.

Provider barriers to clinical trial participation also may be due to a lack of awareness about what is available or appropriate. A physician may be unwilling to let go of control of a person's care because the protocol dictates how treatment and follow-up are conducted. As well, a physician may believe that standard therapy is best; or there may be concern about added administrative burdens for his/her medical staff or additional cost to patients.[49]

Phases of Clinical Trials

Development of pharmaceutical protocols in humans that begins after preliminary laboratory testing has been completed. Four phases of clinical trials exist. In phase I trials, in which few people are enrolled, with the goal is to discover how a particular pharmaceutical acts in a human, these studies look at *pharmacokinetics*. This includes evaluating biophysiologic measures such as study drug levels, vital signs, blood counts, and chemistries to see how these parameters are affected by the new agent and what interactions may be occurring with other drugs a patient may be taking at the same time. Phase I trials also evaluate for all side effects and determine the maximum tolerated dose (MTD) of a drug. Those who participate in phase I cancer clinical trials usually do not have other treatment options.

Phase II trials seek to find out whether the agent or intervention being studied has an effect on a certain type of cancer. In laboratory experiments preceding the trial, the type of cancer in question is identified to be somewhat sensitive to the proposed treatment being tested in humans. The goal of this phase is to determine efficacy and to continue to evaluate the safety and toxicity profile of the treatment. In radiation, this may encompass treatment given in a different way, such as a boost being given concomitantly, or treatment may be delivered using technology that is more sophisticated (e.g., intensity-modulated RT, or radiosurgery techniques). If results are promising, the next phase of study will be pivotal, possibly leading to approval by the Food and Drug Administration (FDA).

Phase III studies are pivotal because they challenge the 'standard of care.' These trials seek to find whether there is equivalence or superiority compared to standard treatment. Participants have an equal chance of being assigned to one of two or more groups. This is called *randomization*. One subject receives the standard treatment, whereas the other gets the new treatment plus the standard treatment, and in other studies standard treatment is compared to a new therapy. Randomization is important because it provides the best way to prove the effectiveness of the new treatment.

Phase IV trials are after-market studies that expand the research on a clinical drug or treatment to determine possible use for other indications or administration schedules. For example, cyclophosphamide, a chemotherapy agent first used in cancer treatment has had the indication expanded to include the treatment of noncancerous diseases such as rheumatoid arthritis and certain other autoimmune disorders. Safety and efficacy data are collected and reported throughout the trial to obtain further approval for expanded indication.

Protection of Human Subjects

At the core of all procedures undertaken in the course of a clinical trial is the protection of human subjects. A human subject is someone who participates in a research study, as either a test article or control and can be either a healthy human or a patient.[50] According to the NIH guidelines for the conduct of research involving human subjects, "A 'human subject' is a living individual about whom the investigator obtains either (1) data through interaction with the individual or (2) identifiable private information."[51] Vulnerable populations are those that are at risk of exploitation from research. They include children, mentally and physically disabled people, prisoners, pregnant women, and ethnic minorities.

Human subject protection is mandated by the United States federal government under the Food and Drug Administration (FDA) of the Department of Health and Human Services. The Code of Federal Regulations (CFR) Title 45 (Public Welfare), Part 46 (Protection of Human Subjects), is the standard for all human subjects research. Good Clinical Practice (GCP) Guidelines and the International Conference on Harmonisation (ICH) for Technical Requirements for Registration of Pharmaceuticals for Human Use as well as CFR, provide the uniformed standard for the design and conduct of ethical research in the United States and the world.[50]

In the past, research subjects have been harmed or used for research without their knowledge or consent; this led to the development of the Nuremberg Code, Declaration of Helsinki, and the Belmont Report.[50,51] The NIH established the Office of Human Subjects Research to assist investigators in clinical trials to understand and act in accordance with regulatory requirements and ethical principles concerning human subjects research.[50,51] The ethical principles of autonomy (self-determination), beneficence (do good), confidentiality (respect privacy), equality (all people are equals), justice (treat all fairly), nonmalfeasance (do no harm), respect for persons, and veracity (truth-telling) need to be followed. The CFR outlines exactly who is in charge and how human research subjects are protected. Two such mechanisms are the Institutional Review Board (IRB) and the informed consent process.

Institutional Review Board

An IRB is composed of at least five members with expertise in science and ethics, as well as other nonscientific areas (e.g., legal or financial), although their primary concerns are in nonscientific areas.[52] This committee provides an objective review of research activities involving human subjects. Members acting within the IRB take into account ethical principles (respect for subjects, beneficence, justice, the fair selection of subjects) contained in the Belmont Report and the requirements laid out in the CFR (45 CFR 46) and follow the policies and procedures per the NIH while reviewing the proposed research. They need to assure that risks to subjects are minimized, that procedures do not expose the subject to unnecessary risk. Anticipated risks should be reasonable and not outweigh potential benefit. Informed consent is obtained from each subject or his or her legal guardian, and the board assures that the research plan provides for data safety monitoring to assure safety and confidentiality.[53] In this way, an IRB assures protection of human subjects during the conduct of a particular study. Investigators must report to the IRB all serious adverse events related to study procedures, as well as report annually to the IRB on the status of all studies for which patients are enrolled. The IRB has the authority to make recommended changes to an informed consent form before approving the opening of a study. Under what is known as the Common Rule, an IRB is required to report clinical investigator misconduct to the institution and the FDA.[52]

Clinical investigator responsibilities include following the current (IRB approved) protocol, personally conducting or supervising the study, ensuring that anyone working with the study understand their duties, ensure informed consent is obtained, report adverse events to sponsor and IRB, maintain accurate documentation, and make it available for inspection, and comply with all requirements from the CFR. The FDA requires the investigator to sign an FDA Form 1572 declaring that he/she understands all responsibilities.

Box 36-3 Elements of an NCI Informed Consent Document

Study title
Purpose
Intended accrual (How many subjects will be enrolled?)
Study procedures; Schedules (What happens if you do take part in the study?)
Eligibility requirements (What is required before enrolling in the study?)
Randomization procedures
Subject responsibilities
Length of study
Withdrawal of consent
Expected risks
Potential benefits of participation
Alternatives to participation in study
Confidentiality
Cost
Instructions regarding injury during study
Discussion of rights
Contact information regarding questions
Signature page

NCI, National Cancer Institute.

Informed Consent

Informed consent is more than a document. It requires a process of explanation that spells out specific details of a protocol. The NCI provides a template of an informed consent document to assure all elements are included (Box 36-3). Informed consent documents should be written in easily understood language, provide explanations, and minimize complicated medical jargon. Potential subjects are allowed to take the consent form home to review and discuss with family before making a decision to participate in the trial by signing the informed consent document. In this manner, the potential subject is protected from possible coercion to participate.[53] Subjects do have the right to decline participation or change their minds and withdraw from a study if they so choose once they have enrolled. Subjects also may be withdrawn from a study if the investigator believes doing so would be in the best interest of the subject (such as when disease progresses or toxicities prevent continuing on study treatment).

Nursing in Clinical Trials

Staff Nurse

Radiation oncology nurses play a valuable role in clinical trials. Staff nurses are often the ones to screen eligible subjects, educate, document, administer study drugs, and manage side effects of therapy. Careful assessment and documentation of side effects and toxicities is a key function that is highly regarded by research investigators and coordinators alike.

The NIH (at the NCI) publishes a booklet of *Common Terminology Criteria for Adverse Events* (CTCAE, Version 3.0) for grading toxicities.[54] Toxicity criteria are spelled out in each of the categories and list specific adverse events. They are graded based on severity of symptoms using a zero (no toxicity) to five (death) scale. Using this CTCAE allows providers to use the same terms and grades so it is easily understood and tracked (much as the TNM system allows for consistency in staging disease). Standardized RT documentation tools such as those designed by ONS make nursing assessments and toxicity grading much more accurate. Communicating frequently with members of the research team assures that protocol procedures and schedules are followed so that any necessary interventions to alleviate adverse events are employed and reported in a timely fashion.

Clinical Trial Nurse

A nurse designated to be responsible for coordinating research-related activities for subjects enrolled in a clinical trial may have variants of the title *Clinical Trial Nurse.* They are responsible for assessing whether a potential subject is actually eligible to enroll in a study. Meticulous review of medical records to screen for eligibility is but the beginning of the role. Often, the clinical trial nurse is the one that conducts the informed consent process. Once a subject enrolls in a study, careful coordination is necessary to make sure all procedures, tests, and treatments (doses and dose modifications) are followed according to the specifications in the protocol.[53] This requires good communication skills, both verbal and written, and patience, to make sure subjects are at their appointed destinations at the correct time. It can be difficult for those subjects participating in a trial and using multimodality treatment (e.g., surgery, chemotherapy/biotherapy and/or radiation) where all must be coordinated within a community setting, not to mention working with healthcare providers and facilities contracted with a subject's insurance company. Data collection, completion, and submission of case report forms are tasks of the clinical trial nurse, although sometimes those responsibilities are delegated. Drug accountability is another responsibility of clinical trial nurses, and strict adherence to guidelines for storage, documentation, and administration are all-important and require close attention to detail. Additionally, clinical trial nurses work to improve enrollment, prevent attrition from studies, and strive to protect their subjects. They certainly contribute to promoting the scientific evidence that leads to better control of cancer.

SUMMARY

As technology continues to evolve and change the practice of radiation oncology, it will be essential that nursing research focus on education, supportive care, and outcomes measurement. The role of clinical trials within the institutional and cooperative group setting provides the nurse with opportunities to promote professional collaboration. Nurses seeking to perform research should build upon the current research foundation and look at the Oncology Nursing Society research priorities.

REFERENCES

1. Nightingale F: *Notes on nursing: what it is and what it is not*, New York, 1969, Dover.
2. Burns N, Grove SK: *The practice of nursing research: conduct, critique, and utilization*, ed 5, St Louis, 2005, WB Saunders.
3. *Nursing's social policy statement*, ed 2, Washington, DC, 2003, American Nurses Association.
4. *University of Minnesota evidence-based nursing* (website): http://evidence.ahc.umn.edu/ebn.htm. Accessed April 20, 2005.
5. *NINR congressional justification for FY 2006*, Washington, DC, 2005, National Institute for Nursing Research.
6. Grant M, Stromborg M: Promoting research collaboration: ONS research committee survey, *Oncol Nurs Forum* 8(2): 48-53, 1981.
7. McGuire D, Stromborg M, Varicchio C: ONS research committee survey of membership's research interests and involvements, *Oncol Nurs Forum* 12(2):99-103, 1985.
8. Grant M: Nursing research. In Dow KH, Hilderly LJ, editors: *Nursing care in radiation oncology*, Philadelphia, 1992, WB Saunders, pp 421-432.
9. Funkhouser SW, Grant MM: 1989 ONS survey of research priorities, *Oncol Nurs Forum* 16(3):413-416, 1989.
10. Mooney K, Ferrell B, Nail L et al: Oncology Nursing Society research priorities survey, *Oncol Nurs Forum* 18(8):1381-1390, 1991.
11. Stetz K, Haberman M, Holcombe J et al: 1994 Oncology Nursing Society research priorities, *Oncol Nurs Forum* 22(5):785-789, 1995.
12. Berger AM, Berry DL, Christopher KA et al: Oncology Nursing Society year 2004 research priorities, *Oncol Nurs Forum* 32(2):281-290, 2005.
13. *Oncology Nursing Society: Radiation therapy (RAD) SIG: about us, 2004* (website): http://radiation.ons.wego.net/index.v3page;jsessionid=1pns5w3csiac7?v2_group=0&p=6657. Accessed April 4, 2005.
14. Shepard N, Kelvin JF: The nursing role in radiation oncology, *Semin Oncol Nurs* 15(4):237-249, 1999.
15. Dow KH: Nursing research in radiation oncology. In Dow KH, Bucholtz JD, Iwamoto R et al, editors: *Nursing care in radiation oncology*, ed 2, Philadelphia, 1997, WB Saunders, pp 421-432.
16. Moore-Higgs G, Watkins-Bruner D, Balmer L et al: The role of licensed nursing personnel in radiation oncology, part A: results of a descriptive study, *Oncol Nurs Soc* 30(1):51-58, 2003.
17. Christman NJ, Oakley MG, Cronin SN: Developing and using preparatory information for women undergoing radiation therapy for cervical or uterine cancer, *Oncol Nurs Forum* 28(1):93-98, 2001.
18. Johnson JE: Coping with radiation therapy: optimism and the effects of preparatory interventions, *Res Nurs Health* 19(1):3-12, 1996.
19. Johnson JE, Lauver DR, Nail LM: Process of coping with radiation therapy, *J Consult Clin Psychol* 57(3):358-364, 1989.
20. Levanthal H, Johnson JE: Laboratory and field experimentation: development of a theory of self-regulation. In Wooldridge PJ, Schmitt MJ, Skipper JK Jr., et al, editors: *Behavioral science and nursing theory*, St Louis, 1983, Mosby, pp 189-262.
21. Velji K, Fitch M: The experience of women receiving brachytherapy for gynecologic cancer, *Oncol Nurs Forum* 28(4):743-751, 2001.
22. Long LE: Being informed: undergoing radiation therapy, *Cancer Nurs* 24(6):463-468, 2001.
23. Christman NJ, Cain LB: The effects of concrete objective information and relaxation on maintaining usual activity during radiation therapy, *Oncol Nurs Forum* 31(2): E39-E45, 2004.
24. King KB, Nail LM, Kreamer K et al: Patients' descriptions of the experience of receiving radiation therapy, *Oncol Nurs Forum* 12(4):55-61, 1985.
25. Johnson JE, Fieler VK, Wlasowicz GS et al: The effects of nursing care guided by self-regulation theory on coping with radiation therapy, *Oncol Nurs Forum* 24(6):1041-1050, 1997.
26. Haylock PJ, Hart LK: Fatigue in patients receiving localized radiation, *Cancer Nurs* 2(6):461-467, 1979.
27. Kubricht DW: Therapeutic self-care demands expressed by outpatients receiving external beam radiation therapy, *Cancer Nurs* 7(1):43-52, 1984.
28. Graydon J: Women with breast cancer: their quality of life following a course of radiation therapy, *J Adv Nurs* 19(4):617-622, 1994.
29. Graydon J, Bubela N, Irvine D et al: Fatigue-reducing strategies used by patients receiving treatment for cancer, *Cancer Nurs* 18(1):23-28, 1995.

30. Mock V, Dow KH, Meares C: *Exercise effects on fatigue, physical functioning, and emotional distress during radiotherapy treatment for breast cancer.* In Proceedings of the 8th International Research Congress, Sigma Theta Tau International, 1996.
31. Erickson JM: Fatigue in adolescents with cancer: a review of the literature, *Clin J Oncol Nurs* 8(2):139-145, 2004.
32. Lovely MP, Miaskowski C, Dodd M: Relationship between fatigue and quality of life in patients with glioblastoma multiforme, *Oncol Nurs Forum* 26(5):921-925, 1999.
33. Mangan MA, Mood DW: The effects of health state, hemoglobin, global symptom distress, mood disturbance, and treatment site on fatigue onset, duration, and distress in patients receiving radiation therapy, *Oncol Nurs Forum* 30(2):E33-E39, 2003.
34. Sarna L, Conde F: Physical activity and fatigue during radiation therapy: a pilot study using actigraph monitors, *Oncol Nurs Forum* 28(6):1043-1046, 2001.
35. Beach P, Siebeneck B, Buderer NF et al: Relationship between fatigue and nutritional status in patients receiving radiation therapy to treat lung cancer, *Oncol Nurs Forum* 28(6):1027-1031, 2001.
36. Armstrong TS: Symptoms experience: a concept analysis, *Oncol Nurs Forum* 30(4):601-606, 2003.
37. Shih A, Miaskowski C, Dodd MJ et al: A research review of the current treatments for radiation-induced oral mucositis in patients with head and neck cancer, *Oncol Nurs Forum* 29(7):1063-1080, 2002.
38. Murphy J, Stacy D, Crook J et al: Testing control of radiation-induced diarrhea with a psyllium bulking agent: a pilot study, *Can Oncol Nurs J* 10(3):96-100, 2000.
39. Berry D, Trigg LJ, Lober WB et al: Computerized symptom and quality-of-life assessment for patients with cancer, part I: development and pilot testing, *Oncol Nurs Forum* 31(5):E75-E83, 2004.
40. Mullen KH, Berry DL, Zierler BK: Computerized symptom and quality-of-life assessment for patients with cancer, part II: acceptability and usability, *Oncol Nurs Forum* 31(5):E84-E89, 2004.
41. Ward-Smith P, Wittkopp D, Sheldon JM: Quality of life among men treated with brachytherapy for prostate cancer, *Urol Nurs* 24(2):95-99, 2004.
42. Overcash JA: Using narrative research to understand the quality of life of older women with breast cancer, *Oncol Nurs Forum* 31(6):1153-1159, 2004.
43. John LD: Quality of life in patients receiving radiation therapy for non-small cell lung cancer, *Oncol Nurs Forum* 28(5):807-813, 2001.
44. Kaasa S, Mastkaasa A, Naess S: Quality of life of lung cancer patients in a randomized clinical trial evaluated by a psychosocial well-being questionnaire, *Acta Oncol* 27(4):335-342, 1988.
45. Sarna L: Women with lung cancer: impact on quality of life, *Qual Life Res* 2(1):13-22, 1993.
46. Given B, Beck S, Etland C et al: *Nursing sensitive outcomes* (website): http://onsopcontent.ons.org/toolkits/evidence/Clinical/outcomes.shtm. Accessed May 24, 2005.
47. Oncology Nursing Society: *9th National Conference on cancer nursing research* (website): www.ons.org/nursingEd/events/research.shtml. Accessed June 4, 2005.
48. National Cancer Institute: *Cancer facts* (website): http://cis.nci.nih.gov/fact/. Accessed June 1, 2005.
49. US Federal Register: *Code of Federal Regulations and ICH Guideline for Good Clinical Practice as adopted by the FDA*, Media, Penn, 2004, Barnett International.
50. National Institutes of Health: *Office of Human Subjects Research, 2005* (website): www.nihtraining.com/ohsrsite. Accessed June 1, 2005.
51. National Institutes of Health: *Guidelines for the conduct of research involving human subjects at the NIH*, Bethesda, Maryland, *2004*, US Dept of Health and Human Services, Public Health Service.
52. Myers LA: IRB regulations and the FDA's mechanisms to assure compliance, *SoCRA SOURCE* 45:20-24, 2005.
53. Klimaszewski AD, Aiken JL, Bacon MA et al, editors: *Manual for clinical trials nursing*, Pittsburgh, 2000, Oncology Nursing Press.
54. Cancer therapy evaluation program: common terminology criteria for adverse events (Version 3.0), Bethesda, Maryland, 2003, National Cancer Institute, National Institutes of Health, Dept of Health and Human Services.

Chapter 37

Advanced Practice Nurses in Radiation Oncology

Colleen K. Lambertz

Global progress in the development of the Advanced Practice Nurse (APN) role marches on! Results of a recent survey conducted by Roodbol[1] revealed that respondents from 68 countries looked favorably upon the concept of the Nurse Practitioner (NP), and 42 countries had programs in place. Nearly half of these programs were at the Master's level. In Malaysia, years of negotiation with university officials led to the development of a clinical specialty program in 1999, and Clinical Nurse Specialist (CNS) status will require a master's degree in 2006. The states and territories of Australia recognize the role of NP/APN with title protection, regulation, and advanced education in all regions, but with differing educational requirements. The Swiss AP/NP role is at the master's level and is still evolving, whereas neighboring Germany has not yet attained the advanced practice role.[2]

Progress in APN role development continues, but the developmental status of the APN role varies widely from country to country around the world. To help reduce that variability, The National Organization of Nurse Practitioner Faculties (NONPF)—well established as the leader in NP education in the United States—has taken measures to influence the implementation of educational guidelines for NPs internationally. In an effort to promote quality education for APNs, its Committee on Global Advancement promotes APN/NP education, fosters understanding of international APN/NP education and practice issues, advocates for quality APN/NP education, and collaborates with other groups involved in APN education and practice.[3] The International Nurse Practitioner/Advanced Practice Nurses (INP/APN) Network, a subgroup of the International Council of Nurses, serves as an international resource for APNs, policy makers, educators, and regulators,[3] while many other organizations join in the effort, as well.

Exciting work to refine the role of the APN internationally continues, while monumental evolution of the role is ongoing in the United States. The earliest pioneers of the APN role in the United States were the Certified Nurse Midwives of the 1920s and the Certified Registered Nurse Anesthetists (CRNAs) of the 1930s, followed by Clinical Nurse Specialists (CNSs) in the 1950s.[4] The first NP program was started in 1965[5] with roots in pediatrics, but with early NP practice concentrating on primary and long-term care. Expansion and blending of the NP and CNS roles into the APN occurred in the 1980s, and the early twenty-first century finds the profession striving to differentiate and strengthen NP and CNS identities and expanding into specialty care. Radiation oncology is one of the newer frontiers being explored by APNs.

It is an exciting time for the APN profession! With over 115,000 NPs and over 14,000 CNSs in the United States,[6] the APN is in demand to fulfill multiple roles across the chronic, acute, primary care, and specialty settings. As America has enjoyed a 20-year increase in the average lifespan over the past 50 years, with another 10 years of longevity expected by 2050, the resultant growing number of older adults continues to increase demands on medical services. The worldwide population of those 65 years or older is projected to nearly double between 2000 and 2030,[7] and the number of Americans age 62 and older is projected to double from 40 million to 80 million in the same period. Meanwhile, the working population is expected to grow by just 12%.[8]

Chronic diseases affect older adults disproportionately and contribute to disability, decreased quality of life, and increased health and long-term care costs.[9] Cancer, also primarily a disease of the elderly, has now surpassed heart disease as the number one killer in all Americans under age 85.[7] With the burgeoning aged population and its health care needs, health analysts predict increased use of NPs as clinicians, team and system leaders, and health promoters.[10] A rise in patient acuity and complex health issues is resulting in growing demand for CNSs, as well. According to the National Association of Clinical Nurse Specialists (NACNS), educational programs for CNSs are reopening and new programs are being developed, with availability of 40 new or revamped programs between 2000 and 2003.[11]

BARRIERS TO APN PRACTICE

Although significant progress was made by APN pioneers of the twentieth century and visions for the future are bright, multiple barriers to current APN practice still exist. An awareness of these barriers is important in order to successfully implement the APN role in any practice arena, including radiation oncology. A recent meta-analysis of APN role development by Lloyd Jones[12] provides an in-depth look at barriers to practice for the interested reader. The following paragraphs explore some of these challenges.

Reimbursement

Many barriers are related to public policy, such as complicated and varied law on APN practice. The federal government regulates parts of APN practice, primarily through reimbursement by Medicare. To define reimbursement parameters, federal regulators must wade through decades of laws written specifically for physicians when they were the only providers of health care. Changes in those laws to reflect APN practice may be slow in coming or may not be made at all unless or until they are challenged successfully.[13]

Further complications arise when the federal government defers to individual state law for licensing and scope of practice decisions that affect reimbursement. Many such state laws were enacted over 30 years ago, yet in some states they are brand new, resulting in inconsistencies in APN practice. Unique societal cultures, governmental personalities, medical and nursing organizations, and patient, provider, and payer needs influence the law-making process and, thereby, influence APN reimbursement for services provided.[13]

Reimbursement is a key driver of APN practice, and confusion about reimbursement issues is pandemic. An American Academy of Nurse Practitioners (AANP) 2003 survey of member NPs indicated that 15.1% of the 5033 responses included in the analysis had difficulty with Medicare reimbursement and 12.8% had difficulty with Medicaid.[14] Referred to as non-physician practitioners (NPPs), NPs, CNSs, and physician assistants (PAs) are considered by the Office of Inspector General—the federal government/Medicare—to be healthcare providers who practice in collaboration with a physician. Prior to the Balanced Budget Act of 1997 (BBA97), Medicare reimbursed NPP services only in rural areas and certain healthcare settings. With enactment of BBA97, Medicare reimbursement for NPPs is allowed in all geographic areas and healthcare settings permitted under state licensing laws if no facility or other provider charges are paid in connection with the service, but discrepancies between NPP and physician reimbursement are inherent within the act.[15]

NPs and CNSs are allowed to bill Medicare directly under Medicare Part B, which provides coverage for non-institutional care such as physician services, outpatient hospital services, medical equipment and supplies, prosthetic devices, radiation therapy, diagnostic x-ray and laboratory tests, ambulance services, home health services, and services provided by NPPs. Physician services include visits to patients in the home, office, hospital, or other institutions.[13,15] The BBA97 set new reimbursement levels for NPPs, allowing payment of the lesser of either 80% of the actual charge or 85% of the scheduled physician fee.[15] The act represented a small improvement in that APNs could bill separately from physicians, but at a reduced rate from physicians for the same services. This sends a message that APNs offer healthcare that is less valuable than that of physicians.

If the NP or CNS bills 'incident-to' the physician, services may be reimbursed at 100% of the Medicare physician fee schedule. 'Incident to' billing may be tricky and places restrictions on where the physician must be located when the APN is seeing the patient. Because little information is available on the types of services being billed in this manner, the Office of the Inspector General's Work Plan for 2004 was to include billing and reimbursement for radiation therapy specifically.[16,17] Other insurers may not require adherence to the 'incident to' rules when billing an APN's work under a physician's name, further confusing this issue.

At this writing, APNs cannot provide the hospice pre-election service to furnish end-of-life evaluation, management, and counseling or certify a patient for home health services and sign for the initial plan of care, even if the APN is the primary provider of care. As of January 2005, however, APNs can perform home health Care Plan Oversight (CPO), which refers to the supervision of patients under Medicare-covered home health or hospice care requiring complex multidisciplinary care modalities, including regular development and review of plans of care. In order to bill for CPO, APNs must have seen and examined the patient and have the 'appropriate' established relationship with the physician who certifies the patient for home health services.[18,19]

The States administer Medicaid, but regulations vary from state to state and from Medicare. States may reimburse NPs in one specialty, but not another. Further complicating the matter, many Medicaid recipients are enrolled in managed care plans whose policies may differ from state and federal rules governing reimbursement for patients not enrolled in managed care.[13] Moreover, private insurers may adopt Medicare's rules and guidelines on billing APN services, or may adopt completely different policies. The rules on APN practice and billing are not found in any one place, but include federal and state law and policies of the insurers.[13,15] Each APN practice must inquire as to each insurer's policies, making practice managers' jobs quite challenging and imputing a burden on the APN in private practice.

SCOPE OF PRACTICE

APNs must practice within state law in order to be reimbursed by Medicare. State scopes of practice are often vague and broad, however, and provide Medicare carriers with insufficient guidance to distinguish between which APN services should be reimbursed and which should not. An initial evaluation of the impact of BBA97 revealed concerns by carrier medical directors that APNs were performing too many complex procedures for which they may not have been adequately trained and were not properly supervised.[15] Furthermore, States may vary from the federal government in educational requirements, because NP curriculum standardization and accreditation standards followed, rather than directed, education. This created potential gaps in competency and further complicated scope of practice development.[20] Variations in scope governing prescriptive authority create the potential for delays in treatment and time constraints for patients, APNs, and physicians by forcing the creation of sophisticated systems for prescription disbursement such as pre-signed prescription pads, call-in services, and prescription writing by providers who have not assessed the client. These barriers create potential weaknesses from payment and quality of care perspectives, and may prompt officials to consider other additional controls for Medicare payments.[15]

CERTIFICATION

Reimbursement from Medicare is tied to certification. Since January 1, 2003, NPs are required to hold a master's degree in nursing, be certified by the American Nurses Credentialing Center (ANCC) or a comparable certifying agency, be licensed as an NP in the state where they practice, and be licensed as registered nurses in order to be reimbursed by Medicare.[15] Dual licensure is a burden that is applied to few other professions! A CNS must be a licensed registered nurse, be certified by the ANCC, and hold a master's degree in a defined clinical area of nursing from an accredited educational institution. NPs and CNSs not so qualified may not garner Medicare reimbursement, hence may find their jobs at risk or be forced to pursue further education.[13,15]

Maintaining certification presents other challenges to the APN. Opportunities for APNs working in specialty practice are increasing, bringing with them questions about whether they are working outside their credentials. A match between credentials and activities is required in order to get a Medicare provider number and reimbursement, and APNs must submit documentation that confirms that they have met requirements for a particular specialty. However, not every specialty has a certification examination available, and it is not economically feasible to develop exams in areas where there are not large numbers of practitioners. Therefore, some CNSs have been forced to take certification exams not reflective of their specialty,[21] and some NPs have been asked to provide extra documentation to maintain certification. APNs must make sure that their credentials meet both the Board of Nursing and certification body's requirements for practice, or risk losing reimbursement for their services or legal authority to practice.[13]

SUPERVISION

The requirement for supervision of APNs by physicians is often a barrier to practice. States vary in their requirements for collaboration or supervision of APNs, but federal law requires that an NP billing Medicare have a collaborative relationship with a physician.[13] Federal law defines 'collaboration' as a process in which an NP works with a physician to deliver healthcare services within the scope of the practitioner's professional expertise, with medical direction and appropriate supervision as provided for in jointly developed guidelines or other mechanism as defined by the law of the State in which the services are performed. Thus, even in states that require no collaborative agreement between NPs and physicians, NPs must establish such a relationship in order to bill Medicare.[13,15]

TITLE PROTECTION

Lack of global title protection presents a challenge for NPs and CNSs. Advanced practice nursing encompasses a variety of roles, each distinct in its own right. The use of global nomenclature such as APN, NPP, APRN, ANP, specialist, expert, and extended class confuses the general public, patients, and healthcare providers including physicians and third-party payers. Rather than using a single designation or title that is recognized universally for a particular role, multiple acronyms and abbreviations to describe advanced nursing practice exist, confusing even members of the Advanced Practice Nursing profession!

It is imperative to clarify titles for reimbursement and professional recognition, but the most important reason to strive for title protection is to protect the public from unqualified practitioners who inappropriately refer to themselves as something that by education, experience, and competence they are not.[22] Establishing parity of terms, competencies, and licensing requirements would also facilitate labor mobility. Fifty of the American nursing boards have language that addresses the advanced practice of nursing, and the National Council of State Boards of Nursing has adopted a nurse licensure compact for advanced practice registered nurses, similar to its compact for RNs and Licensed Practical Nurses (LPNs). States that pursue regulatory approval of the compact can allow APNs who are licensed in any state of the compact to practice in their state.[22] On March 15, 2004, Utah was the first state to pass Advanced Practice Registered Nurse (APRN) compact legislation. On April 25, 2005, Iowa and Utah agreed to mutually recognize APRN licenses, but no date had been set for implementation of the APRN compact.[23]

ATTITUDES OF THE HEALTHCARE COMMUNITY

Attitudes of physicians, patients, other healthcare providers, and institutions about APNs may present barriers to practice. Physicians often express a lack of understanding of Advanced Practice Nursing.[12] Unfamiliar with the APN role, physicians may feel threatened when introduction of APN roles is often characterized by an emphasis on physician replacement or support rather than a patient-centered, health-focused holistic nursing orientation that is complimentary to existing models of care delivery.[24] They may voice concern about their job and financial security, when it is estimated that 30% to 70% of physicians' tasks might be performed by nurses in different roles.[25] Physicians worry about the consequences of a change to their patient mix because of NPs dealing with the 'easy consultations,' which may increase physician stress and resistance to the role.

Such fears raise questions about competency and quality of care provided by APNs and resentment from physicians over differences in training and education. Concerns over competency and quality have been disproved, however, because randomized controlled trial evidence has concluded that NPs and physicians deliver comparable patient outcomes, equal or increased patient satisfaction, high-quality care, and cost-effectiveness.[25-30] CNSs have been found to improve the overall quality of nursing care provided by the staff working with the CNS. Improvements in patient outcomes include less symptom distress, improved pain management practices, decreased emergency room visits, fewer hospital admissions, decreased length of hospital stays and hospital costs, reduced medical complications in hospitalized patients, increased patient satisfaction with nursing care, and increased and earlier return to work after an episode of serious illness.[21]

Resistance to the APN role from nursing staff has been demonstrated. A recent survey of

Registered Nurses in Illinois revealed that RNs in general had strong support of the NP role, but some expressed concern that NPs might not respect or understand the difficulty of the RN role in providing patient care.[31] NPs who have never practiced as an RN may come under heightened scrutiny, because they may have a harder time understanding and appreciating the contribution of the RNs with whom they work. RN resistance to APN orders resulting from the lack of line (managerial) authority between APNs and RNs and a misunderstanding by the RN of the specific components of the APN role have been documented as other reasons for RN resistance to the APN role.[12]

The April 2003 AANP member survey revealed that 41.2% of NPs encountered difficulty with recognition as a primary care provider, with 16.8% reporting difficulty with the receipt of drug samples by pharmaceutical distributors. Difficulty with hospital admissions and privileges was reported by 12% to 13% of NPs, and some had difficulty ordering durable medical equipment (13.4%), ordering long-term care (8.4%), and ordering diagnostics (12.9%).[14]

A review of literature by Gooden and Jackson[32] reported multiple studies that have identified a high level of patient satisfaction with NP delivery of health care in clinic settings in both rural and urban populations, and belief that the quality of health care between NP and physician provider was equivalent. Confidence level among patients not exposed to NPs was questionable, however. Patients who have not previously seen an NP are sometimes hesitant to visit one for the first time, however, the tendency is for patients to want to stay with the NP once they had experienced the level of care provided.[33]

Finally, insufficient organizational planning and preparation for introducing APN roles may lead to underutilization of APNs. Lack of office space, clerical support, communication technology, and educational opportunities result in feelings of isolation and lack of support from the organization. Competing time demands associated with clinical practice and medical functions may prevent participation in education, research, and leadership activities.[24]

OPPORTUNITIES IN ONCOLOGY

Regardless of the barriers to APN practice, unprecedented opportunities for APNs are emerging! More and more APNs are moving from primary provider roles into specialties, including oncology. CNSs have long held a place in oncology, emerging as a specialty when the Oncology Nursing Society (ONS) and the Association of Pediatric Oncology Nurses were founded in the 1970s and oncology nursing developed as a specialty.[34] NPs have been introduced into oncology roles more recently and, of the approximately 106,000 NPs practicing in the United States, about 1% are being used in hematology/oncology centers for episodic and acute care of oncology patients.[14] NPs are also finding a niche in radiation oncology centers, but the role of NP in radiation oncology offers great opportunity for further sculpting.

The ONS is a national organization with more than 32,000 RNs and other healthcare professionals dedicated to excellence in the care of cancer patients.[35] The ONS distinguishes oncology CNSs (OCNS) from oncology NPs (ONP) based on the primary domain of care, scope of practice, and spheres of influence. According to the ONS Position Statement, OCNSs function primarily in the oncology nursing domain as clinical experts within a subspecialty population, type of cancer, type of care, or comprehensive cancer program in hospital-based settings, ambulatory clinics, hospice and home health, and office practices. They work collaboratively with other nurses, health team members, and the cancer care community in promoting health and well being for patients, families, communities, and healthcare systems providing service.[36] The OCNS role may involve activities such as staff education, patient and family education, facilitation of groups to enhance collaboration, development of new clinical programs, policy analysis and development, coordination of research protocols, administration, and supervision and mentoring of staff.[37] In order to remain cost-effective in the changing healthcare environment over the past decade, some OCNSs have assumed additional responsibilities such as utilization review, performance improvement, and case management.[34]

The ONP functions primarily in the medical domain as a clinical expert in oncology by providing direct, episodic health care to prevent and meet the acute, symptomatic, and palliative care needs of patients with cancer.[36] ONPs are qualified to diagnose and manage acute and chronic illness, either independently or collaboratively with physicians. Activities of the ONP could involve obtaining medical histories and conducting physical examinations, ordering and interpreting laboratory, radiologic, and other routine diagnostic tests, prescribing medical interventions, treatments, and medications, and counseling and educating patients and families, either independently or in collaboration with physicians.[36,38]

As illustrated, APN care has been shown to be of comparable quality to physician care and invokes high levels of patient satisfaction. Although fewer in number, studies of OCNS and ONP practice also support that care provided by these professionals is of high quality. Substantial studies have been done in oncology centers to examine the effectiveness of nurse-led care delivered by APNs. These studies suggest that this care is effective, safe, and acceptable to most patients. In fact satisfaction may be higher than with conventional physician-led models of care.[38-48]

Because APN practice is relatively new in radiation oncology, little information is available on APNs in the role. The American Society for Therapeutic Radiology and Oncology (ASTRO) was founded in 1958 with a mission to advance the practice of radiation oncology by promoting excellence in patient care, providing education and research opportunities, and representing radiation oncology in a rapidly evolving socioeconomic healthcare environment.[49] In the late 1990s, changes in reimbursement and a decrease in the number of residents in radiation oncology inspired ASTRO to establish the Joint Committee on Advanced Practice Nursing Roles. Its charge was to find new ways of delivering high quality care in the field, perhaps by utilizing NPPs. In 1997, a multidisciplinary committee of radiation oncology physicians, residents, and nurses conducted the first and only published survey results about NPPs working in radiation oncology, with the goal of delineating and clarifying the roles of CNSs, NPs, and PAs working in the field in the United States. It was unclear as to how many NPPs were actually working in radiation oncology, but mailing lists from ASTRO and ONS were used in an attempt to sample the complete population.[50] It remains the only quantitative look at NPPs in radiation oncology of its kind to date, and these baseline data are presented here for their historical significance.

From the 3529 questionnaires mailed, questionnaires from 86 respondents were selected for analysis consisting of 45 CNSs (52%), 31 NPs (36%), and 10 PAs (12%). The sample had a median of 12 years oncology experience, 5 years radiation oncology experience, and 4 years radiation oncology experience as an APN or PA. This first look at NPPs in radiation oncology found the majority of NPPs working in the northeast and southern United States in private practice versus academic centers with a median number of three physicians, 23% to 30% of NPs and PAs taking call, and 65% of NPs and 80% of PAs reporting directly to a physician. CNSs rarely took call and were more commonly supervised by an administrator or nurse.[50]

Most respondents took patient histories, with NPs and PAs much more likely than CNSs to perform physical examinations. Most practitioners ordered lab tests, but NPs and PAs were more likely to order diagnostic radiology studies (50%) than CNSs (17%), and prescribed medications more than CNSs (NPs 84%, PAs 60%, and CNSs 26%).[50]

Tasks specific to radiation oncology such as simulation, administration of IV contrast, drawing target volumes, two-dimensional treatment planning, writing and signing of treatment prescriptions, verification of patient setup at initiation of treatment, review and signing of initial and weekly beam fields (mostly with supervision and co-signing by physicians) were performed by 10% or less of respondents. Insertion of bladder or rectal catheters and writing and signing of treatment prescriptions with physician co-signatures were performed by 10% to 25% of respondents. Tasks performed frequently by less than three respondents were not included.[50]

Most NPs and PAs were more likely than CNSs to charge for their services, and 86% charged under the physician's name. Thirty-four percent of CNSs charged for their services. Salaries ranged from $30,000 per year to over $70,000, with most NPPs earning $50,000 to $59,000 or more per year. CNSs were much more likely to be involved in development of policies, procedures, and patient education materials, research, support group leadership, and quality improvement activities than NPs or PAs.[50]

Comparatively, ONS membership statistics as of November 2006 indicated that 2971 members held a primary position of CNS (1306) or NP (1665), of which only 137 (4.8%) were in radiation oncology![51] Salaries ranged from $20,000 to more than $90,000 per year, with 36.3% earning $60,000–$79,999. Most APNs worked in patient care (76.1%), with the remaining working in functional areas including administration, education, nursing informatics, research, and 'other' areas. Nearly three-fourths were 40 years old or older (67%), and one-third were at least 50 years old (33.8%).

Only 73 APN members (2.6%) worked in a freestanding or hospital-based outpatient radiation center. Another 677 (24%) worked in outpatient physician offices, but the largest portion reported working in a variety of settings from intensive care to hospice. Sixty-three percent had 16 or more years of nursing experience, whereas 39% had 16 or more years of oncology experience. The median range of oncology experience was 11 to 15 years.[51]

The membership coordinator at ASTRO reports that 386 of its over 7500 members were nurses as of May 2005, but this number was not broken down by APNs. No further demographic information on APN membership was available at this writing.[52]

It is unclear how representative these data were of all NPPs working in radiation oncology, but they represent a baseline with which further research can be compared. Aside from these data, precious little information on the roles, functions, and services provided by APNs in radiation oncology is available, with wide variation in practice across the country based only on anecdotal evidence. The paucity of information along with the barriers common to all APNs compounds the difficulty with which APNs new to the field of radiation oncology realize not only their basic functions but also their full potential in the role.

CREATING A RADIATION ONCOLOGY APN ROLE

Whether an organization is considering incorporation of an APN into a radiation oncology practice, an individual is proposing a new position, or an APN lands in radiation oncology wondering just what the role entails and how to best fulfill it, certain steps may be taken to overcome barriers and improve the likelihood for success in the endeavor. The position may be considered a 'new product'—or in this case, service—and an organized approach to new product development will help minimize uncertainty and confusion and avoid devastating pitfalls. Although the scope of this chapter does not allow a detailed description of new product development, the following paragraphs provide a general framework for bringing the new APN product to market.

New Product Identification

The first step in new product development for the radiation oncology APN is to identify precisely what product—or role—is needed. To make this decision, a look at the organization's strategic management process is necessary. As part of the strategic planning process for radiation oncology, the top management should identify the organizational mission, goals, and objectives. The top management structure will vary depending on the organization and may range from a hospital system's executive staff to a physician in a solo practice.

An environmental analysis will assist in the goal-setting process by providing information on the remote—world and national—and local environments as relates to economic, social, political, technologic, and ecologic factors. Next, the analysis should evaluate the industry environment—health care—and more specifically, the oncology and radiation oncology environments.[53,54] Ideally, the analysis would include a look at many factors, including the community's perceptions of the threats, barriers, and benefits of APN practice, community values, beliefs, norms and standards, cultural practices, customer profiles, human resources, key success factors, and competition among many others.

Next, the information from the environmental analysis would be used to evaluate the organization's external *opportunities* and *threats* compared with its internal *strengths* and *weaknesses*—a SWOT analysis. The SWOT analysis will ascertain a critical view of the organization's internal and external environments and evaluate the fulfillment of its basic mission.[53] The organization then must match what it does well—its strengths—with external opportunities and take steps to minimize the internal weaknesses, which may prevent or limit the organization from taking advantage of opportunities.

Grand Strategy

A synthesis of the information provided by the above analyses provides the infrastructure for selection of one or more organizational grand strategies. An example of a likely strategy in this scenario would be one of growth, which would include market penetration, market development, and product development.[54] Selection of the grand strategy is made simultaneously with development of the organizational long-term goals and objectives.

The grand strategy would drive development of the goals and objectives. From the goals and objectives, the actions through which the organization can attain the objectives and accomplish the goals should be developed. Specific intentions with timetables for achievement should be stated, for example, increase radiation oncology market share by 20% in 3 years, reduce patient wait times by 30% in 2 years, or increase involvement in research protocols by 25% by 2008. This action-planning process generally involves getting input from all levels of the organization and can be quite involved and time-consuming. However, the investment in time up front results in an organized plan for achieving the goals and may save time in the long run, help prevent problems by increasing group-based decision making and employee involvement, and reduce resistance to change.

Marketing Strategy

A marketing strategy would come next, with marketing objectives designed to achieve overall organizational objectives and from which a marketing plan evolves. Marketing strategy development should take into account the competitive, political-legal, economic, technologic, and social-cultural environments, all of which should be continually monitored for trends that may represent opportunities or threats to the organization. A marketing strategy includes identification of target markets and satisfying those markets with a careful balance of the elements of the marketing mix—product, price, distribution, and promotion.[53]

Identification of the target market helps identify what new product—or which APN role—is needed. Gaps in service of the target market can be identified, which help clarify which type of APN will fill those gaps. If the need is for a clinical expert for program development, staff education, policy/procedure development, quality improvement activities, support group facilitation, research protocol involvement, case management, or care coordination, a CNS might be the right fit. Alternatively, if a clinician is needed to take histories, perform physical examinations, diagnose and treat oncology-related medical problems, and prescribe medications, an NP may be the better choice.[38] It is important to realize that, particularly in a small practice, some of these functions may cross over into both roles. Also, the barriers to practice for both roles, such as prescriptive authority, reimbursement, credentialing, privileging, and acceptance in the medical community, must be considered before deciding which service is the correct one.

Once the correct product has been identified, development of a job description can begin. Job descriptions vary widely in nomenclature, but often include general categories such as the following:

- Qualifications: Educational, licensing, and scope of practice
- Job functions: Clinical functions/limitations, education, consultation, research
- Supervision/collaboration: Federal/State requirements, reporting mechanisms
- Performance criteria: Frequency/methods for performance evaluation.[55,56]

For illustration purposes, Box 37-1 contains an example of a job description for an NP position in a private physician radiation oncology practice in Boise, Idaho.

Product Strategy

Having identified the target market and chosen the new APN service to satisfy that market, the product strategy should then be developed. It would include plans for customer service to the target market, such as how the APN would satisfy both internal and external customer needs in the target market. For the APN in radiation oncology, customers could include potential or current patients, collaborating, partnering, and referring physicians, other staff, pharmaceutical and product vendors, the public, and administration, among others.

Along with identification of the target market, consideration of the consumer purchase decision process should occur. This process includes the actions a person takes in purchasing and using products and services. It includes five phases: (1) problem recognition, (2) the information search, (3) an evaluation of alternatives, (4) a purchase decision, and (5) post-purchase behavior.[54] Factors that influence the purchase decision process should be evaluated including motivation and personality of the consumers, perceptions, learning behavior,

Box 37-1 Mountain States Oncology Group, Job Description: Nurse Practitioner

The content of this document is not intended to be an exhaustive list of all responsibilities, duties, and skills required of the Nurse Practitioner.

ESSENTIAL JOB QUALIFICATIONS

1. Graduate of an accredited school of nursing with a Master of Science in Nursing.
2. Completed formal program and awarded certification by the State of Idaho Board of Nursing as a Nurse Practitioner.
3. Current Idaho license.
4. Current license in other states as necessary to provide care for MSOG patients.
5. Knowledge of nursing standards and professional practice as outlined by the Idaho Nurse Practice Act.
6. Skill in collecting and dictating patient histories and physicals, including psychosocial and physical assessments.
7. Skill in collecting data by interview, observation, inspection, auscultation, and palpation.
8. Skill in organizing and reporting data that is accurate, complete, accessible, and confidential to other healthcare team members.
9. State and federal narcotics licenses.

NON-ESSENTIAL JOB QUALIFICATIONS

10. OCN or AOCN.

JOB FUNCTIONS

The Nurse Practitioner:

11. Will primarily be involved in the treatment of stable oncology patients.
12. Will provide follow-up care including acute and routine examinations. Assess progress, identify problems, initiate preventive measures, recognize emergent problems, initiate proper care, while maintaining collaborative contact with physician.
13. Shall consult* with a physician if any of the following conditions apply to a patient:
    - The patient does not respond to treatment plan.
    - The patient presents with an acute unstable condition.
    - The patient presents with a condition that the Nurse Practitioner cannot treat within the scope of Nurse Practitioner training or experience.

*NOTE: Consult shall mean to review in person, by telephone, by chart review, or by recheck with physician.

14. Shall perform procedures consistent with his/her level of experience. New procedures will be validated by demonstration with physician supervision.
15. Shall develop understanding and implementation of dosimetry, radiation therapy, simulation, and radiation prescriptions. Develop skill to implement simple radiation therapy with physician consultation.
16. Shall prescribe treatment within his/her scope of practice and consistent with his/her level of experience. Medical conditions to be managed include but not limited to:
    - Preventive health maintenance
    - Routine health problems
    - Side effect management of cancer and related treatment, including radiation toxicity management
    - Pain management, both chronic and acute
    - Safe effective management of cancer and related treatments including chemotherapy facility management
17. Will order and interpret the following laboratory testing consistent with his/her knowledge and level of experience:
    - Chemistry panels
    - Sedimentation rate (ESR)
    - Liver function tests
    - Gram stain
    - Cultures and sensitivities
    - Serum HCG
    - Hepatitis A, B, C
    - HIV
    - Wet prep

(continued)

Box 37-1 Mountain States Oncology Group, Job Description: Nurse Practitioner—cont'd

- Blood gases
- Tumor markers
- CBC/differential
- Thyroid function tests
- Urinalysis/micro
- Hemoccult
- PAP smear
- PT/PT
- Drug screens/levels
- Glycohemoglobin/hemoglobin AICI on profiles
- Iron profiles
- Arthritis profile
- Others as indicated according to level of experience

18. Will order and interpret the following diagnostic testing consistent with his/her knowledge and level of experience:
    - Chest films
    - Extremity and spinal films
    - Abdominal films
    - KUB
    - EKG
    - Sinus studies
    - Pulmonary function tests
    - CT scans
    - Ultrasounds
    - Dye studies
    - MRI
    - Other studies as indicated according to level of experience.
19. Shall prescribe medications within the guidelines established by the State Board of Nursing and the State Board of Pharmacy.
20. Shall demonstrate positive interpersonal relations in dealing with physicians, patients, patient families, visitors, co-workers, and other medical center employees in a professional and confidential manner.
21. Shall demonstrate the ability to act with sensitivity as a patient advocate.
22. Shall demonstrate accurate documentation of the planned outcomes of care.
23. Shall be responsible for providing relevant education to the patient and persons associated with them, including teaching regarding the plan of care and completion of informed consent.
24. Shall act as a resource and teacher for other members of the healthcare team. Share knowledge and expertise with staff through discussion and participation in educational programs as appropriate.

COLLABORATION

25. The Nurse Practitioner will collaborate with other healthcare providers, including physicians, in providing patient care. This is to include the discussion of patient treatment and the cooperation in the management and delivery of health care.
26. Physician collaboration will be sought when implementing treatments outside the scope of the Nurse Practitioner's knowledge or experience.
27. Monthly chart reviews of three randomly selected Nurse Practitioner charts will be conducted by a collaborating physician.

PERFORMANCE REVIEW

Semi-annual review of the Nurse Practitioner's performance will occur with measurement criteria of:

28. Supervisory observation with examples
29. Multidisciplinary input
30. Chart reviews

The Nurse Practitioner will report to the appropriate physician regarding healthcare matters, and to the medical group administrator regarding matters of personnel, scheduling, billing and policy.

values, beliefs, and attitudes, lifestyles, and the personal influences of market leaders, reference groups, and families. A close evaluation of this process and the factors influencing it as they relate to purchasing APN services would provide clues as to where in the process to provide consumer education, information, and follow-up.[54]

The next element of the marketing mix to consider is packaging, or how to present the APN product to customers and how to position the APN in the organization and the marketplace. Identification of a positioning strategy would determine where the APN product was placed in the consumer's mind relative to competing products. This strategy would position the APN as a desirable alternative to the physician for identified radiation oncology services. Finally, packaging would be considered. In a service-oriented marketing plan, packaging would refer to how the service was offered. This would require a determination of which unique service items would be included in the APN package.

The distribution strategy comes next, which would include development of the place for APN services to occur. Marketing channels make possible the flow of goods from the producer to the buyer. In this situation, services would be provided directly from the producer—the APN—to the buyer of radiation oncology services. This would be referred to as a direct marketing channel, because no intermediaries would be required or even desirable.[54] It would allow consumers to buy the product by interacting with various advertising media without meeting with a sales person. The APN would be acting as his/her own sales person by directly interfacing with the targeted consumers.

The determination would need to be made as to whether the APN would be specified to a single geographic location, as in an exclusive distribution design, or would be available in a few locations, as in a selective distribution design.[53] The placement of the APN in a few different sites would allow customers to be drawn from a wider geographic region and enhance the APN's ability to increase clientele. It would also improve access to these services for the community and improve convenience. This decision would be driven in collaboration with the organization and depends on whether it has a single or multiple locations.

Pricing strategy would be the next element of the marketing mix. Pricing can be difficult, because it is often closely regulated and subject to considerable public scrutiny.[53] Setting the pricing structure for services such as an APN can be especially tricky and will be driven by the APN scope of practice, reimbursement, competition, and the organization's policies and existing fee structures. Important to remember in determining a price for the APN is that price itself could influence the perception of quality and ultimate value to the customer.

Pricing decisions must include consideration of the direct and indirect costs of the APN position. These costs may be estimated in part from the employment contract. Contracts may be organized in a variety of ways, and include information on the following:

- Terms of employment
- Scope of duties
- Exclusive service clauses
- Compensation and benefits, including continuing education
- Revenues and billing
- Confidentiality/medical records
- Liability insurance
- Term and termination
- Management, personnel, and facilities.[57-60]

The contract may or may not cover all the details of employment, and the APN should take a proactive role in negotiating and ensuring that those details are agreed on and perhaps documented in an addendum to the contract in order to ensure the success of the APN/organizational relationship. Other details to consider are the orientation process, securing of privileges, preceptor/mentoring responsibilities and opportunities, and quality improvement responsibilities.

Box 37-2 contains an example of a contract for a radiation oncology NP working in a private physician radiation oncology practice in Boise, Idaho. The AANP also provides NP Tips for Contracting on its website,[60] and a template for an employee contract may be purchased online.[57]

The final element of the marketing mix would be promotion, which is a mix of tools called the *promotional mix*. These tools include advertising, personal selling, sales promotion, and public relations. Promotion is the communication link between the organization and its consumers through advertising, personal selling, sales promotion, and publicity.[54]

Over the last decade, marketing has evolved

Text continued on p. 659

Box 37-2 The Clinic Extended Care Provider Agreement

This Extended Care Provider Agreement ("the Agreement") is made effective this _____ day of ____________, ______ ("the Effective Date"), by and between The Clinic and ____________, NP (Nurse Practitioner).

RECITALS

A. The Clinic is organized to deliver healthcare services at The Clinic that has organized or will organize in the region through its Physicians, in addition to other healthcare providers.
B. Nurse Practitioner is duly licensed by the Idaho State Board of Nursing to practice in the State of Idaho and has satisfied The Clinic's credentialing requirements.
C. The Clinic desires to employ Nurse Practitioner to deliver healthcare services to patients at The Clinic and Nurse Practitioner desires to render healthcare services on behalf of The Clinic, and the parties wish to set forth the terms and conditions of their employment relationship in this Agreement.

NOW, THEREFORE, in consideration of the mutual promises and covenants contained herein and for other good and valuable consideration, the receipt and sufficiency of which are hereby acknowledged, the parties agree as follows:

AGREEMENT

In consideration of the mutual promises, covenants, terms and conditions contained herein, the parties agree as follows:

1. Scope of Employment
Nurse Practitioner shall render professional patient care services, administrative services, and shall perform other duties as may reasonably be requested by The Clinic in accordance with the terms of this Agreement.

2. Scope of Duties
Nurse Practitioner shall devote her professional time and attention in an amount reasonably necessary to carry out her duties hereunder to deliver services on behalf of The Clinic.
Nurse Practitioner shall give The Clinic reasonable prior notice of her intent to schedule time off, including vacation time or time for continuing medical education, consistent with any of Clinic policy or procedure regarding such notification.

3. Non-Discrimination
Nurse Practitioner shall not discriminate in the delivery of care to any patient on the basis of gender, race, color, religion, ethnicity, ability to pay, or manner of payment in rendering professional services pursuant to this Agreement.

4. Fees for Professional Services
Nurse Practitioner shall comply with The Clinic's fee schedules. The fees to be charged for professional services rendered by Nurse Practitioner on behalf of The Clinic shall be determined solely by The Clinic.

5. Exclusive Service
During the term of this Agreement, except as provided below, Nurse Practitioner shall not, without the prior written consent of The Clinic, directly or indirectly provide patient care services to or for any person or firm for compensation, or engage in any professional activity that competes directly or indirectly with or which might be detrimental to the business of The Clinic.

In addition, during the term of this Agreement, Nurse Practitioner shall only engage in other compensated professional activities (apart from the delivery of direct patient care services hereunder), including, by way of example and not limitation, teaching, administrative activities or consultation with hospitals or other healthcare entities or practitioners ("Outside Activities") in a manner subject to the provisions of this Agreement and any applicable to The Clinic's policies issued from time to time. Revenues for such permitted Outside Activities shall be the property of The Clinic as stated in Paragraph 13 herein.

Consistent with the foregoing, Nurse Practitioner shall remain free to render patient care services in emergency situations, to render voluntary medical services on behalf of religious or charitable organizations, to render medical services to any family member or relative, to publish articles in professional journals, or to participate in service or professional organizations, provided that none of these enumerated activities shall interfere with Nurse Practitioner's obligations pursuant to this Agreement.

Box 37-2 The Clinic Extended Care Provider Agreement—cont'd

6. Integrated Operations
Nurse Practitioner shall provide patient care as an integrated participant in The Clinic and in full coordination with the operations of The Clinic. She shall cooperate with and participate in The Clinic's shared systems and infrastructure (*e.g.*, The Clinic's management information system), on an ongoing basis consistent with relevant policies and procedures developed by The Clinic.

7. Professional Contracts
Nurse Practitioner shall provide professional services pursuant to, and in a manner consistent with the provisions of all third party payer contracts, health care benefit plans, and similar arrangements entered into by or on behalf of The Clinic, including, without other limitation, exclusive provider, preferred provider, health maintenance organization, capitate or other "managed care" contracts (collectively referred to as "Health Care Service Contracts"); provided, however, that The Clinic may approve the limited closure of Nurse Practitioner's practice to patients under particular Health Care Service Contracts from time to time in its discretion.

During the term of this Agreement Nurse Practitioner shall not enter individually into any new Health Care Service Contracts, and shall instead refer all such Contracts and contracting opportunities offered to Nurse Practitioner or in which Nurse Practitioner has participated prior to the Effective Date to The Clinic for appropriate action. The Clinic shall proceed to review, negotiate and approve or reject any such Health Care Service Contracts or opportunities on behalf of and in the name of The Clinic.

8. Professional Standards
Nurse Practitioner shall perform her duties under this Agreement in accordance with applicable professional standards and rules of ethics. Nothing in this Agreement shall effect the exercise of Nurse Practitioner's independent professional judgment regarding delivery of services hereunder. Nurse Practitioner will always have a Physician available for consultation.

9. Professional Credentials
Nurse Practitioner shall maintain, during the term of this Agreement, an unrestricted license to practice advanced practice nursing in the State of Idaho, provided, however, that in the case of a restricted license, The Clinic may waive the foregoing requirement to the extent deemed appropriate in The Clinic's sole discretion. Nurse Practitioner shall maintain appropriate membership and the clinical privileges at any other facilities which may be periodically designated by The Clinic. Nurse Practitioner is encouraged to maintain membership in her local society as well as other professional societies as may be necessary or desirable to assist her practice or as otherwise deemed appropriate by The Clinic. Nurse Practitioner shall further adhere to such additional requirements regarding the maintenance of professional credentials, as may be established by The Clinic from time to time.

10. Compliance With Policies
Nurse Practitioner shall comply with all policies and procedures which may be adopted <u>or</u> amended by The Clinic from time to time regarding the practice of medicine or delivery of services hereunder including, but not limited to, policies and procedures relating to quality improvement, clinical competence, interpersonal behavior, peer review and utilization management. Nurse Practitioner additionally shall comply with all applicable laws or regulations relating to the professional medical services to be delivered hereunder. Nurse Practitioner shall, throughout the term of this Agreement, satisfy all continuing medical education requirements as established and modified from time to time by The Clinic and the appropriate regulatory authority. Nurse Practitioner understands and agrees that the development and application of such policies and procedures shall be undertaken by The Clinic in furtherance of its overall business objective of promoting the delivery of good quality health care services at all clinics.

11. Medical Records
Nurse Practitioner shall keep and maintain medical records for each patient receiving professional services pursuant to this Agreement in accordance with customary standards of good medical practice and in compliance with all applicable confidentiality requirements, and shall further comply with any additional documentation procedures established by The Clinic from time to time. All medical records, files, papers, documents and clinical materials ("Records") generated in connection with the delivery of services hereunder shall be the exclusive property of The Clinic. Nurse Practitioner shall give The Clinic access to such Records as may be reasonably requested by The Clinic.

(continued)

Box 37-2 The Clinic Extended Care Provider Agreement—cont'd

Following termination of this Agreement at any time, The Clinic shall, upon reasonable request by Nurse Practitioner and upon Nurse Practitioner's payment of reasonable photocopying or reproduction charges, make available to Nurse Practitioner those Records generated in connection with Nurse Practitioner's delivery of services pursuant to this Agreement which may be necessary for Nurse Practitioner's treatment of patients, preparation of a defense against any malpractice claim, completion of research, response to federal, state or private third party reimbursement investigation or inquiry, or other bona fide purpose. Nurse Practitioner shall secure appropriate patient releases covering the dissemination of such materials when legally required.

12. Physician/Patient Relationship and Patient Confidentiality

Nothing contained in this Agreement, nor in any other agreement to which The Clinic and Nurse Practitioner are parties, is intended to, or shall, modify the physician/patient privilege or the confidential relationship between a patient and physician/health care provider, or is intended in any way to interfere with the delivery of good quality patient care by Nurse Practitioner hereunder.

13. Revenues and Billing for Professional and Other Services

Except as provided below, all income generated by Nurse Practitioner as a result of services payable by a patient and/or a third party payer pursuant to a CPT code, ICD-9 code, or any other patient care coding system, wherever generated, shall be the exclusive property of The Clinic ("Codable Income"). All income generated by Nurse Practitioner through any other professional activity that legally requires a professional medical degree (e.g., medical directorships, outside locum tenens, IMEs) shall be the exclusive property of The Clinic ("Non-Patient Care Income").

Consistent with the foregoing, income generated by Nurse Practitioner which is not Codable Income or Non-Patient Care Income as defined above and which neither involves the expenditure of The Clinic's resources nor interferes with Nurse Practitioner's contractual commitment to The Clinic shall be retained by Nurse Practitioner as her property ("Outside Remuneration"). By way of illustration, Outside Remuneration may include permissible earnings for services or investments (whether or not related to the health care industry) that do not require a professional medical degree to perform or hold.

All Codable Income generated by Nurse Practitioner shall be billed in the name of The Clinic and through The Clinic's group provider number. Nurse Practitioner shall execute in a timely manner all forms, and shall take all other reasonable actions, required by The Clinic which permit The Clinic or its designee to bill and receive payment for services rendered by Nurse Practitioner hereunder. Nurse Practitioner shall additionally endorse and assign to The Clinic any payments for services delivered by Nurse Practitioner pursuant to this Agreement. This Paragraph 13 shall survive termination of this Agreement unless the parties agree otherwise pursuant to Paragraph 13 of this Agreement.

14. Compensation

As full consideration for the professional services performed under this Agreement, including the generation of all Codable Income and all Non-Patient Care Income, The Clinic shall pay to Nurse Practitioner an annual salary as specified in Exhibit A attached hereto and made a part hereof.

15. Benefits

Nurse Practitioner may participate in such benefit programs which are provided to The Clinic employees on the terms and conditions, and subject to the qualification standards which may be established by The Clinic from time to time, in accordance with applicable law. Current benefits are described by Exhibit A attached hereto and incorporated by this reference. The Clinic shall have the right to modify, amend, delete or supplement any such benefits in its direction.

16. Non-Deductible Compensation

If any compensation is paid to, or expense reimbursement is made on behalf of, Nurse Practitioner pursuant to her request which is disallowed in whole or in part as a deductible expense for federal or state income tax purposes, and if The Clinic makes payments to a taxing authority as a result of such disallowance, Nurse Practitioner shall pay to The Clinic an amount equal to the payments, including any interest or penalties.

Box 37-2 The Clinic Extended Care Provider Agreement—cont'd

17. Confidentiality

Nurse Practitioner shall not disclose to any individual or entity not affiliated with The Clinic the following information: (1) the names, addresses, or any other information related to any patient of The Clinic; (2) the techniques used by The Clinic in operating its business generally; (3) any other trade secret or proprietary information of The Clinic including, but not limited to, practice guidelines, medical management protocols, financial data and productivity reports, and other decision-making tools. Information may be disclosed insofar as required by applicable law; provided, however, that Nurse Practitioner agrees to give The Clinic a reasonable prior opportunity to intervene in such legal proceeding pursuant to which such information is sought to seek a protective order or to otherwise lawfully prevent or limit such disclosure or demand. Nurse Practitioner shall not obtain any rights or privileges to any of the confidential information or trade secrets described in this section; all information described herein shall be the exclusive property of The Clinic. Upon termination of this Agreement, Nurse Practitioner shall promptly deliver to The Clinic all documents relating to such information and trade secrets and all of the materials of any kind that are of a proprietary or confidential nature relating to The Clinic's business that are in Nurse Practitioner's possession or under Nurse Practitioner's control. This Paragraph 17 shall survive termination of this Agreement.

18. Insurance Coverage

(a) The Clinic shall during the term of this Agreement maintain on Nurse Practitioner's behalf an appropriate professional liability insurance policy consistent with the provisions of Idaho law.

(b) If the insurance coverage is in the form of Agreement "claims made" policy, the following provisions of this subpart (b) shall also apply: Upon termination of this Agreement, Nurse Practitioner shall, at her own expense, maintain the same or an equivalent professional liability insurance policy or shall obtain prior acts coverage or an extended reporting endorsement (i.e., "tail coverage") or other equivalent coverage in Agreement manner reasonably acceptable to The Clinic. If Nurse Practitioner fails to maintain the coverage required herein reasonably acceptable to The Clinic, then The Clinic may proceed to purchase such other or supplemental liability coverage for claims arising from Nurse Practitioner's practice during the term of this Agreement as is reasonably determined by The Clinic to be necessary and prudent, and may deduct the cost of such coverage from any amounts owed by The Clinic to Nurse Practitioner under this Agreement or any other agreement between the parties or otherwise collect or recover such sums from Nurse Practitioner.

(c) The provisions of this Paragraph 18 shall survive termination of this Agreement.

19. Indemnification

(a) Indemnification by Nurse Practitioner

(i) Nurse Practitioner shall indemnify, defend and hold harmless The Clinic from and against all losses, damages, obligations, liabilities, claims, costs and expenses including, but not limited to, reasonable attorneys' fees and prejudgment interest, arising out of or related to:

(ii) Any liabilities and obligations of and claims against Physician and/or The Clinic relating to the professional or business activities of Nurse Practitioner prior to Nurse Practitioner becoming an employee of The Clinic, including, but not limited to, claims or other professional liability relating to the practice of medicine;

(iii) Any liabilities and obligations of and claims against Nurse Practitioner and/or The Clinic relating to claims of malpractice or professional liability allegedly arising out of his own conduct or omissions occurring during the term of this Agreement;

(iv) The breach by Nurse Practitioner of Services any agreement to which Nurse Practitioner and The Clinic are parties; and

(v) Under any other circumstances provided by law. Notwithstanding any other provision hereof, the indemnity of provisions of Paragraph 19 (in the case of professional liability claims) shall not apply to Nurse Practitioner during any period in which professional liability insurance is in force pursuant to Paragraph 18 hereof, or Nurse Practitioner is otherwise covered for professional liability allegedly occurring during the term of this Agreement pursuant to a policy of professional liability insurance purchased by The Clinic on the Nurse Practitioner's behalf. The indemnification provisions set forth in this Paragraph 19 shall survive the termination of the Nurse Practitioner's employment by The Clinic.

(continued)

Box 37-2 The Clinic Extended Care Provider Agreement—cont'd

(b) Application of Insurance Proceeds
The amount of indemnification owed by the Nurse Practitioner to The Clinic under any circumstances shall be reduced by the amount of insurance proceeds available for the benefit of The Clinic and/or Nurse Practitioner; provided, however, that no provision hereof is intended to, nor shall it have the effect of reducing the amount of available insurance coverage for any party pursuant to any prohibition against contractually assumed liability or otherwise, and shall be construed in a manner to maximize the availability of such coverage for the benefit of The Clinic and/or Nurse Practitioner.
(c) Notice of Claim
As soon as practicable, The Clinic shall provide written notice to Nurse Practitioner as provided in this Agreement of any claim, demand or other matter to which Nurse Practitioner's indemnification obligations may apply, and shall give Nurse Practitioner reasonable opportunity to defend the same at Nurse Practitioner's expense and with counsel of Nurse Practitioner's own selection; provided, however, that The Clinic shall at all times also have the right to participate in the defense at its own expense. If the claim is one that cannot by its nature be defended solely by Nurse Practitioner, The Clinic shall make available all information and assistance that Nurse Practitioner may reasonably request. If Nurse Practitioner shall, within a reasonable time after notice, fail to defend, The Clinic shall have the right, but not the obligation, to undertake the defense of, and to compromise or settle (exercising reasonable business judgment) the claim or other matter on behalf, for the account and the risk of Nurse Practitioner.

TERM AND TERMINATION

20. Term
Unless terminated earlier pursuant to the provisions contained herein, this Agreement shall be for a term of one (1) years, commencing upon the Effective Date and shall automatically renew for one successive one (1) year term unless earlier terminated pursuant to the terms and conditions herein. Not later than six (6) months after this agreement is made and no later than ninety (90) days prior to the annual anniversaries following the effective date hereof, the parties shall discuss in good faith any appropriate revisions to this Agreement, including compensation; provided, however, that all then-existing contract terms shall continue in effect until (and unless) the parties agree in writing to any modification hereof.

21. Immediate Termination
(a) This Agreement shall terminate if Nurse Practitioner:
- (i) becomes disqualified to practice as a Nurse Practitioner in the State of Idaho;
- (ii) becomes unable to perform the services required hereunder for a period of six (6) consecutive months, or for two (2) period of three (3) consecutive months each during any two (2) year interval under this Agreement, including any renewals hereof, as a result of a disability as determined by a physician designated by The Clinic who has no other affiliation with or relationship to The Clinic;
- (iii) dies;
- (iv) accepts other employment that restricts, limits or materially interferes with her continued ability to provide professional patient care under this Agreement;
- (v) becomes uninsurable with The Clinic's insurance carrier for the professional liability coverage required pursuant to Paragraph 18 herein;
- (vi) is convicted of or enters a plea of guilty or *nolo contendere* to any misdemeanor charge related to the delivery of health care services or any felony or otherwise engages in conduct (regardless of the legal consequences of that conduct) which is reasonably determined by The Clinic to be actually or potentially detrimental to the best business, professional, or other interests of The Clinic.

(b) Additionally, this Agreement may be terminated immediately by The Clinic in its discretion if Nurse Practitioner has restrictions imposed upon his license to practice as a Nurse Practitioner by the Idaho State Board of Nursing or otherwise no longer meets the baseline credentialing requirements then applicable.

22. Termination for Cause
Either party may terminate this Agreement upon the other party's material breach of any term or provision of this Agreement which is not cured within thirty (30) days following written notice thereof.

Box 37-2 The Clinic Extended Care Provider Agreement—cont'd

23. Rights Upon Termination

The effective date of Nurse Practitioner's termination shall be the "Termination Date." Unless the parties agree otherwise, upon termination of this Agreement for any reason, The Clinic shall pay to Nurse Practitioner her accrued salary pursuant to Paragraph 14 hereof through the Termination Date, subject to any rights of offset on behalf of The Clinic created by this Agreement or any other agreement between the parties. The amount of compensation shall be calculated by The Clinic and paid to Nurse Practitioner within thirty (30) days after the Termination Date.

24. Post Termination Communication with Patients

The parties shall endeavor, in good faith, to agree upon a mutually acceptable form of communication to patients, consistent with the interests of good quality patient care, upon and after termination of this Agreement.

DISPUTE RESOLUTION

25. Mediation and Arbitration

The parties shall endeavor in good faith to resolve any disputes which may arise regarding this Agreement or any other agreement between them. If they cannot so agree among themselves, they shall initially submit their dispute to mediation by a mutually acceptable third party familiar with business issues in the Boise health care community. If they cannot agree on such a person within ten (10) business days following any such request for mediation or, following such mediation remain in disagreement, then either party may submit all controversies, claims and disputes arising from this Agreement to confidential binding arbitration in Boise, pursuant to the Commercial Arbitration Rules of the American Arbitration Association then in force, or pursuant to such other rules or procedures to which the parties may agree. Each party shall bear his own costs and attorneys' fees with the referenced mediation and any arbitration proceeding hereunder.

MISCELLANEOUS

26. Time of the Essence

Time is of the essence under this Agreement.

27. Governing Law

This Agreement shall be governed by and construed in accordance with the laws of the State of Idaho.

28. Severability

Should any of the provisions of this Agreement to any extent be held to be invalid or unenforceable, the remainder of the Agreement shall continue in full force and effect.

29. Entire Agreement

This Agreement embodies the entire understanding and agreement among the parties regarding the matters contained herein, and supersedes all prior negotiations, understandings or agreements concerning such matters, whether written or oral, including specifically any prior independent contractor arrangements between the parties.

30. Waiver

No provision of this Agreement may be waived, except by an agreement in writing signed by all of the parties hereto. A waiver of any term or provision shall not be construed as a waiver of any other term or provision.

31. Headings

The subject headings used in this Agreement are included for purposes of reference only, and shall not affect the construction or interpretation of any of its provisions.

32. Amendment

This Agreement may be amended by a writing executed by all of the parties to this Agreement or by The Clinic as provided in the following Paragraph of this Agreement. No amendment shall be made to this Agreement which is inconsistent with The Clinic's Operating Agreement.

(continued)

Box 37-2 The Clinic Extended Care Provider Agreement—cont'd

33. Notices

All notices required or permitted by this Agreement shall be in writing and shall be given by personal delivery or sent to the address of the party set forth below by registered or certified mail, postage prepaid, return receipt requested, or by reputable overnight courier, prepaid, receipt acknowledged. Notices shall be deemed received on the earlier of the date of actual receipt or, in the case of notice by mail or overnight courier, the date of receipt marked on the acknowledgment of receipt. Rejection or refusal to accept or the inability to deliver because of change of address of which no notice was given shall not alter the effective receipt date of any such notices.

If to The Clinic:

____

____

____

____

If to Nurse Practitioner:

____

____

____

____

Any party may change its address to which notices should be sent to it by giving the other parties written notice of the new address in the manner set forth in this Paragraph.

34. Construction

Throughout this Agreement, the singular shall include the plural, the plural shall include the singular, and all genders shall be deemed to include other genders, wherever the context so requires.

35. Further Acts

Upon reasonable request from a party hereto, from time to time, each party shall execute and deliver such additional documents and instruments and take such other actions as may be reasonably necessary to give effect to the intents and purposes of this Agreement.

36. Authority

Each of the parties hereto represents to the other that such party has full power and authority to execute, deliver and perform this Agreement, and that the individual executing this Agreement on behalf of the party is fully empowered and authorized to do so.

37. Binding Effect

This Agreement shall be binding upon and inure to the benefit of the parties hereto and their respective successors and permitted assigns.

38. No Beneficiaries

No third parties are intended to benefit by the covenants, agreements, or any other terms or conditions of this Agreement.

39. Counterparts

This Agreement may be executed in any number of counterparts with the same effect as if all parties had signed the same document. All counterparts shall be construed together and shall constitute one agreement.

40. Right of Offset

In determining and paying any amounts owed to Nurse Practitioner under this Agreement, including, but not limited to amounts owed to Nurse Practitioner for professional services rendered hereunder or pursuant to any other agreement with The Clinic, The Clinic shall have a right of offset against any amounts owed by Nurse Practitioner to The Clinic under this Agreement or any other agreement between the parties.

Box 37-2 The Clinic Extended Care Provider Agreement—cont'd

This Agreement is entered into by the parties effective as of the Effective Date, notwithstanding actual signature at a different date.

THE CLINIC

By_______________________________

Its_______________________________

Date_______________________________

NURSE PRACTITIONER

____

Date_______________________________

Reprinted with permission from Mountain States Oncology Group, May 2005.

from transaction-based marketing—an emphasis on production, sales, or customer satisfaction with little or no ongoing relationship—into the relationship era, emphasizing establishment and maintenance of relationships with customers.[53] The realization that establishing and maintaining a relationship with customers is at least as important as attracting new customers drives relationship marketing. It is important to serve internal customers with the same high standards as external customers, because improving customer service inside an organization raises productivity, loyalty, and staff morale, and results in employees who appreciate and value their role in the delivery of superior service to external customers.[53] By converting indifferent customers into loyal ones, the organization and the customers both win. The APN can be instrumental in developing these relationships and enhancing the success of the organization.

Initially, the APN would use a combination of these elements to inform the community about the benefits of his/her services, persuade the members of the community to try them, and remind them later about the benefits they enjoyed. An important promotional method for the APN would be personal selling, entailing that the APN talk personally to prospective internal and external customers. This may require that the target market be further segmented in order to focus the personal selling efforts. Segments could be based on geographic boundaries, professional, educational and economic status, or other pertinent market information obtained in the analyses, but should be sure to include all the stakeholders required for the success of the role implementation.

Promotion of the APN must focus on satisfaction of customers' needs, wants, and expectations, hopefully defined beforehand by the environmental analysis. It is necessary to consider the customers' perceptions of the services they want or need, because many may be unaware of what the APN has to offer and may therefore filter out promotional messages until those perceptions are changed. For example, if customers have experienced only physician services in the past, messages about APN service may not get past their perceptual screen and may go unheeded. Attitudes affect perceptions, and promotional efforts may need to focus on changing customer attitudes by providing evidence of the benefits of APN services and by correcting misconceptions about APNs.[53]

Products are viewed as having a life cycle, much like that of humans. The stages include introduction, growth, maturity, and decline. APN services would likely be viewed as a new product in the introduction stage, at least in radiation oncology. The product would be first entering the market, and the marketing aim would be to gain awareness and stimulate demand by stressing information about its features and merits. This stage is generally associated with slow sales and little profit, a factor that would need to be considered in the budgeting process. Promotions should provide information, differentiate the APN product, and accentuate the APN's value, and should be centered on building primary demand for the product in general. Demand for a particular APN—selective demand—would occur later. If the APN were the only one in the radiation oncology market area initially, he/she would have an opportunity to gain primary and selective demand concurrently.[53,54] Keep in mind that promotional efforts should include internal as well as external customers. Winning the support of internal customers will assist in efforts to attract external customers.

Consideration of the consumer life cycle is necessary, because different promotional techniques would be focused on different groups in the life cycle. Early efforts may want to focus on attracting the consumers most likely to try out the new product—the early adopters. Early adopters tend to be younger, have higher social status, are better educated, enjoy higher incomes than other consumers, and rely more heavily than later adopters on impersonal information sources. More hesitant buyers rely primarily on company-generated promotional information and word-of-mouth communications.[53] Emphasis should be placed on the relative advantages of the APN role and its compatibility with the customers' current values and experiences. The content of personal selling efforts could include the following:

- Definition of an APN practice
- Illumination of APN educational preparation and qualifications
- Licensure and credentialing requirements
- Benefits to consumers
- Scope of APN practice
- Relationship to physicians, delineation of privileges
- Relationship to nursing, radiation therapists, physicists, dosimetrists, other staff
- Reimbursement status and options
- Code of ethics.

Information specific to radiation oncology functions should be included in order to clarify the new APN role for internal and external customers. Functions could include roles in the following:

- Acute and late radiation side-effect management
- Oncologic emergencies
- New and follow-up patient encounters
- Minor surgeries, for example, biopsies
- Simulation
- Administration of IV contrast
- Treatment planning
- Writing and signing of treatment prescriptions
- Verification of patient set-up
- Review/signing of weekly beam fields
- Insertion of bladder or rectal catheters
- Writing/signing of treatment prescriptions
- Physician co-signature requirements
- High- and low-dose brachytherapy procedures
- Administration of radiopharmaceuticals
- Patient/staff education
- Research

Advertising also could be used for promotion of the APN role. Advertising is a non-personal, paid communication used to inform, persuade, and remind consumers of the APN service. Although this form of promotion would not have an immediate feedback loop, as does the personal selling form, it would be attention getting and would communicate specific product benefits to the target market. It would reach large numbers of potential users of APN services and begin to break down barriers in the minds of consumers that typically wait until later in the consumer life cycle to buy the product. As opposed to publicity, it would control what was said, when it was said, and to whom.[53,54]

Web-based marketing is a fast, inexpensive, and efficient method of advertising through organizational websites, online advertisements on other sites, electronic bulletin boards, and online forums or communities.[53] Direct mailing of informational letters or brochures offers advantages such as the ability to select a narrow target market, achieve intensive coverage, send messages quickly, choose from various formats, provide complete information, and personalize each mailing piece.[53] The cost of direct mail may be high, however, and the organization must ensure the quality of its mailing list for it to be effective.

Public relations would be of utmost importance, with either formal or informal campaigns generally being of low cost compared with advertising or direct marketing. One element of public relations is publicity, a non-personal, indirectly paid presentation of an organization, service, or product. The APN could take advantage of publicity in an attempt to create a favorable image of APN practice in the minds of the internal and external consumers. Interviews with the local and regional media would hopefully generate news stories, a documentary, editorials, or public service announcements about APNs and the benefits of their practice. Publicity may add to the credibility of the APN service, increase exposure, and potentially reduce the cost of advertising, but less control is maintained over what is said, to whom, and when.[54] An important part of the public relations campaign would be directed toward the internal customers, because often they will be the ones in direct contact with the external customers, even before the APN.

Although available to the APN, sales promotion techniques generally would not be used. These techniques are often used to support advertising and personal selling by offering incentives such as discounts, deals, and coupons. In this situation, they could be viewed as 'cheapening' the image of APN services.

Together, the components of this planning phase would prepare the APN to begin the process of eliminating misperceptions and reducing the knowledge deficit of the target market. Multiple details for implementation of each element of the marketing plan would need to be further defined. The organization together with the APN could then move forward into the implementation phase of the strategic marketing process that would involve execution of the devised plan. Control, the final phase of the strategic marketing process that would compare the results of the implementation with the goals and act on the deviations, would be implemented as well.

THE FUTURE

Predictions call for increased use of APNs in health care, perhaps especially in radiation oncology. In order to realize these predictions, groups and individuals need to work together to further define the APN roles worldwide and make the changes necessary to overcome barriers to practice and further solidify APNs as anchors in the provision of health care.

What changes will be necessary? To help answer this question, the American Academy of Nurse Practitioners International Think Tank projected that standardized educational curriculum and specialty competencies should be used across all NP educational programs and accrediting and certification bodies. Its vision included adequate funding of graduate nursing education and residency programs by the federal government. It foresaw that consumers will have open access to the services of NPs with reimbursement parity by all health care plans commensurate with the level of services provided, with recognition, titling, and scope of practice being accepted universally.[61]

In order to accomplish these goals, the Think Tank recommended that APNs need to increase their legislative voice by increasing their presence as legislators in all levels of government. Finally, more evidence-based and outcome studies must be done that contribute to NP practice, marketability of NPs, and policy agendas.[61]

As the aged population expands, and with it, the occurrence of chronic illness, the demand for specialty-care physicians is likely to increase, opening the doors for APNs to fulfill the role of primary care provider and migrate into specialty practice. APNs in all settings are charged with the responsibility of documenting the quality of their care through evidence-based medicine, while trying to focus on the inner aspects of the human condition and the art of caring within nursing.[62] Trying to balance technologic approaches to treatment and practices driven by the medical model, APNs must strive to emphasize the holistic, caring practice consistent with the nursing model and with the relationship management era within which they provide care.

The future of APNs in radiation oncology is glowing with potential. As this relatively new specialty evolves, an awareness of the APN customers of today and a thoughtful, proactive approach to role development through the strategic planning and marketing process will help ensure success. APNs in radiation oncology can gain strength and voice by partnering with allies through involvement in specialty organizations like the ONS special interest groups (SIGS) for NPs, CNSs and radiation therapy. The radiation SIG enjoyed 8% growth in 2006, with 1200 members as of October.[63]

Barriers must come down. In 2005, the Oncology Nursing Certification Corporation introduced two role-specific advanced practice oncology nursing certification examinations: The Advanced Oncology Certified Nurse Practitioner (AOCNP) and the Advanced Oncology Certified Clinical Nurse Specialist (AOCNS),[64] which may help minimize the potential for issues with certification, licensing, or reimbursement, and serve to strengthen the image of the radiation oncology APN. Title protection and acceptance of the APN role may be enhanced by converting the advanced practice masters programs to practice doctorates as the entry level for advanced practice nursing. It is clear that current work in NP masters programs is equivalent to that of other doctoral programs such as optometry, pharmacology, medical doctors, and dentists, and work is underway to pursue systematic development of the practice doctorate.[65]

SUMMARY

As the radiation oncology APN role evolves, it is important to be aware of the interweaving of continuity and change. Today's consumers are more sophisticated and are making more educated choices, yet can be reluctant to try new ways of meeting their needs. As this group of consumers ages and requires more health-related services, the radiation oncology APN of the twenty-first century must attract and manage these customers with sharply tuned communication and problem-solving skills and knowledge about their business and their customers.[53]

REFERENCES

1. Roodbol P: NP in global perspective: results of a worldwide study to the nurse practitioner concept. *Program of the 3rd ICN International Nurse Practitioner/Advanced Practice Nursing Network Conference*, June 29–July 2, 2004, Groningen, The Netherlands.
2. Sheer B, Goodyear R: Highlights of the 3rd international council of nurses, nurse practitioner/advanced practice nursing network conference: critical pathways in a global context, *Medscape Nurses* 6(2):1-7, 2004.
3. Beauchesne MA: Global advancement of advanced practice nursing education, *Topics Adv Pract Nurs eJournal* 4(1):1-3, 2004.
4. Murphy-Ende D: Advanced practice nursing: reflections on the past, issues for the future, *Oncol Nurs Forum* 29(1): 106-112, 2002.
5. Silver HK, Ford LC, Stearly SG: A program to increase health care for children: the pediatric practitioner program, *Pediatrics* 39(5):756-760, 1967.
6. Phillips SJ: A comprehensive look at the legislative issues affecting advanced practice, *Nurse Pract Am J Primary Health Care* 30(1):14-47, 2005.
7. Robertson RM, Harmon JE: American Cancer Society and American Heart Association joint statement on cancer statistics report, *PR Newswire* (website): www.sev.prnewswire.com. Accessed January 21, 2005.
8. National Bureau of Economic Research: *NBER Economics of Aging Program program report* (website): www.nber.org/aging. Accessed April 4, 2005.
9. Centers for Disease Control and Prevention: Public health and aging: trends in aging—United States and worldwide, *Morb Mortal Weekly Rep*, 52(6):101-106, 2003.
10. O'Sullivan AL: 20th century nurse practitioners: enduring success, *Top Adv Pract Nurs eJournal* 4(3):1-3, 2004.
11. Nettina S: Opportunities in advanced practice nursing, *Medscape Nurses* 5(1), 2003 (website): www.medscape.com/viewarticle/452771.
12. Lloyd Jones M: Role development and effective practice in specialist and advanced practice roles in acute hospital settings: systematic review and meta-synthesis, *J Adv Nurs* 49(2):191-209, 2005.
13. Buppert C: Billing for nurse practitioner services: guidelines for NPs, physicians, employers, and insurers, *Medscape Nurses* 4(1), 2002 (website): www.medscape.com/viewarticle/422935.
14. *American Academy of Nurse Practitioners 2003-2004 NP practice site survey*. Retrieved 4/4/05 from: www.aanp.org.
15. Department of Health and Human Services Office of Inspector General: *Medicare coverage of non-physician practitioner services, OEI-02-00-00290*, June 2001.
16. Odle TG: Radiation therapy coding and reimbursement, *Radiat Ther* 14(1):27-44, 2005.
17. Centers for Medicare and Medicaid Services: *HHS/OIG fiscal year 2004 work plan*:13, 2004.
18. Centers for Medicare and Medicaid Services: *Home health and hospice consultation and care plan oversight clauses*, ID 92492, 2004.
19. Centers for Medicare and Medicaid Services: *Home health and hospice consultation and care plan oversight clauses*, ID 95770, 2004.
20. Klein TA: Scope of practice and the nurse practitioner: regulation, competency, expansion, and evolution, *Topics Adv Pract Nurs eJournal* 5(2), 2005 (website): www.medscape.com/viewarticle/506277.
21. National Association of Clinical Nurse Specialists: *FAQs* (website): www.nacns.org/faqs. Accessed May 3, 2005.
22. College of Nurses of Ontario: *Acute care/specialty nurse practitioner: policy issues relevant to regulation of the role, October 2003* (website): www.cno.org. Accessed March 9, 2005.
23. National Council of State Boards of Nursing: *Nurse licensure compact, 2005* (website): www.ncsbn.org. Accessed November 20, 2006.
24. Bryant-Lukosius D, DiCenso A, Browne G et al: Advanced practice nursing roles: development, implementation and evaluation, *J Adv Nurs* 48(5):519-529, 2004.
25. Wilson A, Pearson D, Hassey A: Barriers to developing the nurse practitioner role in primary care—the GP perspective, *Fam Pract* 19(6):641-646, 2002.
26. Kinnersley P, Anderson E, Parry K et al: Randomised controlled trial of nurse practitioner versus general practitioner care for patients requesting "same day" consultations in primary care, *BMJ* 320(7241):1043-1048, 2000.
27. Mundinger MO, Kane RL, Lenz ER et al: Primary care outcomes in patients treated by nurse practitioners or physicians, *JAMA* 283(1):59-68, 2000.
28. Lindeke LL, Grabau AM, Jukkala AJ: Rural NP perceptions of barriers to practice, *Nurse Pract* 29(8):50-51, 2004.
29. Hart LG, Salsberg E, Phillips DM et al: Rural health care providers in the United States, *J Rural Health* 18(5): 211-232, 2002.
30. Fulton JS, Baldwin K: An annotated bibliography reflecting

CNS practice and outcomes, *Clin Nurse Spec* 18(1):21-39, 2004.

31. Edmunds MW, Scudder LC: Attitudes of registered nurses toward nurse practitioners, *Medscape Nurses* 6(2) 2004 (website): www.medscape.com/viewarticle/489714.
32. Gooden JM, Jackson E: Attitudes of registered nurses toward nurse practitioners, *J Am Acad Nurs Pract* 16(8): 360-364, 2004.
33. Goolsby MJ: Highlights of the American Academy of Nurse Practitioners 19th annual meeting, *Medscape Nurses* 6(2), 2004 (website): www.medscape.com/viewarticle/483082.
34. McDermott Blackburn K: Roles of advanced practice nurses in oncology, *Oncology* 12(4):591-598, 1998.
35. Oncology Nursing Society: Home page, *May 2005* (website): www.ons.org. Accessed May 25, 2005.
36. Oncology Nursing Society: *The role of the advanced practice nurse in oncology care, position statement, 2003* (website): www.ons.org/publications/positions. Accessed March 15, 2005.
37. Corner J: The role of nurse-led care in cancer management, *Lancet Oncol* 4(10):631-636, 2003.
38. Frankel Kelvin J, Moore-Higgs GJ, Maher KE et al: Non-physician practitioners in radiation oncology: advanced practice nurses and physician assistants, *Int J Radiat Oncol Biol Phys* 45(2):255-263, 1999.
39. McGlynn B: Management of urinary incontinence following radical prostatectomy, *Urol Nurs* 24(6):475-482, 515, 2004.
40. Callahan C: Central line placement for the pediatric oncology patient: a model of advanced practice nurse collaboration, *J Pediatr Oncol Nurs* 21(1):16-21, 2004.
41. McKenna H: The role of an outreach oncology nurse practitioner: a case study evaluation, *Eur J Oncol Nurs* 8(1):66-77, 2004.
42. Garvican L, Grimsey E, Littlejohn P et al: Satisfaction with clinical nurse specialists in a breast care clinic: questionnaire survey, *BMJ* 316(7136):976-977, 1998.
43. Addington-Hall J, MacDonald LD, Anderson HR et al: Randomised controlled trial of co-ordinating care for terminally ill cancer patients, *BMJ* 305(6865):1317-1322, 1992.
44. Raftery JP, Addington-Hall JM, MacDonald LD et al: A randomized controlled trial of the cost-effectiveness of a district co-ordinating service for terminally ill cancer patients, *Palliat Med* 10(2):151-161, 1996.
45. McCorkle R, Benoliel JQ, Donaldson G et al: A randomized clinical trial of home nursing care for lung cancer patients, *Cancer* 64(6):1375-1382, 1989.
46. Corner J, Moore S, Haviland J et al: Nurse led follow up and conventional medical follow up in management of patients with lung cancer: randomized trial, *BMJ* 325(7373): 1145-1147, 2002.
47. Moore S, Corner J, Fuller F: Development of nurse-led follow-up in the management of patients with lung cancer, *NT Res* 4:432-444, 1999.
48. James ND, Guerro D, Brada M: Who should follow-up cancer patients? Nurse specialist based outpatient care and the introduction of a phone clinic system, *Clin Oncol* 6:283-287, 1994.
49. American Society for Therapeutic Radiology and Oncology: About ASTRO: what we do, May 2005 (website): www.astro.org. Accessed April 24, 2005.
50. Frankel Kelvin J, Moore-Higgs GJ: Description of the role of nonphysician practitioners in radiation oncology, *Int J Radiat Oncol Biol Phys* 45(1):163-169, 1999.
51. Oncology Nursing Society: *Membership statistics,* November 20, 2006.
52. American Society for Therapeutic and Radiologic Oncology: *Membership statistics,* May 2005.
53. Boone LE, Kurtz DL: *Contemporary marketing 2005*, Mason, Ohio, 2005, Thomson South-Western.
54. Berkowitz EN, Kerin RA, Rudelius W: *Marketing*, ed 2, Homewood, Ill, 1989, Richard D Irwin.
55. Jones A, Ironside V, Jameson G et al: A job description for the oncology NP, *Nurse Pract* 27(2):61, 2002.
56. Mountain States Oncology Group: *Job description: nurse practitioner,* May 2005.
57. Buppert C: *Employment contract, for purchase (website):* 56. http://www.buppert.com. Accessed May 14, 2005
58. Provenzano R, Nissenson AR: Economics of clinical nephrology practice, *Am J Kidney Dis* 44(1):168-178, 2004.
59. Mountain States Oncology Group: *Extended care provider agreement,* May 2005.
60. American Academy of Nurse Practitioners: *Nurse practitioner tips for contracting* (website): www.aanp.org/practice. Accessed May 14, 2005.
61. Fellows of the American Academy of Nurse Practitioners: *Nurse practitioner practice in 2012, meeting the healthcare needs of tomorrow* (website): www.aanp.org/practice/policy/legislation/regulation. Accessed April 24, 2005.
62. Enzman Hagedorn MI: Caring practices in the 21st century: the emerging role of nurse practitioners, *Topics Adv Pract Nurs eJournal* 4(4) (website): www.medscape.com/viewarticle/496372.
63. Oncology Nursing Society: SIG membership statistics, October 2006.
64. Oncology Nursing Society: *Oncology nursing society strategic plan 2003-2005* (website): www.ons.org. Accessed May 2, 2005.
65. American Academy of Nurse Practitioners Office of Health Policy: Doctor of nursing practice (DNP), *Academy Update*, June 2005.

Chapter 38
Evidence-Based Clinical Guidelines

Judith A. DePalma

In the current healthcare environment clinicians face pressure to reduce cost while continuing to improve quality of care and patient satisfaction. Legally and ethically there is pressure to be delivering the best possible care. Any oncology clinician that is striving for continual quality improvement logically needs to focus on the use of evidence to support clinical decisions. One method of employing evidence is the use of clinical practice guidelines (CPGs) that are based on sound research evidence. CPGs are currently authored by professional associations, healthcare organizations, and government agencies and can be readily accessed through online sources.[1]

CLINICAL PRACTICE GUIDELINES

Clinical practice guidelines are traditionally defined as "systematically developed statements to assist practitioner and patient decisions about appropriate health care for specific clinical circumstances."[2] Guidelines attempt to give the consensus of care and address all the relevant issues to support (1) clinical decisions for a specific patient population, (2) management of a symptom, or (3) the most effective use of a diagnostic or therapeutic procedure. "High quality practice guidelines clarify what interventions are effective in various circumstances and specify the extent of the documentation supporting those interventions."[3] Attributes of good guidelines include validity, reliability, reproducibility, clinical applicability, clinical flexibility, clarity, multidisciplinary process, review of evidence, and documentation.[2,4]

Clinical guidelines can be assigned to one of three general format categories:

1. Algorithms
2. Care pathways
3. Protocol

Algorithms also may be called *flowcharts* or *decision trees*. Pathways are usually day-by-day interdisciplinary guides for the care of a patient with a specific diagnosis, surgery, or diagnostic procedure. Alternative names for pathways may be *care maps*, *critical pathways*, or *patient pathways*. Protocols are usually very detailed, step-by-step instructions for a regimen of care or aspect of care. Some protocols may include algorithms.[5]

USE OF GUIDELINES

Guidelines are, as the term implies, guides to best practice. They should not control practice but should provide a credible framework that allows adaptation to individual patient needs using the clinician's expertise and the resources of the specific practice setting. Guidelines can be used in a variety of ways in practice and education. Guidelines can provide points of reference for clinical practice decisions, orientation of new care providers and clinical education. Several ways that guidelines can address clinical practice decision making are by:

- Implementing a new aspect of care that is evidence-based
- Expanding care across the continuum
- Updating a current standard practice or guideline
- Comparing current care with an established evidence-based guideline

A guideline may be adopted in the current practice for any of the following reasons:

- No standard guide exists for the particular aspect of care
- A credible guideline is currently in place but the plan is to facilitate continuity of care across the continuum, including out-patient and home care and therefore the search is for a comprehensive guideline
- A guideline is needed to compare with the current practice with the goal of either confirming the current level of care or revising the care based on the latest evidence-based guideline

IDEAL GUIDELINES

The ideal guidelines are those that are definitively evidence-based: the references for each aspect of treatment or practice recommendation are clearly cited. The complete citing of evidence allows the reader to locate the original evidence for clarification or further exploration. Aspects of ideal guidelines include the following[6]:

- Development process explained in the document or on the website (Credibility)
- Each step of care or recommendation clearly referenced (Validity, Accuracy)
- Algorithm or step-by-step protocol available that can be easily used by clinicians (Clarity)
- Level of current evidence indicated (Validity)
- Date of development and last update indicated (Currency)[6]
- Reassessment of guidelines for validity is recommended to be done every 3 years[7]

Some guidelines incorporate all aspects of the ideal guideline, whereas others may include only one or more of the factors.

Some guidelines declare that they are evidence-based, but each statement, step of care, or recommendation is not explicitly cited with the source of evidence. Instead, an extensive list of references may be provided, but no clear connection is shown between each fact and reference. Therefore, the reader cannot easily pinpoint the exact source of the original evidence. The difficulty with this type of guideline is that if further clarification is needed because a point is being challenged, the evidence cannot be easily located.

For example, in an acute care setting the practice committee is responsible for changing the clinical setting's policy. They have decided to change practice based on an evidence-based (EB) guideline, but when they locate the guideline, they question some part of the statement. Consequently, before adopting the guideline, it is necessary to locate the original evidence for clarification and further research findings. If the specific statement is not clearly cited, then all the reader knows is that the evidence is located in one of the many references listed at the end of the chapter or section. The evidence can still be located, but only by perusing each reference, which can be overwhelming in regard to time and resources.

It is important to know certain factors about why the guidelines have been developed. These factors are as follows[6]:

- Method used to choose and prioritize the topics
- Guideline development process
- Levels of evidence adopted to support recommendations
- Schedule for regular updating

In a later section of this chapter, websites are reviewed and several examples are given of guidelines that are well evidenced and those that are not.

VALUE OF GUIDELINES

Guidelines, in any of the various formats, have been criticized for imposing external standards on clinicians. Those that pose such an objection do not appreciate the total picture of evidence-based decision making. Evidence-based practice involves problem solving and delivering care based on[8]:

- Best current evidence
- Applied knowledge and individualized care in concert with the clinician's expertise
- An appreciation of the patient's values and expectations

This is extremely relevant to the practice of nursing, where an emphasis on the individualization of quality care has always existed. Nursing needs to move toward making clinical decisions based on evidence rather than taking action based on[9]:

- A response to one research study
- A response to one clinical expert's opinion
- Reliance on intuition
- The rigid maintenance of current practice, merely because it is the way it has always been done

Guidelines have the documented advantages of promoting[6,10]:

- Improved outcomes
- Increased accountability
- Decreased variations in care
- Limited liabilities
- Controlled resource usage
- Increased customer satisfaction
- Enhanced collaboration among caregivers
- Improved comparison of clinical outcomes

Decreased variation in care and controlled resource usage may result in cost savings. Guidelines may be useful in producing better care and decreasing its cost. The advantages listed can be tracked as outcomes of guideline implementation. Outcome data are especially relevant when preimplementation information has been collected as benchmarks to ascertain whether desired outcomes actually did improve.

IMPLEMENTING THE USE OF GUIDELINES

Established evidence-based clinical practice guidelines address the variations in clinical practice and the barriers to interpreting and synthesizing large volumes of scientific studies.[11] Ideally, a tested credible guideline currently exists for the clinicians in a setting to adopt or adapt, rather than needing to develop a new guideline. The process of identifying and implementing guidelines is time consuming, but each step is necessary to assure adoption of the most credible and appropriate guideline and to assure use of the guideline by the clinicians once adopted. (See Box 38-1 for a list of steps to implementing evidence-based decision making and use of guidelines.)

The first project is critical; it sets a positive tone for implementing evidence-based guidelines in any clinical setting. If the first project is successful, resistance and barriers that exist in the clinical setting may diminish. Clinicians who are undecided about the value of guidelines may be convinced to support such an initiative by findings of a successful first project. A system must be put into place to facilitate the implementation steps. Many times a system already exists in the clinical setting for promoting clinical excellence, and that system can be expanded to include guidelines. The choice of the first evidence-based guideline to implement must be taken very seriously. It needs to be a guideline that will have a very positive impact. Ideally, the improved care would impact a high number of clinicians and patients.

Box 38-1 Steps to Implementing Evidence-Based Decision Making and Use of Guidelines

- Assess the readiness of the clinical practice site to adopt evidence-based decision making and guidelines.
- Determine the group who will review practice guidelines.
- Choose the critical clinical issues and needed guidelines.
- Find evidence-based guidelines.
- Evaluate the guidelines for validity and feasibility in the particular clinical setting.
- Develop the implementation and evaluation plans.
- Educate stakeholders about the plans.
- Evaluate outcomes.
- Continually improve guidelines based upon outcome data.

Each of the implementation steps are outlined below:

1. Assess the readiness of the clinical practice site to adopt evidence-based decision making and guidelines.[12]
   - Adopt a process to assess aspects of the clinical practice site that are essential for the successful adoption of guidelines.
   - Review established assessment tools for relevance to the particular clinical site. (Figure 38-1 shows an example of such a tool that can be adapted for use in a variety of clinical settings.)
2. Determine the group who will review practice guidelines.
   - It would be best to use a group that has already been determined as being responsible for clinical excellence.
   - If no such clinical group exists, develop one that includes all stakeholders.
   - Include a few people who have the power to make decisions about changing practice.
   - Include people who are advocates for evidence-based practice and a few who are not.
3. Choose the critical clinical issues and needed guidelines. The stakeholder group should do the following:
   - Brainstorm clinical issues and needed guidelines.
   - Prioritize those that would impact most practitioners or patients.
   - For the first project, choose one that would define a guideline that most likely would receive support for change if the evidence is sufficient.
   - Choose a project that would have the most positive outcomes (clinical, clinician, and organization outcomes).
   - Formulate a statement that will help focus the search for guidelines. The statement should include the following:
     - Type of patient
     - Aspect of care
     - Timing of care

An example of such a statement is "a guideline is needed for skin care of radiation patients both during and after treatment regimen."

1. What is the purpose stated for initiating an evidence-based practice program?
   - ☐ Increase quality
   - ☐ Decrease cost
   - ☐ Other, specify ____________

2. Who is driving the initiation of this program?
   - ☐ Executive administration (CEO, Vice President)
   - ☐ Medical staff administration (Department Head)
   - ☐ Nursing administration
   - ☐ Particular service ____________
   - ☐ Other, specify ____________

3. Rate the level of support/commitment within the organization:

	High	Moderate	Minimal	None
Administration	☐	☐	☐	☐
Medical staff	☐	☐	☐	☐
Nursing	☐	☐	☐	☐
Support services	☐	☐	☐	☐
Few key individuals	☐	☐	☐	☐

4. Who will facilitate such a program in your organization?
   - ☐ Key individual(s); specify ____________
   - ☐ Groups such as team or unit(s); specify ____________
   - ☐ Other, specify ____________

5. What barriers do you anticipate?
   - ☐ Lack of support
   - ☐ Not seen as a priority
   - ☐ Resistance from key areas or key individuals
   - ☐ Too few resources to support
   - ☐ Lack of expertise in some areas to accomplish
   - ☐ Competing processes
   - ☐ Other, specify ____________

6. What structures are already in place within the organization to facilitate? (Check all that apply)
   - ☐ Established committees or groups that could assume this responsibility (i.e., quality improvement teams, service specific clinical groups)
   - ☐ Educational resources
   - ☐ Informatics/computer support
   - ☐ Library resources
   - ☐ Other, specify ____________

7. What processes are already in place within the organization to facilitate?
   - ☐ Quality improvement
   - ☐ Clinical review
   - ☐ Benchmarking
   - ☐ Human resource incentives (Job descriptions, performance evaluations)
   - ☐ Other, specify ____________

8. What would be the best scope to begin this process at this time?
   - ☐ Limit to a particular team, specify ____________
   - ☐ Limit to a particular service, specify ____________
   - ☐ Limit to a particular physician or practice, specify ____________
   - ☐ Limit to a specific patient population
   - ☐ Implement throughout the total organization
   - ☐ Other level, specify ____________

9. Check any of the following items that you believe would be a good starting focus. Provide the best example for each that you check.
   - ☐ High volume case type ____________
   - ☐ High cost case type ____________
   - ☐ New patient population ____________
   - ☐ Organization "Known for" ____________
   - ☐ Problem case type ____________
   - ☐ Cases with great variation in outcomes ____________
   - ☐ Other, specify ____________

10. What idea(s) do you have for a good initial project? Use examples from question 9. Choose the two that you know would have the greatest support and could be successful.

    Idea ____________ ☐ Guidelines already in place
    ____________ ☐ Guidelines need updated
    ☐ No guidelines

    Idea ____________ ☐ Guidelines already in place
    ____________ ☐ Guidelines need updated
    ☐ No guidelines

11. What is unique in the organization that might impact the implementation of evidence-based guidelines or practice? (include positive and negative aspects)

    ____
    ____
    ____

12. What is a realistic overall timeframe for implementation? ______ months

13. What else is going on within the organization that would impede this process or compete for resources? (i.e., JCAHO visit pending, union activities)

14. Check all of the following individuals who would be vital on the initial planning group. If you have specific individuals in mind, list their names.
    - ☐ Administrator
    - ☐ Physician(s)
    - ☐ Nurses (APN and staff)
    - ☐ Support services (PT, OT)
    - ☐ Pharmacist
    - ☐ Librarian
    - ☐ Informatics/Computer/Technical support
    - ☐ Clergy
    - ☐ Researcher (nurse researcher, statistician)
    - ☐ Other, specify ____________

15. What external individuals, organizations, or resources would you suggest be involved in the planning and implementation of the project?
    - ☐ Faculty of collaborating university
    - ☐ Librarian (none at organization)
    - ☐ Informatics/computer/technical support (none at organization)
    - ☐ Researcher (none at organization)
    - ☐ Clergy
    - ☐ Other, specify ____________

Figure 38-1 Evidence-Based Practice (EBP) Organizational Assessment (Acute Care Version).
Copyright© 2002, J. DePalma.

4. Find evidence-based guidelines.
   - Search literature for evidence-based guidelines.
   - Search online sites for evidence-based guidelines.
   - Search professional organizations for evidence-based guidelines.
   - Focus or expand the search.
   - Search for literature that supports use of guidelines, describes the implementation process in a specific setting, or proposes outcomes to be gained from the use of a specific guideline.
5. Evaluate the guidelines for validity and feasibility in the particular clinical setting.
   - Identify an evaluation instrument that is feasible to use.
   - Evaluate the credibility of the guideline based on the factors in the instrument.
   - Determine the feasibility of using the guideline in the clinical setting.
     - Consider supporting factors.
     - Consider barriers.
   - Accept, by consensus, a guideline or revise a guideline to increase the feasibility of acceptance.
   - Possibly secure feedback from a broader group, if deemed necessary.
6. Develop the Implementation and Evaluation Plans.
   - Write out a step-by-step plan for the implementation of the guideline.
     - Include a time line.
     - Include education of clinicians.
     - Include development of patient education materials.
     - Secure all approvals that are needed.
     - Pilot test the implementation plan with one unit or at least a few clinicians.
   - Based upon desired outcomes, formulate a detailed evaluation plan while writing the implementation plan.
     - Ascertain what benchmark data are available.
     - Determine what systems are in place or need to be developed to monitor outcomes.
     - Develop any data collection tools that need to be added to point-of-care documentation in order to track outcomes.
     - Ideally modify point-of-care documentation to include all outcomes data needed.
     - Test the evaluation plan with a small group of patients to determine whether adequate data are being collected and the tracking system is working.
7. Educate stakeholders about the plans.
   - Include education in the implementation plan.
   - Recognize the need for reeducation at key times in the process.
   - Use the continuing education resources that are available, when possible.
8. Evaluate outcomes.
   - Based on the evaluation plan and the test of the plan, track desired outcomes.
   - Review the data at regular intervals.
   - Planning group reviews the data to determine whether any changes are needed.
   - Submit summary reports to other appropriate groups for review.
   - Disseminate the positive outcomes internally and to the public.
9. Continually improve guidelines based on outcome data.
   - Based on the outcome tracking, confirm the appropriateness of the guideline, or revise the guideline.
   - Establish a schedule for continual review of outcomes.

FINDING PRACTICE GUIDELINES

One of the crucial skills that is needed to effectively implement evidence-based guidelines is the ability to find valid and appropriate practice guidelines. Clinical guidelines can be accessed online from the websites of government agencies and professional organizations. Guidelines from such credible sources vary in presentation format and availability. Some guidelines incorporate all aspects of the ideal guideline whereas others only include one or more of the aspects. Some guidelines are available in abstract and full-text format online, for example, those on the federal websites. Guidelines of some professional organizations have to be purchased.

A number of websites that are credible and relevant to radiation therapy practice were accessed and the evidence-based guidelines presented therein were reviewed as information was gathered for this textbook. (Box 38-2 contains a list of those websites.) A variety of sites were included to give

Box 38-2 Websites for Guidelines

National Guidelines Clearinghouse (NGC)
www.guideline.gov

National Comprehensive Cancer Network (NCCN)
www.nccn.org

The American Society of Clinical Oncology (ASCO)
www.asco.org

American College of Radiology (ACR)
www.acr.org

Oncology Nursing Society (ONS)
www.ons.org

American Cancer Society (ACS)
www.cancer.org

American Society for Therapeutic Radiology and Oncology (ASTRO)
www.astro.org

a representative sample of the range of both federal government and professional organization–sponsored sites. The review of each website included the following aspects, as available:

- Purpose of the developing organization
- Guideline development process
- Range of guidelines, with a focus on relevant radiation therapy (RT) guidelines
- Comparison of a guideline with the aspects of an ideal guideline

National Guidelines Clearinghouse (NGC)

The National Guidelines Clearinghouse (NGC) was established through a collaboration with the Agency for Health Care Research and Quality (AHRQ) of the U.S. Department of Health and Human Services and the American Medical Association and the American Association of Health Plans in 1998.[13]

The mission of the NGC is "to provide physicians, nurses, and other health professionals, healthcare providers, health plans, integrated delivery systems, purchasers, and others an accessible mechanism for obtaining objective, detailed information on clinical practice guidelines and to further their dissemination, implementation, and use" (NGC). Guidelines on this site originate from a variety of federal and professional organizations. A few of the oncology-specific organizations whose guidelines are listed at www.ngc.gov/browse/guideline_index.aspx include the following:

- American College of Radiology
- American Society for Blood & Marrow Transplantation
- American Society of Breast Disease
- American Society of Clinical Oncology
- Canadian Breast Cancer Initiative
- Oncology Nursing Society

The guidelines on this website include the following key components:

- Structured abstracts (summaries) about the guideline and its development
- Links to full-text guidelines, where available, and/or ordering information for print copies
- Palm-based PDA downloads of the *Complete NGC Summary* for all guidelines represented in the database
- A guideline comparison utility that gives users the ability to generate side-by-side comparisons for any combination of two or more guidelines
- An annotated bibliography database where users can search for citations for publications and resources about guidelines, including guideline development and methodology, structure, evaluation, and implementation

The NGC guidelines are indexed primarily according to the contributing professional organization, but they also can be searched by disease, condition, or treatment/intervention. When a search was done using 'oncology' and 'radiation' as the keywords, a list of 89 guidelines resulted, dating from the mid-1990s to 2005. These were mostly oriented toward medical diagnosis and treatment for specific neoplasms, such as gliomas, advanced squamous cell carcinoma of the head and neck, brain metastases, and unresectable non-small cell lung cancer. Some of the guidelines were non-U.S., which might limit the usability of the guideline.

When the list of 89 guidelines was limited with 'nursing' as a keyword, only 20 items remained in the list, including:

- Chemotherapy and Biotherapy: Guidelines and Recommendations for Practice From the Oncology Nursing Society[14]
- Cancer Pain From the Singapore Ministry of Health[15]
- Management of Patients With Lung Cancer. a National Clinical Guideline From the Scottish Intercollegiate Guidelines Network[16]

- Cancer: Nutrition Management for Older Adults From the American Academy of Family Physicians—Medical Specialty Society, American Dietetic Association, and Nutrition Screen Initiative[17]

Each guideline's brief summary included the following:

- Major recommendations
- Clinical algorithm, if available
- Type of evidence supporting the recommendation
- Bibliographic source (citation for reference list)
- Date released
- Guideline developers
- Source of funding
- Guideline committee
- Guideline availability (electronic and print copies)
- Availability of companion documents

Although the NGC is a credible and reputable website, the guidelines themselves need to be assessed individually for the level of evidence that is used and the manner in which the evidence is cited because of the wide variety of sources of guidelines. For example, the full document of *Management of Brain Metastases: Role of Radiotherapy Alone or in Combination With Other Treatment Modalities*[18] prepared by the Neuro-oncology Disease Site Group, has recommendations and evidence that supports the recommendations, but each recommendation is not cited with the evidence source. When searching a large, broad-based database such as the NGC, it is important that the most complete copy of the guideline is accessed, because some of the first formats accessed are merely summaries.

National Comprehensive Cancer Network (NCCN)

The National Comprehensive Cancer Network (NCCN) began in 1995 and consists of 19 hospitals. The purpose of NCCN is to develop a comprehensive set of evidence-based diagnostic, treatment, and supportive care guidelines designed to guide medical decisions in cancer care. The guidelines exist in the categories of treatment by cancer site, detection, prevention, risk reduction, and supportive care. Each guideline has an extensive bibliography of all studies that are included in the meta-analysis conducted in the process of developing the guideline. Guidelines are listed according to the site of the cancer, detection, prevention and risk reduction of cancer, and supportive care. Supportive care refers primarily to symptom management. All guidelines are available in full text online.

The *Cancer-related Fatigue Guideline*[19] was revised in 2005 and authored by a panel of notable nurses and physicians. The guideline is detailed with algorithms, decision-making models, and narrative to support the assessment and treatment recommendations. The guideline includes the following:

- A definition of cancer-related fatigue
- Standards of care for both adults and children
- Screening techniques
- Primary evaluation
- Interventions for active treatment
- Interventions for long-term follow-up
- Interventions for end-of-life

References are cited throughout the narrative, and a reference list is included at the end of the document. The NCCN guidelines are extremely credible and reliable to use. On the other hand, the NCCN guidelines are so detailed and comprehensive that they may be intimidating or overwhelming to a group of clinicians who are beginning to implement guidelines. A way to approach the guidelines in this situation would be to look at one aspect of fatigue management rather than the total guideline to be implemented. The guideline could be implemented in stages as the clinical group has had an opportunity to study the details of the guideline and establish the processes needed to implement guidelines in the clinical setting.

The American Society of Clinical Oncology

The American Society of Clinical Oncology (ASCO) is the world's leading professional organization representing physicians who treat people with cancer. ASCO's members set the standard for patient care worldwide and lead the fight for more effective cancer treatments, increased funding for clinical and translational research, and cures for the many different cancers that strike millions of people around the world every year.

Twenty-seven guidelines were indexed according to types of cancer and one general category of supportive care and quality of life. Guidelines are developed by a panel of experts consisting of the following:

- Disease experts
- Methodology experts
- Patient representative
- Fellow representative

- Representative of the Health Services Research Committee of ASCO

Drafts of the guidelines that are developed from the research literature are peer reviewed and ultimately approved by the ASCO Board of Directors.

The guideline entitled *Postmastectomy Radiotherapy*[4] was reviewed. An abstract was available that summarized the purpose, the level of evidence found related to the topic, and whether recommendations were made. The date of adoption by ASCO is listed, as are those of any updates.

The full text of the guidelines are available online and as articles in the *Journal of Clinical Oncology*. The full text articles include the following:

- Abstract
- Introduction
- Practice guidelines
- Method
- References

Each recommendation that was made in the practice guidelines section was clearly referenced, and the level of evidence and level of recommendation was indicated. Both of these levels are explained in a table within the article. Levels of evidence range from I to IV, with level I being the best evidence. The levels of recommendations range from A to D, with the A level being the most desirable and D signifying little or no empirical evidence.

As an example, in the *Postmastectomy Radiotherapy* (PMRT) guideline,[4] one of the practice recommendations is that such therapy is appropriate for patients with four or more positive axillary lymph nodes. The level of evidence for this recommendation is level II, which means the evidence is from at least one well-designed randomized trial. The grade of recommendation is a B, which means the findings are generally consistent and the level of evidence ranges from II to IV.

American College of Radiology

The American College of Radiology (ACR), a nonprofit professional society, focuses on advancing the science of radiology, improving radiologic services to the patient, studying socioeconomic aspects of radiology, and encouraging continuing education of clinicians. Its membership includes radiologists, radiation oncologists, medical physicists, interventional radiologists, and nuclear medicine physicians. ACR develops scientifically based appropriateness criteria to assist radiologists, radiation oncologists, and referring physicians in making appropriate imaging decisions for given patient clinical conditions.

The ACR periodically defines new practice guidelines and technical standards for radiologic practice to help advance the science of radiology and to improve the quality of service to patients throughout the United States. Existing practice guidelines and technical standards are reviewed for revision or renewal, as appropriate, every 5 years. Each practice guideline and technical standard, representing a policy statement by ACR, has undergone a thorough consensus process in which it has been subjected to extensive review, requiring the approval of the Commission on Quality and Safety and the ACR Board of Chancellors, the ACR Council Steering Committee, and the ACR Council.

A lengthy list of practice guidelines is available on the website, categorized by anatomic site and specialty type of radiology. Thirteen guidelines are listed for radiation oncology. Several of the guidelines are related to brachytherapy, one deals with total body irradiation, and another with informed consent. The *Compliance Program Guidelines for Radiologists and Radiation Oncologists* is available for purchase from the ACR store on the website. The *ACR Practice Guideline for Radiation Oncology*[20] was available in full text on the website. This guideline was designed to provide appropriate radiologic care for oncology patients. The preamble to the document warns that the guidelines are not a legal standard of care but are just recommendations. The Guideline addresses the following:

- Process of radiation therapy
- Qualifications and responsibilities of personnel
- Equipment specifications
- Patient and personnel safety
- Quality improvement

Recommendations are listed under each heading, but no references are cited for each recommendation. This guideline was originally authored in 1990 and revised every 5 years, with the last revision in 2004.

Oncology Nursing Society

The Oncology Nursing Society (ONS) is a nonprofit professional organization of registered nurses and other healthcare providers dedicated to excellence in patient care, education, research, and administration in oncology nursing.

Guidelines and standards of practice are listed under publications on the website. There is free access to a description of the publication and an excerpt, but the full text must be purchased. Guidelines published as of 2004 are evidence-based. The guidelines are authored by experts in the oncology nursing field and are peer-reviewed by content and evidence-based experts before publication.

The *Manual for Radiation Oncology Nursing Practice and Education*[21] is evidence-based with citations for each practice recommendation. The guideline provides current evidence on patient assessment, symptom management, documentation, radiation protection, and quality improvement. It is written in outline form and lists references for each content area.

American Cancer Society

The American Cancer Society (ACS) is the nationwide community-based voluntary health organization dedicated to eliminating cancer as a major health problem by preventing cancer, saving lives, and diminishing suffering from cancer, through research, education, advocacy, and service. ACS concentrates on developing cancer societies and on collaboration with other cancer-related organizations throughout the world in carrying out shared strategic directions.

A primary focus is to provide information for consumers; therefore any information that could be identified as a guideline was for patients, survivors, and families. Under *Coping With Physical and Emotional Changes* on the website, symptoms and side effects were addressed for radiation therapy. Commonly asked question were addressed, such as:

- What can I do about skin problems?
- What can I do about hair loss?
- Will I develop eating problems?

The answers are provided as a bulleted list of recommendations, with no cited references. For the eating problems question the user is referred to the *NCCN Nausea and Vomiting Treatment Guidelines for Patients With Cancer.*

American Society for Therapeutic Radiology and Oncology

The American Society for Therapeutic Radiology and Oncology (ASTRO) is dedicated to advancing the practice of radiation oncology by promoting excellence in patient care, providing opportunities for educational and professional development, promoting research and disseminating research results, and representing radiation oncology in a rapidly evolving socioeconomic healthcare environment.

Although no actual guidelines are listed on the website, in the research area, under Clinical Practice Tools, there is a list of organizations with evidence-based and consensus-based practice tools. Each site is concisely described, and access is available through a link with the resource sites.

Literature Search

Besides the search of the aforementioned websites, a literature search was done using OVID to search the MEDLINE and CINAHL databases. Several relevant guidelines that were accessed in this manner include the following:

- Antiemetic guidelines—a collaborative effort to simplify the available guidelines and provide an easy-to-use reference for the practitioner[22]
- Evidence-based oncology oral care guideline—multidisciplinary work group at the University of Pennsylvania Health System formulated a guideline based on the current evidence[23]
- RT protectants—update of the American Society of Clinical Oncology guidelines[24]

EVALUATING GUIDELINES

Ideally, a guideline evaluation should involve a critique of the credibility of the guideline and then a judgment of the level of feasibility of implementing the guideline in the particular clinical setting. Several instruments currently exist to help evaluate important attributes of guidelines. All of them address both broad areas of credible development and appropriateness to the individual clinical situation.

As a general overview, the discussion points that Sackett and colleagues[8] designed can be used to evaluate a guideline for validity and applicability. The recommended questions to ask include the following:

- Evaluating for validity:
  - Did the developers do a comprehensive literature review within the past 12 months?
  - Are each of the recommendations linked with the level of evidence and a specific criterion?
- Evaluating for applicability:
  - Are there sufficient patient numbers to warrant implementation of the guideline?

- Are the beliefs of individual patients and the community of health care providers compatible with the guideline?
- How much energy and resources would be required in order to implement the guideline?
- What are the geographic, organizational, traditional, authoritarian, legal, or behavioral barriers to implementing the guideline?

Appraisal of Guidelines for Research & Evaluation Instrument

The Appraisal of Guidelines for Research & Evaluation (AGREE)[25] was designed to provide a framework for assessing the quality of clinical practice guidelines; this instrument consists of 23 key items in six domains:

1. Scope and purpose
2. Stakeholder involvement
3. Rigor of development
4. Clarity and presentation
5. Applicability
6. Editorial independence

The user responds on a 4-point Likert scale to each of 13 items with the range being strongly disagree to strongly agree. For example, under the Scope and Purpose section, one of the items is "The clinical questions covered by the guideline are specifically described." Ten of the items require short answer responses to a statement about what a quality guideline should include.

The recommended number of appraisers for each guideline is two at a minimum, with the ideal of four to increase the reliability of the assessment. Scoring is done by section or domain, resulting in a percentage of agreement.

Cluzeau Appraisal Instrument

The purpose of the Cluzeau Appraisal Instrument[26] is to assess the quality of a clinical guideline, especially to identify guidelines that lack rigorous development standards. The instrument has been tested and has been described as reliable and valid.[27] The instrument consists of 37 items that are scored as 'yes,' 'no,' 'not sure,' or 'not applicable.' The items are categorized into three dimensions:

- Rigor of development, which includes the development process and methods of including evidence
- Context and content, which includes clarity, readability, and cost/benefit
- Application, which focuses on implementation and application strategies

Numerous appraisers are recommended so that the mean scores can be compared and consensus can be reached.

SUBSTITUTES FOR GUIDELINES

If no guidelines are available for the specific clinical topic or aspect of care that is of interest to the clinical group, other options are available that promote the use of best evidence. These include the following:

- Systematic reviews or meta-analyses of research studies that conclude with recommendations for practice based on the results of the studies
- Consensus statements that usually originate from professional organizations or national conferences

Systematic Reviews

An integrated, or systematic, review is a summary of evidence on a particular topic that uses a rigorous process to identify, appraise, and synthesize research studies to answer a specific clinical question. Such a review is usually conducted by a panel of experts, and the synthesis results in recommendations for best practice based on the evidence that is currently available.[28] A meta-analysis goes beyond a mere review and synthesis of quantitative research findings. In a meta-analysis, statistical analyses are done combining the data from already published studies[29] to calculate measures such as effect sizes. A meta-analysis may confirm existing findings from individual studies or clarify conflicting findings.

The Cochrane Library has set the gold standard for systematic reviews. The Cochrane Database of Systematic Reviews is published quarterly as part of The Cochrane Library and is available at www.cochrane.org/reviews/index.htm. The database consists of a set of high-quality literature reviews that are highly structured summaries of carefully selected articles on health-related topics—randomized controlled trials are a major emphasis of the database.[30] It includes over 1600 completed reviews and many protocols of reviews under preparation, and therefore is a good starting point when conducting the literature search to identify the evidence on a particular intervention. Abstracts can be searched and viewed free of charge, but full text of the reviews can be accessed online only if the library facility subscribes to the Cochrane Library service or the reviews can be purchased individually.[31]

A search of the Cochrane Database of Systematic Reviews resulted in several reviews relevant to radiation therapy for the patient with cancer. The specific topics include the following:

- Chemotherapy, RT, and combined modality for Hodgkin's disease, with emphasis on second cancer risk[32]
- Combined chemotherapy and RT (without surgery) compared with RT alone in localized carcinoma of the esophagus[33]
- Hyperbaric oxygen therapy for late radiation tissue injury[34]

Each of the reviews included the following elements:

- Background
- Objectives
- Search strategy
- Selection criteria
- Main results
- Conclusions

Cochrane reviews are generally well accepted by physicians because of the known credibility. This fact further emphasizes the value of searching the Cochrane database early in any clinical search.

Consensus Statements

Consensus statements may originate from a panel of experts that is selected to discuss best practice. Often such statements are developed during discussions at a national conference. Various levels of evidence can be used during the discussion of what is the current best practice, with the ideal being to include relevant research studies. The practice recommendations are presented to the conference attendees for discussion and clarification and finally acceptance by the majority.

Several examples of consensus statements from the literature include the following:

- Brachytherapy for localized prostate cancer—professional organizations in Germany formulated a consensus statement with recommendations and guidelines for the indications, planning, implementation, and follow-up of permanent interstitial brachytherapy[35]
- Radiation therapy of benign disease—German Working Group on Radiotherapy initiated a consensus process with an expert panel. The final statement was discussed and agreed upon at a national conference[36]
- High-dose intensity-modulated radiation therapy for prostate cancer—use of consensus statement of the American Society of Therapeutic Radiation Oncology to guide the treatment of 772 patients with prostate cancer[37]
- Postmastectomy radiation therapy for breast cancer patients with limited lymph node involvement—panel recommendation[38]
- Workshop on partial breast irradiation to determine the state of the art and the science[39]

Other Literature

Other literature that may support adoption of guidelines are articles published in professional journals that address how guidelines were developed, how existing guidelines were used by specific groups, or the outcomes of compliance with practice guidelines with a specific patient population. A search of the literature resulted in the following examples relevant to radiation therapy:

- An update and expansion of published clinical practice guidelines for the treatment of cancer treatment–induced diarrhea[40]
- A study to determine patterns and predictors aligned with institutional treatment guidelines for older women with breast cancer[41]
- A testimony to the importance of treatment guideline for high dose rate brachytherapy[42]
- Development of evidence-based practice guidelines for radiation skin care in British Columbia[43]
- Women with breast cancer participating in the development of psychosocial clinical practice guidelines[44]
- Discussion of NCCN breast cancer guidelines related to use of radiation for older women undergoing breast conservation[45]
- Outcomes of the use of the American Cancer Society and the National Comprehensive Cancer Network's guidelines for prostate cancer screening[46]
- Comparison of outcomes with patients with soft tissue sarcomas who were treated with evidence-based practice guidelines[47]
- Critique of the American Cancer Society's guidelines for breast cancer screening[48]
- Using long-term follow-up guidelines to facilitate the care of childhood cancer survivors[49]

- A 10-year review of chronic radiation enteritis[50]
- Assessment of the scope and quality of guidelines in lung cancer[51]
- Method for lung cancer evidence review and guideline development[52]
- Developing guidelines for end-of-life decision making by adolescents[53]

All of these could be used in conjunction with the actual guidelines to support the adoption or adaptation of guidelines.

EXAMPLE OF USE OF A GUIDELINE

As previously mentioned, a guideline may be adopted because in the current practice setting no standard protocol exists for the particular aspect of care of interest or a credible guideline is currently in place but there is a need to update or expand the perspective of care and therefore a revision of the guideline is needed.

The following is an example of the process used by one radiation therapy (RT) clinical site in adopting a guideline to manage treatment-related fatigue:

Setting: Free-standing RT center associated with several community hospitals

Group: Biweekly meeting of all clinical care providers to discuss clinical issues

Problem: Noted in chart review that majority of patients experience fatigue during treatment but no plan of care or protocol exists in this setting.

Decisions: A sub-group of the clinical group was formed with one representative from each category of healthcare providers. The charge to this group was to search and review available guidelines and bring a recommendation and implementation plan to the total group.

Planning

Once the total clinical group determined that a guideline for management of fatigue would be feasible to implement, members of the group made recommendations as to where guidelines might be found that would be credible. A thorough online search was then conducted by the sub-group for existing fatigue guidelines. After reviewing the literature and websites, the National Comprehensive Cancer Network's (NCCN) Fatigue Guideline[19] was determined to be the most comprehensive and the most likely to be accepted at the clinical site.

The sub-group brought the NCCN Fatigue Guideline to the total group with the following recommendations:

1. Adopt the NCCN guideline.
2. Implement a portion of the guideline first and then evolve to adopting all aspects of the guideline that are relevant to the Center's practice.
3. The first aspects of the guideline to be implemented should be
   - Screening
   - Interventions for patients on active treatment

After a review of the NCCN Fatigue Guideline by all members of the clinical group, all of the sub-group's recommendations were accepted. The sub-group was then charged with designing detailed implementation and evaluation plans. During this process, key individuals in administration were kept apprised of the progress in order to secure administrative support and needed resources for implementation and maintenance of the guideline and evaluation of clinical outcomes resulting from the guideline.

Implementation

The implementation plan that was outlined, based on the NCCN guideline,[19] was written as follows:

1. All patients will be screened for fatigue as a vital sign on a 0–10 scale.
   a. Mild fatigue (1–3)
   b. Moderate (4–6)
   c. Severe (7–10)
2. Documentation forms will be edited to include:
   a. Fatigue level
   b. Interventions taken or discussed with patient regarding fatigue
3. Initial interventions will be recommended based upon level of fatigue
   a. Mild—
      i. Educate about usual pattern and cause of fatigue
      ii. Teach how to self-monitor between treatments
      iii. Introduce possible coping strategies
      iv. Clinicians will do reevaluation each visit
   b. Moderate or Severe—do further assessment including:
      i. Onset, pattern, duration
      ii. Change over time
      iii. Factors that aggravate or alleviate

iv. Other possible causes, that is, recurrence of malignancy, pain, anemia

4. Evidence-based interventions for patients on active treatment with Moderate or Severe levels of fatigue should focus on the following (all are expanded upon in detail in the NCCN guideline[19]:
   a. Energy conservation
   b. Activity enhancement, including a progressive exercise regimen
   c. Distraction
   d. Restorative therapy
   e. Nutrition consultation
   f. Sleep therapy
   g. Family support
   h. Psychosocial interventions
   i. Pharmacologic treatment, if necessary
      i. Psychostimulants
      ii. Antidepressants
5. Evaluation of outcomes will be done and tracked over time to determine trend.
   a. Baseline data on fatigue will be collected either from chart review or real-time data collection for a period of time prior to implementing the new guideline.
   b. Data regarding fatigue will be collected and analyzed once guideline in place.
      i. Occurrence of fatigue
      ii. Levels of fatigue
      iii. Duration of fatigue
      iv. Effective strategies used by patients
      v. Patient satisfaction with strategies
      vi. Process should be evaluated by the data to show what percentage of clinicians are following guideline.
   c. Baseline and current data will be compared to determine whether outcomes are improving in the areas of screening and interventions.

Once the guideline has been implemented and evaluated, the results need to be reviewed by the total clinical group and distributed to all appropriate individuals and groups. Clinicians and the public should be made aware of the positive outcomes that occur or the need for revision of the guidelines based on patient data. In this particular situation, the first phase of the guideline worked well with a few adjustments, especially in the documentation forms to prompt clinicians to assess and follow the intervention recommendations. Evaluation was a time-consuming process, and so a collaboration was formed with university colleagues. Whenever possible, professional students were given access to the data to do the data analysis and summarize the results for their academic scholarly projects.

SUMMARY

Adopting an evidence-based approach to clinical decision making is time consuming and demands many resources, but the benefits usually outweigh the risks and resources. Positive outcomes usually can be expected at the patient, caregiver, and organizational level. A practice environment that fosters inquiry and pursuit of the best current evidence is one that promotes professional development and ownership of practice. In the current healthcare environment with the nursing shortage and the emphasis on cost containment while improving quality of care, reliance on evidence-based decision making through the use of guidelines fosters positive outcomes.

REFERENCES

1. Goolsby MJ: Evaluating and applying clinical practice guidelines, *J Am Acad Nurse Pract* 13(1):3-6, 2001.
2. Institute of Medicine, Committee to Advise the Public Health Service on Clinical Practice Guidelines. In Field MJ, Lohr KN, editors: *Clinical practice guidelines: directions of a new program*, Washington, DC, 1990, National Academy Press, p 39.
3. Cates JR, Young DN, Guerriero DJ et al: Evaluating the quality of clinical practice guidelines, *J Manipulative Physiol Ther* 24(3):170-176, 2001.
4. Recht A, Edge SB, Solin LJ et al: Postmastectomy radiotherapy: clinical practice guidelines of the American Society of Clinical Oncology, *J Clin Oncol* 19(5):1539-1569, 2001.
5. DePalma JA: Evidence-based clinical practice guidelines, *Semin Perioper Nurs* 9(3):115-120, 2000.
6. Thomas L, Hotchkiss R: Evidence-based guidelines. In Craig JV, Smyth RL, editors: *The evidence-based practice manual for nurses*, Philadelphia, 2002, Churchill Livingstone, p 222.
7. Shekelle PG, Ortiz E, Rhodes S et al: Validity of the Agency for Healthcare Research and Quality clinical practice guidelines, *JAMA* 286(12):1461-1467, 2001.
8. Sackett, DL, Straus SE, Richardson WS et al: *Evidence-based medicine: how to practice and teach EBM*, Edinburgh, 2002, Churchill Livingstone.
9. DePalma J: Evidence-based practice. In Bruner DW, Haas ML, Gosselin-Acomb TK, editors: *Manual for radiation oncology nursing practice and education*, ed 3, Pittsburgh, 2005, Oncology Nursing Society, pp 5-8.
10. Mead P: Clinical guidelines: promoting clinical effectiveness or a professional minefield? *J Adv Nurs* 31(1):110-116, 2000.

11. Slutsky J: Using evidence-based practice guidelines: tools for improving practice. In Melnyk BM, Fineout-Overhold E, editors: *Evidence-based practice in nursing & healthcare*, Philadelphia, 2005, Lippincott Williams & Wilkins, pp 221-236.
12. Pravikoff DS, Tanner AB, Pierce ST: Readiness of US nurses for evidence-based practice, *Am J Nurs* 105(9): 40-51, 2005.
13. Agency for Health Care Policy and Research: Invitation to submit guidelines to the National Guideline Clearinghouse, *Fed Reg* 63:18027, 1998.
14. *Chemotherapy and biotherapy: guidelines and recommendations for practice*, Pittsburgh, 2001, Oncology Nursing Society.
15. *Cancer pain*, Singapore, 2003, Singapore Ministry of Health.
16. *Management of lung cancer: a national clinical guideline recommended for use in Scotland by the Scottish Intercollegiate Guidelines Network*, Edinburgh, 1998, Scottish Intercollegiate Guidelines Network.
17. Barrocas A, Purdy D, Brady P et al: *Cancer: nutrition management for older adults*, Washington, DC, 2002, Nutrition Screening Initiative.
18. Tsao MN, Laetsch NS, Wong RKS et al: *Management of brain metastases: role of radiotherapy alone or in combination with other treatment modalities*, Ontario, 2004, Cancer Care (website): www.guideline.gov/summary/pdf.aspx?doc_id=4983&stat=1&string=radiation+AND+therapy. Accessed December 12, 2005.
19. *Cancer-related fatigue guidelines*, Version 2, 2005, National Comprehensive Cancer network (website): www.nccn.org/professionals/physicians_glsPDF/fatigue/pdf. Accessed December 14, 2005.
20. American College of Radiology: *The ACR practice guideline for* radiation oncology: 2004 (website): www.acr.org/s_acr/bin.asp?TrackID=&SID=1&DID=12276&CID=1075&VID=2&DOC=File.PDF. Accessed December 15, 2005.
21. Bruner DW, Haas ML, Gosselin-Acomb TK: *Manual for radiation oncology nursing practice and education*, ed 3, Pittsburgh, 2005, Oncology Nursing Society.
22. Koeller JM, Aapro MS, Gralla RJ et al: Antiemetic guidelines: creating a more practical treatment approach, *Support Care Cancer* 10(7):519-522, 2002.
23. Stricker CT, Sullivan J: Evidence-based oncology oral care clinical practice guidelines: development, implementation and evaluation, *Clin J Oncol Nurs* 7(2):222-227, 2003.
24. Schuchter LM, Hensley ML, Meropol NJ et al: 2002 update of recommendations for the use of chemotherapy and radiotherapy protectants: clinical practice guidelines of the American Society of Clinical Oncology, *J Clin Oncol* 20(12):2895-2903, 2002.
25. AGREE Collaboration: *Appraisal of guidelines for research & evaluation instrument: 2001* (website): www.agreecollaboration.org/instrument/. Accessed December 12, 2005.
26. Cluzeau F, Littlejohns P, Grimshaw J et al: *Appraisal instrument for clinical guideline*, London, 1997, St George's Hospital Medical School.
27. Graham ID, Calder LA, Hebert PC et al: A comparison of clinical practice guideline appraisal instruments, *Int J Technol Assess Health Care* 16(4):1024-1038, 2000.
28. Melnyk BM, Fineout-Overhold E, editors: *Evidence-based practice in nursing & healthcare*, Philadelphia, 2005, Lippincott Williams & Wilkins.
29. LoBiondo-Wood G, Haber J: *Nursing research: methods, critical appraisal & utilization*, ed 5, New York, 2002, Mosby.
30. White PJ: Evidence-based medicine for consumers: a role for the Cochrane collaboration, *J Med Libr Assoc* 90(2): 218-222, 2002.
31. Vrabel M: Searching for evidence: the value of a librarian-clinician collaboration–the librarian's role, *Home Health Care Manage Pract* 17(4):186-192, 2005.
32. Franklin JG, Paus MD, Pluetschow A et al: Chemotherapy, radiotherapy and combined modality for Hodgkin's disease, with emphasis on second cancer risk, *Cochrane Database Syst Rev* (4):CD003187, 2005.
33. Cochrane Upper Gastrointestinal and Pancreatic Diseases Group: Combined chemotherapy and radiotherapy (without surgery) compared with radiotherapy alone in localized carcinoma of the esophagus, *Cochrane Database Syst Rev* (4):2005.
34. Bennett MH, Feidmeir J, Hampson N et al: Hyperbaric oxygen therapy for late radiation tissue injury, *Cochrane Database Syst Rev* (4):2005.
35. Hakenberg OW, Wirth MP, Hermann T et al: Recommendations for the treatment of localized prostate cancer by permanent interstitial brachytherapy, *Urol Int* 70(1): 15-20, 2003.
36. Micke O, Seegenschmiedt MH, German Working Group on Radiotherapy in Germany: Consensus guidelines for radiation therapy of benign diseases: a multicenter approach in Germany, *Int J Radiat Oncol Biol Phys* 52(2):496-513, 2002.
37. Zelefsky MJ, Fuks Z, Hunt M et al: High-dose intensity modulated radiation therapy for prostate cancer: early toxicity and biochemical outcome in 772 patients, *Int J Radiat Oncol Biol Phys* 53(5):1111-1116, 2002.
38. Rollins G: Amid controversy, panel recommends postmastectomy radiation therapy for breast cancer patients with limited lymph node involvement, *Rep Med Guidel Outcomes Res* 12(3):1-2, 5, 2001.
39. Wallner P, Arthur D, Bartelink H et al: Workshop on partial breast irradiation: state of the art and the science, *J Natl Cancer Inst* 96(3):175-184, 2004.
40. Benson AB, Ajani JA, Catalano RB et al: Recommended guidelines for the treatment of cancer treatment-induced diarrhea, *J Clin Oncol* 22(14):2918-2926, 2004.
41. Giordano SH, Hortobagylo GN, Kau SW et al: Breast cancer treatment guidelines in older women, *J Clin Oncol* 23(4):783-791, 2005.
42. Nag S: High dose rate brachytherapy: its clinical applications and treatment guidelines, *Technol Cancer Res Treat* 3(3):269-287, 2004.
43. Nystedt KE, Hill JE, Mitchell AM et al: The standardization of radiation skin care in British Columbia: a collaborative approach, *Oncol Nurs Forum* 32(6):1199-1205, 2005.
44. Rankin N, Newell S, Sanson-Fisher R et al: Consumer participation in the development of psychosocial clinical practice guidelines: opinions of women with breast cancer, *Eur J Cancer Care (Engl)* 9(2):97-104, 2000.
45. Susman E: In latest NCCN breast cancer guidelines, radiation remains option for older women undergoing breast conservation, *Oncol Times* 27(10):10, 2005.
46. Grubb RL, Roehl KA, Antenor JA et al: Results of

compliance with prostate cancer screening guidelines, *J Urol* 174(2):668-672, 2005.

47. Ray-Coquard I, Thiesse P, Ranchere-Vince D et al: Conformity to clinical practice guidelines, multidisciplinary management and outcome of treatment for soft tissue sarcomas, *Ann Oncol* 15(2):307-315, 2004.
48. Goolsby MJ, Ricalde L: Critique of the American Cancer Society guidelines for breast cancer screening: update 2003, *J Am Acad Nurse Pract* 16(18):322-325, 2003.
49. Eshelman D, Landier W, Sweeney T et al: Facilitating care for childhood cancer survivors: integrating children's oncology group long-term follow-up guidelines and health links in clinical practice, *J Pediatr Oncol Nurs* 21(5): 271-280, 2004.
50. Jain G, Scolapio J, Wasserman E et al: Chronic radiation enteritis: a ten-year follow-up, *J Clin Gastroenterol* 35(3): 214-217, 2002.
51. Harpole LH, Kelley MJ, Schreiber G et al: Assessment of the scope and quality of clinical practice guidelines in lung cancer, *Chest* 123(1 suppl):7S-20S, 2003.
52. McCrory DC, Colice GL, Lewis SZ et al: Overview of methodology for lung cancer evidence review and guideline development, *Chest* 123(1 suppl):3S-6S, 2003.
53. Hinds, PS, Oakes L, Furman W et al: End-of-life decision making by adolescents, parents and healthcare providers in pediatric oncology: research to evidence-based practice guidelines, *Cancer Nurs* 24(2):122-134, 2001.

Chapter 39

Clinical Outcomes and Documentation

Dianna Wellen Traylor

Oncology nursing documentation is an essential and legally required component of radiation oncology nursing practice. Nurses communicate patient status and record patients' responses to both their illness and care. An entire team of healthcare providers including therapists, radiation and medical oncologists, nutritionists, and social workers rely on accurate and comprehensive nursing documentation. Precise, timely, and appropriate documentation enables the radiation oncology department to provide legal proof of actions that meet patient care standards required for quality treatment, improved performance, continued accreditation, licensing, and certification. Moreover, in today's economic healthcare market, an accurate medical record is necessary for reimbursement and unequivocally links the department to the viability of the institution.

In today's healthcare data environment, technology plays a strategic role in the rapid and efficient documentation of patient care. When using an electronic medical record (EMR), cancer diagnosis, stage, radiation prescription site, pain level, laboratory values, chemotherapy, current medication and family history, psychosocial information, patient and family education, emergency room and hospital admissions, successful self-care measures, and patients' responses to their treatment can all be documented and instantly retrieved by multiple staff.

This chapter discusses leveraging the EMR in order to comply with nursing documentation principles, standards, and legalities. This chapter also describes clinical patient outcome data that collects as a direct by-product of the use of electronic documentation tools, toxicity measurements, and additional patient care items.

Author's note: Electronic medical records (EMRs) are now in use extensively throughout the healthcare system to document the clinical and business aspects of patient care. The following chapter works on the assumption that the radiation oncology clinician is using an EMR; however, this content can and should be leveraged for paper-based systems.

EVOLVING DOCUMENTATION PRINCIPLES

In an environment beleaguered with litigation and documentation seemingly required just to "pass inspection," paper nursing notes are often viewed as a perfunctory, laborious, and time-consuming activity with little clinical return on investment. Provided, of course, that the chart can even be obtained, frustration with documentation compounds because clinicians find themselves duplicating existing data not easily viewable from other sections of the patient chart. In the hospital setting, shadow charts or manila treatment folders are not the appropriate place for the oncology clinician to chart. The clinician should file the original hard copy within the primary hospital record. In addition, if hospital policy specifically allows, keep a copy within the patient's shadow chart. Thankfully, given the current realities of documentation in an EMR, clinicians practicing in radiation oncology may no longer find it such an onerous responsibility.

Thorough and legal documentation within a radiation oncology department includes a great deal of information from therapy, dosimetry, medical physics, and oncology. It contains unique and mathematically complex data such as intensity-modulated radiation therapy (IMRT) calibration, three-dimensional treatment plans and ongoing port-film verification. Although clinicians outside of the department rarely comprehend the physics and mathematical intricacies of radiation oncology charting, all documentation entered and stored in the patient's EMR is a permanent and legal part of the record and may not be deleted.[1] Consequently, documentation within an EMR offers many advantages.

Advantages of documentation in an EMR:

1. Immediate access to essential information such as pain level, laboratory results, dramatic weight loss, concurrent chemotherapy treatment, or clinical trial enrollment

2. Wireless notebooks and PDAs facilitate the speed and timeliness of documentation
3. Alert messaging for elevated toxicity scores and out-of-range lab values
4. Elimination of redundant charting, consequently saving time for all clinical staff
5. Effective communication by way of providing concurrent patient chart access to multiple members of the healthcare team, regardless of their physical location
6. Store and retrieve information in real time while consistently updating patient information
7. Efficiencies gained by knowing patient schedules, arrivals, and cancellations
8. Provide legible documentation with a higher percentage rate of maintaining patient confidentially than a paper-based chart
9. Rapid accumulation of de-identified patient outcome data that can be used nation wide to support oncology nursing research
10. Support to maintain Health Information Portability and Accountability Act (HIPAA) compliance via role and security driven chart access

In litigation cases, chart documentation confirms that the standard of care was delivered. Standards established by the American Nurses Association (ANA) and the Joint Commission on Accreditation of Healthcare Facilities (JCAHO) are the accepted set of guiding principles. The department will need to provide copies of flowsheets, medication administration records, procedure notes, treatment plans, assessment values, and the nursing plan of care. As long as documentation policies and guidelines have been followed, the data contained within will be satisfactory.

DOCUMENTATION

Fortunately, oncology clinicians are not restricted to one basic format for communication. Many methods are acceptable to accreditation agencies, insurance companies, Medicare, and the medical legal system. Most prevalent in the oncology literature are tools to assist medical oncology clinicians, specifically paper forms for documenting chemotherapy administration and education.[2-5] Documentation tools to expedite intake of basic health history and psychosocial information are also available.[6] More recently, computerized assessment tools for consistent data collection and graphing have been made available. Consequently, it is much easier and faster for a clinician to recognize patient trends developing over time. Electronic medical records encourage a standardized range of responses, and these responses should be guided by evidence-based practice.

Documentation of Evidence-Based Practice

Evidence-based practice (EBP) is the delivery of care framed around the best and most current evidence for action. It considers the patient's values, attitudes, beliefs, and expectations, and it is applied with clinical expertise.[7] There is a hierarchical level of evidence within EBP. The relative hierarchy ranges from strong to weak, with strong being the meta-analysis of multiple controlled clinical trials; weak evidence includes expert opinions, practice guidelines, and practice standards.

Nursing documentation forms can prompt the clinician to consider optimal evidence-based best practice. However, the application of EBP is not legally implicit unless documentation exists to substantiate the assessment and care given to the patient or family. It is the role of the advanced practice nurse to be a strong consumer of nursing research, and their contribution to EBP documentation should rightfully be expected. Forms can be created to reflect the patient's response to questions that imply EBP recommended interventions or evaluations. For example, to choose or develop an oral assessment guide, the advanced practice nurse would review the existing literature to discover that a valid tool and frequently used oral assessment guide has existed since 1988.[8] This Oral Assessment Guide (Table 39-1) promotes the creation of an assessment with three consistent levels of response. The guide prompts the clinician to consider the eight basic categories needed to perform a thorough oral assessment. When documenting in an electronic format, prior assessment results are available for the clinician to instantly identify dramatic changes in the patient's condition. The EBP loop then closes with the documentation of the oral assessment and nursing interventions. Additionally, the electronic data can be reviewed retrospectively to answer questions concerning severity of oral symptoms related to diagnosis, types of treatment, and the success of nursing education and treatment interventions.

Table 39-1 Oral Assessment Guide

Category	1	2	3
Voice	Normal	Deeper or raspy	Difficulty talking or painful
Swallow	Normal swallow	Some pain on swallow	Unable to swallow
Lips	Smooth, pink, and moist	Dry or cracked	Ulcerated or bleeding
Tongue	Pink, moist, and papillae present	Coated or loss of papillae with a shiny appearance with or without redness	Blistered or cracked
Saliva	Watery	Thick or ropey	Absent
Mucous membranes	Pink and moist	Reddened or coated Increased whiteness without ulcerations	Ulcerations with or without bleeding
Gingiva	Pink, stippled, and firm	Edematous with or without redness	Spontaneous bleeding or bleeding with pressure
Teeth or dentures	Clean and no debris	Plaque or debris in localized areas between teeth if present	Plaque or debris generalized along gum line or denture bearing area

Documentation in Radiation Oncology

Radiation oncology nursing is a unique and diverse specialty. The roles, practice parameters, and responsibilities of radiation oncology clinicians vary based on the clinical setting.[9-12] Clinicians may work within an academically affiliated university, National Cancer Institute (NCI)-designated cancer center, a community hospital, a private clinic, or a freestanding comprehensive center. As a result, a variety of documentation formats have evolved. These may include handwritten narrative notes, computerized flow sheets, dictated progress notes, and research protocol forms.

In 2005, the Oncology Nursing Society published the third edition of a *Manual for Radiation Oncology Nursing Practice and Education.*[9] This manual provides radiation oncology clinicians with evidence-based nursing documentation guidelines related to general symptoms, site-specific, and disease-specific management.

The Radiation Oncology Special Interest Group (RO SIG) of the Oncology Nursing Society is the largest professional organization available to oncology clinicians to discuss and discover evidence-based practices. Additionally, in 2002 the Radiation Oncology SIG released the second edition of *Radiation Therapy Patient Care Record: a Tool for Documenting Nursing Care.*[13] The short-term goals are to improve and standardize the documentation of nursing care provided to patients receiving radiation therapy and improve the documentation of side effect management and patient education. The forward-thinking long-term goal of the RO SIG is to roll up data and provide radiation oncology clinicians nationwide with a de-identified database to be used for nursing research and patient care evaluation.

Using the RT Patient Care Record in a paper-based format prevents nationwide data collection and roll-up. However, with standard use of an EMR, valuable projects such as this have a strong possibility of execution and completion.

Continuity of care and consistency in nursing assessment, intervention, and evaluation can easily be recognized through well-designed and organized documentation tools.[14] The next step for radiation oncology nursing is to identify the pertinent outcomes to monitor while using the tools provided by their professional organization. This challenge is coupled with the need to provide documentation that reflects JCAHO, professional, and institution-specific standards of care in a way that results in clarity and efficiency and eliminates redundant data entry.

DOCUMENTATION AND QUALITY ASSURANCE IN RADIATION ONCOLOGY

The Joint Commission on Accreditation of Healthcare Organizations (JCAHO) was established in 1953 and has been a motivating force in regulating the standard of care delivered by healthcare organizations. A recent shift has taken place within quality focused accreditation bodies. Instead of determining whether an organization's documentation can assure quality care, JCAHO now focuses on whether an organization is consistently making efforts to improve the care it provides (quality improvement).[9] The JCAHO provides national standards of care to guide and instruct organizations in developing quality improvement (QI) programs. Accreditation is taken very seriously and can impact on malpractice insurance rates, private and Medicare insurance contracts, recruitment, funding eligibility, and research grant opportunities.

The JCAHO relies on experts within each professional domain to advise on best practice standards. In oncology nursing practice, the Oncology Nursing Society has established standards of care to serve as the basic units of measurement and evaluation of clinical nursing practice.[5] In addition, healthcare facilities often develop institution-specific standards of care for managers to use in monitoring and evaluating nursing practice and clinical outcomes. Regulatory agencies demand that the quality and appropriateness of patient care be monitored and evaluated.[15] Standards of care can guide clinicians in developing consistent systems and tools to meet these regulatory requirements.

Electronic documentation rapidly facilitates the reporting of data to support target areas for continuous quality improvement. For example, if department compliance with pain level documentation and subsequent intervention is found to be below standard, increased awareness of expected performance can be communicated to the staff and a variety of charting options for data entry can be made available. The department can then derive an electronic report alerting the staff to their increased level of compliance on a weekly or monthly basis. It is precisely in this way that an electronic medical record can rapidly record, report, and subsequently contribute to the quality of care delivered to patients.

Given its multidisciplinary nature and its existence in a highly technical and data-rich environment, software applications offer particular benefits to clinicians working in radiation oncology. Highly specialized software now commonly links to linear accelerators to verify and record treatment data and simultaneously capture treatment-related charges. Acknowledging warnings and mandating co-signatures for specific functions are two examples of using the software tool as a means to minimize human error and improve quality treatment outcomes. Combined with scheduling, billing, complete diagnosis and staging information, imaging, assessments, automated weekly treatment notes, and laboratory information, it is not unusual for radiation therapy centers to completely eliminate paper within the department.

Achieving paperless status for its own sake should be discouraged. Being paperless is not the goal; yet becoming a paperless department can definitely be a positive outcome. If the department wisely uses software tools to facilitate processes and deliver efficiencies, then the outcome will inevitably be paperless. However, it is also possible to be a paperless department that still creates miscommunication, frustration, and errors. The question is not, "How can we become paperless?" Rather, the question is, "How can we get better at something by using the software tools that we have in place today?"

FUTURE TRENDS IN DOCUMENTATION

Future documentation trends in oncology nursing will directly reflect the increasing power and use of electronic technology. Some of the trends that adhere to all patient privacy and data security regulations include the following:

- Wireless laptops used for data entry throughout the radiation oncology department
- PDA used to obtain patient information while outside of the department setting
- Voice recognition software used to instantly dictate and correct patient notes without the use of a transcriptionist or a keyboard
- Waiting room kiosks with private touch-screen technology that allows the patient to answer questions related to pain and symptom management. These answers instantly become a part of the patient chart, and staff can review them before seeing the patient.
- Secure e-mail communications with the patient that do not pertain to an acute episode or an emergency event
- Electronic generation of medication prescriptions to a local pharmacy

As the ability to communicate and collect data becomes faster and easier, data expectations evolve. EMR use will increase exponentially, along with the value it can bring to the radiation oncology clinicians.

REFERENCES

1. Mureth ER: Computer-based patient records. In Meiner S, editor: *Nursing documentation: legal focus across practice settings*, Thousand Oaks, Calif, 2002, Sage Publications, pp 29-40.
2. Cushman KE: A tool for documenting chemotherapy administration quickly and completely, *Oncol Nurs Forum* 18(3):599-600, 1991.
3. Moore JM, Knobf MT: A nursing flow sheet for documentation of ambulatory oncology, *Oncol Nurs Forum* 18(5): 933-939, 1991.
4. Pfeifer P: Documentation of care in an oncology outpatient setting, *Oncol Nurs Forum* 19(5):809-818, 1992.
5. Pickett RR: Outpatient oncology chemotherapy documentation tool, *Oncol Nurs* Forum 19(3):515-517, 1992.
6. Skinn B, Stacey D: Establishing an integrated framework for documentation: use of a self-reporting health history and outpatient oncology record, *Oncol Nurs Forum* 21(9):1557-1566, 1994.
7. Sackett DL, Strauss SE, Richardson WS: *Evidence-based medicine: how to practice and teach EBM*, ed 2, London, 2000, Churchill Livingstone.
8. Eilers J, Berger AM, Petersen MC et al: Development, testing, and application of the oral assessment guide, *Oncol Nurs Forum* 15:325-330, 1988.
9. Bruner DW, Haas ML, Gosselin-Acomb TK: *Manual for radiation oncology nursing practice and education*, ed 3, Pittsburgh, 2005, Oncology Nursing Society.
10. Bucholtz J: Radiation therapy. In Ziegfeld C, editor: *Core curriculum for oncology nursing*, Philadelphia, 1987, WB Saunders, pp 207-224.
11. Lynch M, Vanes L: Flow sheet documentation of chemotherapy administration and patient teaching, *Oncol Nurs Forum* 18(4):777-783, 1991.
12. Strohl R: The nursing role in radiation oncology: symptom management and chronic reactions, *Oncol Nurs Forum* 15(4):429-434, 1991.
13. Catlin-Huth C, Haas ML, Pollock V: *Radiation therapy patient care record: a tool for documenting nursing care*, ed 2, Pittsburgh, 2002, Oncology Nursing Society.
14. Pevny V: Outcome of a quality assurance review: development of a documentation tool for chemotherapy administration, *Oncol Nurs Forum* 20(3):535-541, 1993.
15. Thomas D: Quality assessment and improvement via the ten-step model, *Oncol Issues* 9(2):21-23, 1994.

Chapter 40

Geriatric Considerations in Radiation Oncology Nursing

Sarah H. Kagan and Mary Longnecker Garrett

Older adults who undergo radiation therapy have apparent and numerous nursing care needs. Radiation therapy offers important curative and palliative treatment options for older adults who have cancer. These options are balanced against logistic challenges in performing treatment, managing radiation toxicities, and supporting psychosocial experiences. These challenges are typically amplified by comorbid disease and functional changes common to late life. Consequently, individual and family needs arise in decision making and expectation of treatment, treatment and toxicity, and self-care and adherence. Literature that directly addresses the nursing needs of older adults treated with radiation therapy is sparse and scientifically unsophisticated. Extrapolation from existing literature in gerontology and in radiation therapy in the context of sound clinical analysis and judgment must direct care of these older adults and their families and direct future research.

This chapter outlines key aspects of nursing care for older adults treated with radiation therapy. Existing scientific evidence is integrated with clinical analysis to synthesize recommendations for practice and research. A brief review of the demography of cancer and aging and chronic illness and aging, essential gerontologic and geriatric principles, and selected systemic and organ aging changes outline the significance of geriatric considerations in radiation oncology nursing. Clinical practice is addressed through integration of aging content in the context of radiation oncology nursing. Decision making and clinical expectations, treatment and toxicity, and self-care and adherence are delineated with reference to fundamental issues such as ageism and functional reserve and practical considerations such as adaptation of teaching materials. Suggestions for future research and education to improve practice conclude the chapter.

DEMOGRAPHY OF CANCER AND AGING

The common adage that advancing age is the single greatest risk factor for cancer is particularly meaningful for radiation oncology nurses.[1] Approximately 60% to 70% of people diagnosed with cancer are older than age 65.[1,2] Few credible statistics delimit how many of those individuals diagnosed with cancer are treated primarily or in combination with radiation therapy.[3] Nonetheless, clinical consideration of standard treatment protocols for the most common cancers, which primarily affect individuals over 65 years of age—prostate, breast, lung, and colorectal cancers—suggests radiation therapy plays a prominent role overall in cancer therapy for older adults.[3] Paradoxically, ageism in cancer care generally may foment perceptions that radiation therapy is better tolerated by older adults who are physically fragile and could not withstand the rigors of chemotherapy or surgery. Such beliefs may result in greater representation of older adults in radiation therapy when compared with younger peers.[4-7] Radiation oncology nurses are likely to care for a disproportionately larger number of older adults than their colleagues in many medical and surgical oncology settings.

Radiation oncologists—as primary clinical partners with radiation oncology nurses—are beginning to evince substantial interest in treating older adults commensurate with current cancer demographics and clinical needs. Biomedical literature documenting clinical utility of radiation therapy in treating older adults with curative or palliative intent has expanded significantly over three decades.[8,9] Evidence documented in that literature now encompasses age-related analyses of radiation therapy for central nervous system, head and neck, genitourinary, and bronchogenic malignancies among others.[8-27] Almost uniformly, older adults are shown to be able to tolerate radiation therapy and receive clinical benefit from it. Further, more sophisticated theoretical and evidence-based analyses of senescent—loss of replicative function over time—cells response to radiation are being presented to complement more clinical papers.[28-31] Salvi and colleagues,[3,28] in particular, explore issues of aging biology, cellular senescence and radiation dose in the context of effective treatment.[30,31] Despite the theoretical explorations offered by Salvi and colleagues[3,28] and more numerous age-related analyses of treatment trials, scientific and clinical understanding of treatment response, experience, and toxicity for older adults lags sharply behind this literature.

The multifaceted impact of providing radiation therapy to older adults is poorly defined. Outcomes of the interaction of aging, age-related disease, and late life functional decline with radiation therapy, for example, are not well investigated. However, consideration of lessons from gerontology and geriatric literature with attached issues such as functional decline offers insight into enhancing radiation therapy nursing practice, education, and research. Clinical aspects of the demography of aging and chronic illness interface with fundamentals of gerontology and geriatrics and the principles of aging in place, functional reserve, and age related change to outline means to infuse radiation oncology nursing with aging knowledge to achieve best practices.

DEMOGRAPHY OF AGING AND CHRONIC ILLNESS

The American population is aging, with those age 65 and over expected to account for 15% of the general population by 2015.[32] Those older than age 85 currently comprise the most rapidly growing group, although speculation grows regarding centenarians overtaking them in this demographic race.[33] Although this increase is mild compared to those faced by other societies, including Italy, Japan and Australia, societal problems of care needs, work force preparation, and generational burden emerge nonetheless.[33,34] As the age groups typically defined as older grows larger, those generally defined as younger—the putative caregivers for older adults in need of supportive and skilled care—are declining in number.[33] A stable birth rate, among other factors, accounts for this increasingly large inverse pyramid of age distribution in our population.[33] Our aging population and adherent issues of age distribution intersect with current trends in age-related disease and disability to shape implications for nursing care.

The risk of age-related comorbid illness rises with chronologic age. Wolff and colleagues[35] note that, in 1999, 82% of Medicare beneficiaries had one or more chronic conditions. In their sample of over 1.2 million, prevalence of chronic conditions rose as expected with advancing chronologic age. More than 30% of those aged over 85 years had more than four comorbid conditions as opposed to 15.7% of those 65–69 years.[35] Notably, in a study reported by Fillenbaum and colleagues,[36] cancer seemed not to be associated with comorbid disease at baseline as are hypertension, diabetes, coronary artery disease, and cerebrovascular disease among older community dwelling adults. This pattern of comorbid disease implies clinical differences in groups of older adults who have cancer. Those older adults who have cancer may be less ill in a global sense than peers who have hypertension, diabetes, coronary artery disease, and cerebrovascular disease.

Functional status decline is associated with advancing age. Some of that association may be spuriously conjoined with images of age-predicated disease prevalent in late life. Freedman and Martin and Schoeni[37,38] examined national trends in two papers using a national data set[37] and systematic review.[38] Functional status change, assessed in 1984 and 1993, was measured by Freedman and Martin[37] as in difficulty "seeing words in a newspaper," "lifting and carrying ten pounds," "climbing a flight of stairs," and "walking a quarter mile." Functional status improved most markedly for those over 80 years of age and was attributed at least in part to improved health status nationally. Improvements in physical function for older adults occurred over time in systematic review of eight surveys completed by other authors as well.[38] Physical function, despite demographic trends in aging, may shift rapidly as that older population becomes healthier and relatively more functional by age over time.

Our aging population and increasingly inverse age distribution combines with age-related disease and functional disability to present expected issues opposed against surprising changes. Although our society is aging rapidly, disease treatment and health status may be improving, enabling longevity with better function. The juxtaposition conflicts with common images of aging that reinforce frailty, illness, and neediness. Older adults treated for cancer with radiation and other therapies who may be less ill when compared with age-matched peers contradicts common stereotypes.[36] Those being treated with radiation therapy may fulfill this contradiction in varied ways. Radiation oncology nurses must then be prepared with knowledge of aging, disease, and function and intersections of radiation therapy with age-related changes and principles to support comprehensive care of older adults and avoid stereotypes and misinformation.

FUNDAMENTALS OF GERONTOLOGY AND GERIATRICS

Radiation oncology nursing, like most other specialties relies heavily on language as an element of communication, a primary tool used in assessment, intervention, and continuity.[39-44] Language used in describing and discussing matters pertaining to the age of a patient, to groups of patients considered older, and to clinical challenges associated with aging and late life is critical to precise delineation and clear communication around such topics.[45] Confusion around accurate language in care of older adults is common where even the labels for the specialty itself seem to vary.

Although the specialty of caring for older adults and the science pertaining to that care is generally termed geriatrics—and is in fact the choice for the title of this chapter—the term *gerontology* is often also used particularly by nurses. The distinction is an important one because geriatrics is defined as a branch of medicine or, less commonly, of social science that focuses on the health of older people.[46] Cohen[47] noted that the etymology of the word merged roots for old age and physician, connoting then health and illness within a medical focus. Gerontology is a broader label for all science pertaining to study of aging and being old.[46] It encompasses health and illness, implied by geriatrics, and adds study of philosophical, psychological, sociological, and economic facets of aging and old age. Hence, although much of this chapter is focused on implications of physical aging for radiation oncology nursing, attention to economic, social, emotional, and cognitive issues is necessary to a comprehensive understanding of intersections of gerontology, geriatrics, and oncology. Critical issues in cancer and aging are easily framed through application of major principles in gerontology.

Aging in Place

Aging in place is the gerontologic principle by which America hopes to experience old age. Simply, aging in place is the principle of living within a community without the segregation of an institutional residence. Despite often significant comorbid disease, most older adults live in their communities rather than in residential facilities like nursing homes.[48] This ability to maintain residence typifies aspirations to live in a community, surrounded by familiar people, activities, and institutions. Acute and chronic illnesses beget needs for varying instrumental, functional, and emotional supports to compensate for functional decline. Those needs are—although mediated at the individual, family, and cultural levels—often weighed against concerns for welfare of younger family members and fears of becoming a burden. Individual, familial, cultural, and other patterns and life ways bear tremendous influence on expression of aging in place, support and systems for informal care, and perceptions of filial responsibility and family burden. Careful investigation of an older adult's place of residence and meanings attached to it underlie effective nursing assessment with skillful referral to resources such as social work and resources for family and other informal caregiving.

Functional Reserve

Maintenance of function is a cardinal principle applied in direct care of older adults undergoing radiation therapy.[49] Function fundamentally supports radiation therapy because patients must maintain physical and mental capacity to adhere to treatment. Older adults may evince functional decline as levels of toxicity are reached. Declining functional reserve becomes the leverage point for assessing alterations in capacity and intervening to limit decline and rehabilitate baseline function.[50,51] It represents decreased reserve with which to respond to change despite the ability to maintain homeostasis under accustomed physiologic, psychologic, and social conditions.[51] Such decline is revealed in the case of an older patient who has been living alone without difficulty but lacks additional reserve to continue living alone during the final weeks of radiation therapy because of increasing fatigue and fewer social supports to compensate for impaired activities of daily living and instrumental activities of daily living.

Functional capacity often can be preserved through functional exercise, activities deliberately used to mimic or repeat necessary daily activities.[52] Functional exercise, for maintenance of mental function, generally includes cognitively intense activities such as completing crossword puzzles or other skills requiring attention, memory, and fund of knowledge.[53] Physical functional exercise quite simply mimics daily activities.[52] For example, arising from a chair for an established number of repetitions helps maintain sit to stand capacity. Mental functional exercise uses varied cognitive skills in manipulation of instrumental activities of daily life.[53] Use of such exercises in care planning operationalizes gerontologic principles of function and functional status in care of older adults undergoing radiation therapy.

Aging Changes

Understanding tissue, organ, and system tolerances to radiation therapy with advancing age is difficult. Incomplete knowledge of how tumor and normal tissue sensitivity, resistance, and repair change with age hinders practice development. Although age-related changes in target organs are often summarized to guide expectations for acute and late radiation toxicity in older adults, science that directly investigates the interaction of cellular and tissue level aging changes with radiation is nearly absent, sharply limiting clinical application.[54] Thoughtful consideration of possible ramifications arising from age-related changes and influence of comorbid acute and chronic illness better guides individualized assessment, planning, and evaluation and makes use of available evidence and best practices.[55] Most broadly in advancing age, tissue and organ function are stable with declining reserve. Apparent functional decline, however, may be inextricable from subclinical or actual disease.[51,54] These compound changes may result in tissue fragility, organ dysfunction, and functional impairment in the context of radiation therapy, especially when comorbid disease is present.[50,51,54,56] The precise range of toxicity onset and severity within parameters of age- and disease-related functional decline, however, remains unclear. Adaptation of existing practice guidelines for treatment toxicity based on supposition about tissue and organ changes is less than secure.

Cutaneous aging offers a paradigm through which radiation oncology nurses can see possible consequences of age-related changes and radiation therapy. The skin is subject to extrinsic forces, most prominently solar exposure, that compound and obscure intrinsic age-related changes.[54,57] Grossly, the skin becomes thinner, less elastic, and less able to maintain homeostasis with age.[57] Importantly in radiation therapy, cellular production also slows with advancing age so that fibroblast migration, in wound healing for example, is likely delayed. Solar aging creates further structural changes, such as those seen in increased collagen cross-linking and hypovascularity, and alters cellular activity in other cellular groups—melanocytes, for example—leading to adherent functional changes such as problems in pigmentation. Consequently, although individual presentation varies, older adults may have earlier, more pronounced cutaneous acute and chronic radiation toxicities.[57,58] Research to guide prospective prediction and prevention is nonetheless absent. Therefore, careful baseline assessment including solar exposure and other pertinent history such as skin disease forms the foundation for continuous assessment and proactive intervention where available scientific and experiential evidence allow.

Knowledge of interaction between discrete aging changes in other organ systems and radiation is similarly based on extrapolation of available evidence of senescent cells, radiation injury, and functional change.[3,54,58] Acute and late toxicities particular to specific systems have yet to be investigated directly. They may be postulated generally, extrapolating from known changes with age, to shape clinical expectations.[54] Patients should then be evaluated individually, estimating biologic age—sometimes called *physiological age*—using available markers of organ function and global patient function to refine clinical judgment.[3,54,59-61] Aging changes in the gastrointestinal tract are, for example, of great clinical concern because they play out in treatment of specific cancers where the field includes organs within the system. The risk of acute treatment toxicities such as stomatitis or radiation-induced diarrhea can tax an older adult's functional reserve, create a cascade of related symptoms, and result in delay or cessation of treatment. Here again, functional reserve is almost certainly the operant issue because gastrointestinal changes with age are minimal or of little effect in homeostatic function.[62-64] The influence of comorbid illness and its treatment, however, confounds this clinical picture and warrants specific assessment. Clinical effects of individual pathologies may be difficult to discern against the backdrop of aging changes.[65]

Functional Changes

Implications of gross functional changes associated with age-related disease or geriatric syndromes, as opposed to discrete organ or tissue changes, are likely critical in treatment adherence, self-care, and survival.[3,66,67] Alterations in cognition, posture and gait, as well as coping, caregiving, and social support are readily apparent influences on treatment decisions, tolerance, and adherence in radiation therapy. Working backward from baseline presentation to disentangle normal aging changes, age-related disease, and geriatric syndromes offers an effective clinical strategy to improve and individualize care with or without direct generalizeable evidence.[55] Geriatric syndromes are those that are prevalent in late life, are attributes to interactions of aging changes and disease, and are posited to have multiple morbidities involved.[50,52,68] Table 40-1 lists examples of common geriatric syndromes.

Cognition

Normal aging does not affect general overall cognitive function.[53] Functional cognitive reserve does, however, decline with advancing chronologic age. Homeostatic alterations such as metabolic or fluid balance shifts, and environmental influences including multiple personal losses may tax that declining functional reserve. Delirium and depression are among the most concerning geriatric syndromes resulting from and influencing decompensated cognitive and emotional reserve.[50,69] Further, advancing age is associated with the onset of diseases—most prominently Alzheimer's dementia—that directly affect cognitive capacity.

Table 40-1 Common Geriatric Syndromes

Geriatric syndrome	Functional impairment
Delirium	Cognition
Urinary incontinence	Micturition
Repeated falls	Ambulation
Failure to thrive	Nutrition and global function

Data from Phillips EM, Bodenheimer CF, Roig RL, Cifu DX: *Arch Phys Med Rehabil* 85(7 suppl3):S18-S22, 2004, and Flacker JM: *J Am Geriatr Soc* 51(4):574-576, 2003.

Interjecting cancer and radiation therapy into the complex picture of cognition in late life adds uncharted complexity and unknown clinical ramifications. Early work in cognition and chemotherapy reflects a likely relationship between cancer treatment and cognition in the exemplar cases of breast and prostate cancers.[70,71] Nuances in the association between treatment and cognition remain unclear. As a result, local or systemic responses to radiation therapy echoed in the phenomenon of fatigue, which might contribute to impaired cognition, remain equally unclear. Whether radiation therapy might create primary triggers for impairment or whether responses such as fatigue might be secondary influences on cognition require further exploration. Nonetheless, careful attention to baseline cognition with screening assessment and specialist referrals as indicated by on-going assessment data furnishes a structure within which to track functional change and optimize outcomes based on available scientific and clinical data.

Cognition and learning extend the significance of cognitive function in care of older adults undergoing radiation therapy. Radiation therapy is generally provided on an outpatient basis, and thus older adults and their caregivers are called upon to learn, retain, and apply complicated information as they make decisions and engage in self-care during treatment. Research in information needs, provision, and outcomes in cancer care and specifically in radiation therapy suggests a truly complex phenomenon.[41,42] There is significant variation among patients with respect to information needs and information seeking and little guarantee of information retention and positive effects on outcomes of care.[40-42] Adapting information and educational materials for generational influences such as familiarity with technologic devices and for sensory-perceptual changes such as decreased visual acuity necessitates more individualized approaches to providing information to older patients and their families. These adaptations refine more typical strategies to increase readability, including using large font sizes and lowering reading level.[72,73] Alternate forms to convey and maintain information also offer advantages as in the care diary reported by Sharp and colleagues.[44]

Posture and Gait

Posture and gait are commonly overlooked in assessments for radiation therapy. Although independent ambulation is not generally requisite to tolerate and complete a course of radiation therapy, significant changes in ability to move among positions from sit to stand and especially to tolerate therapeutic positions needed for daily therapy may prevent completion of simulation and treatment. Most fundamentally, even mild kyphotic changes along with pain or other associated distress such as respiratory symptoms may often preclude supine positioning necessary to treatment unless thorough assessment and creative intervention are undertaken.

Assessment of posture attends to underlying etiologies, most commonly osteoporosis, vertebral compression fractures, and more obscure disease and associated geriatric and other syndromes such as repeated falls and deconditioning.[74] Careful initial assessment of posture, with appropriate referral to physical therapy for further more sophisticated assessment, enables judgment of possibilities for postural correction, positioning during treatment, and implications for dosing. For example, patients being treated for head and neck cancer using a mask will require team consideration of kyphotic and other anatomic changes of the upper torso and neck. Treatment of these patients may also prompt re-examination of institutional practice variations around use of long and short masks to address needs of an aging patient population.

Patients who may be able to assume supine positioning may nonetheless endure musculoskeletal pain or respiratory and associated symptoms in that position. Such pain warrants inquiry into existing pain regimens for musculoskeletal pain, adaptation to encompass strategies such as pretreatment pain medication, and judicious referral to physical therapy for conditioning and corrective exercises. Respiratory symptoms, such as shortness of breath and dyspnea, demand investigation of sometimes subtle initial presentation, patterns, and risk of decompensation. Discerning physiologic decompensation, behavioral responses and anxiety, and interactions among them may require referrals for consultation and monitoring depending on severity. Developing and implementing nursing plans that prescribe baseline and periodic reassessment and clearly outlined interventions to maintain continuity then become critical to treatment tolerance and adherence.

Gait changes are less influential in radiation therapy because the environment and care procedures are easily adapted to allow for limited or absent independent ambulation. Nonetheless, baseline assessment and follow-up of gait changes may prove valuable to monitoring treatment tolerance and anticipating home caregiving needs. Etiologies of gait change encompass an exhaustive list of factors related to the individual's tumor and comorbid disease, which are not specifically related to advancing age, seen easily in care of a younger patient with a central nervous system malignancy.[75] Gait changes may be associated with geriatric syndromes such as repeated falls. Subtle changes from baseline also may indicate early changes in status that could signal tumor response or impending complications as part of atypical response depending on tumor presentation.

Psychosocial Function

Psychosocial, emotional, and spiritual capacity and patterns accumulated through decades of adult activities necessarily influence responses to the experience of cancer and radiation therapy.[76-79] Older adults live in a psychologic, social, and cultural milieu nuanced by their life experiences and relationships. Life in this intricate milieu is balanced against older adults' particular life ways, preferences and desires, needs, and resources. The diagnosis of a particular cancer and assent to treatment with radiation layers meaning, concerns, and perceived susceptibilities.[80,81] Consequently, radiation oncology nurses who attend to these issues in assessment build individualized care plans with greater opportunity to anticipate problems and develop mutual goals with patients.[55]

The personal social import of cancer and its treatment in general and radiation therapy in particular may hold special meaning for the current cohort of older adults. Their lifetimes traverse the clinical introduction of radiation as a therapeutic modality and the everyday use of high technology such as high-speed personal computers, the World Wide Web, and voice technologies including messaging and paging. Introduction to the radiation therapy unit as an environment for care may provoke a range of responses from marked aversion through full engagement. These responses are predicated on life experiences, previous encounters, and individual, familial, and cultural belief systems. Inquiry into beliefs, concerns, and fears held by older adults and their family members and other significant supports warrants insightfully questioning to avoid preconception.[55]

Older adults are commonly supported by a group of loved ones who, as family or other significant people in a particular older adult's life, offer functional, instrumental, and existential care and support. Older adults who have measurable decrements in activities of daily living or in instrumental activities of daily living are thought to have congruent compensatory care needs. Table 40-2 lists activities of daily living and instrumental activities of daily living. Personal experiences of caregiving and its receipt also may include less tangible care involving emotional and spiritual support.

Table 40-2 Activities of Daily Living and Instrumental Activities of Daily Living

Activities of daily living*	Instrumental activities of daily living†
Bathing	Telephone use
Tub versus shower	Considered essential for living alone
Dressing	Transportation
Selecting clothing	Automobile
Donning clothing	May be generationally specific for women
	Public transit
Toileting	Shopping
	Food
	Other
Transferring	Meal preparation
Chair or bed to different locale	Food selection
	Food storage
Continence	Housework
Bladder	
Bowel	
Feeding	Medication use
Utensil manipulation	Correct medication
Chewing and swallowing	Correct dose
Meal completion	Correct time
	Financial management
	May be generationally specific for women

*Data from Shelkey M, Wallace M: Katx index of independence in activities of daily living (ADL), *Try this: best practices in nursing care to older adults from the Hartford Institute for Geriatric Nursing*, 1998 (website): www.hartfordign.org/publications/trythis/issue02.pdf.

†Data from Moses S: Instrumental activities of daily living, *Family practice notebook.com*, 2000 (website): www.fpnotebook.com/GER3.htm.

Caregivers are also affected by the experience of cancer and the rigors of radiation therapy.[84] Primary caregivers may feel strain or burden that antedates radiation therapy or begins with onset of toxicity, functional decline, or worsening prognosis. The relationship of the caregiver to the recipient—the patient receiving radiation therapy—is a determining factor in both perceived benefits and stressors in caregiving.

Adult children—almost always daughters or daughters-in-law—may, for instance, feel competing demands of childrearing and parent care. Those feeling opposing care responsibilities are commonly termed the "sandwich generation."[85] Benefits of transcending generational boundaries and recasting relationships are often overlooked in daily pressures of achieving caregiving tasks.

Spouses or life partners often experience different stressors in caregiving that emerge from long-held images of aging, relationship dynamics, and behaviors imbedded in shifting needs.[84,86] Further, the often invisible factor of spousal or life partner functional status—as opposed to patient functional status—may determine success and satisfaction in informal caregiving for older adults undergoing radiation therapy. Successful completion of radiation therapy may hinge on care provided to older adults by those individuals most important to them, often necessitating investigation of that caregiving relationship.

Somewhat counterintuitively, older adults who are being treated for cancer may in fact be caregivers themselves. In an aging society, an older adult may be the primary caregiver for an adult relative of the same—as with a spouse or life partner—or younger generation—as with an adult child who has diminished functional capacity. More popularly, older adults and especially older women may be caring for grandchildren or other young relatives. These caregiving responsibilities often influence access to care, decision making, and self-care. Further, such responsibilities may shift the older person's overarching priorities away from treatment of the cancer to maintaining role function at home. This shift may then not match priorities around cancer treatment assumed by radiation oncology nurses and their team colleagues.

Alternatively, many old-old adults—those older than age 85—may have outlived their family and social cohort incurring cumulative loss exacerbated by cancer and its treatment. These older adults may be at risk for functional compromise and sharply limited support as fatigue and associated symptoms increase their care needs over the course of radiation therapy. Careful baseline and follow-up assessment of perceived loss, psychologic and spiritual health with associated problems such as depression and existential crisis, related functional needs, and available support undergirds successful treatment and care planning.

Clinical assessment of functional alterations and needs in older adults is complex and must be individualized to the person and the treatment modality.[55] Effective assessment for radiation therapy requires baseline knowledge of normal aging and comorbid disease. Appraisal of alteration in cognition, posture and gait, and psychologic, emotional, and social function refines baseline and follow-up assessment by addressing functional areas at risk during radiation therapy.[67,69,87-89] Periodic screening and targeted intervention throughout treatment and during posttreatment follow-up optimize treatment process and outcomes for older adults, their caregivers, and other concerned family and loved ones.

ASSESSMENT AND INTERVENTION IN PRACTICE

Integrating gerontologic and geriatric principles into established radiation therapy practice presents challenges in learning new content and finding precious time in already established patterns of clinical encounters. Many authors have written about the virtues of comprehensive geriatric assessment versus more stratified or abbreviated assessment to improve care for older adults with cancer.[50,69,88-90]

Comprehensive Geriatric Assessment

Comprehensive geriatric assessment, or CGA as it is abbreviated, offers extensive screening and detailed assessment of function and geriatric syndromes.[87-89] Focused, detailed assessment of functional ability, physical health, cognitive and mental health, and socioenvironmental situation is accomplished through application of standardized instruments like the Katz Activities of Daily Living Scale and the Lawton Instrumental Activities of Daily Living Scale.[82,83,87] The process is time and skill intensive; needing hours to complete and requiring specialized training. Although the information gleaned in CGA is clearly advantageous in an ideal scenario, CGA in cancer practice is marked by the disadvantages of time and training generally unavailable in most radiation oncology units. Further, CGA may be ineffective in cancer practice where comorbid disease and performance status rather than age and global function better reflect likelihood of successful treatment.[20,89,91,92] Recent investigations support integration of gerontologic principles in gero-oncology assessment through adaptation. Overcash and colleagues[67] offer an abbreviated CGA, whereas Ingram and colleagues[89] show that abbreviated self-report format may be successfully employed in assessment of older adults.

Integrating Aging into Radiation Oncology

Radiation oncology nurses face increased needs for aging-specific knowledge and confront selection of appropriate tools and avenues for collaboration given growing evidence supporting abbreviated formats for geriatric assessment.[67,89,93,94] The necessity of interdisciplinary team practice in gero-oncology is underscored by available data and is simultaneously limited by availability of established geriatric interdisciplinary teams in many institutions. Table 40-3 enumerates typical members of an interdisciplinary geriatric team and examples of clinical foci of their practices to illustrate how referral to individual clinicians may be of use to radiation oncology nurses in creating and implementing plans of care for older adults.

Many institutions may have representatives of these disciplines available but not integrated into a geriatric team. Others may have some but not all of these clinicians on staff. Radiation oncology nurses must avail their patients of available services to provide necessary care. Clinicians who may offer overlapping services such as geriatric advanced practice nurses and geriatrician may substitute for each other in certain clinical settings and situations. Similarly, clinicians already involved in care may offer skills duplicated by adding another member to the patient's care team. For example, both occupational therapists and speech language pathologists have considerable skill in cognitive assessment. Collaborating with a speech language pathologist (SLP) about oral care for an older adult who has head and neck cancer may avoid initial duplication of assessment by a mental health clinician or occupational therapist if the SLP has an existing relationship with the patient.

Table 40-3 Core Geriatric Team Members and Examples of Clinical Foci

Team member	Clinical focus
Geriatric Advanced Practice Nurse	Geriatric assessment Care coordination Referral identification Care management
Geriatric physician	Geriatric assessment Geriatric syndrome management Chronic illness management
Social worker	Individual/family therapy Family assessment and intervention Community services referral Institutional placement
Physical therapist	Assessment and intervention in: Ambulation/gross motor function Environmental mobility
Occupational therapist	Assessment and intervention in: Environmental manipulation Device and tool use Cognitive function for ADL/IADL
Speech language pathologist	Assessment and intervention in: Communication Swallowing Cognitive function for communication/swallowing
Registered dietician	Assessment and intervention in: Nutrition assessment IADLs related to food intake
Mental health clinician Psychiatric advanced practice nurse Psychiatrist Psychologist Pastoral counselor	Cognitive and mental assessment Cognitive therapies Mental health intervention Spiritual and existential assessment Grief, loss, and support therapies

ADLs, Activities of daily living; *IADLs*, intermediate activities of daily living.

In addition to institutional resources and clinical colleagues, familiarity with community-based services for older adults enhances the scope of radiation oncology nursing practice. Although referral to social work is essential for access to many community services, time and effort can be saved with basic knowledge of services designed to aid both well and ill elders who remain in the community or transition to more sheltered residential facilities. Although many nurses are familiar with services such as "Meals on Wheels"—in-home meal delivery for income-eligible older adults—few know that most such services are administered under a county-based system called Area Agencies on Aging. Table 40-4 lists examples of community-based programs and services typical to them.

Integration of any aging knowledge and adherent issues of assessment, referral, and intervention in radiation therapy must be precisely targeted using current evidence and best practices. As a result, nursing practice is enhanced through judicious use of electronic, print, and personal resources as individual clinicians build knowledge and skill. Although access to electronic databases such as PubMed and Medline is increasingly widespread, access to appropriate assessment tools and to gerontologic and geriatric specialists is less common. Resources on the World Wide Web offer access to current tools and expert advice when they are not available in the clinical setting.

The John A. Hartford Institute of Geriatric Nursing offers the best options for comprehensive geriatric nursing resources (www.hartfordign.org/)

Table 40-4 Community-Based Programs for Older Adults and Services Typically Provided

Program	Typical services	Contact
Area Agency on Aging	Nursing home grants Elder neglect/abuse reporting In-home meals Homemaker services	Telephone book government pages World wide web search for county of residence
American Cancer Society	Chapter specific Geriatric or family grants Transportation Caregiving assistance	www.cancer.org
Visiting Nursing Associations Home Nursing Agencies	Medicare skilled care Nursing Physical therapy Care assistance Nursing aide requires nurse oversight	Referral from social work or nursing to contracting agency
For-fee Geriatric Case Management	Coordination of care in absence of family caregiver Determination of private service eligibility Location of private services	Area Agency on Aging Local telephone book World wide web search
The Center for Advocacy for the Rights and Interests of the Elderly	Networking Advocacy	www.carie.org
Medicare	Information about Medicare benefits	www.medicare.gov

because it incorporates the new interactive site www.GeroNurseOnline.org and the Try This Series of clinical tools (www.hartfordign.org/resources/education/tryThis.html) among other features. There are over 30 Try This issues available. Issues 1–4, 6–9, 13, 14, 16, 17, and 23 are invaluable to improving radiation oncology nursing for older adults. Table 40-5 lists the topics and tools in these issues of the Try This Series. Composition of each tool is noted to indicate time general commitment. Referrals indicate possible sources for further assessment and intervention.

The Merck Institute of Health and Aging Practicing Physician Education Project Toolkits (www.miahonline.org/tools/index.html) offer additional resources with the dual advantage of clinical utility and opportunities to collaborate with physician colleagues. The Merck Falls Toolkit, for example, is especially useful in radiation oncology practice and contains the "get up and go" test, which is quickly and easily administered by a nurse or physician with little training. In this test, patient ability to get up from a chair and walk forward independently is evaluated. The assessment is valuable in fall risk and other mobility concerns. The results of "get up and go" in radiation oncology nursing could be used to trigger referrals to geriatric services from a physician or nurse practitioner or rehabilitation services from a physiatrist or physical therapist. Bookmarking such electronic resources on unit computer workstations and including them in educational programs and practice guidelines offers the opportunity to include current, peer-reviewed knowledge and tools for better care of older adults who have cancer.

AGE, AGEISM, AND CLINICAL DECISION MAKING

Gerontologic principles and knowledge of aging and disease, no matter how extensive, are successfully applied only within a context of understanding what it means to be old. Perception of aging and late life in a particular society, such as the United States, is predicated on shared and individual values and meaning.[78,79] Such perception then influences decisions in health and social care.

Ageism, or the discriminations made on the basis of advancing chronologic age, often is imbedded within values and meaning, thus delimiting choice and option in decisions.[95-97] Ageism is most commonly and pervasively constructed as negative

Table 40-5 Examples of Issues from the John A. Hartford Foundation Institute of Geriatric Nursing Try This Assessment Series*

Topic	Tool	Composition	Referral
Overall geriatric nursing assessment	Fulmer SPICES	6 general items	Advanced practice nurse
Activities of daily living	Katz ADL Index	6 items scored 0 or 1	Physical therapy Occupational therapy
Depression	Geriatric depression scale	30 items with leveled scoring	Mental health clinician
Sleeplessness	Pittsburgh Sleep Quality Index	9 items 1 item with multiple parts	Advanced practice nurse Geriatrician Sleep specialist
Sleepiness	Epworth Sleepiness Scale	8 items scored 0 (never doze) to 3 (high chance of dozing)	Advanced practice nurse Geriatrician Sleep specialist
Pain	FACES scale Visual analog	Single item ranking	Advanced practice nurse Pain specialist
Fall risk	Fall Assessment Tool	12 patient characteristics 2 environmental characteristics	Physical therapy Occupational therapy
Malnutrition	Mini-Nutritional Assessment	Screening 6 items Assessment 12 items	Dietician
Acute confusion	Confusion Assessment Methods	4 features present or absent	Advanced practice nurse Mental health clinician
Caregiver burden	Caregiver Strain Index	13 items	Advanced practice nurse Mental health clinician Social worker
Family preferences for participation in care of hospitalized older adults	Family Preferences Index	15 items scored yes or no Item 15 is "other" allowing for individualized assessment	Advanced practice nurse Mental health clinician Social worker Pastoral counselor
Elder neglect and abuse	Elder Assessment Instrument	6 domains items easily assessed	Mental health clinician Social worker Advanced practice nurse
Medication misuse	Beer's Criteria	Drug list	Advanced practice nurse Geriatrician
Pain in dementia	Checklist of Non-Verbal Pain Indicators	6 items	Advanced practice nurse Pain specialist Mental health clinician

*Data from ***Try This*** is a publication of the John A. Hartford Foundation Institute for Geriatric Nursing. ***Try This*** issues are available at www.hartfordign.org.

external stereotypes of older adults often with attached questions of social or economic value.[97,98] More insidiously, positively intended ageism—or parentalism on the part of younger clinicians or family members—may jeopardize decision making with misinformation or misrepresentation of the older person's wishes.[99] Finally, and most subtly, older adults—as products of their own social environments—may stereotype themselves. Self-stereotyping emerges in conversations where older adults verbally or nonverbally express the sense that they are "too old" for a particular treatment or activity.[100,101] Ageism, whether it arises from the older person or the social environment, has potentially deleterious effects directly on health and function and negative consequences for effective decision making in radiation therapy and cancer care for older adults.[95,102]

Ageism is likely common in cancer care and influences decision making in myriad and invisible ways. Assumptions about treatment preferences, treatment tolerance, end-of-life wishes, and priority-accorded cancer and its treatment are clearly reflected in clinical discourse. That reflection, however, may be obscured as clinicians participate in that discourse with patients, family members, and one another using those assumptions to delineate assessment, identification, and intervention. For example, chronologic age often shapes the very identity of patients as one of the first demographic variables employed in patient presentation. Decisions may proceed from that point of age to limitations in treatment options, expectations, and even outcomes. Multiple effects of ageism on decisions in cancer care documented in a growing literature simultaneously argue for further exploration as the demographics of aging, healthcare technologies, and social mores shift.[99,103-105]

Radiation oncology nurses may witness two primary influences of ageism as they care for older patients. First, radiation oncology nurses may see explicit evidence of ageism that avoids patient voice, desire, and capacity either by diminishing or amplifying patient characteristics. This ageism generally is used in clinical situations where the patient is interviewed very little, where family members may speak for the patient without specific cultural permission to do so, and where clinicians perform inadequate assessment and rely instead on practice preferences. Second, radiation oncology nurses also may treat older patients who have had insufficient assessment and who are summarily referred for radiation therapy with the belief that it will be better tolerated than other options.[3,20,28,106] Best practices to subvert ageism with older adults who have cancer generally rely on awareness. Although radiation oncology nurses may not be able to abolish ageism in their practice settings, awareness and sensitivity to these issues coupled with thoughtful assessment and dialogue with patients, family, and colleagues may avoid negative consequences and support communication and decision making.

SUMMARY

Infusing radiation oncology nursing with gerontologic knowledge is an evolving process of balancing ever evolving knowledge against available best practices to create practices of screening, referral, intervention, and follow-up. Most adults diagnosed with cancer in our society are over age 65. Age older than 65 is inadequate as a representation of clinical concern; biologic age, comorbid disease, and functional decline portray areas of concern with greater precision. Nevertheless, these bounding demographics mandate increasing sophistication in knowledge of aging and related topics, greater focus on older adults and their families, and more precise referral and collaboration. Radiation oncology nursing and patient process and outcomes improve with application of gerontologic and geriatric principles, aging changes, geriatric assessment, and best practices. Attention to physical and cognitive function, gait and posture, and psychologic, emotional, social, and spiritual function reveals nuanced change that may influence radiation therapy. Use of geriatric assessment, referral sources, and intervention in these areas underpins best geriatric nursing and interdisciplinary practice in radiation therapy. Conversely, assumption about senescent tissue interactions with various forms of radiation and influence on early and late effects and toxicities should be avoided given a current lack of specific evidence. Investigation of a range of topics from cellular senescence and biomarkers of aging and cancer through meaning and experience specific to older adults undergoing radiation therapy is necessary to move practice forward. In the interim, incorporation of gerontologic and geriatric knowledge that focuses on function not specifically attached to disease or diagnosis provides avenues to improve assessment and intervention for older adults undergoing radiation therapy. Awareness of the social context of aging and being old is requisite to productively infusing radiation oncology nursing practice with gerontologic knowledge.

REFERENCES

1. Edwards BK, Howe HL, Ries LA et al: Annual report to the nation on the status of cancer, 1973–1999, featuring implications of age and aging on US cancer burden, *Cancer* 94(10):2766-2792, 2002.
2. Jemal A, Murray T, Ward E et al: Cancer statistics, 2005, *CA Cancer J Clin* 55(1):10-30, 2005.
3. Salvi G, Bavasso A, Frascino V et al: Biological optimization of the dose in elderly patients, *Rays* 29(3): 327-332, 2005.
4. Momm F, Becker G, Bartelt S et al: The elderly, fragile tumor patient: radiotherapy as an effective and most feasible treatment modality, *J Pain Sympt Manage* 27(1): 3-4, 2004.
5. Bouchardy C, Rapiti E, Fioretta G et al: Undertreatment

strongly decreases prognosis of breast cancer in elderly women, *J Clin Oncol* 21(19):3580-3587, 2003.
6. Gajdos C, Tartter PI, Bleiweiss IJ et al: The consequence of undertreating breast cancer in the elderly, *J Am Coll Surg* 192(6):698-707, 2001.
7. Langer CJ: Elderly patients with lung cancer: biases and evidence, *Curr Treat Options Oncol* 3(1):85-102, 2002.
8. Badib AO, Kurohara SS, Webster JH: Radiotherapy of carcinoma of the uterine cervix in the aged, *Geriatrics* 25(1):108-112, 1970.
9. Uno T, Isobe K, Kawakami H et al: Efficacy and toxicities of concurrent chemoradiation for elderly patients with esophageal cancer, *Anticancer Res* 24(4):2483-2486, 2004.
10. Agranovich A, Czaykowski P, Hui D et al: Radiotherapy for muscle-invasive urinary bladder cancer in elderly patients, *Can J Urol* 10(6):2056-2061, 2003.
11. Allal AS, Maire D, Becker M et al: Feasibility and early results of accelerated radiotherapy for head and neck carcinoma in the elderly, *Cancer* 88(3):648-652, 2000.
12. Brada M, Stenning SP: Radiotherapy for malignant gliomas in the elderly, *Semin Oncol* 30(6 suppl 19):63-67, 2003.
13. Brandes AA, Monfardini S: The treatment of elderly patients with high-grade gliomas, *Semin Oncol* 30(6 suppl 19):58-62, 2003.
14. Brandes AA, Rigon A, Monfardini S: Radiotherapy of the brain in elderly patients, *Eur J Cancer* 36(4):447-451, 2000.
15. Brandes AA, Vastola F, Basso U et al: A prospective study on glioblastoma in the elderly, *Cancer* 97(3):657-662, 2003.
16. Chen SW, Liang JA, Yang SN et al: High dose-rate brachytherapy for elderly patients with uterine cervical cancer, *Jpn J Clin Oncol* 33(5):221-228, 2003.
17. Chinot OL: Should radiotherapy be standard therapy for brain tumors in the elderly? Cons, *Semin Oncol* 30 (6 suppl 19):68-71, 2003.
18. Extermann M: Management issues for elderly patients with breast cancer, *Curr Treat Options Oncol* 5(2):161-169, 2004.
19. Ghosh S, Sujendran V, Alexiou C et al: Long term results of surgery versus continuous hyperfractionated accelerated radiotherapy (CHART) in patients aged >70 years with stage 1 non-small cell lung cancer, *Eur J Cardiothorac Surg* 24(6):1002-1007, 2003.
20. Patterson CJ, Hocking M, Bond M et al: Retrospective study of radiotherapy for lung cancer in patients aged 75 years and over, *Age Ageing* 27(4):515-518, 1998.
21. Pignon T, Gregor A, Schaake Koning C et al: Age has no impact on acute and late toxicity of curative thoracic radiotherapy, *Radiother Oncol* 46(3):239-248, 1998.
22. Pignon T, Scalliet P: Radiotherapy in the elderly, *Eur J Surg Oncol* 24(5):407-411, 1998.
23. Sakurai H, Mitsuhashi N, Takahashi M et al: Radiation therapy for elderly patient with squamous cell carcinoma of the uterine cervix, *Gynecol Oncol* 77(1):116-120, 2000.
24. Schofield CP, Sykes AJ, Slevin NJ et al: Radiotherapy for head and neck cancer in elderly patients, *Radiother Oncol* 69(1):37-42, 2003.
25. Ulutin HC, Pak Y, Dede M: Can radiotherapy be a treatment option for elderly women with invasive vulvar carcinoma without radical surgery? *Eur J Gynaecol Oncol* 23(5):426-428, 2002.
26. Uno T, Kawakami H, Funami Y et al: Chemoradiation for patients with esophageal cancer aged 80 and older, *Anticancer Res* 21(6A):4095-4097, 2001.
27. Zachariah B, Balducci L, Venkattaramanabalaji GV et al: Radiotherapy for cancer patients aged 80 and older: a study of effectiveness and side effects, *Int J Radiat Oncol Biol Phys* 39(5):1125-1129, 1997.
28. Salvi G, Dinapoli N, Maronta D: Clinical target volume definition in the elderly patient, *Rays* 28(3):343-344, 2003.
29. Baumann M: Is curative radiation therapy in elderly patients limited by increased normal tissue toxicity? *Radiother Oncol* 46(3):225-227, 1998.
30. Bringold F, Serrano M: Tumor suppressors and oncogenes in cellular senescence, *Exp Gerontol* 35(3):317-329, 2000.
31. Cristofalo VJ, Lorenzini A, Allen RG et al: Replicative senescence: a critical review, *Mech Ageing Dev* 125 (10-11):827-848, 2004.
32. Kovner CT, Mezey M, Harrington C: Who cares for older adults? Workforce implications of an aging society, *Health Aff (Millwood)* 21(5):78-89, 2002.
33. Anderson GF, Hussey PS: Population aging: a comparison among industrialized countries, *Health Aff (Millwood)* 19(3):191-203, 2000.
34. Palacios R: The future of global ageing, *Int J Epidemiol* 31(4):786-791, 2002.
35. Wolff JL, Starfield B, Anderson G: Prevalence, expenditures, and complications of multiple chronic conditions in the elderly, *Arch Intern Med* 162(20):2269-2276, 2002.
36. Fillenbaum GG, Pieper CF, Cohen HJ et al: Comorbidity of five chronic health conditions in elderly community residents: determinants and impact on mortality, *J Gerontol A Biol Sci Med Sci* 55(2):M84-M89, 2000.
37. Freedman VA, Martin LG: Understanding trends in functional limitations among older Americans, *Am J Pub Health* 88(10):1457-1462, 1998.
38. Freedman VA, Martin LG, Schoeni RF: Recent trends in disability and functioning among older adults in the United States: a systematic review, *JAMA* 288(24): 3137-3146, 2002.
39. McKinstry A, Perry A: Evaluation of speech in people with head and neck cancer: a pilot study, *Int J Lang Commun Disord* 38(1):31-46, 2003.
40. Semple CJ, McGowan B: Need for appropriate written information for patients, with particular reference to head and neck cancer, *J Clin Nurs* 11(5):585-593, 2002.
41. Barnett GC, Charman SC, Sizer B et al: Information given to patients about adverse effects of radiotherapy: a survey of patients' views, *Clin Oncol (R Coll Radiol)* 16(7):479-484, 2004.
42. Czaja R, Manfredi C, Price J: The determinants and consequences of information seeking among cancer patients, *J Health Comm* 8(6):529-562, 2003.
43. Koedoot CG, Oort FJ, de Haan RJ et al: The content and amount of information given by medical oncologists when telling patients with advanced cancer what their treatment options are: palliative chemotherapy and watchful waiting, *Eur J Cancer* 40(2):225-235, 2004.
44. Sharp L, Laurell G, Tiblom Y et al: Care diaries: a way of increasing head and neck cancer patients' involvement in

Q

R

their own care and the communication between clinicians, *Cancer Nurs* 27(2):119-126, 2004.
45. Brown A, Draper P: Accommodative speech and terms of endearment: elements of a language mode often experienced by older adults, *J Adv Nurs* 41(1):15-21, 2003.
46. *Oxford English dictionary*, ed 2, Oxford, England, 2005, Oxford University Press.
47. Cohen HJ: The origin of the word geriatrics, *J Am Geriatr Soc* 51(11):1676-1677, 2003.
48. Jones A: The National Nursing Home survey: 1999 summary, *Vital Health Stat* 13(152):1-116, 2002.
49. Garman KS, Cohen HJ: Functional status and the elderly cancer patient, *Crit Rev Oncol Hematol* 43(3):191-208, 2002.
50. Ferrucci L, Guralnik JM, Cavazzini C et al: The frailty syndrome: a critical issue in geriatric oncology, *Crit Rev Oncol Hematol* 46(2):127-137, 2003.
51. Shlipak MG, Stehman-Breen C, Fried LF et al: The presence of frailty in elderly persons with chronic renal insufficiency, *Am J Kidney Dis* 43(5):861-867, 2004.
52. Phillips EM, Bodenheimer CF, Roig RL et al: Geriatric rehabilitation: 4—physical medicine and rehabilitation interventions for common age-related disorders and geriatric syndromes, *Arch Phys Med Rehabil* 85(7 suppl 3):S18-S22, 2004.
53. Fillit HM, Butler RN, O'Connell AW et al: Achieving and maintaining cognitive vitality with aging, *Mayo Clin Proc* 77(7):681-696, 2002.
54. Haas ML: Utilizing geriatric skills in radiation oncology, *Geriatr Nurs* 25(6):355-360, 2004.
55. Happ MB, Williams CC, Strumpf NE et al: Individualized care for frail elders: theory and practice, *J Gerontol Nurs* 22(3):6-14, 1996.
56. Klein BE, Klein R, Knudtson MD et al: Frailty, morbidity and survival, *Arch Gerontol Geriatr* 41(2):141-149, 2005.
57. Gosain A, DiPietro LA: Aging and wound healing, *World J Surg* 28(3):321-326, 2004.
58. Mendelsohn FA, Divino CM, Reis ED et al: Wound care after radiation therapy, *Adv Skin Wound Care* 15(5):216-224, 2002.
59. MacDonald SW, Dixon RA, Cohen AL et al: Biological age and 12-year cognitive change in older adults: findings from the Victoria Longitudinal Study, *Gerontology* 50(2):64-81, 2004.
60. Jackson SH, Weale MR, Weale RA: Biological age—what is it and can it be measured? *Arch Gerontol Geriatr* 36(2):103-115, 2003.
61. Farquharson SM, Gupta R, Heald RJ et al: Surgical decisions in the elderly: the importance of biological age, *J R Soc Med* 94(5):232-235, 2001.
62. Madsen JL, Graff J: Effects of ageing on gastrointestinal motor function, *Age Ageing* 33(2):154-159, 2004.
63. Bourdiol P, Mioche L, Monier S: Effect of age on salivary flow obtained under feeding and non-feeding conditions, *J Oral Rehabil* 31(5):445-452, 2004.
64. Xue SA, Hao GJ: Changes in the human vocal tract due to aging and the acoustic correlates of speech production: a pilot study, *J Speech Lang Hear Res* 46(3):689-701, 2003.
65. Ship JA, Pillemer SR, Baum BJ: Progress in geriatrics: xerostomia and the geriatric patient, *J Am Geriatr Soc* 50(3):535-543, 2002.
66. Goodwin J, Samet J, Hunt W: Determinants of survival in older cancer patients, *J Natl Cancer Inst* 88(15):1031-1038, 1996.
67. Overcash JA, Beckstead J, Extermann M et al: The abbreviated comprehensive geriatric assessment (aCGA): a retrospective analysis, *Crit Rev Oncol Hematol* 54(2):129-136, 2005.
68. Flacker JM: What is a geriatric syndrome anyway? *J Am Geriatr Soc* 51(4):574-576, 2003.
69. Balducci L, Carreca I: Supportive care of the older cancer patient, *Crit Rev Oncol Hematol* 48(suppl):S65-S70, 2003.
70. Salminen E, Portin R, Korpela J et al: Androgen deprivation and cognition in prostate cancer, *Br J Cancer* 89(6):971-976, 2003.
71. Shilling V, Jenkins V, Fallowfield L et al: The effects of hormone therapy on cognition in breast cancer, *J Steroid Biochem Mol Biol* 86(3-5):405-412, 2003.
72. Dunn J, Steginga SK, Rose P et al: Evaluating patient education materials about radiation therapy, *Patient Educ Couns* 52(3):325-332, 2004.
73. Monsivais D, Reynolds A: Developing and evaluating patient education materials, *J Contin Educ Nurs* 34(4):172-176, 2003.
74. Puche RC, Morosano M, Masoni A et al: The natural history of kyphosis in postmenopausal women, *Bone* 17(3):239-246, 1995.
75. Aapro MS: Progress in the treatment of breast cancer in the elderly, *Ann Oncol* 4(13 suppl 4):207-210, 2002.
76. Levy B, Ashman O, Dror I: To be or not to be: the effects of aging stereotypes on the will to live, *Omega (Westport)* 40(3):409-420, 1999-2000.
77. Maclean N, Pound P: A critical review of the concept of patient motivation in the literature on physical rehabilitation, *Soc Sci Med* 50(4):495-506, 2000.
78. Paulson S: How various 'cultures of fitness' shape subjective experiences of growing older, *Ageing Soc* 25(2):229-244, 2005.
79. Poortman A-R, Van Tilburg TG: Past experiences and older adults' attitudes: a life course perspective, *Ageing Soc* 25(2):19-39, 2005.
80. Chapple A, Ziebland S: Prostate cancer: embodied experience and perceptions of masculinity, *Sociol Health Illness* 24(6):820-841, 2002.
81. Wells M: The hidden experience of radiotherapy to the head and neck: a qualitative study of patients after completion of treatment, *J Adv Nurs* 28(4):840-848, 1998.
82. Shelkey M, Wallace M: Katz index of independence in activities of daily living (ADL), *Try this: best practices in nursing care to older adults from the Hartford Institute for Geriatric Nursing*, 1998 (website): www.hartfordign.org/publications/trythis/issue02.pdf. Accessed May 31, 2005.
83. Moses S: Instrumental activities of daily living, *Family practice notebook.com*, 2000 (website): www.fpnotebook.com/GER3.htm. Accessed May 31, 2005.
84. Nijboer C, Tempelaar R, Sanderman R et al: Cancer and caregiving: the impact on the caregiver's health, *Psychooncology* 7(1):3-13, 1998.

85. Spillman BC, Pezzin LE: Potential and active family caregivers: changing networks and the 'sandwich generation,' *Milbank Q* 78(3):347-374, 2000.
86. Ingersoll-Dayton B, Raschick M: The relationship between care-recipient behaviors and spousal caregiving stress, *Gerontologist* 44(3):318-327, 2004.
87. Beers MH: Comprehensive geriatric assessment. In Beers MH, editor: *The Merck manual of geriatrics*, ed 3, 2005, Merck (online): www.merck.com/mrkshared/mmg/home.jsp.
88. Chen CC-H, Kenefick AL, Tang ST et al: Utilization of comprehensive geriatric assessment in cancer patients, *Crit Rev Oncol Hematol* 49(1):53-67, 2004.
89. Ingram SS, Seo PH, Martell RE et al: Comprehensive assessment of the elderly cancer patient: the feasibility of self-report methodology, *J Clin Oncol* 20(3):770-775, 2002.
90. Balducci L, Lyman GH, Fabri PJ: Management of cancer in the aged, *Comprehens Ther* 22(2):88-93, 1996.
91. Garman KS, Pieper CF, Seo P et al: Function in elderly cancer survivors depends on comorbidities, *J Gerontol A Biol Sci Med Sci* 58(12):M1119-M1124, 2003.
92. Yamazaki H, Inoue T, Yoshida K et al: Changes in performance status of elderly patients after radiotherapy, *Radiat Med* 19(1):9-18, 2001.
93. Bourbonniere M, Kagan SH: Nursing intervention and older adults who have cancer: specific science and evidence based practice, *Nurs Clin North Am* 39(3):529-543, 2004.
94. Scholder J, Kagan S, Jean Schumann M: Nurse competence in aging overview, *Nurs Clin North Am* 39(3):429-442, 2004.
95. Levy BR: Eradication of ageism requires addressing the enemy within, *Gerontologist* 41(5):578-579, 2001.
96. Palmore E: The ageism survey: first findings, *Gerontologist* 41(5):572-575, 2001.
97. Cohen ES: The complex nature of ageism: what is it? Who does it? Who perceives it? *Gerontologist* 41(5): 576-577, 2001.
98. Tsuchiya A, Dolan P, Shaw R: Measuring people's preferences regarding ageism in health: some methodological issues and some fresh evidence, *Soc Sci Med* 57(4): 687-696, 2003.
99. Austin D, Russell EM: Is there ageism in oncology? *Scot Med J* 48(1):17-20, 2003.
100. Levy B: Improving memory in old age through implicit self-stereotyping, *J Pers Soc Psych* 71(6):1092-1107, 1996.
101. Levy BR: Mind matters: cognitive and physical effects of aging self-stereotypes, *J Gerontol B Psychol Sci Soc Sci* 58(4):P203-P211, 2003.
102. Hausdorff JM, Levy BR, Wei JY: The power of ageism on physical function of older persons: reversibility of age-related gait changes, *J Am Geriatr Soc* 47(11):1346-1349, 1999.
103. Aapro MS: The frail are not always elderly, *J Clin Oncol* 23(17-18):2121-2122, 2005.
104. Kearney N, Miller M: Elderly patients with cancer: an ethical dilemma, *Crit Rev Oncol Hematol* 33(2):149-154, 2000.
105. Murthy VH, Krumholz HM, Gross CP: Participation in cancer clinical trials: race-, sex-, and age-based disparities, *JAMA* 291(22):2720-2726, 2004.
106. Goffin JR, Rajan R, Souhami L: Tolerance of radiotherapy and chemotherapy in elderly patients with bladder cancer, *Am J Clin Oncol* 27(2):172-177, 2004.

Chapter 41

Influence of Complementary and Alternative Medicine

Georgia M. Decker

Numerous definitions of complementary and alternative medicine (CAM), all referring to a broad range of philosophies, approaches, and applications, have evolved over time.[1] The term *alternative* has been used as an umbrella term to describe therapies not taught in medical schools in the United States (U.S.) or provided in U.S. hospitals.[2,3] Eisenberg[4] was among the first to note that the term *alternative* was no longer accurate because many medical schools (now) include these therapies in their curricula, and some therapies are provided to interested patients in hospitals and cancer centers. Segen[5] reported that alternative healthcare systems constitute an array of treatments and ideologies that are based on no common or consistent philosophy. Micozzi[6] maintains that CAM covers a broad range of health and medical systems often derived from ancient societies with the common theme that the body has energy along with material aspects, can heal itself, and healing comes from the inner resources of the body. It has been maintained that unproven methods (alternative therapies for cancer treatment) should be distinguished from complementary methods applied to mainstream care for symptom management and to enhance quality of life (QOL).[3,7] It is, therefore, the interchangeable use and presumed understanding of the terms *complementary* and *alternative* that has contributed to miscommunication and misunderstanding between patients and healthcare professionals, as well as *among* healthcare professionals.[1] Communication is key. Conventional therapies or approaches, also known as *standard*, *traditional*, or *biomedical*, are those that have been used in Western medicine.[8] Complementary and alternative medicine (CAM) is referred to as *alternative* or *unconventional* when these therapies are used in lieu of conventional approaches. When combined with conventional methods, the terms *integrative*, *integrated*, or *complementary* are used. It is the *intent* with which a therapy is used that describes it.[9] The Oncology Nursing Society (ONS) position on "The Use of Complementary and Alternative Therapies in Cancer Care" promotes standardizing terminology to enhance communication.[9] For the purpose of this chapter, the acronym *CAM* will be used when referencing these therapies, and the term *conventional* is used when referring to traditional or standard approaches.

In the United States, patients seeking CAM have not been discouraged from using it by public education, legislative action, and medical advances in the mid 1970s to 1980s.[10] National surveys reinforce the notion that there is an enduring interest in and use of CAM in the United States and Europe.[4,11] Initial surveys regarding CAM use in the United States were not disease or population specific. However, by the end of the 1990s and early 2000, knowledge about the use of CAM by specific populations with cancer, including cancer site and ethnicity, had emerged.[12,13] Additional studies have reported CAM use specific to those in urban, suburban, and rural areas and by the elderly. When compared with non-CAM users, individuals who use CAM are more likely to be female, better educated, and have higher incomes.[13] The quality and quantity of information about CAM therapies use has increased; however, there remains much to be learned about the indications, contraindications, potential benefits, and adverse effects of specific therapies when used in specific clinical situations.

The Office of Alternative Medicine (OAM) was established in 1992 in response to the continued use of and issues surrounding CAM therapies. This office became the National Center for Complementary and Alternative Medicine (NCCAM) in 1998.

NCCAM is one of the 27 institutes and centers that make up the National Institutes of Health (NIH). NCCAM has four primary focus areas: research (clinical and basic science research), training and career development (predoctoral, postdoctoral, and career researchers), outreach (conferences, educational programs, and exhibits, information clearinghouse), and integration of scientifically proven CAM practices into conventional medicine.[14]

In an effort to increase quality cancer research and information about CAM use, the National Cancer Institute (NCI) established the Office of Cancer Complementary and Alternative Medicine (OCCAM). The OCCAM promotes and supports research within CAM disciplines and therapies as they relate to the prevention, diagnosis, and treatment of cancer, cancer-related symptoms, and side effects of conventional treatment. OCCAM coordinates the NCI CAM research and informational activities, collaboration with other governmental and nongovernmental organizations on cancer CAM issues, and liaison with health practitioners and researchers regarding cancer CAM issues.[15,16]

The White House Commission on Complementary and Alternative Medicine Policy (WHC-CAMP) was established in March 2000 to address issues related to access and delivery of CAM, priorities for research, and to identify the need for consumer and healthcare professional education.[17] In 2003 to 2004, the Institutes of Medicine (IOM) of the National Academies sponsored seven committee meetings to investigate scientific, policy, and practice questions that occur from the increasing use of CAM. The IOM is a nongovernment agency established in 1970 that guarantees unbiased, evidenced-based information and advice concerning health and science policy to policy makers, healthcare professionals, and the public.[18]

CATEGORIES OF COMPLEMENTARY AND ALTERNATIVE MEDICINE

Currently, there are two main approaches to categorizing CAM therapies. The National Center for Complementary and Alternative Medicine (NCCAM) classifies CAM therapies into five domains: (1) alternative medical systems, (2) mind-body interventions, (3) biologically based therapies, (4) manipulative and body-based methods, and (5) energy therapies. The NCI OCCAM expanded the NCCAM domains with additional categories for clarification: movement therapy and pharmacologic and biologic treatments with a subcategory of complex natural products.[19]

- *Alternative medical systems* are built on complete systems of theory and practice.
- *Mind-body interventions* uses a variety of techniques designed to enhance the mind's capacity to affect bodily function and symptoms.
- *Biologically based therapies* in CAM use substances found in nature, such as herbs, foods, and vitamins.
- *Manipulative and body-based methods* in CAM are based on manipulation and/or movement of one or more parts of the body.
- *Energy therapies* involve the use of energy field and are of two types: biofield therapies and bioelectromagnetic-based therapies.
- *Movement therapies* are modalities used to improve patterns of bodily movement.
- *Pharmacologic and biologic therapies* are drugs, vaccines, off-label use of prescription drugs, and other biologic interventions not yet accepted in mainstream medicine.
- *Complex natural products*, a subcategory of pharmacologic and biologic therapies, consist of crude natural substances and unfractionated extracts from marine organisms used for healing and treatment of disease.[15] Table 41-1 provides examples and describes the domains as defined by the OCCAM.

USE BY CANCER PATIENTS

In 2000, a survey reported that Americans with cancer who were participating in clinical trials used spirituality (94%), imagery (86%), massage (80%), lifestyle, diet, and nutrition (60%), herbal/botanical (20%), and high-dose vitamins (14%).[20] Other surveys report use by patients with cancer at 50% to 83%.[21,22] Another study reported that characteristics associated with CAM use by females with gynecologic cancer, except cancer of the cervix, include annual incomes greater than $30,000 and use of CAM before cancer diagnosis. Respondents in this same study reported their reasons for using CAM as (1) hope of improved well-being and (2) possible anticancer effects of the particular CAM modalities used.[13] Some of the reported reasons for seeking CAM therapies have remained consistent: philosophical similarity (active patient

Table 41-1 NCI OCCAM Domains of CAM and Modalities in Clinical Trials

Domain	Definition	Examples	Modality in clinical trials
Alternative medical systems	Systems built upon completed systems of theory and practice	Traditional Chinese medicine (acupuncture), Ayurveda, homeopathy, naturopathy, Tibetan medicine	Acupuncture Acupressure Electroacupuncture Traumeel S
Manipulative and body-based methods	Methods based on manipulation and/or movement of one or more parts of the body	Chiropractic, therapeutic massage, osteopathy, reflexology	Distance healing Exercise-based counseling Group therapy Healing touch Music therapy Spirituality, religiosity Standard counseling Stress management training
Energy therapies	Therapies involving the use of energy fields	Reiki, therapeutic touch, pulsed fields, magnet therapy	Energy healing Energy therapy Reiki Touch
Mind-body interventions	Techniques designed to enhance the mind's capacity to affect bodily function and symptoms	Meditation, hypnosis, art therapy, biofeedback, mental healing, imagery, relaxation therapy, support groups, music therapy, cognitive-behavioral therapy, prayer, dance therapy, psychoneuroimmunology, aromatherapy, animal-assisted therapy	Distance healing, exercise-based counseling, group therapy, healing touch, music therapy, spirituality and religiosity
Movement therapy	Modalities used to improve patterns of bodily movement	Tai chi, Feldenkrais, Hatha yoga, Alexander technique, dance therapy, qi gong, Rolfing, Trager method, applied kinesiology	None
Biologically based (nutritional) therapeutics`	Assortment of nutrients and nonnutrient and bioactive food components that are used as chemopreventative agents, and the use of specific foods or diets as cancer prevention or treatment strategies	Dietary regimens such as macrobiotics, vegetarian, Gerson therapy, Kelley/Gonzalez regimen, vitamins, dietary macronutrients, supplements, antioxidants, melatonin, selenium, coenzyme Q10, ephedrine, orthomolecular medicine	Black cohosh Creatine Curcumin Flax seed Folic acid Fruit and vegetable extracts Garlic Ginger Herbal therapy Juven L-carnitine Low-fat diet Lycopene Macrobiotic diet Noni fruit extract

(continued)

Table 41-1 NCI OCCAM Domains of CAM and Modalities in Clinical Trials—cont'd

Domain	Definition	Examples	Modality in clinical trials
			Nutritional supplements Pomegranate juice Selenium Soy protein isolate Valerian officinalis Vitamins C and E Zinc sulfate
Pharmacologic and biologic treatments	Drugs, complex natural products, vaccines, and other biologic interventions not yet accepted in mainstream medicine, off-label use of prescription drugs	Antineoplastons, products from honey bees, 714-X, low-dose naltrexone, met-enkephalin, immunoaugmentative therapy, laetrile, hydrazine sulfate, New Castle virus, melatonin, ozone therapy, thymus therapy, enzyme therapy, high-dose vitamin C	Antineoplastons Pancreatic proteolytic enzymes
Complex natural products	Subcategory of pharmacologic and biologic treatments consisting of an assortment of plant samples (botanicals), extracts of crude natural substances, and unfractionated extracts from marine organisms used for healing and treatment of disease	Herbs and herbal extracts, mixtures of tea polyphenols, shark cartilage, Essiac tea, cordyceps, Sun Soup, MGN-3	Chinese herbal extract Green tea extract (Polyphenon E) Kanglaite injection Milk thistle Mistletoe Pycnogeno Shark cartilage St. John's wort Virulizin

Data from Decker G, Lee, C: Complementary and alternative medicine (CAM) therapies. In Yarbro CH, Frogge MH, Goodman M, editors: *Cancer nursing principles and practice*, ed 6, Sudbury, Mass, 2005, Jones and Bartlett, pp 590-620.
NIC, National Cancer Institute; *OCCAM*, Office of Cancer Complementary and Alternative Medicine.

role, natural, less toxic treatments, spiritual elements), personal control over treatment, positive relationship with CAM therapy provider, and increased sense of well-being.[23] Other factors that have been reported as contributing to the increased use of CAM include dissatisfaction with the contemporary healthcare system because of what are perceived to be ineffective therapies, adverse effects, poor communication, insufficient time with and insufficient access to healthcare professionals, rejection if or when an anti-science viewpoint is expressed, desperation, and cost of care.[23] Stevinson[23] and Furnham[24] reported that patients have consistently expressed a desire to take control of their own health, actively participate in decisions related to health and wellness, and choose treatment plans involving solely conventional, solely CAM, or a combination of both.

EVIDENCE-BASED PRACTICE

Evidence-based practice (EBP) is the care of patients using the best available evidence from the results of research to guide clinical decision making. This includes defining the question, accessing the information, judging the credibility of the results, and applying these results to the care of patients.[25] Defining EBP for certain CAM therapies is similar to conventional medicine, and it comes about as a result of integrating clinical expertise, epidemiologic studies, and anecdotal evidence. Some authors assert that there cannot be two kinds of medicine—conventional and alternative.[26] That is, there can only be one type of medicine: one that is adequately tested versus one that has not been tested, reasoning that once a treatment has been tested rigorously, it no longer matters whether it was considered "alternative" at the outset. When a modality is determined to be reasonable, safe, and effective, it may be accepted into clinical practice.[26]

Levels of evidence in CAM must be generated in the same fashion as that of conventional medicine. This begins with clinical trials involving CAM modalities for the treatment of cancer and/or cancer-related side effects. The results of these trials will establish a foundation for the development of evidence-based practice, research utilization, evidence-based health care, and practice guidelines. Levels of evidence are often used by organizations such as the NCI (clinical trials), ONS (Priority Symptom Management [PRISM] project), and in databases such as Natural Medicine Comprehensive Database[27] and the Natural Standard Database.[28] Table 41-2 provides examples and comparisons of the strength of study design, endpoints measured, and level of evidence scoring employed by several of these databases.

In spite of increasing use of CAM therapies in the United States and abroad, there remains limited data on safety, efficacy, and mechanism of action of many individual therapies. Many CAM approaches are already in use with little or no preclinical or clinical research support, and therefore, case reports or case series may be the only data available.[16] The NCI Best Case Series Program provides a pathway for the review of fully documented case reports of cancer patients treated with alternative medical approaches. The program goal is to identify alternative approaches to cancer treatment that warrant NCI-initiated prospective research. A credible case is one that meets *all* of the following criteria: (1) a pathologic diagnosis of cancer from a tissue specimen obtained before an alternative medicine intervention and after any conventional anticancer therapy, (2) documentation that a patient used the alternative medicine intervention under evaluation, (3) documentation of tumor regression appropriate for the disease type and location, and (4) absence of confounding and/or concurrent anticancer therapies.[29]

Because the concept of an evidence-based approach to CAM is still in early development, recommending CAM therapies remains a challenge for healthcare professionals. Several authors have provided information to assist in this process. Eisenberg[30] provides an algorithm for physicians advising patients regarding CAM therapies, whereas Decker[31] offers an algorithm for advising cancer patients regarding CAM therapies and CAM practitioners (Figure 41-1). Ernst and colleagues[32,33] strove to establish a base of evidence for CAM and offered a direction-of-evidence model. Now, professionals often have patients who request information regarding CAM therapies for prevention or treatment of medical conditions. Ernst maintains that this interest may intensify when traditional therapies are not providing the desired result.[32]

PATIENT DECISION MAKING

The desire for CAM therapies can be complicated by the amount of (often inaccurate) information available from a variety of sources including the internet and well-meaning friends and family.[32] Professional opinions differ, and methods for rating CAM therapies vary even among experts. Ernst[32] uses "direction of evidence" and "weight of evidence" (low, moderate, and high), whereas Eisenberg and colleagues use "recommend," "tolerate," and "avoid."

Many patients want to participate in medical decision making. A partnering relationship with one's healthcare professional is replacing the dated, paternalistic one between physicians and their patients.[34] Participation in treatment decisions allows patients the opportunity to reclaim autonomy and a sense of control.[35,36] This process requires time to acquire and evaluate accurate and sufficient information about a particular diagnosis and existing treatments and standards of care. There are a variety of other factors that may influence patients' participation in a collaborative approach. These factors include the patient's age, educational level, the social structure of the family, influences of relatives and friends, financial concerns, and insurance coverage. It has been an accepted belief that a patient's initial priority should focus only on a chance of cure and prevention of possible spread of disease.[37,38]

Mastaglia and Kristjanson[39] describe a demonstrated age difference in the perceived locus of control based on age. Age-related differences in

Table 41-2 Common Levels of Evidence in Cancer CAM

	Strength of study design	Strength of endpoints measured	Level of evidence score
Physician data query[130]	1, RCT (DB/NB) 2, Non-RCT 3, Case series 4, Best case series	A, Total mortality B, CS-mortality C, QOL D, Indirect surrogates	1–4 joined with A-D Joining score for study design with strength of endpoints measured
Natural standards database[28]	A, Strong scientific evidence B, Good scientific evidence C, Unclear or conflicting scientific evidence D, Fair negative scientific evidence F, Strong negative scientific evidence Lack of evidence, unable to evaluate efficacy because of lack of adequate human data	Quality of study 0–2 Poor 3–4 Good 5 Excellent	A B C D F Lack of evidence
Natural medicines comprehensive database[27]	Weight of evidence □ Low; □ □ Moderate; □ □ □ High Direction of evidence ↑ Clearly positive; ⇗ Tentatively positive; □ Uncertain ⇘ Tentatively negative; ↓ Clearly negative Serious safety concerns YES, Serious events have been reported or are considered possible NO, Reports of serious events were not located and are considered unlikely		Weight of evidence Direction of evidence Serious safety concerns
Priority Symptom PRISM Project[83]	1, SR or MA of multiple RCTs 2, > 1 RCT N>100 3, > 1 non-RCT 4, Qualitative SR nonexperimental 5, Case controlled 6, Correlational study or case series 7, NIH consensus reports, practice guidelines 8, Qualitative designs, expert opinion		I, Level of evidence 1–3 II, Level of evidence 4–7 III, Level of evidence 8

Adapted from Decker G, Lee C: Complementary and alternative medicine (CAM) therapies. In Yarbro CH, Frogge MH, Goodman M, editors: *Career nursing: principles and practice*, ed 6, pp 590-620, 2005: Jones and Bartlett Publishers, Sudbury, Mass., www.jbpub.com. Reprinted with permission.

CAM, Complementary and alternative medicine; *RCT*, randomized controlled trial; *DB/NB*, Double Blind/nonblinded; *CS*, case series; *QOL*, quality of life; *SR*, systematic review; *MA*, meta-analysis; *NIH*, National Institutes of Health.

coping/control strategies are described by Baltes.[40] Age-related cognitive weakening limits processing and memorizing information and therefore the aging patient may not seek additional information.[41] Making treatment decisions is often difficult and fraught with anxiety and fear. Cancer treatment decisions must sometimes be made within a short time interval, and feeling forced to quickly make these decisions may diminish a patient's ability to participate in the decision.[42] Making the decision to integrate a CAM modality can make this process even more complex. Brett describes the variability in an individual's response to the subject of CAM modalities and suggests that culture, religion, and age influence a person's perceptions. These perceptions can range from the therapy being considered essential to expressing cynicism.[43] It is not unusual for CAM users of all

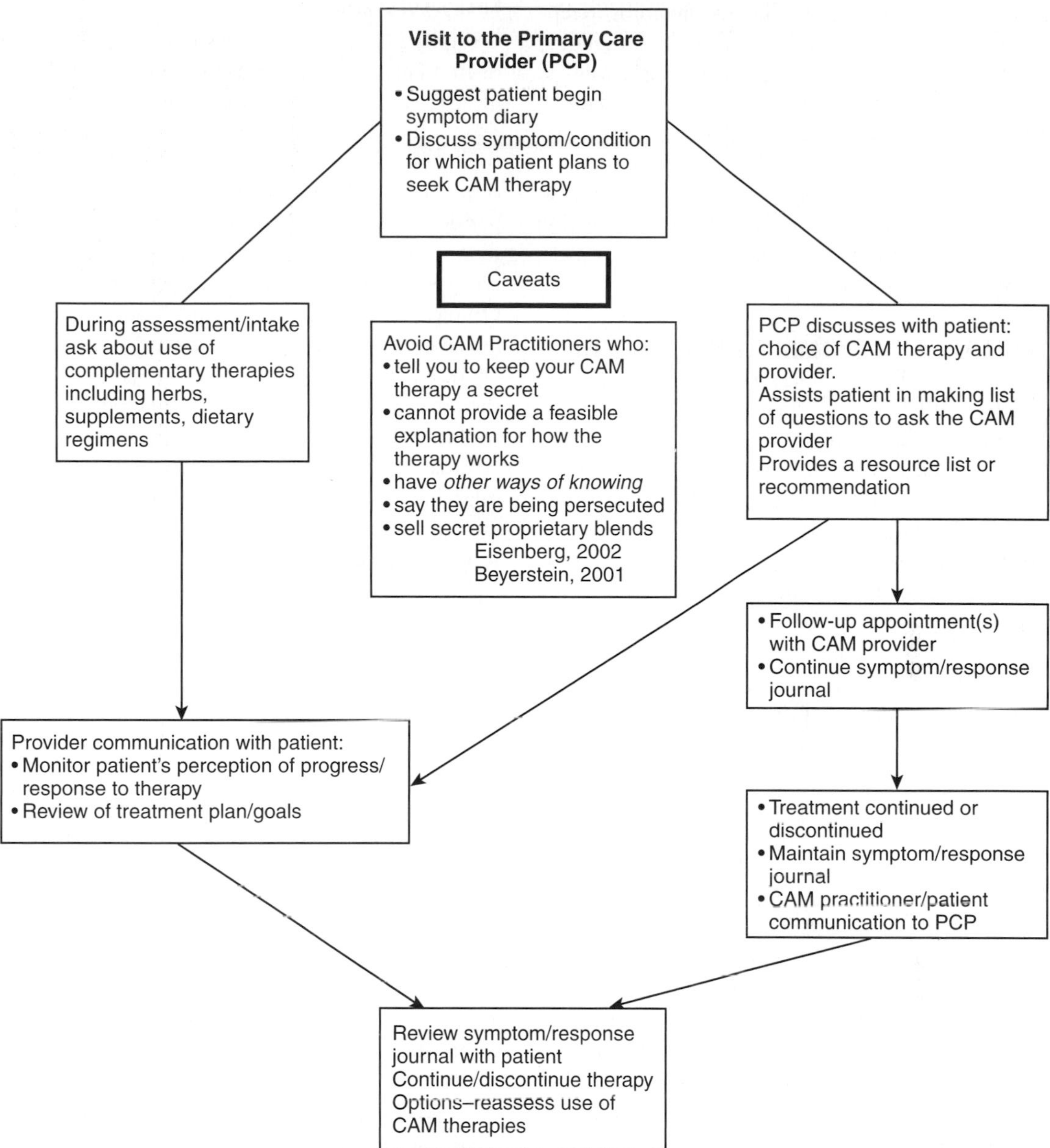

Figure 41-1 Discussing CAM Therapies With Patients.
From Buchsel P, Yarbro CH: Oncology nursing in the ambulatory setting, 2005: Jones and Bartlett Publishers, Sudbury, Mass., www.jbpub.com. Reprinted with permission.

ages to believe that a CAM therapy used for their heart condition or depression cannot or will not have any impact on their cancer or cancer therapy. That is they may believe that an herb or supplement is diagnosis specific.

It is important to note that Downer and colleagues[44] discovered that even when a chosen complementary therapy had little influence on a patient's illness, the patient still reported satisfaction with that particular therapy. The toxic effects of conventional therapy and the lack of hope provided the dissatisfaction reported. According to Kassab and Stevensen,[45] misinformation about CAM therapies may arise from word of mouth and speculation. For example, even among experts, opinions vary regarding the belief that massage spreads cancer. Some current recommendations include avoiding deep tissue massage over tumor sites and contiguous lymph glands and over irradiated fields because the skin is fragile.[46,47] Consequently, a recommendation or decision to use a particular CAM therapy might not be an unequivocal "yes" or "no." The answer might vary from *not during radiation therapy but OK afterward* or *you must take a multiple vitamin supplement with this particular therapy* to *do not use this during or after cancer therapy*.

EXAMPLES OF COMMON MODALITIES

Acupuncture

Acupuncture has been used by many Americans and performed by many physicians, dentists, and acupuncturists for a variety of health conditions, particularly pain. This treatment typically involves insertion of a needle into the skin in specific sites (acupoints) for therapeutic purposes. Acupoint stimulation also may be achieved via electrical current, laser, moxibustion, pressure, ultrasound, and vibration and of Japanese, Korean, or Chinese types. The underlying principle is that *qi* (pronounced 'chee' and translated as meaning *energy*) is present at birth and maintained throughout life. It circulates throughout the body, and 12 meridians provide a major path for the flow of *qi*. There are approximately 350 acupoints along the 12 meridians, with additional acupoints that lie outside the meridian pathways. Health is a balance of yin and yang (opposite forces present in everyone). Disease or any medical condition is a result of imbalance, usually a result of a blockage or deficiency of energy. Acupuncture theory embraces the belief that stimulating the appropriate acupoints aids the body in the ability to correct any imbalance in the flow of energy, thus restoring balance. It is also held that changes in the balance of energy and flow of *qi* may be identified before disease has developed, and therefore, acupuncture has a role in the prevention of illness and maintenance of health. It has been and is still routinely used in Eastern countries. It has also been integrated with allopathic and osteopathic medicine in the United States.[32,48] Acupuncture has been and continues to be used for pain and other disorders of the musculoskeletal system; headaches; stress; ear, nose, and throat (ENT) conditions including sinusitis, tinnitus and vertigo; allergies; dental pain; addictions; and immune system disorders, among others.

Strength of Evidence

Over 30 meta-analyses or systematic reviews conducted between 1996 and 2004 examined the use of acupuncture for symptom management mostly related to pain. Nearly 400 randomized controlled trials (RCT) results are reported in Medline® (www.ncbi.nlm.nih.gov/entrez) for the same time period. There is no evidence of the physical existence of *qi* or meridian. The effects of acupuncture are reportedly better than placebo in most trials.[32] Opioid peptides, serotonin, and other neurotransmitters are released by acupuncture.[49,50] Conclusive evidence exists that acupuncture is effective in the treatment of dental pain[51] and postoperative nausea.[52] Efficacy of acupuncture in relief from asthma, back pain, drug dependency, fibromyalgia, migraine and tension headaches, neck pain, osteoarthritis, and stroke is considered inconclusive by some authors.[53] Others suggest the evidence is equivocal and/or promising for some indications including addiction, stroke rehabilitation, postoperative- and chemotherapy-related nausea and vomiting, tennis elbow, carpal tunnel syndrome, and asthma.[48]

Contraindications

The "needling" technique is contraindicated in those patients with severe bleeding disorders or who are at increased risk for infection as in neutropenia, during the first trimester of pregnancy, with the exception of treatment for nausea,[54] and in patients with cardiac pacemakers, who should not be treated with electrical stimulation.[55] Caution is advised for the first treatment and some authors recommend that this treatment be administered with a patient supine. Some patients become drowsy, so care should be taken by these patients regarding operating machinery, including driving. Needles should not be reused and strict asepsis is mandatory.[55] Side effects include bleeding, bruising, pain with needling, and worsening of symptoms. Reported adverse events are rare but include pneumothorax and death.[55]

Opportunities

The following are recent studies of acupuncture:

Randomized Study of Acupuncture to Improve End-of-Life Symptom Distress in Patients With Metastatic Colorectal Cancer UPITTS-010901

Acupuncture to Improve Quality of Life in

Patients With Advanced Cancer 1 R21 AT01010-01

Acupuncture for Shortness of Breath in Cancer Patients 1 R21 AT010290-01

Practitioners

Nationally, acupuncturists can be certified in two ways. They can complete a formal, full-time educational program that includes both classroom and clinical hours or participate in an apprenticeship program. Acupuncturists also must complete a "Clean Needle Technique" approved course. Medical doctors with training in acupuncture also may obtain board certification. The National Certification Commission of Acupuncture and Oriental Medicine (NCCAOM) established standards for certification that are accepted by some states for licensure. Medical doctors must possess a valid medical license and be certified through the American Academy of Medical Acupuncture (www.medicalacupuncture.org). Some states re-quire medical referral whereas others allow nonmedical practitioners to see patients without referral (www.nccaom.org). A comparison of licensed versus certified acupuncturists is available at www.asny.org.

Qi Gong

Qi gong (chi kung) means "energy cultivation," and refers to movements that are believed to improve health, longevity, and harmony within oneself and the world.[56] There are thousands of such movements, and qi gong may include any done with the intention of enhancing energy. It is based on four common principles, sometimes referred to as the "secrets" of qi gong: mind (the presence of intention), eyes (the focus of intention), movement (the action of intention), and breath (the flow of intention). Numerous styles exist and may include meditation, exercise, and self-massage.[32] Mastery in qi gong is the achievement of the ultimate goal—harmonious existence and action in all situations. Mastery is not exhibited as someone knowing everything, but rather, regardless of a level of achievement, mastery includes a willingness to continue learning. Elements that define this level of expertise include curiosity, ease in action, and clarity of focus and intention, perseverance, nonattachment, resilience, openness, creativity, responsiveness, and fluid balance. Numerous books and teachers profess to teach the secrets of qi gong and the power of the possibility of its applications. Authors agree that it is actually defined by a person's willing to practice and experience, that is, the availability to learn.[32,56]

Strength of Evidence

A 1-hour session of qi gong resulted in improved hemodynamics in patients with congestive heart failure in a small (n = ?) uncontrolled study.[32,57]

Contraindications

Psychosis has been reported in patients using qi gong. It is not known whether a latent condition was involved.[32,58]

Opportunities

Ernst[32] suggested that qi gong can be used for health promotion, functional disorders, and symptom control. Yang[57] predicts use in the treatment of arthritis.

Practitioners

Because it is considered a form of Chinese medicine, acupuncturists and those appropriately credentialed in acupuncture and/or Oriental medicine are typically the practitioner of qi gong. The Directory of Information Resources Online (DIRLINE) is compiled by the National Library of Medicine (www.dirline.nlm.nih.gov/dirlineb.htm). It contains information about a variety of health organizations, including CAM associations and organizations.

Reiki

Reiki means "universal life energy." It is an ancient form of healing. The practitioner is the conduit for the movement of energy. It is the energy—not the healer—that influences healing. In this respect, Reiki differs from other healing systems. That is, energy travels through the healing, *not* from the healer. Reiki is said to alleviate physical, emotional, and spiritual blockages.[5] The five premises of Reiki include (1) an energy of unique properties exists that is applicable to physical and psychologic conditions, (2) the energy has a source, (3) this source can be tapped, (4) a person can be taught to use this energy, and (5) the effects of this energy are palpable and subjective. The energy is considered pure because it is not influenced by the practitioner's faith or religion.[5] The practitioner gently places his or her hands on the client, in a particular series of positions. Typically, 5 minutes are spent on each of 12 positions although this may vary based on the needs of the client. The client remains fully clothed at all times and there is no pressure, massage, or manipulation applied to the client. The environment is kept quiet and soothing, and the client should emerge feeling relaxed.

Strength of Evidence

Two meta-analyses examining Reiki (with therapeutic touch) were reported between 1999 and 2004. More than 20 RCTs are reported in Medline for the same time period. Reiki may be helpful in the treatment of pain,[59] mood changes,[60] and fatigue.[61] Mansour and colleagues[62] tested a standardization procedure for placebo Reiki in an effort to provide a foundation for a subsequent randomized and placebo-controlled Reiki efficacy study. Based on results, authors plan a randomized three-arm Reiki efficacy clinical trial.

Contraindications

None known.[32]

Opportunities

Reiki appears to have few adverse effects and can eventually be self-administered. Ongoing study: ACTIVE CLINICAL TRIAL: Reiki/Energy Healing in Prostate Cancer NCCAM, R21AT1120.

Practitioners

Typically, Reiki is taught in three parts. Reiki I includes history of Reiki, the Reiki hand positions, and Reiki symbols and their names (drawn and used for specific conditions), and meditation manifestation. Reiki II involves intense training focusing on advanced techniques and includes a review of Reiki I. The training for Reiki II involves knowledge of long distance healing, scanning techniques, and the long distance Reiki symbols and their names. Typically, there are two USUI-REIKI-Tibetan attunements at intervals throughout the course. Reiki III (master level) includes a review of previous training and practice and brings to the student knowledge for long distance healing, scanning techniques, more meditation techniques, and an additional Reiki symbol. Typically, there is a Reiki attunement at the end of the course.

Aromatherapy

Aromatherapy is the controlled use of plant essences for therapeutic purposes.[63] *Essential oil* is the aromatic essence of a plant in the form of an oil or resin derived from plant leaf, stalk, bark, root, flower, fruit, or seed. The *carrier* is the diluent(s) used to dilute a concentrated essential oil for application. The *neat* is the direct application of the essential oil compound (essential oil plus carrier) to the skin. The *note* is the unique aromatic variable of an essential oil used when blending combinations of essential oil compounds: the *top note* is bright, the *middle note* is lingering, and the *base note* is grounding.[64] Essential oils can be applied directly to the skin through a compress or massage, inhaled via a diffuser or steaming water, or added directly to bath water. At the present time, there are about 150 essential oils.[65] The hypothesized mechanism of action in the use of essential oils begins with the olfactory sense.[32] After sensing the smell, the limbic system is activated in retrieving learned memories. Essential oils are also absorbed via the dermal route and subcutaneous fat into the bloodstream. Entry into the body via the oral route into the digestive system is not recommended. Often, aromatherapy is practiced with massage. Aromatherapy massage is used in palliative care settings to improve quality of life for patients with cancer. Published data on dosing, comparative methods of administration, and therapeutic outcomes in the use of essential oils in aromatherapy are limited.

Strength of Evidence

A 2003 Cochrane Database systematic review was performed involving aromatherapy for dementia. Nearly 20 RCTs are reported in Medline, conducted between 1998 and 2004, for the use of aromatherapy in various clinical settings, of which four involve patients with cancer. Cook and Ernst[66] reviewed 12 trials in a systematic review; six trials suggested that aromatherapy massage has a relaxing effect.[66] Louis and Kowalski[67] measured the responses of 17 patients with cancer to humidified essential lavender oil and noted a positive change in blood pressure, pulse, pain, anxiety, depression, and sense of well-being after both the humidified water treatment and lavender treatment. Olleveant and colleagues[68] compared drop size among six different essential oils and reported that the bottles differed in their method of delivery; they recommended a universal standardization of measure to ensure equity and safety in administration. Massage and aromatherapy massage offer short-term benefits for psychologic well-being, with the effect on anxiety being supported by limited evidence.[69] Evidence is mixed as to whether aromatherapy enhances the effects of massage. Replication, longer follow-up, and larger trials are needed to accrue the necessary evidence.[69] Graham and colleagues[70] reported negative results in 313 patients who were randomly assigned inhalation aromatherapy concurrently with radiation treatment.

Contraindications

Contraindications to the use of essential oils are pregnancy, contagious disease, epilepsy, venous thrombosis, varicose veins, open wounds or skin sites, and recent surgeries of any type. Essential oils should not be administered orally or applied undiluted on the skin. Possible adverse events associated with the use of essential oils are photosensitivity, allergic reactions, nausea, and headache. Many essential oils have the potential to either enhance or reduce the effects of prescribed medications including antibiotics, tranquilizers, antihistamines, anticonvulsants, barbiturates, morphine, and quinidine.[32] Cases of potentially serious reactions involving the use of essential oils have been reported in two individuals without known allergies or sensitivities prior to exposure.[71]

Opportunities

Campbell and colleagues[72] and Avis[73] suggest safe methods of integration of aromatherapy in clinical practice: Identify certified staff to serve as resources and educators. Conduct patient assessment. Select essential oils with low known risk potential. Choose one supplier with stringent product testing. Develop a range of oils and methods of application that can be used consistently. When blending oils, consider symptoms, patient allergies, and preference of aroma. Obtain a verbal consent. Place oil on tissue for patients in semi-private rooms. Document outcome of intervention. Avoid vaporizers in clinical settings.

Practitioners

The practice of aromatherapy can be used in combination with massage therapy and holistic nursing care programs. Certification is available through the National Association for Holistic Aromatherapy Standards of Aromatherapy Training (NAHA, www.naha.org). Schools must provide 200 hours of training and practical tuition in the fields of aromatherapy, essential oil studies, anatomy, and physiology. In addition, students must submit a research paper, 10 case histories, and pass a written examination. Holistic nursing certification is available through the American Holistic Nurses' Certification Corporation (AHNCC, http://ahna.org/edu/certification.html). Requirements include a bachelor of science degree (BSN), continuing education, 1 year of practice, and passing a written exam. Certification in aromatherapy or holistic nursing does not qualify a nurse to work independently nor does it necessarily meet institutional requirements for practice.[74]

Antioxidants

Antioxidant vitamins—E, C, and beta-carotene—are believed to have health-promoting properties. Coenzyme Q10 (CoQ10, ubiquinone) is an antioxidant found in all living cells, is involved in the production of energy within cells, and is believed to have powerful antioxidant effects. Although the data are incomplete, it appears that up to 30% of Americans are taking some form of antioxidant supplement. Research has shown that patients with cancer take antioxidants, typically at doses higher than recommended daily allowances.[75] Antioxidants act by scavenging free radicals. The debate that surrounds antioxidants and chemotherapy has focused on cancer therapy that creates free radicals through their cytotoxic mechanism, such as alkylating agents, antimetabolites, and radiation therapy. Limited research supports the belief that chemotherapy diminishes total antioxidant status,[76] but inconsistencies based on cancer site, cancer therapy, research methodologies, patient populations, variability in doses, duration of supplementation, and timing of interventions prevent formulation of conclusions.[77] For example, vitamin C is often publicized for its benefit to patients with cancer. And yet an increasing number of patients have been told by their oncologists to avoid vitamins and herbs, that is, *anything* with antioxidant potential while they are undergoing certain cancer therapies. This is difficult for patients to understand because foods contain some antioxidants, vitamins and minerals, and most fruits, vegetables, beans, and nuts differ only slightly from commonly used herbs.[78] The first of several recent studies that addressed taking high doses of vitamin C was carried out at Memorial Sloan-Kettering Cancer Center in New York City.[79] Human cancer cells were transplanted into mice, the mice were injected with vitamin C, and then the amount of vitamin C in the cells was measured. Cancer cells appeared to absorb large amounts of vitamin C by converting it into a more absorbable form. Once inside the cell, it is converted to ascorbic acid. These results, according to David Golde[79] raised the possibility that cancer cells may use vitamin C to shield themselves against radiation and chemotherapy. Other researchers say it's far too early to make that recommendation. There is no evidence yet that vitamin C actually shields cancer cells from treatment, says Mark Levine, MD, an endocrinologist and vitamin C expert at the National Institutes of Health. The cancers tested in Golde's research, he says, may simply have grown from tissues that normally take in large amounts of the vitamin.[80] In spring of 2000, the worry about antioxidants and cancer therapies grew, despite several warnings about the interpretation of these studies. John Russo, Jr.,[81] (a pharmacist) wrote a caution to the readers of his newsletter about the possible interference of antioxidants with brachytherapy for prostate cancer. His cautions were built upon the research of David Golde. However, what cancer cells do with the vitamin C after it is absorbed remains unknown.[78] Furthermore, the concept that tumor cells can be protected is largely based on the assumption that antioxidants are extremely efficient.[78]

Strength of Evidence

Over 45 meta-analyses or systematic reviews reviewing antioxidants (of which five involved patients with cancer) were reported between 1994 and 2004. Over 2000 randomized clinical trials (RCTs) that may spell out involvement of antioxidants are reported in Medline for this same time period. Belief that antioxidants may interfere with the efficacy of cancer therapy is not new. The association between beta-carotene and increased risk of lung cancer in smokers is well known.[82,83] However, it has been suggested that selective inhibition of tumor cell growth is an action of antioxidants and that antioxidants may also promote cellular differentiation with enhanced cytotoxic effects.[84] Ray and colleagues[85] suggest that typically recommended doses may be insufficient to combat the higher production of reactive oxygen metabolites. It has also been argued that inadequate coverage may actually contribute to malignant cell proliferation.[84] Researchers have been concerned that although antioxidants may decrease some kinds of toxicity associated with cancer chemotherapy, the therapeutic benefit of the cancer therapy may be compromised. Ladas and colleagues[77] reviewed more than 100 citations on antioxidant status and cancer outcomes and antioxidant use among patients receiving chemotherapy with or without radiation therapy; of the 52 that met their research criteria, 31 were observational studies and 21 were intervention trials. Their findings showed a decline in the total antioxidant status of patients receiving cancer therapy but conflicting and inconsistent results regarding the effect of chemotherapy on antioxidant status in patients receiving cancer therapy.[77] Lenzhofer and colleagues[86] found supplementation with vitamin E altered the metabolism of doxorubicin. Ladas and colleagues[77] question whether this means decreased treatment efficacy, arguing that adjunctive agents such as mesna and amifostine are used to reduce free radicals and do not appear to interfere in therapeutic benefit.[77] Among patients receiving chemotherapy for bone marrow transplant and total-body irradiation, serum vitamin E levels decreased even among those receiving total parenteral nutrition.[87] Two randomized studies treating patients with gynecologic cancers with doxorubicin, cyclophosphamide, cisplatin with folfiri or melphalan and selenium, vitamin E or selenium and vitamin E or placebo demonstrated increased serum selenium levels but not vitamin E levels after supplementation.[88] Studies among patients with breast cancer reveal a possible direct effect of selenium supplementation on serum and whole blood selenium.[77] The recommended daily allowances (RDAs) appear to be inadequate for maintaining plasma antioxidant levels in patients receiving high-dose chemotherapy before stem-cell transplant). Antioxidants may have a role in cancer prevention. Holm and colleagues[89] and Ingram[90] suggest that high vitamin C intake before diagnosis of breast cancer has a positive effect on mortality. Brawley and Parnes[91] report that selenium and vitamin E supplementation may reduce the risk of prostate cancer. Variability in doses, duration of supplementation, and timing of interventions prevent formulation of conclusions in this area of research as well.[77]

Contraindications

Contraindications for specific antioxidants are related to those known, for example, beta-carotene and lung cancer risk among smokers.

- Potential interactions with vitamin C include aluminum antacids, cyclosporine, statins, calcium channel blockers and protease inhibitors, iron, and vitamin E.[92]
- Potential interactions with vitamin E include cholestyramine, colestipol, mineral oil, anticonvulsants, anticoagulants, and verapamil.[92]
- Potential interactions with beta-carotene include cholestyramine, colestipol, mineral oil, and orlistat.[92]

Opportunities

The following study is being conducted:

Phase III Randomized Study of Selenium and Vitamin E for the Prevention of Prostate Cancer (SELECT Trial), NCCAM, NCI, SWOG-S0000.

Practitioners

Registered dieticians (RDs) have a minimum of a bachelors degree in dietetics.

The certified nutritionist (CN) has education and training in clinical nutrition and may be a nurse or other healthcare professional. Caution should be taken when choosing a nutrition practitioner to be certain that he or she has expertise in cancer care and supplements and nutrition.

St. John's Wort

St. John's wort has been proven to interfere with chemotherapy and has been implicated in lowering the dose of a wide range of drugs because it strongly activates the drug-metabolizing enzyme cytochrome P450 CYP3A4, *not* because of antioxidant activity.[93] St. John's wort was commonly used for treating depression during the 1990s but has since been used less often because of the concerns regarding drug interactions.[93] No other herb has been definitively identified as an inhibitor of chemotherapy drugs. Consider that the widespread use of herbs and herb extracts to minimize cancer therapy side effects in the Orient is accompanied by extensive favorable reports. Although many herbs have some antioxidant potential, their influence over oxidative reactions is low because of the low dosage commonly employed. Unlike vitamin C, which is presented as a pure or nearly pure compound in dietary supplements, herbs contain little vitamin C (in relation to Dr. Golde's concern) and low levels of antioxidant substances.[78,93] They also contain little, if any, of the substances that appeared to inhibit cisplatin cytotoxicity in cultured glioma cells.[94]

St. John's wort is also known as amber touch-and-heal, devil's scourge, goatweed, hypericum, Klamath weed, millepertuis, rosin rose, Tipton weed, and witch's herb. St. John's wort (SJW) is a member of the *Hypericaceae* family and contains naphthodianthrones, flavonoids, bioflavonoids, phloroglucinols, tannins, volatile oils, and xanthones. The chemical composition depends on the harvesting and drying processes and storage. The biologic activity of St. John's wort is believed to be caused by several of its components, not a single component.[95] St John's wort has been used topically and systemically for its medicinal properties for centuries. Uses have included wound healing, burns, as a diuretic, melancholia, pain, gastritis malaria, hemorrhoids, and mental illness, among others.[96] Contemporary use is almost exclusively as an antidepressant.[97] The pharmacologic actions of this herb include antiretroviral and antidepressant. The mechanism of action is not definitively known. Possibilities include modulation of interleukin-6 and GABA receptor binding, inhibition of serotonin reuptake, noradrenaline, and dopamine. There is some question regarding action as a monoamine oxidase (MAO) inhibition. The active ingredients have not been identified and therefore when considering safety, the entire extract must be taken under consideration.[95] Some authors believe hypericin and hyperforin to be the active constituents.[97]

Strength of Evidence

Six meta-analyses reviewed the efficacy in SJW in treating mild to moderate depression.[97-101] Over 50 RCTs are reported in Medline that were conducted between 1994 and 2004. A number of comparative RCTs have suggested this herb to be as effective as pharmaceutical antidepressants.[101-104] SJW has been shown to be equally as effective as light therapy in the treatment of seasonal affective disorder.[105] One study identified no antiretroviral effects on patients who were HIV-positive.[106] There have been positive results reported with premenstrual syndrome,[23] menopausal symptoms,[105] and fatigue.[107] In an open label crossover study design, six healthy men and six healthy women ages 22 to 38 years measured plasma pharmacokinetics of alprazolam as a probe for CYP3A4 activity before and after 14 days of SJW administration.

A significant decrease in CYP3A4 activity as measured by alterations in alprazolam pharmacokinetics suggest that long-term therapy with SJW may cause diminished clinical impact or increased dose requirements for all CYP3A4 substrates. This represents approximately 50% of all available medications.[108] As monotherapy, SJW has a respectable safety profile considered superior to conventional antidepressants.[97,109]

Contraindications

SJW is contraindicated during pregnancy and lactation. It causes photosensitivity, gastrointestinal symptoms, fatigue, and anxiety. Cases of mania, subacute toxic neuropathy, and breakthrough bleeding (in patients taking oral contraceptives) have been reported. Concurrent use of SJW with serotonin reuptake inhibitors can result in serotonin syndrome. An episode of transplant rejection was reported in a patient receiving cyclosporine. Additional research suggests that use of SJW reduced plasma levels of medications metabolized by hepatic cytochrome P450, including anticoagulants, anticonvulsants, digoxin, theophylline, and protease inhibitors. A single study indicated no interaction with alcohol.[97] There is inadequate evidence to support use in treatment of severe depression.[32,95]

Opportunities

The following study is ongoing:

Phase III Randomized Study of Sertraline (Zoloft) Versus Hypericum Perforatum (St. John's Wort) in Cancer Patients With Mild to Moderate Depression, CCCWFU-98101, CCCWFU-BGOI-152.

Practitioners

Practitioners should be pharmacists and other healthcare providers who have knowledge of both prescription and over-the-counter (OTC) medications, as well as herbal preparations.

SYMPTOM MANAGEMENT

Symptom management in cancer care includes the time from diagnosis to survivorship. Tremendous advances have been made in offering relief from the minor inconveniences to the major debilitating aspects of symptoms associated with the disease process, its treatment, and the possible physical, emotional, spiritual, and psychologic long-term consequences. Oncology nurses are experts in cancer symptom management, reducing the overall impact of symptoms on health outcomes.[110] Quality cancer care, as identified by the Oncology Nursing Society (ONS), embraces appropriate symptom management as a supportive care component.[9] The Priority Symptom Management (PRISM) project developed by the ONS Foundation Center for Leadership, Information, and Research (CLIR) in 2000 focused on six primary symptoms: anorexia, cognitive dysfunction, depression, fatigue, neutropenia, and pain.[111] Conventional approaches to symptom management have been enhanced in the past several years by the popularity and availability of CAM therapies. Critical appraisal of the quality of CAM approaches in symptom management is available for a limited number of symptoms at this time because of evolving approaches and pending clinical trials.[1]

Anorexia

Anorexia is defined as the loss of the compensatory increase in feeding.[112-114] Anorexia, involuntary weight loss, tissue wasting, poor performance, and ultimately death characterize the condition of advanced protein calorie malnutrition, also referred to as *cachexia*. The cancer anorexia-cachexia syndrome is multidimensional, maladapted, and involves physiologic and behavioral components that correlate with compromised quality of life and poor outcomes.[1] Aspects contributing to the anorexia-cachexia syndrome include abnormalities in the mouth and digestive tract, changes in taste and smell, learned aversion to specific foods, and cancer treatment. Traditional approaches for cachexia include (1) curing the cancer, (2) increasing nutritional intake, (3) inhibiting muscle and fat wasting, and (4) identifying the causes of reduced food intake.[112] First-line traditional interventions are glucocorticoids and progesterones. Second-line traditional interventions are cannabinoids, antiserotonergic drugs, and metoclopramide. CAM modalities in use or under review are eicosapentaenoic acid, melatonin, and hydrazine sulfate.[1]

Depression

Depression is frequent, highly treatable, and too often an unrecognized source of distress among patients with cancer. Cancer or other medical illnesses, cancer therapy, or side effects of other treatments or adjunctive medications used in cancer care may cause symptoms of depression or psychologic responses to the cancer experience. Many of the symptoms of depression, including changes in appetite, weight, and/or sleep patterns, fatigue, and loss of energy are not reliable indicators of depression in people with cancer. Surveys have identified depression as one of the most common reasons for using CAM.[115] The most popular therapies include exercise, herbal medicine, and relaxation.[11,115] Tricyclic antidepressants and selective serotonin reuptake inhibitors (SSRIs) are examples of traditional approaches to depression and demonstrate efficacy in the treatment of depression and are often coupled with counseling and psychotherapy.

Pain

The symptom of pain is known as the fifth vital sign. Patients may experience noncancer pain through comorbidities or injury predating a cancer diagnosis, further complicating management. Consultation frequency between healthcare provider and patients that focuses on pain and pain-related concerns has been measured.[116] Regimens can be individually tailored to enable patients to meet preferences, lifestyle, and desired outcome goals. Traditional approaches with known effectiveness in pain management include antitumor therapy,[117,118] nonsteroidal antiinflammatory drugs,[119] opioids, adjuvant agents (biphosphonates,[120] antidepressants,[121]), and transcutaneous electrical nerve stimulation.[122] Potentially effective CAM approaches include acupuncture,[48] cognitive-behavioral therapy,[123] massage,[124] and relaxation with guided imagery.[125,126] CAM approaches with variable efficacy are topical capsaicin,[127] chiropractic manipulation,[124] music,[128] and distraction.[128,129] Given the various types and causes of pain associated with cancer, multiple approaches to pain relief are needed and remain a challenge for clinicians and patients.

REFERENCES

1. Decker G, Lee C: Complementary and alternative medicine (CAM) therapies. In Yarbo CH, Frogge MH, Goodman M, editors: *Cancer nursing: principles and practice*, ed 6, Sudbury, Mass, 2005, Jones and Bartlett, pp 590-620.
2. Cassileth BR: Overview of alternative/complementary medicine, *Cancer Pract* 6(4):243-245, 1998.
3. Vickers AJ, Cassileth BR: Unconventional therapies for cancer and cancer-related symptoms, *Lancet Oncol* 2(4):226-232, 2001.
4. Eisenberg DM, Kessler RC, Foster C et al: Unconventional medicine in the United States: prevalence, costs, and patterns of use, *N Engl J Med* 328(4):246-252, 1993.
5. Segen JC: *Dictionary of alternative medicine*, Stamford, Conn, 1998, Appleton & Lange.
6. Micozzi MS: *Fundamentals of Complementary and Alternative Medicine*, New York, 1996, Churchill-Livingstone.
7. Cassileth BR, Vickers AJ: Complementary and alternative therapies, *Urol Clin North Am* 30(2):369-376, 2003.
8. Cancer facts: complementary and alternative medicine in cancer treatment: questions and answers. In *Fact sheet*, Bethesda, 2003, National Cancer Institute, www.cancer.gov/cancertopics/factsheet.
9. *The use of complementary and alternative therapies in cancer care*, Pittsburgh, 2002, Oncology Nursing Society.
10. Antman K, Benson MC, Chabot J et al: Complementary and alternative medicine: the role of the cancer center, *J Clin Oncol* 19(18[Suppl]):55S-60S, 2001.
11. Eisenberg DM, Davis RB, Ettner SL et al: Trends in alternative medicine use in the United States, 1990-1997: results of a follow-up national survey, *JAMA* 280(18): 1569-1575, 1998.
12. Ashikaga T, Bosompra K, O'Brien P et al: Use of complementary and alternative medicine by breast cancer patients: prevalence, patterns and communication with physicians, *Support Care Cancer* 10(7):542-548, 2002.
13. Swisher EM, Cohn DE, Goff BA et al: Use of complementary and alternative medicine among women with gynecologic cancers, *Gynecol Oncol* 84(3):363-367, 2002.
14. National Center for Complementary and Alternative Medicine (website home page): http://nccam.nih.gov. Accessed November, 2006.
15. Office of Cancer Complementary and Alternative Medicine: National Cancer Institute (website home page): www.nih.gov/news/NIH. Accessed November, 2006.
16. White JD: Complementary and alternative medicine research: a National Cancer Institute perspective, *Semin Oncol* 29(6):546-551, 2002.
17. White House Commission on Complementary and Alternative Medicine Policy: Washington, DC, 2003, US Department of Health and Human Services (website): www.whccamp.hhs.gov/es.html.
18. *Use of complementary and alternative medicine (CAM) by the American public*, 2004, Institute of Medicine of the National Academies.
19. White JD: The National Cancer Institute's perspective and agenda for promoting awareness and research on alternative therapies for cancer, *J Altern Complement Med* 8(5):545-550, 2002.
20. Sparber A, Bauer L, Curt G et al: Use of complementary medicine by adult patients participating in cancer clinical trials, *Oncol Nurs Forum* 27(4):623-630, 2000.
21. Ernst E, Cassileth BR: The prevalence of complementary/alternative medicine in cancer: a systematic review, *Cancer* 83(4):777-782, 1998.
22. Basch E, Ulbricht C: Prevalence of CAM use among US cancer patients: an update, *J Cancer Integrat Med* 2(1): 13-14, 2004.
23. Stevinson C: Why patients use complementary and alternative medicine. In Ernst E, editor: *The desktop guide to complementary and alternative medicine: an evidence-based approach*, Edinburgh, 2001, Harcourt, pp 395-403.

24. Furnham A: Why do people choose and use complementary therapies? In Ernst E, editor: *Complementary medicine: an objective appraisal*, Oxford, 1996, Butterworth Heinemann, pp 71-88.
25. Fletcher RH: Clinical practice guidelines. In *UpToDate*, 2004 (website): www.utdol.com. Accessed November, 2006.
26. Angell M, Kassirer JP: Alternative medicine—the risks of untested and unregulated remedies, *N Engl J Med* 339(12):839-841, 1998.
27. *Natural Medicines Comprehensive Database*, 2004 (website): www.naturaldatabase.com. Accessed November, 2006.
28. *Natural standard database*, Houston, 2004, University of Texas, MD Anderson Cancer Center (website): www.naturalstandard.com. Accessed November, 2006.
29. White JD: The National Cancer Institute's perspective and agenda for promoting awareness and research on alternative therapies for cancer, *J Altern Complement Med* 8(5):545-550, 2002.
30. Eisenberg DM: Advising patients who seek alternative medical therapies, *Ann Intern Med* 127(1):61-69, 1997.
31. Decker G: Integrating complementary and alternative medicine therapies into an oncology practice. In Buchsel PC, Yarbro CH, editors: *Oncology nursing in the ambulatory setting: issues and models of care*, Sudbury, Mass, 2005, Jones and Bartlett, pp 355-376.
32. Ernst E, editor: *The desktop guide to complementary and alternative medicine: an evidence-based approach*, Edinburgh, 2001, Mosby.
33. Ernst E: Research into complementary/alternative medicine: an attempt to dispel the myths, *Int J Clin Pract* 55(6): 376-379, 2001.
34. Pinquart MD, Duberstein PR: Information needs and decision-making processes in older cancer patients, *Crit Rev Oncol Hematol* 51(1):69-80, 2004.
35. Llewelyn-Thomas HA, McGreal MJ, Theil EC: Cancer patients' decision making and trial entry preferences: the effects of framing information about short-term toxicity and long-term survival, *Med Decision Making* 15(1):4-12, 1995.
36. Truant TB, Bottorff JL: Decision making related to complementary therapies: a process of regaining control, *Patient Educ Couns* 38(2):131-142, 1999.
37. Davison BJ, Degner LF, Morgan TR: Information and decision-making preferences in men with prostate cancer, *Oncol Nurs Forum* 22(8):1402-1408, 1995.
38. Degner LF, Kristjanson LJ, Bowman D et al: Information needs and decision making preferences in women with breast cancer, *JAMA* 277(18):1485-1492, 1997.
39. Mastaglia MK, Kristjanson LJ: Factors influencing women's decisions for choice of surgery for stage I and stage II breast cancer in western Australia, *J Adv Nurs* 35(6):836-847, 2001.
40. Baltes M, Staudiner P: *Interactive minds: lifespan perspectives on the social foundation of cognition*, New York, 1996, Cambridge University Press.
41. Polsky D, Keating NL, Weeks JC et al: Patient choice of breast cancer treatment: impact on health state preferences, *Med Care* 40(11):1068-1079, 2002.
42. Elit L, Charles C, Gold I et al: Women's perceptions about treatment decision making for ovarian cancer, *Gynecol Oncol* 88(2):89-95, 2003.
43. Brett H: *Complementary therapies in the care of older people*, Philadelphia, 2002, LoHurr Publishers.
44. Downer SM, Cody MM, McVluskey P et al: Pursuit and practice of complementary therapies by cancer patients receiving complementary therapies alongside conventional therapies, *BMJ* 309(6947):86-89, 1994.
45. Kassab S, Stevensen C: Common misunderstandings about complementary therapies for patients with cancer, *Complement Ther Nurs Midwifery* 2(3):62-65, 1996.
46. Decker GC, Cleveland MJ: Complementary and alternative therapies. In Gate RA, Fink RM, editor: *Oncology nursing secrets*, Philadelphia, 2001, Hanley and Belfus, pp 144-152.
47. Tisserand R, Balacs T: *Essential oil safety: a guide for health-care professionals*, New York, 1995, Churchill Livingstone.
48. Mayer DJ: Acupuncture: an evidence-based review of the clinical literature, *Ann Rev Med* 51:49-63, 2000.
49. Han JS, Terenius L: Neurochemical basis of acupuncture analgesia, *Ann Rev Pharmacol Toxicol* 22:193-220, 1982.
50. Andersson S, Lundeberg T: Acupuncture—from empiricism to science: functional background to acupuncture effects in pain and disease, *Med Hypoth* 45(3):271-281, 1995.
51. Ernst E, Pittler MH: The effectiveness of acupuncture in treating acute dental pain: a systematic review, *Br Dent J* 184(9):443-447, 1998.
52. Vickers AJ: Can acupuncture have specific effects on health? A systematic review of acupuncture antiemesis trials, *J R Soc Med* 89(6):303-311, 1996.
53. Melchart D, Linde K, Fischer P et al: Acupuncture for recurrent headaches: a systematic review of randomized controlled trials, *Cephalalgia* 19(9):779-786, 1999; discussion 765.
54. Aikins Murphy P: Alternative therapies for nausea and vomiting of pregnancy, *Obstet Gynecol* 91(1):149-155, 1998.
55. Ernst E, White A: Life-threatening adverse reactions after acupuncture? A systematic review, *Pain* 71(2): 123-126, 1997.
56. Eichelberger B: *Qi gong basics* (website): acupuncture.com/education/tcmbasics/whatisqigong.htm. Accessed November 20, 2006.
57. Yang JM: *A brief history of qigong* (website): acupuncture.com/qigong_tuina/qigonghistory.htm. Accessed April 26, 2006.
58. Wu CY: Spontaneous dynamic qigong and mental disorders, *Zhong Xi Yi Jie He Za Zhi* 10(8):497-498, 1990.
59. Olson K, Hanson J: Using Reiki to manage pain: a preliminary report, *Cancer Prev Control* 1(2):108-113, 1997.
60. Lafreniere KD et al: Effects of therapeutic touch on biochemical and mood indicators in women, *J Altern Complement Med* 5(4):367-370, 1999.
61. Post-White J, Kinney ME, Savik K et al: Therapeutic massage and healing touch improve symptoms in cancer, *Integr Cancer Ther* 2(4):332-344, 2003.
62. Mansour AA, Beuche M, Laing G et al: A study to test the effectiveness of placebo Reiki standardization procedures developed for a planned Reiki efficacy study, *J Altern Complement Med* 5(2):153-164, 1999.
63. Ernst E: The current position of complementary/alternative medicine in cancer, *Eur J Cancer* 39(16):2273-2277, 2003.

64. Perez C: Clinical aromatherapy, part I: an introduction into nursing practice, *Clin J Oncol Nurs* 7(5):595-596, 2003.
65. Thomas DV: Aromatherapy: mythical, magical, or medicinal? *Holist Nurs Pract* 16(5):8-16, 2002.
66. Cooke B, Ernst E: Aromatherapy: a systematic review, *Br J Gen Pract* 50(455):493-496, 2000.
67. Louis M, Kowalski SD: Use of aromatherapy with hospice patients to decrease pain, anxiety, and depression and to promote an increased sense of well-being, *Am J Hosp Palliat Care* 19(6):381-386, 2002.
68. Olleveant NA, Humphris G, Roe B: How big is a drop? A volumetric assay of essential oils, *J Clin Nurs* 8(3): 299-304, 1999.
69. Fellowes D, Barnes K, Wilkinson S: Aromatherapy and massage for symptom relief in patients with cancer, *Cochrane Database Syst Rev* (2):CD002287, 2004.
70. Graham PH, Browne L, Cox H et al: Inhalation aromatherapy during radiotherapy: results of a placebo-controlled double-blind randomized trial, *J Clin Oncol* 21(12):2372-2376, 2003.
71. Maddocks-Jennings W: Critical incident: idiosyncratic allergic reactions to essential oils, *Complement Ther Nurs Midwifery* 10(1):58-60, 2004.
72. Campbell L, Pollard A, Roeton C: The development of clinical practice guidelines for the use of aromatherapy in a cancer setting, *Aust J Holist Nurs* 8(1):14-22, 2001.
73. Avis A: Aromatherapy in practice, *Nurs Stand* 13(24): 14-15, 1999.
74. Lee CO: Clinical aromatherapy, part II: safe guidelines for integration into clinical practice, *Clin J Oncol Nurs* 7(5):597-598, 2003.
75. VandeCreek L, Rogers E, Lester J: Use of alternative therapies among breast cancer outpatients compared with the general population, *Altern Ther Health Med* 5(1): 71-76, 1999.
76. Durken M, Herrnring C, Finckh B et al: Impaired plasma antioxidative defense and increased nontrans-ferrin-bound iron during high-dose chemotherapy and radiochemotherapy preceding bone marrow transplantation *Free Radic Biol Med* 28(6):887-894, 2000.
77. Ladas EJ, Jacobson JS, Kennedy DD et al: Antioxidants and cancer therapy: a systematic review, *J Clin Oncol* 22(3):517-528, 2004.
78. Dharmananda S: *Do herbs, vitamins, and antioxidants adversely affect cancer therapies?* (website): www.itmonline.org/arts/antioxidants.htm. Accessed July 10, 2005.
79. Golde DM: Cancer tumors shown to consume large amounts of vitamin C—researchers are cautious about cancer patients taking vitamin C supplements, *News@MSKCC* (online serial): www.mskcc.org. Accessed April 26, 2006.
80. Levine M, Rumsey RS, Daruwala R et al: Criteria and recommendations for vitamin C intake, *JAMA* 281: 1415-1423, 1999.
81. Russo JJPD: Potential interaction between antioxidants and cancer treatment. In *The MedCom Resource*, 2000 (website): www.medcomres.com. Accessed November, 2006.
82. Omenn GS, Goodman GE, Thornquist MD et al: Effects of a combination of beta carotene and vitamin A on lung cancer and cardiovascular disease, *N Engl J Med* 334(18):1150-1155, 1996.
83. Albanes D, Heinonen OP, Huttunen JK et al: Effects of alpha-tocopherol and beta-carotene supplements on cancer incidence in the Alpha-Tocopherol Beta-Carotene Cancer Prevention Study, *Am J Clin Nutr* 62(6[suppl]): 1427S-1430S, 1995.
84. Conklin KA: Dietary antioxidants during cancer chemotherapy: impact on chemotherapeutic effectiveness and development of side effects, *Nutr Cancer* 37(1):1-18, 2000.
85. Ray SD, Patel D, Wong V et al: In vivo protection of DNA damage associated apoptotic and necrotic cell deaths during acetaminophen-induced nephrotoxicity, amiodarone-induced lung toxicity and doxorubicin-induced cardiotoxicity by a novel IH636 grape seed proanthocyanidin extract, *Res Commun Mol Pathol Pharmacol* 107(1-2):137-166, 2000.
86. Lenzhofer R, Ganzinger U, Rameis H et al: Acute cardiac toxicity in patients after doxorubicin treatment and the effect of combined tocopherol and nifedipine pretreatment, *J Cancer Res Clin Oncol* 106(2):143-147, 1983.
87. Jonas CR, Puckett AB, Jones DP et al: Plasma antioxidant status after high-dose chemotherapy: a randomized trial of parenteral nutrition in bone marrow transplantation patients, *Am J Clin Nutr* 72(1):181-189, 2000.
88. Sundstrom H, Korpela H, Sajanti E et al: Supplementation with selenium, vitamin E and their combination in gynaecological cancer during cytotoxic chemotherapy, *Carcinogenesis* 10(2):273-278, 1989.
89. Holm LE, Nordevang E, Hjalmar ML et al: Treatment failure and dietary habits in women with breast cancer, *J Natl Cancer Inst* 85(1):32-36, 1993.
90. Ingram D: Diet and subsequent survival in women with breast cancer, *Br J Cancer* 69(3):592-595, 1994.
91. Brawley OW, Parnes H: Prostate cancer prevention trials in the USA, *Eur J Cancer* 36(10):1312-1315, 2000.
92. *PDR for nutritional supplements*, Montvale, NJ, 2001, Medical Economics, Thomson Healthcare.
93. Mathijssen RH: Effects of St. John's wort on irinotecan metabolism, *J Natl Cancer Inst* 94(16):1187-1188, 2002.
94. Roller A, Weller M: Antioxidants specifically inhibit cisplatin cytotoxicity of human malignant glioma cells, *Anticancer Res* 18(6A):4493-4497, 1998.
95. Fetrow C, Avila A: *A professional's handbook of complementary and alternative medicines*, Philadelphia, 1999, Springhouse.
96. Ernst E: Harmless herbs? A review of the recent literature, *Am J Med* 104(2):170-178, 1998.
97. Ernst E: The risk-benefit profile of commonly used herbal therapies: ginkgo, St. John's Wort, ginseng, echinacea, saw palmetto, and kava, *Ann Intern Med* 136(1):42-53, 2002.
98. Kasper S, Dienel A: Cluster analysis of symptoms during antidepressant treatment with *Hypericum* extract in mildly to moderately depressed out-patients: a meta-analysis of data from three randomized, placebo-controlled trials, *Psychopharmacology* (Berl) 164(3):301-308, 2002.
99. Linde K, Ramirez G, Mulrow CD et al: St John's wort for depression—an overview and meta-analysis of randomised clinical trials, *BMJ* 313(7052):253-258, 1996.
100. Whiskey E, Werneke U, Taylor D: A systematic review

and meta-analysis of *Hypericum perforatum* in depression: a comprehensive clinical review, *Int Clin Psychopharmacol* 16(5):239-252, 2001.

101. Harrer G, Schmidt U, Kuhn U et al: Comparison of equivalence between the St. John's wort extract LoHyp-57 and fluoxetine, *Arzneimittelforschung* 49(4): 289-296, 1999.
102. Philipp M, Kohnen R, Hiller KO: *Hypericum* extract versus imipramine or placebo in patients with moderate depression: randomised multicentre study of treatment for eight weeks, *Br Med J* 319(7224):1534-1538, 1999.
103. Schrader E: Equivalence of St John's wort extract (Ze 117) and fluoxetine: a randomized, controlled study in mild-moderate depression, *Int Clin Psychopharmacol* 15(2):61-68, 2000.
104. Woelk H: Comparison of St John's wort and imipramine for treating depression: randomised controlled trial, *Br Med J* 321(7260):536-539, 2000.
105. Wheatley D: *Hypericum* in seasonal affective disorder (SAD), *Curr Med Res Opin* 15(1):33-37, 1999.
106. Gulick RM, McAuliffe V, Holden-Wiltse J et al: Phase I studies of hypericin, the active compound in St. John's Wort, as an antiretroviral agent in HIV-infected adults: AIDS Clinical Trials Group Protocols 150 and 258, *Ann Intern Med* 130(6):510-514, 1999.
107. Stevinson C, Ernst E: A pilot study of *Hypericum perforatum* for the treatment of premenstrual syndrome, *Br J Gynaecol* 107(7):870-876, 2000.
108. Markowitz JS, Donovan JL, DeVane CL et al: Effect of St John's wort on drug metabolism by induction of cytochrome P450 3A4 enzyme, *JAMA* 290(11): 1500-1504, 2003.
109. Ernst E, Rand JI, Stevinson C: Complementary therapies for depression: an overview, *Arch Gen Psychiatry* 55(11):1026-1032, 1998.
110. Ropka ME, Spencer-Cisek P: PRISM: Priority Symptom Management Project phase I: assessment, *Oncol Nurs Forum* 28(10):1585-1594, 2001.
111. PRISM (Priority Symptom Management) Project, Oncology Nursing Society Foundation, 2004 (website): www.ons.org/publications.
112. Inui A: Cancer anorexia-cachexia syndrome: current issues in research and management, *CA Cancer J Clin* 52(2):72-91, 2002.
113. Inui A: Cancer anorexia-cachexia syndrome: are neuropeptides the key? *Cancer Res* 59(18):4493-4501, 1999.
114. Inui A, Meguid MM: Cachexia and obesity: two sides of one coin? *Curr Opin Clin Nutr Metab Care* 6(4):395-399, 2003.
115. Astin JA, Shapiro SL, Eisenberg DM et al: Mind-body medicine: state of the science, implications for practice, *J Am Board Fam Pract* 16(2):131-147, 2003.
116. Rogers MS, Todd CJ: The 'right kind' of pain: talking about symptoms in outpatient oncology consultations, *Palliat Med* 14(4):299-307, 2000.
117. Paice JA: Pain. In Yarbro CH, Grogge MH, Goodman M, editors: *Cancer symptom management*, Sudbury, Mass, 2004, Jones and Bartlett.
118. Simmonds PC: Palliative chemotherapy for advanced colorectal cancer: systematic review and meta-analysis: Colorectal Cancer Collaborative Group, *Br Med J* 321(7260):531-535, 2000.
119. McNicol E, Strassels S, Goudas L et al: Nonsteroidal anti-inflammatory drugs, alone or combined with opioids, for cancer pain: a systematic review, *J Clin Oncol* 22(10):1975-1992, 2004.
120. Mannix K, Admedzai SH, Anderson H et al: Using bisphosphonates to control the pain of bone metastases: evidence-based guidelines for palliative care, *Palliat Med* 14(6):455-461, 2000.
121. McQuay HJ, Tramer M, Nye BH et al: A systematic review of antidepressants in neuropathic pain, *Pain* 68 (2-3):217-227, 1996.
122. Martin LA, Hagen NA: Neuropathic pain in cancer patients: mechanisms, syndromes, and clinical controversies, *J Pain Symptom Manage* 14(2):99-117, 1997.
123. Dalton JA, Keefe FJ, Carlson J et al: Tailoring cognitive-behavioral treatment for cancer pain, *Pain Manage Nurs* 5(1):3-18, 2004.
124. Ernst E: Manual therapies for pain control: chiropractic and massage, *Clin J Pain* 20(1):8-12, 2004.
125. *Pain*, 2004, National Cancer Institute (website): http://www.cancer.gov/cancertopics/pdq. Accessed November 2006.
126. Pan CX, Morrison RS, Ness J et al: Complementary and alternative medicine in the management of pain, dyspnea, and nausea and vomiting near the end of life: a systematic review, *J Pain Symptom Manage* 20(5):374-387, 2000.
127. Mason L, Moore RA, Derry S et al: Systematic review of topical capsaicin for the treatment of chronic pain, *Br Med J* 328(7446):991, 2004.
128. Kwekkeboom KL: Music versus distraction for procedural pain and anxiety in patients with cancer, *Oncol Nurs Forum* 30(3):433-440, 2003.
129. Terkelsen AJ, Andersen OK, Molgaard H et al: Mental stress inhibits pain perception and heart rate variability but not a nociceptive withdrawal reflex, *Acta Physiol Scand* 180(4):405-414, 2004.
130. *Levels of evidence for human studies of cancer complementary and alternative medicine*, Bethesda, 2004, National Cancer Institute.

Index

A

D

E

F

G

H

I

J

T

X

Y

Z